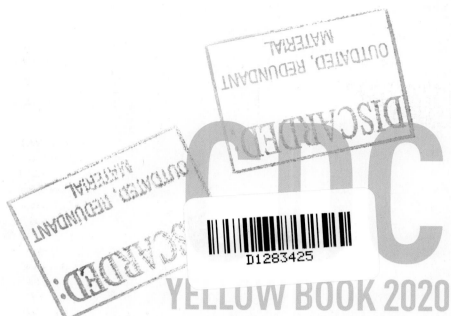

# CDC
## YELLOW BOOK 2020

# Health Information for International Travel

# CDC

## YELLOW BOOK 2020

# Health Information for International Travel DISCARD

Editors in Chief Gary W. Brunette, MD, MS
and Jeffrey B. Nemhauser, MD

**CHIEF MEDICAL EDITOR**
Phyllis E. Kozarsky, MD

**MEDICAL EDITORS**
Kristina M. Angelo, DO, MPH&TM
Nicole J. Cohen, MD, MS
Douglas H. Esposito, MD, MPH
Stephen M. Ostroff, MD
Edward T. Ryan, MD
David R. Shlim, MD
Richard W. Steketee, MD, MPH
Michelle Weinberg, MD, MPH
Mary Elizabeth Wilson, MD

**MANAGING EDITOR**
Jenique Meekins

**TECHNICAL EDITOR**
Ronnie Henry

US DEPARTMENT OF HEALTH AND
HUMAN SERVICES

PUBLIC HEALTH SERVICE

CENTERS FOR DISEASE CONTROL AND
PREVENTION

NATIONAL CENTER FOR EMERGING AND
ZOONOTIC INFECTIOUS DISEASES

DIVISION OF GLOBAL MIGRATION AND
QUARANTINE

ATLANTA, GEORGIA

**OXFORD**
UNIVERSITY PRESS

Oxford University Press is a department of the University of Oxford. It furthers
the University's objective of excellence in research, scholarship, and education
by publishing worldwide. Oxford is a registered trade mark of Oxford University
Press in the UK and certain other countries.

Published in the United States of America by Oxford University Press
198 Madison Avenue, New York, NY 10016, United States of America.

CIP data is on file at the Library of Congress
ISBN 978–0–19–092893–3 (pbk.)
ISBN 978–0–19–006597–3 (hbk.)

9 8 7 6 5 4 3 2 1
Paperback and Hardback printed by LSC Communications, United States of America

Oxford University Press is proud to pay a portion of its sales for this book to the CDC Foundation.
Chartered by Congress, the CDC Foundation began operations in 1995 as an independent,
nonprofit organization fostering support for CDC through public-private partnerships. Further
information about the CDC Foundation can be found at www.cdcfoundation.org. The CDC
Foundation did not prepare any portion of this book and is not responsible for its contents.

**Suggested Citation**

Centers for Disease Control and Prevention. CDC Yellow Book 2020: Health Information for International Travel. New York: Oxford University Press; 2017.

Readers are invited to send comments and suggestions regarding this publication to Gary W. Brunette, Editor-in-Chief, Centers for Disease Control and Prevention, Division of Global Migration and Quarantine), Travelers' Health Branch (proposed), 1600 Clifton Road NE, Mail Stop E-28, Atlanta, GA 30333, USA.

**Disclaimers**

Both generic and trade names (without trademark symbols) are used in this text. In all cases, the decision to use one or the other was made based on recognition factors and was done for the convenience of the intended audience. Therefore, the use of trade names and commercial sources in this publication is for identification only and does not imply endorsement by the US Department of Health and Human Services, the Public Health Service, or CDC. Descriptions of drugs, biologics, or medical products used for an indication not in the approved labeling or packaging ("off-label" uses) do not constitute official HHS approval or endorsement of those products or uses. The uses described in this publication have been identified by subject-matter experts on the basis of published evidence and clinical experience. Clinicians who use a product for an off-label use should be well informed about the product, base its use on firm scientific rationale and sound medical evidence, and maintain records of the product's use and effects.

References to non-CDC Internet sites are provided as a service to readers and do not constitute or imply endorsement of these organizations or their programs by the US Department of Health and Human Services, the Public Health Service, or CDC. CDC is not responsible for the content of these sites. URL addresses were current as of the date of publication.

Boundaries and labels shown on maps are not necessarily authoritative.

**Notice**

This material is not intended to be, and should not be considered, a substitute for medical, legal, or other professional advice. Treatment for the conditions described in this material is highly dependent on the individual circumstances. While this material is designed to offer accurate information with respect to the subject matter covered and to be current as of the time it was written, research and knowledge about medical, legal, and health issues are constantly evolving, and dose schedules for medications and vaccines are being revised continually, with new side effects recognized and accounted for regularly. Therefore, readers must always check the product information and clinical procedures with the most up-to-date published product information and data sheets provided by the manufacturers and the most recent codes of conduct and safety regulation. Oxford University Press and the authors make no representations or warranties to readers, express or implied, as to the accuracy or completeness of this material, including without limitation that they make no representations or warranties as to the accuracy or efficacy of the drug dosages mentioned in the material. The authors and the publishers do not accept, and expressly disclaim, any responsibility for any liability, loss, or risk that may be claimed or incurred as a consequence of the use and/or application of any of the contents of this material.

The Publisher is responsible for author selection, and the Publisher and the Author(s) make all editorial decisions, including decisions regarding content. The Publisher and the Author(s) are not responsible for any product information added to this publication by companies purchasing copies of it for distribution to clinicians.

For additional copies, please contact Oxford University Press. Order online at www.oup.com/us.

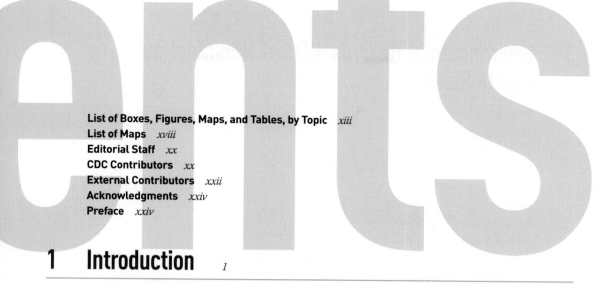

# 1 Introduction  *1*

# 2 Preparing International Travelers  *9*

# 3 Environmental Hazards & Other Noninfectious Health Risks *125*

# 4 Travel-Related Infectious Diseases *169*

# 5  Travelers with Additional Considerations  *395*

# 6  Health Care Abroad  *421*

# 7  Family Travel  *435*

# 8  Travel by Air, Land & Sea  *465*

# 9  Travel for Work & Other Reasons  *485*

# 10  Popular Itineraries  *535*

# 11  Posttravel Evaluation   *603*

# List of Boxes, Figures, Maps, and Tables, by Topic

## DISEASES, CONDITIONS & VACCINES

## RESOURCES

### General Resources

### Insect Avoidance

### Pretravel Consultation

### Water Treatment

## SELECTED POPULATIONS

### Cruise Ship Passengers

### Health Care Workers

### Immigrants & Migrants

### Immunocompromised Travelers

# List of Maps

## DESTINATION AND REFERENCE MAPS

# Editorial Staff

**Editors in Chief:** Gary W. Brunette and Jeffrey B. Nemhauser

**Chief Medical Editor:** Phyllis E. Kozarsky

**Medical Editors:** Kristina M. Angelo, Nicole J. Cohen, Douglas H. Esposito, Stephen M. Ostroff, Edward T. Ryan, David R. Shlim, Richard W. Steketee, Michelle Weinberg, and Mary Elizabeth Wilson

**Managing Editor:** Jenique Meekins

**Technical Editor:** Ronnie Henry

**Cartographer:** R. Ryan Lash

**Assistant Cartographer:** C. Virginia Lee

# CDC Contributors

Abe, Karon

Acosta, Anna

Ali, Ibne

Alvarado-Ramy, Francisco

Angelo, Kristina

Ansari, Armin

Anstey, Erica

Appiah, Grace

Arboleda, Nelson

Arguin, Paul M.

Baggett, Henry C.

Ballesteros, Michael F.

Barton Behravesh, Casey

Beavers, Suzanne

Beckman, Michele G.

Benedict, Katherine

Benowitz, Isaac

Biggs, Holly

Blaney, David D.

Bonilla, Luis
Brogdon, William G.
Brooks, John T.
Brown, Clive M.
Bruce, Beau
Brunette, Gary W.
Cantey, Paul T.
Cardemil, Cristina V.
Chatham-Stevens, Kevin
Chiller, Tom M.
Choi, Mary Joung
Clemmons, Nakia S.
Cooley, Laura
Cope, Jennifer
Czarkowski, Alan G.
Dionne-Odom, Jodie
Dubray, Christine
Duong, Krista Kornylo
Edelson, Paul
Eichwald, John
Erskine, Stefanie K.
Esposito, Douglas H.
Estivariz, Concepcion
Fischer, Marc
Francois Watkins,
Louise K.
Friedman, Cindy R.
Fry, Alicia
Gaines, Joanna
Galland, G. Gale
Galloway, Renee L.
Gastañaduy, Paul A.
Gee, Jay E.
Geissler, Aimee L.
Gerber, Susan I.
Gershman, Mark D.
Goodson, James L.
Goswami, Neela
Gould, Carolyn
Green, Michael D.

Griffin, Patricia M.
Hall, Aron J.
Hall, Rebecca
Ham, David
Harris, Aaron
Harvey, Pauline
Hawley, William A.
Healy, Jessica
Hendricks Walters, Kate
Henry, Ronnie
Herwaldt, Barbara L.
Hill, Vincent
Hills, Susan L.
Hinton, Cindy
Hlavsa, Michele C.
Hughes, Mike
Hunter, Jennifer C.
Jackson, Brendan
Jentes, Emily S.
Jones, Jeffrey L.
Jungerman, Robynne M.
Kersh, Gilbert J.
Kharod, Grishma A.
Knust, Barbara
Kozarsky, Phyllis E.
Kroger, Andrew T.
Lanzieri, Tatianna
Laughlin, Mark
Lee, Keun
Lessa, Fernanda C.
Lindsey, Nichole
LoBue, Philip
Lopez, Adriana S.
Lutgring, Joseph
MacArthur, John
Maloney, Susan A.
Marano, Nina
Marin, Mona
Marlow, Mariel A.
Marston, Chung K.

Martin, Diana L.
Martin, Stacey
McCollum, Andrea M.
McCotter, Orion Z.
McFarland, Jeffrey
McNamara, Lucy
Mead, Paul S.
Meyer, Sarah A.
Mintz, Eric D.
Montgomery, Susan
Montiel, Sonia H.
Moore, Matt
Morales, Michelle
Morof, Diane F.
Moser, Kathleen
Mott, Joshua
Mounts, Anthony
Mullan, Robert J.
Mutebi, John-Paul
Ncho, Hammad
Negron, Maria E.
Nelson, Christina A.
Nelson, Noele P.
Nicholson, William L.
Paddock,
Christopher D.
Park, Benjamin
Patel, Manisha
Patimeteeporn, Calvin
Perez-Padilla, Janice
Peters, Philip J.
Peterson, Brett W.
Powers, Ann M.
Rabold, Elizabeth
Raczniak, Gregory A.
Reef, Susan E.
Reyes, Nimia L.
Robinson, Candice
Roellig, Dawn
Roguski, Katherine

Rollin, Pierre E.
Routh, Janell
Roy, Sharon
Russell, Michelle
Santelli, Ana Carolina
Sauber-Schatz, Erin K.
Schafer, Ilana J.
Schmid, D. Scott
Sharp, Tyler M.
Shoemaker, Trevor
Skoff, Tami H.
Sleet, David A.
Sotir, Mark J.
Spradling, Phil
Staples, J. Erin
Stauffer, Kendra
Stoddard, Robyn A
Stoney, Rhett J
Straily, Anne
Tan, Kathrine R.
Tardivel, Kara
Teshale, Eyasu
Tiller, Rebekah
Tiwari, Tejpratap S. P.
Uribe, Carolina
Vieira, Antonio
Villarino, Margarita E.
Walker, Allison Taylor
Wallace, Ryan M.
Wassilak, Steven G. F.
Waterman, Stephen H.
Watson, John T.
Weinberg, Michelle S.
White, Stephanie
Wien, Simone
Winstead, Allison
Wong, Karen K.
Workowski, Kimberly

# External Contributors

| | |
|---|---|
| Ansdell, Vernon E. | University of Hawaii, Honolulu, HI |
| Atkinson, Gregory | Teesside University, Middlesbrough, UK |
| Backer, Howard D. | California Emergency Medical Services Authority, Sacramento, CA |
| Barbeau, Deborah Nicolls | Tulane University, New Orleans, LA |
| Barkati, Sapha | McGill University, Centre for Tropical Disease, Montreal, Canada |
| Barnett, Elizabeth D. | Boston University School of Medicine and Boston Medical Center, Boston, MA |
| Batterham, Alan M. | Teesside University, Middlesbrough, UK |
| Boggild, Andrea K. | University of Toronto, Toronto, Canada |
| Borwein, Sarah T. | TravelSafe Medical Centre, Hong Kong, China |
| Bozkurt, Taylan | JMS Burn Centers, Inc., Augusta, GA |
| Bunn, Bill | Medical University of South Carolina; Navistar International Corporation |
| Carroll, I. Dale | The Pregnant Traveler, Spring Lake, MI |
| Changizi, Roohollah | United Family Hospital, subsidiary of United Family Healthcare, Beijing, China |
| Chen, Lin H. | Mount Auburn Hospital—Travel Medicine Center, Cambridge, MA, and Harvard Medical School, Boston, MA |
| Chimiak, James M. | Divers Alert Network, Durham, NC |
| Connor, Bradley A. | Weill Medical College of Cornell University, New York, NY |
| DeRomaña, Inés | University of California System, Education Abroad Program, Santa Barbara, CA |
| Ejike-King, Lacreisha | US Food and Drug Administration, US Department of Health and Human Services, Rockville, MD |
| Fairley, Jessica K. | Emory University School of Medicine, Atlanta, GA |
| Florez-Arango, Jose F. | Biomedical Informatics, College of Medicine, Texas A&M Health Science Center, College Station, TX |
| Forgione, Michael | Keesler Medical Center, Keesler AFB, Mississippi |
| Franco-Paredes, Carlos | Division of Infectious Diseases, University of Colorado at Denver, School of Medicine, Aurora, CO; Hospital Infantil de México Federico Gómez, Mexico City, Mexico |
| Freedman, David O. | Shoreland, Inc., Milwaukee, WI |
| Gracia, J. Nadine | Office of Minority Health, US Department of Health and Human Services, Rockville, MD |
| Hackett, Peter H. | Institute for Altitude Medicine, Telluride, CO, and Altitude Research Center, University of Colorado Denver School of Medicine, Denver, CO |
| Hamer, Davidson H. | Center for Global Health and Development Boston University; Department of Global Health, Boston University School of Public Health and Section of Infectious Diseases, Boston Medical Center, Boston, MA |
| Henao-Martinez, Andres | Division of Infectious Diseases, University of Colorado at Denver, School of Medicine, Aurora, CO |
| Henderson, John | United Nations consultant, Burma |
| Hochberg, Natasha S. | Section of Infectious Diseases, Boston University School of Medicine, Boston, MA |
| Javed, Uzma | Office of American Citizens Services |
| Kain, Kevin C. | University of Toronto, Toronto, Canada |
| Kayden, Stephanie | Harvard Humanitarian Initiative, Cambridge, MA; Harvard Medical School, Boston, MA; Brigham and Women's Hospital, Boston, MA |
| Keystone, Jay S. | University of Toronto, Toronto, Canada |

| | |
|---|---|
| Kotton, Camille Nelson | Massachusetts General Hospital and Harvard University, Boston, MA |
| LaRocque, Regina C. | Massachusetts General Hospital and Harvard Medical School, Boston, MA |
| Law, Catherine | National Center for Complementary and Integrative Health, National Institutes of Health, Bethesda, MD |
| Levi, Matt | CHI Franciscan Health, Tacoma, WA |
| Libman, Michael | McGill University, Centre for Tropical Disease, Montreal, Canada |
| McDevitt, Sue Ann | New York, NY |
| Neumann, Karl | Weill Medical College of Cornell University and New York Presbyterian Hospital/Cornell Medical Center, New York, NY |
| Nilles, Eric J. | Harvard Humanitarian Initiative, Cambridge, MA; Harvard Medical School, Boston, MA; Brigham and Women's Hospital, Boston, MA |
| Nord, Daniel A. | Divers Alert Network, Durham, NC |
| Norton, Scott | Children's National Medical Center, Washington, DC |
| Parker, Salim | Dee Bee Medical Centre, Cape Town; South African Society of Travel Medicine, Johannesburg, South Africa |
| Pogemiller, Hope | University of Minnesota Medical School, Minneapolis, MN |
| Rhodes, Gary | Center for Global Education, University of California, Los Angeles, CA |
| Riddle, Mark S. | Naval Medical Research Center, Silver Spring, MD |
| Rosselot, Gail A. | Travel Well of Westchester, Briarcliff Manor, NY |
| Ryan, Edward T. | Massachusetts General Hospital and Harvard University, Boston, MA |
| Sampson, Dana M. | Office of Minority Health, US Department of Health and Human Services, Rockville, MD |
| Shlim, David R. | Jackson Hole Travel and Tropical Medicine, Jackson Hole, WY |
| Shurtleff, David | National Center for Complementary and Integrative Health, National Institutes of Health, Bethesda, MD |
| Staat, Mary Allen | International Adoption Center, Cincinnati Children's Hospital Medical Center, Cincinnati, OH |
| Taggart, Linda R. | University of Toronto, Toronto, Canada |
| Thompson, Andrew | University of Liverpool, Liverpool, UK |
| Valk, Thomas H. | VEI Inc., Marshall, VA |
| Van Tilburg, Christopher | Providence Hood River Memorial Hospital, Hood River, OR |
| Waggoner, Jesse | Department of Medicine, Division of Infectious Diseases, Emory University School of Medicine, Atlanta, GA |
| Wanat, Karolyn | Medical College of Wisconsin, Milwaukee, WI |
| Wangu, Zoon | Department of Pediatric Infectious Diseases, Boston Medical Center, Boston, MA |
| Weinberg, Nicholas | Geisel School of Medicine, Dartmouth College, Hanover, NH |
| Wilson, Mary Elizabeth | Harvard School of Public Health, Boston, MA |
| Wu, Henry M. | Emory University, Department of Medicine, Atlanta, GA |
| Youngster, Ilan | Children's Hospital Boston and Harvard University, Boston, MA |

All contributors have signed a statement indicating that they have no conflicts of interest with the subject matter or materials discussed in the document(s) that they have written or reviewed for this book and that the information that they have written or reviewed for this book is objective and free from bias.

# Acknowledgments

The *CDC Yellow Book 2020: Health Information for International Travel* editorial team gratefully acknowledges all the authors and reviewers for their commitment to this new edition. We extend sincere thanks to the following people for their contributions to the production of this book:

- Kelly M. Winter for serving in the role of managing editor and guiding this edition through the first half of production.

- Elise Beltrami, Nicole Cohen, Rachel Eidex, and Scott Santibanez for their extensive review of the text.

- Maeghan Dessecker, Johanzynn Gatewood, and Calvin Patimeteeporn for their assistance in preparing the text for publication.

# Preface

To stay on the cutting edge of travel health information, this latest edition of the *CDC Yellow Book: Health Information for International Travel* has been extensively revised. The book serves as a guide to the practice of travel medicine, as well as the authoritative source of US government recommendations for immunizations and prophylaxis for foreign travel. As international travel continues to become more common in the lives of US residents, having at least a basic understanding of the medical problems that travelers face has become a necessary aspect of practicing medicine. The goal of this book is to be a comprehensive resource for clinicians to find the answers to their travel health–related questions.

**Centers for Disease Control and Prevention**
Robert R. Redfield, MD, Director
**National Center for Emerging and Zoonotic Infectious Diseases**
Rima Khabbaz, MD, Director
**Division of Global Migration and Quarantine**
Martin S. Cetron, MD, Director
Gary W. Brunette, MD, MS, Chief, Travelers' Health Branch
Jeffrey B. Nemhauser, MD, Chief Medical Officer, Travelers' Health Branch
Jenique Meekins, Health Communications Specialist, Travelers' Health Branch

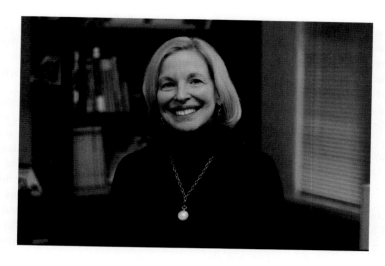

## With Gratitude to Phyllis E. Kozarsky

**Phyllis E. Kozarsky, MD,** is the longest serving member of the Travelers' Health Branch at the Centers for Disease Control and Prevention (CDC). More than 25 years ago, she came to the branch, bringing with her extensive experience in travel medicine and infectious diseases. Over the years, Phyllis has helped elevate the quality of the work performed by branch epidemiologists, public health advisors, medical officers, and communicators thanks to her generously shared clinical insight. Phyllis has also served as an editor of CDC's *Yellow Book* since 1999. *Yellow Book 2020* will be her final one as Chief Medical Editor, and it is to her great legacy and contribution to travel medicine that we gratefully and fondly dedicate this edition.

It is difficult to imagine the field of travel medicine without Phyllis Kozarsky. A wealth of knowledge and critical judgment in all areas of travel medicine—she really is one of the best in the world—Phyllis is remarkably humble and naturally reticent by nature, qualities that have prevented many of the members of our community from fully appreciating the key role she has played in developing this specialty. In 1991, after helping to create the International Society of Travel Medicine (ISTM), she then managed the organization for several years until it gained its footing. She was also instrumental in creating ISTM's Certificate of Travel Health exam. An infectious disease specialist, Phyllis started and ran the travel medicine clinic at Emory University in Atlanta, while simultaneously serving as a stable and knowledgeable presence in the travel medicine section of the CDC.

**David R. Shlim, MD**

When I think of Phyllis Kozarsky, it is her big beautiful smile and her willingness to pitch in and work as part of a team to solve problems that first come to mind.

Phyllis shaped travel medicine as it exists today. Masterful in bringing evidence to practice and policy, she led efforts to define a core body of knowledge for the specialty. She then developed the examination that awards clinicians who pass it, a certificate recognizing their expertise, according to internationally established standards. She has provided crucial support to the GeoSentinel surveillance network and the Global TravEpiNet (GTEN) consortium, and translated the data each provides into sensible guidance for travel medicine practitioners. Her many experiences—as a professor in an academic institution, as an expert consultant in CDC's Division of Global Migration and Quarantine, and her work with industry—have provided Phyllis with the multiple perspectives she uses to develop her sound, workable recommendations.

Practical, pragmatic, resourceful, deeply knowledgeable, and highly connected to colleagues throughout the world, Phyllis has a deft touch when dealing with controversial and complicated issues. Her many publications include guidelines and useful advice for common as well as emerging problems, including Zika and Ebola. She has written about vulnerable populations and business and corporate travelers. She has communicated information to the public through interviews and other media outlets, and as Chief Medical Editor for multiple editions of the *Yellow Book*, Phyllis has reached the global community of travel medicine practitioners.

**Mary E. Wilson, MD**

A clade of scholars currently focuses on virtual or counterfactual history. So let us ask, hypothetically, "What if in the late 1980's there would have been no Phyllis Kozarsky at Emory University to collaborate mainly with the CDC in the project for the 1991 Atlanta Travel Medicine Conference?" The simple answer is that there would have been no meeting, and the International Society of Travel Medicine (ISTM) would not have been founded!

Over the decades, Phyllis has continued to contribute as a top leader in crucial projects whenever needed, forging compromises and building bridges. On the surface, soft as velvet, but—when necessary—convincing colleagues with hard facts and her little smile, up to the final success. Phyllis has been one of the main travel medicine achievers in many functions both inside and outside the CDC and the ISTM.

**Robert Steffen, MD**

Few others in my experience have Phyllis Kozarsky's common sense and wisdom, two of her strongest personal qualities. Wise beyond her years, she is also a caretaker: a compassionate, thoughtful and nurturing individual, always sensitive to the needs of others, an excellent team player and peacemaker. She has never sought the limelight in terms of her work with ISTM, preferring instead to be in the background, letting others take credit even when she was very much involved in the work and its accomplishments. She preferred to be, as I saw it, 'the power behind the throne'. She has carved out her many successes with a quiet determination.

Phyllis is a remarkably bright, innovative leader in the field of travel medicine. A visionary, not a follower, her accomplishments are a testament to her desire to make the world a better place. Her

tremendous interpersonal skills have made her an effective, innovative leader in the field of travel medicine and a beloved friend.

**Jay S. Keystone, MD**

Phyllis Kozarsky has played a critical role in defining, nurturing, and holding to high standards the field of travel medicine. Her depth of expertise is unsurpassed, but more importantly, she has been amazingly adept at linking the fields of clinical medicine and public health. She has facilitated countless connections, bringing together disparate groups, topics, and nations. With regard to CDC's *Yellow Book*, Phyllis' input has ensured it has remained the authoritative travel medicine reference, enabling countless providers to render outstanding care and advice. We will miss her knowledge, counsel, wit and graciousness as she steps down as Chief Medical Editor.

**Edward T. Ryan, MD**

I have known my friend and colleague Dr. Phyllis Kozarsky for over 25 years and I cannot think of a single person who has had as much influence on the field of travel medicine as she has. An advocate for public and professional education in travel medicine, Phyllis was a founding member of the International Society of Travel Medicine (ISTM), served as its first Secretary Treasurer, and organized its first conference in 1991; she chaired its first Professional Education Committee and created the ISTM Certification Examination. She has also served as editor of the premier textbook in travel medicine. Her accomplishments—clinical, educational and organizational—set her apart from virtually everyone else in the field. And matched by her accomplishments and intelligence (perhaps even exceeding them) are her warmth, compassion and generosity of spirt, her kindness, empathy and true respect of others.

**Bradley A. Connor, MD**

The CDC *Yellow Book* first appeared in 1967. Originally a thin pamphlet, it presented to readers some specific provisions of the International Health Regulations.

For the last 11 editions (over the past 20 years), Phyllis Kozarsky has guided the transformation of the *Yellow Book* into the comprehensive travel medicine reference by which all other sources of travel medicine information are now judged. Its guidelines and recommendations articulate the evidence-base in the US-context as determined by the CDC and its various advisory bodies. And while a number of other national and international resources are available, experienced clinicians outside the United States continue to refer to the *Yellow Book* as a mandatory pillar of consultation for all matters of clinical decision support to safeguard the health of their travelers.

Phyllis, who directed her own travel clinic at Emory University where she had an enviable publication record as a Professor of Medicine, has been steadfast in ensuring that the *Yellow Book* be written primarily for practicing clinicians. Over the years, she assembled a cadre of expert co-editors and contributors from outside the agency (mainly experts from GeoSentinel and ISTM) who themselves had day-to-day experience in the practice of travel medicine, helping make each edition come to life.

Phyllis' vision and soft-spoken subject-matter mastery—combined with her dogged diligence up until the last possible publication deadline—has allowed her to bring together experts from inside and outside the CDC. Experts who craft language that provides readers with a comprehensive understanding of a topic, and a best-possible, very practical solution to any clinical scenario that might walk into the travel clinic. The qualifications for Phyllis' successor should simply include the attributes mentioned in this dedication piece; one should ask for no more and no less.

**David O. Freedman, MD**

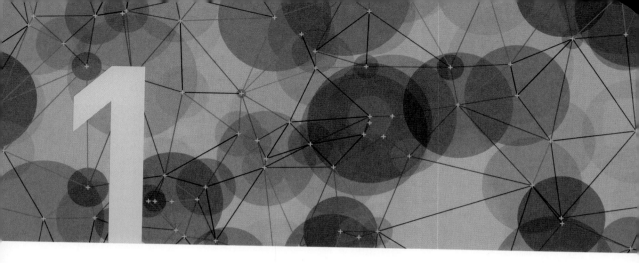

# Introduction

## INTRODUCTION TO TRAVEL HEALTH & THE CDC YELLOW BOOK

Phyllis E. Kozarsky, Ronnie Henry

### TRAVEL HEALTH

The number of people traveling internationally continues to grow. According to the World Tourism Organization, there were 1.33 billion worldwide international tourist arrivals in 2017, an increase of 88% from 2015. International arrivals increased 6% in January–April 2018 compared to the same period in 2017. In 2017, US residents made nearly 88 million trips with at least 1 night outside the United States.

The importance of protecting the health of individual travelers, as well as safeguarding the health of the communities to which they return, cannot be overstated. People travel internationally for many reasons, including tourism, business, study abroad, research, visiting friends and relatives, ecotourism, adventure, medical tourism, mission work, and international disaster response. Travelers are as unique as their itineraries, covering all age ranges and having a variety of preexisting health concerns and conditions. The infectious disease risks that travelers face are dynamic—some travel destinations have become safer, while in other areas new diseases have emerged, and other diseases have reemerged.

The risk of becoming ill or injured during international travel depends on many factors, such as the region of the world visited, a traveler's age and health status, the length of the trip, and the diversity of planned activities. CDC provides international travel health information that covers the range of health risks travelers may face, with the aim of assisting travelers and clinicians to better understand the measures necessary to prevent illness and injury during international travel. This publication and the CDC Travelers' Health website (www.cdc.gov/travel) are 2 primary avenues of communicating CDC's travel health recommendations.

# BOX 1-1. CDC contact information for clinicians

## CDC-INFO NATIONAL CONTACT CENTER

All topics for clinicians and general public *(English and Spanish)*

- 8 am to 8 pm Eastern, M–F: toll-free at 800-CDC-INFO (800-232-4636)
- Email form: www.cdc.gov/info

## CDC EMERGENCY OPERATIONS CENTER

Emergency or urgent patient care assistance *(Note: This line is not intended for public inquiries.)*

- Available 24 hours per day, 7 days per week: 770-488-7100
- Email: eocreport@cdc.gov

## CDC DRUG SERVICE

Distribution of special biologic agents and drugs

- Formulary: www.cdc.gov/laboratory/drugservice/formulary.html
- 8 am to 4:30 pm Eastern, M–F: 404-639-3670
- After hours/weekends/holidays: 770-488-7100
- Email: drugservice@cdc.gov

## CHIKUNGUNYA, JAPANESE ENCEPHALITIS, TICKBORNE ENCEPHALITIS, AND YELLOW FEVER

Diagnostic testing assistance and for questions about antibody response to yellow fever vaccination

- 8 am to 4:30 pm Mountain, M–F: 970-221-6400 (Division of Vectorborne Diseases)
- Viral Special Pathogens Branch can also assist with tickborne encephalitis, 8:30 am to 5:30 pm Eastern, M–F: 404-639-1115
- After hours/weekends/holidays: 770-488-7100
- State or local health departments may be able to assist: www.cdc.gov/ncezid/dhcpp/vspb/specimens.html

## DENGUE

Diagnostic testing assistance

- 8 am to 5 pm Atlantic (office in Puerto Rico), M–F: 787-706-2399
- After hours/weekends/holidays: 770-488-7100
- Clinical/laboratory guidance: www.cdc.gov/Dengue/clinicalLab/index.html

## MALARIA

Diagnosis and management assistance

- 9 am to 5 pm Eastern, M–F: 770-488-7788 or toll-free at 855-856-4713
- Emergency consultation after hours/weekends/holidays: 770-488-7100, ask for a Malaria Branch clinician

## PARASITIC DISEASES (OTHER THAN MALARIA)

*Live Support*

Evaluation and management assistance for patients suspected to have a parasitic disease

- 8 am to 4 pm Eastern, M–F: 404-718-4745
- Emergency consultation after hours/weekends/holidays: 770-488-7100, ask for an on-call clinician in Parasitic Diseases
- Email: parasites@cdc.gov

*Online Support (DPDx)*

Online diagnostic assistance service for laboratorians, pathologists, and other health professionals developed and maintained by CDC's Division of Parasitic Diseases and Malaria (DPDM)

- www.cdc.gov/dpdx/contact.html

## RICKETTSIAL DISEASES

Diagnosis and management assistance

- 8:30 am to 4:30 pm Eastern, M–F: 404-639-1075
- Emergency consultation after hours/weekends/holidays: 770-488-7100, ask for an on-call clinician in Rickettsial Diseases

## VIRAL HEMORRHAGIC FEVERS

*Diagnosis*

Consultation for diagnosis and reporting suspected cases in or requiring evacuation to the United States

- 8:30 am to 5:30 pm Eastern, Eastern, M–F: 404-639-1115
- Emergency consultation after hours/weekends/holidays: 770-488-7100

*Treatment*

Requests for ribavirin from Valeant Pharmaceuticals through the Food and Drug Administration (FDA)

- FDA Provider Request Line: 301-736-3400
- Simultaneously notify Valeant at 800-548-5100, ext. 5 (domestic) or 949-461-6971 (international)

# HISTORY AND ROLES OF THE YELLOW BOOK

*CDC Health Information for International Travel* ("The Yellow Book") has been a trusted resource for over 50 years. In 1967, CDC published the first Yellow Book, a small pamphlet intended to satisfy the International Sanitary Regulations requirements (1951) and later, the International Health Regulations (IHR). Adopted by the World Health Organization (WHO) in 1969 and completely revised in 2005, the IHR are designed to ensure maximum security against the international spread of diseases, with minimum interference with world travel and commerce. A copy of the current IHR and supporting information can be found on the WHO website (www.who.int/csr/ihr/en).

In addition to reporting public health events of international concern, the United States must also inform the public about health requirements for entering or leaving other countries, such as the need to be vaccinated against yellow fever. The Yellow Book and the CDC Travelers' Health website aim to communicate these requirements under the IHR (2005).

The Yellow Book has expanded significantly in breadth and depth over the years. It is written primarily for clinicians, including physicians, nurses, and pharmacists. Others, such as people in the travel industry, multinational corporations, missionary and volunteer organizations, and individual travelers, can also find a wealth of information here.

Authored by subject-matter experts both within and outside CDC, the guidelines presented in this book are evidence-based and supported by best practices. Internal text citations have not been included; however, a bibliography is appended to the end of each section for those interested in more detailed information. The CDC Travelers' Health program and the CDC Foundation are pleased to partner with Oxford University Press, Inc., to publish the 2020 edition. In addition to the printed copy, a searchable, online version of the Yellow Book can be found on the CDC Travelers' Health website (www.cdc.gov/yellowbook).

Although this publication includes the most current information available at the time of printing, requirements and recommendations can change. Check the CDC Travelers' Health website (www.cdc.gov/travel) and the online Yellow Book for regularly updated information on requirements for international travel.

## CONTACT INFORMATION FOR CDC

Questions, comments, and suggestions for CDC Travelers' Health, including comments about this publication, may be made through the CDC-INFO contact center, toll-free at 800-CDC-INFO (800-232-4636) 8 AM to 8 PM Eastern Time (Monday–Friday, closed on holidays) or by visiting www.cdc.gov/info to submit your question through an online form.

### Pretravel or Posttravel Clinical Questions

The CDC is not a medical facility. Clinicians needing assistance with preparing patients for international travel should consider a referral to a travel clinic or a clinic listed on the International Society of Travel Medicine (ISTM) website (www.istm.org).

Clinicians with posttravel health questions regarding their patients may refer to a clinic listed on the ISTM website, the American Society of Tropical Medicine and Hygiene website (www.astmh.org), or a medical university with specialists in infectious diseases.

State and local health departments may also be useful resources.

Because of the complexity of some travel-related diseases, Box 1-1 lists contact information for providers needing clinical assistance.

## BIBLIOGRAPHY

1. United Nations World Tourism Organization. UNWTO World Tourism Barometer, Vol. 16 (June 6). Madrid: United Nations World Tourism Organization; 2018 [cited 2018 Jul 12]. Available from: www.e-unwto.org/doi/abs/10.18111/wtobarometereng.2018.16.1.3.

2. US Department of Commerce, Office of Travel and Tourism Industries. 2017 US Citizen Travel to International Regions. Washington, DC: US Department of Commerce; 2018 [cited 2018 Jul 12]. Available from: https://travel.trade.gov/view/m-2017-O-001/index.html.

3. World Health Organization. International Health Regulations (2005). Geneva: World Health Organization; 2008 [cited 2018 Jul 12]; 2nd edition. Available from: www.who.int/ihr/publications/9789241596664/en/.

# TRAVEL EPIDEMIOLOGY

Allison Taylor Walker, Regina C. LaRocque, Mark J. Sotir

**1**

Travelers are an epidemiologically important population because of their mobility, their potential for exposure to diseases outside their home country, and the possibility that they may serve as a conduit for disease from one country to another. In the past 10 years, for example, travelers have faced newly emerging threats, including Ebola, chikungunya, and Zika. Evolving epidemiology of disease, the increasing prevalence of antimicrobial drug resistance, and the development of new vaccines and prophylactic treatments have each contributed to create the ongoing need for surveillance of international travelers.

The risk of travel-related illness varies depending on destination and traveler characteristics. Existing information regarding the actual risk for travelers (often expressed as number of events per 100,000 travelers) is limited for several reasons. It is difficult to obtain an accurate numerator (number of cases of disease among travelers) and denominator (number of travelers overall or travelers to a specific destination who are susceptible to infection). To calculate a true risk for a traveler, scientific studies would have to document the number of travelers susceptible to that disease or condition and the number of those affected during a specific period of time. If the illness is mild, the traveler may never seek health care, or clinicians might not perform diagnostic tests to identify the cause accurately. Furthermore, because travelers often visit multiple destinations, it could be difficult to determine the location where the exposure occurred and attribute risk to that location.

Frequently quoted studies on the incidence of infection in travelers use a variety of methodologic designs, each with its own strengths and weaknesses, making findings difficult to compare or combine. These studies have examined, for the most part, only a few key diseases or conditions, combining all travelers regardless of destination. Many have been single-clinic or single-destination studies that lead to conclusions that are not generalizable to groups of travelers with different local, national, or cultural backgrounds.

Health care providers must understand the epidemiologic features of the traveling population to guide pretravel recommendations and posttravel evaluations. The characteristics of travel-related diseases must be considered, including mode of transmission, incubation period, signs and symptoms, duration of illness, and diagnostic testing. The presence, frequency, seasonality, and geographic distribution of the disease need to be assessed; these might change over time because of outbreaks, emergence or reemergence in new areas or populations, successful public health interventions, or other factors.

Data on disease incidence in local populations could identify the most important diseases to monitor within a country, but the relevance of such data to travelers—who have different risk behaviors, eating habits, accommodations, knowledge of preventive measures, and activities—is usually limited. Surveillance data that focus on travelers or on illnesses that affect travelers are therefore more useful in describing travel-related disease patterns and risks.

Two existing networks provide data on the demographics of US international travelers and the acquisition of travel-related illness. Global TravEpiNet (GTEN) is a consortium of health clinics across the United States that provide pretravel health consultations; data from GTEN provide a snapshot of the types of travelers seeking pretravel health care and their travel practices, as well as longitudinal cohort data on risk and acquisition of travel-associated conditions. The GeoSentinel Global Surveillance Network, a worldwide data collection and communication network composed of International Society of Travel Medicine (ISTM) travel and tropical medicine clinics, collects posttravel illness surveillance data. GeoSentinel analyzes this data to describe the relationships between travel and travel-related illness in specific subpopulations of travelers.

Familiarity with the epidemiology and prevalence of travel-related infections, coupled with demographic information on travelers and their particular travel details, can help clinicians provide optimal health-related information and advice. Clinical networks and surveillance systems provide epidemiologic data on new and prevalent global infectious disease threats. Improved collaboration between travel health providers and the travel health clinical networks is needed to further expand and develop the evidence base in this field; this will allow for better-informed preparation before travel and enhanced clinical awareness of travel epidemiology for clinicians seeing patients before and after travel.

## BIBLIOGRAPHY

1. Adachi K, Coleman MS, Khan N, Jentes ES, Arguin P, Rao SR, et al. Economics of malaria prevention in US travelers to West Africa. Clin Infect Dis. 2014 Jan;58(1):11–21.

2. CDC. Malaria surveillance—United States, 2011. MMWR Surveill Summ. 2013 Nov 1;62(5):1–17.

3. Esposito DH, Stich A, Epelboin L, Malvy D, Han PV, Bottieau E, et al. Acute muscular sarcocystosis: an international investigation among ill travelers returning from Tioman Island, Malaysia, 2011–2012. Clin Infect Dis. 2014 Nov 15;59(10):1401–10.

4. Harvey K, Esposito DH, Han P, Kozarsky P, Freedman DO, Plier DA, et al. Surveillance for travel-related disease—GeoSentinel Surveillance System, United States, 1997–2011. MMWR Surveill Summ. 2013 Jul. 19;62:1–23.

5. LaRocque RC, Rao SR, Lee J, Ansdell V, Yates JA, Schwartz BS, et al. Global TravEpiNet: a national consortium of clinics providing care to international travelers—analysis of demographic characteristics, travel destinations, and pretravel healthcare of high-risk US international travelers, 2009–2011. Clin Infect Dis. 2012 Feb. 15;54(4):455–62.

6. Leder K, Torresi J, Libman MD, Cramer JP, Castelli F, Schlagenhauf P, et al. GeoSentinel surveillance of illness in returned travelers, 2007–2011. Ann Intern Med. 2013 Mar. 19;158(6):456–68.

7. Millman AJ, Esposito DH, Biggs HM, Decenteceo M, Klevos A, Hunsperger E, et al. Chikungunya and dengue virus infections among United States community service volunteers returning from the Dominican Republic. Am J Trop Med Hyg. 2014 Mar. 14;64(6):1336–41.

8. Sharp TM, Pillai P, Hunsperger E, Santiago GA, Anderson T, Vap T, et al. A cluster of dengue cases in American missionaries returning from Haiti. Am J Trop Med Hyg. 2010 Jan.;86(1):6–22.

9. Sotir M, Freedman D. Basic epidemiology of infectious diseases, including surveillance and reporting. In: Zuckerman J, Leggat P, Brunette G, editors. Essential Travel Medicine. Chichester (UK): John Wiley & Sons; 2015.

10. United Nations World Tourism Organization. UNWTO Tourism Highlights, 2016 ed. [Internet]. Madrid: World Tourism Organization; 2016 [cited 2018 Mar. 26]. Available from: http://media.unwto.org/press-release/2016-01-18/international-tourist-arrivals-4-reachrecord-12-billion-2015.

# WHY GUIDELINES DIFFER

David R. Shlim

## INTRODUCTION

Numerous international, national, and professional organizations publish guidelines and recommendations for travelers, including the CDC Yellow Book. Travel health providers should be aware of these recommendations, even though they may not follow them in every instance. This way they can explain to their patients how their recommendations, and their patients' choices, may be at odds with what others recommend. It can be unsettling for patients to receive travel medicine advice, vaccines, or an antimalarial drug prescription from a provider, only to find that what has been advised or prescribed is contradicted by what other professionals, friends, or destination-country nationals have to say. The skillful travel health provider will be able to help the traveler reconcile seemingly conflicting advice.

## HOW GUIDELINES ARE CREATED

In the United States, the Food and Drug Administration (FDA) approves standards for how to use a vaccine or medication, including dosages, ages for which the product is approved, and booster recommendations. Recommendations about when to use a product may come from a separate body, such as the Advisory Committee on Immunization Practices (ACIP). To give ACIP the best possible information on which to base their recommendations, working groups of experts may hold meetings to review the literature and new studies. CDC Yellow Book travel advice will always be compatible with ACIP recommendations but may, on occasion, offer country- and situation-specific guidelines for vaccine use.

International organizations such as the World Health Organization (WHO) and national committees of other countries, as well as medical organizations such as the International Society of Travel Medicine (ISTM) or the Infectious Diseases Society of America, may each promote their own sets of guidance. Other professional organizations may create consensus clinical practice guidelines based on published medical literature and expert opinion. Travel medicine–specific paid subscription services employ travel medicine experts to organize and present guidelines for health care providers who see international travelers in their practice but who may lack expertise in the subject. Guidance provided about vaccines and malaria prophylaxis can differ from CDC advice.

Guidelines put forward by different countries and organizations may differ in substantial ways. Reasons for this include differing licensure and availability of products, cultural perceptions of risk, lack of definitive evidence, and differences of opinion among experts.

### Availability of Products

Travel health providers can only use the products available to them. Availability is determined by the regulatory approval status of the product and, to a lesser extent, the marketing and distribution plan of the manufacturer. Regulatory approval processes vary greatly by country. For example, registering a new vaccine or antimalarial drug in the United States is a costly and rigorous process. If the market in a particular country is insufficient to justify the expense of registration, a commercial company may not seek it.

Standards for licensure also vary. What may be sufficient for one regulatory authority may not suffice for another. For example, primaquine, an option for malaria prophylaxis in the United States, is not registered or commercially available in Switzerland. Atovaquone-proguanil was available for malaria prophylaxis in the United States before many other countries. Four Japanese encephalitis vaccines are available in the world, but only 1 is licensed in the United States.

Even when the same products are available, recommendations for use may not be the same in all countries. The injectable capsular polysaccharide typhoid vaccine and the oral typhoid vaccine are examples. In the United States, a booster of the polysaccharide vaccine is recommended after 2 years, but in most European countries, a booster is recommended after 3 years. In the United States, a packet of 4 oral typhoid vaccine capsules is dispensed, whereas in Europe, 3 doses are considered adequate. The regulatory agencies may have reviewed the same data and drawn different conclusions, or they may have reviewed different data at separate times. Regulatory submissions to various agencies rarely occur at the same time; therefore, the data available for review by each agency may not be the same, for legitimate reasons.

## Perception of Risk

People from varying backgrounds can view the same risk data and come to very different conclusions as to the cost and benefit of minimizing that risk to what they consider to be an acceptable level. For example, recommendations to prevent malaria during travel to India vary widely. Germany does not recommend using standard prophylaxis for any travel to an Indian destination; standby emergency treatment (SBET) or self-treatment) only is the recommendation for identified risk destinations. Guidelines from the United Kingdom recommend only awareness and mosquito bite prevention for more than half the Indian subcontinent, including large cities and popular tourist destinations in the north and south, while suggesting prophylaxis consideration for some travelers or for those visiting higher-risk areas. By contrast, CDC recommends malaria prophylaxis for any Indian destination (except for some mountainous areas of northern states) for all travelers.

## Lack of Evidence

In many cases, limited or no data are available to inform an evidence-based assessment. Travel health providers must then defer to expert opinion or extrapolate from limited data in conjunction with expert opinion. In travel medicine, it is rare to have numerator and denominator data on the risk of any disease. For example, any new data on the risk of hepatitis A in travelers would have to account for the high immunization rate with hepatitis A vaccine. Because such data are rarely available, travel health providers often rely on historical data that captured few actual cases.

## CAN WE HARMONIZE GUIDELINES?

The complex nature of how health organizations

(continued)

# WHY GUIDELINES DIFFER (CONTINUED)

obtain, evaluate, and verify data, combined with fundamental differences in risk perception, makes it likely that multiple, overlapping, and at times conflicting guidelines will continue to exist. However, conflicting guidelines have decreased in the past decade due to the efforts of several organizations. A recent example has been the collaboration among the WHO, US CDC, and the European Centre for Disease Prevention and Control (ECDC) to develop consistency and clarity in defining the risk of Zika infection for travelers so that providers can more clearly relay traveler risk, particularly to those who are pregnant or planning pregnancy.

In summary, the role of the travel health provider is to understand the various differences in guidelines, interpret this information, and convey tailored and informed advice in an assured and comforting manner to travelers.

## BIBLIOGRAPHY

1. CDC. Malaria surveillance—United States, 2015. MMWR Surveill Summ. 2018 May 4;67(7):1–28.

2. CDC. Advisory Committee on Immunization Practices (ACIP). Atlanta: CDC; 2018 [cited 2018 Sep 12]. Available from: www.cdc.gov/vaccines/acip/.

3. Chiodini PL, Field VK, Whitty CJM, Lalloo DG. Guidelines for malaria prevention in travellers from the UK: 2017. London: Public Health England; 2017 [cited 2018 Sep 12]. Available from: https://assets.publishing.service.gov.uk/government/uploads/system/uploads/attachment_data/file/660051/Guidelines_for_malaria_prevention_in_travellers_from_the_UK_2017.pdf.

4. Committee to Advise on Tropical Medicine and Travel (CATMAT). Canadian recommendations for the prevention and treatment of malaria. Ottawa: Public Health Agency of Canada; 2014 [cited 2018 Sep 12]. Available from: http://publications.gc.ca/collections/collection_2014/aspc-phac/HP40-102-2014-eng.pdf.

5. German Society for Tropical Medicine and International Health Association (DTG). [Recommendations for the prophylaxis and treatment of malaria of DTG 2018]. 2018 [cited 2018 Sep 12]. Available from: www.dtg.org/empfehlungen-und-leitlinien/empfehlungen/malaria.html.

6. Hill DR, Ericsson CD, Pearson RD, Keystone JS, Freedman DO, Kozarsky PE, et al. The practice of travel medicine: guidelines by the Infectious Diseases Society of America. Clin Infect Dis. 2006 Dec 15;43(12):1499–539.

7. World Health Organization. International Health Regulations (2005). Geneva: World Health Organization; 2016 [cited 2018 Sep 12]. Available from: www.who.int/ihr/publications/9789241580496/en.

8. World Health Organization. International Travel and Health. Geneva: World Health Organization; 2012 (with 2016 updates) [cited 2016 June 14]. Available from: www.who.int/ith/en/.

*Perspectives* sections are editorial discussions written to add depth and clinical perspective to the official recommendations contained in the book. The views and opinions expressed in this section are those of the authors and do not necessarily represent the official position of CDC.

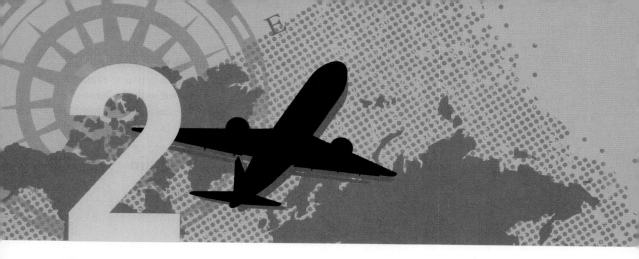

# Preparing International Travelers

## THE PRETRAVEL CONSULTATION

Lin H. Chen, Natasha S. Hochberg

The pretravel consultation offers a dedicated time to prepare travelers for the health concerns that might arise during their trips. The objectives of the pretravel consultation are to:

1. Perform an individual risk assessment.
2. Communicate to the traveler anticipated health risks.
3. Provide risk management measures, including immunizations, malaria prophylaxis, and other medications as indicated.

### THE TRAVEL MEDICINE SPECIALIST

Travel medicine specialists have in-depth knowledge of immunizations, risks associated with specific destinations, and the implications of traveling with underlying conditions. Therefore, a comprehensive consultation with a travel medicine expert is indicated for all travelers, and is particularly important for those with a complicated health history, special risks (such as traveling at high altitudes or working in refugee camps), or exotic or complicated itineraries. Clinicians who wish to be travel medicine providers are encouraged to join the International Society of Travel Medicine (ISTM) and consider specialty training and certification.

### COMPONENTS OF A PRETRAVEL CONSULTATION

Effective pretravel consultations require attention to the health background of the traveler and incorporate the itinerary, trip duration, travel purpose, and activities, all of which determine health risks (Table 2-1). The pretravel consultation is the major opportunity to educate the traveler about health risks at the destination and how to mitigate them. The typical pretravel consultation does not include a physical examination; a separate appointment with the same or a different provider may be necessary to assess a

## Table 2-1. Information necessary for a risk assessment during pretravel consultations

| Health Background | |
| --- | --- |
| Past medical history | Age<br>Sex<br>Underlying conditions<br>Allergies (especially any pertaining to vaccines, eggs, or latex)<br>Medications |
| Special conditions | Pregnancy (including trimester)<br>Breastfeeding<br>Disability or handicap<br>Immunocompromising conditions or medications<br>Older age<br>Psychiatric condition<br>Seizure disorder<br>Recent surgery<br>Recent cardiopulmonary event<br>Recent cerebrovascular event<br>History of Guillain-Barré syndrome<br>Severe allergies |
| Immunization history | Routine vaccines<br>Travel vaccines |
| Prior travel experience | Experience with malaria chemoprophylaxis<br>Experience with altitude<br>Illnesses related to prior travel |
| **Trip Details** | |
| Itinerary | Countries and specific regions, including order of countries if >1 country<br>Rural or urban |
| Timing | Trip duration<br>Season of travel<br>Time to departure |
| Reason for travel | Tourism<br>Business<br>Visiting friends and relatives<br>Volunteer, missionary, or aid work<br>Research or education<br>Adventure<br>Pilgrimage<br>Adoption<br>Seeking health care (medical tourism) |

## Table 2-1. Information necessary for a risk assessment during pretravel consultations (continued)

| | |
|---|---|
| Travel style | Independent travel or package tour<br>Propensity for "adventurous" eating<br>Traveler risk tolerance<br>General hygiene standards at destination<br>Modes of transportation<br>Accommodations (such as tourist or luxury hotel, guest house, hostel or budget hotel, dormitory, local home or host family, or tent) |
| Special activities | Disaster relief<br>Medical care (providing or receiving)<br>High altitude<br>Diving<br>Cruise ship<br>Rafting or other water exposure<br>Cycling<br>Extreme sports<br>Spelunking<br>Anticipated interactions with animals<br>Anticipated sexual encounters |

person's fitness to travel. Because travel medicine clinics are not available in some communities, primary care physicians should seek guidance (by phone or other communication, if available) from travel medicine specialists to address areas of uncertainty.

Travel health advice should be personalized, highlighting the likely exposures and also reminding the traveler of ubiquitous risks, such as injury, foodborne and waterborne infections, vectorborne disease, respiratory tract infections, and bloodborne and sexually transmitted infections. Balancing the cautions with an appreciation of the positive aspects of the journey leads to a more meaningful pretravel consultation. Attention to the cost of recommended interventions may be critical. Some travelers may not be able to afford all of the recommended immunizations and medications, a situation that requires prioritizing interventions. (See Prioritizing Care for the Resource-Limited Traveler later in this chapter.)

## Assess Individual Risk

Many elements merit consideration in assessing a traveler's health risks (Table 2-1). Certain travelers may confront special risks. Recent hospitalization for serious problems may lead the travel health provider to recommend delaying travel. Air travel is contraindicated for certain conditions, such as <3 weeks after an uncomplicated myocardial infarction and <10 days after thoracic or abdominal surgery. The travel health provider and traveler should consult with the relevant health care providers most familiar with the underlying illnesses. Other travelers with specific risks include travelers who are visiting friends and relatives, long-term travelers, travelers with small children, travelers with chronic illnesses, immunocompromised travelers, and pregnant travelers. More comprehensive discussion on advising travelers who have additional health considerations is available in Chapter 5. Providers should determine whether recent outbreaks or other safety notices have been posted for the traveler's destination; information is available on the CDC and US Department of State websites, and in various other resources.

In addition to recognizing the traveler's characteristics, health background, and destination-specific risks, the exposures related to special activities also merit discussion. For example, river rafting could expose a traveler to schistosomiasis or leptospirosis, and spelunking in Central America could put the traveler at risk of histoplasmosis. Flying from lowlands to high-altitude areas and trekking or climbing in mountainous regions introduces the risk of altitude illness. Therefore, the provider should inquire about plans for specific leisure, business, and health care–seeking activities.

## Communicate Risk

Once destination-specific risks for a particular itinerary have been assessed by the provider, they should be clearly communicated to the traveler. The process of risk communication is a 2-way exchange of information between the clinician and traveler, in which they discuss potential health hazards at the destination and the effectiveness of preventive measures, with the goal of improving understanding of risk and promoting more informed decision making. Risk communication is among the most challenging aspects of a pretravel consultation, because travelers' perception of and tolerance for risk can vary widely. For a more detailed discussion, see *Perspectives*: Travelers' Perception of Risk in this chapter.

## Manage Risk

Immunizations are a crucial component of pretravel consultations, and the risk assessment forms the basis of recommendations for travel vaccines. For example, providers should consider whether there is sufficient time before travel to complete a vaccine series; the purpose of travel and specific destination within a country will inform the need for particular vaccinations. At the same time, the pretravel consultation presents an opportunity to update routine vaccines (Table 2-2). Particular attention

## Table 2-2.  Vaccines to update or consider during pretravel consultations

| VACCINE | TRAVEL-RELATED OCCURRENCES AND RECOMMENDATIONS |
|---|---|
| **Routine Vaccines** (Vaccination considerations should be based on ACIP guidelines.) | |
| *Haemophilus influenzae* type b | No report of travel-related infection, although organism is ubiquitous. |
| Hepatitis B | Recommended for travelers visiting countries where HBsAg prevalence is ≥2%. Vaccination may be considered for all international travelers, regardless of destination, depending upon the traveler's behavioral risk and potential for exposure as determined by the provider and traveler. |
| Human papillomavirus (HPV) | No report of travel-acquired infection; however, sexual activity during travel may lead to HPV and other sexually transmitted infections. |
| Influenza | Year-round transmission may occur in tropical areas. Outbreaks have occurred on cruise ships, and 2009 influenza A (H1N1) illustrated the rapidity of spread via travel. Novel influenza viruses such as avian influenza H5N1 and H7N9 can be transmitted to travelers visiting areas with circulation of these viruses. |
| Measles, mumps, rubella | Infections are common in countries and communities that do not immunize children routinely, including Europe. Outbreaks have occurred in the United States as a result of infection in returning travelers. |
| Meningococcal | Outbreaks occur regularly in sub-Saharan Africa in the "meningitis belt" during the dry season, generally December through June, although transmission may occur at other times for those with close contact with local populations. Outbreaks have occurred with Hajj pilgrimage, and the Kingdom of Saudi Arabia requires the quadrivalent vaccine for pilgrims. |

# Table 2-2. Vaccines to update or consider during pretravel consultations (continued)

| VACCINE | TRAVEL-RELATED OCCURRENCES AND RECOMMENDATIONS |
|---|---|
| Pneumococcal | Organism is ubiquitous, and causal relationship to travel is difficult to establish. |
| Polio | Unimmunized or underimmunized travelers can become infected with either wild poliovirus or vaccine-derived poliovirus. Because the international spread of wild poliovirus in 2014 was declared a Public Health Emergency of International Concern under the International Health Regulations, temporary recommendations for polio vaccination are in place for countries with wild poliovirus circulation for their residents, long-term visitors, and international travelers. |
| Rotavirus | Common in developing countries, although not a common cause of travelers' diarrhea in adults. The vaccine is only recommended in young children. |
| Tetanus, diphtheria, pertussis | Rare cases of diphtheria have been attributed to travel. Pertussis has occurred in travelers, recently in adults whose immunity has waned. |
| Varicella | Infections are common in countries that do not immunize children routinely, as in most developing countries. Naturally occurring disease tends to affect adults. |
| Zoster | Travel (a form of stress) may trigger varicella zoster reactivation, but causal relationship is difficult to establish. |
| **Travel Vaccines** | |
| Cholera | Cases in travelers have occurred in association with travel to Haiti. |
| Hepatitis A | Prevalence of hepatitis A virus infection may vary among regions within a country. Serologic testing may be considered in travelers from highly endemic countries since they may be immune. Some travel health providers advise people traveling outside the United States to consider hepatitis A vaccination regardless of their country of destination. |
| Japanese encephalitis | Rare cases have occurred, estimated at <1 case/1 million travelers to endemic countries. However, the severe neurologic sequelae and high fatality rate warrant detailed review of trip plans to assess the level of risk. |
| Rabies | Rabies preexposure immunization simplifies postexposure immunoprophylaxis, as adequately screened immunoglobulin may be difficult to obtain in many destinations. |
| Tickborne encephalitis (vaccine not available in the United States) | Cases have been identified in travelers with an estimated risk of 1/10,000 person-months in travelers. Endemic areas are expanding in Europe. |
| Typhoid | UK surveillance found the highest risk to be travel to India (6 cases/100,000 visits), Pakistan (9 cases/100,000 visits), and Bangladesh (21 cases/100,000 visits), although risk is substantial in many destinations. |
| Yellow fever | Risk occurs mainly in defined areas of sub-Saharan Africa and the Amazonian regions of South America. Some countries require proof of vaccination for entry. For travelers visiting multiple countries, order of travel may make a difference in the requirements. |

Abbreviation: HBsAg, hepatitis B surface antigen.

should be paid to vaccines for which immunity may have waned over time or following a recent immunocompromising condition (such as after a hematopoietic stem cell transplant). Asking the question, "Do you have any plans to travel again in the next 1–2 years?" may help the traveler justify an immunization for travel over a number of years rather than only the upcoming trip, such as rabies preexposure or Japanese encephalitis. Travelers should receive a record of immunizations administered and instructions to follow up as needed to complete a vaccine series.

Another major focus of pretravel consultations for many destinations is the prevention of malaria. Malaria continues to cause substantial morbidity and mortality in travelers. Since 1973, the annual number of US malaria cases reported to CDC has shown an increasing trend; therefore, pretravel consultation must carefully assess travelers' risk for malaria and recommend preventive measures. For travelers going to malaria-endemic countries, it is imperative to discuss malaria transmission, ways to reduce risk, recommendations for prophylaxis, and symptoms of malaria.

Travelers with underlying health conditions require attention to their health issues as they relate to the destination and activities. For example, a traveler with a history of cardiac disease should carry medical reports, including a recent electrocardiogram. Asthma may flare in a traveler visiting a polluted city or from physical exertion during a hike; travelers should be encouraged to discuss with their primary care provider how to plan for treatment and bring necessary medication in case of asthma exacerbation. Travelers should be counseled on how to obtain travel medical insurance and how they can find reputable medical facilities at their destination, such as using the ISTM website (www.istm.org), the American Society of Tropical Medicine and Hygiene website (www.astmh.org), or the State Department Travel website (https://travel.state.gov/content/travel/en/international-travel/before-you-go/your-health-abroad.html). Any allergies or serious medical conditions should be identified on a bracelet or a card to expedite medical care in emergency situations.

The pretravel consultation also provides another setting to remind travelers of basic health practices during travel, including frequent handwashing, wearing seatbelts, using car seats for infants and children, and safe sexual practices. Topics to be explored are numerous and could be organized into a checklist, placing priority on the most serious and frequently encountered issues (Table 2-3, Box 2-1). General issues such as preventing injury and sunburn also deserve mention. Written information is essential to supplement oral advice and enable travelers to review the instructions from their clinic visits; educational material is available on the CDC Travelers Health webpage (www.cdc.gov/travel). Advice on self-treatable conditions may minimize the need for travelers to seek medical care while abroad and possibly lead to faster return to good health.

## Self-Treatable Conditions

Despite providers' best efforts, some travelers will become ill. Obtaining reliable and timely medical care during travel can be problematic in many destinations. As a result, prescribing certain medications in advance can empower the traveler to self-diagnose and treat common health problems. With some activities in remote settings, such as trekking, the only alternative to self-treatment would be no treatment. Pretravel counseling may result in a more accurate self-diagnosis and treatment than relying on local medical care in some areas. In addition, the increasing awareness of substandard and counterfeit drugs in pharmacies in the developing world makes it more important for travelers to bring quality manufactured drugs with them from a reliable supplier in their own country (see Chapter 6, *Perspectives*: Avoiding Poorly Regulated Medicines and Medical Products during Travel).

Travel health providers need to recognize the conditions for which the traveler may be at risk, and educate the traveler about the diagnosis and treatment of those conditions. The keys to successful self-treatment strategies are providing a simple disease or condition definition, providing a treatment, and educating the traveler about the expected outcome of treatment. Using travelers'

## Table 2-3. Major topics for discussion during pretravel consultations

| | |
|---|---|
| Immunizations | Review routine immunizations and those travel immunizations indicated for the specific itinerary and based on the traveler's medical history. |
| | Discuss utility of titers when records are unavailable or unreliable, particularly for measles, mumps, rubella, hepatitis A, and varicella. |
| | Screen for chronic hepatitis B for people born in countries with HBsAg prevalence ≥2% (see Map 4-4). |
| | Discuss indications for, effectiveness of, and adverse reactions to immunizations. |
| Malaria chemoprophylaxis | Determine if there is a risk of malaria. |
| | Discuss personal protective measures. |
| | Discuss risks and benefits of chemoprophylaxis and recommended choices of chemoprophylaxis for the itinerary. |
| Other vectorborne diseases | Define risk of disease in specific itinerary and insect precautions needed. |
| Respiratory illnesses | Discuss areas of particular concern (such as avian influenza in Asia or MERS in the Arabian Peninsula). |
| | Consider influenza self-treatment for high-risk travelers. |
| Travelers' diarrhea | Recommend strategies to decrease risk of diarrhea. |
| | Discuss antibiotics for self-treatment, adjunct medications such as loperamide, and staying hydrated. |
| Altitude illness | Determine if the itinerary puts the traveler at risk of altitude illness. |
| | Discuss preventive measures such as gradual ascent, adequate hydration, and medications to prevent and treat. |
| Other environmental hazards | Caution travelers to avoid contact with animals to reduce the potential for bites and scratches that can transmit rabies. |
| | Advise travelers to avoid walking barefoot to avoid certain parasitic infections. |
| | Advise travelers to avoid wading or swimming in freshwater where there is risk for schistosomiasis or leptospirosis. |
| | Remind travelers to apply sunscreen to skin exposed to the sun. |
| Personal safety | Discuss precautions travelers can take to minimize risks, such as traffic accidents, alcohol excess, personal assault, robbery, or drowning. |
| | Provide information on travel health and medical evacuation insurance. |
| | Advise travelers to look for security bulletins related to their destination and consider areas to avoid. |
| Bloodborne pathogens | Inform travelers who will provide health care overseas what to do in case of needlestick or bloodborne pathogen exposure. |
| | Discuss use of postexposure prophylaxis for HIV. |
| | See Box 2-1 for summary on sexual health recommendations for travelers. |
| Disease-specific counseling | Remind travelers to keep medications and supplies in carry-on luggage. |
| | Advise travelers to prepare for exacerbations or complications from underlying disease. |

Abbreviations: HBsAg, hepatitis B surface antigen; MERS, Middle East respiratory syndrome.

## BOX 2-1. Summary of sexual health recommendations for travelers

**BEFORE TRAVEL**

- Obtain recommended vaccinations, including those that protect against sexually transmitted infections.
- Get recommended tests for HIV and treatable STDs. Be aware of STD symptoms in case any develop.
- Check condom packaging and expiration dates.
- Review local laws about sexual practices and obtain contact information for medical and law enforcement services.

- If pregnant or considering pregnancy, review whether Zika virus infection is a risk at destination.

**DURING TRAVEL**

- Use good judgment in choosing consensual adult sex partners.
- Use condoms consistently and correctly to decrease the risk of HIV and STDs.
- If indicated, be prepared to start taking medications for HIV postexposure prophylaxis or unintended pregnancy within 72

hours after a high-risk sexual encounter.
- Never engage in sex with a minor (<18 years old), child pornography, or trafficking activities in any country.
- Report suspicious activity to US and local authorities as soon as it occurs.

**AFTER TRAVEL**

- To avoid exposing sex partners at home, see a clinician to get recommended tests for HIV and treatable STDs.

---

diarrhea as an example, a practitioner could provide the following advice:

- "Travelers' diarrhea" is the sudden onset of abnormally loose, frequent stools.

- Most cases will resolve within 2–5 days, and symptoms can be managed with loperamide or bismuth subsalicylate.

- For diarrhea severe enough to interrupt travel plans, an antibiotic can be prescribed that travelers can carry with them (see Travelers' Diarrhea section in this chapter).

- The traveler should feel better within 6–24 hours.

- If symptoms persist for 24–36 hours despite self-treatment, it may be necessary to seek medical attention.

To minimize the potential negative effects of a self-treatment strategy, the recommendations should follow a few key points:

- Drugs recommended must be safe, well tolerated, and effective for use as self-treatment.

- A drug's toxicity or potential for harm, if used incorrectly or in an overdose situation, should be minimal.

- Simple and clear directions are critical. Consider providing handouts describing how to use the drugs. Keeping the directions simple will increase the effectiveness of the strategy.

The following are some of the most common situations in which people would find self-treatment useful. The extent of self-treatment recommendations offered to the traveler should reflect the remoteness and difficulty of travel and the availability of reliable medical care at the destination. The recommended self-treatment options for each disease are provided in the designated section of the Yellow Book or discussed below.

- Travelers' diarrhea (Chapter 2, Travelers' Diarrhea)

- Altitude illness (Chapter 3, High-Altitude Travel & Altitude Illness)

- Jet lag (Chapter 8, Jet Lag)

- Motion sickness (Chapter 8, Motion Sickness)

- Respiratory infections (Chapter 11, Respiratory Infections)

- Skin conditions such as allergic reactions or superficial fungal infections (Chapter 11, Skin & Soft Tissue Infections)

- Urinary tract infections: common among many women; carrying an antibiotic for empiric treatment may be valuable

- Vaginal yeast infections: self-treatment course of patient's preferred antifungal medication can be prescribed for women who are prone to infections, sexually active, or who may be receiving antibiotics for other reasons (including doxycycline for malaria chemoprophylaxis)

- Occupational exposure to HIV (Chapter 9, Health Care Workers, Including Public Health Researchers and Laboratorians)

- Malaria self-treatment (see Chapter 4, Malaria)

In sum, travelers should be encouraged to carry a travel health kit with prescription and nonprescription medications. Providers should review medication lists for possible drug interactions. More detailed information for providers and travelers is given in Chapter 6, Travel Health Kits; supplementary travel health kit information for travelers with specific needs is given in Chapter 5.

## BIBLIOGRAPHY

1. Freedman DO, Chen LH, Kozarsky P. Medical considerations before travel. N Engl J Med. 2016 July 21;375:247–60.

2. Hatz CFR, Chen LH. Pre-travel consultation. In: Keystone JS, Freedman DO, Kozarsky PE, Connor BA, Nothdurft HD, editors. Travel Medicine. 3rd ed. Philadelphia: Saunders Elsevier; 2013. pp. 31–6.

3. Hill DR, Ericsson CD, Pearson RD, Keystone JS, Freedman DO, Kozarsky PE, et al. The practice of travel medicine: guidelines by the Infectious Diseases Society of America. Clin Infect Dis. 2006 Dec 15;43(12):1499–539.

4. International Society of Travel Medicine. Body of knowledge for the practice of travel medicine—2012. Atlanta: International Society of Travel Medicine; 2012 [cited 2018 Feb 18]. Available from: www.istm.org/bodyofknowledge.

5. Kozarsky PE, Steffen R. Travel medicine education—what are the needs? J Travel Med. 2016 Jul 4;23(5).

6. Leder K, Chen LH, Wilson ME. Aggregate travel vs. single trip assessment: arguments for cumulative risk analysis. Vaccine. 2012 Mar 28;30(15):2600–4.

7. Leder K, Torresi J, Libman MD, Cramer JP, Castelli F, Schlagenhauf P, et al. GeoSentinel surveillance of illness in returned travelers, 2007–2011. Ann Intern Med. 2013 Mar 19;158(6):456–68.

8. Schwartz BS, Larocque RC, Ryan ET. In the clinic: travel medicine. Ann Intern Med. 2012 Jun 5;156(11):ITC6:1–16.

9. Steffen R, Behrens RH, Hill RD, Greenaway C, Leder K. Vaccine-preventable travel health risks: what is the evidence—what are the gaps? J Travel Med. 2015;22(1):1–12.

10. Riddle MS, Connor BA, Beeching NJ, DuPont HL, Hamer DH, Kozarsky P, et al. Guidelines for the prevention and treatment of travelers' diarrhea: a graded expert panel report. J Travel Med. 2017 Apr 1;24(suppl_1):S57–S74.

# TRAVELERS' PERCEPTION OF RISK

David R. Shlim

**2**

Travel medicine is based on the concept of risk reduction. In the context of travel medicine, "risk" refers to the possibility of harm occurring during the course of a trip. Some risks may be avoidable, while others may not. For example, vaccine-preventable diseases may be mostly avoidable, depending on the protective efficacy of the vaccine. Perception of risk is a subjective evaluation of whether a risk is considered large or small; is 1 in 10,000 a large risk or a small risk? Tolerance refers to acknowledging a risk and accepting it; a risk of 1 in 100,000 may be tolerable for one traveler but not for another.

For many years, travel medicine practitioners have felt that statistics for a given risk could help them objectively advise travelers about that risk. However, the rates of diseases in a particular country or location, such as typhoid fever, malaria, or Japanese encephalitis (JE), may not help clinicians or travelers determine the threshold for making a decision based on those statistics alone. With risks of diseases ranging from 1 in 500 (an estimate of the risk of typhoid in unvaccinated travelers in Nepal), to 1 in 1,000,000 (an assessment of the risk of JE in travelers to Asia), travelers still need to determine what these statistics mean. Additional information to help make an informed decision may include length of travel, type of travel, and proposed accommodations.

Even when risk is low, travelers' decisions will still reflect their perception and tolerance of risk. When told that the risk of JE is 1 in 1,000,000, one traveler might reply, "Then I guess I don't have to worry about it," while another traveler might say, "That one traveler will be me!" Each traveler will have ideas about the risks, benefits, and costs of vaccines and drug prophylaxis, and these should be discussed in detail with their clinician.

Perception and tolerance of risk are connected to the concept of commitment, particularly in regards to remote, adventurous travel. Commitment refers to the fact that certain parts of a journey may not easily be reversed once entered upon. For example, a traveler trekking into a remote area may need to accept that rescue, if available at all, may be delayed for days. A traveler who has a myocardial infarction in a country with no advanced cardiac services may have a difficult time obtaining definitive medical care. If the traveler has already contemplated these concerns and accepted them, it will be easier to deal with them if they occur.

The goal of travel medicine should be to assess the risks for the traveler, and educate the traveler to skillfully manage and minimize risk rather than try to eliminate it. Travel medicine practitioners should discuss available risk statistics and assess their clients' perception and tolerance of risk. Once this is done, the provider can then help travelers find their individual comfort level when making decisions about destinations, activities, and prophylactic measures.

*Perspectives* sections are written as editorial discussions aiming to add depth and clinical perspective to the official recommendations contained in the book. The views and opinions expressed in this section are those of the author and do not necessarily represent the official position of CDC.

# LAST-MINUTE TRAVELERS

Gail A. Rosselot

Although all travelers are encouraged to access pretravel services at least 1 month before departure, clinicians can provide pretravel care to those leaving on short notice, even within days or sometimes hours of departure. The category of "last-minute travelers" can include people who are leaving on short notice (such as humanitarian aid workers) or people who have planned a trip for some time but delayed receiving pretravel care.

Providing complete pretravel services to last-minute travelers can be challenging and there is typically time for only a single encounter.

## VACCINATIONS

Consider the traveler's itinerary, trip activities, and risk of infection at the destination. Note that immunity varies by vaccine, so emphasize preventive behaviors for travelers who might not be adequately protected if they are vaccinated immediately before travel.

### Routine Vaccinations

Most travelers who attended school in the United States have received standard routine vaccinations. If the traveler is not up-to-date, even when departure is imminent, provide the first or additional doses of routine vaccines, including a seasonal influenza vaccination, if needed.

### Recommended Vaccinations: Single-Dose Protection

Even when a traveler has limited time before departure, research supports the use of certain single-dose vaccines, if indicated, to initiate protection. These include hepatitis A (monovalent), typhoid (injectable), polio (inactivated), cholera, and quadrivalent (ACWY) meningococcal meningitis vaccines (see the respective disease sections in Chapter 4 for indications and dosing).

### Recommended Vaccinations: Multiple Doses Needed

Last-minute travelers often cannot complete the full course of vaccines that require multiple doses to induce full protection. If a traveler needs protection against hepatitis B, Japanese encephalitis, or rabies, the clinician can consider approved accelerated schedules or information on resources for vaccination at the destination. It is unclear what level of protection any given traveler will have if he or she does not complete a full series of multi-dose vaccination.

### HEPATITIS B

As time allows, the traveler should receive the accelerated monovalent hepatitis B (Engerix-B) schedule (0, 1, and 2 months, plus a 12-month booster) or the super-accelerated combination hepatitis A/B (Twinrix) schedule (0, 7, 21–30 days, plus a 12-month booster). If an accelerated schedule cannot be completed before travel, start the vaccination series and schedule a follow-up visit to complete it or, for extended-stay travelers or expatriates, help them identify resources at the destination to complete the series.

### JAPANESE ENCEPHALITIS

Japanese encephalitis vaccine is administered as 2 doses on days 0 and 7–28 (see Chapter 4, Japanese Encephalitis). A study of adults given 2 doses of Ixiaro 7 days apart found that 99% were protected. However, people who receive only a single dose may have a suboptimal response and may not be protected. Travelers who cannot complete the primary vaccine series ≥1 week before travel should be counseled to adhere rigidly to mosquito precautions if they will be at risk for Japanese encephalitis. Alternatively, the clinician can help them identify resources for vaccination with Ixiaro or several alternative vaccines that may be available at their destination, particularly if they will be long-stay travelers (Imojev Sanofi, SA14-14-2 Chengdu). However, travelers should be aware that vaccines received in some countries may be of substandard quality (see Chapter 6, *Perspectives*: Avoiding Poorly Regulated Medicines and Medical Products during Travel).

### RABIES

Because of the multiple immunizations required to complete a primary rabies vaccine series (0, 7, and 21 or 28 days), last-minute travelers may not be able to complete the series before departure. A person who starts but does not complete a primary series and is exposed should receive the same postexposure prophylaxis as a completely unimmunized person. Counsel travelers on animal avoidance and the need to seek care urgently after an exposure. Travelers should consider purchasing travel health insurance to pay for care and medical evacuation insurance in case evacuation is needed to receive timely postexposure prophylaxis.

## Required Vaccinations

Yellow fever vaccination certificates are valid 10 days after vaccine administration (the length of time considered necessary for immunity to develop). If a traveler plans to visit a country with a yellow fever vaccine requirement within this 10-day window, it may be necessary to rearrange the order of travel or reschedule the trip. Otherwise, the traveler risks being denied entry at the country's border and would be at risk for yellow fever. Travelers for whom the yellow fever vaccination is contraindicated can be issued a medical waiver letter if a country entry requirement (and not risk of yellow fever infection) is the only reason to vaccinate.

Quadrivalent (ACWY) meningococcal vaccine is required of all travelers to Saudi Arabia for religious pilgrimage, including Hajj. Hajj visas cannot be issued without proof that applicants received meningococcal vaccine ≥10 days and ≤3 years (≤5 years for conjugate vaccine) before arriving in Saudi Arabia.

Certain countries require departing travelers to show proof of polio vaccination if they have been in the country >4 weeks. This requirement should not present a problem to travelers receiving the vaccine at the last minute. Countries with this requirement can change. Consult the CDC website (wwwnc.cdc.gov/travel/news-announcements/polio-guidance-new-requirements) for a current list. For more information, see Chapter 4, Poliomyelitis.

## MALARIA

The choice of malaria prophylaxis for last-minute travelers must factor in time until departure. For travelers leaving in <2 weeks, doxycycline, atovaquone-proguanil, or, when appropriate, primaquine should be used.

## HEALTH COUNSELING

Pretravel counseling is critical for last-minute travelers. During your risk assessment, determine prior knowledge and experience with travel health risks. Focus on major risks of the trip, and deliver simple messages about prevention and self-care. Provide travelers with education and prescriptions for travelers' diarrhea and, if indicated, altitude illness. Encourage last-minute travelers to purchase all medications in the United States before departure to avoid buying medications that may be of poor quality or counterfeit. As time allows, provide counseling on topics such as preventing injuries, adhering to food and water precautions, and insect bite prevention (see The Pretravel Consultation in this chapter).

## SPECIAL CHALLENGES AND ADDITIONAL CONSIDERATIONS

### The Traveler Leaving in a Few Hours

If time does not permit an appointment, the clinician can still provide general prevention messages and recommendations for care by telephone or secure digital messaging. Refer the traveler to useful websites such as CDC (www.cdc.gov/travel), the Department of State (www.travel.state.gov), the Heading Home Healthy Program (www.headinghomehealthy.org), and the International Society of Travel Medicine clinic directory (www.istm.org). Emphasize and reassure the traveler that many travel health risks can be prevented by adhering to healthy behaviors.

### The Traveler with Preexisting Medical Conditions

These patients may be at increased risk for travel-related illness if they have inadequate time for preparation. They should consider purchasing travel health insurance, trip insurance, and medical evacuation insurance, and should carry an extra supply of all medications and a portable medical record. Emphasize the importance of a pretravel appointment or conversation with their treating clinician. Some conditions, such as pregnancy and immunosuppression, often require additional discussion and advance planning and may warrant delaying departure.

## The Last-Minute, Extended-Stay Traveler

Advise these travelers to arrange an early visit with a qualified clinician at their destination for additional evaluation and education. A last-minute consultation does not provide an expatriate with adequate time for a full medical and psychological evaluation.

## Recurring Last-Minute Travelers

Any clinic that frequently sees last-minute travelers may want to address this as an administrative issue. Consider building flexibility into the clinic schedule and proactively identifying people likely to travel at the last minute (such as college students and corporate employees). For these travelers, preemptive vaccinations for certain itineraries might also be considered.

### BIBLIOGRAPHY

1. Centers for Disease Control and Prevention. Epidemiology and Prevention of Vaccine-Preventable Diseases. Hamborsky J, Kroger A, Wolfe S, eds. 13th ed. Washington D.C. Public Health Foundation; [cited 2018 Apr]. Available from: www.cdc.gov/vaccines/pubs/pinkbook/index.html.

2. Chen LH, Leder K, Wilson ME. Business travelers: vaccination considerations for this population. Expert Rev Vaccines. 2013; 12(4):453–66.

3. Cramer JP, Jelninek T, Paulke-Korinek M, Reisinger EC, Dieckmann S, Alberer M, et al. One-year immunogenicity kinetics and safety of a purified chick embryo cell rabies vaccine and inactivated Vero cell-derived Japanese encephalitis vaccine administered concomitantly according to a new, 1-week, accelerated primary series. J Travel Med. 2016; 23 (3):1–8.

4. Sanford CA and EC Jong. Immunizations. Med Clin N Am. 2016; 100: 247–59.

5. Wong C and Scotland L. The last minute traveller. In: Shaw M, Wong C, editors. The Practical Compendium of Immunisations for International Travel. Auckland (NZ): Adis; 2015. pp. 117–23.

6. Zuckerman JN, Van Damme P, Van Herck K, Loscher T. Vaccination options for last-minute travellers in need of travel-related prophylaxis against hepatitis A and B and typhoid fever: a practical guide. Travel Med Infect Dis. 2003 Nov;1(4):219–26.

# COMPLEMENTARY & INTEGRATIVE HEALTH APPROACHES

David Shurtleff, Kathleen Meister, Catherine Law

Travelers often ask their health care providers about the use of complementary or integrative health approaches for travel-related illnesses and conditions. This should come as no surprise, given that many people—approximately 1 in 3 American adults—report using these types of products and practices. Some complementary approaches for travel-related health problems are promoted widely, especially on the Internet. However, little of the promotional material is supported by research evidence, and some of it is misleading or false. This section focuses on claims that have been made about alleged benefits of complementary approaches for travel-related health problems and what the science says about some of the herbal products, dietary supplements (see Box 2-2), and other complementary approaches suggested for travel-related ailments and hazards.

## COMPLEMENTARY APPROACHES TO TRAVEL WELLNESS: CLAIMS VS. SCIENCE

### Malaria Prophylaxis and Treatment

#### CLAIMS

Many consumer websites promote "natural" ways to prevent or treat malaria, which often involve dietary changes or herbal products, such as quinine from the cinchona tree (*Cinchona* spp.) or extracts and material from the artemisia plant (*Artemisia annua* L. or sweet wormword).

# About dietary supplements and unproven therapies

- The Food and Drug Administration (FDA) regulates dietary supplements, but the regulations are different and generally less strict than those for prescription or over-the-counter drugs. Learn more at https://nccih.nih.gov/health/supplements/wiseuse.htm.
- Two major safety concerns about dietary supplements are potential drug interactions and product contamination. Analyses of supplements sometimes find differences between labeled and actual ingredients. For example, products marketed as dietary supplements have been found to contain illegal hidden ingredients such as prescription drugs.

  Consult the FDA's safety advisories to learn the latest regarding product recalls and safety alerts: www.fda.gov/Food/RecallsOutbreaksEmergencies/SafetyAlertsAdvisories/default.htm.
- Unproven therapies are discussed in this section only for educational purposes and are not recommended for use. CDC endorses only FDA-approved therapies.

## WHAT THE SCIENCE SAYS

Urge patients to follow official recommendations and not rely on unproven "natural" approaches in an attempt to prevent or treat such a serious disease. Recommended drugs to prevent and treat malaria are described in Chapter 4, Malaria.

## Zika Prophylaxis and Treatment

### CLAIMS

Consumer websites and online videos have claimed, without credible evidence, that various herbs or other natural products will protect against or treat the Zika virus.

### WHAT THE SCIENCE SAYS

There is no evidence that any of these products can prevent or treat Zika virus infection. For more information see Chapter 4, Zika.

## Travelers' Diarrhea Prevention and Treatment

### CLAIMS

It has been claimed that a variety of products, including probiotics, goldenseal, activated charcoal, and grapefruit seed extract, can prevent or treat travelers' diarrhea (TD).

### WHAT THE SCIENCE SAYS
#### PROBIOTICS

Using probiotics for the prevention of TD is controversial. Although some studies have had promising results, meta-analyses have reached conflicting conclusions. It is difficult to interpret the evidence because studies have used a variety of microbial strains, some studies were not well controlled, and the optimal dose and duration of use have not been defined. For more information, see Traveler's Diarrhea in this chapter.

#### GOLDENSEAL

No high-quality research on goldenseal for TD has been published. Studies show that goldenseal inhibits cytochrome P450 enzymes, raising concerns that it may increase the toxicity or alter the effects of drugs.

#### ACTIVATED CHARCOAL

No solid evidence supports claims that activated charcoal helps with TD, bloating, stomach cramps, or gas. The side effects of activated charcoal have not been well documented but were mild when it was tested on healthy people. **Warning:** Children should not be given activated charcoal for diarrhea and dehydration. It may absorb nutrients, enzymes, and antibiotics in the intestine and mask the severity of fluid loss.

#### GRAPEFRUIT SEED EXTRACT

Claims that grapefruit seed extract can prevent bacterial foodborne illnesses are unfounded and not supported by research. People who need to avoid grapefruit because it interacts with medicine that they are taking should also avoid grapefruit seed extract.

## Altitude Illness Prevention and Treatment

### CLAIMS

A variety of natural products, including coca, garlic, *Ginkgo biloba*, and vitamin E, have been promoted for the prevention or treatment of altitude illness.

### WHAT THE SCIENCE SAYS

#### COCA

Coca tea has been used for altitude illness, but there is no strong evidence on whether it works or has adverse effects. It will result in a positive drug test for cocaine metabolites. For more information, see Chapter 10, Peru: Cusco, Machu Picchu & Other Regions.

#### GARLIC

There is no evidence supporting claims that garlic helps reduce altitude illness. Garlic supplements appear safe for most adults. Possible side effects include breath and body odor, heartburn, and upset stomach. Some people have allergic reactions to garlic. Short-term use of most commercially available garlic supplements poses only a limited risk of drug interactions.

#### GINKGO BILOBA

Studies of ginkgo for preventing altitude illness have had inconsistent but mostly negative results. Whether the differences in results relate to the different preparations used in the studies has not been determined. Products made from standardized ginkgo leaf extracts appear to be safe when used as directed. However, ginkgo may increase the risk of bleeding in some people and interact with anticoagulants. In addition, studies by the National Toxicology Program showed that rodents developed liver and thyroid tumors after being given a ginkgo extract for up to 2 years.

#### VITAMIN E

One study investigated vitamin E, in combination with other antioxidants, for altitude illness; the results were negative.

For more information on altitude illness, see Chapter 3, High-Altitude Travel & Altitude Illness.

## Motion Sickness

### CLAIMS

Complementary approaches advocated for preventing or treating motion sickness include acupressure, magnets, ginger, pyridoxine (vitamin $B_6$), and homeopathic remedies.

### WHAT THE SCIENCE SAYS

#### ACUPRESSURE AND MAGNETS

Research does not support the use of acupressure or magnets for motion sickness.

#### GINGER

Although some studies have shown that ginger may ease pregnancy-related nausea and vomiting and may help control nausea related to cancer chemotherapy when used in addition to conventional medication, there is no strong evidence that ginger helps with motion sickness. In some people, ginger can have mild side effects such as abdominal discomfort. Research has not definitively shown whether ginger interacts with medications, but concerns have been raised that it might interact with anticoagulants. The effect of using ginger supplements with common over-the-counter drugs for motion sickness (such as dimenhydrinate [Dramamine]) is unknown.

#### PYRIDOXINE (VITAMIN $B_6$)

Although an American Congress of Obstetrics and Gynecology 2015 Practice Bulletin Summary recommends pyridoxine (vitamin $B_6$) alone or in combination with doxylamine (an antihistamine) as a safe and effective treatment for nausea and vomiting associated with pregnancy, there is no evidence supporting claims that pyridoxine prevents or alleviates motion sickness. Taking excessive doses of pyridoxine supplements for long periods of time can affect nerve function.

#### HOMEOPATHIC PRODUCTS

There is no evidence supporting claims that homeopathic products prevent or alleviate motion sickness.

## Jet Lag/Sleep Problems

### CLAIMS

Complementary approaches that have been suggested for jet lag or other sleep problems include the dietary supplement melatonin; relaxation techniques and other mind and body practices; aromatherapy; and herbs such as chamomile, kava, and valerian.

## WHAT THE SCIENCE SAYS
### MELATONIN

Some evidence suggests that melatonin supplements may help with sleep problems caused by jet lag. Recent systematic reviews indicate that it may be of some benefit for people traveling in either an eastward or westward direction. Before suggesting melatonin to your patients, consider the following:

- People with epilepsy or who take an oral anticoagulant should **never** use melatonin without medical supervision.

- Melatonin supplements appear to be safe for most people when used short-term; less is known about their long-term safety. Side effects from melatonin are uncommon but can include drowsiness, headache, dizziness, or nausea.

- Melatonin should not be taken early in the day, as it may cause sleepiness and delay adaptation to local time.

- Melatonin is sold as a dietary supplement. Dietary supplements are regulated less strictly than drugs. The amounts of ingredients in dietary supplements may vary, and product contamination is a potential concern. A 2017 analysis of melatonin supplements sold in Canada found that their actual melatonin content ranged from −83% to +478% of the labeled content and that there was substantial lot-to-lot variation. Also, 26% of products contained serotonin as a contaminant.

### RELAXATION TECHNIQUES AND OTHER MIND AND BODY PRACTICES

Relaxation techniques, such as progressive relaxation, and other mind and body practices, such as mindfulness-based stress reduction, may help with insomnia, but it has not been established whether they are effective for jet lag.

### AROMATHERAPY AND HERBS

There is very little evidence that aromatherapy or the herbs chamomile or valerian help with insomnia. Significant side effects are uncommon, but chamomile can cause allergic reactions. Another herb, kava, is also promoted for sleep but good research on its effectiveness is lacking. More importantly, kava supplements have been linked to a risk of severe liver damage.

## Colds and Flu
### CLAIMS

Although colds and flu are not uniquely travel-related hazards, many people are concerned about trying to avoid these illnesses during a trip. They may turn to complementary health approaches that have been advocated for preventing or treating colds or flu, including zinc products, neti pots and other forms of saline nasal irrigation, vitamin C, probiotics, echinacea, and others.

### WHAT THE SCIENCE SAYS
### ZINC

Zinc taken orally (often in the form of lozenges) may reduce the duration of a cold. Zinc, particularly in large doses, can have side effects including nausea and diarrhea. The intranasal use of zinc can cause anosmia (loss of sense of smell), which may be long-lasting or permanent.

### SALINE IRRIGATION

Nasal saline irrigation, such as with neti pots, may be useful and safe for chronic sinusitis. However, even in places where tap water is safe to drink, people should use only sterile, distilled, boiled-then-cooled, or specially filtered water for nasal irrigation to avoid the risk of introducing waterborne pathogens. Nasal saline irrigation may help relieve the symptoms of acute upper respiratory tract infections, but the evidence is not definitive.

### VITAMIN C

Taking vitamin C supplements regularly reduces the risk of catching a cold among people who perform intense physical exercise but not in the general population. Taking vitamin C on a regular basis may lead to shorter colds, but taking it only after a cold starts does not. Vitamin C supplements appear safe, even at high doses.

**PROBIOTICS**

Probiotics might reduce susceptibility to colds or other upper respiratory tract infections and the duration of the illnesses, but the quality of the evidence is low or very low.

**ECHINACEA**

Numerous studies have tested the herb echinacea to see whether it can prevent colds or relieve cold symptoms. A 2014 systematic review concluded that echinacea has not been convincingly shown to be effective; however, a weak effect has not been ruled out.

**OTHER**

There is no strong evidence that garlic, Chinese herbs, oil of oregano, or eucalyptus essential oil prevent or treat colds, or that the homeopathic product Oscillococcinum prevents or treats influenza or influenzalike illness.

## Insect Protection: Botanical Repellents

### CLAIMS

Many products are promoted as "natural" insect repellents, and their use may appeal to people who prefer not to use synthetic products. Products promoted as natural mosquito repellents include citronella products, oil of lemon eucalyptus (OLE), and neem oil (a component of agricultural insecticide products that is promoted on some websites for home use). Essential oils and other natural products are promoted to repel bed bugs.

### WHAT THE SCIENCE SAYS

**MOSQUITOES**

Laboratory-based studies found that botanicals, including citronella products, worked for shorter periods than products containing DEET. For people wishing to use botanicals, CDC recommends Environmental Protection Agency (EPA)–registered products containing OLE. There are no high-quality studies on the effectiveness or safety of neem oil for preventing

mosquito bites (see Chapter 3, Mosquitoes, Ticks & Other Arthropods).

**BED BUGS**

There is no evidence that the natural products marketed to repel bed bugs are effective. Instead, travelers should be encouraged to follow steps to detect and avoid bed bugs, such as inspecting their mattresses and keeping their luggage off the floor or bed. Information is available on CDC's website at www.cdc.gov/parasites/bedbugs and Box 3-2, Bed bugs and international travel.

## Sun Protection

### CLAIMS

Many "natural" sunscreen products are promoted online, as are recipes for making your own and advice on consuming dietary supplements or drinking teas to protect against sun damage.

### WHAT THE SCIENCE SAYS

Studies have not proven that any herbal product or dietary supplement, including aloe vera, beta carotene, selenium, or epigallocatechin gallate (EGCG), an extract from green tea, reduces the risk of skin cancer or sun damage. For more information, see Chapter 3, Sun Exposure.

## Homeopathic Vaccines

### CLAIMS

Proponents of homeopathy claim that products called "nosodes" or homeopathic vaccines are effective substitutes for conventional immunizations.

### WHAT THE SCIENCE SAYS

There is no credible scientific evidence or plausible scientific rationale to support these claims. For more information, see Vaccination & Immunoprophylaxis: General Recommendations in this chapter.

## UNTESTED THERAPIES IN OTHER COUNTRIES

CDC does not recommend traveling to other countries for untested medical interventions or to buy medications that are not approved in the United States. For more information see Medical Tourism in Chapter 9.

## TALKING TO TRAVELERS ABOUT COMPLEMENTARY HEALTH APPROACHES

Given the vast number of complementary or integrative interventions and the wealth of potentially misleading information about them that can be found on the internet, discussing the use of these approaches with patients may seem daunting. However, it is important to be proactive, as surveys show that many patients are reluctant to raise the topic with their health care providers. Federal agencies, such as the National Center for Complementary and Integrative Health (NCCIH), offer evidence-based resources (nccih.nih.gov/health/providers) to help you and your patients have a meaningful discussion about complementary approaches.

## ACKNOWLEDGMENTS

The authors thank Mr. Philip Kibak of ICF for his editorial assistance.

### BIBLIOGRAPHY

1. Erland LA, Saxena PK. Melatonin natural health products and supplements: presence of serotonin and significant variability of melatonin content. J Clin Sleep Med. 2017 Feb 15;13(2):275–81.

2. Giddings SL, Stevens AM, Leung DT. Traveler's diarrhea. Med Clin North Am. 2016 Mar;100(2):317–30.

3. Hao Q, Lu Z, Dong BR, Huang CQ, Wu T. Probiotics for preventing acute upper respiratory tract infections. Cochrane Database Syst Rev. 2015 Feb 3(2):CD006895.

4. Herxheimer A. Jet lag. BMJ Clin Evid. 2014 Apr 29;2014:2303.

5. Is it really "FDA approved"? US Food and Drug Administration; 2017. [cited 2018 Mar 20]. Available from: www.fda.gov/forconsumers/consumerupdates/ucm047470.htm.

6. Is rinsing your sinuses with neti pots safe? US Food and Drug Administration; 2017. [cited 2018 Mar 20]. Available from: www.fda.gov/ForConsumers/ConsumerUpdates/ucm316375.htm.

7. Karsch-Völk M, Barrett B, Kiefer D, Bauer R, Ardjomand-Woelkart K, Linde K. Echinacea for preventing and treating the common cold. Cochrane Database Syst Rev. 2014 Feb 20;(2):CD000530.

8. Wang C, Lü L, Zhang A, Liu C. Repellency of selected chemicals against the bed bug (Hemiptera: Cimicidae). J Econ Entomol. 2013 Dec;106(6):2522–9.

# PRIORITIZING CARE FOR THE RESOURCE-LIMITED TRAVELER

Zoon Wangu, Elizabeth D. Barnett

Travelers seen in pretravel clinic consultations often have financial constraints and must pay out of pocket for pretravel care, as many health insurance plans provide no or limited coverage for travel immunizations and prophylactic medications. The variety of insurance plans, number of travelers without adequate insurance coverage, and number of student and budget travelers challenges even the most savvy travel medicine clinicians. As an example, the estimated cost of a US pretravel consultation for a backpacker planning a 4-week trip to West Africa may be as high as $1,400 for the initial consultation and vaccinations, excluding malaria prophylaxis.

Travelers with limited budgets may be at higher risk for travel-associated infections, as they often visit remote areas, stay in more modest accommodations, and eat in restaurants with lower hygiene standards. The total cost of a becoming ill with a vaccine- or prophylaxis-preventable disease (e.g., hospitalization, treatment, lost wages) may, in many cases, outweigh the initial cost of vaccination and prophylaxis, making a pretravel consultation particularly important. The cost and benefit of obtaining travel health insurance and evacuation insurance before travel must also be considered (see Chapter 6, Travel Insurance, Travel Health Insurance & Medical Evacuation Insurance). The goal of this section is to guide travel health recommendations for travelers with financial constraints.

## VACCINES

### Required Vaccines

Only 2 vaccines are required categorically for some travelers: meningococcal vaccine for pilgrims traveling to Mecca during the Hajj and yellow fever vaccine for travelers to certain countries in Africa and South America (see Yellow Fever Vaccine & Malaria Prophylaxis Information, by Country in this chapter). Prioritize these vaccines, since the traveler may be denied entry to the country without proof of vaccination. Note that those staying in a yellow fever–endemic country only briefly (such as during an airport layover) may still need evidence of vaccination to enter other countries on their itinerary.

In a few specific circumstances, travelers to polio-affected countries may be asked to show proof of polio vaccination before departure if their duration of stay is >4 weeks (see Chapter 4, Poliomyelitis). Travelers and clinicians are advised to check the latest recommendations for their destinations.

### Routine Vaccines

All travelers should be up-to-date with routine vaccines before international travel, regardless of destination. The benefits of these vaccines extend beyond the travel period, and in many cases lifelong immunity is achieved. Since these vaccines are mass-produced as part of the scheduled national childhood and adult vaccination programs, associated costs are generally low, and many insurance companies reimburse the patient for the cost of administration. Travelers can also obtain these vaccines in a health department or primary care setting, where costs may be lower than those at a travel clinic. Prioritize the routine vaccines that protect against diseases for which the traveler is most likely to be at general risk, for example influenza, measles, and hepatitis A.

Some travelers may be immune to the disease for which immunization is being considered. Pretravel antibody testing may be covered by insurance when vaccines are not. The decision to test rather than vaccinate will also depend on time to departure.

### Recommended Vaccines

Consider time until departure, risk of disease at the destination, effectiveness and safety of vaccine, and likelihood of repeat travel. For example, although currently not a routine vaccine for US adults, hepatitis A vaccine can provide lifelong immunity and should be considered for travel to all destinations. On the other hand, hepatitis B (also not a routine vaccine for US adults) is not as significantly associated with travel, and vaccination may be a lower priority. Typhoid vaccine for both adults and children has limited effectiveness, and protection lasts only 2–5 years depending on formulation, thus making it more valuable just for higher-risk destinations or those where typhoid is more likely to be acquired (such as the Indian subcontinent).

Review the itinerary in detail to determine need for Japanese encephalitis vaccine. Some travelers may be able to obtain single-dose vaccine at a much lower cost outside the United States, bearing in mind issues surrounding quality of vaccines in many countries (see Chapter 6, *Perspectives*: Avoiding Poorly Regulated Medicines and Medical Products during Travel). Those who decline vaccine should have a clear understanding of when and how to use insect repellents and other measures to prevent mosquito bites.

When considering rabies vaccine for resource-limited travelers, consider the risk of animal exposure, access to local health care, and availability of rabies immune globulin and rabies vaccine at the traveler's destination. Travelers who decline pre-exposure immunization should have a plan of action if an exposure occurs. In many areas, rabies vaccine or immune globulin are difficult or impossible to obtain, and travelers may need to be evacuated to receive postexposure prophylaxis.

## MALARIA PROPHYLAXIS

Every pretravel consultation should include detailed advice about preventing mosquito bites (see Chapter 3, Mosquitoes, Ticks & Other Arthropods). The risk of acquiring malaria varies widely depending on destination, accommodations, and activities during travel. Costs associated with the different regimens vary widely. Providers should stay up-to-date on the usual cost of antimalarial medications in their region and at the pharmacies used by their travelers so that the most cost effective drug can be recommended to the traveler for their itinerary. Travelers who raise the question of purchasing antimalarial drugs at their destination should be advised about the risk of inappropriate, substandard, and counterfeit medications and discouraged from this practice (see Chapter 6, *Perspectives*: Avoiding Poorly Regulated Medicines and Medical Products during Travel).

## TRAVELERS' DIARRHEA

Travelers' diarrhea (TD) is among the most common travel-related illnesses. Antibiotics to treat moderate to severe diarrhea should be considered; prophylaxis may be indicated only in select cases of patients at high risk for TD-related complications (see Travelers' Diarrhea later in this chapter). As with antimalarial drugs purchased at the destination, advise travelers about the risk of purchasing counterfeit antibiotics overseas.

## PREVENTIVE BEHAVIORS

Budget travelers and those who cannot afford travel vaccines will continue to challenge travel medicine practitioners. When immunization or prophylactic medications cannot be given because of financial constraints, educate travelers about alternative ways to reduce risk. For example, advise travelers to avoid animal bites, use insect precautions, follow safe sex practices, wash their hands or use alcohol-based hand sanitizer frequently, and observe food and water precautions to the best of their ability.

Travelers can be reassured that the actions they take to avoid these preventable hazards may, in the long run, protect against travel-associated risks that are more prevalent than certain vaccine-preventable diseases.

### BIBLIOGRAPHY

1. Adachi K, Coleman MS, Khan N, Jentes ES, Arguin P, Rao SR, et al. Economics of malaria prevention in US travelers to West Africa. Clin Infect Dis. 2014 Jan;58(1):11–21.

2. Jentes ES, Blanton JD, Johnson KJ, Petersen BW, Lamias MJ, Robertson K, et al. The global availability of rabies immune globulin and rabies vaccine in clinics providing indirect care to travelers. J Travel Med. 2014 Jan–Feb;21(1):62–6.

3. Johnson DF, Leder K, Torresi J. Hepatitis B and C infection in international travelers. J Travel Med. 2013 May–Jun;20(3):194–202.

4. Mangtani P, Roberts JA. Economic evaluations of travelers' vaccinations. In: Zuckerman JN, Jong EC, editors. Travelers' Vaccines. 2nd ed. Shelton, CT: People's Medical Publishing House; 2010. pp. 553–67.

5. REDBOOK® System (electronic version). Truven Health Analytics, Greenwood Village, Colorado, USA. [cited 2018 Mar 5]. Available from: www.micromedexsolutions.com/.

6. Riddle MS, Connor BA, Beeching NJ, DuPont HL, Hamer DH, Kozarsky P et al. Guidelines for the prevention and treatment of travelers' diarrhea: a graded expert panel report. J Travel Med. 2017;24(1):S63–80.

7. Steffen R, Connor BA. Vaccines in travel health: from risk assessment to priorities. J Travel Med. 2005 Jan–Feb;12(1):26–35.

8. Wu D, Guo CY. Epidemiology and prevention of hepatitis A in travelers. J Travel Med. 2013 Nov–Dec;20(6):394–9.

# TELEMEDICINE

Taylan Bozkurt, Jose F. Flórez-Arango, Matt Levi

## WHAT IS TELEMEDICINE?

Telemedicine is commonly referred to as providing diagnostics and therapeutic services via information and communication technologies. Telemedicine interventions can be as simple as 2 doctors discussing a case over the phone to decide on an intervention or as complex as real-time monitoring of astronauts at the International Space Station.

Benefits of telemedicine include reducing cost and time associated with unnecessary transportation of patients, quicker access to care with minimized waiting time, access to subspecialty care, and maintaining patients in familiar environments. Telemedicine has benefits in both rural and urban areas, but it is not always a viable option. In remote rural areas, there may not be the bandwidth and connectivity capable of supporting the communication technologies. In the urban setting, users may contend with internal firewalls and security settings.

Telemedicine can serve as an alternative to a pretravel clinical visit. It can be used directly with patients when traveling to answer questions or provide guidance to distant clinicians in case of emergencies, which can help maintain continuity of care. In addition, it may be used to assist clinicians with posttravel evaluations when there are unusual clinical findings and subspecialty assistance is needed.

## CONDUCTING A REMOTE PRETRAVEL CONSULTATION

Telemedicine enables a convenient method to deliver pretravel consultations with the same elements as in an in-person visit. Providers should continue to follow the professional standards as with in-person consultations, including the same code of ethics, security and privacy practices, and adherence to clinical guidelines. What can and can't be done in a remote consultation varies by state, so providers will need to check with their state medical boards about any restrictions. A valuable resource on telemedicine, including requirements by state, is available at https://prognocis.com/wp-content/uploads/2017/01/Telemedicine-Whitepaper.pdf.

Practices should provide patients with a resource that outlines the expectations and outcomes of telemedicine before they schedule the consultation, including the limitations of a remote consultation. Intake information, including medical history, prior medical records, or diagnostic information, may be requested of the patient and made available to the provider in advance. Patients are encouraged to set up in advance and test their connections to the telemedicine software or equipment.

At the time of the consultation, it is important to establish informed consent with the patient and ensure that the patient is in an appropriate care setting (for example, depending on the state, the patient may need to physically be in a location where the provider is licensed to practice medicine at the time of the consultation). Depending on the circumstances, a telepresenter (such as another health care provider or even a translator) may need to be present with the patient to assist with the intake and exam.

## PRESCRIPTION MEDICATIONS AND VACCINES

Medications and vaccinations can be prescribed during a telemedicine encounter. Remote vaccine prescriptions are allowed in several states. Pharmacies receive the prescription electronically or over the phone, and the pharmacist may be able to administer any injectable vaccines (see www.pharmacist.com/article/pharmacist-administered-immunizations-what-does-your-state-allow). Yellow fever vaccine can only be administered at specially registered clinics, so a traveler may need a separate clinic visit to receive this vaccine. For medications and vaccines that may not be routinely stocked in a traveler's local pharmacy, such as malaria prophylaxis, the traveler should allow time for the pharmacy to order them.

## WHEN A TRAVELER IS OVERSEAS

A travel medicine provider may be called on to provide a consultation for a traveler overseas for any number of reasons. The provider's willingness and ability to provide a remote overseas consultation will vary with type of question or the nature of the problem, willingness to work pro bono (or ability to charge for services), and perhaps the time of day, but it is important to remember that the same security and privacy practices apply as in a domestic consultation. In the case of lost medication, CDC does not endorse procuring medication or filling prescriptions overseas because of the risk of counterfeit drugs. However, in an emergency, such as with lost or stolen antimalarial drugs, a provider may be able to help a traveler locate a reputable source for replacing them.

## TECHNOLOGY REQUIREMENTS

When communicating with patients abroad, legal obligations under the Health Insurance Portability and Accountability Act ("HIPAA") remain relevant. Providers must also ensure that the chosen technology to conduct telemedicine encounters, whether store-and-forward or live-video, is HIPAA compliant. Although encryption is not specifically addressed under HIPAA, it would be best to ensure technology is encrypted because of requirements to safeguard patient health information.

Providers must also consider bandwidth and connectivity. In the United States today, connectivity in some rural communities is often inadequate, and accessing websites is often difficult because of internal firewalls. Mobile hotspots may be used in some situations in lieu of dial-up or Ethernet connections.

Certain telemedicine vendors have optimized software to work in a low-bandwidth setting, while others have focused on targeted, established markets. Discuss needs with telemedicine vendors to understand the minimum bandwidth at which their software will meet expectations.

## LEGAL ISSUES

The Health Insurance Portability and Accountability Act (HIPAA) must be taken into account in discussions about patient data in health care today, and conversations around telemedicine will certainly include HIPAA compliance. When beginning to provide remote pretravel consultations, providers should use video software that already is HIPAA compliant. Providers should investigate specific legal requirements of the country where the traveler is located, as well as maintain compliance with federal and state privacy and security laws. In the United States, each state medical board has its own telemedicine regulations. Some states do not permit providers to practice telemedicine across state lines; some do not permit the prescribing of certain medications. It is critical that the travel clinic carefully read these medical board regulations before embarking on telemedicine consults.

In addition, particularly if providers are not part of a larger system or they are sole practitioners, they should explore whether or not there is a need for a business associate agreement or business associate contract.

When working with international partners, such as companies based outside the country in which the provider practices, additional legal issues may arise and should be considered.

## REIMBURSEMENT

Much like reimbursement for face-to-face encounters, providers need to ensure that the clinic meets certain legal requirements and payer guidelines. In the United States, the pretravel consultation is generally not reimbursed by health insurance companies, so a telemedicine practice may be primarily fee-for-service. If corporate personnel are traveling and their companies are paying for the service, it is wise to make sure the company is willing to permit their employees to engage in telemedicine and that they will reimburse for this service.

For during- and posttravel consults, issues such as eligibility for payment and licensure may surface. The provider's medical board and the traveler's payer may have to be queried as to whether teleconsultation is permissible, and which current procedural terminology (CPT) codes are usable.

## TELEMEDICINE RESOURCES

Additional information relating to telemedicine standards, guidelines, and practice may be available through the following resources:

- American Telemedicine Association, Practice Guidelines and Resources: http://thesource.americantelemed.org/resources/telemedicine-practice-guidelines#

- American Telemedicine Association, Glossary of Terms: http://thesource.americantelemed.org/resources/telemedicine-glossary

- American Medical Association: www.ama-assn.org/delivering-care/telemedicine-mobile-apps

- Center for Connected Health Policy: www.telehealthpolicy.us/resources

- Centers for Medicare & Medicaid Services: www.cms.gov/Outreach-and-Education/Medicare-Learning-Network-MLN/

MLNProducts/downloads/
TelehealthSrvcsfctsht.pdf; www.cms.gov/
Medicare/Medicare-General-Information/
Telehealth

- Federation of State Medical Boards: www.
  fsmb.org/Media/Default/PDF/FSMB/
  Advocacy/FSMB_Telemedicine_Policy.pdf

- Health Insurance Portability and
  Accountability Act (HIPAA): www.hhs.gov/
  hipaa/index.html

- Institute of Medicine: www.nationalacademies.
  org/hmd/Reports/2012/The-Role-of-
  Telehealth-in-an-Evolving-Health-Care-
  Environment.aspx

- Strengths and Limitations of Telemedicine:
  https://academic.oup.com/jtm/article/
  23/5/taw048/2579370; www.ncbi.nlm.nih.
  gov/pmc/articles/PMC4895094; www.
  acha.org/documents/Programs_Services/
  webhandouts_2016/WE1-146_Neighbor.pdf

2

# LEGAL ISSUES IN TRAVEL MEDICINE

Andrés F. Henao-Martínez, Carlos Franco-Paredes

**2**

Travel medicine providers—as in other medical specialties—are at risk of legal action. Claims for medical negligence may involve any of the following: 1) failure of duty of care; 2) failure to uphold the standard of practice; 3) care resulting in physical, financial or psychological loss; and 4) failure to reach the standard of care directly caused this loss.

Although travel medicine practitioners come from many backgrounds, in the travel medicine arena they are preventive medicine specialists. As such, in giving advice, they provide education and not generally "hands on" patient care. Although misunderstandings and legal action may occur despite best efforts, certain guidance is helpful.

**Communication.** The likelihood of a lawsuit is lessened by good communication between the provider and the traveler patient. All elements of a pretravel consultation must be covered either verbally during the visit or given as written material for the patient to take home. Since time is a limitation, clinics need to provide handouts on how to avoid common health problems not discussed during the consultation. It is also is helpful to provide written information about medications and vaccinations (see below) that are being given or prescribed.

**Documentation.** Clinics should have a method for documenting all aspects of the consultation as well as an area within the record for the provider to comment on the patient's questions or responses to recommendations. Many electronic medical records enable the provider to add items unique to travel health and to add comments regarding the consultation.

**Identification of problems.** Providers are encouraged to consult with their risk management personnel or legal advisors in the event of a contentious office visit or exchange after the visit. Good documentation of all communications in a nonjudgmental fashion between traveler patient and provider is critical.

## EXAMPLES OF LEGAL ISSUES IN TRAVEL MEDICINE

### Prescription Medications

#### FLUOROQUINOLONES

Fluoroquinolone use is sometimes associated with tendinitis, tendon rupture, peripheral neuropathy, and central nervous system adverse events. Lawsuits regarding these problems continue, and it is unknown whether a single dose of a fluoroquinolone used for the self-treatment of travelers' diarrhea can lead to such events. Thus, despite the fact that prescriptions come from pharmacies with directions and adverse event information, providers should also discuss potential adverse events with their patients.

#### MEFLOQUINE

Mefloquine may cause serious neuropsychiatric adverse events, including visual hallucinations, psychosis, insomnia, seizures, nightmares, neuropathies (motor and sensory), and dizziness. These adverse events can persist after discontinuation of the drug. Providers should not prescribe mefloquine to patients with a seizure disorder or a psychiatric disorder (depression, generalized anxiety disorder, psychosis, or schizophrenia). CDC also recommends against its use in patients with cardiac conduction abnormalities. Travelers receiving a prescription for mefloquine should receive a copy of the US Food and Drug Administration (FDA) medication guide (www.accessdata. fda.gov/drugsatfda_docs/ label/2008/019591s023lbl.pdf).

Because of its low cost and convenient weekly dosing, however, mefloquine remains an attractive option for some travelers. Therefore, providers recommending mefloquine for malaria prophylaxis should document clearly and carefully why they selected this drug over other antimalarial drugs; a notation that the provider reviewed the medical history for potential contraindications should also be included as part of the patient record.

### PRIMAQUINE AND TAFENOQUINE

These drugs may cause potentially fatal hemolysis in G6PD-deficient patients. Thus, clinicians should screen anyone receiving a prescription for either of these medications for G6PD deficiency.

### DRUG INTERACTIONS

Drug interactions may occur among medications prescribed for a traveler. Medication reconciliation is an essential part of the travel history. Electronic medical records and other pharmacy aids are useful to alert clinicians of drug interactions in real time, when decisions are being made about travel medication prescriptions. Use fluoroquinolones and macrolides with caution in traveler patients taking other QT interval–prolonging agents. Concurrent use of antibiotics with cholera or oral typhoid vaccines may produce a reduced vaccine immune response. Antibody-containing products may affect live attenuated vaccines.

### OFF-LABEL USE

Sometimes providers find it useful to recommend to travelers medications not approved by FDA for that specific purpose. Examples include use of primaquine alone for malaria prophylaxis and rifaximin to prevent travelers' diarrhea. However, advisors will sometimes recommend medication uses other than those considered standard of care, and these should be discussed with the traveler prior to prescribing and be documented along with the traveler's acceptance.

## Vaccine Side Effects and Contraindications

To deliver effective and safe vaccinations, travel health providers should review carefully the patient's past medical history, allergies, and vaccination history. Failure to administer a vaccine correctly can cause an adverse event or result in a traveler acquiring a preventable disease abroad. Travel health providers should discuss and then document any relevant conversations regarding the risk of acquiring a disease, should the patient refuse a vaccine. Travelers known to be immunocompromised, whose immune status may preclude a robust, protective antibody response to vaccination, should be made aware of such.

Serious vaccine-associated adverse events may be due to a variety of causes. Allergic reactions to vaccine components are common. Immunocompromised travelers may particularly suffer adverse events after receiving live vaccines. Eliciting a history of pregnancy, breastfeeding status, immunosuppressive medications, immunocompromised status, and allergies becomes crucial to minimizing vaccine-associated adverse events. Vaccine information statements should be available in the clinic and reviewed with the traveler patient (www.cdc.gov/vaccines/hcp/vis/index.html).

It is essential to document a patient's history and the data used in decision making, especially when a vaccine is not given or when a provider administers a vaccine despite precautions about its use. It is critical that patients understand (and clinicians document the discussion) about any risks associated with non–FDA-approved dosing schedules, such as those used for the accelerated delivery of some vaccines.

## Deep Vein Thrombosis (DVT)

Long-distance travel increases the risk of DVT and pulmonary embolism by approximately 3-fold. The association is stronger with flights (continued)

of longer duration. Travel medicine providers should counsel patients about DVT and recommend measures to decrease its risk (occasional walking, aisle seat selection, and exercises), and document this discussion in the medical record (see Chapter 8, Deep Vein Thrombosis & Pulmonary Embolism).

## SUMMARY AND RECOMMENDATIONS

Maintaining a standard of care in one's practice is important not only for the patient's protection but for the provider as well. This section gives examples of issues that may bring legal action in the travel medicine arena. Clinic providers should have adequate training in travel medicine and engage in continuing education. It is wise for at least 1 provider at each location to have earned the Certificate in Travel Health (CTH), awarded by the International Society of Travel Medicine (ISTM) upon successful completion of the CTH examination. It is also advisable for providers to remain current in the field by accessing continuing education programs offered by CDC and ISTM.

### BIBLIOGRAPHY

1. Burton B. Australian army faces legal action over mefloquine. BMJ. 2004;329(7474):1062.

2. Hinrichs-Krapels S, Bussmann S, Dobyns C, Kácha O, Ratzmann N, Holm Thorvaldsen J, et al. Key considerations for an economic and legal framework facilitating medical travel. Front Public Health. 2016;4:47.

3. Kahn SR, Lim W, Dunn AS, Cushman M, Dentali F, Akl EA, et al. Prevention of VTE in nonsurgical patients. Chest. 2012 Feb;141(2):e195S–226S.

4. Kennedy KM, Flaherty GT. Medico-legal risk, clinical negligence and the practice of travel medicine. J Travel Med. 2016;23(5):doi: 10.1093/jtm/taw048.

5. Lapostolle F, Surget V, Borron SW, Desmaizières M, Sordelet D, Lapandry C, et al. Severe pulmonary embolism associated with air travel. N Engl J Med. 2001;345(11):779–83.

*Perspectives* sections are written as editorial discussions aiming to add depth and clinical perspective to the official recommendations contained in the book. The views and opinions expressed in this section are those of the authors and do not necessarily represent the official position of CDC.

# VACCINATION & IMMUNOPROPHYLAXIS: GENERAL RECOMMENDATIONS

Andrew T. Kroger, Candice L. Robinson

Evaluation of people before travel should include a review and provision of routine vaccines recommended based on age and other individual characteristics. Additionally, some routine vaccines are recommended at earlier ages for international travelers. For example, MMR (measles-mumps-rubella) vaccine and hepatitis A vaccine are recommended for infants aged 6–11 months who travel abroad. Recommendations for specific vaccines related to travel will depend on itinerary, duration of travel, and host factors. Vaccinations against diphtheria, tetanus, pertussis, measles, mumps, rubella, varicella, poliomyelitis, hepatitis A, hepatitis B, *Haemophilus influenzae* type b (Hib), rotavirus, human papillomavirus (HPV), and pneumococcal and meningococcal invasive disease are routinely administered in the United States, usually in childhood or adolescence. Influenza vaccine is routinely recommended for all people aged ≥6 months, each year. Herpes zoster (shingles) vaccine is recommended for adults aged ≥50 years.

If a person does not have a history of adequate protection against these diseases, immunizations appropriate to age and previous immunization status should be obtained, whether or not international travel is planned. A visit to a clinician for travel-related immunizations should be seen as an opportunity to bring an incompletely vaccinated person up-to-date on his or her routine vaccinations. For additional details on specific vaccines' and toxoids' recommendations, backgrounds, adverse reactions, precautions, and contraindications, refer to the respective ACIP recommendations (www.cdc.gov/vaccines/acip/index.html). For information on vaccinating travelers with altered immune function, see Chapter 5, Immunocompromised Travelers.

## SPACING OF IMMUNOBIOLOGICS

### Simultaneous Administration

With some exceptions (such as PCV13 and PPSV23, PCV13 and MenACWY-D [Menactra], and Menactra and DTaP), all commonly used vaccines can safely and effectively be given simultaneously (on the same day) at separate sites without impairing antibody responses or increasing rates of adverse reactions. This knowledge is particularly helpful for international travelers, for whom exposure to several infectious diseases might be imminent. Simultaneous administration of all indicated vaccines is encouraged for people who are the recommended age to receive these vaccines and for whom no contraindications exist. With the same exceptions as listed above for simultaneous vaccination, if not administered on the same day, an inactivated vaccine may be given at any time before or after a different inactivated vaccine or a live-virus vaccine. PCV13 and PPSV23 should be administered 8 weeks apart. PCV13 and Menactra should be administered 4 weeks apart in some high-risk groups. Menactra and DTaP should be administered 6 months apart in some high-risk groups.

The immune response to an injected or intranasal live-virus vaccine (such as MMR, varicella, or live attenuated influenza vaccines) might be impaired if administered within 28 days of another live-virus vaccine. Typically, the immune response is impaired only for the live-virus vaccine administered second. Whenever possible, injected or intranasal live-virus vaccines administered on different days should be given ≥28 days apart. If 2 injected or intranasal live-virus vaccines are not administered on the same day but <28 days apart, the second vaccine should be repeated in ≥28 days.

No evidence exists that inactivated vaccines interfere with the immune response to yellow fever vaccine. Therefore, inactivated vaccines can be administered either simultaneously or at any time before or after yellow fever vaccination. ACIP recommends that yellow fever vaccine be given at the same time as other live-virus vaccines.

Limited data suggest that coadministration of yellow fever vaccine with measles-rubella or MMR vaccines might decrease the immune response. One study involving the simultaneous administration of yellow fever and MMR vaccines and a second involving simultaneous administration of yellow fever and measles-rubella vaccines in children demonstrated a decreased immune response against all antigens except measles when the vaccines were given on the same day versus 30 days apart. Additional studies are needed to confirm these findings, but they suggest that, if possible, yellow fever and MMR should be given 30 days apart.

Additional data suggest that oral Ty21a typhoid vaccine, a live bacterial vaccine, can be administered simultaneously or at any interval before or after yellow fever vaccine. There are no data on the immune response to live attenuated oral cholera vaccine (Vaxchora) or nasally administered live attenuated influenza vaccine administered simultaneously with yellow fever vaccine. However, data from live attenuated influenza and MMR vaccines found no evidence of interference. If yellow fever vaccine and another injectable live-virus vaccine are not administered either simultaneously or ≥30 days apart, providers may consider measuring the patient's neutralizing antibody response to vaccination before travel. Contact the state health department or the CDC Arboviral Disease Branch (970-221-6400) to discuss serologic testing.

No data are available on concomitant administration of the currently available formulation of oral cholera vaccine with other vaccines, including the enteric-coated oral typhoid vaccine. Based on expert opinion of how oral cholera vaccine buffer might interfere with the enteric-coated oral typhoid vaccine formulation, taking the first oral typhoid vaccine dose ≥8 hours after ingestion of oral cholera vaccine might decrease potential interference of the vaccine buffer with oral typhoid vaccine.

Measles and other live-virus vaccines may interfere with the response to tuberculin skin testing and the interferon-γ release assay. Tuberculin testing, if otherwise indicated, can be done either on the same day that live-virus vaccines are administered or 4–6 weeks later. Tuberculin skin testing is not a prerequisite for administration of any vaccine. Neither oral typhoid vaccine nor oral cholera vaccine have been associated with suppressing the response to tuberculosis testing.

## Missed Doses and Boosters

In some cases, a scheduled dose of vaccine may not be given on time. If this occurs, the dose should be given at the next visit. However, travelers may forget to return to complete a series or for a booster at the specified time. Available data indicate that intervals between doses longer than those routinely recommended do not affect seroconversion rate or titer when the schedule is completed. Consequently, it is not necessary to restart the series or add doses of any vaccine because of an extended interval between doses. There are some exceptions to this rule. Some experts recommend repeating the series of oral typhoid vaccine if the 4-dose series is extended to more than 3 weeks. If an extended interval passes between doses of the preexposure rabies vaccine series, immune status should be assessed by serologic testing 7–14 days after the final dose in the series.

## Antibody-Containing Blood Products

Antibody-containing blood products from the United States, such as immune globulin (IG) products, do not interfere with the immune response to yellow fever vaccine and are not believed to interfere with the response to live typhoid, live attenuated influenza, rotavirus, or zoster vaccines. When MMR and varicella vaccines are given shortly before, simultaneously with, or after an antibody-containing blood product, response to the vaccine can be diminished. The duration of inhibition of MMR and varicella vaccines is related to the dose of IG in the product. MMR and varicella vaccines either should be administered ≥2 weeks before receipt of a blood product or should be delayed 3–11 months after receipt of the blood product, depending on the dose and type of blood product (Table 2-4).

## Table 2-4. Recommended intervals between administration of antibody-containing products and measles-containing vaccine or varicella-containing vaccine[1]

| INDICATION | DOSE AND ROUTE | RECOMMENDED INTERVAL BEFORE MEASLES OR VARICELLA VACCINATION |
|---|---|---|
| **Blood transfusion** | | |
| Red blood cells (RBCs), washed | 10 mL/kg (negligible IgG/kg) IV | None |
| RBCs, adenine-saline added | 10 mL/kg (10 mg IgG/kg) IV | 3 months |
| Packed RBCs (hematocrit 65%)[2] | 10 mL/kg (60 mg IgG/kg) IV | 6 months |
| Whole blood (hematocrit 35%–50%)[2] | 10 mL/kg (80–100 mg IgG/kg) IV | 6 months |
| Plasma/platelet products | 10 mL/kg (160 mg IgG/kg) IV | 7 months |
| Botulism immune globulin, intravenous (human) | 1.0 mL/kg (50 mg IgG/kg) IV | 6 months |
| Cytomegalovirus prophylaxis (CMV IGIV) | 150 mg/kg IV (maximum) | 6 months |
| **Hepatitis A (IG), duration of international travel** <2-month stay ≥2-month stay | 0.1 mL/kg (3.3 mg IgG/kg) IM 0.2 mL/kg (10 mg IgG/kg) IM | 3 months 3 months |

# Table 2-4. Recommended intervals between administration of antibody-containing products and measles-containing vaccine or varicella-containing vaccine[1] (continued)

| INDICATION | DOSE AND ROUTE | RECOMMENDED INTERVAL BEFORE MEASLES OR VARICELLA VACCINATION |
|---|---|---|
| **Hepatitis B prophylaxis (HBIG)** | 0.06 mL/kg (10 mg IgG/kg) IM | 3 months |
| **Intravenous immune globulin (IVIG)** Replacement therapy[3] Immune thrombocytopenic purpura (ITP) Postexposure measles prophylaxis (for immunocompromised people) Postexposure varicella prophylaxis[5] Kawasaki disease | 300–400 mg/kg IV[3] 400 mg/kg IV or 1 g/kg IV 400 mg/kg IV 400 mg/kg IV 2 mg/kg IV | 8 months 8 months or 10 months[4] 8 months 8 months 11 months |
| **Measles prophylaxis (IG)** Immunocompetent contact | 0.5 mL/kg (80 mg IgG/kg) IM | 6 months |
| **Monoclonal antibody to respiratory syncytial virus (RSV) F protein (Synagis [MedImmune])**[6] | 15 mg/kg IM | None |
| **Rabies prophylaxis (HRIG)** | 20 IU/kg (22 mg IgG/kg) IM | 4 months |
| **Tetanus (TIG)** | 250 units (10 mg IgG/kg) IM | 3 months |
| **Varicella zoster immune globulin**[4,5] | 125 units/10 kg (60–200 mg IgG/kg) IM (maximum 625 units) | 5 months |

Abbreviations: IG, immune globulin; IM, intramuscular; IV, intravenous.

[1] Adapted from Table 3.5, Kroger AT, Duchin J, Vázquez M. General best practice guidelines for immunization. Best practices guidance of the Advisory Committee on Immunization Practices (ACIP). Atlanta, GA: CDC [cited 2018 Jan 18]. Available from: www.cdc.gov/vaccines/hcp/acip-recs/general-recs/downloads/general-recs.pdf. This table is not intended for determining the correct indications and dosage for the use of IG preparations. Unvaccinated people may not be fully protected against measles during the entire recommended interval, and additional doses of IG or measles vaccine may be indicated after measles exposure. Concentrations of measles antibody in an IG preparation can vary by manufacturer's lot. For example, more than a 4-fold variation in the amount of measles antibody titers has been demonstrated in different IG preparations. Rates of antibody clearance after receipt of an IG preparation can also vary. Recommended intervals are extrapolated from an estimated half-life of 30 days for passively acquired antibody and an observed interference with the immune response to measles vaccine for 5 months after a dose of 80 mg IgG/kg (Source: Mason W, Takahashi M, Schneider T. Persisting passively acquired measles antibody following gamma globulin therapy for Kawasaki disease and response to live virus vaccination [abstract 311]. Presented at the 32nd meeting of the Interscience Conference on Antimicrobial Agents and Chemotherapy, Los Angeles, California, October 1992). Does not include zoster vaccine. Zoster vaccine may be given with antibody-containing products.

[2] Assumes a serum IgG concentration of 16 mg/mL.

[3] Measles vaccination is recommended for children with mild or moderate immunosuppression from HIV infections and varicella vaccination may be considered for children with mild or moderate immunosuppression from HIV infections, but both are contraindicated for people with severe immunosuppression from HIV, with any other immunosuppressive disorder, or on immunosuppressive medications.

[4] Recommendation adapted from Neunert C, Lim W, Crowther M, Cohen A, Solberg L, Crowther MA. The American Society of Hematology 2011 evidence-based practice guideline for immune thrombocytopenia. Blood. 2011;117(16):4190–207.

[5] If varicella zoster immune globulin is not available, IVIG can be used. The recommendation for use of IVIG is based on best judgment of experts and is supported by reports comparing varicella IgG titers measured in both IVIG and varicella zoster immune globulin preparations and patients given IVIG and varicella zoster immune globulin. Although licensed IVIG preparations contain antivaricella antibodies, the titer of any specific lot of IVIG is uncertain, because IVIG is not tested routinely for antivaricella antibodies. No clinical data demonstrating effectiveness of IVIG for postexposure prophylaxis of varicella are available. The recommended IVIG dose for postexposure prophylaxis of varicella is 1 dose of 400 mg/kg, intravenously (see http://redbook.solutions.aap.org/chapter.aspx?sectionid=88187270&bookid=1484).

[6] Contains only antibody to respiratory syncytial virus.

IG administration may become necessary for another indication after MMR or varicella vaccines have been given. In such a situation, the IG may interfere with the immune response to the MMR or varicella vaccines. Vaccine virus replication and stimulation of immunity usually occur 2–3 weeks after vaccination. If the interval between administration of 1 of these vaccines and the subsequent administration of an IG preparation is ≥14 days, the vaccine need not be readministered. If the interval is <14 days, the vaccine should be readministered after the interval shown in Table 2-4, unless serologic testing indicates that antibodies have been produced. Such testing should be performed after the interval shown in Table 2-4, to avoid detecting antibodies from the IG preparation.

When IG is given with the first dose of hepatitis A vaccine, the proportion of recipients who develop a protective level of antibody is not affected, but antibody concentrations are lower. Because the final concentrations of antibody are many times higher than those considered protective, this reduced immunogenicity is not expected to be clinically relevant. However, the effect of reduced antibody concentrations on long-term protection is unknown.

IG preparations interact minimally with other inactivated vaccines and toxoids. Other inactivated vaccines may be given simultaneously or at any time interval before or after an antibody-containing blood product is used. However, such vaccines should be administered at different sites from the IG.

## VACCINATING PEOPLE WITH ACUTE ILLNESSES

Every opportunity should be taken to provide needed vaccinations. The decision to delay vaccination because of a current or recent acute illness depends on the severity of the symptoms and their cause. Although a moderate or severe acute illness is sufficient reason to postpone vaccination, minor illnesses (such as diarrhea, mild upper respiratory infection with or without low-grade fever, or other low-grade febrile illness) are not contraindications to vaccination.

Antimicrobial therapy is not a contraindication to vaccination, with several exceptions:

- Antibiotics may interfere with the response to oral typhoid vaccine and oral cholera vaccine.

- Antiviral agents active against herpes viruses (such as acyclovir) may interfere with the response to varicella-containing vaccines.

- Antiviral agents active against influenza virus (such as zanamivir and oseltamivir) may interfere with the response to live attenuated influenza vaccine.

## VACCINATION SCHEDULING FOR SELECTED TRAVEL VACCINES

Table 2-5 lists the minimum age and minimum interval between doses for vaccines routinely recommended in the United States.

## ALLERGY TO VACCINE COMPONENTS

Vaccine components can cause allergic reactions in some recipients. These reactions can be local or systemic and can include anaphylaxis or anaphylacticlike responses. The vaccine components responsible can include the vaccine antigen, animal proteins, antibiotics, preservatives (such as thimerosal), or stabilizers (such as gelatin). The most common animal protein allergen is egg protein in vaccines prepared by using embryonated chicken eggs (influenza and yellow fever vaccines). People with a history of egg allergy who have experienced only hives after exposure to egg should receive influenza vaccine. Any licensed inactivated influenza vaccine that is otherwise appropriate for the recipient's age and health status may be used.

People who report having had reactions to egg involving symptoms other than hives, such as angioedema, respiratory distress, lightheadedness, or recurrent emesis, or who required epinephrine or another emergency medical intervention, may similarly receive any licensed inactivated influenza vaccine that is otherwise appropriate for the recipient's age and health status. If a person has a severe egg sensitivity or has a positive skin test to yellow fever vaccine but the vaccination is recommended because of their travel destination–specific risk, desensitization can be performed under direct supervision of a physician experienced in the management of anaphylaxis. In such circumstances, both yellow fever and influenza vaccines should be administered

## Table 2-5. Recommended and minimum ages and intervals vaccine doses[1,2]

| VACCINE AND DOSE NUMBER | RECOMMENDED AGE FOR THIS DOSE | MINIMUM AGE FOR THIS DOSE | MINIMUM INTERVAL TO NEXT DOSE[3] |
|---|---|---|---|
| Japanese encephalitis, Vero cell (Ixiaro)-1[4] | 2 months - 17 years<br>18–65 years | ≥2 months<br>≥18 years | 28 days<br>7 days |
| Ixiaro-2 | 2 months -17 years: 28 days after dose 1<br>18–65 years: 7 days after dose 1 | 28 days after dose 1<br>7 days after dose 1 | NA |
| Live cholera vaccine (Vaxchora)<br>Rabies-1 (preexposure) | 18–64 years<br>See footnote 5 | 18 years | NA |
| Rabies-2 | 7 days after dose 1 | 7 days after dose 1 | 14 days |
| Rabies-3 | 21 days after dose 1 | 21 days after dose 1 | NA |
| Typhoid, inactivated (ViCPS) | ≥2 years | ≥2 years | NA |
| Typhoid, live attenuated (Ty21a) | ≥6 years | ≥6 years | See footnote 6 |
| Yellow fever | ≥9 months[7] | ≥9 months[7] | 10 years |

[1] Adapted from Table 1, CDC. General recommendations on immunization: recommendations of the Advisory Committee on Immunization Practices (ACIP). MMWR Recomm Rep. 2011 Jan 28;60(RR-2):1–61.
[2] Combination vaccines are available. Use of licensed combination vaccines is generally preferred over separate injections of their equivalent component vaccines (CDC. Combination vaccines for childhood immunization. MMWR Recomm Rep. 1999 May 14;48[RR-5]:1–14.). When administering combination vaccines, the minimum age for administration is the oldest age for any of the individual components (exception: the minimum age for the first dose of MenHibrix is 6 weeks); the minimum interval between doses is equal to the largest interval of any of the individual components.
[3] See www.cdc.gov/vaccines/schedules for recommended revaccination (booster) schedules.
[4] Ixiaro is approved by the Food and Drug Administration for people aged ≥2 months.
[5] There is no minimum age for preexposure immunization for rabies (CDC. Human rabies prevention—United States, 2008: recommendations of the Advisory Committee on Immunization Practices. MMWR Recomm Rep. 2008 May 23;57[RR-3]:1–28).
[6] Oral typhoid vaccine is recommended to be administered 1 hour before a meal with a cold or lukewarm drink (temperature not to exceed body temperature—98.6°F [37°C]) on alternate days, for a total of 4 doses.
[7] Yellow fever vaccine may be administered to children aged <9 months in certain situations (CDC. Yellow fever vaccine: recommendations of the Advisory Committee on Immunization Practices [ACIP]. MMWR Recomm Rep. 2010 Jul 30;59[RR-7]:1–27.).

in an inpatient or outpatient medical setting. Vaccine administration should be supervised by a health care provider who is able to recognize and manage severe allergic reactions. A previous severe allergic reaction to any vaccine, regardless of the component suspected of being responsible for the reaction, is a contraindication to future receipt of the vaccine.

Some vaccines contain a preservative or trace amounts of antibiotics to which people might be allergic. Providers administering the vaccines should carefully review the prescribing information before deciding if the rare person with such an allergy should receive the vaccine. No recommended vaccine contains penicillin or penicillin derivatives.

Some vaccines (MMR vaccine, inactivated polio vaccine [IPV], hepatitis A vaccine, some hepatitis B vaccines, some influenza vaccines, rabies vaccine, varicella vaccine, and smallpox vaccine) contain trace amounts of neomycin or other antibiotics; the amount is less than would normally be used for the skin test to determine hypersensitivity. However, people who have experienced anaphylactic reactions to this antibiotic generally should not receive these vaccines. Most often, neomycin allergy is a contact dermatitis— a manifestation of a delayed-type (cell-mediated) immune response rather than anaphylaxis. A history of delayed-type reactions to neomycin is not a contraindication to receiving these vaccines.

Thimerosal, an organic mercurial compound in use since the 1930s, has been added to certain immunobiologic products as a preservative. Thimerosal is present at preservative concentrations in multidose vials of some brands of vaccine. Receiving thimerosal-containing vaccines has been postulated to lead to induction of allergy. However, there is limited scientific evidence for this assertion. Allergy to thimerosal usually consists of local delayed-type hypersensitivity reactions. Thimerosal elicits positive delayed-type hypersensitivity patch tests in 1%–18% of people tested, but these tests have limited or no clinical relevance. Most people do not experience reactions to thimerosal administered as a component of vaccines, even when patch or intradermal tests for thimerosal indicate hypersensitivity. A localized or delayed-type hypersensitivity reaction to thimerosal is not a contraindication to receipt of a vaccine that contains thimerosal.

Since mid-2001, vaccines routinely recommended for infants have been manufactured without thimerosal as a preservative. Vaccines that still contain thimerosal as a preservative include some influenza vaccines, DT, and 1 Td vaccine. Additional information about thimerosal and the thimerosal content of vaccines is available on the FDA website (www.fda.gov/cber/vaccine/thimerosal.htm).

## REPORTING ADVERSE EVENTS AFTER IMMUNIZATION

Modern vaccines are extremely safe and effective. Benefits and risks are associated with the use of all immunobiologics—no vaccine is completely effective or completely safe for all recipients. Adverse events after immunization have been reported with all vaccines, ranging from frequent, minor, local reactions to extremely rare, severe, systemic illness, such as that associated with yellow fever vaccine. Adverse events following specific vaccines and toxoids are discussed in detail in each ACIP statement. In the United States, clinicians are required by law to report selected adverse events occurring after vaccination with any vaccine in the recommended childhood series. In addition, CDC strongly recommends that all vaccine adverse events be reported to the Vaccine Adverse Event Reporting System (VAERS), even if a causal relation to vaccination is not certain. VAERS reporting forms and information are available electronically at www.vaers.hhs.gov, or they may be requested by telephone: 800-822-7967 (toll-free). Clinicians are encouraged to report electronically at https://vaers.hhs.gov/esub/step1.

## INJECTION ROUTE AND INJECTION SITE

Injectable vaccines are administered by intramuscular, intradermal, and subcutaneous routes. The method of administration of injectable vaccines depends in part on the presence of an adjuvant in some vaccines. The term *adjuvant* refers to a vaccine component distinct from the antigen, which enhances the immune response to the antigen. Vaccines containing an adjuvant (DTaP, DT, HPV, RZV, Td, Tdap, pneumococcal conjugate, Hib, hepatitis A, hepatitis B) should be injected into a muscle mass, because administration subcutaneously or intradermally can cause local irritation, induration, skin discoloration, inflammation, and granuloma formation. Detailed discussion and recommendations about vaccination of people with bleeding disorders or receiving anticoagulant therapy are available in the ACIP general best practices guidelines for immunization.

Routes of administration are recommended by the manufacturer for each immunobiologic. Deviation from the recommended route of administration may reduce vaccine efficacy or increase local adverse reactions. Detailed recommendations on the route and site for all vaccines have been published in ACIP recommendations; a compiled list of these publications is available on the CDC website at www.cdc.gov/vaccines/hcp/acip-recs (also see Appendix B).

BIBLIOGRAPHY

1. CDC. Human rabies prevention—United States, 2008: recommendations of the Advisory Committee on Immunization Practices. MMWR Recomm Rep. 2008 May 23;57(RR-3):1–28.

2. CDC. Updated recommendations for use of tetanus toxoid, reduced diphtheria toxoid, and acellular pertussis (Tdap) vaccine in adults aged 65 years and older—Advisory Committee on Immunization Practices

(ACIP), 2012. MMWR Morb Mortal Wkly Rep. 2012 Jun 29;61(25):468–70.

3. Cohn AC, MacNeil JR, Clark TA, Ortega-Sanchez IR, Briere EZ, Meissner HC, et al. Prevention and control of meningococcal disease: recommendations of the Advisory Committee on Immunization Practices (ACIP). MMWR Recomm Rep. 2013 Mar 22;62(2):1–28.

4. Grohskopf LA, Sokolow LZ, Broder KR, et al. Prevention and control of seasonal influenza with vaccines: recommendations of the Advisory Committee on Immunization Practices— United States, 2017–2018 influenza season. MMWR Recomm Rep. 2017;66(RR-2):1–22.

5. Kobayashi M, Bennett NM, Gierke R, Almendares O, Moore MR, Whitney CG, et al. Intervals between PCV13 and PPSV23 vaccines: recommendations of the Advisory Committee on Immunization Practices (ACIP). MMWR Morb Mortal Wkly Rep. 2015 Sep 4;64(64):944–7.

6. Kroger AT, Duchin J, Vázquez M. General best practice guidelines for immunization. Best practices guidance of the Advisory Committee on Immunization Practices

(ACIP). Atlanta, GA: CDC [cited 2018 Jan 18]. Available from: www.cdc.gov/vaccines/hcp/acip-recs/general-recs/downloads/general-recs.pdf.

7. McLean HQ, Fiebelkorn AP, Temte JL, Wallace GS, CDC. Prevention of measles, rubella, congenital rubella syndrome, and mumps, 2013: summary recommendations of the Advisory Committee on Immunization Practices (ACIP). MMWR Recomm Rep. 2013 Jun 14;62(RR-04):1–34.

8. Neunert C, Lim W, Crowther M, Cohen A, Solberg L, Crowther MA. The American Society of Hematology 2011 evidence-based practice guideline for immune thrombocytopenia. Blood. 2011;117(16):4190–207.

9. Shimabukuro TT, Nguyen M, Martin D, DeStefano F. Safety monitoring in the Vaccine Adverse Event Reporting System (VAERS). Vaccine. 2015 Aug 26;33(36):4398–405.

10. Staples JE, Gershman M, Fischer M, CDC. Yellow fever vaccine: recommendations of the Advisory Committee on Immunization Practices (ACIP). MMWR Recomm Rep. 2010 Jul 30;59(RR-7):1–27.

**2**

# INTERACTIONS BETWEEN TRAVEL VACCINES & DRUGS

Ilan Youngster, Elizabeth D. Barnett

Potential interactions between vaccines and medications, including those already taken by the traveler, must be considered during pretravel consultations. The importance of this topic is highlighted by a study identifying potential drug–drug interactions with travel-related medications in 45% of travelers using chronic medications, and 3.5% of interactions are potentially serious. Interactions of commonly used travel-related vaccines and medications are discussed here.

## INTERACTIONS BETWEEN VACCINES

Concomitant administration of multiple vaccines, including live attenuated vaccines, generally is safe and effective. However, the spacing between the administration of some vaccines that are not given at the same time needs consideration.

A single study suggested that in adults, concomitant administration of the 13-valent pneumococcal conjugate vaccine (PCV13) with

the trivalent inactivated influenza vaccine results in lower immunogenicity to the PCV13 components. The clinical significance of this observation is uncertain, as responses still met FDA criteria of noninferiority. Infants given PCV13 and inactivated influenza vaccine concomitantly had a slightly increased risk of fever and febrile seizure, but this risk must be weighed against the need for both vaccines before travel and the time available to separate them.

Administering a live-virus vaccine within 4 weeks after administration of another live-virus vaccine can decrease immunogenicity to the second administered vaccine; therefore, live-virus vaccines should be administered the same day or ≥4 weeks apart. If the 4-week span is not achievable, the second vaccine may be administered sooner to afford some protection, but should be readministered ≥4 weeks later if the traveler is at continued risk. A study examining concurrent administration of the yellow fever vaccine with the measles-mumps-rubella (MMR) vaccine in 12-month-old children showed slightly reduced immunogenicity to yellow fever and mumps components, compared with responses following separate vaccination with MMR and yellow fever vaccines 30 days apart. (See "Simultaneous Administration" in Chapter 4, Yellow Fever.) Similarly, risk for varicella vaccine failure among people who received varicella vaccine within 28 days of MMR vaccination was 3-fold higher than among people who received varicella vaccine >28 days after MMR vaccination.

Concerns about spacing between doses of live vaccines not given at the same visit applies only to live injectable or intranasal vaccines, so live oral cholera vaccine (CVD 103-HgR, Vaxchora, PaxVax) may be administered simultaneously or at any interval before or after administration of most other vaccines. One exception to this rule is the Ty21a oral typhoid vaccine. Oral cholera vaccine should be administered before Ty21a vaccine, and 8 hours should separate the cholera vaccine and the first dose of Ty21a.

## INTERACTIONS BETWEEN TRAVEL VACCINES AND DRUGS

### Live Attenuated Oral Typhoid and Cholera Vaccines

Live attenuated vaccines generally should be avoided in immunocompromised travelers, including those taking immunomodulators, calcineurin inhibitors, cytotoxic agents, antimetabolites, and high-dose steroids (see Table 5-2).

Antimicrobial agents may be active against the vaccine strains in the oral typhoid and cholera vaccines and may prevent adequate immune response to these vaccines. Vaccination with oral typhoid vaccine should be delayed for >72 hours and with oral cholera vaccine for >14 days after administration of antimicrobial agents. Parenteral typhoid vaccine is an alternative to oral vaccine, but there is no parenteral cholera vaccine currently available, and no killed oral cholera vaccines are licensed in the United States.

Chloroquine and atovaquone-proguanil at doses used for malaria chemoprophylaxis may be given concurrently with oral typhoid vaccine. Data from an older formulation of the CVD 103-HgR oral cholera vaccine suggest that the immune response to the vaccine may be diminished when it is given concomitantly with chloroquine. Live attenuated oral cholera vaccine should be given at least 10 days before beginning antimalarial prophylaxis with chloroquine. A study in children using oral cholera vaccine suggested no decrease in immunogenicity when given with atovaquone-proguanil.

### Rabies Vaccine

Concomitant use of chloroquine may reduce the antibody response to intradermal rabies vaccine administered for preexposure vaccination. The intramuscular route should be used for people taking chloroquine concurrently. (Currently, intradermal administration of rabies vaccine is not approved in the United States.)

## INTERACTIONS BETWEEN ANTIMALARIALS AND SELECTED OTHER DRUGS

This section describes some of the more commonly encountered drug interactions. Any time a new medication is prescribed, clinicians should check for any interactions and inform the traveler of the potential risk.

### Mefloquine

Mefloquine may interact with several categories of drugs, including other antimalarial drugs, drugs that alter cardiac conduction, and anticonvulsants. Mefloquine is associated with increased toxicities of the antimalarial drug lumefantrine (available in the United States in fixed combination to treat people with uncomplicated *Plasmodium falciparum* malaria), potentially causing fatal prolongation of the QTc interval. Lumefantrine should therefore be avoided or used with caution in patients taking mefloquine prophylaxis. Although no conclusive data are available with regard to coadministration of mefloquine and other drugs that may affect cardiac conduction, mefloquine should be used with caution or avoided in patients taking antiarrhythmic or β-blocking agents, calcium-channel blockers, antihistamines, H$_1$-blocking agents, tricyclic antidepressants, selective serotonin reuptake inhibitors (SSRIs), or phenothiazines. Mefloquine may also lower plasma levels of a number of anticonvulsants, such as valproic acid, carbamazepine, phenobarbital, and phenytoin; concurrent use of mefloquine with these agents should be avoided. In general, mefloquine should be avoided in travelers with a history of seizures, mood disorders, or psychiatric disease. Mefloquine can also lead to increased levels of calcineurin inhibitors and mTOR inhibitors (tacrolimus, cyclosporine A, and sirolimus). Potent CYP3A4 inhibitors such as macrolides (azithromycin, clarithromycin, erythromycin), azole antifungals (ketoconazole, voriconazole, posaconazole and itraconazole), SSRIs (fluoxetine, sertraline, fluvoxamine), antiretroviral protease inhibitors (ritonavir, lopinavir, darunavir, atazanavir, saquinavir), and cobicistat (available in a combination with elvitegravir) may increase levels of mefloquine, increasing the risk for QT prolongation. CYP3A4 inducers such as efavirenz, nevirapine, etravirine, rifampin, rifabutin, St John's wort, and glucocorticoids may reduce plasma concentrations of mefloquine, and concurrent use should be avoided. Concurrent use of mefloquine with the direct-acting protease inhibitors boceprevir and telaprevir used to treat hepatitis C should also be avoided. The newer direct-acting protease inhibitors (grazoprevir, paritaprevir, simeprevir) are believed to be associated with fewer drug–drug interactions, but as safety data are lacking, alternatives to mefloquine should be considered pending additional data.

## Chloroquine

Chloroquine may increase risk of prolonged QTc interval when given with other QT-prolonging agents (such as sotalol, amiodarone, and lumefantrine), and the combination should be avoided. The antiretroviral rilpivirine has also been shown to prolong QTc, and coadministration should be avoided. Chloroquine inhibits CYP2D6; when given concomitantly with substrates of this enzyme (such as metoprolol, propranolol, fluoxetine, paroxetine, flecainide), increased monitoring for side effects may be warranted. Chloroquine absorption may be reduced by antacids or kaolin; ≥4 hours should elapse between doses of these medications. Concomitant use of cimetidine and chloroquine should be avoided, as cimetidine can inhibit the metabolism of chloroquine and may increase drug levels. CYP3A4 inhibitors such as ritonavir, ketoconazole, and erythromycin may also increase chloroquine levels, and concomitant use should be avoided. Chloroquine inhibits bioavailability of ampicillin, and 2 hours should elapse between doses. Chloroquine is also reported to decrease the bioavailability of ciprofloxacin and methotrexate. Chloroquine may increase digoxin levels; increased digoxin monitoring is warranted. Use of chloroquine could possibly also lead to increased levels of calcineurin inhibitors and should be used with caution.

## Atovaquone-Proguanil

Tetracycline, rifampin, and rifabutin may reduce plasma concentrations of atovaquone and should not be used concurrently with atovaquone-proguanil. Metoclopramide may reduce bioavailability of atovaquone; unless no other antiemetics are available, this antiemetic should not be used to treat the vomiting that may accompany use of atovaquone at treatment doses. Atovaquone-proguanil should not be used with other medications that contain proguanil. Patients on warfarin may need to reduce their anticoagulant dose or monitor their prothrombin time more closely while taking atovaquone-proguanil, although coadministration of these drugs is not contraindicated. The use of novel oral anticoagulants (dabigatran, rivaroxaban and apixaban) is not expected to cause significant interactions, and their use has been suggested as an alternative in patients in need of anticoagulation. Atovaquone-proguanil may interact with the antiretroviral protease inhibitors ritonavir, darunavir, atazanavir, indinavir, and lopinavir, in addition to the nonnucleoside reverse transcriptase inhibitors nevirapine, etravirine, and efavirenz, resulting in decreased levels of atovaquone-proguanil. Despite the potential for interactions, atovaquone-proguanil is well tolerated in most patients receiving these antivirals and is the preferred antimalarial for short-term travel. Cimetidine and fluvoxamine interfere with the metabolism of proguanil and should therefore be avoided.

## Doxycycline

Phenytoin, carbamazepine, and barbiturates may decrease the half-life of doxycycline. Patients on anticoagulants may need to reduce their anticoagulant dose while taking doxycycline because of its ability to depress plasma prothrombin activity. Absorption of tetracyclines may be impaired by bismuth subsalicylate, preparations containing iron, and antacids containing calcium, magnesium, or aluminum; these preparations should not be taken within 3 hours of taking doxycycline. Doxycycline may interfere with the bactericidal activity of penicillin, so in general, these drugs should not be taken together. Doxycycline has no known interaction with antiretroviral agents, but concurrent use may lead to increased levels of calcineurin inhibitors and mTOR inhibitors (sirolimus).

## INTERACTIONS WITH DRUGS USED TO TREAT TRAVELERS' DIARRHEA

### Azithromycin

Close monitoring for side effects of azithromycin is recommended when azithromycin is used with nelfinavir. Increased anticoagulant effects have been noted when azithromycin is used with warfarin; monitoring prothrombin time is recommended for people taking these drugs concomitantly. Additive QTc prolongation may occur when azithromycin is used with the antimalarial artemether, and concomitant therapy should be avoided. Drug interactions have been reported with macrolides and antiretroviral protease inhibitors, as well as efavirenz and nevirapine, and can increase risk of QTc prolongation, though a short treatment course is not contraindicated for those without an underlying cardiac abnormality. Concurrent use with macrolides may lead to increased levels of calcineurin inhibitors.

### Fluoroquinolones

Increase in the international normalized ratio (INR) has been reported when levofloxacin and warfarin are used concurrently. Concurrent administration of ciprofloxacin and antacids that contain magnesium or aluminum hydroxide may reduce bioavailability of ciprofloxacin. Ciprofloxacin decreases clearance of theophylline and caffeine; theophylline levels should be monitored when ciprofloxacin is used concurrently. Ciprofloxacin and other fluoroquinolones should not be used with tizanidine. Sildenafil should not be used in patients on ciprofloxacin, as concomitant use is associated with increased rates of adverse effects. Fluoroquinolones have no known interaction with antiretroviral agents, but concurrent use may increase levels of calcineurin inhibitors and fluoroquinolone levels, and use should reflect renal function.

### Rifaximin

Rifaximin is not absorbed in appreciable amounts by intact bowel, and no clinically significant drug interactions have been reported to date with rifaximin except for minor changes in INR when used concurrently with warfarin.

#### RIFAMYCIN SV

No clinical drug interactions have been studied. Because of minimal systemic rifamycin concentrations observed after the recommended dose, clinically relevant drug interactions are not expected.

## INTERACTIONS WITH DRUGS USED FOR TRAVEL TO HIGH ALTITUDES

### Acetazolamide

Acetazolamide produces alkaline urine that can increase the rate of excretion of barbiturates and salicylates and may potentiate salicylate toxicity, particularly if taking a high dose of aspirin. Decreased excretion of dextroamphetamine, anticholinergics, mecamylamine, ephedrine, mexiletine, or quinidine may also occur. Hypokalemia caused by corticosteroids may be potentiated by concurrent use of acetazolamide. Acetazolamide should not be given to patients taking the anticonvulsant topiramate, as concurrent use is associated with increased toxicity. Increased monitoring of cyclosporine, tacrolimus, and sirolimus is warranted if these drugs are given with acetazolamide. Concurrent administration of metformin and acetazolamide should be done with caution, as there may be an additive risk for lactic acidosis. Acetaminophen and diclofenac sodium form complex bonds with acetazolamide in the stomach's acidic environment, impairing absorption. These agents should not be taken within 30 minutes of acetazolamide.

## Dexamethasone

Dexamethasone interacts with multiple classes of drugs. Using this drug to treat altitude illness may, however, be lifesaving. Interactions may occur with dexamethasone and the following drugs and drug classes: macrolide antibiotics, anticholinesterases, anticoagulants, hypoglycemic agents, isoniazid, digitalis preparations, oral contraceptives, and phenytoin.

## DRUG INTERACTIONS IN PATIENTS ON HIV MEDICATIONS

Patients with HIV can be a challenge in the pretravel consultation (See Chapter 5, Immuno-compromised Travelers). A study in Europe showed that as many as 29% of HIV-positive travelers do not disclose their disease and medication status when seeking pretravel advice. Antiretroviral medications have multiple drug interactions, especially through activation or inhibition of CYP3A4 and CYP2D6. There are several

reports of antimalarial treatment failure and prophylaxis failure in patients on protease inhibitors and both nucleoside and nonnucleoside reverse transcriptase inhibitors, whereas entry and integrase inhibitors are not a common cause of drug–drug interactions with commonly administered travel-related medications. A number of the potential interactions are listed above, and 2 excellent resources for HIV medication interactions can be found at www.hiv-druginteractions.org and at www.aidsinfo.nih.gov. Preexposure prophylaxis with emtricitabine/tenofovir is not a contraindication for any of the commonly used travel-related medications.

## INTERACTIONS WITH HERBAL OR NUTRITIONAL SUPPLEMENTS

As many as 30% of travelers take herbal or nutritional supplements, and many consider them to be of no clinical relevance and will not disclose their use unless specifically asked during the pretravel consultation. Special attention should be given to supplements that activate or inhibit CYP2D6 or CYP3A4 like ginseng, hypericum, St. John's wort, and grapefruit extract. Coadministration with medications that are substrates of CYP2D6 or 3A4 should be avoided (chloroquine, mefloquine, macrolides).

## BIBLIOGRAPHY

1. Frenck RW Jr, Gurtman A, Rubino J, Smith W, van Cleeff M, Jayawardene D, et al. Randomized, controlled trial of a 13-valent pneumococcal conjugate vaccine administered concomitantly with an influenza vaccine in healthy adults. Clin Vaccine Immunol. 2012 Aug;19(8):1296–303.

2. Jabeen E, Qureshi R, Shah A. Interaction of antihypertensive acetazolamide with nonsteroidal anti-inflammatory drugs. J Photochem Photobiol B. 2013 Aug 5;125:155–63.

3. Kollaritsch H, Que JU, Kunz C, Wiedermann G, Herzog C, Cryz SJ Jr. Safety and immunogenicity of live oral cholera and typhoid vaccines administered alone or in combination with antimalarial drugs, oral polio vaccine, or yellow fever vaccine. J Infect Dis. 1997 Apr;175(4):871–5.

4. Nascimento Silva JR, Camacho LA, Siqueira MM, Freire Mde S, Castro YP, Maia Mde L, et al. Mutual interference on the immune response to yellow fever vaccine and a combined vaccine against measles, mumps and rubella. Vaccine. 2011 Aug 26;29(37):6327–34.

5. Nielsen US, Jensen-Fangel S, Pedersen G, Lohse N, Pedersen C, Kronborg G, et al. Travelling with HIV: a cross sectional analysis of Danish HIV-infected patients. Travel Med Infect Dis. 2014 Jan–Feb;12(1):72–8.

6. Ridtitid W, Wongnawa M, Mahatthanatrakul W, Raungsri N, Sunbhanich M. Ketoconazole increases plasma concentrations of antimalarial mefloquine in healthy human volunteers. J Clin Pharm Ther. 2005 Jun;30(3):285–90.

7. Sbaih N, Buss B, Goyal D, Rao SR, Benefield R, Walker AT, et al. Potentially serious drug interactions resulting from the pre-travel health encounter. Open Forum Infect Dis. 2018 Oct 22;5(11):ofy266.

8. Stienlauf S, Meltzer E, Kurnik D, Leshem E, Kopel E, Streltsin B, et al. Potential drug interactions in travelers with chronic illnesses: a large retrospective cohort study. Travel Med Infect Dis. 2014 Sep–Oct;12(5):499–504.

# YELLOW FEVER VACCINE & MALARIA PROPHYLAXIS INFORMATION, BY COUNTRY

Mark D. Gershman, Emily S. Jentes, Rhett J. Stoney (Yellow Fever)
Kathrine R. Tan, Paul M. Arguin (Malaria)

The following pages present country-specific information on yellow fever (YF) vaccine requirements and recommendations (Table 2-6) and malaria transmission information and prophylaxis recommendations. Country-specific maps of malaria transmission areas, country-specific maps depicting yellow fever vaccine recommendations, and a reference map of China are included to aid in interpreting the information. The information was accurate at the time of publication; however, this information is subject to change at any time as a result of changes in disease transmission or, in the case of YF, changing country entry requirements. Updated information reflecting changes since publication can be found in the online version of this book (www.cdc.gov/yellowbook) and on the CDC Travelers' Health website (www.cdc.gov/travel). General recommendations for other vaccines to consider during the pretravel consultation can be found on the CDC Travelers' Health website (www.cdc.gov/travel).

## YELLOW FEVER

Since publication of the 2018 edition of the CDC Yellow Book, large YF outbreaks occurred in eastern Brazil in 2017 and 2018, involving states where YF was not previously considered endemic. Notably, human YF cases occurred within the greater metropolitan area of São Paulo City and not far from the metropolitan limits of Rio de Janeiro City. In response, the Brazil Ministry of Health conducted mass vaccination campaigns in the newly affected areas. Based on a review of the situation by the World Health Organization (WHO) Scientific and Technical Advisory Group on Geographical Yellow Fever Risk Mapping, in which CDC participates, preliminary expanded YF vaccination recommendations were made for international

## Table 2-6. Categories of recommendations for yellow fever (YF) vaccination

| YF VACCINATION CATEGORY | RATIONALE FOR RECOMMENDATION |
| --- | --- |
| Recommended | Vaccination recommended for all travelers ≥9 months of age to areas with endemic or transitional YF risk, as determined by persistent or periodic YF virus transmission. |
| Generally not recommended | Vaccination generally not recommended in areas where the potential for YF virus exposure is low, as determined by absence of reports of human YF and past evidence suggestive of only low levels of YF virus transmission. However, vaccination might be considered for a small subset of travelers who are at increased risk for exposure to YF virus because of prolonged travel, heavy exposure to mosquitoes, or inability to avoid mosquito bites. |
| Not recommended | Vaccination not recommended in areas where there is no risk of YF virus transmission, as determined by absence of past or present evidence of YF virus circulation in the area or environmental conditions not conducive to YF virus transmission. |

travelers to the eastern and southeastern states of Brazil. Given that the Brazil Ministry of Health has initiated its plan to vaccinate the entire population of Brazil against YF by mid-2019, these preliminary vaccination recommendations for international travel will likely be made permanent by the advisory group.

Revaccination against yellow fever was previously required by certain countries at 10-year intervals to comply with International Health Regulations (IHR). In 2014, the World Health Assembly (of WHO) adopted the recommendation to amend the IHR by removing the 10-year booster dose requirement, and stipulated a 2-year transition period for this change. Consequently, as of July 11, 2016, a completed International Certificate of Vaccination or Prophylaxis (ICVP) is valid for the lifetime of the vaccinee. Moreover, countries cannot require proof of revaccination (booster) against yellow fever as a condition of entry, even if the last vaccination was >10 years prior.

In the United States, the Advisory Committee on Immunization Practices (ACIP) published a new recommendation in 2015 that 1 dose of yellow fever vaccine provides long-lasting protection and is adequate for most travelers. The recommendation also identifies specific groups of travelers who should receive additional doses and others for whom additional doses may be considered. For details, see Chapter 4, Yellow Fever. For the most up-to-date information about yellow fever vaccine boosters, consult the CDC Travelers' Health website or the specific publication posted on the ACIP website (www.cdc.gov/mmwr/pdf/wk/mm6423.pdf).

Ultimately, the clinician's decision whether or not to vaccinate any traveler must take into account the traveler's risk of being infected with YF virus, country entry requirements, and individual risk factors for serious adverse events after YF vaccination (such as age and immune status). For a thorough discussion of YF and guidance for vaccination, see Chapter 4, Yellow Fever.

NOTE: Despite the recent changes to the IHR regarding YF vaccine boosters, it is uncertain whether all countries with YF vaccination entry requirements will fully adopt this change. Even if countries modify their official policies to extend the validity period of the ICVP from 10 years to the lifetime of the vaccinee, there is no guarantee that all national border officials will be aware of such policy change or be able to enforce it. CDC obtains information yearly from WHO about official country entry requirements. WHO likely will not be asking countries about YF vaccine booster entry requirements in the yearly questionnaires, because it will be assumed that countries are complying with the amended IHR. This could leave a gap in the foreseeable future in accurate published information about entry requirements for YF vaccine boosters for certain countries. Past experience has demonstrated that information given by consulates and embassies about vaccination requirements is often not accurate. Therefore, providers and travelers should not rely solely on such information when determining current YF vaccination entry requirements for specific destinations. With the caveats described above, readers should refer to the online version of this book (www.cdc.gov/yellowbook) and the CDC Travelers' Health website (www.cdc.gov/travel) for any reported updates to country entry requirements since publication of this edition.

## MALARIA

The following recommendations to protect travelers from malaria were developed by using the best available data from multiple sources. Countries are not required to submit malaria surveillance data to CDC. On an ongoing basis, CDC actively solicits data from multiple sources, including WHO (main and regional offices); national malaria control programs; international organizations, such as the International Society of Travel Medicine; CDC overseas staff; US military; academic, research, and aid organizations; and published records from the medical literature. The reliability and accuracy of those data are also assessed. If the information is available, trends in malaria incidence and other data are considered in the context of malaria control activities within a given country or other mitigating factors such as natural disasters, wars, and other events that may affect the ability to control malaria or accurately count and report it. Factors such as the volume of travel to that country and the number of acquired cases reported in the US surveillance system are also examined. Based on all those considerations, recommendations are developed to try to accurately describe areas of the country where transmission occurs, substantial occurrences of antimalarial drug resistance, the proportions of species present, and the recommended prophylaxis options.

These recommendations should be used in conjunction with an individual risk assessment, taking into account not only the destination country but also the detailed itinerary including specific cities, types of accommodation, season, and style of travel, as well as special health conditions such as pregnancy.

Several medications are available for malaria prophylaxis. When deciding which drug to use, clinicians should consider the specific itinerary, length of trip, drug costs, previous adverse reactions to antimalarials, drug allergies, and medical history.

For a thorough discussion of malaria and guidance for prophylaxis, see Chapter 4, Malaria.

# COUNTRY-SPECIFIC INFORMATION

## AFGHANISTAN

**YELLOW FEVER**

**Requirements:** Required if traveling from a country with risk of YF virus transmission and ≥9 months of age.[1]
**Recommendations:** None

MALARIA

**Areas with malaria:** April–December in all areas <2,500 m (8,202 ft).
**Drug resistance**[3]: Chloroquine.
**Malaria species:** *P. vivax* 95%, *P. falciparum* 5%.
**Recommended chemoprophylaxis:** Atovaquone-proguanil, doxycycline, mefloquine, or tafenoquine.[4]

## ALBANIA

**YELLOW FEVER**

**Requirements:** Required if traveling from a country with risk of YF virus transmission and ≥1 year of age.[1]
**Recommendations:** None

MALARIA
No malaria transmission.

## ALGERIA

**YELLOW FEVER**

**Requirements:** Required if traveling from a country with risk of YF virus transmission and ≥1 year of age, including transit >12 hours in an airport located in a country with risk of YF virus transmission.[1]
**Recommendations:** None

MALARIA
No malaria transmission.

## AMERICAN SAMOA (US)

**YELLOW FEVER**

**Requirements:** None
**Recommendations:** None

MALARIA
No malaria transmission.

## ANDORRA

**YELLOW FEVER**

**Requirements:** None
**Recommendations:** None

MALARIA
No malaria transmission.

## ANGOLA

**YELLOW FEVER**

**Requirements:** Required for arriving travelers from all countries if traveler is ≥9 months of age.

**Recommendations:** *Recommended* for all travelers ≥9 months of age.

MALARIA

**Areas with malaria:** All.
**Drug resistance**[3]: Chloroquine.
**Malaria species:** *P. falciparum* 90%, *P. ovale* 5%, *P. vivax* 5%.
**Recommended chemoprophylaxis:** Atovaquone-proguanil, doxycycline, mefloquine, or tafenoquine.[4]

## ANGUILLA (UK)

**YELLOW FEVER**

**Requirements:** None
**Recommendations:** None

MALARIA
No malaria transmission.

## ANTARCTICA

**YELLOW FEVER**

**Requirements:** None
**Recommendations:** None

MALARIA
No malaria transmission.

## ANTIGUA AND BARBUDA

**YELLOW FEVER**

**Requirements:** Required if traveling from a country with risk of YF virus transmission and ≥1 year of age.[1]
**Recommendations:** None

MALARIA
No malaria transmission.

## ARGENTINA

**YELLOW FEVER**

**Requirements:** None
**Recommendations:**
*Recommended* for travelers ≥9 months of age going to Corrientes and Misiones Provinces.
*Generally not recommended* for travelers going to Formosa Province and designated areas of Chaco, Jujuy, and Salta Provinces (Map 2-1).
*Not recommended* for all travelers whose itineraries are limited to areas and provinces not listed above.

MALARIA
No malaria transmission.

## ARMENIA

**YELLOW FEVER**

**Requirements:** None
**Recommendations:** None

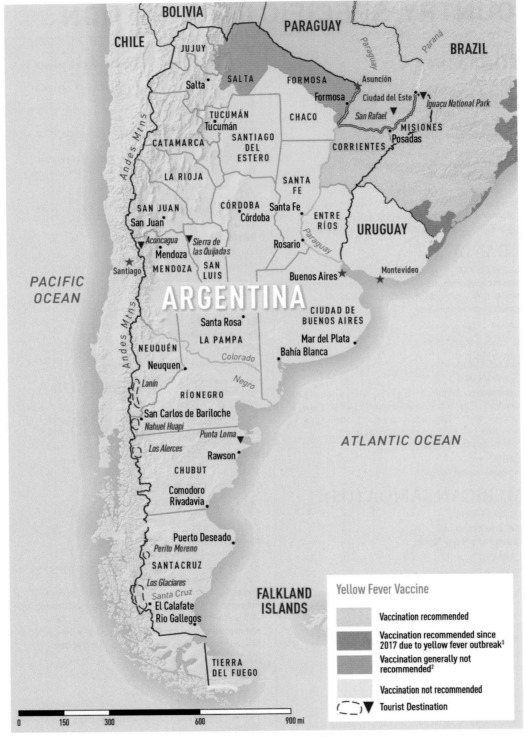

**MAP 2-1.** Yellow fever vaccine recommendations in Argentina[1]

[1,2,3] See footnotes on page 101

Within the map:

BOLIVIA

PARAGUAY

CHILE

JUJUY

Salta

SALTA

FORMOSA

Asunción

BRAZIL

Formosa

Ciudad del Este

Iguaçu National Park

TUCUMÁN

CHACO

San Rafael

MISIONES

Tucumán

Posadas

CATAMARCA

SANTIAGO DEL ESTERO

CORRIENTES

LA RIOJA

SANTA FE

SAN JUAN

CÓRDOBA

Santa Fe

San Juan

Córdoba

ENTRE RÍOS

Aconcagua

Sierra de las Quijadas

URUGUAY

Mendoza

Rosario

MENDOZA

SAN LUIS

Buenos Aires

Montevideo

PACIFIC OCEAN

Santiago

ARGENTINA

CIUDAD DE BUENOS AIRES

Santa Rosa

LA PAMPA

Mar del Plata

NEUQUÉN

Colorado

Bahía Blanca

Neuquen

Negro

Lanín

RÍONEGRO

San Carlos de Bariloche

Nahuel Huapi

Punta Loma

ATLANTIC OCEAN

Los Alerces

Rawson

CHUBUT

Comodoro Rivadavia

Puerto Deseado

Perito Moreno

SANTACRUZ

Los Glaciares

FALKLAND ISLANDS

Santa Cruz

El Calafate

Rio Gallegos

Andes Mtns

Paraná

Paraguay

TIERRA DEL FUEGO

**Yellow Fever Vaccine**

Vaccination recommended

Vaccination recommended since 2017 due to yellow fever outbreak[3]

Vaccination generally not recommended[2]

Vaccination not recommended

Tourist Destination

0    150    300    600    900 mi

**MALARIA**
No malaria transmission.

# ARUBA

**YELLOW FEVER**

**Requirements:** Required if traveling from a country with risk of YF virus transmission and ≥9 months of age, including transit >12 hours in an airport located in a country with risk of YF virus transmission.[1]
**Recommendations:** None

**MALARIA**
No malaria transmission.

# AUSTRALIA

**YELLOW FEVER**

**Requirements:** Required if traveling from a country with risk of YF virus transmission and ≥1 year of age, including transit >12 hours in an airport located in a country with risk of YF virus transmission. This requirement excludes Galápagos Islands in Ecuador and the island of Tobago; it is limited to Misiones Province in Argentina.
**Recommendations:** None

**MALARIA**
No malaria transmission.

# AUSTRIA

**YELLOW FEVER**
**Requirements:** None
**Recommendations:** None

**MALARIA**
No malaria transmission.

# AZERBAIJAN

**YELLOW FEVER**
**Requirements:** None
**Recommendations:** None

**MALARIA**
No malaria transmission.

# AZORES (PORTUGAL)

**YELLOW FEVER**
**Requirements:** None
**Recommendations:** None

**MALARIA**
No malaria transmission.

# BAHAMAS, THE

**YELLOW FEVER**

**Requirements:** Required if traveling from a country with risk of YF virus transmission and ≥1 year of age, including transit >12 hours in an airport located in a country with risk of YF virus transmission.[1]
**Recommendations:** None

**MALARIA**
No malaria transmission.

# BAHRAIN

**YELLOW FEVER**

**Requirements:** Required if traveling from a country with risk of YF virus transmission and ≥9 months of age, including transit >12 hours in an airport located in a country with risk of YF virus transmission.[1]
**Recommendations:** None

**MALARIA**
No malaria transmission.

# BANGLADESH

**YELLOW FEVER**

**Requirements:** Required if traveling from a country with risk of YF virus transmission and ≥1 year of age.[1]
**Recommendations:** None

**MALARIA**

**Areas with malaria:** All areas, except in the city of Dhaka.
**Drug resistance**[3]: Chloroquine.
**Malaria species:** *P. falciparum* 90%, *P. vivax* 10%, and *P. malariae* rare.
**Recommended chemoprophylaxis:** Atovaquone-proguanil, doxycycline, mefloquine, or tafenoquine.[4]

# BARBADOS

**YELLOW FEVER**

**Requirements:** Required if traveling from a country with risk of YF virus transmission and ≥1 year of age.[1] This requirement excludes Guyana and the island of Trinidad.
**Recommendations:** None

**MALARIA**
No malaria transmission.

# BELARUS

**YELLOW FEVER**
**Requirements:** None
**Recommendations:** None

**MALARIA**
No malaria transmission.

# BELGIUM

**YELLOW FEVER**
**Requirements:** None
**Recommendations:** None

**MALARIA**
No malaria transmission.

# BELIZE

**YELLOW FEVER**

**Requirements:** Required if traveling from a country with risk of YF virus transmission and ≥1 year of age, including transit in an airport located in a country with risk of YF virus transmission.[1]

**Recommendations:** None

### MALARIA

**Areas with malaria:** Rare locally transmitted cases. None in Belize City and islands frequented by tourists, such as Ambergris Caye.

**Drug resistance[3]:** None.

**Malaria species:** *P. vivax* 100%.

**Recommended chemoprophylaxis:** None (practice mosquito avoidance).

# BENIN

### YELLOW FEVER

**Requirements:** Required if traveling from a country with risk of YF virus transmission and ≥1 year of age, including transit in an airport located in a country with risk of YF virus transmission.[1]

**Recommendations:** *Recommended* for all travelers ≥9 months of age.

### MALARIA

**Areas with malaria:** All.

**Drug resistance[3]:** Chloroquine.

**Malaria species:** *P. falciparum* >85%, *P. ovale* 5%–10%, *P. vivax* rare.

**Recommended chemoprophylaxis:** Atovaquone-proguanil, doxycycline, mefloquine, or tafenoquine.[4]

# BERMUDA (UK)

### YELLOW FEVER

**Requirements:** None

**Recommendations:** None

### MALARIA

No malaria transmission.

# BHUTAN

### YELLOW FEVER

**Requirements:** Required if traveling from a country with risk of YF virus transmission, including transit in an airport located in a country with risk of YF virus transmission.[1]

**Recommendations:** None

### MALARIA

**Areas with malaria:** Rare cases in rural areas <1,700 m (5,577 ft) in districts along the southern border shared with India. Rare seasonal cases May–September in Ha, Lhuentse, Monggar, Punakha, Trashigang, Trongsa, Tsirang, Yangtse, and Wangdue. None in districts of Bumthang, Gaza, Paro, and Thimphu.

**Drug resistance[3]:** Chloroquine.

**Malaria species:** *P. falciparum* 70%, *P. vivax* 30%.

**Recommended chemoprophylaxis:** None (practice mosquito avoidance).

# BOLIVIA

### YELLOW FEVER

**Requirements:** Required if traveling from a country with risk of YF virus transmission and ≥1 year of age.[1]

**Recommendations:**

*Recommended* for all travelers ≥9 months of age traveling to the following areas <2,300 m (7,546 ft) in elevation and east of the Andes Mountains: the entire departments of Beni, Pando, Santa Cruz, and designated areas (Map 2-2) of Chuquisaca, Cochabamba, La Paz, and Tarija departments.

*Not recommended* for travelers whose itineraries are limited to areas >2,300 m (7,546 ft) in elevation and all areas not listed above, including the cities of La Paz and Sucre.

### MALARIA

**Areas with malaria:** All areas <2,500 m (8,202 ft). None in the city of La Paz (Map 2-3).

**Drug resistance[3]:** Chloroquine.

**Malaria species:** *P. vivax* 93%, *P. falciparum* 7%.

**Recommended chemoprophylaxis:** Atovaquone-proguanil, doxycycline, mefloquine, primaquine[4], or tafenoquine.[4]

# BONAIRE

### YELLOW FEVER

**Requirements:** Required if traveling from a country with risk of YF virus transmission and ≥9 months of age, including transit >12 hours in an airport located in a country with risk of YF virus transmission.[1]

**Recommendations:** None

### MALARIA

No malaria transmission.

# BOSNIA AND HERZEGOVINA

### YELLOW FEVER

**Requirements:** None

**Recommendations:** None

### MALARIA

No malaria transmission.

# BOTSWANA

### YELLOW FEVER

**Requirements:** Required if traveling from or having passed through a country with risk of YF virus transmission and ≥1 year of age, including transit in an airport located in a country with risk of YF virus transmission.[1]

**Recommendations:** None

### MALARIA

**Areas with malaria:** Present in the following subdistricts: Botete, Chobe (including Chobe National Park), Ngami, Okavango, and Tuteme. Also present in

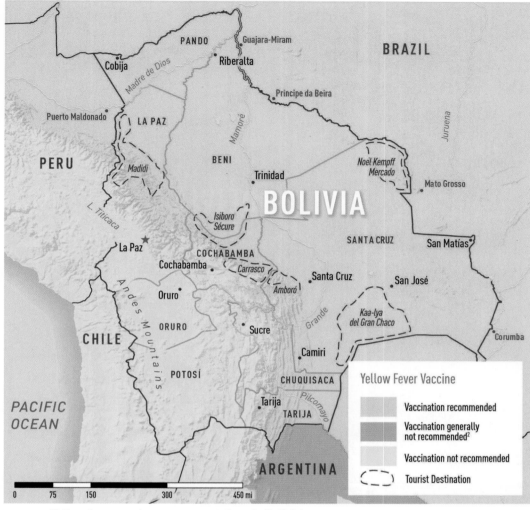

**MAP 2-2.** Yellow fever vaccine recommendations in Bolivia[1]

[1,2] See footnotes on page 101

the following districts: Bobirwa, Northeast (including Francistown), Ghanzi, Mahalapaye, and Serowe Palapye. Rare cases in the districts of Kgalagadi North, Keneng West, and Southern. None in the city of Gaborone (Map 2-4).

**Drug resistance**[3]: Chloroquine.

**Malaria species:** *P. falciparum* 90%, *P. vivax* 5%, *P. ovale* 5%.

**Recommended chemoprophylaxis:** Subdistricts of Botete, Chobe (including Chobe National Park), Ngami, Okavango, and Tuteme and districts or Bobirwa, Northeast (including Francistown), Ghanzi, Mahalapaye, and Serowe Palapye: Atovaquone-proguanil, doxycycline, mefloquine, or tafenoquine.[4] Areas with rare cases: None (practice mosquito avoidance).

# BRAZIL

**YELLOW FEVER**

**Requirements:** None

**Recommendations:**

***Recommended*** for all travelers ≥9 months of age going to the following areas: the entire states of Acre, Amapá, Amazonas, Distrito Federal (including the capital city of Brasília), Espirito Santo,* Goiás, Maranhão, Mato Grosso, Mato Grosso do Sul, Minas Gerais, Pará, Paraná,* Rio de Janeiro (including the city of Rio de Janeiro and all coastal islands),* Rio Grande do Sul,* Rondonia, Roraima, Santa Catarina,* São Paulo (including the city of São Paulo and all coastal islands),* and Tocantins and designated

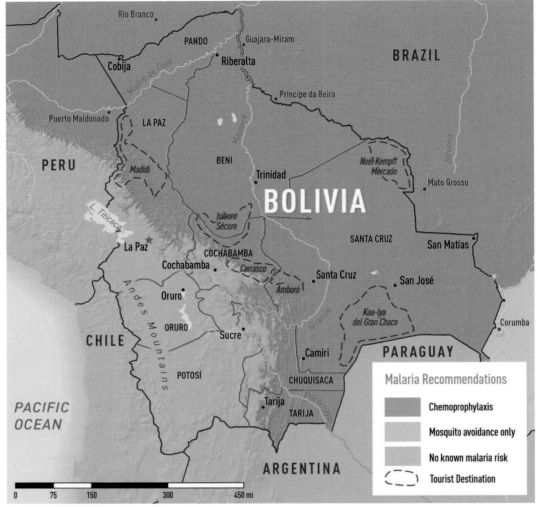

MAP 2-3. Malaria in Bolivia

areas (Map 2-5) of the following states: Bahia* and Piauí. Vaccination is also recommended for travelers visiting Iguaçu Falls.

***Not recommended*** for travelers whose itineraries are limited to areas not listed above, including the cities of Fortaleza and Recife (Map 2-5).

***Note:** In 2017, CDC expanded YF vaccination recommendations for travelers to Brazil in response to a large YF outbreak in multiple eastern states. A list of areas in Bahia state for which vaccination is now recommended can be found at www.who.int/ith/ith-country-list.pdf. The expanded YF vaccination recommendations for these states are preliminary. For updates, refer to the CDC Travelers' Health website at www.cdc.gov/travel.

## MALARIA

**Areas with malaria:** All areas of the states of Acre, Amapá, Amazonas, Rondonia, and Roraima. Also present in the states of Maranhão, Mato Grosso, and Para, but rare cases in their capital cities. Rare cases in the rural areas of the states of Espirito Santo, Goiás, Mato Grosso do Sul, Piauí, and Tocantins. Rare cases in the rural forested areas of the states of Rio de Janeiro and São Paolo. No malaria in the cities of Brasilia, Rio de Janeiro, São Paolo, and none at Iguaçu Falls (Map 2-6).

**Drug resistance**[3]: Chloroquine.

**Malaria species:** *P. vivax* 85%, *P. falciparum* 15%.

**Recommended chemoprophylaxis:** States of Acre, Amapá, Amazonas, Rondonia, and Roraima. States of

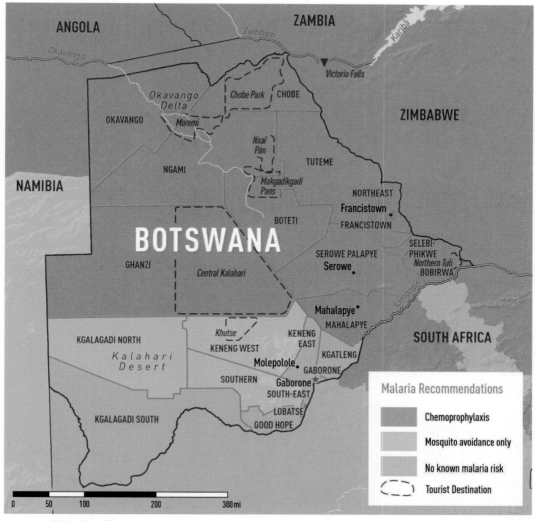

MAP 2-4. Malaria in Botswana

Maranhão, Mato Grosso, and Para (but not their capital cities): Atovaquone-proguanil, doxycycline, mefloquine, or tafenoquine.[4] Areas with rare cases: None (practice mosquito avoidance).

# BRITISH INDIAN OCEAN TERRITORY; INCLUDES DIEGO GARCIA (UK)

## YELLOW FEVER
**Requirements:** None
**Recommendations:** None

## MALARIA
No malaria transmission.

# BRUNEI

## YELLOW FEVER
**Requirements:** Required if traveling from a country with risk of YF virus transmission and ≥9 months of age, including transit >12 hours in an airport located in a country with risk of YF virus transmission.[1]
**Recommendations:** None

## MALARIA
No malaria transmission.

# BULGARIA

## YELLOW FEVER
**Requirements:** None
**Recommendations:** None

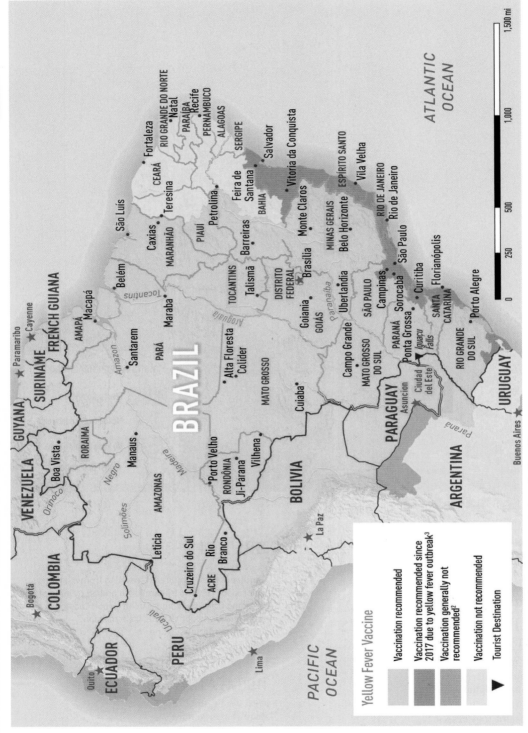

**MAP 2-5. Yellow fever vaccine recommendations in Brazil[1]**

[1,2,3] See footnotes on page 101

Yellow Fever Vaccine

- Vaccination recommended
- Vaccination recommended since 2017 due to yellow fever outbreak[3]
- Vaccination generally not recommended[2]
- Vaccination not recommended
- ▶ Tourist Destination

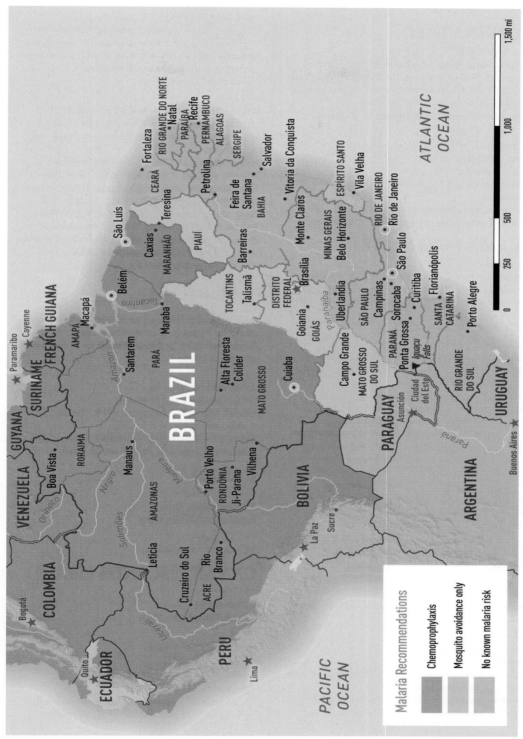

MAP 2-6. Malaria in Brazil

**Malaria Recommendations**

- Chemoprophylaxis
- Mosquito avoidance only
- No known malaria risk

**MALARIA**
No malaria transmission.

# BURKINA FASO

**YELLOW FEVER**

**Requirements:** Required if traveling from a country with risk of YF virus transmission and ≥9 months of age, including transit in an airport located in a country with risk of YF virus transmission.

**Recommendations:** *Recommended* for all travelers ≥9 months of age.

**MALARIA**

**Areas with malaria:** All.

**Drug resistance**[3]: Chloroquine.

**Malaria species:** *P. falciparum* >80%, *P. ovale* 5%–10%, *P. vivax* rare.

**Recommended chemoprophylaxis:** Atovaquone-proguanil, doxycycline, mefloquine, or tafenoquine.[4]

# BURMA (MYANMAR)

**YELLOW FEVER**

**Requirements:** Required if traveling from a country with risk of YF virus transmission and ≥1 year of age, including transit >12 hours in an airport located in a country with risk of YF virus transmission.[1]

**Recommendations:** None

**MALARIA**

**Areas with malaria:** Present at altitudes <1,000 m (3,281 ft), including Bagan. Rare transmission above 1,000 m (3,281 ft) (Map 2-7).

**Drug resistance**[3]: Chloroquine and mefloquine.

**Malaria species:** *P. falciparum* 60%, *P. vivax* 35%, *P. malariae, P. ovale,* and *P. knowlesi* rare.

**Recommended chemoprophylaxis:** In the provinces of Bago, Kachin, Kayah, Kayin, Shan, and Tanintharyi <1,000 m (3,281 ft): Atovaquone-proguanil, doxycycline, or tafenoquine.[4]

All other areas <1,000 m (3,281 ft): Atovaquone-proguanil, doxycycline, mefloquine, or tafenoquine.[4]

Above 1,000 m (3,281 ft): None (practice mosquito avoidance).

# BURUNDI

**YELLOW FEVER**

**Requirements:** Required for arriving travelers from all countries if traveler is ≥9 months of age.

**Recommendations:** *Recommended* for all travelers ≥9 months of age.

**MALARIA**

**Areas with malaria:** All.

**Drug resistance**[3]: Chloroquine.

**Malaria species:** *P. falciparum* 86%, *P. malariae, P. ovale,* and *P. vivax* 14% combined.

**Recommended chemoprophylaxis:** Atovaquone-proguanil, doxycycline, mefloquine, or tafenoquine.[4]

# CAMBODIA

**YELLOW FEVER**

**Requirements:** Required if traveling from a country with risk of YF virus transmission and ≥1 year of age, including transit >12 hours in an airport located in a country with risk of YF virus transmission.[1]

**Recommendations:** None

**MALARIA**

**Areas with malaria:** Present throughout the country, including Siem Reap city. None in the city of Phnom Penh and at the temple complex at Angkor Wat.

**Drug resistance**[3]: Chloroquine and mefloquine.

**Malaria species:** *P. falciparum* 60%, *P. vivax* 40%.

**Recommended chemoprophylaxis:** In the provinces of Banteay Meanchey, Battambang, Kampot, Koh Kong, Odder Meanchey, Pailin, Preah Vihear, Pursat, and Siem Reap bordering Thailand: Atovaquone-proguanil, doxycycline, or tafenoquine.[4] All other areas with malaria: Atovaquone-proguanil, doxycycline, mefloquine, or tafenoquine.[4]

# CAMEROON

**YELLOW FEVER**

**Requirements:** Required for arriving travelers from all countries if traveler is ≥9 months of age.

**Recommendations:** *Recommended* for all travelers ≥9 months of age.

**MALARIA**

**Areas with malaria:** All.

**Drug resistance**[3]: Chloroquine.

**Malaria species:** *P. falciparum* >85%, *P. ovale* 5%–10%, *P. vivax* rare.

**Recommended chemoprophylaxis:** Atovaquone-proguanil, doxycycline, mefloquine, or tafenoquine.[4]

# CANADA

**YELLOW FEVER**

**Requirements:** None

**Recommendations:** None

**MALARIA**
No malaria transmission.

# CANARY ISLANDS (SPAIN)

**YELLOW FEVER**

**Requirements:** None

**Recommendations:** None

**MALARIA**
No malaria transmission.

# CAPE VERDE

**YELLOW FEVER**

**Requirements:** Required if traveling from a country with risk of YF virus transmission and ≥1 year of age,

2

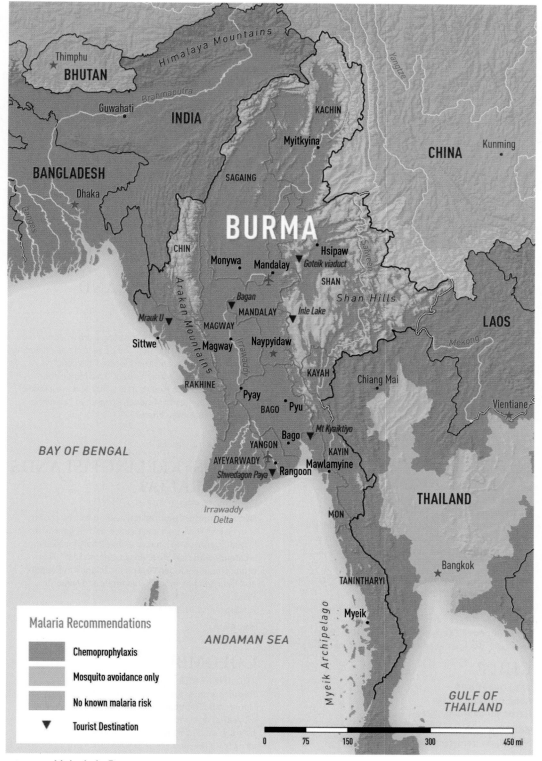

MAP 2-7. **Malaria in Burma**

including transit >12 hours in an airport located in a country with risk of YF virus transmission.[1]

**Recommendations:** None

#### MALARIA

**Areas with malaria:** Rare cases in São Tiago Island.
**Drug resistance[3]:** Chloroquine.
**Malaria species:** Primarily *P. falciparum*.
**Recommended chemoprophylaxis:** None (practice mosquito avoidance).

# CAYMAN ISLANDS (UK)

### YELLOW FEVER

**Requirements:** None
**Recommendations:** None

#### MALARIA

No malaria transmission.

# CENTRAL AFRICAN REPUBLIC

### YELLOW FEVER

**Requirements:** Required for arriving travelers from all countries if traveler is ≥9 months of age.
**Recommendations:** *Recommended* for all travelers ≥9 months of age.

#### MALARIA

**Areas with malaria:** All.
**Drug resistance[3]:** Chloroquine.
**Malaria species:** *P. falciparum* 85%, *P. malariae, P. ovale,* and *P. vivax* 15% combined.
**Recommended chemoprophylaxis:** Atovaquone-proguanil, doxycycline, mefloquine, or tafenoquine.[4]

# CHAD

### YELLOW FEVER

**Requirements:** Required for arriving travelers from all countries if traveler is ≥9 months of age.
**Recommendations:**
*Recommended* for all travelers ≥9 months of age traveling to areas south of the Sahara Desert (Map 4-13).
*Not recommended* for travelers whose itineraries are limited to areas in the Sahara Desert (Map 4-13).

#### MALARIA

**Areas with malaria:** All.
**Drug resistance[3]:** Chloroquine.
**Malaria species:** *P. falciparum* 85%, *P. malariae, P. ovale,* and *P. vivax* 15% combined.
**Recommended chemoprophylaxis:** Atovaquone-proguanil, doxycycline, mefloquine, or tafenoquine.[4]

# CHILE

### YELLOW FEVER

**Requirements:** None
**Recommendations:** None

#### MALARIA

No malaria transmission.

# CHINA *(Map 2-8)*

### YELLOW FEVER

**Requirements:** Required if traveling from a country with risk of YF virus transmission and ≥9 months of age, including transit >12 hours in an airport located in a country with risk of YF virus transmission.[1] This requirement does not apply to travelers whose itineraries are limited to Hong Kong Special Administrative Region (SAR) and Macao SAR.
**Recommendations:** None

#### MALARIA

**Areas with malaria:** Rare cases in the counties along the China-Burma (Myanmar) border in Yunnan Province and Motuo County in Tibet. No malaria in areas where most major river cruises pass.
**Drug resistance[3]:** Chloroquine and mefloquine.
**Malaria species:** Primarily *P. vivax; P. falciparum* in Yunnan Province.
**Recommended chemoprophylaxis:** None (practice mosquito avoidance).

# CHRISTMAS ISLAND (AUSTRALIA)

### YELLOW FEVER

**Requirements:** Required if traveling from a country with risk of YF virus transmission and ≥1 year of age, including transit >12 hours in an airport located in a country with risk of YF virus transmission.[1] This requirement excludes Galápagos Islands in Ecuador and the island of Tobago; it is limited to Misiones Province in Argentina.
**Recommendations:** None

#### MALARIA

No malaria transmission.

# COCOS (KEELING) ISLANDS (AUSTRALIA)

### YELLOW FEVER

**Requirements:** Required if traveling from a country with risk of YF virus transmission and ≥1 year of age, including transit >12 hours in an airport located in a country with risk of YF virus transmission.[1] This requirement excludes Galápagos Islands in Ecuador and the island of Tobago; it is limited to Misiones Province in Argentina.
**Recommendations:** None

#### MALARIA

No malaria transmission.

# COLOMBIA

### YELLOW FEVER

**Requirements:** Required if arriving from Angola, Brazil, Democratic Republic of the Congo, or Uganda and ≥1 year of age and for travelers who have transited >12 hours in an airport located in a country with risk of YF virus transmission.[1]

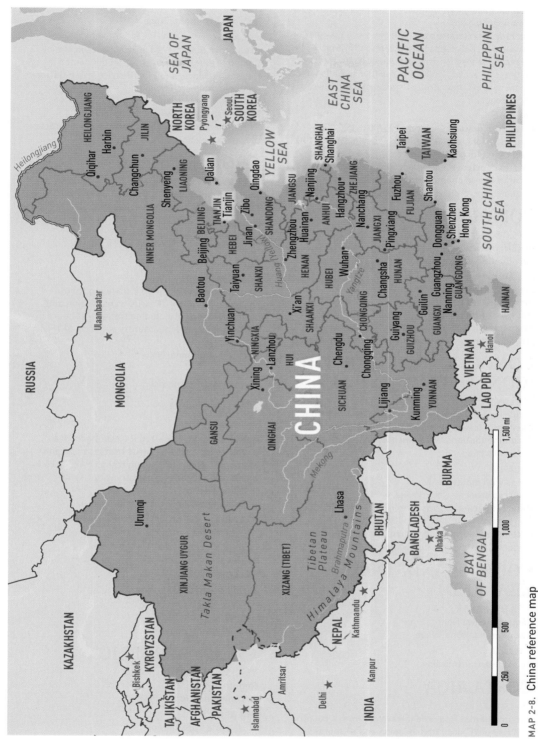

MAP 2-8. China reference map

**Recommendations:**
*Recommended* for all travelers ≥9 months of age except as mentioned below.
*Generally not recommended* for travelers to the cities of Barranquilla, Cali, Cartagena, and Medellín (Map 2-9).
*Not recommended* for travelers whose itineraries are limited to all areas >2,300 m (7,546 ft) in elevation, the department of San Andrés y Providencia, and the capital city of Bogotá.

MALARIA
**Areas with malaria:** All areas <1,700 m (5,577 ft). None in Bogotá, Cartagena, and Medellín. (Map 2-10).
**Drug resistance**[3]: Chloroquine.
**Malaria species:** *P. falciparum* 50%, *P. vivax* 50%.
**Recommended chemoprophylaxis:** Atovaquone-proguanil, doxycycline, mefloquine, or tafenoquine.[4]

# COMOROS

YELLOW FEVER
**Requirements:** None
**Recommendations:** None

MALARIA
**Areas with malaria:** All.
**Drug resistance**[3]: Chloroquine.
**Malaria species:** Primarily *P. falciparum*.
**Recommended chemoprophylaxis:** Atovaquone-proguanil, doxycycline, mefloquine, or tafenoquine.[4]

# CONGO, REPUBLIC OF THE (CONGO-BRAZZAVILLE)

YELLOW FEVER
**Requirements:** Required for arriving travelers from all countries if traveler is ≥9 months of age.
**Recommendations:** *Recommended* for all travelers ≥9 months of age.

MALARIA
**Areas with malaria:** All.
**Drug resistance**[3]: Chloroquine.
**Malaria species:** *P. falciparum* 90%, *P. ovale* 5%–10%, *P. vivax* rare.
**Recommended chemoprophylaxis:** Atovaquone-proguanil, doxycycline, mefloquine, or tafenoquine.[4]

# COOK ISLANDS (NEW ZEALAND)

YELLOW FEVER
**Requirements:** None
**Recommendations:** None

MALARIA
No malaria transmission.

# COSTA RICA

YELLOW FEVER
**Requirements:** Required if traveling from a country with risk of YF virus transmission and ≥9 months of age.[1] This requirement excludes Argentina and Panama.
**Recommendations:** None

MALARIA
**Areas with malaria:** Rare local cases in Matina Canton in Limón Province, Sarapiquí Canton in Heredia Province, and Pital District in San Carlos Canton in Alajuela Province.
**Drug resistance**[3]: None.
**Malaria species:** *P. vivax*.
**Recommended chemoprophylaxis:** None (practice mosquito avoidance).

# CROATIA

YELLOW FEVER
**Requirements:** None
**Recommendations:** None

MALARIA
No malaria transmission.

# CUBA

YELLOW FEVER
**Requirements:** Required if traveling from a country with risk of YF virus transmission and ≥9 months of age, including transit >12 hours in an airport located in a country with risk of YF virus transmission.[1]
**Recommendations:** None

MALARIA
No malaria transmission.

# CURAÇAO

YELLOW FEVER
**Requirements:** Required if traveling from a country with risk of YF virus transmission and ≥9 months of age, including transit >12 hours in an airport located in a country with risk of YF virus transmission.[1]
**Recommendations:** None

MALARIA
No malaria transmission.

# CYPRUS

YELLOW FEVER
**Requirements:** None
**Recommendations:** None

MALARIA
No malaria transmission.

# CZECH REPUBLIC

YELLOW FEVER
**Requirements:** None
**Recommendations:** None

MALARIA
No malaria transmission.

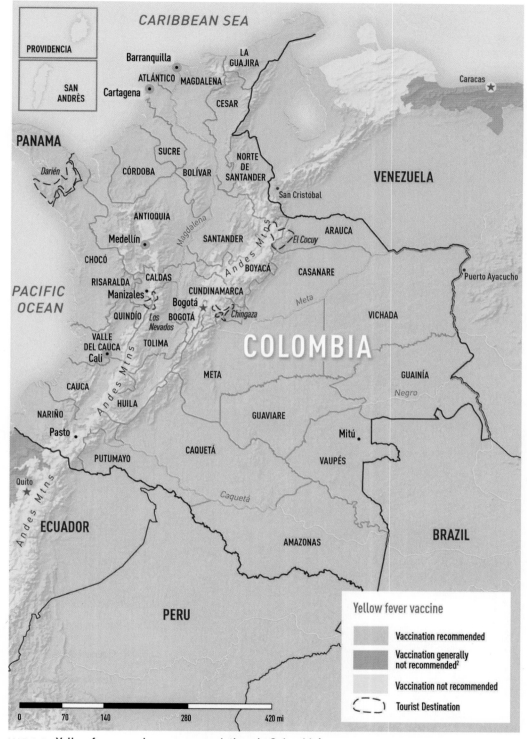

MAP 2-9. **Yellow fever vaccine recommendations in Colombia**[1]

[1,2] See footnotes on page 101

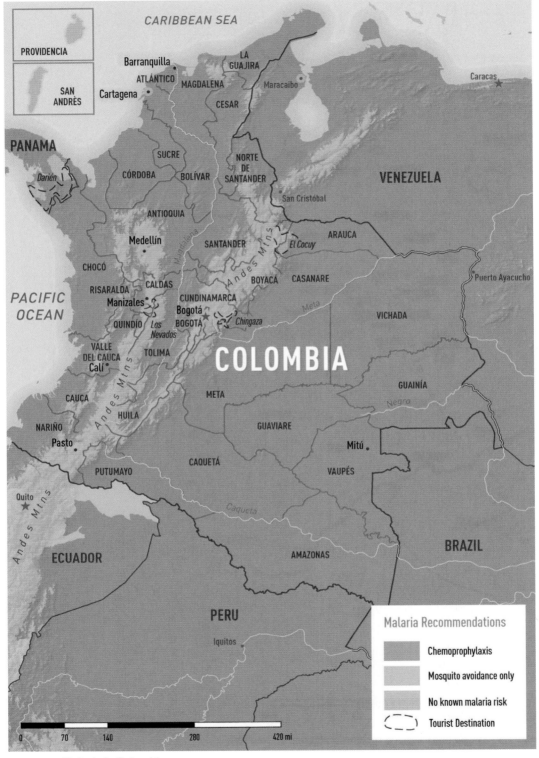

MAP 2-10. **Malaria in Colombia**

## CÔTE D'IVOIRE (IVORY COAST)

**YELLOW FEVER**

**Requirements:** Required for arriving travelers from all countries if traveler is ≥9 months of age.
**Recommendations:** *Recommended* for all travelers ≥9 months of age.

**MALARIA**

**Areas with malaria:** All.
**Drug resistance[3]:** Chloroquine.
**Malaria species:** *P. falciparum* 85%, *P. ovale* 5%–10%, *P. vivax* rare.
**Recommended chemoprophylaxis:** Atovaquone-proguanil, doxycycline, mefloquine, and tafenoquine.[4]

## DEMOCRATIC REPUBLIC OF THE CONGO (CONGO-KINSHASA)

**YELLOW FEVER**

**Requirements:** Required for arriving travelers from all countries if traveler is ≥9 months of age.
**Recommendations:** *Recommended* for all travelers ≥9 months of age

**MALARIA**

**Areas with malaria:** All.
**Drug resistance[3]:** Chloroquine.
**Malaria species:** *P. falciparum* >90%, *P. ovale* 5%, *P. vivax* rare.
**Recommended chemoprophylaxis:** Atovaquone-proguanil, doxycycline, mefloquine, or tafenoquine.[4]

## DENMARK

**YELLOW FEVER**

**Requirements:** None
**Recommendations:** None

**MALARIA**

No malaria transmission.

## DJIBOUTI

**YELLOW FEVER**

**Requirements:** Required if traveling from a country with risk of YF virus transmission and ≥1 year of age, including transit in an airport located in a country with risk of YF virus transmission.[1]
**Recommendations:** None

**MALARIA**

**Areas with malaria:** All.
**Drug resistance[3]:** Chloroquine.
**Malaria species:** *P. falciparum* 90%, *P. vivax* 5%–10%.
**Recommended chemoprophylaxis:** Atovaquone-proguanil, doxycycline, mefloquine, or tafenoquine.[4]

## DOMINICA

**YELLOW FEVER**

**Requirements:** Required if traveling from a country with risk of YF virus transmission and ≥1 year of age, including transit >12 hours in an airport located in a country with risk of YF virus transmission.[1]
**Recommendations:** None

**MALARIA**

No malaria transmission.

## DOMINICAN REPUBLIC

**YELLOW FEVER**

**Requirements:** None
**Recommendations:** None

**MALARIA**

**Areas with malaria:** Primarily in the provinces by the border with Haiti, and the provinces (including resort areas) of Santo Domingo and La Altagracia. Rare locally transmitted cases in the city of Santo Domingo (Distrito Nacional) and other provinces.
**Drug resistance[3]:** None.
**Malaria species:** *P. falciparum* 100%
**Recommended chemoprophylaxis:** Provinces bordering Haiti, and provinces of Santo Domingo (except Santo Domingo city [Distrito Nacional]) and La Altagracia: Atovaquone-proguanil, chloroquine, doxycycline, mefloquine, or tafenoquine.[4] Santo Domingo (Distrito Nacional) city and other provinces: None (practice mosquito avoidance).

## EASTER ISLAND (CHILE)

**YELLOW FEVER**

**Requirements:** This country has not stated its YF vaccination certificate requirements.
**Recommendations:** None

**MALARIA**

No malaria transmission.

## ECUADOR, INCLUDING THE GALÁPAGOS ISLANDS

**YELLOW FEVER**

**Requirements:** Required if traveling from a country with risk of YF virus transmission and ≥1 year of age.[1]
**Recommendations:**
*Recommended* for all travelers ≥9 months of age traveling to areas <2,300 m (7,546 ft) in elevation in the following provinces east of the Andes Mountains: Morona Santiago, Napo, Orellana, Pastaza, Sucumbios, and Zamora-Chinchipe (Map 2-11).
*Generally not recommended* for travelers whose itineraries are limited to areas <2,300 m (7,546 ft) in elevation in the following provinces west of the Andes mountains: Esmeraldas,* Guayas, Los Rios, Santa

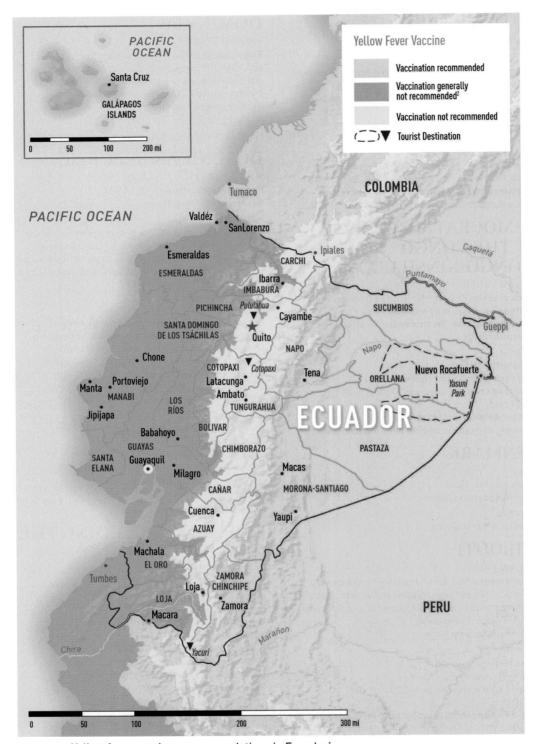

MAP 2-11. **Yellow fever vaccine recommendations in Ecuador**[1]

[1,2] See footnotes on page 101

Elena, Santo Domingo de los Tsachilas, and designated areas of Azuay, Bolivar, Canar, Carchi, Chimborazo, Cotopaxi, El Oro, Imbabura, Loja, Pichincha, and Tungurahua (Map 2-11).

**Not recommended** for travelers whose itineraries are limited to all areas >2,300 m (7,546 ft) in elevation, the cities of Guayaquil and Quito, or the Galápagos Islands (Map 2-11).

*The CDC vaccination recommendation for Esmeraldas Province differs from that published on the WHO International Travel and Health website.

### MALARIA

**Areas with malaria:** Areas at altitudes <1,500 m (4,921 ft) in the provinces of Carchi, Esmeraldas, Morona Santiago, Orellana, and Pastaza. Rare cases in other provinces in areas <1,500 m (4,921 ft). Not present in the cities of Guayaquil and Quito or the Galápagos Islands (Map 2-12).

**Drug resistance**[3]: Chloroquine.

**Malaria species:** *P. vivax* 72%, *P. falciparum* 28%.

**Recommended chemoprophylaxis:** Areas with malaria in Carchi, Esmeraldas, Morona Santiago, Orellana, and Pastaza Provinces: Atovaquone-proguanil, doxycycline, mefloquine, or tafenoquine.[4] Other areas with rare cases of malaria: None (practice mosquito avoidance).

# EGYPT

### YELLOW FEVER

**Requirements:** Required if traveling from a country with risk of YF virus transmission and ≥9 months of age, including transit >12 hours in an airport located in a country with risk of YF virus transmission. This includes Eritrea, Rwanda, Somalia, Tanzania, and Zambia.[1] In the absence of a vaccination certificate, the person will be detained in quarantine for up to 6 days after departure from an area at risk of YF virus transmission.

**Recommendations:** None

### MALARIA

No malaria transmission.

# EL SALVADOR

### YELLOW FEVER

**Requirements:** Required if traveling from a country with risk of YF virus transmission and ≥1 year of age, including transit >12 hours in an airport located in a country with risk of YFV transmission.[1]

**Recommendations:** None

### MALARIA

**Areas with malaria:** Rare cases along Guatemalan border.

**Drug resistance**[3]: None.

**Malaria species:** *P. vivax* 99%, *P. falciparum* <1%.

**Recommended chemoprophylaxis:** None (practice mosquito avoidance).

# EQUATORIAL GUINEA

### YELLOW FEVER

**Requirements:** Required if traveling from a country with risk of YF virus transmission and ≥6 months of age.[1]

**Recommendations:** **Recommended** for all travelers ≥9 months of age.

### MALARIA

**Areas with malaria:** All.

**Drug resistance**[3]: Chloroquine.

**Malaria species:** *P. falciparum* 85%; *P. malariae, P. ovale,* and *P. vivax* 15% combined.

**Recommended chemoprophylaxis:** Atovaquone-proguanil, doxycycline, mefloquine, or tafenoquine.[4]

# ERITREA

### YELLOW FEVER

**Requirements:** Required if traveling from a country with risk of YF virus transmission and ≥9 months of age, including transit >12 hours in an airport located in a country with risk of YF virus transmission.[1]

**Recommendations:**

**Generally not recommended** for travelers going to the following states: Anseba, Debub, Gash Barka, Mae Kel, and Semenawi Keih Bahri.

**Not recommended** for all areas not listed above, including the Dahlak Archipelago (Map 4-13).

### MALARIA

**Areas with malaria:** All areas <2,200 m (7,218 ft). None in Asmara.

**Drug resistance**[3]: Chloroquine.

**Malaria species:** *P. falciparum* 85%, *P. vivax* 10%–15%, *P. ovale* rare.

**Recommended chemoprophylaxis:** Atovaquone-proguanil, doxycycline, mefloquine, or tafenoquine.[4]

# ESTONIA

### YELLOW FEVER

**Requirements:** None

**Recommendations:** None

### MALARIA

No malaria transmission.

# ESWATINI (SWAZILAND)

### YELLOW FEVER

**Requirements:** Required if traveling from a country with risk of YF virus transmission.[1]

**Recommendations:** None

### MALARIA

**Areas with malaria:** Present in eastern areas bordering Mozambique and South Africa, including all of Lubombo district and the eastern half of Hhohho, Manzini, and Shiselweni districts.

**Drug resistance**[3]: Chloroquine.

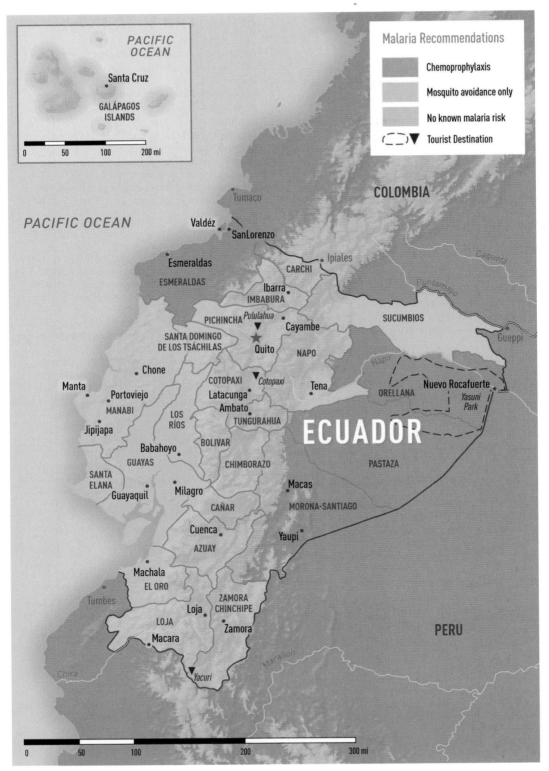

MAP 2-12. Malaria in Ecuador

**Malaria species:** *P. falciparum* 90%, *P. vivax* 5%, *P. ovale* 5%.
**Recommended chemoprophylaxis:** Atovaquone-proguanil, doxycycline, mefloquine, or tafenoquine.[4]

# ETHIOPIA

### YELLOW FEVER

**Requirements:** Required if traveling from a country with risk of YF virus transmission and ≥9 months of age, including transit >12 hours in an airport located in a country with risk of YF virus transmission.[1]
**Recommendations:**
***Recommended*** for all travelers ≥9 months of age, except as mentioned below.
***Generally not recommended*** for travelers whose itinerary is limited to the Afar and Somali Provinces (Map 2-13).

### MALARIA

**Areas with malaria:** All areas below 2,500 m (8,202 ft), except none in the city of Addis Ababa (Map 2-14).
**Drug resistance[3]:** Chloroquine.
**Malaria species:** *P. falciparum* 60%–70%, *P. vivax* 30%–40%, *P. malariae* and *P. ovale* rare.
**Recommended chemoprophylaxis:** Atovaquone-proguanil, doxycycline, mefloquine, or tafenoquine.[4]

# FALKLAND ISLANDS (ISLAS MALVINAS)

### YELLOW FEVER

**Requirements:** None
**Recommendations:** None

### MALARIA

No malaria transmission.

# FAROE ISLANDS (DENMARK)

### YELLOW FEVER

**Requirements:** None
**Recommendations:** None

### MALARIA

No malaria transmission.

# FIJI

### YELLOW FEVER

**Requirements:** Required if traveling from a country with risk of YF virus transmission and ≥1 year of age, including transit >12 hours in an airport located in a country with risk of YF virus transmission.[1]
**Recommendations:** None

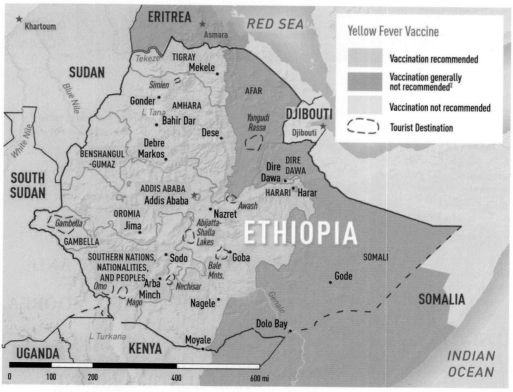

**MAP 2-13. Yellow fever vaccine recommendations in Ethiopia[1]**

[1,2] See footnotes on page 101

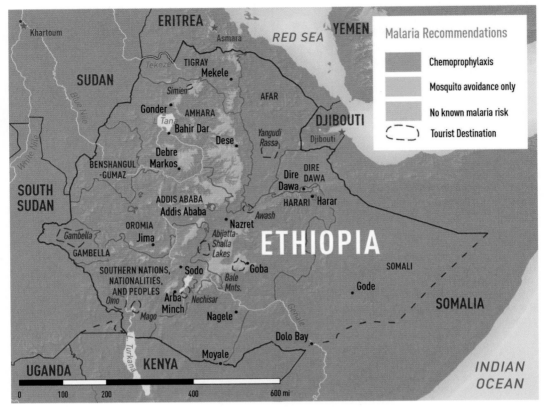

MAP 2-14. Malaria in Ethiopia

MALARIA
No malaria transmission.

# FINLAND

YELLOW FEVER
**Requirements:** None
**Recommendations:** None

MALARIA
No malaria transmission.

# FRANCE

YELLOW FEVER
**Requirements:** None
**Recommendations:** None

MALARIA
No malaria transmission.

# FRENCH GUIANA

YELLOW FEVER
**Requirements:** Required for arriving travelers from all countries if traveler is ≥1 year of age.
**Recommendations:** *Recommended* for all travelers ≥9 months of age.

MALARIA
**Areas with malaria:** All areas, including Matoury, Macouria, and Kourou, except none in coastal areas west of Kourou and Cayenne City.
**Drug resistance**[3]: Chloroquine.
**Malaria species:** *P. vivax* >70%, *P. falciparum* 20%–30%, *P. malariae* rare.
**Recommended chemoprophylaxis:** Atovaquone-proguanil, doxycycline, mefloquine, or tafenoquine.[4]

# FRENCH POLYNESIA, INCLUDING THE ISLAND GROUPS OF SOCIETY ISLANDS (TAHITI, MOOREA, AND BORA-BORA); MARQUESAS ISLANDS (HIVA OA AND UA HUKA); AND AUSTRAL ISLANDS (TUBUAI AND RURUTU)

**YELLOW FEVER**

**Requirements:** Required if traveling from a country with risk of YF virus transmission and ≥1 year of age, including transit >12 hours in an airport located in a country with risk of YF virus transmission.[1]
**Recommendations:** None

**MALARIA**
No malaria transmission.

# GABON

**YELLOW FEVER**

**Requirements:** Required for arriving travelers from all countries if traveler is ≥1 year of age.
**Recommendations:** *Recommended* for all travelers ≥9 months of age.

**MALARIA**
**Areas with malaria:** All.
**Drug resistance**[3]: Chloroquine.
**Malaria species:** *P. falciparum* 90%, *P. malariae*, *P. ovale*, and *P. vivax* 10% combined.
**Recommended chemoprophylaxis:** Atovaquone-proguanil, doxycycline, mefloquine, or tafenoquine.[4]

# GAMBIA, THE

**YELLOW FEVER**

**Requirements:** Required if traveling from a country with risk of YF virus transmission and ≥9 months of age.[1]
**Recommendations:** *Recommended* for all travelers ≥9 months of age.

**MALARIA**
**Areas with malaria:** All.
**Drug resistance**[3]: Chloroquine.
**Malaria species:** *P. falciparum* ≥85%, *P. ovale* 5%–10%, *P. malariae* and *P. vivax* rare.
**Recommended chemoprophylaxis:** Atovaquone-proguanil, doxycycline, mefloquine, or tafenoquine.[4]

# GEORGIA

**YELLOW FEVER**

**Requirements:** None
**Recommendations:** None

**MALARIA**
No malaria transmission.

# GERMANY

**YELLOW FEVER**

**Requirements:** None
**Recommendations:** None

**MALARIA**
No malaria transmission.

# GHANA

**YELLOW FEVER**

**Requirements:** Required for arriving travelers from all countries if traveler is ≥9 months of age.

**Recommendations:** *Recommended* for all travelers ≥9 months of age.

**MALARIA**
**Areas with malaria:** All.
**Drug resistance**[3]: Chloroquine.
**Malaria species:** *P. falciparum* 90%, *P. ovale* 5%–10%, *P. vivax* rare.
**Recommended chemoprophylaxis:** Atovaquone-proguanil, doxycycline, mefloquine, or tafenoquine.[4]

# GIBRALTAR (UK)

**YELLOW FEVER**

**Requirements:** None
**Recommendations:** None

**MALARIA**
No malaria transmission.

# GREECE

**YELLOW FEVER**

**Requirements:** None
**Recommendations:** None

**MALARIA**
**Areas with malaria:** Rare local transmission May–November associated with imported malaria cases, in agricultural areas. None in tourist areas.
**Drug resistance**[3]: Not applicable.
**Malaria species:** *P. vivax* 100%.
**Recommended chemoprophylaxis:** None.

# GREENLAND (DENMARK)

**YELLOW FEVER**

**Requirements:** None
**Recommendations:** None

**MALARIA**
No malaria transmission.

# GRENADA

**YELLOW FEVER**

**Requirements:** Required if traveling from a country with risk of YF virus transmission and ≥1 year of age, including transit >12 hours in an airport located in a country with risk of YF virus transmission.[1]
**Recommendations:** None

**MALARIA**
No malaria transmission.

# GUADELOUPE

**YELLOW FEVER**

**Requirements:** Required if traveling from a country with risk of YF virus transmission and ≥1 year of age, including transit >12 hours in a country with risk of YF virus transmission.[1]
**Recommendations:** None

**MALARIA**
No malaria transmission.

# GUAM (US)

YELLOW FEVER

**Requirements:** None
**Recommendations:** None

MALARIA

No malaria transmission.

# GUATEMALA

YELLOW FEVER

**Requirements:** Required if traveling from a country with risk of YF virus transmission and ≥1 year of age, including transit >12 hours in an airport located in a country with risk of YF virus transmission.[1]
**Recommendations:** None

MALARIA

**Areas with malaria:** Rural areas only at altitudes <1,500 m (4,921 ft). None in Antigua, Guatemala City, or Lake Atitlán.
**Drug resistance[3]:** None.
**Malaria species:** *P. vivax* 97%, *P. falciparum* 3%.
**Recommended chemoprophylaxis:** Escuintla Province: Atovaquone-proguanil, chloroquine, doxycycline, mefloquine, or tafenoquine.[4] All other areas with malaria: Atovaquone-proguanil, chloroquine, doxycycline, mefloquine, primaquine,[4] or tafenoquine.[4]

# GUINEA

YELLOW FEVER

**Requirements:** Required if traveling from a country with risk of YF virus transmission and ≥1 year of age.[1]
**Recommendations:** *Recommended* for all travelers ≥9 months of age.

MALARIA

**Areas with malaria:** All.
**Drug resistance[3]:** Chloroquine.
**Malaria species:** *P. falciparum* >85%, *P. ovale* 5%–10%, *P. vivax* rare.
**Recommended chemoprophylaxis:** Atovaquone-proguanil, doxycycline, mefloquine, or tafenoquine.[4]

# GUINEA-BISSAU

YELLOW FEVER

**Requirements:** Required for arriving travelers from all countries if traveler is ≥1 year of age.
**Recommendations:** *Recommended* for all travelers ≥9 months of age.

MALARIA

**Areas with malaria:** All.
**Drug resistance[3]:** Chloroquine.
**Malaria species:** *P. falciparum* >85%, *P. ovale* 5%–10%, *P. vivax* rare.
**Recommended chemoprophylaxis:** Atovaquone-proguanil, doxycycline, mefloquine, or tafenoquine.[4]

# GUYANA

YELLOW FEVER

**Requirements:** Required if traveling from a country with risk of YF virus transmission and ≥1 year of age, including transit in an airport located in a country with risk of YF virus transmission.[1]
**Recommendations:** *Recommended* for all travelers ≥9 months of age.

MALARIA

**Areas with malaria:** All areas. Rare cases in the cities of Amsterdam and Georgetown.
**Drug resistance[3]:** Chloroquine.
**Malaria species:** *P. falciparum* 50%, *P. vivax* 50%.
**Recommended chemoprophylaxis:** Areas with malaria except cities of Amsterdam and Georgetown: Atovaquone-proguanil, doxycycline, mefloquine, or tafenoquine.[4] Cities of Georgetown and Amsterdam: None (practice mosquito avoidance).

# HAITI

YELLOW FEVER

**Requirements:** Required if traveling from a country with risk of YF virus transmission and ≥1 year of age.[1]
**Recommendations:** None

MALARIA

**Areas with malaria:** All (including Port Labadee).
**Drug resistance[3]:** None.
**Malaria species:** *P. falciparum* 99%, *P. malariae* rare.
**Recommended chemoprophylaxis:** Atovaquone-proguanil, chloroquine, doxycycline, mefloquine, or tafenoquine.[4]

# HONDURAS

YELLOW FEVER

**Requirements:** Required if traveling from a country with risk of YF virus transmission and ≥1 year of age, including transit >12 hours in an airport located in a country with risk of YF virus transmission.[1]
**Recommendations:** None

MALARIA

**Areas with malaria:** Present throughout the country and in Roatán and other Bay Islands. None in San Pedro Sula and Tegucigalpa.
**Drug resistance[3]:** None.
**Malaria species:** *P. vivax* 93%, *P. falciparum* 7%.
**Recommended chemoprophylaxis:** Atovaquone-proguanil, chloroquine, doxycycline, mefloquine, primaquine,[4] or tafenoquine.[4]

# HONG KONG SAR (CHINA)

YELLOW FEVER

**Requirements:** None
**Recommendations:** None

MALARIA

No malaria transmission.

## HUNGARY

**YELLOW FEVER**
**Requirements:** None
**Recommendations:** None

MALARIA
No malaria transmission.

## ICELAND

**YELLOW FEVER**
**Requirements:** None
**Recommendations:** None

MALARIA
No malaria transmission.

## INDIA

**YELLOW FEVER**
**Requirements:** Any traveler (except infants <9 months old) arriving by air or sea without a yellow fever vaccination certificate is detained in isolation for up to 6 days if that person

- arrives within 6 days of departure from an area with risk of YF virus transmission,
- has been in such an area in transit (except those passengers and members of flight crews who, while in transit through an airport in an area with risk of YF virus transmission, remained in the airport during their entire stay and the health officer agrees to such an exemption),
- arrives on a ship that started from or touched at any port in an area with risk of YF virus transmission up to 30 days before its arrival in India, unless such a ship has been disinsected in accordance with the procedure recommended by WHO, or
- arrives on an aircraft that has been in an area with risk of YF virus transmission and has not been disinsected in accordance with the Indian Aircraft Public Health Rules, 1954, or as recommended by WHO.

1) The following are regarded as countries and areas with risk of YF virus transmission:
2) **Africa:** Angola, Benin, Burkina Faso, Burundi, Cameroon, Central African Republic, Chad, Congo, Côte d'Ivoire, Democratic Republic of the Congo, Equatorial Guinea, Ethiopia, Gabon, The Gambia, Ghana, Guinea, Guinea-Bissau, Kenya, Liberia, Mali, Mauritania, Niger, Nigeria, Rwanda, Senegal, Sierra Leone, South Sudan, Sudan, Togo, and Uganda.
3) **Americas:** Argentina, Bolivia, Brazil, Colombia, Ecuador, French Guiana, Guyana, Panama, Paraguay, Peru, Suriname, Trinidad and Tobago (Trinidad only), and Venezuela.
4) **Note:** When a case of yellow fever is reported from any country, that country is regarded by the government of India as a country with risk of YF virus transmission and is added to the above list.

**Recommendations:** None

MALARIA
**Areas with malaria:** All areas throughout the country, including cities of Bombay (Mumbai) and Delhi, except none in areas >2,000 m (6,562 ft) in Himachal Pradesh, Jammu and Kashmir, and Sikkim (Map 2-15).
**Drug resistance[3]:** Chloroquine.
**Malaria species:** *P. vivax* 50%, *P. falciparum* >40%, *P. malariae* and *P. ovale* rare.
**Recommended chemoprophylaxis:** Atovaquone-proguanil, doxycycline, mefloquine, or tafenoquine.[4]

## INDONESIA

**YELLOW FEVER**
**Requirements:** Required if traveling from a country with risk of YF virus transmission and ≥9 months of age.[1]
**Recommendations:** None

MALARIA
**Areas with malaria:** All areas of eastern Indonesia (provinces of Maluku, Maluku Utara, Nusa Tenggara Timur, Papua, and Papua Barat), including the town of Labuan Bajo and Komodo Islands in the Nusa Tenggara region. Rural areas of Kalimantan (Borneo), Nusa Tenggara Barat (includes the island of Lombok), Sulawesi, and Sumatra. Low transmission in rural areas of Java, including Pangandaran, Sukalumi, and Ujung Kulong. None in cities of Jakarta and Ubud, resort areas of Bali and Java, and Gili Islands and the Thousand Islands (Pulau Seribu).
**Drug resistance[3]:** Chloroquine (*P. falciparum* and *P. vivax*).
**Malaria species:** *P. falciparum* 57%, *P. vivax.* 43%, *P. malariae*, *P. knowlesi*, *P. ovale* rare.
**Recommended chemoprophylaxis:** Atovaquone-proguanil, doxycycline, mefloquine, or tafenoquine.[4]

## IRAN

**YELLOW FEVER**
**Requirements:** Required if traveling from a country with risk of YF virus transmission and ≥9 months of age, including transit >12 hours in an airport located in a country with risk of YF virus transmission.[1]
**Recommendations:** None

MALARIA
**Areas with malaria:** March–November in rural areas of Fars Province, Sistan-Baluchestan Province, and southern, tropical parts of Hormozgan and Kerman Provinces.
**Drug resistance[3]:** Chloroquine.
**Malaria species:** *P. vivax* 93%, *P. falciparum* 7%.
**Recommended chemoprophylaxis:** Atovaquone-proguanil, doxycycline, mefloquine, or tafenoquine.[4]

## IRAQ

**YELLOW FEVER**
**Requirements:** Required if traveling from to a country with risk of YF virus transmission and ≥9 months of age,

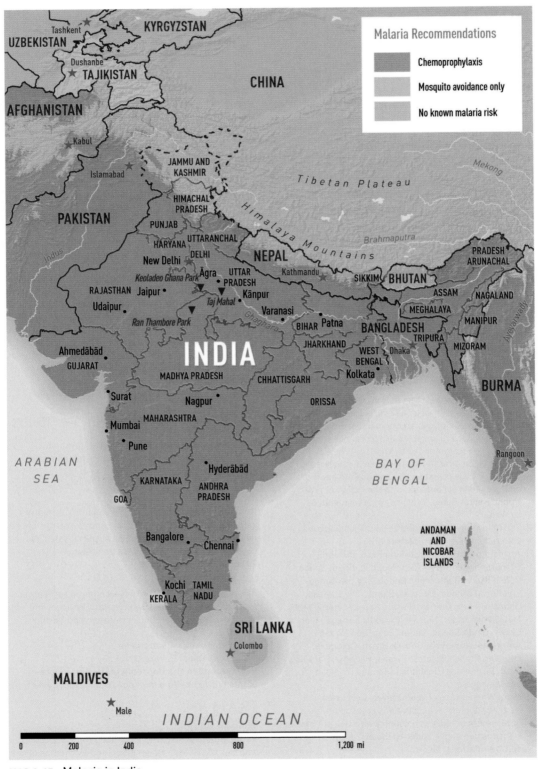

**MAP 2-15. Malaria in India**

including transit >12 hours in an airport located in a country with risk of YF virus transmission.[1]
**Recommendations:** None

MALARIA
No malaria transmission.

# IRELAND

YELLOW FEVER
**Requirements:** None
**Recommendations:** None

MALARIA
No malaria transmission.

# ISRAEL

YELLOW FEVER
**Requirements:** None
**Recommendations:** None

MALARIA
No malaria transmission.

# ITALY INCLUDING HOLY SEE (VATICAN CITY)

YELLOW FEVER
**Requirements:** None
**Recommendations:** None

MALARIA
No malaria transmission.

# JAMAICA

YELLOW FEVER
**Requirements:** Required if traveling from a country with risk of YF virus transmission and ≥1 year of age, including transit >12 hours in an airport located in a country with risk of YF virus transmission.[1]
**Recommendations:** None

MALARIA
No malaria transmission.

# JAPAN

YELLOW FEVER
**Requirements:** None
**Recommendations:** None

MALARIA
No malaria transmission.

# JORDAN

YELLOW FEVER
**Requirements:** Required if traveling from a country with risk of YF virus transmission and ≥1 year of age, including transit >12 hours in an airport located in a country with risk of YF virus transmission.[1]
**Recommendations:** None

MALARIA
No malaria transmission.

# KAZAKHSTAN

YELLOW FEVER
**Requirements:** None
**Recommendations:** None

MALARIA
No malaria transmission.

# KENYA

YELLOW FEVER
**Requirements:** Required if traveling from a country with risk of YF virus transmission and ≥1 year of age.[1]
**Recommendations:**
*Recommended* for all travelers ≥9 months of age, except as mentioned below.
*Generally not recommended* for travelers whose itinerary is limited to the following areas: the entire North Eastern Province; the states of Kilifi, Kwale, Lamu, Malindi, and Tanariver in the Coast Province; and the cities of Mombasa and Nairobi (Map 2-16).

MALARIA
**Areas with malaria:** Present in all areas (including game parks) at altitudes <2,500 m (8,202 ft), including the city of Nairobi (Map 2-17).
**Drug resistance**[3]: Chloroquine.
**Malaria species:** *P. falciparum* >85%, *P. vivax* 5%–10%, *P. ovale* rare.
**Recommended chemoprophylaxis:** Atovaquone-proguanil, doxycycline, mefloquine, or tafenoquine[4]

# KIRIBATI (FORMERLY GILBERT ISLANDS), INCLUDES TARAWA, TABUAERAN (FANNING ISLAND), AND BANABA (OCEAN ISLAND)

YELLOW FEVER
**Requirements:** Required if traveling from a country with risk of YF virus transmission and ≥1 year of age.[1]
**Recommendations:** None

MALARIA
No malaria transmission.

# KOSOVO

YELLOW FEVER
**Requirements:** None
**Recommendations:** None

MALARIA
No malaria transmission.

# KUWAIT

YELLOW FEVER
**Requirements:** None
**Recommendations:** None

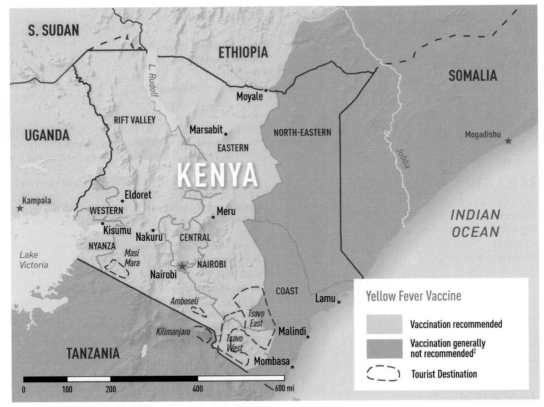

MAP 2-16. Yellow fever vaccine recommendations in Kenya[1]

[1,2] See footnotes on page 101

MALARIA
No malaria transmission.

# KYRGYZSTAN

### YELLOW FEVER
**Requirements:** Required if traveling from a country with risk of YF virus transmission and ≥1 year of age, including transit >12 hours in an airport located in a country with risk of YF virus transmission.[1]
**Recommendations:** None

### MALARIA
No malaria transmission.

# LAOS

### YELLOW FEVER
**Requirements:** Required if traveling from a country with risk of YF virus transmission.[1]
**Recommendations:** None

### MALARIA
**Areas with malaria:** All, except none in the city of Vientiane.
**Drug resistance**[3]: Chloroquine and mefloquine.
**Malaria species:** *P. falciparum* 65%, *P. vivax* 34%, *P. malariae* and *P. ovale* 1% combined.

**Recommended chemoprophylaxis:** Along the Laos-Burma (Myanmar) border in the provinces of Bokeo and Louang Namtha and along the Laos-Thailand border in the province of Champasak and Saravan, along the Laos-Cambodia border, and along the Laos-Vietnam border: Atovaquone-proguanil, doxycycline, or tafenoquine.[4] All other areas with malaria: Atovaquone-proguanil, doxycycline, mefloquine, or tafenoquine.[4]

# LATVIA

### YELLOW FEVER
**Requirements:** None
**Recommendations:** None

### MALARIA
No malaria transmission.

# LEBANON

### YELLOW FEVER
**Requirements:** None
**Recommendations:** None

### MALARIA
No malaria transmission.

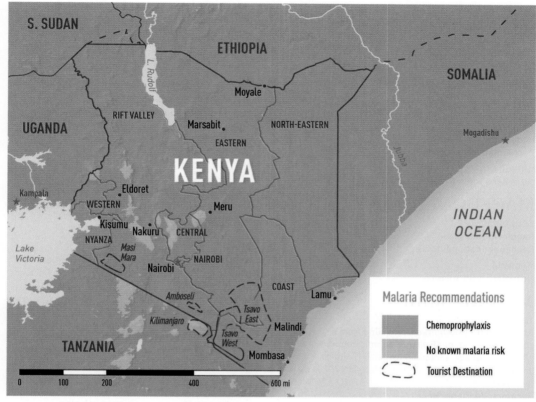

MAP 2-17. Malaria in Kenya

Malaria Recommendations
- Chemoprophylaxis
- No known malaria risk
- Tourist Destination

# LESOTHO

### YELLOW FEVER
**Requirements:** Required if traveling from a country with risk of YF virus transmission and ≥6 months of age, including transit >12 hours in an airport located in a country with risk of YF virus transmission.[1]
**Recommendations:** None

### MALARIA
No malaria transmission.

# LIBERIA

### YELLOW FEVER
**Requirements:** Required if traveling from a country with risk of YFV transmission and ≥9 months of age.[1]
**Recommendations: *Recommended*** for all travelers ≥9 months of age.

### MALARIA
**Areas with malaria:** All.
**Drug resistance**[3]**:** Chloroquine.
**Malaria species:** *P. falciparum* >85%, *P. ovale* 5%–10%, *P. vivax* rare.
**Recommended chemoprophylaxis:** Atovaquone-proguanil, doxycycline, mefloquine, or tafenoquine.[4]

# LIBYA

### YELLOW FEVER
**Requirements:** Required if traveling from a country with risk of YF virus transmission and ≥1 year of age, including transit in an airport located in a country with risk of YF virus transmission.[1]
**Recommendations:** None

### MALARIA
No malaria transmission.

# LIECHTENSTEIN

### YELLOW FEVER
**Requirements:** None
**Recommendations:** None

### MALARIA
No malaria transmission.

# LITHUANIA

### YELLOW FEVER
**Requirements:** None
**Recommendations:** None

### MALARIA
No malaria transmission.

## LUXEMBOURG

**YELLOW FEVER**
**Requirements:** None
**Recommendations:** None

**MALARIA**
No malaria transmission.

## MACAU SAR (CHINA)

**YELLOW FEVER**
**Requirements:** None
**Recommendations:** None

**MALARIA**
No malaria transmission.

## MACEDONIA

**YELLOW FEVER**
**Requirements:** None
**Recommendations:** None

**MALARIA**
No malaria transmission.

## MADAGASCAR

**YELLOW FEVER**
**Requirements:** Required if traveling from a country with risk of YF virus transmission and ≥9 months of age, including transit >12 hours in an airport located in a country with risk of YF virus transmission.[1]
**Recommendations:** None

**MALARIA**
**Areas with malaria:** All areas, except rare cases in the city of Antananarivo.
**Drug resistance**[3]**:** Chloroquine.
**Malaria species:** *P. falciparum* 85%, *P. vivax* 5%–10%, *P. ovale* 5%.
**Recommended chemoprophylaxis:** All areas except the city of Antananarivo: Atovaquone-proguanil, doxycycline, mefloquine, or tafenoquine.[4] Antananarivo: None (practice mosquito avoidance).

## MADEIRA ISLANDS (PORTUGAL)

**YELLOW FEVER**
**Requirements:** None
**Recommendations:** None

**MALARIA**
No malaria transmission.

## MALAWI

**YELLOW FEVER**
**Requirements:** Required if traveling from a country with risk of YF virus transmission and ≥1 year of age, including transit >12 hours in an airport located in a country with risk of YF virus transmission.[1]
**Recommendations:** None

**MALARIA**
**Areas with malaria:** All.
**Drug resistance**[3]**:** Chloroquine.
**Malaria species:** *P. falciparum* 90%; *P. malariae, P. ovale,* and *P. vivax* 10% combined.
**Recommended chemoprophylaxis:** Atovaquone-proguanil, doxycycline, mefloquine, or tafenoquine.[4]

## MALAYSIA

**YELLOW FEVER**
**Requirements:** Required if traveling from a country with risk of YF virus transmission and ≥1 year of age, including transit >12 hours in an airport located in a country with risk of YF virus transmission.[1]
**Recommendations:** None

**MALARIA**
**Areas with malaria:** Present in rural areas. None in Georgetown, Kuala Lumpur, and Penang State (includes Penang Island).
**Drug resistance**[3]**:** Chloroquine.
**Malaria species:** *P. falciparum, P. vivax, P. Knowlesi, P. malariae,* and *P. ovale.*
**Recommended chemoprophylaxis:** Rural areas: Atovaquone-proguanil, doxycycline, mefloquine, or tafenoquine.[4]

## MALDIVES

**YELLOW FEVER**
**Requirements:** Required if traveling from a country with risk of YF virus transmission and ≥1 year of age, including transit >12 hours in an airport located in a country with risk of YF virus transmission.[1]
**Recommendations:** None

**MALARIA**
No malaria transmission.

## MALI

**YELLOW FEVER**
**Requirements:** Required for arriving travelers from all countries if traveler is ≥1 year of age.
**Recommendations:**
***Recommended*** for all travelers ≥9 months of age going to areas south of the Sahara Desert (Map 4-13).
***Not recommended*** for travelers whose itineraries are limited to areas in the Sahara Desert (Map 4-13).

**MALARIA**
**Areas with malaria:** All.
**Drug resistance**[3]**:** Chloroquine.
**Malaria species:** *P. falciparum* >85%, *P. ovale* 5%–10%, *P. vivax* rare.
**Recommended chemoprophylaxis:** Atovaquone-proguanil, doxycycline, mefloquine, or tafenoquine.[4]

## MALTA

**YELLOW FEVER**

**Requirements:** Required if traveling from a country with risk of YF virus transmission and ≥9 months of age, including transit >12 hours in an airport located in a country with risk of YF virus transmission.[1] If indicated on epidemiologic grounds, infants <9 months of age are subject to isolation or surveillance if coming from an area with risk of YF virus transmission.
**Recommendations:** None

MALARIA
No malaria transmission.

## MARSHALL ISLANDS

**YELLOW FEVER**

**Requirements:** None
**Recommendations:** None

MALARIA
No malaria transmission.

## MARTINIQUE (FRANCE)

**YELLOW FEVER**

**Requirements:** Required if traveling from a country with risk of YF virus transmission and ≥1 year of age, including transit >12 hours in an airport located in a country with risk of YF virus transmission.[1]
**Recommendations:** None

MALARIA
No malaria transmission.

## MAURITANIA

**YELLOW FEVER**

**Requirements:** Required if traveling from a country with risk of YF virus transmission and ≥1 year of age.[1]
**Recommendations:**
*Recommended* for all travelers ≥9 months of age traveling to areas south of the Sahara Desert (Map 4-13).
*Not recommended* for travelers whose itineraries are limited to areas in the Sahara Desert (Map 4-13).

MALARIA
**Areas with malaria:** All areas except Dakhlet-Nouadhibou and Tiris-Zemour in the north.
**Drug resistance[3]:** Chloroquine.
**Malaria species:** *P. falciparum* >85%, *P. ovale* 5%–10%, *P. vivax* rare.
**Recommended chemoprophylaxis:** Atovaquone-proguanil, doxycycline, mefloquine, or tafenoquine.[4]

## MAURITIUS

**YELLOW FEVER**

**Requirements:** Required if traveling from a country with risk of YF virus transmission and ≥1 year of age, including transit >12 hours in an airport located in a country with risk of YF virus transmission.[1]

**Recommendations:** None

MALARIA
No malaria transmission.

## MAYOTTE (FRANCE)

**YELLOW FEVER**

**Requirements:** Required if traveling from a country with risk of YF virus transmission and ≥1 year of age, including transit >12 hours in an airport located in a country with risk of YF virus transmission.[1]
**Recommendations:** None

MALARIA
**Areas with malaria:** Rare cases.
**Drug resistance[3]:** Chloroquine.
**Malaria species:** *P. falciparum* 93%, *P. vivax* 5%, *P. malariae* and *P. ovale* 2%.
**Recommended chemoprophylaxis:** None (practice mosquito avoidance).

## MEXICO

**YELLOW FEVER**

**Requirements:** None
**Recommendations:** None

MALARIA
**Areas with malaria:** Present in Chiapas and southern part of Chihuahua. Rare cases in Campeche, Durango, Jalisco, Nayarit, Quintana Roo, San Luis Potosi, Sinaloa, Sonora, and Tabasco. No malaria along the US-Mexico border (Map 2-18).
**Drug resistance[3]:** None.
**Malaria species:** *P. vivax* 100%.
**Recommended chemoprophylaxis:** States of Chiapas and southern part of Chihuahua: Atovaquone-proguanil, chloroquine, doxycycline, mefloquine, primaquine,[4] or tafenoquine.[4] States of Campeche, Durango, Jalisco, Nayarit, Quintana Roo, San Luis Potosi, Sinaloa, Sonora, and Tabasco: None (practice mosquito avoidance).

## MICRONESIA, FEDERATED STATES OF; INCLUDES YAP ISLANDS, POHNPEI, CHUUK, AND KOSRAE

**YELLOW FEVER**

**Requirements:** None
**Recommendations:** None

MALARIA
No malaria transmission.

## MOLDOVA

**YELLOW FEVER**

**Requirements:** None
**Recommendations:** None

MALARIA
No malaria transmission.

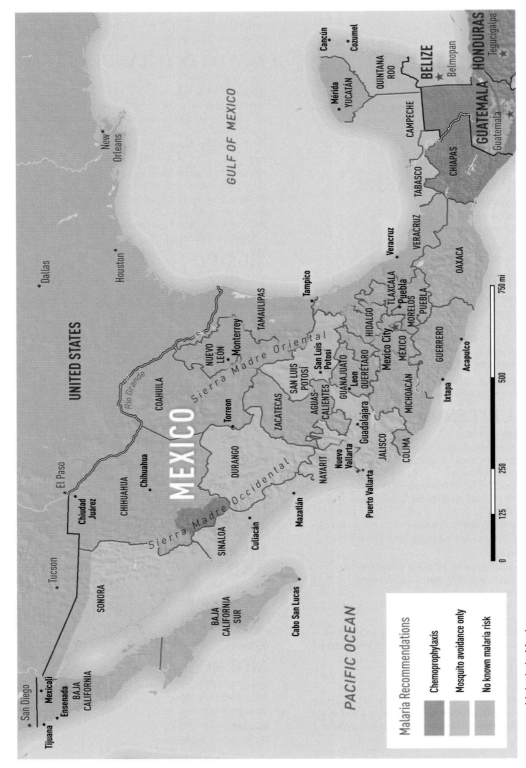

**Malaria Recommendations**

Chemoprophylaxis

Mosquito avoidance only

No known malaria risk

MAP 2-18. Malaria in Mexico

## MONACO

**YELLOW FEVER**

**Requirements:** None
**Recommendations:** None

MALARIA
No malaria transmission.

## MONGOLIA

**YELLOW FEVER**

**Requirements:** None
**Recommendations:** None

MALARIA
No malaria transmission.

## MONTENEGRO

**YELLOW FEVER**

**Requirements:** None
**Recommendations:** None

MALARIA
No malaria transmission.

## MONTSERRAT (UK)

**YELLOW FEVER**

**Requirements:** Required if traveling from a country with risk of YF virus transmission and ≥1 year of age, including transit in an airport located in a country with risk of YF virus transmission.[1]
**Recommendations:** None

MALARIA
No malaria transmission.

## MOROCCO

**YELLOW FEVER**

**Requirements:** None
**Recommendations:** None

MALARIA
No malaria transmission.

## MOZAMBIQUE

**YELLOW FEVER**

**Requirements:** Required if traveling from a country with risk of YF virus transmission and ≥9 months of age, including transit >12 hours in an airport located in a country with risk of YF virus transmission.[1]
**Recommendations:** None

MALARIA
**Areas with malaria:** All.
**Drug resistance[3]:** Chloroquine.
**Malaria species:** *P. falciparum* >90%, *P. malariae*, *P. ovale*, and *P. vivax* rare.
**Recommended chemoprophylaxis:** Atovaquone-proguanil, doxycycline, mefloquine, or tafenoquine.[4]

## NAMIBIA

**YELLOW FEVER**

**Requirements:** Required if traveling from a country with risk of YF virus transmission and ≥9 months of age, including transit >12 hours in an airport located in a country with risk of YF virus transmission.[1]
**Recommendations:** None

MALARIA
**Areas with malaria:** Present in the regions of Kavango (East and West), Kunene, Ohangwena, Omusati, Oshana, Oshikoto, Otjozondjupa, and Zambezi. Rare cases in other parts of the country. No malaria in city of Windhoek (Map 2-19).
**Drug resistance[3]:** Chloroquine.
**Malaria species:** *P. falciparum* >90%; *P. malariae*, *P. ovale*, and *P. vivax* rare.
**Recommended chemoprophylaxis:** Kavango (East and West), Kunene, Ohangwena, Omusati, Oshana, Oshikoto, Otjozunupa, and Zambezi: Atovaquone-proguanil, doxycycline, mefloquine, or tafenoquine.[4] Other parts of the country with rare cases: None (practice mosquito avoidance).

## NAURU

**YELLOW FEVER**

**Requirements:** Required if traveling from a country with risk of YF virus transmission and ≥1 year of age.[1]
**Recommendations:** None

MALARIA
No malaria transmission.

## NEPAL

**YELLOW FEVER**

**Requirements:** Required if traveling from a country with risk of YF virus transmission and ≥1 year of age, including transit >12 hours in an airport located in a country with risk of YF virus transmission.[1]
**Recommendations:** None

MALARIA
**Areas with malaria:** Present throughout the country at altitudes <2,000 m (6,562 ft). None in Kathmandu and on typical Himalayan treks.
**Drug resistance[3]:** Chloroquine.
**Malaria species:** *P. vivax* 85%, *P. falciparum* 15%.
**Recommended chemoprophylaxis:** Atovaquone-proguanil, doxycycline, mefloquine, or tafenoquine.[4]

## NETHERLANDS

**YELLOW FEVER**

**Requirements:** None
**Recommendations:** None

MALARIA
No malaria transmission.

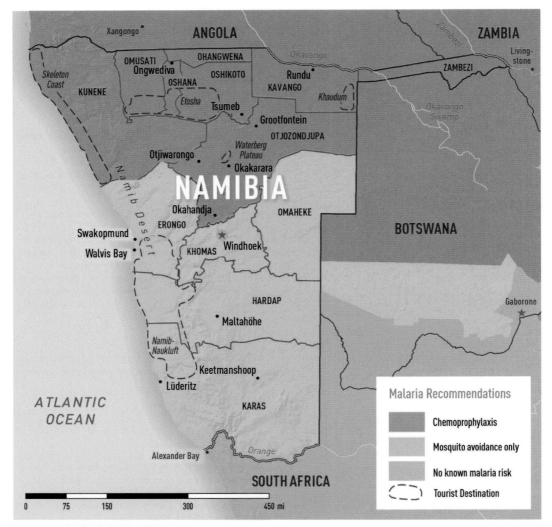

MAP 2-19. Malaria in Namibia

# NEW CALEDONIA (FRANCE)

**YELLOW FEVER**

**Requirements:** Required if traveling from a country with risk of YF virus transmission and ≥1 year of age, including transit >12 hours in an airport located in a country with risk of YF virus transmission.[1] **Note:** In the event of an epidemic threat to the territory, a specific vaccination certificate may be required.
**Recommendations:** None

MALARIA
No malaria transmission.

# NEW ZEALAND

**YELLOW FEVER**

**Requirements:** None
**Recommendations:** None

MALARIA
No malaria transmission.

# NICARAGUA

**YELLOW FEVER**

**Requirements:** Required if traveling from a country with risk of YF virus transmission and ≥1 year of age.
**Recommendations:** None

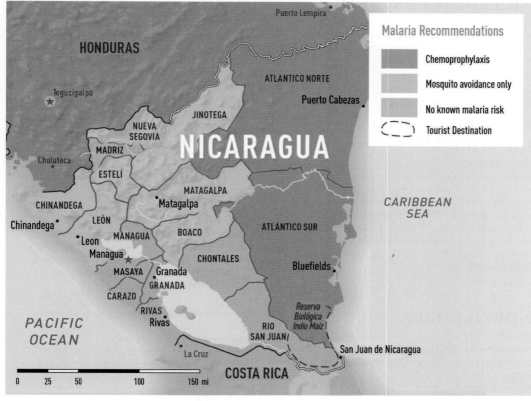

MAP 2-20. Malaria in Nicaragua

## MALARIA

**Areas with malaria:** Present in Región Autónoma Atlántico Norte (RAAN) and Región Autónoma Atlántico Sur (RAAS). Rare cases in Boaco, Chinandega, Esteli, Jinotega, Leon, Matagalpa, and Nueva Segovia. No malaria in the city of Managua (Map 2-20).
**Drug resistance[3]:** None.
**Malaria species:** *P. vivax* 90%, *P. falciparum* 10%.
**Recommended chemoprophylaxis:** Región Autónoma Atlántico Norte (RAAN) and Región Autónoma Atlántico Sur (RAAS): Atovaquone-proguanil, chloroquine, doxycycline, mefloquine, or tafenoquine.[4] Other areas with malaria: None (practice mosquito avoidance).

# NIGER

## YELLOW FEVER

**Requirements:** Required for arriving travelers from all countries if traveler is ≥1 year of age. The government of Niger recommends vaccine for travelers departing Niger.
**Recommendations:**
*Recommended* for all travelers ≥9 months of age traveling to areas south of the Sahara Desert (Map 4-13).

*Not recommended* for travelers whose itineraries are limited to areas in the Sahara Desert (Map 4-13).

## MALARIA

**Areas with malaria:** All.
**Drug resistance[3]:** Chloroquine.
**Malaria species:** *P. falciparum* 85%, *P. ovale* 5%–10%, *P. vivax* rare.
**Recommended chemoprophylaxis:** Atovaquone-proguanil, doxycycline, mefloquine, or tafenoquine.[4]

# NIGERIA

## YELLOW FEVER

**Requirements:** Required if traveling from a country with risk of YF virus transmission and ≥1 year of age.[1]
**Recommendations:** *Recommended* for all travelers ≥9 months of age.

## MALARIA

**Areas with malaria:** All.
**Drug resistance[3]:** Chloroquine.
**Malaria species:** *P. falciparum* >85%, *P. ovale* 5%–10%, *P. vivax* rare.
**Recommended chemoprophylaxis:** Atovaquone-proguanil, doxycycline, mefloquine, or tafenoquine.[4]

## NIUE (NEW ZEALAND)

YELLOW FEVER

**Requirements:** Required if traveling from a country with risk of YF virus transmission and ≥9 months of age.[1]
**Recommendations:** None

MALARIA
No malaria transmission.

## NORFOLK ISLAND (AUSTRALIA)

YELLOW FEVER

**Requirements:** Required if traveling from a country with risk of YF virus transmission and ≥1 year of age, including transit >12 hours in an airport located in a country with risk of YF virus transmission. This requirement excludes Galápagos Islands in Ecuador and the island of Tobago; it is limited to Misiones Province in Argentina.[1]
**Recommendations:** None

MALARIA
No malaria transmission.

## NORTH KOREA

YELLOW FEVER

**Requirements:** Required if traveling from a country with risk of YF virus transmission and ≥1 year of age.[1]
**Recommendations:** None

MALARIA
**Areas with malaria:** Present in southern provinces.
**Drug resistance**[3]**:** None.
**Malaria species:** Presumed to be 100% *P. vivax.*
**Recommended chemoprophylaxis:** Atovaquone-proguanil, chloroquine, doxycycline, mefloquine, primaquine,[4] or tafenoquine.[4]

## NORTHERN MARIANA ISLANDS (US), INCLUDES SAIPAN, TINIAN, AND ROTA ISLAND

YELLOW FEVER

**Requirements:** None
**Recommendations:** None

MALARIA
No malaria transmission.

## NORWAY

YELLOW FEVER

**Requirements:** None
**Recommendations:** None

MALARIA
No malaria transmission.

## OMAN

YELLOW FEVER

**Requirements:** Required if traveling from a country with risk of YF virus transmission and ≥9 months of age, including transit >12 hours in an airport located in a country with risk of YF virus transmission.[1]
**Recommendations:** None

MALARIA
**Areas with malaria:** Sporadic transmission in Dakhliyah, North Batinah, and North and South Sharqiyah.
**Drug resistance**[3]**:** Chloroquine
**Malaria species:** *P. falciparum* and *P. vivax*
**Recommended chemoprophylaxis:** None (practice mosquito avoidance).

## PAKISTAN

YELLOW FEVER

**Requirements:** Required if traveling from a country with risk of YF virus transmission and ≥1 year of age, including transit >12 hours in an airport located in a country with risk of YF virus transmission.[1]
**Recommendations:** None

MALARIA
**Areas with malaria:** All areas (including all cities) <2,500 m (<8,202 ft).
**Drug resistance**[3]**:** Chloroquine.
**Malaria species:** *P. vivax* 70%, *P. falciparum* 30%.
**Recommended chemoprophylaxis:** Atovaquone-proguanil, doxycycline, mefloquine, or tafenoquine.[4]

## PALAU

YELLOW FEVER

**Requirements:** None
**Recommendations:** None

MALARIA
No malaria transmission.

## PANAMA

YELLOW FEVER

**Requirements:** Required if traveling from a country with risk of YF virus transmission and ≥1 year of age.[1]
**Recommendations:**
***Recommended*** for all travelers ≥9 months of age traveling to all mainland areas east of the area surrounding the canal (the entire provinces of Darién, Emberá, and Kuna Yala [also spelled Guna Yala] and areas of the provinces of Colón and Panama that are east of the canal) (Map 2-21).
***Not recommended*** for travelers whose itineraries are limited to areas west of the canal, the city of Panama, the canal area itself, and the Balboa Islands (Pearl Islands) and San Blas Islands (Map 2-21).

MALARIA
**Areas with malaria:** Present in the provinces of Darién, Kuna Yala (also spelled Guna Yala), Ngäbe-Buglé, and eastern Panama province. None in Panama Oeste, the Canal Zone, and Panama City (Map 2-22).

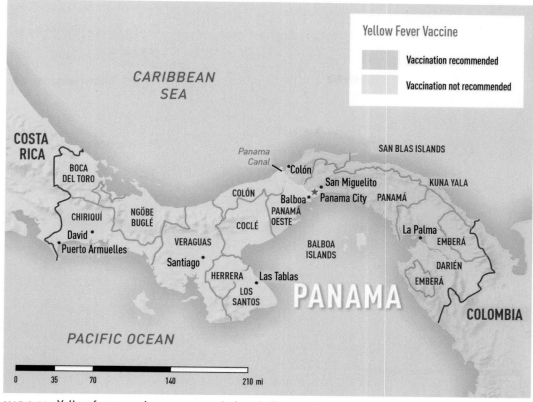

**MAP 2-21. Yellow fever vaccine recommendations in Panama[1]**

[1] See footnotes on page 101

**Drug resistance[3]:** Chloroquine (east of the Panama Canal).
**Malaria species:** *P. vivax* 99%, *P. falciparum* 1%.
**Recommended chemoprophylaxis:** Provinces of Darién, Guna Yala, and eastern Panama province: Atovaquone-proguanil, doxycycline, mefloquine, primaquine,[4] or tafenoquine.[4]
Ngäbe-Buglé: Atovaquone-proguanil, chloroquine, doxycycline, mefloquine, primaquine,[4] or tafenoquine.[4]

# PAPUA NEW GUINEA

### YELLOW FEVER

**Requirements:** None
**Recommendations:** None

### MALARIA

**Areas with malaria:** Present throughout the country at altitudes <2,000 m (6,561 ft).
**Drug resistance[3]:** Chloroquine (both *P. falciparum* and *P. vivax*).
**Malaria species:** *P. falciparum* 65%–80%, *P. vivax* 10%–30%, *P. malariae* and *P. ovale* rare.
**Recommended chemoprophylaxis:** Atovaquone-proguanil, doxycycline, mefloquine, or tafenoquine.[4]

# PARAGUAY

### YELLOW FEVER

**Requirements:** Required if traveling from a country with risk of YF virus transmission and ≥1 year of age.[1]
**Recommendations:**
***Recommended*** for all travelers ≥9 months of age, except as mentioned below.
Generally not recommended for travelers whose itinerary is limited to the city of Asunción.

### MALARIA
No malaria transmission.

# PERU

### YELLOW FEVER

**Requirements:** None
**Recommendations:**
***Recommended*** for all travelers ≥9 months of age going to areas at elevations <2,300 m (7,546 ft) in the regions of Amazonas, Loreto, Madre de Dios, San Martin, Ucayali, Puno, Cusco, Junín, Pasco, and Huánuco, and designated areas (Map 2-23) of the

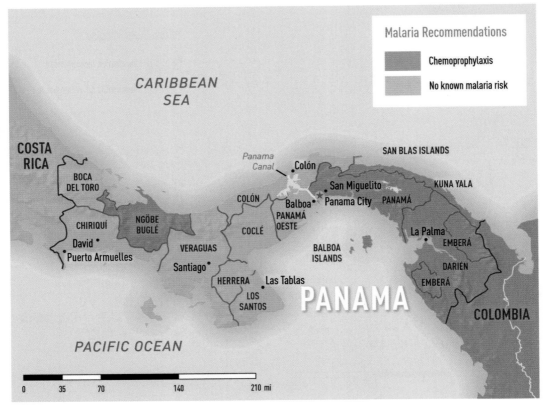

MAP 2-22. Malaria in Panama

following regions: far north of Apurimac, far northern Huancavelica, far northeastern Ancash, eastern La Libertad, northern and eastern Cajamarca, northern and northeastern Ayacucho, and eastern Piura. **Generally not recommended** for travelers whose itineraries are limited to the following areas west of the Andes: regions of Lambayeque and Tumbes and the designated areas (Map 2-23) of western Piura and south, west, and central Cajamarca. **Not recommended** for travelers whose itineraries are limited to the following areas: all areas >2,300 m (7,546 ft) in elevation, areas west of the Andes not listed above, the city of Cusco, the capital city of Lima, Machu Picchu, and the Inca Trail (Map 2-23).

### MALARIA
**Areas with malaria:** All departments <2,000 m (6,562 ft), including the cities of Iquitos and Puerto Maldonado and only the remote eastern regions of La Libertad and Lambayeque. None in the following areas: Lima Province; the cities of Arequipa, Ica, Moquegua, Nazca, Puno, and Tacna; the highland tourist areas (Cusco, Machu Picchu, and Lake Titicaca); and along the Pacific Coast (Map 2-24).
**Drug resistance**[3]: Chloroquine.
**Malaria species:** *P. vivax* 85%, *P. falciparum* 15%.

**Recommended chemoprophylaxis:** Atovaquone-proguanil, doxycycline, mefloquine, or tafenoquine.[4]

## PHILIPPINES

### YELLOW FEVER
**Requirements:** Required if traveling from a country with risk of YF virus transmission and ≥1 year of age, including transit in an airport located in a country with risk of YF virus transmission.[1]
**Recommendations:** None

### MALARIA
**Areas with malaria:** Present in Palawan and Mindanao Islands. None in metropolitan Manila and other urban areas.
**Drug resistance**[3]: Chloroquine.
**Malaria species:** *P. falciparum* 70%–80%, *P. vivax* 20%–30%, *P. knowlesi* rare.
**Recommended chemoprophylaxis:** Atovaquone-proguanil, doxycycline, mefloquine, or tafenoquine.[4]

## PITCAIRN ISLANDS (UK)

### YELLOW FEVER
**Requirements:** Required if traveling from a country with risk of YF virus transmission and ≥1 year of age,

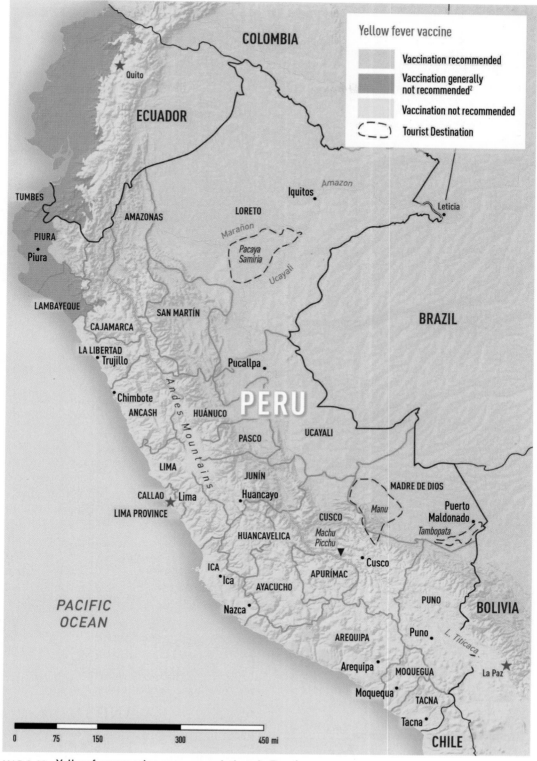

**MAP 2-23.** Yellow fever vaccine recommendations in Peru[1]

[1,2] See footnotes on page 101

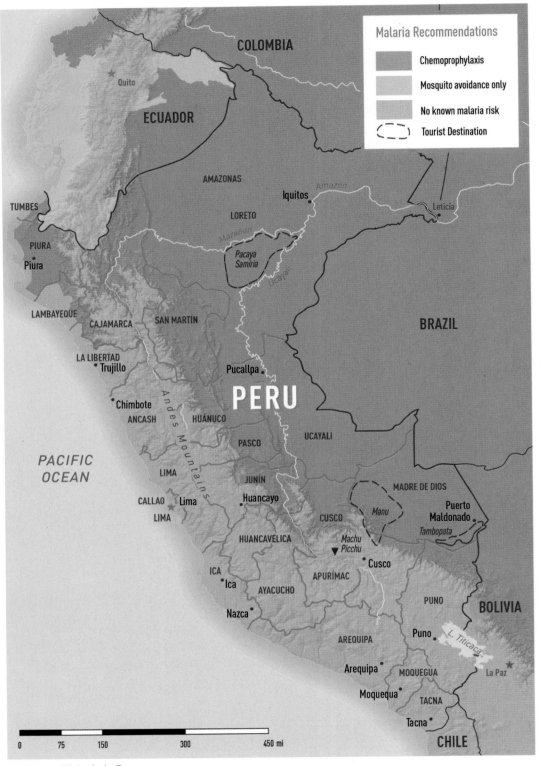

MAP 2-24. Malaria in Peru

including transit in an airport located in a country with risk of YF virus transmission.[1]
**Recommendations:** None

**MALARIA**
No malaria transmission.

# POLAND

**YELLOW FEVER**
**Requirements:** None
**Recommendations:** None

**MALARIA**
No malaria transmission.

# PORTUGAL

**YELLOW FEVER**
**Requirements:** None
**Recommendations:** None

**MALARIA**
No malaria transmission.

# PUERTO RICO (US)

**YELLOW FEVER**
**Requirements:** None
**Recommendations:** None

**MALARIA**
No malaria transmission.

# QATAR

**YELLOW FEVER**
**Requirements:** None
**Recommendations:** None

**MALARIA**
No malaria transmission.

# ROMANIA

**YELLOW FEVER**
**Requirements:** None
**Recommendations:** None

**MALARIA**
No malaria transmission.

# RUSSIA

**YELLOW FEVER**
**Requirements:** None
**Recommendations:** None

**MALARIA**
No malaria transmission.

# RWANDA

**YELLOW FEVER**
**Requirements:** Required if traveling from a country with risk of YF virus transmission and ≥1 year of age.
**Recommendations:** *Generally not recommended* for travelers to Rwanda.

**MALARIA**
**Areas with malaria:** All.
**Drug resistance[3]:** Chloroquine.
**Malaria species:** *P. falciparum* 90%, *P. vivax* 5%, *P. ovale* 5%.
**Recommended chemoprophylaxis:** Atovaquone-proguanil, doxycycline, mefloquine, or tafenoquine.[4]

# RÉUNION (FRANCE)

**YELLOW FEVER**
**Requirements:** Required if traveling from a country with risk of YF virus transmission and ≥1 year of age, including transit >12 hours in an airport located in a country with risk of YF virus transmission.[1]
**Recommendations:** None

**MALARIA**
No malaria transmission.

# SABA

**YELLOW FEVER**
**Requirements:** None
**Recommendations:** None

**MALARIA**
No malaria transmission.

# SAINT BARTHELEMY

**YELLOW FEVER**
**Requirements:** Required if traveling from a country with risk of YF virus transmission and ≥1 year of age, including transit >12 hours in an airport located in a country with risk of YF virus transmission.[1]
**Recommendations:** None

**MALARIA**
No malaria transmission.

# SAINT HELENA (UK)

**YELLOW FEVER**
**Requirements:** Required if traveling from a country with risk of YF virus transmission and ≥1 year of age.[1]
**Recommendations:** None

**MALARIA**
No malaria transmission.

# SAINT KITTS (SAINT CHRISTOPHER) AND NEVIS (UK)

**YELLOW FEVER**
**Requirements:** Required if traveling from a country with risk of YF virus transmission and ≥1 year of age.[1]
**Recommendations:** None

**MALARIA**
No malaria transmission.

## SAINT LUCIA

YELLOW FEVER

**Requirements:** Required if traveling from a country with risk of YF virus transmission and ≥9 months of age.[1]
**Recommendations:** None

MALARIA

No malaria transmission.

## SAINT MARTIN

YELLOW FEVER

**Requirements:** Required if traveling from a country with risk of YF virus transmission and ≥1 year of age, including transit >12 hours in an airport located in a country with risk of YF virus transmission.[1]
**Recommendations:** None

MALARIA

No malaria transmission.

## SAINT PIERRE AND MIQUELON (FRANCE)

YELLOW FEVER

**Requirements:** None
**Recommendations:** None

MALARIA

No malaria transmission.

## SAINT VINCENT AND THE GRENADINES

YELLOW FEVER

**Requirements:** Required if traveling from a country with risk of YF virus transmission and ≥1 year of age.[1]
**Recommendations:** None

MALARIA

No malaria transmission.

## SAMOA (FORMERLY WESTERN SOMOA)

YELLOW FEVER

**Requirements:** Required if traveling from a country with risk of YF virus transmission and ≥1 year of age, including transit >12 hours in an airport located in a country with risk of YF virus transmission.[1]
**Recommendations:** None

MALARIA

No malaria transmission.

## SAN MARINO

YELLOW FEVER

**Requirements:** None
**Recommendations:** None

MALARIA

No malaria transmission.

## SÃO TOMÉ AND PRÍNCIPE

YELLOW FEVER

**Requirements:** Required if traveling from a country with risk of YF virus transmission and ≥1 year of age, including transit in an airport located in a country with risk of YF virus transmission.[1]
**Recommendations: Generally not recommended** for travelers to São Tomé and Príncipe.

MALARIA

**Areas with malaria:** All.
**Drug resistance**[3]**:** Chloroquine.
**Malaria species:** *P. falciparum* 85%; *P. malariae*, *P. ovale*, *P. vivax* 15% combined.
**Recommended chemoprophylaxis:** Atovaquone-proguanil, doxycycline, mefloquine, or tafenoquine.[4]

## SAUDI ARABIA

YELLOW FEVER

**Requirements:** Required if traveling from a country with risk of YF virus transmission and ≥1 year of age, including transit >12 hours in an airport located in a country with risk of YF virus transmission.[1]
**Recommendations:** None

MALARIA

**Areas with malaria:** Asir and Jizan emirates by border with Yemen. None in the cities of Jeddah, Mecca, Medina, Riyadh, and Ta'if.
**Drug resistance**[3]**:** Chloroquine.
**Malaria species:** *P. falciparum* predominantly.
**Recommended chemoprophylaxis:** Atovaquone-proguanil, doxycycline, mefloquine, or tafenoquine.[4]

## SENEGAL

YELLOW FEVER

**Requirements:** Required if traveling from a country with risk of YF virus transmission and ≥9 months of age, including transit in an airport located in a country with risk of YF virus transmission.[1]
**Recommendations: *Recommended*** for all travelers ≥9 months of age.

MALARIA

**Areas with malaria:** All.
**Drug resistance**[3]**:** Chloroquine.
**Malaria species:** *P. falciparum* >85%, *P. ovale* 5%–10%, *P. vivax* rare.
**Recommended chemoprophylaxis:** Atovaquone-proguanil, doxycycline, mefloquine, or tafenoquine.[4]

## SERBIA

YELLOW FEVER

**Requirements:** None
**Recommendations:** None

MALARIA

No malaria transmission.

## SEYCHELLES

### YELLOW FEVER
**Requirements:** Required if traveling from a country with risk of YF virus transmission and ≥1 year of age, including transit >12 hours in an airport located in a country with risk of YF virus transmission.[1]
**Recommendations:** None

### MALARIA
No malaria transmission.

## SIERRA LEONE

### YELLOW FEVER
**Requirements:** Required for arriving travelers from all countries.
**Recommendations:** *Recommended* for all travelers ≥9 months of age.

### MALARIA
**Areas with malaria:** All.
**Drug resistance**[3]**:** Chloroquine.
**Malaria species:** *P. falciparum* >85%, *P. ovale* 5%–10%, *P. malariae* and *P. vivax* rare.
**Recommended chemoprophylaxis:** Atovaquone-proguanil, doxycycline, mefloquine, or tafenoquine.[4]

## SINGAPORE

### YELLOW FEVER
**Requirements:** Required if traveling from a country with risk of YFV transmission and ≥1 year of age, including transit >12 hours in an airport located in a country with risk of YFV transmission.[1]
**Recommendations:** None

### MALARIA
No malaria transmission.

## SINT EUSTATIUS

### YELLOW FEVER
**Requirements:** Required if traveling from a country with risk of YF virus transmission and ≥6 months of age.[1]
**Recommendations:** None

### MALARIA
No malaria transmission.

## SINT MAARTEN

### YELLOW FEVER
**Requirements:** Required if traveling from a country with risk of YF virus transmission and ≥6 months of age.[1]
**Recommendations:** None

### MALARIA
No malaria transmission.

## SLOVAKIA

### YELLOW FEVER
**Requirements:** None
**Recommendations:** None

### MALARIA
No malaria transmission.

## SLOVENIA

### YELLOW FEVER
**Requirements:** None
**Recommendations:** None

### MALARIA
No malaria transmission.

## SOLOMON ISLANDS

### YELLOW FEVER
**Requirements:** Required if traveling from a country with risk of YF virus transmission.[1]
**Recommendations:** None

### MALARIA
**Areas with malaria:** All.
**Drug resistance**[3]**:** Chloroquine.
**Malaria species:** *P. falciparum* 60%, *P. vivax* 35%–40%, *P. ovale* <1%.
**Recommended chemoprophylaxis:** Atovaquone-proguanil, doxycycline, mefloquine, or tafenoquine.[4]

## SOMALIA

### YELLOW FEVER
**Requirements:** Required if traveling from a country with risk of YF virus transmission and ≥9 months of age, including transit >12 hours in an airport located in a country with risk of YF virus transmission.[1]
**Recommendations:**
Generally not recommended for travelers going to the following regions: Bakool, Banaadir, Bay, Galguduud, Gedo, Hiiraan, Lower Juba, Lower Shabelle, Middle Juba, and Middle Shabelle (Map 4-13).
***Not recommended*** for all other areas not listed above.

### MALARIA
**Areas with malaria:** All.
**Drug resistance**[3]**:** Chloroquine.
**Malaria species:** *P. falciparum* 90%, *P. vivax* 5%–10%, *P. malariae* and *P. ovale* rare.
**Recommended chemoprophylaxis:** Atovaquone-proguanil, doxycycline, mefloquine, or tafenoquine.[4]

## SOUTH AFRICA

### YELLOW FEVER
**Requirements:** Required if traveling from a country with risk of YF virus transmission and ≥1 year of age, including transit >12 hours in an airport located in a country with risk of YF virus transmission.[1]
**Recommendations:** None

### MALARIA
**Areas with malaria:** Present along the border with Zimbabwe and Mozambique. Specifically in Mopani, Vhembe, and Waterberg district municipalities of Limpopo Province; Ehlanzeni district municipality in

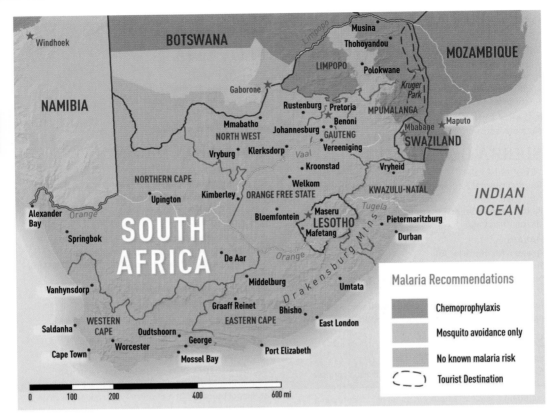

MAP 2-25. **Malaria in South Africa**

Mpumalanga Province; and Umknanyakude in Kwazulu-Natal Province. Present in Kruger National Park (Map 2-25)

**Drug resistance**[3]: Chloroquine.

**Malaria species:** *P. falciparum* 90%, *P. vivax* 5%, *P. ovale* 5%.

**Recommended chemoprophylaxis:** Areas in Limpopo, Mpumalanga, and Kwazulu-Natal Provinces with malaria: Atovaquone-proguanil, doxycycline, mefloquine, or tafenoquine.[4]

# SOUTH GEORGIA AND THE SOUTH SANDWICH ISLANDS

**YELLOW FEVER**

**Requirements:** This country has not stated its yellow fever vaccination certificate requirements.

**Recommendations:** None

**MALARIA**

No malaria transmission.

# SOUTH KOREA

**YELLOW FEVER**

**Requirements:** None

**Recommendations:** None

**MALARIA**

**Areas with malaria:** Limited to the months of March–December in rural areas in the northern parts of Incheon, Kangwon-do, and Kyônggi-do Provinces, including the demilitarized zone (DMZ).

**Drug resistance**[3]: None.

**Malaria species:** *P. vivax* 100%.

**Recommended chemoprophylaxis:** Atovaquone-proguanil, chloroquine, doxycycline, mefloquine, primaquine,[4] or tafenoquine.[4]

# SOUTH SUDAN, REPUBLIC OF

**YELLOW FEVER**

**Requirements:** Required for arriving travelers from all countries if traveler is ≥9 months of age.

**Recommendations: *Recommended*** for all travelers ≥9 months of age.

MALARIA

**Areas with malaria:** All.
**Drug resistance**[3]: Chloroquine.
**Malaria species:** *P. falciparum* 90%, *P. vivax* 5%–10%, *P. malariae* and *P. ovale* rare.
**Recommended chemoprophylaxis:** Atovaquone-proguanil, doxycycline, mefloquine, or tafenoquine.[4]

# SPAIN

YELLOW FEVER

**Requirements:** None
**Recommendations:** None

MALARIA

No malaria transmission.

# SRI LANKA

YELLOW FEVER

**Requirements:** Required if traveling from a country with risk of YF virus transmission and ≥9 months of age, including transit >12 hours in an airport located in a country with risk of YF virus transmission.[1]
**Recommendations:** None

MALARIA

No malaria transmission.

# SUDAN

YELLOW FEVER

**Requirements:** Required if traveling from a country with risk of YF virus transmission and ≥1 year of age, including transit >12 hours in an airport located in a country with risk of YF virus transmission.[1] A certificate may be required for travelers departing Sudan.
**Recommendations:**

***Recommended*** for all travelers ≥9 months of age traveling to areas south of the Sahara Desert (Map 4-13).

***Not recommended*** for travelers whose itineraries are limited to areas in the Sahara Desert and the city of Khartoum (Map 4-13).

MALARIA

**Areas with malaria:** All.
**Drug resistance**[3]: Chloroquine.
**Malaria species:** *P. falciparum* 90%, *P. vivax* 5%–10%, *P. malariae* and *P. ovale* rare.
**Recommended chemoprophylaxis:** Atovaquone-proguanil, doxycycline, mefloquine, or tafenoquine.[4]

# SURINAME

YELLOW FEVER

**Requirements:** Required if traveling from a country with risk of YF virus transmission and ≥1 year of age, including transit >12 hours in an airport located in a country with risk of YF virus transmission.[1]

**Recommendations: *Recommended*** for all travelers ≥9 months of age.

MALARIA

**Areas with malaria:** Present in the municipality of Tapanahony in Sipaliwini Province. Rare cases in Brokopondo Province, Marowijne Province, and Boven Saramacca municipality in Sipaliwini Province. No malaria in Paramaribo.
**Drug resistance**[3]: Chloroquine.
**Malaria species:** *P. falciparum* 70%, *P. vivax* 15%–20%.
**Recommended chemoprophylaxis:** Tapanahony municipality in Sipaliwini Province: Atovaquone-proguanil, doxycycline, mefloquine, or tafenoquine.[4] Other areas with malaria: None (practice mosquito avoidance).

# SWEDEN

YELLOW FEVER

**Requirements:** None
**Recommendations:** None

MALARIA

No malaria transmission.

# SWITZERLAND

YELLOW FEVER

**Requirements:** None
**Recommendations:** None

MALARIA

No malaria transmission.

# SYRIA

YELLOW FEVER

**Requirements:** None
**Recommendations:** None

MALARIA

No malaria transmission.

# TAIWAN

YELLOW FEVER

**Requirements:** None
**Recommendations:** None

MALARIA

No malaria transmission.

# TAJIKISTAN

YELLOW FEVER

**Requirements:** None
**Recommendations:** None

MALARIA

**Areas with malaria:** Rare indigenous cases.
**Drug resistance**[3]: Chloroquine.
**Malaria species:** *P. vivax* 90%, *P. falciparum* 10%.
**Recommended chemoprophylaxis:** None (practice mosquito avoidance).

# TANZANIA

**YELLOW FEVER**

**Requirements:** Required if traveling from a country with risk of YF virus transmission and ≥1 year of age, including transit >12 hours in an airport located in a country with risk of YF virus transmission.[1]

**Recommendations:** *Generally not recommended* for travelers to Tanzania.

**MALARIA**

**Areas with malaria:** All areas <1,800 m (5,906 ft).
**Drug resistance**[3]: Chloroquine.
**Malaria species:** *P. falciparum* >85%, *P. ovale* >10%, *P. malariae* and *P. vivax* rare.
**Recommended chemoprophylaxis:** Atovaquone-proguanil, doxycycline, mefloquine, or tafenoquine.[4]

# THAILAND

**YELLOW FEVER**

**Requirements:** Required if traveling from a country with risk of YF virus transmission and ≥9 months of age, including transit in an airport located in a country with risk of YF virus transmission.[1]

**Recommendations:** None

**MALARIA**

**Areas with malaria:** Primarily in provinces that border Burma (Myanmar), Cambodia, and Laos and the provinces of Kalasin, Krabi (Plai Phraya district), Nakhon Si Thammarat, Narathiwat, Pattani, Phang Nga (including Phang Nga City), Rayong, Sakon Nakhon, Songkhla, Surat Thani, and Yala, especially the rural forest and forest fringe areas of these provinces. Rare to few cases in other parts of Thailand, including other parts of Krabi Province and the cities of Bangkok, Chiang Mai, Chiang Rai, Koh Phangan, Koh Samui, and Phuket. None in the islands of Krabi Province (Koh Phi, Koh Yao Noi, Koh Yao Yai, and Ko Lanta) and Pattaya City (Map 2-26).
**Drug resistance**[3]: Chloroquine and mefloquine.
**Malaria species:** *P. falciparum* 50% (up to 75% in some areas), *P. vivax* 50% (up to 60% in some areas), *P. ovale* and *P. knowlesi* rare.
**Recommended chemoprophylaxis:** Provinces that border Burma (Myanmar), Cambodia, and Laos, the provinces of Kalasin, Plai Phraya district of Krabi, Nakhon Si Thammarat, Narathiwat, Pattani, Phang Nga (including Phang Nga City), Rayong, Sakon Nakhon, Songkhla, Surat Thani, and Yala: Atovaquone-proguanil, doxycycline, or tafenoquine.[4] All other areas of Thailand with malaria including the cities of Bangkok, Chiang Mai, Chiang Rai, Koh Phangan, Koh Samui, and Phuket: None (practice mosquito avoidance).

# TIMOR-LESTE

**YELLOW FEVER**

**Requirements:** Required if traveling from a country with risk of YF virus transmission and ≥1 year of age, including transit in an airport located in a country with risk of YF virus transmission.[1]

**Recommendations:** None

**MALARIA**

**Areas with malaria:** Present in Oecusse District. Rare cases in other districts.
**Drug resistance**[3]: Chloroquine.
**Malaria species:** *P. falciparum* 50%, *P. vivax* 50%, *P. ovale* <1%, *P. malariae* <1%.
**Recommended chemoprophylaxis:** Oecusse District: Atovaquone-proguanil, doxycycline, mefloquine, or tafenoquine.[4] Other districts: None (practice mosquito avoidance).

# TOGO

**YELLOW FEVER**

**Requirements:** Required for arriving travelers from all countries if traveler is ≥9 months of age.
**Recommendations:** *Recommended* for all travelers ≥9 months of age.

**MALARIA**

**Areas with malaria:** All.
**Drug resistance**[3]: Chloroquine.
**Malaria species:** *P. falciparum* 85%, *P. ovale* 5%–10%, remainder *P. vivax*.
**Recommended chemoprophylaxis:** Atovaquone-proguanil, doxycycline, mefloquine, or tafenoquine.[4]

# TOKELAU (NEW ZEALAND)

**YELLOW FEVER**

**Requirements:** None
**Recommendations:** None

**MALARIA**

No malaria transmission.

# TONGA

**YELLOW FEVER**

**Requirements:** None
**Recommendations:** None

**MALARIA**

No malaria transmission.

# TRINIDAD AND TOBAGO

**YELLOW FEVER**

**Requirements:** Required if traveling from a country with risk of YF virus transmission and ≥1 year of age, including transit in an airport located in a country with risk of YF virus transmission.[1]

**Recommendations:**
*Recommended* for all travelers ≥9 months of age traveling to densely-forested areas on the island of Trinidad.
*Not recommended* for cruise ship passengers and airplane passengers in transit, or travelers whose itineraries are limited to the island of Tobago.

**MALARIA**

No malaria transmission.

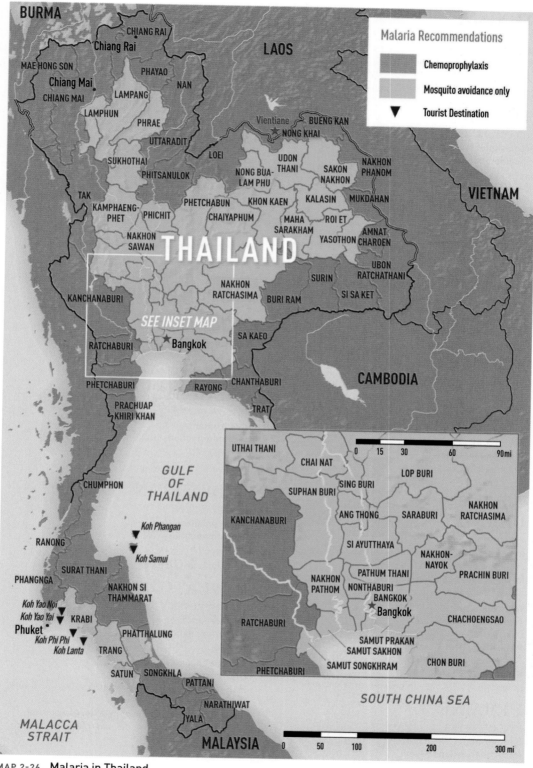

MAP 2-26. **Malaria in Thailand**

## TUNISIA
YELLOW FEVER
**Requirements:** None
**Recommendations:** None

MALARIA
No malaria transmission.

## TURKEY
YELLOW FEVER
**Requirements:** None
**Recommendations:** None

MALARIA
No malaria transmission.

## TURKMENISTAN
YELLOW FEVER
**Requirements:** None
**Recommendations:** None

MALARIA
No malaria transmission.

## TURKS AND CAICOS ISLANDS (UK)
YELLOW FEVER
**Requirements:** None
**Recommendations:** None

MALARIA
No malaria transmission.

## TUVALU
YELLOW FEVER
**Requirements:** None
**Recommendations:** None

MALARIA
No malaria transmission.

## UGANDA
YELLOW FEVER
**Requirements:** Required for arriving travelers from all countries if traveler is ≥1 year of age.
**Recommendations:** *Recommended* for all travelers ≥9 months of age.

MALARIA
**Areas with malaria:** All.
**Drug resistance**[3]: Chloroquine.
**Malaria species:** *P. falciparum* >85%; remainder *P. malariae*, *P. ovale*, and *P. vivax*.
**Recommended chemoprophylaxis:** Atovaquone-proguanil, doxycycline, mefloquine, or tafenoquine.[4]

## UKRAINE
YELLOW FEVER
**Requirements:** None
**Recommendations:** None

MALARIA
No malaria transmission.

## UNITED ARAB EMIRATES
YELLOW FEVER
**Requirements:** None
**Recommendations:** None

MALARIA
No malaria transmission.

## UNITED KINGDOM (WITH CHANNEL ISLANDS AND ISLE OF MAN)
YELLOW FEVER
**Requirements:** None
**Recommendations:** None

MALARIA
No malaria transmission.

## UNITED STATES
YELLOW FEVER
**Requirements:** None
**Recommendations:** None

MALARIA
No malaria transmission.

## URUGUAY
YELLOW FEVER
**Requirements:** None
**Recommendations:** None

MALARIA
No malaria transmission.

## UZBEKISTAN
YELLOW FEVER
**Requirements:** None
**Recommendations:** None

MALARIA
No malaria transmission.

## VANUATU
YELLOW FEVER
**Requirements:** None
**Recommendations:** None

MALARIA
**Areas with malaria:** All.
**Drug resistance**[3]: Chloroquine.
**Malaria species:** *P. falciparum* 60%, *P. vivax* 35%–40%, *P. ovale* <1%.
**Recommended chemoprophylaxis:** Atovaquone-proguanil, doxycycline, mefloquine, or tafenoquine.[4]

# VENEZUELA

**YELLOW FEVER**

**Requirements:** Required if traveling from Brazil and ≥1 year of age, including transit >12 hours in an airport located in Brazil.

**Recommendations:**

***Recommended*** for all travelers ≥9 months of age, except as mentioned below.

***Generally not recommended*** for travelers whose itineraries are limited to the following areas: the states of Aragua, Carabobo, Miranda, Vargas, and Yaracuy, and the Distrito Capital (Map 2-27).

***Not recommended*** for travelers whose itineraries are limited to the following areas: all areas >2,300m (7,546 ft) in elevation in the states of Merida, Tachira, and Trujillo; the states of Falcón and Lara; Margarita Island; the capital city of Caracas; and the city of Valencia (Map 2-27).

**MALARIA**

**Areas with malaria:** All areas <1,700m (5.577 ft). Present in Angel Falls (Map 2-28).

**Drug resistance**[3]: Chloroquine.

**Malaria species:** *P. vivax* 83%, *P. falciparum* 17%.

**Recommended chemoprophylaxis:** Atovaquone-proguanil, doxycycline, mefloquine, or tafenoquine.[4]

# VIETNAM

**YELLOW FEVER**

**Requirements:** None
**Recommendations:** None

**MALARIA**

**Areas with malaria:** Rural areas only. Rare cases in the Mekong and Red River Deltas. None in the cities of Da Nang, Haiphong, Hanoi, Ho Chi Minh (Saigon), Nha Trang, and Qui Nhon.

**Drug resistance**[3]: Chloroquine and mefloquine.

**Malaria species:** *P. falciparum* 50%–90%, *P. vivax.* 10%–50%, *P. knowlesi* rare.

**Recommended chemoprophylaxis:** Southern part of the country in the provinces of Dac Lac, Gia Lai, Khanh Hoa, Kon Tum, Lam Dong, Ninh Thuan, Song Be, Tay Ninh: Atovaquone-proguanil doxycycline, or tafenoquine.[5] Other areas with malaria except Mekong and Red River Deltas: Atovaquone-proguanil, doxycycline, omefloquine, or tafenoquine.[4] Mekong and Red River Deltas: None (practice mosquito avoidance).

# VIRGIN ISLANDS, BRITISH

**YELLOW FEVER**

**Requirements:** None
**Recommendations:** None

**MALARIA**

No malaria transmission.

# VIRGIN ISLANDS, US

**YELLOW FEVER**

**Requirements:** None
**Recommendations:** None

**MALARIA**

No malaria transmission.

# WAKE ISLAND, US

**YELLOW FEVER**

**Requirements:** None
**Recommendations:** None

**MALARIA**

No malaria transmission.

# WESTERN SAHARA

**YELLOW FEVER**

**Requirements:** This territory has not stated its yellow fever vaccination certificate requirements.

**Recommendations:** None

**MALARIA**

**Areas with malaria:** Rare cases.

**Drug resistance**[3]: Chloroquine.

**Malaria species:** Unknown.

**Recommended chemoprophylaxis:** None (practice mosquito avoidance).

# YEMEN

**YELLOW FEVER**

**Requirements:** None
**Recommendations:** None

**MALARIA**

**Areas with malaria:** All areas <2,000 m (6,562 ft). None in Sana'a.

**Drug resistance**[3]: Chloroquine.

**Malaria species:** *P. falciparum* 95%; *P. malariae, P. vivax,* and *P. ovale* 5% combined.

**Recommended chemoprophylaxis:** Atovaquone-proguanil, doxycycline, mefloquine, or tafenoquine.[4]

# ZAMBIA

**YELLOW FEVER**

**Requirements:** Required if traveling from a country with risk of YF virus transmission and ≥1 year of age, including transit >12 hours in an airport located in a country with risk of YF virus transmission.[1]

**Recommendations:**

***Generally not recommended*** for travelers going to the North West and Western Provinces (Map 2-29).

***Not recommended*** in all other areas not listed above.

**MALARIA**

**Areas with malaria:** All.

**Drug resistance**[3]: Chloroquine.

**Malaria species:** *P. falciparum* >90%, *P. vivax* up to 5%, *P. ovale* up to 5%.

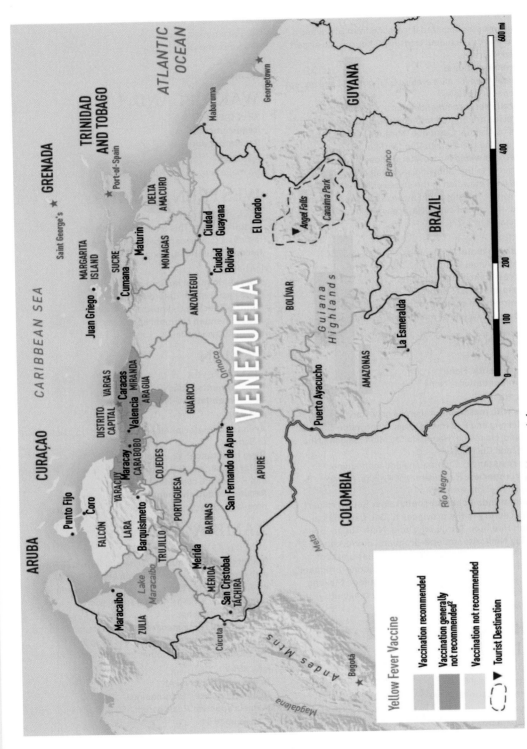

MAP 2-27. Yellow fever vaccine recommendations in Venezuela[1]

[1,2] See footnotes on page 101

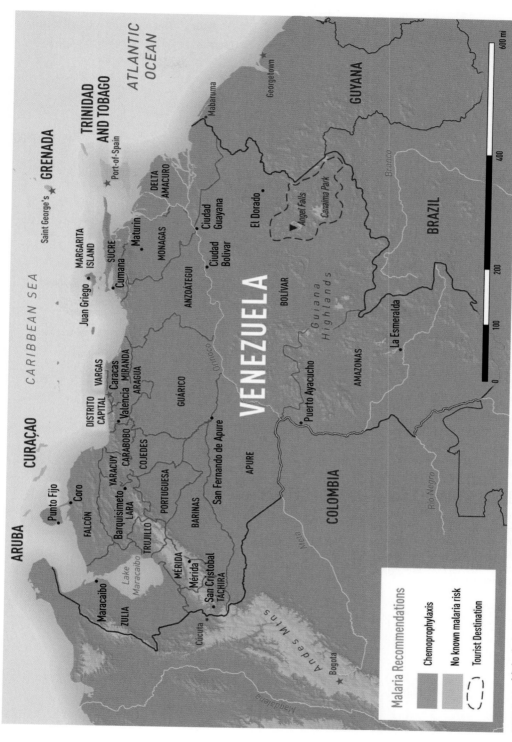

MAP 2-28. Malaria in Venezuela

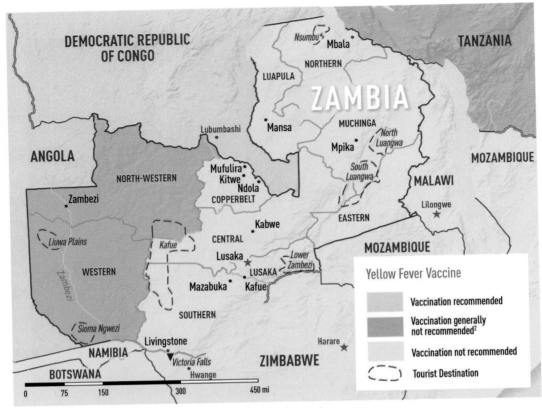

MAP 2-29. Yellow fever vaccine recommendations in Zambia[1]

[1,2] See footnotes on page 101

**Recommended chemoprophylaxis:** Atovaquone-proguanil, doxycycline, mefloquine, or tafenoquine.[4]

# ZIMBABWE

### YELLOW FEVER

**Requirements:** Required if traveling from a country with risk of YF virus transmission and ≥9 months of age, including transit >12 hours in an airport located in a country with risk of YF virus transmission.[1]
**Recommendations:** None

### MALARIA

**Areas with malaria:** All.
**Drug resistance**[3]**:** Chloroquine.
**Malaria species:** *P. falciparum* >90%, *P. vivax* up to 5%, *P. ovale* up to 5%.
**Recommended chemoprophylaxis:** Atovaquone-proguanil, doxycycline, mefloquine, or tafenoquine.[4]

# FOOTNOTES

## Yellow Fever

[1] The official WHO list of countries with risk of YF virus transmission can be found in Table 4-23. Proof of yellow fever vaccination should be required only if traveling from a country on the WHO list, unless otherwise specified. The following countries, containing only areas with low potential for exposure to YF virus, are not on the WHO list: Eritrea, Rwanda, São Tomé and Príncipe, Somalia, Tanzania, Zambia.

[2] An elevation of 2,300 m is equivalent to 7,546 ft.

## Malaria

[3] Refers to *P. falciparum* malaria unless otherwise noted.

[4] Primaquine and tafenoquine can cause hemolytic anemia in people with G6PD deficiency. Patients must be screened for G6PD deficiency before starting primaquine or tafenoquine.

## Yellow Fever Maps

[1] Current as of August 2018. This map is an updated version of the 2010 map created by the Informal WHO Working Group on the Geographic Risk of Yellow Fever.

[2] Yellow fever (YF) vaccination is generally not recommended in areas where there is low potential for YF virus exposure. However, vaccination might be considered for a small subset of travelers to these areas who are at increased risk for exposure to YF virus because of prolonged travel, heavy exposure to mosquitoes, or inability to avoid mosquito bites. Consideration for vaccination of any traveler must take into account the traveler's risk of being infected with YF virus, country entry requirements, and individual risk factors for serious vaccine-associated adverse events (such as age or immune status).

[3] In 2017, CDC expanded yellow fever vaccination recommendations for travelers to Brazil because of a large outbreak of yellow fever in multiple states in that country. Please refer to the CDC Travelers' Health website (www.cdc.gov/travel) for more information and updated recommendations.

# FOOD & WATER PRECAUTIONS

Patricia M. Griffin, Vincent Hill

Contaminated food and water often pose a risk for travelers. Many of the infectious diseases associated with contaminated food and water are caused by pathogens transmitted via the fecal–oral route. Swallowing, inhaling aerosols of, or coming in contact with contaminated water—including natural freshwater, marine water, or the water in inadequately treated swimming pools, water playgrounds (splash parks or splash pads), or hot tubs and spas—can transmit pathogens that can cause diarrhea, vomiting, or infection of the ears, eyes, skin, or the respiratory or nervous system.

## FOOD

Advise travelers to select food with care. Raw food is especially likely to be contaminated. Raw or undercooked meat, fish, and shellfish can carry various intestinal and systemic pathogens. (Some fish harvested from tropical waters can transmit toxins that survive cooking; see Food Poisoning from Marine Toxins in this chapter.) In areas where hygiene and sanitation are inadequate or unknown, travelers should avoid consuming salads; uncooked vegetables; raw, unpeeled fruits; and unpasteurized fruit juices. Fruits that can be peeled are safest when peeled by the person who eats them. Produce should be rinsed with safe water (see Water Disinfection in this chapter). Foods of animal origin, including meat and eggs, should be thoroughly cooked; milk and milk products, including milk used in soft cheese, should be pasteurized. In restaurants, inadequate refrigeration and lack of food safety training among staff can result in transmission of pathogens. Consumption of food and beverages obtained from street vendors has been associated with an increased risk of illness. In general, foods that are fully cooked and served hot are safest, as are foods people carefully prepare themselves.

Travelers should wash their hands with soap and water before preparing food, before eating, after using the bathroom or changing diapers, before and after caring for someone who is ill, and after contact with animals or their environments. If soap and water are not available, use an alcohol-based hand sanitizer (with ≥60% alcohol) and wash hands with soap and water as soon as they become available. Hand sanitizer is not very effective against *Cryptosporidium* or norovirus and does not work well when hands are visibly dirty or greasy.

The safest way to feed an infant aged <6 months is to breastfeed exclusively. If the infant is fed formula prepared from commercial powder, the powder should be reconstituted with hot water at a temperature of ≥158°F (≥70°C). This precaution will kill most pathogens with which the infant formula may have been contaminated during manufacturing or through handling after opening. To ensure that the water is hot enough, travelers should prepare formula within 30 minutes after boiling the water (see Water Disinfection in this chapter). The prepared formula should be cooled to a safe temperature for feeding (for example, by placing the bottle upright in a bath of safe water and safe ice [see below], keeping the bath water below the nipple ring) and used within 2 hours of preparation. Bottles and nipples should be washed and then sterilized (in boiling water or in an electric sterilizer). Travelers may wish to pack enough formula for their trip, because manufacturing standards vary widely around the world.

Tell travelers not to bring perishable food from high-risk areas back to their home country without refrigeration. Moreover, travelers should exercise the same cautions about food and water served on flights that they do for restaurants.

## WATER

### Drinking Water and Other Beverages

In many parts of the world, particularly where water treatment, sanitation, and hygiene are inadequate, tap water may contain disease-causing agents, including viruses, bacteria, and parasites, or chemical contaminants. As a result, tap water in some places may be unsafe for drinking, preparing food and beverages, making ice, cooking, and brushing teeth. Infants, young children, pregnant women, the elderly, and people whose immune systems are compromised (for example, because of HIV, chemotherapy, or transplant medications) may be especially susceptible to illness.

Travelers should avoid drinking or putting into their mouths tap water unless they are reasonably certain it is safe. Many people choose to disinfect or filter their water when traveling to destinations where safe tap water may not be available. Tap water that is safe for drinking is still not sterile and should not be used for sinus or nasal irrigation or rinsing, including use in neti pots and for ritual ablution unless it is further disinfected by the traveler. Tap water should never be used to clean or rinse contact lenses. Water that looks cloudy or colored may be contaminated with chemicals and will not be made safe by boiling or disinfection. In these situations, travelers should use bottled water if it is available.

In areas where tap water may be unsafe, only commercially bottled water from an unopened, factory-sealed container or water that has been adequately disinfected should be used for drinking, preparing food and beverages, making ice, cooking, and brushing teeth. (See Water Disinfection in this chapter for proper disinfection techniques.)

Beverages made with water that has just been boiled, such as tea and coffee, are generally safe to drink. When served in unopened, factory-sealed cans or bottles, carbonated beverages, commercially prepared fruit drinks, water, alcoholic beverages, and pasteurized drinks generally can be considered safe. Because water on the outside of cans and bottles may be contaminated, they should be wiped clean and dried before opening or drinking directly from the container.

Beverages that may not be safe for consumption include fountain drinks or other drinks made with tap water and iced drinks. Because ice might be made from contaminated water, travelers in areas with unsafe tap water should request that beverages be served without ice.

## Recreational Water

Pathogens that cause gastrointestinal, respiratory, skin, ear, eye, and neurologic illnesses can be transmitted by contaminated recreational water in inadequately treated pools, water playgrounds (splash pads or spray parks) or hot tubs/spas, or in freshwater or marine water. Recreational water contaminated by human feces from swimmers, sewage, animal waste, or wastewater runoff can appear clear but still contain disease-causing infectious or chemical agents. Ingesting even small amounts of such water can cause illness. To protect other people, children and adults with diarrhea should not enter recreational water. Infectious pathogens, such as *Cryptosporidium*, can survive for days even in well-maintained pools, water playgrounds, and hot tubs/spas.

Maintaining proper pH and free chlorine or bromine concentration is necessary to prevent transmission of most infectious pathogens in water in pools, water playgrounds, and hot tubs/spas. If travelers would like to test recreational water before use, CDC recommends pH 7.2–7.8 and a free available chlorine concentration of 2–4 ppm in hot tubs/spas (4–6 ppm if bromine is used) and 1–3 ppm in pools and water playgrounds. Test strips may be purchased at most superstores, hardware stores, and pool supply stores. *Pseudomonas*, which can cause "hot tub rash" or "swimmer's ear," and *Legionella* (see Chapter 4, Legionellosis) can multiply in hot tubs and spas in which chlorine or bromine concentrations are not adequately maintained. Travelers at increased risk for legionellosis, such as the elderly and those with immunocompromising conditions, may choose to avoid entering or walking near higher-risk areas such as hot tubs/spas. Travelers should avoid pools, water playgrounds, and hot tubs/spas where bather limits are not enforced or where the water is cloudy. Additional guidance can be found at www.cdc.gov/healthywater/swimming.

Travelers should not swim or wade 1) near storm drains; 2) in water that may be contaminated with sewage, human or animal feces, or wastewater runoff; 3) in lakes or rivers after heavy rainfall; 4) in freshwater streams, canals, and lakes in schistosomiasis-endemic areas of the Caribbean, South America, Africa, and Asia (see Chapter 4, Schistosomiasis); 5) in water that might be contaminated with urine from animals infected with *Leptospira* (see Chapter 4, Leptospirosis); or 6) in warm seawater or brackish water (mixture of fresh and sea water) when they have wounds.

A traveler with an open wound should consider staying out of the water or covering the wound with a water-repellent bandage (often labeled "waterproof"), as seawater and brackish water can contain germs, such as *Vibrio* spp., that can cause wound infections. If a sore or open wound comes into contact with untreated recreational water, it should be washed thoroughly with soap and water to reduce the chance of infection.

*Naegleria fowleri* (www.cdc.gov/parasites/naegleria) is a parasite found in warm freshwater around the world. To help prevent a rare but fatal infection caused by this parasite, travelers should hold their nose shut or wear a nose clip when swimming, diving, or participating in similar activities in warm freshwater (including lakes, rivers, ponds, hot springs, or locations with water warmed by discharge from power plants and industrial complexes). They should also avoid digging in or stirring up sediment, especially in warm water. This infection has also been linked to use of contaminated tap water for sinus and nasal irrigation.

BIBLIOGRAPHY

1. CDC. Notes from the field: primary amebic meningo-encephalitis associated with ritual nasal rinsing—St. Thomas, US Virgin Islands, 2012. MMWR Morb Mortal Wkly Rep. 2013 Nov 15;62(45):903.

2. Drinking Water: Camping, Hiking, Travel. CDC; 2016. [cited 2016 Apr 15]. Available from: www.cdc.gov/healthywater/drinking/travel/index.html.

3. Eberhart-Phillips J, Besser RE, Tormey MP, Koo D, Feikin D, Araneta MR, et al. An outbreak of cholera from food served on an international aircraft. Epidemiol Infect. 1996 Feb;116(1):9–13.

4. Food Safety. CDC; 2018. [cited 2018 Mar 4]. Available from: www.cdc.gov/foodsafety/index.html.

5. Healthy Swimming: Ear Infections. CDC; 2016. [cited 2016 Apr 15]. Available from: www.cdc.gov/healthywater/swimming/swimmers/rwi/ear-infections.html.

6. Healthy Swimming: Rashes. CDC; 2016. [cited 2016 Apr 15]. Available from: www.cdc.gov/healthywater/swimming/swimmers/rwi/rashes.html.

7. *Legionella* (Legionnaires' Disease and Pontiac Fever). CDC; 2017. [cited 2018 Mar 4]. Available from: www.cdc.gov/legionella/index.html.

8. Parasites—*Naegleria fowleri*—Primary amebic meningoencephalitis (PAM) - Amebic Encephalitis. CDC; 2017. [cited 2016 Apr 15]. Available from: www.cdc.gov/parasites/naegleria/index.html.

9. Traveler's Health: Food and Water Safety. CDC; 2018. [cited 2018 Mar 4]. Available from: wwwnc.cdc.gov/travel/page/food-water-safety.

10. Yoder JS, Straif-Bourgeois S, Roy SL, Moore TA, Visvesvara GS, Ratard RC, et al. Primary amebic meningoencephalitis deaths associated with sinus irrigation using contaminated tap water. Clin Infect Dis. 2012 Nov;55(9):e79–85.

# WATER DISINFECTION

Howard D. Backer, Vincent Hill

## RISK FOR TRAVELERS

Waterborne disease is a risk for international travelers who visit countries that have poor hygiene and inadequate sanitation, and for wilderness visitors who rely on surface water in any country, including the United States. The list of potential waterborne pathogens is extensive and includes bacteria, viruses, protozoa, and parasitic helminths. Most of the organisms that can cause travelers' diarrhea can be waterborne. Many types of bacteria and viruses can cause intestinal (enteric) infection through drinking water. Protozoa that are commonly waterborne include *Cryptosporidium*, *Giardia*, and *Entameba histolytica* (the cause of amebic dysentery). Parasitic worms are not commonly transmitted through drinking water, but it is a potential means of transmission for some.

Where treated tap water is available, aging or inadequate water treatment infrastructure may not effectively disinfect water or maintain water quality during distribution. Some larger hotels and resorts may provide additional onsite water treatment to provide potable water. Travelers can ask the facility manager about safety of their water; however, if there is concern, it may be easiest for travelers to treat the water themselves. Where untreated surface or well water is used and there is no sanitation infrastructure, the risk of waterborne infection is high.

Bottled water has become the convenient solution for most travelers, but in some places it may not be superior to tap water. Moreover, the plastic bottles create an ecological problem, since most developing countries do not recycle plastic bottles. All international travelers, especially long-term travelers or expatriates, should become familiar with and use simple methods to ensure safe drinking water. Several methods are scalable and some can be improvised from local resources, allowing adaptation to disaster relief and refugee situations. Table 2-7 compares benefits and limitations of different methods. Additional information on water treatment and disinfections methods can be found at www.cdc.gov/healthywater/drinking/travel.

## FIELD TECHNIQUES FOR WATER TREATMENT

### Heat

Common intestinal pathogens are readily inactivated by heat. Microorganisms are killed in a shorter time at higher temperatures, whereas temperatures as low as 140°F (60°C) are effective with a longer contact time. Pasteurization uses this principle to kill foodborne enteric pathogens and spoilage-causing organisms at temperatures between 140°F (60°C) and 158°F (70°C), well below the boiling point of water (212°F [100°C]).

Although boiling is not necessary to kill common intestinal pathogens, it is the only easily recognizable end point that does not require a thermometer. All organisms except bacterial spores, which are rarely waterborne enteric pathogens, are killed in seconds at boiling temperature. In addition, the time required to heat

the water from 60°C to boiling works toward heat disinfection. Any water that is brought to a boil should be adequately disinfected; however, if fuel supplies are adequate, travelers should consider boiling for 1 minute to allow for a margin of safety. Although the boiling point decreases with altitude, at common terrestrial travel elevations it is still well above the temperature required to inactivate enteric pathogens (for example, at 16,000 ft [4,877 m] the boiling temperature of water is 182°F [84°C]). In hot climates with sunshine, a water container placed in a simple reflective solar oven can reach pasteurization temperature of 65°C. Travelers with access to electricity can bring a small electric heating coil or a lightweight beverage warmer to boil water.

### Filtration and Clarification

Portable hand-pump or gravity-drip filters with various designs and types of filter media are commercially available to international travelers. Filter pore size is the primary determinant of a filter's effectiveness, unless the filter is designed to remove microbes by electrochemical attachment to filter media. Filter pore size will be described as being "absolute" or "nominal": absolute pore size filters will remove all microbes of the identified pore size or larger, whereas nominal pore size filters allow 20%–30% of particles or microorganisms of the pore size to pass through. Progressively smaller pore size filters require higher pressure to push water through the filter, often at a slower rate and higher cost. Filters that claim Environmental Protection Agency (EPA) designation of water "purifier" undergo company-sponsored testing to demonstrate removal of at least $10^6$ bacteria (99.9999%), $10^4$ viruses (99.99%), and $10^3$ *Cryptosporidium* oocysts or *Giardia* cysts (99.9%). (EPA does not independently test the validity of these claims.)

Filters with absolute pore size of 1 μm or smaller should effectively remove protozoan parasites like Cryptosporidium and Giardia. Microfilters with "absolute" pore sizes of 0.1–0.4 μm are usually effective at removing bacteria as well as cysts but may not adequately remove enteric viruses, like norovirus (Table 2-8). Water in remote alpine areas with little human and animal activity generally has little contamination with

# Table 2-7. Comparison of water disinfection techniques

| TECHNIQUE | ADVANTAGES | DISADVANTAGES |
|---|---|---|
| Heat | • Does not impart additional taste or color<br>• Single step that inactivates all enteric pathogens<br>• Efficacy is not compromised by contaminants or particles in the water as for chemical disinfection and filtration | • Does not improve taste, smell, or appearance of source water<br>• Fuel sources may be scarce, expensive, or unavailable<br>• Does not prevent recontamination during storage |
| Filtration | • Simple to operate<br>• Requires no holding time for treatment<br>• Large choice of commercial product designs<br>• Adds no unpleasant taste and often improves taste and appearance of water<br>• Can be combined with chemical disinfection to increase microbe removal | • Adds bulk and weight to baggage<br>• Many filters do not reliably remove viruses<br>• More expensive than chemical treatment<br>• Eventually clogs from suspended particulate matter and may require some field maintenance or repair<br>• Does not prevent recontamination during storage |
| Chlorine, iodine, electrolytic solutions | • Inexpensive and widely available in liquid or tablet form<br>• Taste can be removed by simple techniques<br>• Flexible dosing<br>• Equally easy to treat large and small volumes<br>• Will preserve microbiologic quality of stored water | • Impart taste and odor to water<br>• Flexible dosing requires understanding of principles<br>• Iodine is physiologically active, with potential adverse effects<br>• Not readily effective against *Cryptosporidium* oocysts<br>• Efficacy decreases with cloudy water<br>• Corrosive and stains clothing |
| Chlorine dioxide | • Low doses have no taste or color<br>• Simple to use and available in liquid or tablet form<br>• More potent than equivalent doses of chlorine<br>• Effective against all waterborne pathogens, including *Cryptosporidium* | • Volatile and sensitive to sunlight: do not expose tablets to air, and use generated solutions rapidly<br>• No persistent residual concentration, so does not prevent recontamination during storage |
| Ultraviolet (UV) | • Imparts no taste<br>• Portable battery-operated devices now available<br>• Effective against all waterborne pathogens<br>• Extra doses of UV can be used for added assurance and with no side effects | • Requires clear water<br>• Does not improve taste or appearance of water<br>• Relatively expensive (except solar disinfection [SODIS])<br>• Requires batteries or power source (except SODIS)<br>• Cannot know if devices are delivering required UV doses<br>• No persistent residual concentration, so does not prevent recontamination during storage |

enteric pathogens, so microfilters with ceramic, synthetic fiber, compressed carbon, or large-pore hollow-fiber filter elements are sufficient to remove bacteria and protozoan cysts, the primary pathogens.

For areas with high levels of human and animal activity in the watershed or developing areas with poor sanitation, higher levels of filtration discussed below or other techniques to remove viruses are preferred. If using a microfilter,

## Table 2-8. Microorganism size and susceptibility to filtration

| ORGANISM | AVERAGE SIZE (μM) | MAXIMUM RECOMMENDED FILTER RATING (μM ABSOLUTE) |
|---|---|---|
| Viruses | 0.03 | Not specified (optimally 0.01, ultrafiltration) |
| Enteric bacteria (such as *Escherichia coli*) | 0.5 × 2–8 | 0.2–0.4 (microfiltration) |
| *Cryptosporidium* oocyst | 4–6 | 1 (microfiltration) |
| *Giardia* cyst | 8 × 19 | 3.0–5.0 (microfiltration) |
| Helminth eggs | 30 × 60 | Not specified; any microfilter |
| Schistosome larvae | 50 × 100 | Not specified; any microfilter |

one option to remove viruses is pretreatment with chlorine. Progressively finer levels of filtration known as ultrafiltration, nanofiltration, and reverse osmosis can remove particles of 0.01, 0.001, and 0.0001 μm, respectively. All of these filters can remove viruses. Portable ultrafilters are the most commonly available "purifying" filters and may operate by gravity, hand-pump, or drink-through. Ultrafilter-based filters will have a rated pore size of 0.01 μm, and should be effective for removing viruses, bacteria, and parasites. All are effective, although drink-through is least practical because of the negative pressure required to draw water through the filter.

Nanofilters will have rated pore sizes of 0.001 μm and thus will remove chemicals and organic molecules. Reverse osmosis filters (having pore sizes of 0.0001 μm [0.1 nm] and smaller) will remove monovalent salts and dissolved metals, thus achieving desalination. The high price and slow output of small hand-pump reverse osmosis units prohibit use by land-based travelers; however, they are survival aids for ocean voyagers, and larger powered devices are used for military and refugee situations.

In resource-limited international settings, filters may be used in the communities and households that are made from ceramic clay or simple sand and gravel (slow sand or biosand). Gravel and sand filters can be improvised in remote or austere situations when no other means of disinfection is available.

Water can be clarified by using chemical products that coagulate and flocculate (clump together) suspended particles that cause a cloudy appearance and bad taste and do not settle by gravity. This process removes many but not all microorganisms, unless the product also contains a disinfectant. Alum, an aluminum salt that is widely used in food, cosmetic, and medical applications, is the principal agent for coagulation/flocculation, but many other natural substances are used throughout the world. When using alum, a one-fourth teaspoon of alum powder can be added to a quart of cloudy water and the water stirred frequently for a few minutes. The process can be repeated, if necessary, until clumps form. The clumped material is allowed to settle, and then the water is poured through a coffee filter or clean, fine cloth to remove the sediment. Most microbes are removed, but not all, so a second disinfection step is necessary. Tablets or packets of powder that combine flocculant and a chemical disinfectant are available commercially (for example, Chlor-floc and P&G Purifier of Water).

Granular-activated carbon (GAC) treats water by adsorbing organic and inorganic chemicals (including chlorine or iodine compounds) and most heavy metals, thereby improving odor, taste, and safety. GAC is a common component of household and field filters. It may trap microorganisms, but GAC filters are generally not designed or rated for microbe removal and do not kill microorganisms.

## Chemical Disinfection

### LIQUID AND TABLET PRODUCTS

Chemical disinfectants for drinking water treatment, including chlorine compounds, iodine, and chlorine dioxide, are commonly available as commercial products. Sodium hypochlorite, the active ingredient in common household bleach, is the primary disinfectant promoted by CDC and the World Health Organization. Other chlorine-containing compounds such as calcium hypochlorite and sodium dichloroisocyanurate, available in granular or tablet formulation, are equally effective for water treatment. An advantage of chemical water disinfection products is flexible dosing that allows use by individual travelers, small or large groups, or communities. In emergency situations, or when other commercial chemical disinfection water treatment products are not available, household bleach can be used for flexible dosing based on water volume and clarity. Refer to CDC guidelines at www.cdc.gov/healthywater/emergency/drinking/making-water-safe.html.

Given adequate concentrations and length of exposure (contact time), chlorine and iodine have similar activity and are effective against bacteria and viruses (www.cdc.gov/safewater/effectiveness-on-pathogens.html). *Giardia* cysts are more resistant to chemical disinfection; however, field-level concentrations are effective with longer contact times. For this reason, dosing and concentrations of chemical disinfection products are generally targeted to the cysts. Some common waterborne parasites, such as *Cryptosporidium* and possibly *Cyclospora*, are poorly inactivated by chlorine- and iodine-based disinfection at practical concentrations, even with extended contact times.

Chemical disinfection may be supplemented with filtration to remove resistant oocysts from drinking water. Cloudy water contains substances that will neutralize disinfectant, so it will require higher concentrations or contact times or, preferably, clarification through settling, coagulation/flocculation, or filtration before disinfectant is added.

Because iodine has physiologic activity, WHO recommends limiting iodine water disinfection to a few weeks. Iodine use is not recommended for people with unstable thyroid disease or known iodine allergy. In addition, pregnant women should not use iodine to disinfect water over the long term because of the potential effect on the fetal thyroid. Pregnant travelers who have other options should use an alternative means such as heat, chlorine, or filtration.

Some prefer the taste of iodine to chlorine, but neither is appealing in doses often recommended for field use. The taste of halogens in water can be improved by running water through a filter containing activated carbon or adding a 25-mg tablet of vitamin C, a tiny pinch of powdered ascorbic acid, or a small amount of hydrogen peroxide (5–10 drops of 3% peroxide per quart), then stir or shake. Repeat until taste of chlorine or iodine is gone.

### CHLORINE DIOXIDE

Chlorine dioxide ($ClO_2$) can kill most waterborne pathogens, including *Cryptosporidium* oocysts, at practical doses and contact times. Tablets and liquid formulations are commercially available to generate chlorine dioxide in the field for personal use.

### SALT (SODIUM CHLORIDE) ELECTROLYSIS

Electrolytic water purifiers generate a mixture of oxidants, including hypochlorite, by passing an electrical current through a simple brine salt solution. Purifier products sold for personal and group travel use produce an oxidant solution that can be added to water to kill microorganisms. This technique has been engineered into portable, battery-powered products that are commercially available.

## Ultraviolet (UV) Light

UV light kills bacteria, viruses, and *Cryptosporidium* oocysts in water. The effect depends on UV dose and exposure time. Portable battery-operated units that deliver a metered, timed dose of UV are an effective way to disinfect small quantities of clear water in the field. Larger units with higher output are available where a power source is available. These units have limited effectiveness in water with high levels of suspended solids and turbidity, because suspended particles can shield microorganisms from UV light.

## Solar Irradiation and Heating

UV irradiation of water using sunlight (solar disinfection or SODIS) can improve the microbiologic quality of water and may be used in austere emergency situations. Solar disinfection is not effective on turbid water. If the headlines in a newspaper cannot be read through the bottle of water, then the water must be clarified before solar irradiation is used. Under cloudy weather conditions, water must be placed in the sun for 2 consecutive days. (See www.sodis.ch/index_EN for further information.)

## Silver and Other Products

Silver ion has bactericidal effects in low doses, and some attractive features include lack of color, taste, and odor, and the ability of a thin coating on the container to maintain a steady, low concentration in water. Silver is widely used by European travelers as a primary drinking water disinfectant. In the United States, silver is approved only for maintaining microbiologic quality of stored water because its concentration can be strongly affected by adsorption onto the surface of the container, and there has been limited testing on viruses and cysts. Silver is available alone or in combination with chlorine in tablet formulation.

Several other common products, including hydrogen peroxide, citrus juice, and potassium permanganate, have antibacterial effects in water and are marketed in commercial products for travelers. None have sufficient data to recommend them for primary water disinfection at low doses in the field.

## Photocatalytic Disinfection

Advanced oxidation processes use UV light or natural sunlight to catalyze the production of potent disinfectants for microorganisms and can break down complex organic contaminants and even most heavy metals into nontoxic forms. Titanium dioxide ($TiO_2$) is the most effective substance, but other metal oxides, chitins, and nanoparticles also have oxidative potential. A $TiO_2$-impregnated membrane incorporated into a portable bag is available commercially.

## CHOOSING A DISINFECTION TECHNIQUE

Table 2-9 summarizes advantages and disadvantages of field water disinfection techniques and their microbicidal efficacy. It is advisable to test a method before travel.

## Table 2-9. Summary of field water disinfection techniques

| | BACTERIA | VIRUSES | PROTOZOAN CYSTS (GIARDIA/AMEBAS) | CRYPTOSPORIDIA | HELMINTHS/ SCHISTOSOMES |
|---|---|---|---|---|---|
| Heat | + | + | + | + | + |
| Filtration | + | +/−[1] | + | + | + |
| Halogens | + | + | +[2] | − | +/−[3] |
| Chlorine dioxide | + | + | + | + | + |

[1] Most filters make no claims for viruses. Hollow-fiber filters with ultrafiltration pore size and reverse osmosis are effective.
[2] Require higher concentrations and contact time than for bacteria or viruses.
[3] Eggs are not very susceptible to chlorine or iodine, but risk of waterborne transmission is very low.

## BIBLIOGRAPHY

1. Backer H. Field water disinfection. In: Auerbach PS, editor. Wilderness Medicine. 7th ed. Philadelphia: Mosby Elsevier; 2017. pp. 1985–2030.

2. Backer H, Hollowell J. Use of iodine for water disinfection: iodine toxicity and maximum recommended dose. Environ Health Perspect. 2000 Aug;108(8):679–84.

3. Bielefeldt AR. Appropriate and sustainable water disinfection methods for developing communities. In: Buchaman K, editor. Water Disinfection. New York City: Nova Science; 2011. pp. 41–75.

4. CDC. Safe water systems for the developing world: a handbook for implementing household-based water treatment and safe storage projects. Atlanta: CDC, 2000 [cited 2016 Sep 19]. Available from: www.cdc.gov/safewater/pdf/sws-for-the-developing-world-manual.pdf.

5. Clasen T, Roberts I, Rabie T, Schmidt W, Cairncross S. Interventions to improve water quality for preventing diarrhoea. Cochrane Database Syst Rev. 2006;(3):CD004794.

6. Ciochetti DA, Metcalf RH. Pasteurization of naturally contaminated water with solar energy. Appl Environ Microbiol. 1984 Feb;47(2):223–8.

7. Sobsey MD, Stauber CE, Casanova LM, Brown JM, Elliott MA. Point of use household drinking water filtration: a practical, effective solution for providing sustained access to safe drinking water in the developing world. Environ Sci Technol. 2008 Jun 15;42(12):4261–7.

8. Swiss Federal Institute of Aquatic Science and Technology. SODIS method. Dübendorf, Switzerland: Swiss Federal Institute of Aquatic Science and Technology; 2012 [cited 2016 Sep 21]. Available from: www.sodis.ch/methode/index_EN.

9. Wilhelm N, Kaufmann A, Blanton E, Lantagne D. Sodium Hypochlorite Dosage for Household and Emergency Water Treatment: updated recommendations. J Water Health. 2018;16:112–25.

10. World Health Organization. Boil water. Technical Brief. WHO; 2015 [cited 2016 Mar 13]. Available from: http://apps.who.int/iris/bitstream/10665/155821/1/WHO_FWC_WSH_15.02_eng.pdf?ua=1.

11. World Health Organization. Guidelines for drinking-water quality. WHO; 2011 [cited 2016 Mar 13]. Available from: http://apps.who.int/iris/bitstream/10665/44584/1/9789241548151_eng.pdf.

# FOOD POISONING FROM MARINE TOXINS

Vernon E. Ansdell

Poisoning from ingested marine toxins is an underrecognized hazard for travelers, particularly in the tropics and subtropics. Furthermore, the risk is increasing because of climate change, coral reef damage, and spread of toxic algal blooms (Map 2-30).

## CIGUATERA FISH POISONING

Ciguatera fish poisoning occurs after eating reef fish contaminated with toxins such as ciguatoxin or maitotoxin. These potent toxins originate from *Gambierdiscus toxicus*, a small marine organism (dinoflagellate) that grows on and around coral reefs. Dinoflagellates are ingested by herbivorous fish. The toxins produced by *G. toxicus* are then modified and concentrated as they pass up the marine food chain to carnivorous fish and finally to humans. Ciguatoxins are concentrated in fish liver, intestines, roe, and heads.

*G. toxicus* may proliferate on dead coral reefs more effectively than other dinoflagellates. The risk of ciguatera poisoning is likely to increase as coral reefs deteriorate because of climate change, ocean acidification, offshore construction, and nutrient runoff.

### Risk for Travelers

Up to 50,000 cases of ciguatera poisoning get reported annually worldwide. Because the disease is underrecognized and underreported, this is likely a significant underestimate. The incidence in travelers to highly endemic areas has been estimated as high as 3 per 100. Ciguatera

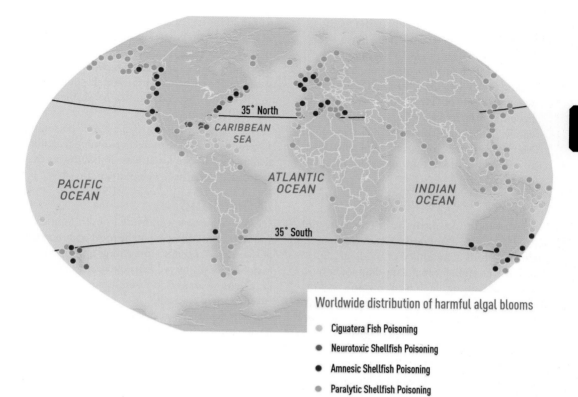

Worldwide distribution of harmful algal blooms

- Ciguatera Fish Poisoning
- Neurotoxic Shellfish Poisoning
- Amnesic Shellfish Poisoning
- Paralytic Shellfish Poisoning

**MAP 2-30. Areas reporting select harmful algal blooms**

Harmful algal blooms occur widely and contribute to seafood toxicity. Risk of poisoning in humans depends on the particular seafood consumed, where it was caught or harvested, and—in some instances—the exposure of that seafood to a harmful algal bloom.

Harmful algal bloom data from Woods Hole Oceanographic Institution, Woods Hole, MA: 2015. [cited 2018 Aug 28]. Available from: www.whoi.edu/redtide/regions/world-distribution.

is widespread in tropical and subtropical waters, usually between the latitudes of 35°N and 35°S; it is particularly common in the Pacific and Indian Oceans and the Caribbean Sea. The incidence and geographic distribution of ciguatera poisoning are increasing. Newly recognized areas of risk include the Canary Islands, the eastern Mediterranean, and the western Gulf of Mexico. Medical practitioners must be aware that cases of ciguatera fish poisoning acquired by travelers in endemic areas may present in nonendemic (temperate) areas. In addition, cases of ciguatera fish poisoning are seen with increasing frequency in nonendemic areas as a result of the increasing global trade in seafood products.

Fish that are most likely to cause ciguatera poisoning are large carnivorous reef fish, such as barracuda, grouper, moray eel, amberjack, sea bass, or sturgeon. Omnivorous and herbivorous fish such as parrot fish, surgeonfish, and red snapper can also be a risk.

## Clinical Presentation

Ciguatera poisoning may cause gastrointestinal, cardiovascular, neurologic, and neuropsychiatric illness. The first symptoms usually develop within 3–6 hours after eating contaminated fish but may be delayed for up to 30 hours. Adverse health effects referable to the above-named organ systems include:

- Diarrhea, nausea, vomiting, and abdominal pain

- Bradycardia, heart block, hypotension

- Paresthesias, weakness, pain in the teeth or a sensation that the teeth are loose, burning or metallic taste in the mouth, generalized itching, sweating, and blurred vision. Cold allodynia (abnormal sensation when touching cold water or objects) has been reported as characteristic, but there can be acute sensitivity to both hot and cold. Neurologic symptoms usually last a few days to several weeks but may persist for months or even years.

- Fatigue, general malaise, insomnia

The overall death rate from ciguatera poisoning is <0.1% but varies according to the toxin dose and availability of medical care to deal with complications. The diagnosis of ciguatera poisoning is based on the characteristic signs and symptoms and a history of eating fish species known to carry ciguatera toxin. Fish testing can be done by the US Food and Drug Administration (FDA) in their laboratory at Dauphin Island. There is no readily available test for ciguatera toxins in human clinical specimens.

## Prevention

Travelers can take the following precautions to prevent ciguatera fish poisoning:

- Avoid or limit consumption of reef fish.

- Never eat high-risk fish such as barracuda or moray eel.

- Avoid eating the parts of the fish that concentrate ciguatera toxin: liver, intestines, roe, and head.

Ciguatera toxins do not affect the texture, taste, or smell of fish, nor are they destroyed by gastric acid, cooking, smoking, freezing, canning, salting, or pickling.

## Treatment

There is no specific antidote for ciguatoxin or maitotoxin poisonings. Symptomatic treatment may include gabapentin or pregabalin (neuropathic symptoms), amitriptyline (chronic paresthesias, depression, and pruritus), fluoxetine (chronic fatigue), and nifedipine or acetaminophen (headaches). Intravenous mannitol has been reported in uncontrolled studies to reduce the severity and duration of neurologic symptoms, particularly if given within 48 hours of the appearance of symptoms. It should only be given to hemodynamically stable, well-hydrated patients.

After recovering from ciguatera poisoning, patients may want to avoid consuming fish, nuts, alcohol, or caffeine for at least 6 months, as they may cause a relapse in symptoms.

## SCOMBROID

Scombroid occurs worldwide in both temperate and tropical waters. One of the most common fish poisonings, it occurs after eating improperly refrigerated or preserved fish containing high levels of histamine and often resembles a moderate to severe allergic reaction.

Fish typically associated with scombroid have naturally high levels of histidine in the flesh and include tuna, mackerel, mahi mahi (dolphin fish), sardine, anchovy, herring, bluefish, amberjack, and marlin. Histidine is converted to histamine by bacterial overgrowth in fish improperly stored after capture. Histamine and other scombrotoxins are resistant to cooking, smoking, canning, or freezing.

### Clinical Presentation

Scombroid poisoning resembles an acute allergic reaction, usually appearing 10–60 minutes after eating contaminated fish. Symptoms include flushing of the face and upper body (resembling sunburn), severe headache, palpitations, itching, blurred vision, abdominal cramps, and diarrhea. Untreated, symptoms usually resolve within 12 hours but may last up to 48 hours. Rarely, there may be respiratory compromise, malignant arrhythmias, and hypotension requiring hospitalization. There are no long-term sequelae. Diagnosis is usually clinical. Clustering of cases helps exclude the possibility of true fish allergy.

### Prevention

Fish contaminated with histamine may have a peppery, sharp, salty, taste or "bubbly" feel but will usually look, smell, and taste normal. The key to prevention is to make sure that the fish is properly iced or refrigerated at temperatures <38°F (<3.3°C) or immediately frozen after being caught. Cooking, smoking, canning, or freezing will not destroy histamine in contaminated fish.

## Treatment

Scombroid poisoning usually responds well to antihistamines ($H_1$-receptor blockers, although $H_2$-receptor blockers may also provide some benefit).

## SHELLFISH POISONING

Several forms of poisoning may occur after ingesting toxin-containing shellfish, including filter-feeding bivalve mollusks (mussels, oysters, clams, scallops, and cockles), gastropod mollusks (abalone, whelks, and moon snails), or crustaceans (Dungeness crab, shrimp, and lobster). Toxins originate in small marine organisms (dinoflagellates or diatoms) that are ingested and are concentrated by shellfish.

## Risk for Travelers

Contaminated (toxic) shellfish may be found in temperate and tropical waters, typically during or after phytoplankton blooms, also called harmful algal blooms (HABs). One example of a HAB is the Florida red tide caused by *Karenia brevis*.

## Clinical Presentation

Poisoning results in gastrointestinal and neurologic illness of varying severity. Symptoms typically appear 30–60 minutes after ingesting toxic shellfish but can be delayed for several hours. Diagnosis is usually one of exclusion and typically is made clinically in patients who have recently eaten shellfish.

### PARALYTIC SHELLFISH POISONING

Paralytic shellfish poisoning (PSP) is the most common and most severe form of shellfish poisoning. PSP is caused by eating shellfish contaminated with saxitoxins. These potent neurotoxins are produced by various dinoflagellates. A wide range of shellfish may cause PSP, but most cases occur after eating mussels or clams.

PSP occurs worldwide but is most common in temperate waters, especially off the Pacific and Atlantic Coasts of North America, including Alaska. The Philippines, China, Chile, Scotland, Ireland, New Zealand, and Australia have all reported cases.

Symptoms usually appear 30–60 minutes after eating toxic shellfish and include numbness and tingling of the face, lips, tongue, arms, and legs. There may be headache, nausea, vomiting, and diarrhea. Severe cases are associated with ingestion of large doses of toxin and clinical features such as ataxia, dysphagia, mental status changes, flaccid paralysis, and respiratory failure. The case-fatality ratio is dependent on the availability of modern medical care, including mechanical ventilation. The death rate may be particularly high in children.

### NEUROTOXIC SHELLFISH POISONING

Neurotoxic shellfish poisoning (NSP) is caused by eating shellfish contaminated with brevetoxins produced by the dinoflagellate *K. brevis*. Predominately an illness of the Western Hemisphere (southeastern coast of the United States, the Gulf of Mexico, and the Caribbean), there are also reports of the disease from New Zealand.

NSP usually presents as a gastroenteritis accompanied by neurologic symptoms resembling mild ciguatera or paralytic shellfish poisoning, 30 minutes to 3 hours after a shellfish meal. A syndrome known as aerosolized red tide respiratory irritation (ARTRI) occurs when aerosolized brevetoxins are inhaled in sea spray. This has been reported in association with a red tide (*K. brevis* HAB) in Florida. It can induce bronchoconstriction and may cause acute, temporary respiratory discomfort in healthy people. People with asthma may experience more severe and prolonged respiratory effects.

### DIARRHEIC SHELLFISH POISONING

Diarrheic shellfish poisoning (DSP) is caused by eating shellfish contaminated with toxins such as okadaic acid. It occurs worldwide, with outbreaks reported from China, Japan, Scandinavia, France,

Belgium, Spain, Chile, Uruguay, Ireland, the United States, and Canada.

Most cases result from eating toxic bivalve mollusks such as mussels and scallops. Symptoms usually occur within 2 hours of eating contaminated shellfish and include chills, diarrhea, nausea, vomiting, and abdominal pain. Symptoms usually resolve within 2–3 days. No deaths have been reported.

### AMNESIC SHELLFISH POISONING

Amnesic shellfish poisoning (ASP) is a rare form of shellfish poisoning caused by eating shellfish contaminated with domoic acid, produced by the diatom *Pseudonitzchia* spp. Outbreaks of ASP have been reported in Canada, Scotland, Ireland, France, Belgium, Spain, Portugal, New Zealand, Australia, and Chile. Implicated shellfish include mussels, scallops, razor clams, and other crustaceans.

In most cases, gastrointestinal symptoms such as diarrhea, vomiting, and abdominal pain develop within 24 hours of eating toxic shellfish, followed by headache, memory loss, and cognitive impairment. In severe cases there may be hypotension, arrhythmias, ophthalmoplegia, coma, and death. Survivors may have severe anterograde, short-term memory deficits.

## Prevention

Shellfish poisoning can be prevented by avoiding potentially contaminated shellfish. This is particularly important in areas during or shortly after algal blooms, which may be locally referred to as "red tides" or "brown tides." Shellfish also carry a significant risk of infection from various viral and bacterial infections, for example hepatitis A virus, norovirus, *Vibrio vulnificus*, *Vibrio parahaemolyticus*, and several *Salmonella* and *Shigella* species. Ideally, travelers to developing countries should avoid eating all shellfish. Marine shellfish toxins cannot be destroyed by cooking or freezing.

## Treatment

Treatment is symptomatic and supportive. Severe cases of paralytic shellfish poisoning may require mechanical ventilation.

### BIBLIOGRAPHY

1. Chan TY. Ciguatera fish poisoning in East Asia and Southeast Asia. Mar Drugs. 2015 Jun 2;13(6):3466–78.

2. Friedman MA, Fleming LE, Fernandez M et al. Ciguatera fish poisoning: treatment, prevention and management. Mar Drugs. 2008;6:456–79.

3. Hungerford JM. Scombroid poisoning: a review. Toxicon. 2010 Aug 15;56(2):231–43.

4. Isbister GK, Kiernan MC. Neurotoxic marine poisoning. Lancet Neurol. 2005 Apr;4(4):219–28.

5. Palafox NA, Buenoconsejo-Lum LE. Ciguatera fish poisoning: review of clinical manifestations. J Toxicol Toxin Rev. 2001 May;20(2):141–60.

6. Schnorf H, Taurarii M, Cundy T. Ciguatera fish poisoning: a double-blind randomized trial of mannitol therapy. Neurology. 2002 Mar 26;58(6):873–80.

7. Sobel J, Painter J. Illnesses caused by marine toxins. Clin Infect Dis. 2005 Nov 1;41(9):1290–6.

# TRAVELERS' DIARRHEA

Bradley A. Connor

Travelers' diarrhea (TD) is the most predictable travel-related illness. Attack rates range from 30% to 70% of travelers, depending on the destination and season of travel. Traditionally, it was thought that TD could be prevented by following simple recommendations such as "boil it, cook it, peel it, or forget it," but studies have found that people who follow these rules may still become ill. Poor hygiene practice in local restaurants is likely the largest contributor to the risk for TD.

TD is a clinical syndrome that can result from a variety of intestinal pathogens. Bacterial pathogens are the predominant risk, thought to account for up to 80%–90% of TD. Intestinal viruses may account for at least 5%–15% of illnesses, although multiplex molecular diagnostic assays increase their detection. Infections with protozoal pathogens are slower to manifest symptoms and collectively account for approximately 10% of diagnoses in longer-term travelers. What is commonly known as "food poisoning" involves the ingestion of preformed toxins in food. In this syndrome, vomiting and diarrhea may both be present, but symptoms usually resolve spontaneously within 12 hours.

## INFECTIOUS AGENTS

Bacteria are the most common cause of TD. Overall, the most common pathogen identified is enterotoxigenic *Escherichia coli*, followed by *Campylobacter jejuni*, *Shigella* spp., and *Salmonella* spp. Enteroaggregative and other *E. coli* pathotypes are also commonly found in cases of TD. There is increasing discussion of *Aeromonas* spp., *Plesiomonas* spp., and newly recognized pathogens (*Acrobacter, Larobacter*, enterotoxigenic *Bacteroides fragilis*) as potential causes of TD as well. Viral diarrhea can be caused by a number of pathogens, including norovirus, rotavirus, and astrovirus.

*Giardia* is the main protozoal pathogen found in TD. *Entamoeba histolytica* is a relatively uncommon cause of TD, and *Cryptosporidium* is also relatively uncommon. The risk for *Cyclospora* is highly geographic and seasonal: the most well-known risks are in Nepal, Peru, Haiti, and Guatemala. *Dientamoeba fragilis* is a flagellate occasionally associated with diarrhea in travelers. Most of the individual pathogens are discussed in their own sections in Chapter 4, and diarrhea in returned travelers is discussed in Chapter 11.

## RISK FOR TRAVELERS

TD occurs equally in male and female travelers and is more common in young adult travelers than in older travelers. In short-term travelers, bouts of TD do not appear to protect against future attacks, and >1 episode of TD may occur during a single trip. A cohort of expatriates residing in Kathmandu, Nepal, experienced an average of 3.2 episodes of TD per person in their first year. In more temperate regions, there may be seasonal variations in diarrhea risk. In south Asia, for example, much higher TD attack rates are reported during the hot months preceding the monsoon.

In environments in warmer climates where large numbers of people do not have access to plumbing or latrines, the amount of stool contamination in the environment will be higher and more accessible to flies. Inadequate electrical capacity may lead to frequent blackouts or poorly functioning refrigeration, which can result in unsafe food storage and an increased risk for disease. Lack of safe water may lead to contaminated foods and drinks prepared with such water; inadequate water supply may lead to shortcuts in cleaning hands, surfaces, utensils, and foods such as fruits and vegetables. In addition, handwashing may not be a social norm and could be an extra expense; thus there may be no handwashing stations in food preparation areas. In destinations in which effective food handling courses have been provided, the risk for TD has been demonstrated to decrease. However, even in developed countries, pathogens such as *Shigella sonnei* have caused TD linked to handling and preparation of food in restaurants.

## CLINICAL PRESENTATION

Bacterial and viral TD presents with the sudden onset of bothersome symptoms that can range from mild cramps and urgent loose stools to severe abdominal pain, fever, vomiting, and bloody diarrhea, although with norovirus vomiting may be more prominent. Protozoal diarrhea, such as that caused by *Giardia intestinalis* or *E. histolytica*, generally has a more gradual onset of low-grade symptoms, with 2–5 loose stools per day. The incubation period between exposure and clinical presentation can be a clue to the etiology:

- Bacterial toxins generally cause symptoms within a few hours.

- Bacterial and viral pathogens have an incubation period of 6–72 hours.

- Protozoal pathogens generally have an incubation period of 1–2 weeks and rarely present in the first few days of travel. An exception can be *Cyclospora cayetanensis*, which can present quickly in areas of high risk.

Untreated bacterial diarrhea usually lasts 3–7 days. Viral diarrhea generally lasts 2–3 days. Protozoal diarrhea can persist for weeks to months without treatment. An acute bout of gastroenteritis can lead to persistent gastrointestinal symptoms, even in the absence of continued infection (see Chapter 11, Persistent Diarrhea in Returned Travelers). This presentation is commonly referred to as postinfectious irritable bowel syndrome. Other postinfectious sequelae may include reactive arthritis and Guillain-Barré syndrome.

## PREVENTION

For travelers to high-risk areas, several approaches may be recommended that can reduce, but never completely eliminate, the risk for TD. These include following instructions regarding food and beverage selection, using agents other than antimicrobial drugs for prophylaxis, using prophylactic antibiotics, and carefully washing hands with soap where available. Carrying small containers of alcohol-based hand sanitizers (containing ≥60% alcohol) may make it easier for travelers to clean their hands before eating when handwashing is not possible. No vaccines are available for most pathogens that cause TD, but travelers should refer to the Cholera, Hepatitis A, and Typhoid & Paratyphoid Fever sections in Chapter 4 regarding vaccines that can prevent other foodborne or waterborne infections to which travelers are susceptible.

### Food and Beverage Selection

Care in selecting food and beverages can minimize the risk for acquiring TD. See the Food & Water Precautions section in this chapter for CDC's detailed food and beverage recommendations. Although food and water precautions continue to be recommended, travelers may not always be able to adhere to the advice. Furthermore, many of the factors that ensure food safety, such as restaurant hygiene, are out of the traveler's control.

## Nonantimicrobial Drugs for Prophylaxis

The primary agent studied for prevention of TD, other than antimicrobial drugs, is bismuth subsalicylate (BSS), which is the active ingredient in adult formulations of Pepto-Bismol and Kaopectate. Studies from Mexico have shown that this agent (taken daily as either 2 oz. of liquid or 2 chewable tablets 4 times per day) reduces the incidence of TD by approximately 50%. BSS commonly causes blackening of the tongue and stool and may cause nausea, constipation, and rarely tinnitus.

Travelers with aspirin allergy, renal insufficiency, and gout, and those taking anticoagulants, probenecid, or methotrexate should not take BSS. In travelers taking aspirin or salicylates for other reasons, the use of BSS may result in salicylate toxicity. BSS is not generally recommended for children aged <12 years; however, some clinicians use it off-label with caution to avoid administering BSS to children aged ≤18 years with viral infections, such as varicella or influenza, because of the risk for Reye syndrome. BSS is not recommended for children aged <3 years or pregnant women. Studies have not established the safety of BSS use for periods >3 weeks. Because of the number of tablets required and the inconvenient dosing, BSS is not commonly used as prophylaxis for TD.

The use of probiotics, such as *Lactobacillus* GG and *Saccharomyces boulardii*, has been studied in the prevention of TD in small numbers of people. Results are inconclusive, partially because standardized preparations of these bacteria are not reliably available. Studies are ongoing with prebiotics to prevent TD, but data are insufficient to recommend their use. There have been anecdotal reports of beneficial outcomes after using bovine colostrum as a daily prophylaxis agent for TD. However, commercially sold preparations of bovine colostrum are marketed as dietary supplements that are not Food and Drug Administration (FDA) approved for medical indications. Because no data from rigorous clinical trials demonstrate efficacy, there is insufficient information to recommend the use of bovine colostrum to prevent TD.

## Prophylactic Antibiotics

Although prophylactic antibiotics can prevent some TD, the emergence of antimicrobial resistance has made the decision of how and when to use antibiotic prophylaxis for TD difficult. Controlled studies have shown that use of antibiotics reduces diarrhea attack rates by 90% or more. The prophylactic antibiotic of choice has changed over the past few decades as resistance patterns have evolved. Fluoroquinolones have been the most effective antibiotics for the prophylaxis and treatment of bacterial TD pathogens, but increasing resistance to these agents among *Campylobacter* and *Shigella* species globally limits their potential use. In addition fluoroquinolones are associated with tendinitis and an increased risk of *Clostridioides difficile* infection, and current guidelines discourage their use for prophylaxis. Alternative considerations include azithromycin, rifaximin, and rifamycin SV.

At this time, prophylactic antibiotics should not be recommended for most travelers. Prophylactic antibiotics afford no protection against nonbacterial pathogens and can remove normally protective microflora from the bowel, increasing the risk of infection with resistant bacterial pathogens. Travelers may become colonized with extended-spectrum β-lactamase (ESBL)–producing bacteria, and this risk is increased by exposure to antibiotics while abroad. Additionally, the use of antibiotics may be associated with allergic or adverse reactions, and prophylactic antibiotics limit the therapeutic options if TD occurs; a traveler relying on prophylactic antibiotics will need to carry an alternative antibiotic to use if severe diarrhea develops despite prophylaxis.

The risks associated with the use of prophylactic antibiotics should be weighed against the benefit of using prompt, early self-treatment with antibiotics when moderate to severe TD occurs, shortening the duration of illness to 6–24 hours in most cases. Prophylactic antibiotics may be considered for short-term travelers who are high-risk hosts (such as those who are immunosuppressed or with significant medical comorbidities) or those who are taking critical trips (such as engaging in a sporting event) without the opportunity for time off in the event of sickness.

## TREATMENT

### Oral Rehydration Therapy

Fluids and electrolytes are lost during TD, and replenishment is important, especially in young children or adults with chronic medical illness. In adult travelers who are otherwise healthy, severe dehydration resulting from TD is unusual unless vomiting is prolonged. Nonetheless, replacement of fluid losses remains an adjunct to other therapy and helps the traveler feel better more quickly. Travelers should remember to use only beverages that are sealed, treated with chlorine, boiled, or are otherwise known to be purified.

For severe fluid loss, replacement is best accomplished with oral rehydration solution (ORS) prepared from packaged oral rehydration salts, such as those provided by the World Health Organization. ORS is widely available at stores and pharmacies in most developing countries. ORS is prepared by adding 1 packet to the indicated volume of boiled or treated water—generally 1 liter. Travelers may find most ORS formulations to be relatively unpalatable due to their saltiness. In mild cases, rehydration can be maintained with any palatable liquid (including sports drinks), although overly sweet drinks, such as sodas, can cause osmotic diarrhea if consumed in quantity.

### Antimotility Agents

Antimotility agents provide symptomatic relief and are useful therapy in TD. Synthetic opiates, such as loperamide and diphenoxylate, can reduce frequency of bowel movements and therefore enable travelers to ride on an airplane or bus. Loperamide appears to have antisecretory properties as well. The safety of loperamide when used along with an antibiotic has been well established, even in cases of invasive pathogens; however, acquisition of ESBL-producing pathogens may be more common when loperamide and antibiotics are coadministered. Antimotility agents alone are not recommended for patients with bloody diarrhea or those who have diarrhea and fever. Loperamide can be used in children, and liquid formulations are available. In practice, however, these drugs are rarely given to small children (aged <6 years).

## Antibiotics

Antibiotics are effective in reducing the duration of diarrhea by about a day in cases caused by bacterial pathogens that are susceptible to the particular antibiotic prescribed. However, there are concerns about adverse consequences of using antibiotics to treat TD. Travelers who take antibiotics may acquire resistant organisms such as ESBL-producing organisms, resulting in potential harm to travelers—particularly those who are immunosuppressed or women who may be prone to urinary tract infections—and the possibility of introducing these resistant bacteria into the community. In addition, there is concern about the effects of antibiotic use on travelers' microbiota and the potential for adverse consequences such as *Clostridioides difficile* infection as a result. These concerns have to be weighed against the consequences of TD and the role of antibiotics in shortening the acute illness and possibly preventing postinfectious sequelae (see Chapter 11, Persistent Diarrhea in Returned Travelers).

Primarily because of these concerns, an expert advisory panel was convened in 2016 to prepare consensus guidelines on the prevention and treatment of TD. A classification of TD using functional impact for defining severity (Box 2-3) was suggested rather than the frequency-based algorithm that has traditionally been used. The guidelines suggest an approach that matches therapeutic intervention with severity of illness, in terms of both safety and effectiveness (Table 2-10).

The effectiveness of a particular antimicrobial drug depends on the etiologic agent and its antibiotic sensitivity (Table 2-11). As empiric therapy or to treat a specific bacterial pathogen, first-line antibiotics have traditionally been the fluoroquinolones, such as ciprofloxacin or levofloxacin. Increasing microbial resistance to the fluoroquinolones, especially among *Campylobacter* isolates, may limit their usefulness in many destinations, particularly South and Southeast Asia, where both *Campylobacter* infection and fluoroquinolone resistance is prevalent. Increasing fluoroquinolone resistance has been reported from other destinations and in other bacterial pathogens, including in *Shigella* and *Salmonella*. In addition, the use of fluoroquinolones has been associated with tendinopathies and the development of *C. difficile* infection. FDA warns that the potentially serious side effects of fluoroquinolones may outweigh their benefit in treating uncomplicated respiratory and urinary tract infections; however, because of the short duration of therapy for TD, these side effects are not believed to be a significant risk.

A potential alternative to fluoroquinolones is azithromycin, although enteropathogens with decreased azithromycin susceptibility have been documented in several countries. Rifaximin has been approved to treat TD caused by noninvasive strains of *E. coli*. However, since it is often difficult for travelers to distinguish between invasive and noninvasive diarrhea, and since they would have to carry a backup drug in the event of invasive diarrhea, the overall usefulness of

---

BOX 2-3. Travelers' diarrhea definitions

**Mild (acute):** diarrhea that is tolerable, is not distressing, and does not interfere with planned activities.

**Moderate (acute):** diarrhea that is distressing or interferes with planned activities.

**Severe (acute):** diarrhea that is incapacitating or completely prevents planned activities; all dysentery is considered severe.

## Table 2-10. Travelers' diarrhea treatment recommendations

**Therapy of mild travelers' diarrhea**
- Antibiotic treatment is not recommended in patients with mild travelers' diarrhea.
- Loperamide or BSS may be considered in the treatment of mild travelers' diarrhea.

**Therapy of moderate travelers' diarrhea**
- Antibiotics may be used to treat cases of moderate travelers' diarrhea.
- Fluoroquinolones may be used to treat moderate travelers' diarrhea.
- Azithromycin may be used to treat moderate travelers' diarrhea.
- Rifaximin may be used to treat moderate, noninvasive travelers' diarrhea.
- Loperamide may be used as adjunctive therapy for moderate to severe travelers' diarrhea. Antimotility agents alone are not recommended for patients with bloody diarrhea or those who have diarrhea and fever.
- Loperamide may be considered for use as monotherapy in moderate travelers' diarrhea.

**Therapy of severe travelers' diarrhea**
- Antibiotics should be used to treat severe travelers' diarrhea.
- Azithromycin is preferred to treat severe travelers' diarrhea.
- Fluoroquinolones may be used to treat severe, nondysenteric travelers' diarrhea.
- Rifaximin may be used to treat severe, nondysenteric travelers' diarrhea.[1]
- Single-dose antibiotic regimens may be used to treat travelers' diarrhea.

[1] These treatment recommendations were developed prior to the approval of rifamycin SV in the United States. Because it is in the same category of antimicrobial drug as rifaximin and because they have the same mechanism of action, rifamycin SV can be considered as an alternative to rifaximin.

## Table 2-11. Acute diarrhea antibiotic treatment recommendations

| ANTIBIOTIC[1] | DOSE | DURATION |
|---|---|---|
| Azithromycin[2,3] | 1,000 mg | Single or divided dose[4] |
|  | 500 mg daily | 3 days |
| Levofloxacin | 500 mg daily | 1–3 days[4] |
| Ciprofloxacin | 750 mg | Single dose[4] |
|  | 500 mg bid | 3 days |
| Ofloxacin | 400 mg bid | 1–3 days[4] |
| Rifamycin SV[5] | 388 mg bid | 3 days |
| Rifaximin[5] | 200 mg tid | 3 days |

[1] Antibiotic regimens may be combined with loperamide 4 mg initially followed by 2 mg after each loose stool, not to exceed 16 mg in a 24-hour period.
[2] Use empirically as first-line in Southeast Asia or other areas if fluoroquinolone-resistant bacteria are suspected.
[3] Preferred regimen for dysentery or febrile diarrhea.
[4] If symptoms are not resolved after 24 hours, continue daily dosing for up to 3 days.
[5] Do not use if clinical suspicion for *Campylobacter, Salmonella, Shigella*, or other causes of invasive diarrhea. Use may be reserved for patients unable to receive fluoroquinolones or azithromycin.

rifaximin as empiric self-treatment remains to be determined.

Single-dose regimens are equivalent to multi-dose regimens and may be more convenient for the traveler. Single-dose therapy with a fluoroquinolone is well established, both by clinical trials and clinical experience. The best regimen for azithromycin treatment may also be a single dose of 1,000 mg, but side effects (mainly nausea) may limit the acceptability of this large dose. Giving azithromycin as 2 divided doses on the same day may limit this adverse event.

## Treatment of TD Caused by Protozoa

The most common parasitic cause of TD is *Giardia intestinalis*, and treatment options include metronidazole, tinidazole, and nitazoxanide (see Chapter 4, Giardiasis). Although cryptosporidiosis is usually a self-limited illness in immunocompetent people, nitazoxanide can be considered as a treatment option. Cyclosporiasis is treated with trimethoprim-sulfamethoxazole. Treatment of amebiasis is with metronidazole or tinidazole, followed by treatment with a luminal agent such as iodoquinol or paromomycin.

A new therapeutic option is rifamycin SV, which was approved by FDA in November 2018 to treat TD caused by noninvasive strains of *E. coli* in adults. Rifamycin SV is a nonabsorbable antibiotic in the ansamycin class of antibacterial drugs formulated with an enteric coating that targets delivery of the drug to the distal small bowel and colon. Two randomized clinical trials showed that rifamycin SV was superior to placebo and noninferior to ciprofloxacin in the treatment of TD.

## Treatment for Children

Children who accompany their parents on trips to high-risk destinations can contract TD as well, with elevated risk if they are visiting friends and family. Causative organisms include bacteria responsible for TD in adults, as well as viruses including norovirus and rotavirus. The main treatment for TD in children is ORS. Infants and younger children with TD are at higher risk for dehydration, which is best prevented by the early initiation of oral rehydration. Empiric antibiotic therapy should be considered if there is bloody or severe watery diarrhea or evidence of systemic infection. In older children and teenagers, treatment recommendations for TD follow those for adults, with possible adjustments in the dose of medication. Among younger children, macrolides such as azithromycin are considered first-line antibiotic therapy, although some experts now use short-course fluoroquinolone therapy (despite its not being FDA-approved for this indication in children) for travelers aged <18 years. Rifaximin is approved for use in children aged ≥12 years. Rifamycin SV is approved for use only in adults.

Breastfed infants should continue to nurse on demand, and bottle-fed infants can continue to drink formula. Older infants and children should be encouraged to eat and may consume a regular diet. Children in diapers are at risk for developing diaper rash on their buttocks in response to the liquid stool. Barrier creams, such as zinc oxide or petrolatum, could be applied at the onset of diarrhea to help prevent and treat rash. Hydrocortisone cream is the best treatment for an established rash. More information about diarrhea and dehydration is discussed in Chapter 7, Traveling Safely with Infants & Children.

## BIBLIOGRAPHY

1. Black RE. Epidemiology of travelers' diarrhea and relative importance of various pathogens. Rev Infect Dis. 1990 Jan–Feb;12(Suppl 1):S73–9.

2. DeBruyn G, Hahn S, Borwick A. Antibiotic treatment for travelers' diarrhea. Cochrane Database Syst Rev 2000;3:1–21.

3. DuPont HL, Ericsson CD, Farthing MJ, Gorbach S, Pickering LK, Rombo L, et al. Expert review of the evidence base for prevention of travelers' diarrhea. J Travel Med. 2009 May–Jun;16(3):149–60.

4. Farthing M, Salam MA, Lindberg G, Dite P, Khalif I, Salazar-Lindo E, et al. Acute diarrhea in adults and children: a global perspective. J Clin Gastroenterol. 2013 Jan;47(1):12–20.

5. Kantele A, Lääveri T, Mero S, Vilkman K, Pakkanen S, Ollgren J, et al. Antimicrobials increase travelers' risk of colonization by extended-spectrum betalactamase producing Enterobacteriaceae. Clin Infect Dis. 2015 Mar 15;60(6):837–46.

6. Kendall ME, Crim S, Fullerton K, Han PV, Cronquist AB, Shiferaw B, et al. Travel-associated enteric infections diagnosed after return to the United States, Foodborne Diseases Active Surveillance Network (FoodNet), 2004–2009. Clin Infect Dis. 2012 Jun;54(Suppl 5):S480–7.

7. Mcfarland LV. Meta-analysis of probiotics for the prevention of travelers' diarrhea. Cochrane Database Syst Rev 2010;Cd003048.

8. Raja MK, Ghosh AR. Laribacter hongkongensis: an emerging pathogen of infectious diarrhea. Folia Microbiol. (Praha) 2014 Jul;59 (4):341–7.

9. Riddle MS, Connor BA, Beeching NJ, DuPont HL, Hamer DH, Kozarsky PE et al. Guidelines for the prevention and treatment of travelers' diarrhea: a graded expert panel report. J Travel Med. 2017;24(Suppl 1):S2–S19.

10. Riddle MS, DuPont HL, Connor BA. ACG clinical guideline: diagnosis, treatment, and prevention of acute diarrheal infections in adults. Am J Gastroenterol. 2016 May;111(5):602–22.

11. Shlim DR. Looking for evidence that personal hygiene precautions prevent travelers' diarrhea. Clin Infect Dis. 2005 Dec 1;41(Suppl 8):S531–5.

12. Steffen R, Hill DR, DuPont HL. Traveler's diarrhea: a clinical review. JAMA. 2015 Jan 6;313(1):71–80.

13. Zboromyrska Y, Hurtado JC, Salvador P, Alvarez-Martinez MJ, Valls ME, Marcos MA, et al. Aetiology of travelers' diarrhea: evaluation of a multiplex PCR tool to detect different enteropathogens. Clin Microbiol Infect. 2014;20:O753–9.

**2**

# ANTIBIOTICS IN TRAVELERS' DIARRHEA—BALANCING THE RISKS & BENEFITS

Mark S. Riddle, Bradley A. Connor

For the past 30 years, randomized controlled trials have consistently and clearly demonstrated that antibiotics shorten the duration of illness and alleviate the disability associated with travelers' diarrhea (TD). Treatment with an effective antibiotic shortens the average duration of a TD episode by about a day, and if the traveler combines an antibiotic with an antimotility agent such as loperamide, the duration of illness is shortened even further. Emerging data on the potential long-term health consequences of TD, such as irritable bowel syndrome, dyspepsia, and chronic constipation, might suggest a benefit of early antibiotic therapy given the association between more severe and longer disease and risk of postinfectious consequences.

Although these clinical results are impressive, antibiotics, like any drug, are not without consequences. Each of the antibiotics commonly used to treat TD have side effects, but these are generally mild and self-limiting, and the benefits appear to outweigh the risks. More recently, however, there has been concern that antibiotics used by travelers might result in significant changes in the host microbiome as well as the acquisition of multidrug-resistant bacteria. Multiple observational studies have found that those people who travel (in particular to regions of Asia), develop TD, and take antibiotics are at incrementally increasing risk for colonization with extended-spectrum β-lactamase–producing Enterobacteriaceae (ESBL-PE). The direct effects of colonization on the average traveler appears limited; carriage is most often transient but does persist in a small percentage of those who are colonized. However, international travel by a household member is associated with ESBL-PE colonization among close-living contacts, which suggests potential larger public health consequences from acquiring ESBL-PE during travel.

The challenge that we face as providers and travelers is how to balance the risk of colonization and the global spread of resistance with the health benefits of antibiotic treatment of TD. Although the role of travelers in the translocation of infectious disease and resistance cannot be ignored, the ecology of ESBL-PE infections is complex and includes environmental, diet, immigration, and local nosocomial transmission dynamics. ESBL-PE infections are an emerging health threat, and addressing this complex problem will require multiple strategies.

How, then, to prepare a traveler with a prescription for empiric self-treatment before a trip? There needs to be a conversation with the traveler about the multilevel (individual, community, global) risks of travel, travelers' diarrhea, preventing TD through hand hygiene and careful selection of foods and beverages, and antibiotic treatment. Reserving antibiotics for moderate to severe TD should be emphasized strongly, and using antimotility agents alone may be suggested for mild TD. Elderly travelers (because of the serious consequences of bloodstream infections in this population) or those with recurrent urinary tract infections (because *Escherichia coli* is a common cause) may be at higher risk of health consequences as a result of ESBL-PE colonization. At a minimum these travelers should be made aware of this risk, and should be counseled to convey their travel exposure history to their treating providers if they become ill after travel. Though further studies are needed (and many are underway), a rational approach is advised to decrease exposure by using single-dose regimens and selecting an antibiotic agent that minimizes microbiome disruption and risk of colonization. Additionally, as travel and untreated TD independently increase the risk of ESBL-PE colonization, nonantibiotic chemoprophylactic strategies, such as the use of bismuth subsalicylate, may decrease both the acute and posttravel risk concerns. Strengthening the resilience of the host microbiota to prevent infection and unwanted colonization, as with the use of prebiotics or probiotics, are promising potential strategies but need further investigation.

Finally, we must be cognizant of the fact that we expect the traveler to be the diagnostician, practitioner, and patient when it comes to managing TD. For even the most astute traveler, making such learned decisions can be challenged by the anxiety-provoking onset of that first abdominal cramp in sometimes austere and inconvenient settings. Providing prospective travelers with clear written guidance about TD prevention and step-by-step instructions about how and when to use medications for TD is crucial.

## BIBLIOGRAPHY

1. Arcilla MS, van Hattem JM, Haverkate MR, Bootsma MCJ, van Genderen PJJ, Goorhuis A, et al. Import and spread of extended-spectrum β-lactamase-producing Enterobacteriaceae by international travellers (COMBAT study): a prospective, multicentre cohort study. Lancet Infect Dis. 2017 Jan;17(1):78–85.

2. Riddle MS, Connor BA, Beeching NJ, DuPont HL, Hamer DH, Kozarsky P, et al. Guidelines for the prevention and treatment of travelers' diarrhea: a graded expert panel report. J Travel Med. 2017 Apr 1;24(Suppl 1):S57–S74.

*Perspectives* sections are written as editorial discussions aiming to add depth and clinical perspective to the official recommendations contained in the book. The views and opinions expressed in this section are those of the authors and do not necessarily represent the official position of CDC.

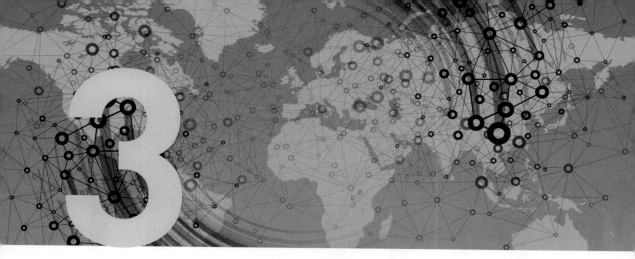

# 3

# Environmental Hazards & Other Noninfectious Health Risks

## INJURY & TRAUMA

Erin M. Parker, Erin K. Sauber-Schatz, David A. Sleet, Michael F. Ballesteros

In 2015 and 2016, more than 1,700 US citizens died from nonnatural causes in foreign countries, excluding deaths in the wars in Iraq and Afghanistan. Motor vehicle crashes—not crime or terrorism—are the number 1 cause of nonnatural deaths among US citizens living, working, or traveling abroad (Figure 3-1). In 2015 and 2016, 484 Americans died in vehicle crashes in foreign countries (28% of nonnatural deaths). Another 312 died of suicide (18%); 309 were victims of homicide (18%), and 307 drowned or died as a result of a boating incident (17%).

Countries may lack emergency care that approximates US standards; trauma centers

capable of providing optimal care for serious injuries are uncommon outside urban areas, if they exist at all. Travelers should be aware of the increased risk of certain injuries while traveling or residing internationally, particularly in low- and middle-income countries, and take preventive steps to reduce the chances of serious injury. (For information on motor vehicle crashes and road safety, see Chapter 8, Road & Traffic Safety.)

## VIOLENCE-RELATED INJURIES

Violence, including suicide and homicide, is a leading worldwide public health problem that affects US citizens traveling, working, or residing

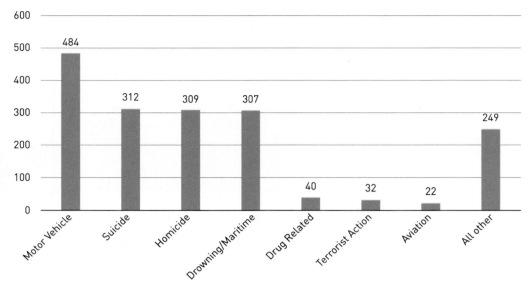

**FIGURE 3-1.** Leading causes of injury death for US citizens in foreign countries, 2015 & 2016[1,2,3,4]

[1] Data from US Department of State. Deaths of US citizens in foreign countries by nonnatural causes. Washington, DC: US Department of State; [cited 2018 Mar 1]. Available from: https://travel.state.gov/content/travel/en/international-travel/while-abroad/death-abroad1/death-statistics.html.

[2] Excludes deaths of US citizens fighting wars in Afghanistan or Iraq, and deaths that were not reported to the US embassy or consulate.

[3] "Motor Vehicle" includes deaths classified as "vehicle accidents," including the following subcategories: auto, bus, motorcycle, pedestrian, train, and other.

[4] "All Other" includes deaths classified as armed conflict, disaster, hostage-related, natural disaster, other accident, and undetermined/unknown.

internationally. Each year >1.6 million people lose their lives to violence; only one-fifth of the total are casualties due to armed conflict. Rates of violent deaths in low- and middle-income countries are 3 times those in higher-income countries, although variations exist within countries. For longer-term travelers, social isolation and substance abuse, particularly in areas of poverty and rigid gender roles, may increase the risk of depression and suicide. See Mental Health later in this chapter for more detailed information on suicide prevention.

Mexico, the Philippines, Jamaica, and Haiti have the highest number of homicide deaths among US travelers; Mexico accounts for 50% of all homicide deaths in US citizens living or traveling in foreign countries. Criminals may view travelers to their country as wealthy, naïve targets, inexperienced and unfamiliar with the culture and less able to seek assistance once victimized.

Traveling in high-poverty areas or regions of civil unrest, using alcohol or drugs, and visiting unfamiliar environments (particularly at night) each increase the likelihood that a traveler becomes a victim of violence (see Safety & Security Overseas in this chapter for more information).

## WATER AND AQUATIC INJURIES

Drowning is often the leading cause of injury death to US citizens visiting countries where water recreation is a major activity. Although risk factors remain to be defined clearly, lack of familiarity with local water currents and conditions, inability to swim, and absence of lifeguards on duty likely contribute to drowning deaths. Rip currents can be especially dangerous. Diving into shallow water is a risk factor for head and spinal cord injuries, with young men affected disproportionately. Alcohol or drug use is a factor in some cases.

Boating can be a hazard, especially if boaters are unfamiliar with the equipment they are using, do not know proper boating etiquette or rules for watercraft navigation, or are new to the water environment in a foreign country. Many boating fatalities result from inexperience or failure to wear a personal flotation device (lifejacket); travelers should have enough lifejackets on board for all passengers. Children and weak swimmers should wear a lifejacket at all times while boating. Advise travelers not to ride in boats operated by obviously inexperienced, uncertified, or intoxicated drivers.

Scuba diving is a frequent pursuit of travelers to coastal destinations. Researchers estimate the death rate among divers worldwide to be approximately 16 deaths per 100,000 divers per year. Travelers should either be experienced divers or dive with a reputable dive shop and instructors. See Scuba Diving: Decompression Illness & Other Dive-Related Injuries later in this chapter for a more detailed discussion about diving risks and preventive measures.

Travelers should not swim alone or in unfamiliar waters and should wear appropriately sized and US Coast Guard–approved lifejackets whenever participating in water recreation activities. If travel includes planned water activities, travelers should consider bringing their own lifejackets with them. Improving swimming skills, learning safe rescue techniques (such as use of poles or ropes as rescue aids so responders can avoid entering the water), and taking cardiopulmonary resuscitation (CPR) classes can substantially increase the likelihood of survival in an emergency. See the World Health Organization drowning resources (www. who.int/violence_injury_prevention/drowning/ en) and the International Life Saving Federation (https://ilsf.org) for more information.

## OTHER UNINTENTIONAL INJURIES

In developing countries where building codes are not enforced or do not exist, fires represent a substantial risk to traveler health and safety. Often there are no smoke alarms or access to emergency services, and the fire department's focus is on putting out fires rather than on fire prevention or victim rescue.

To prevent fire-related injuries, travelers should select accommodations no higher than the sixth floor (fire ladders generally cannot reach higher than the sixth floor) and confirm that hotels have smoke alarms and, preferably, sprinkler systems. Travelers may want to bring their own smoke alarms with them, and they should always identify at least 2 escape routes from buildings. Crawling low under smoke and covering one's mouth with a wet cloth are helpful in escaping a fire. Families should agree on a meeting place outside the building in case of a fire. The National Fire Protection Association has additional guidance on hotel fire safety for domestic travel that may also be useful internationally: see www.nfpa.org/Public-Education/By-topic/ Property-type-and-vehicles/Hotels-and-motels/ Hotel-fire-safety-tips.

Carbon monoxide (CO) inhalation, poisoning, and death can occur during fires but may also be the result of exposure to improperly vented heating devices. Travelers may want to bring a personal CO detector that can sound an alert in the presence of this lethal gas. Engine exhaust is a dangerous, unanticipated source of CO; remind travelers to avoid diving and swimming off the back of boats where exhaust fumes typically discharge.

Adventure activities such as mountain climbing, skydiving, whitewater rafting, off-roading, kayaking, skiing, and snowboarding are popular with travelers. A lack of rapid emergency trauma response, inadequate trauma care in remote locations, and sudden, unexpected weather changes compromise safety and hamper rescue efforts, delay care, and reduce survivability. For recreational activities with a risk of falling, helmet use is strongly encouraged; if helmets are unlikely to be available at the destination, travelers should bring them from home.

In 2017, 15 US citizens abroad died in aircraft crashes. Travel by local, lightweight aircraft in many countries can be risky. Travel on unscheduled flights, in small aircraft, at night, in inclement weather, and with inexperienced pilots carries the highest risk. Travelers should avoid using local, unscheduled, small aircraft, and refrain if possible from flying in bad weather and at night. If available, choose larger aircraft (>30 seats), as they are more likely to have undergone more strict and regular safety inspections. Larger aircraft also provide more protection in the event of a crash.

## TRAVEL PREPARATION TIPS

Health care providers, vendors of travel services, and travelers themselves should consider taking the following actions when planning for a trip outside the United States:

- Purchase special travel health and medical evacuation insurance if destinations include countries where there may not be access to good medical care (see Chapter 6, Travel Insurance, Travel Health Insurance & Medical Evacuation Insurance).

- Learn basic first aid and CPR before traveling internationally with another person.

- Bring a travel health kit, customized to anticipated itinerary and activities.

- Review US State Department travel advisories and alerts (www.travel.state.gov/destination), and check the US embassy or consulate (www.usembassy.gov) for country-specific personal security risks and safety tips.

- Enroll in the US State Department's Smart Traveler Enrollment Program (https://step.state.gov/step). Enrolled travelers receive emails about safety conditions at their destination and direct embassy contact in case of natural disasters and man-made emergencies, such as political unrest, rioting, and terrorist activity.

### BIBLIOGRAPHY

1. Balaban V, Sleet DA. Pediatric travel injuries: risk, prevention, and management. In: Kamat DM, Fischer PR, editors. American Academy of Pediatrics Textbook of Global Child Health. 2nd ed. Elk Grove Village (IL): American Academy of Pediatrics; 2015.

2. Cortés LM, Hargarten SW, Hennes HM. Recommendations for water safety and drowning prevention for travelers. J Travel Med. 2006; 13(1):21–34.

3. Guse CE, Cortes LM, Hargarten SW, Hennes HM. Fatal injuries of US citizens abroad. J Travel Med. 2007; 14(5):279–87.

4. Krug EG, Mercy JA, Dahlberg LL, Zwi AB. The world report on violence and health. Lancet. 2002; 360(9339):1083–8.

5. McInnes RJ, Williamson LM, Morrison A. Unintentional injury during foreign travel: A review. J Travel Med. 2002; 9:297–307.

6. Traveler's Checklist. US Department of State. [cited 2018 Mar 1]. Available from: https://travel.state.gov/content/travel/en/international-travel/before-you-go/travelers-checklist.html.

7. Vann RD, Lang MA, eds. Recreational diving fatalities. In: Proceedings of the Divers Alert Network 2010 April 8–10 Workshop. Durham (NC): Divers Alert Network; 2011.

8. World Health Organization. Global health estimates 2015: Deaths by cause, age, sex, by country and by region, 2000–2015. Geneva; 2016.

9. World Health Organization. Global report on drowning: preventing a leading killer. World Health Organization. Geneva; 2014. [cited 1 Apr 2019]. Available from: https://www.who.int/violence_injury_prevention/global_report_drowning/en/.

# MENTAL HEALTH

Thomas H. Valk

International travel is stressful. Stressors vary to some extent with the type of travel: short-term tourist travel likely creates the least stress, whereas frequent travel, humanitarian and disaster work, and expatriation cause the most.

Given the stressors of travel, preexisting psychiatric disorders can recur, latent or undiagnosed problems can become apparent, and new problems can arise. In addition, jet lag, fatigue, and work or family pressures can trigger anxiety and aggravate depressive symptoms in short-term travelers.

## OCCURRENCE IN TRAVELERS

Incidence data based on population surveys of travelers are nonexistent. Data from clinical populations include the following:

- In a study of British diplomats, 11% of medical evacuations were "nonphysical," or psychological in nature. Of those evacuated for psychological reasons, 71% were in their 20s. There was an overall incidence of 0.3% for psychological evacuations. Of these, 41% were for depression.

- In a study of the US Foreign Service from 1982 through 1986, the incidence of psychiatric evacuations was 0.2%. Of these, 50% were for substance abuse or affective disorder. Evacuations for mania and hypomanic states accounted for 3%.

- A study of psychiatric emergencies in travelers to Hawaii estimated a rate of 0.2% for tourists and 2% for transient travelers (those arriving in Hawaii with no immediate plans to leave) versus 1% for residents. In order of decreasing frequency, diagnoses in this population were schizophrenia, alcohol abuse, anxiety reaction, and depression.

## THE PRETRAVEL CONSULTATION AND MENTAL HEALTH EVALUATION

Any pretravel consultation should include a mental health screening, especially for the following groups: those planning extended or frequent travel; participants in humanitarian or disaster relief work; and anyone intending to take up long-term or semipermanent residence in another country. As travel medicine specialists rarely have mental health credentials, a brief inquiry aimed at eliciting previously diagnosed psychiatric disorders should be undertaken. To introduce this portion of the consultation and to elicit the most cooperation, practitioners can enumerate these facts:

- International travel is stressful for everyone and has been associated with the emergence or reemergence of mental health problems.

- The availability of culturally compatible mental health services varies widely.

- Laws regarding the use of illicit substances can be severe in some countries.

The practitioner should then ask about indicators of overt or underlying mental health problems:

- Previously treated or diagnosed psychiatric disorders (including any associated with prior travel) and the type of treatment involved (inpatient, outpatient, medications)

- Current psychiatric disorders and treatment

- Current or past use of illicit substances

- Substance use disorder (formally diagnosed) or suggestions from health care providers, friends, or family that the traveler might be using alcohol or other substances to excess

- Serious mental health problems in the immediate family

In general, any history of inpatient treatment, psychotic episodes, violent or suicidal behavior, affective disorder (including mania, hypomania, or major depression), any treatment for substance use problems, and any current treatments would warrant further evaluation by a mental health professional, preferably one experienced in handling problems related to international travel. On occasion, a patient's mental status during the pretravel consultation may be notably abnormal, which would also warrant a referral.

People with mental health issues may face several challenges and barriers to healthy travel. Pretravel health care providers should be prepared to discuss the following topics:

- **Mental health treatment.** Culturally compatible mental health treatment for long-term travelers or expatriates may be difficult to find in the destination country, requiring assistance from a mental health professional with overseas experience.

- **Importation of psychotropic medications.** Customs regulations in some countries prohibit importation of medications used to treat mental health disorders. Officials may confiscate schedule II drugs such as narcotics or stimulants (including amphetamines and methylphenidate) commonly used to treat attention deficit disorder. Rules vary by country and travelers should check with the host country's embassy in advance of travel. Health care providers (including pharmacists) in the destination country may be able to provide guidance to colleagues about medication restrictions. Advise travelers to carry medications in their original containers, along with a letter from the prescribing physician indicating the medical reason for the prescription. Remind them that even if they adhere to these guidelines, customs officials may seize their medication.

- **Refilling prescriptions.** Obtaining refills of psychotropic medications while living overseas can be problematic, as availability or even legality of these drugs varies from country to country. Again, checking with the country's embassy may be helpful, as would checking with a reputable in-country pharmacy or health care provider. Sometimes visiting friends or relatives or other members of the company or organization traveling can bring additional medication.

- **Laboratory monitoring of medication levels.** Locating in-country laboratory facilities capable of measuring levels of lithium or other mood-stabilizing medications can be challenging. Travelers should not assume stability of levels, particularly in environments with high ambient temperatures. Increased perspiration can lead to lithium toxicity, even on a consistent dose.

- **Contraindicated medications.** Because of its potential for neuropsychiatric side effects, patients with mental health issues should not take mefloquine for malaria prophylaxis. Please see the discussion of mefloquine in Chapter 4, Malaria.

- **Support groups.** Currently sober patients with substance use disorders may wish to attend Alcoholics Anonymous (AA) and Narcotics Anonymous (NA) meetings while overseas. AA and NA maintain lists of meetings, by country, on their websites. Travelers should confirm availability and language of meetings in advance.

- **Medical evacuation insurance.** Travelers with mental health problems should consider purchasing international travel health and medical evacuation policies that include coverage for psychiatric emergencies.

## STRESSORS AND COUNTERMEASURES

Jet lag is a common, manageable stressor for most international travelers. Readers can find more details about this condition—and what to do about it—in Chapter 8, Jet Lag. Almost anyone visiting a foreign culture can experience culture shock. With culture shock, travelers lose their sense of mastery over their environment, and even routine tasks of everyday life become a challenge. Separation from family and support systems, unfamiliar behavior and language, and new threats to health and safety can aggravate this condition. Foreknowledge of the phenomenon will help minimize the stress experienced, as will advance study of the culture, language, health and security threats, and their countermeasures. Fortunately, for most travelers culture shock is a limited syndrome that does not usually go beyond variations in mood, energy, sleep, and attitudes toward the host country culture as might be seen in an adjustment disorder. Symptoms lasting beyond 12 months may require assessment.

Regular exercise, moderation in the use of intoxicants, adequate sleep and nutrition, and use of relaxation techniques such as meditation, yoga, or biofeedback can be useful methods to reduce the stress associated with international travel.

## POSTTRAVEL MENTAL HEALTH ISSUES

Travelers who witness traumatic and life-threatening events can experience acute stress disorder (ASD) or posttraumatic stress disorder (PTSD). The work performed by humanitarian aid or disaster relief workers or war correspondents increases their risk of developing subclinical or outright ASD or PTSD. If a traveler has had traumatic experiences, clinicians should inquire about:

- Recurrent, intrusive recollections, distressing dreams, and feeling as if the event is happening repeatedly

- Avoiding thoughts, feelings, activities, places, or people that lead to memories of the event

- Diminished interest in activities, inability to experience positive emotions, or an inability to remember significant details of the event

- Difficulty sleeping or concentrating, irritability, or an exaggerated startle response

As symptoms of PTSD may occur months or even years after an event, education about the possibility of having such symptoms in the future is worthwhile. If there is any concern about a possible reaction to a traumatic event, referral to a mental health professional is warranted.

**3**

## BIBLIOGRAPHY

1. American Psychiatric Association. Diagnostic and Statistical Manual of Mental Disorders. 5th ed. Arlington, VA: American Psychiatric Association; 2013.

2. Benedek DM, Wynn GH. Clinical manual for management of PTSD. Arlington, VA: American Psychiatric Publishing, Inc.; 2011.

3. Bonny-Noach H, Sagiv-Alayoff M. Rescuing Israeli travellers: effects of substance abuse, mental health, geographic region of rescue, gender and age of rescuees. J Travel Med. 2017 Sep 1;24(5).

4. Feinstein A, Owen J, Blair N. A hazardous profession: war, journalists, and psychopathology. Am J Psychiatry. 2002 Sep; 159(9):1570–5.

5. Felkai P, Kurimay T. Patients with mental problems—the most defenseless travellers. J Travel Med. 2017 Sep 1;24(5).

6. Felkai P, Debreceni EO, Kurimay T. Travelers with mental problems—the most defenseless travelers. J Travel Med. 2017 Sep 1; 24(5).

7. Liese B, Mundt KA, Dell LD, Nagy L, Demure B. Medical insurance claims associated with international business travel. Occup Environ Med. 1997 Jul; 54(7):499–503.

8. Patel D, Easmon CJ, Dow C, Snashall DC, Seed PT. Medical repatriation of British diplomats resident overseas. J Travel Med. 2000 Mar–Apr; 7(2):64–9.

9. Streltzer J. Psychiatric emergencies in travelers to Hawaii. Compr Psychiatry. 1979 Sep–Oct; 20(5): 463–8.

10. Valk TH. Psychiatric medical evacuations within the Foreign Service. Foreign Serv Med Bull. 1988; 268: 9–11.

# SAFETY & SECURITY OVERSEAS

Uzma Javed

Violence is a leading worldwide public health problem and a concern of US citizens traveling, working, or residing abroad. International terrorism and crime are risks anywhere in the world, but international travelers operating in unfamiliar environments face particular hurdles. Travelers overseas, particularly tourists, may not have an immediately accessible network of friends or family to assist them in an emergency. Local government responses to violent activities and crime may not be what US residents expect; an effective local government may not exist to respond at all. Language barriers, unanticipated costs, or different cultural mores can compound an already challenging situation. US travelers should research conditions at their destination to learn what risks they are likely to face and have plans to mitigate those risks while they are abroad.

## BEFORE TRAVEL

Travelers need clear, timely, and reliable safety and security information to make decisions about travel plans. This information is available from the Bureau of Consular Affairs (BCA) in the Department of State, the organization charged with protecting US citizens abroad.

BCA assigns every country a travel advisory level ranging from 1 (Exercise Normal Precautions) to 4 (Do Not Travel). Travel advisories describe the risks found in a country and the actions US citizens should take to mitigate those risks. US embassies and consulates abroad may also issue alerts, which inform US citizens of specific safety, security, or health concerns in a country, such as demonstrations, crime trends, weather events, and health events. For more details, see http://travel.state.gov/travelsafely.

The Department of State also releases an annual worldwide caution that provides information on universal travel risks, including the threat of terrorism against US citizens and its interests abroad. The country information pages on the BCA website provide all available travel information, including details about entry and exit requirements, local laws and customs, health conditions, transportation, and other relevant topics.

US citizens should enroll with the Department of State's Smart Traveler Enrollment Program (http://STEP.state.gov) before traveling abroad. A free service, STEP allows enrollees to receive information from the local US embassy or consulate about safety, security, or health conditions at their destination. It also assists the embassy or consulate to locate missing US citizens or contact them in an emergency, such as a natural disaster, civil unrest, or family emergency.

## CRISES ABROAD

Whether traveling or living outside the United States, US citizens should prepare for a potential crisis. The Department of State is committed to assisting US citizens who become victims of crime, need assistance during a crisis or a natural disaster, or who need consular services (such as replacing a lost or stolen passport) or financial assistance to return to the United States. The State Department can also support locating missing US citizens abroad.

US citizens should research the country they are visiting or residing in, stay connected with the nearest US embassy or consulate, and create personal safety plans. For more information about what travelers can do to prepare, or how the Department of State can assist US citizens, visit https://travel.state.gov/content/travel/en/international-travel/before-you-go/crisis-abroad-be-ready.html.

## CRIME

One of the most common threats to the safety of US citizens abroad comes from criminal activity. Encourage travelers to research crime trends and patterns at their destination using the Overseas Security Advisory Council website (www.osac.gov). Common-sense strategies to avoid becoming a crime victim are, for the most part, the same everywhere, but the following should be stressed with international travelers:

- Limit travel at night; travel with a companion, and vary routine travel habits.

- Do not wear expensive clothing or accessories.

- Avoid accommodations on the ground floor or immediately next to the stairs, and lock all windows and doors.

- Take only recommended, safe modes of local transportation.

- If confronted in a robbery, give up all valuables and do not resist attackers. Resistance can escalate to violence and result in injury or death.

Crime victims overseas should contact the nearest US embassy, consulate, or consular agency. The Department of State can help replace stolen passports, contact family and friends, identify health care providers, explain the local criminal justice process, and connect victims of crime with available resources. However, they do not have the legal authority to conduct a criminal investigation or prosecute crimes.

## TERRORISM

Terrorist attacks against Western interests in multiple regions, including Europe, Asia, Africa, and the Middle East threaten US citizens living and traveling abroad. Potential targets include high-profile sporting events, public transportation systems, residential areas, business offices, hotels, clubs, restaurants, places of worship, schools, shopping malls, and other tourist destinations where US citizens gather in large numbers. Past attacks have ranged from assassinations and kidnappings to suicide operations, hijackings, and bombings.

Despite being a worldwide threat and cause for concern, terrorist attacks have involved relatively few international travelers. From June 2016 through June 2017, only 10 US citizens were killed in terrorist attacks overseas. Travelers can reduce their chances of becoming victims of terrorism by:

- Looking out for unattended packages or bags in public places and other crowded areas

- Being cautious of unexpected packages

- Choosing to wear clothing that does not identify them as a tourist (such as T-shirts bearing the US flag or the logos of a favorite, US-based sports team)

- Trying to blend in with the locals

These strategies incorporate the same defensive alertness and good judgment that people should use to keep safe from crime. Awareness is key—taking precautions to be aware of surroundings and adopting protective measures.

## LOCAL LAWS AND SPECIAL CIRCUMSTANCES

US citizens are subject to local laws, and if they violate those laws—even unknowingly—may face arrest, imprisonment, or deportation. In addition, some crimes are prosecutable both in the United States as well as in the country where the crime was committed. US citizens arrested or detained abroad should ask local law enforcement and/or

prison officials to notify the US embassy or consulate immediately.

Lesbian, gay, bisexual, transgender, and intersex (LGBTI) travelers can face unique challenges traveling abroad. Laws and attitudes in some countries may affect safety and ease of travel. Legal protections vary from country to country. Many countries do not legally recognize same-sex marriage. More than 70 countries consider consensual same-sex sexual relations a crime, sometimes carrying severe punishment. US citizens should review the Human Rights Report (www.state.gov/j/drl/rls/hrrpt) for further details.

For specific information about local laws and special circumstances in specific destinations, visit https://travel.state.gov/content/travel/en/international-travel/International-Travel-Country-Information-Pages.html.

## USEFUL WEBSITES
Department of State

- International Travel: https://travel.state.gov/content/travel/en/international-travel.html

- Country Information:

- Travel Advisories: https://travel.state.gov/content/travel/en/traveladvisories/traveladvisories.html/

- US Embassies or Consulates: www.usembassy.gov

- Smart Traveler Enrollment Program: https://step.state.gov/step

**Overseas Security Advisory Council**: www.osac.gov/Pages/Home.aspx

# MOSQUITOES, TICKS & OTHER ARTHROPODS

John-Paul Mutebi, John E. Gimnig

Because vector control programs vary in coverage and effectiveness, travel health practitioners should advise travelers to use

repellents and other general protective measures against biting arthropods. Although prophylactic drugs are available to protect against malaria, the effectiveness is variable depending on patterns of drug resistance, bioavailability, and compliance with medication. And while vaccines are available for diseases such as yellow fever and Japanese encephalitis, there are no available vaccines or chemoprophylaxis for other mosquitoborne diseases such as dengue, chikungunya, Zika, filariasis, and West Nile encephalitis; for tickborne diseases such as Lyme borreliosis, tickborne encephalitis, and relapsing fever; for sand fly–borne diseases such as visceral and cutaneous leishmaniasis; and for black fly–borne diseases such as onchocerciasis (river blindness).

The Environmental Protection Agency (EPA) regulates repellent products in the United States. CDC recommends that consumers use only those repellent products registered by the EPA. Registration indicates that the EPA has determined that the product is both efficacious and safe for human use, when applied according to the instructions on the label.

## GENERAL PROTECTIVE MEASURES

**Avoid outbreaks.** As much as possible, travelers should avoid known foci of epidemic arthropodborne disease transmission. The CDC Travelers' Health website provides updates on regional disease transmission patterns and outbreaks (www.cdc.gov/travel).

**Wear appropriate clothing.** Travelers can minimize areas of exposed skin by wearing long-sleeved shirts, long pants, boots, and hats. Tucking in shirts, tucking pants into socks, and wearing closed shoes instead of sandals may help reduce risk. Application of repellents or insecticides, such as permethrin, to clothing and gear can provide an added layer of protection. Remind travelers to always follow instructions on the label when applying repellents to clothing. (Additional information on clothing repellents and their proper use is included below.)

**Check for ticks.** Travelers should inspect themselves and their clothing for ticks during outdoor activity and at the end of the day. Prompt removal of attached ticks can prevent some infections. Showering soon after leaving a tick-infested area

may prevent ticks from attaching or facilitate detection of recently attached ticks.

**Bed nets.** Bed nets provide essential protection to travelers staying in accommodations lacking adequate window screens and air conditioning. Bed nets that do not reach the floor should be tucked under mattresses. Treating bed nets with a pyrethroid insecticide helps maximize their efficacy. Travelers may opt to buy a pretreated net or, as an alternative, apply the insecticide after purchase. Nets treated with a pyrethroid insecticide will be effective for several months if not washed. Long-lasting pretreated nets may be effective for much longer.

**Insecticides and spatial repellents.** Active ingredients in these products, metofluthrin and allethrin, provide protection from mosquito bites over a wide area. Spray aerosols can clear rooms or areas of mosquitoes; coils, vaporizing mats, and spatial repellents repel mosquitoes from a circumscribed area. Use insecticides and repellent products with caution, avoiding direct inhalation of spray or smoke.

Although many of these products demonstrate insecticidal or repellent activity under particular conditions, their efficacy in preventing vectorborne disease has not been evaluated adequately in peer-reviewed studies. For this reason, reliance on these products alone may afford insufficient protection from bites. Encourage travelers to apply an EPA-registered repellent to their skin and/or clothing and to use bed nets wherever vectorborne diseases are a risk.

Optimum protection can be provided by applying the repellents described in the following sections to clothing and to exposed skin (Box 3-1).

## REPELLENTS FOR USE ON SKIN AND CLOTHING

CDC has evaluated information published in peer-reviewed scientific literature and data available from EPA to identify several types of EPA-registered products that provide repellent activity sufficient to help people reduce the bites of disease-carrying insects. Products containing the following active ingredients typically provide reasonably long-lasting protection:

BOX 3-1. Maximizing protection from mosquitoes and ticks

To optimize protection against mosquitoes and tick bites:

- Wear a long-sleeved shirt, long pants, and socks.
- Treat clothing with permethrin or purchase pretreated clothing.
  > Permethrin-treated clothing will retain repellent activity through multiple washes.

> Repellents used on skin can also be applied to clothing but provide shorter duration of protection (same duration as on skin) and must be reapplied after laundering.
- Apply lotion, liquid, or spray repellent to exposed skin.

- Use repellent whenever outdoors (or indoors if mosquitoes can get inside); mosquitoes can bite any time of day or night.
- Check yourself during and after outdoor activity (your entire body); remove any attached ticks promptly.

**3**

- **DEET** (chemical name: *N,N*-diethyl-*m*-toluamide or *N,N*-diethyl-3-methyl-benzamide). Products containing DEET include, but are not limited to, Off!, Cutter, Sawyer, and Ultrathon.

- **Picaridin** (KBR 3023 [Bayrepel] and icaridin outside the US; chemical name: 2-(2-hydroxyethyl)-1-piperidinecarboxylic acid 1-methylpropyl ester). Products containing picaridin include, but are not limited to, Cutter Advanced, Skin So Soft Bug Guard Plus, and Autan (outside the United States).

- **Oil of lemon eucalyptus (OLE) or PMD** (chemical name: para-menthane-3,8-diol), the synthesized version of OLE. Products containing OLE and PMD include, but are not limited to, Repel and Off! Botanicals. This recommendation refers to EPA-registered products containing the active ingredient OLE (or PMD). CDC does not recommend using "pure" oil of lemon eucalyptus (essential oil not formulated) as a repellent. It has not undergone similar, validated testing for safety and efficacy and is not registered with EPA as an insect repellent.

- **IR3535** (chemical name: 3-[*N*-butyl-*N*-acetyl]-aminopropionic acid, ethyl ester). Products containing IR3535 include, but are not limited to, Skin So Soft Bug Guard Plus Expedition and SkinSmart.

- **2-undecanone** (chemical name: methyl nonyl ketone). The product BioUD contains 2-undecanone.

EPA characterizes the active ingredients DEET and picaridin as "conventional" repellents. Biopesticide repellents—OLE, PMD, IR3535, and 2-undecanone—are derived from, or are synthetic versions of, natural materials.

## Repellent Efficacy

Published data indicate that repellent efficacy and duration of protection vary considerably among products and among mosquito and tick species. Ambient temperature, level of activity, perspiration, water exposure, abrasive removal, and other factors affect efficacy and duration of protection. In general, higher concentrations of active ingredients provide longer duration of protection, regardless of the active ingredient. Products with <10% active ingredient may offer only limited protection, often 1–2 hours. Products that offer sustained-release or controlled-release (microencapsulated) formulations, even with lower active ingredient concentrations, may provide longer protection times. Studies suggest that concentrations of DEET above approximately 50% do not offer a marked increase in protection time against mosquitoes; DEET efficacy tends to plateau at a concentration of approximately 50%. CDC recommends using products with ≥20% DEET on exposed skin to reduce biting by insects that may spread disease.

Recommendations regarding use of repellents are based on peer-reviewed scientific studies and data submitted to regulatory agencies. People may experience some variation in protection from different products. Regardless of the product used, travelers getting insect bites should reapply the repellent according to the label instructions, try a different product, or, if possible, leave the area.

Ideally, travelers should purchase repellents before traveling. They are sold online as well as in hardware stores, drug stores, supermarkets, camping, sporting goods, and military surplus stores. When purchasing repellents overseas, look for the active ingredients specified above on the product labels.

## Repellency Awareness Graphic

A new graphic appearing on the label of insect repellents applied to the skin helps consumers more easily identify for how long the repellent is effective against mosquitoes and ticks (Figure 3-2). Use of this graphic by manufacturers is voluntary. Companies that apply to the EPA for permission to use the graphic must first provide data documenting their current testing protocols and standard evaluation practices.

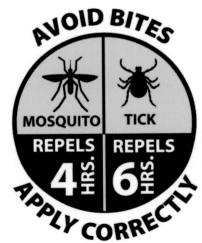

FIGURE 3-2. Sample repellency awareness graphic for skin-applied insect repellents[1]

[1] Image from: www.epa.gov/insect-repellents/repellency-awareness-graphic

## Repellents and Sunscreen

Combined sunscreen/repellents are not recommended. Advise travelers to use separate products, applying sunscreen first, followed by repellent. Repellents applied according to label instructions may be used with sunscreen with no reduction in repellent activity. Limited data show that DEET-containing insect repellents applied over sunscreen decrease the sun protection factor of the sunscreen by one-third; travelers using both products may therefore need to reapply sunscreen more frequently. In general, travelers typically need to apply sun protection more often and in larger amounts than they do insect repellent.

## Repellents and Insecticides for Use on Clothing

Travelers can apply permethrin to clothing, hats, shoes, bed nets, jackets, and camping gear for added protection. Products such as Permanone and Sawyer, Permethrin, Repel, and Ultrathon Permethrin Clothing Treatment are EPA-registered specifically to treat clothing and gear. Alternatively, commercially available clothing pretreated with permethrin is marketed to consumers in the United States as Insect Shield, BugsAway, or Insect Blocker.

Permethrin is a highly effective insecticide, acaricide (pesticide that kills ticks and mites), and repellent. Permethrin-treated clothing repels and kills ticks, chiggers, mosquitoes, and other biting and nuisance arthropods. Clothing and other items must be treated 24–48 hours in advance of travel to allow them to dry. As with all pesticides, follow the label instructions when using permethrin clothing treatments.

Permethrin-treated materials retain their ability to repel or kill insects after repeated launderings. To provide continued protection, travelers should retreat their clothing and gear as described on the product label. Clothing treated before purchase is labeled for efficacy through 70 launderings. Clothing treated with the other repellent products described above (such as DEET) provides protection from biting arthropods but will not last through washing and will require more frequent application.

## Precautions when Using Insect Repellents

Instruct travelers to take the following precautions when using repellents:

- Apply only to exposed skin or clothing, as directed on the product label. Do not apply to skin covered by clothing.

- Never use on cuts, wounds, or irritated skin.

- When using sprays, do not spray directly on face—spray on hands first and then apply to face. Do not apply to eyes or mouth, and only sparingly around ears.

- Wash hands after application to avoid accidental exposure to eyes or ingestion.

- Children should not handle repellents. Instead, adults should apply to their own hands first and then gently spread on the child's exposed skin. Avoid applying directly to children's hands. After returning indoors, wash children's treated skin and clothing with soap and water or give the child a bath.

- Use just enough to cover exposed skin or clothing. Heavy application and saturation are generally unnecessary for effectiveness. If biting insects do not respond to a thin film of repellent, apply a bit more.

- After returning indoors, wash repellent-treated skin with soap and water, or bathe. Wash treated clothing before wearing it again. This precaution may vary with different products—be sure to check the label.

If travelers experience a rash or other reaction (itching or swelling) from an insect repellent, they should wash off the product using mild soap and water and discontinue its use. For severe reactions, call a local poison-control center for further guidance. Travelers seeking health care because of a reaction to a repellent should bring the product container with them to show the doctor. Never apply permethrin to skin but only to clothing, bed nets, or other fabrics as directed on the product label.

## BOX 3-2. Bed bugs and international travel

Bed bugs are small, flat insects that are reddish-brown in color, wingless, and range from 1 to 7 mm in length. Although bed bugs have not been shown to transmit disease, their bites can produce strong allergic reactions and considerable emotional stress.

A recent resurgence in bed bug infestations worldwide, particularly in developed countries, is thought to be related to the increase in international travel, pest control strategy changes in travel lodgings, and insecticide resistance. Bed bug infestations have been reported increasingly in hotels, theaters, and any locations where people congregate, including the workplace, dormitories, and schools. Travelers may transport bed bugs in luggage and on clothing.

Personal belongings transported in vehicles infested with bed bugs is another means of spreading these insects.

### PROTECTIVE MEASURES AGAINST BED BUGS

Encourage travelers to take the following precautions to avoid or reduce their exposure to bed bugs:

- Inspect the premises of hotels or other sleeping locations for bed bugs on mattresses, box springs, bedding, and furniture, particularly built-in furniture with the bed, desk, and closets as a continuous structural unit. Travelers who observe evidence of bed bug activity—whether it is the bugs themselves or physical signs such as blood-spotting on linens—should seek alternative lodging.

- Keep suitcases closed when they are not in use and keep them off the floor.
- Remove clothing and personal items (such as toiletry bags and shaving kits) from the suitcase only when they are in use.
- Carefully inspect clothing and personal items before returning them to the suitcase.
- Keep in mind that bed bug eggs and nymphs are very small and can be overlooked easily.

Prevention is by far the most effective and inexpensive way to protect oneself from these pests. The cost of ridding a personal residence of these insects is considerable, and efforts at control are often not immediately successful even when conducted by professionals.

## Children and Pregnant Women

Most repellents can be used on children aged >2 months. Protect infants aged <2 months from mosquitoes by using an infant carrier draped with mosquito netting with an elastic edge for a tight fit. Products containing OLE specify that they should not be used on children aged <3 years. Other than the safety tips listed above, EPA does not recommend any additional precautions for using registered repellents on children or on pregnant or lactating women.

## USEFUL LINKS

- Find the Repellent that is Right for You (EPA): www.epa.gov/insect-repellents/find-repellent-right-you

- Using Insect Repellents Safely (EPA): www.epa.gov/insect-repellents/

using-insect-repellents-safely-and-effectively

- West Nile Virus: Prevention (CDC): www.cdc.gov/westnile/faq/repellent.html

- Choosing and Using Insect Repellents (National Pesticide Information Center): http://npic.orst.edu/ingred/ptype/repel.html

## BED BUGS

The recent resurgence in bed bug infestations worldwide, particularly in developed countries, is giving travelers cause for concern. Although bed bugs do not transmit diseases, their bites may be a nuisance. Travelers can take measures to avoid bed bug bites and avoid transporting them in luggage and clothing (Box 3-2).

BIBLIOGRAPHY

1. Barnard DR, Xue RD. Laboratory evaluation of mosquito repellents against *Aedes albopictus*, *Culex nigripalpus*, and *Ochlerotatus triseriatus* (Diptera: Culicidae). J Med Entomol. 2004 Jul; 41(4):726–30.

2. Fradin MS, Day JF. Comparative efficacy of insect repellents against mosquito bites. N Engl J Med. 2002 Jul 4; 347(1):13–18.

3. Goodyer LI, Croft AM, Frances SP, Hill N, Moore SJ, Onyango SP, et al. Expert review of the evidence base for arthropod bite avoidance. J Travel Med. 2010 May–Jun; 17(3):182–92.

4. Lupi E, Hatz C, Schlagenhauf P. The efficacy of repellents against *Aedes*, *Anopheles*, *Culex* and *Ixodes* spp.—a literature review. Travel Med Infect Dis. 2013 Nov–Dec; 11(6):374–411.

5. Montemarano AD, Gupta RK, Burge JR, Klein K. Insect repellents and the efficacy of sunscreens. Lancet. 1997 Jun 7; 349(9066):1670–1.

6. Murphy ME, Montemarano AD, Debboun M, Gupta R. The effect of sunscreen on the efficacy of insect repellent: a clinical trial. J Am Acad Dermatol. 2000 Aug; 43(2 Pt 1):219–22.

7. Pages F, Dautel H, Duvallet G, Kahl O, de Gentile L, Boulanger N. Tick repellents for human use: prevention of tick bites and tick-borne diseases. Vector Borne Zoonotic Dis. 2014 Feb; 14(2): 85–93.

8. Strickman D, Frances, SP, Debboun M. Prevention of bug bites, stings, and disease. Fla Entomol. 2009; 92(4):677–8.

# SUN EXPOSURE

Karolyn A. Wanat, Scott A. Norton

When international travelers engage in outdoor activities, they may be exposed to more ultraviolet (UV) radiation than usual, particularly in sunny locations or at high elevations. Even winter activities, such as snow skiing, can result in significant UV exposure. Short bursts of high-intensity UV radiation (such as the occasional beach vacation) as well as frequent, prolonged, cumulative UV exposure can cause acute effects, such as sunburn and phototoxic medication reactions, and delayed effects, such as sun damage, premature aging, and skin cancers.

## RISK FACTORS

Time of year, time of day, and location of exposure influence the amount of UV exposure a traveler receives. Most UV light reaches the earth's surface during summer months. UVB, which is more carcinogenic than UVA, is most intense between the hours of 10 AM and 4 PM, at higher elevations, and in locations closer to the equator. Water, sand, and snow reflect UV light and therefore increase UVB exposure.

People with certain medical conditions are at increased risk for adverse effects of UV exposure. Solid-organ transplant recipients, for example, are at much higher risk for UVB-induced skin cancers. People with autoimmune connective tissue diseases (such as systemic lupus erythematosus) exhibit heightened photosensitivity. These patients should receive counseling about how best to protect themselves during hours of maximal exposure. Moreover, many medications, including several prescribed specifically for travelers, can lead to photosensitivity reactions:

- Acetazolamide

- Antibiotics, including doxycycline (and other tetracyclines to a lesser degree), fluoroquinolones, sulfonamides

- Nonsteroidal anti-inflammatory drugs (NSAIDs), especially naproxen, piroxicam, ketoprofen

- Other common medications, such as furosemide, thiazide diuretics, methotrexate, and sulfonylureas

## CONSEQUENCES

### Sunburn

Sunburn is a common and self-limited condition. Clinical features vary from mild pink to painful red skin with edema and blistering on exposed surfaces. Systemic symptoms may include headache, fever, nausea, vomiting, and myalgia. Management involves symptomatic pain relief. People rarely notice they are developing a sunburn as the burn occurs. Cool compresses and bland topical emollients (such as petrolatum or zinc oxide) may be applied. Refrigerating topical emollients before application can provide added relief. Aloe vera is used commonly as a sunburn remedy, but studies are equivocal regarding its benefit.

Intact blisters should not be ruptured intentionally. Topical corticosteroids (such as hydrocortisone 1% cream or ointment) or diclofenac gel may decrease pain and inflammation. Patients typically derive benefit from oral pain relievers such as acetaminophen, aspirin, or other NSAIDs. Systemic steroids do not improve symptoms or hasten recovery.

Severe or extensive sunburns may cause fever, headache, vomiting, or dehydration; treatment includes avoidance of further sun exposure, rest in a cool setting, fluid replacement, and NSAIDs. For severe, blistering cases, it may be necessary to hospitalize the patient for fluid replacement (oral or intravenous) and pain control, similar to burn victims. It is important to maintain clean skin with gentle cleansing and treatment with emollients.

### Sun Damage and Skin Cancer

High-intensity or chronic exposure to UV radiation causes permanent loss of skin elasticity, wrinkling, and solar lentigines (brown macules with irregular borders), especially in fair-skinned people. Preventing sunburn and sun overexposure is the best way to avoid these changes.

Development of skin cancers (basal and squamous cell carcinomas [BCCs and SCCs]) is linked closely to UV exposure. BCCs typically appear as pearly or bleeding papules or ulcers or ulcerated papules, often on sun-exposed areas. These tumors rarely metastasize and can be cured with excision or other methods.

SCCs present on sun-exposed areas as scaling or bleeding papules or plaques. SCCs are 10 times more likely to metastasize than are BCCs. Solid-organ transplant patients receiving immunosuppressive therapy and patients with chronic lymphocytic leukemia are at increased risk of SCC.

Only approximately 5% of skin cancers are melanomas, although the incidence is increasing in most populations. In addition to fair skin and genetics, having had blistering sunburns before the age of 18 also is a risk factor. Melanomas are associated with the highest rates of morbidity and mortality, but early detection and treatment ensure nearly complete recovery. Melanomas can have a variety of clinical presentations, the most common of which is an irregularly bordered macule or papule. Depending on the tumor stage, surgical excision with adjuvant therapy may be required.

Intermittent intense sun exposure and blistering sunburns are associated with the development of BCC and cutaneous melanoma, whereas chronic and cumulative sun exposure is more associated with SCC. This explains the observation that people with infrequent vacations spent sunbathing in tropical areas are at greatly increased risk for melanoma.

## Other Photosensitive Disorders

Increased sun exposure can exacerbate existing skin conditions and can unmask photosensitive disorders, such as polymorphous light eruption, solar urticaria, porphyrias, and autoimmune connective tissue diseases such as dermatomyositis or systemic lupus erythematosus. If sun exposure causes prolonged or severe symptoms (such as swelling, pruritus, arthralgias, fever), medical evaluation is warranted.

**Phytophotodermatitis** is a noninfectious condition that results from interaction of natural psoralens, most commonly found in the juice of tropical limes, and UVA radiation from the sun. The result is an exaggerated sunburn that creates a painful line of blisters, followed by asymptomatic hyperpigmented lines that may take weeks or months to resolve.

**Photo-onycholysis,** a separation or lifting of the nail plate from the nail bed, is described in people taking doxycycline after a day of intense sun exposure. The most common setting is someone taking doxycycline for malaria prophylaxis during a trip to a tropical location.

## PREVENTION

Travel preparation should include planning to prevent sun overexposure. Awareness that UVB radiation is highest during midday and that UV exposure still occurs in cooler weather and on overcast days is necessary to guide general safe sun behaviors. UV exposure increases with travel to lower latitudes (closer to the equator) or to higher elevations.

## Sunscreens

Sunscreens are topical preparations that can reflect or absorb UV radiation. They may contain organic substances that filter (absorb or capture) UV radiation, inorganic products that reflect UV radiation, or both. Inorganic agents contain micropulverized metallic nanoparticles of zinc oxide or titanium dioxide, which both reflect and absorb UV radiation.

The most effective sunscreens are "broad spectrum," combining agents capable of reflecting and filtering both UVA and UVB radiation. The US Food and Drug Administration's current labeling guidelines, adopted in 2010, indicate that broad-spectrum sunscreen products with a sun protection factor (SPF) ≥15 may state, "If used as directed with other sun-protection measures, [this product] decreases the risk of skin cancer and early skin aging caused by the sun." The same labeling guidelines do not permit manufacturers to claim that products are waterproof or sweatproof; sunscreens may be labeled "water resistant" (up to either 40 or 80 minutes).

Recommendations for sunscreen use include:

- Before going outside, apply broad-spectrum sunscreen (SPF ≥15) to protect skin from both UVA and UVB, even on cloudy or cool days. Some professional organizations, such as the American Academy of Dermatology, recommend using sunscreens with an SPF ≥30. Apply sunscreen liberally to create a thin film on all exposed body surface areas, obtaining assistance to apply to difficult-to-reach areas.

- Reapply every 2–3 hours and promptly after sweating or being in the water, as sunscreens are neither waterproof nor sweatproof.

- Make sure that the sunscreen is not past its expiration date.

- When also using insect repellent, apply sunscreen first, let it dry, then apply repellent. Very limited data suggest that DEET-containing insect repellents can attenuate the UVB protection provided by sunscreen, by as much as one-third of the reported SPF. Sunscreens may increase the absorption of DEET through the skin.

- Avoid products that contain both sunscreen and insect repellent.

Inorganic sunscreens cover a broad spectrum of UV radiation and are associated with a reduced risk of allergic or irritant contact dermatitis. Although they may leave a thin, white film on the skin, they are cosmetically more acceptable than the thick, opaque pastes associated with older products. By contrast, organic sunscreens are easier to apply and less likely to leave a visible film but may trigger a sensitivity or allergic reaction. If this happens, using an inorganic sunscreen may be an alternative.

Travelers may also opt (or be required, in some locations) to use inorganic sunscreens due to the reported adverse environmental effects of the organic sunscreens: oxybenzone, 4-methylbenzylidene camphor, octocrylene, and octinoxate. In 2018, for example, Hawaii passed a law banning sunscreens containing octinoxate and oxybenzone in response to evidence of their toxicity to coral marine life.

Babies <6 months of age should have only minimal exposure to direct sunlight. Protect infants by using covered strollers, umbrellas/parasols, and hats, rather than by applying sunscreen.

## Protective Clothing

Sun-protective garments (for example, pants, long-sleeved shirts, and hats) can protect against UV radiation. Efficacy depends on the fabric. A cotton t-shirt (SPF ≤15) affords even less protection when the shirt is wet. Thicker fabrics with tighter weaves, such as denim, offer high SPF protection. Travelers can treat lighter-weight fabrics (nylon and cotton) with UV-filtering dyes and other products to enhance UV protection.

Other protective measures include hats and sunglasses. Hats with a wide circumferential brim (at least 3 inches in diameter) that shades the face, neck, and ears are ideal. Lightweight *kepi*-style ("French Foreign Legion") sunhats, with a flap to cover the neck and ears, are quite effective, especially for children. These protect the skin much more than a baseball cap. Wrap-around sunglasses or those with sun-blocking sidepieces provide the best UV protection.

## Sun Avoidance

If possible, avoiding direct sun during peak hours (10 AM to 4 PM) will decrease UV exposure. Seeking shade under trees, umbrellas, or other structures will also reduce UV exposure, although UV rays can still reflect off substances such as water, snow, and sand.

## BIBLIOGRAPHY

1. American Cancer Society. Skin cancer. [cited 2018 Mar 17]. Available from: www.cancer.org/cancer/skin-cancer.html.

2. Diaz JH, Nesbitt Jr. T. Sun exposure behavior and protection: recommendations for travelers. J Travel Med. 2013; 20(2):108–118.

3. Monteiro AF, Rato M, Martins C. Drug-induced photosensitivity: photoallergic and phototoxic reactions. Clin Dermatol 2016; 34:571.

4. Skin Cancer Foundations. Sun protection. [cited 2018 Mar 17]. Available from: www.skincancer.org/prevention/sun-protection.

5. Young AR, Claveau J, Rossi AB. Ultraviolet radiation and the skin: photobiology and sunscreen photoprotection. J Am Acad Dermatol 2017; 76:S100.

# EXTREMES OF TEMPERATURE

Howard D. Backer, David R. Shlim

International travelers encounter extremes of climate to which they are not accustomed. Exposure to heat and cold can result in serious injury or death. Travelers should investigate the climate extremes they will face during their journey and prepare with proper clothing, equipment, and knowledge.

## PROBLEMS ASSOCIATED WITH HOT CLIMATES

### Risk for Travelers

Many of the most popular travel destinations are tropical or desert areas. Travelers who sit on the beach or by the pool and do only short walking tours incur minimal risk of heat illness. Those participating in strenuous hiking, biking, or work in the heat are at risk, especially travelers coming from cool or temperate climates who are not in good physical condition and not acclimatized to the heat.

### Clinical Presentations

#### PHYSIOLOGY OF HEAT INJURIES

Unlike in the cold, where adaptive behaviors play a more important role in body heat conservation, tolerance to heat depends largely on physiologic factors. The major means of heat dissipation are radiation (while at rest) and evaporation of sweat (during exercise), both of which become minimal with air temperatures above 95°F (35°C) and high humidity.

Two major organs are involved in temperature regulation: the cardiovascular system, which must increase blood flow to shunt heat from the core to the surface, while meeting the metabolic demands of exercise; and the skin, where sweating and heat exchange take place. Cardiovascular status and conditioning are the major physiologic variables affecting the response to heat stress at all ages. Many chronic illnesses (in particular, those involving the cardiovascular system or the skin) limit tolerance to heat and predispose to heat illness; these include cardiovascular disease, diabetes, renal disease, and extensive skin disorders or scarring that limits sweating.

Apart from environmental conditions and intensity of exercise, dehydration is the most important predisposing factor in heat illness. Dehydration also reduces exercise performance, decreases time to exhaustion, and increases internal heat load. Temperature and heart rate increase in direct proportion to the level of dehydration. Sweat is a hypotonic fluid containing sodium and chloride. Sweat rates commonly reach 1 L per hour or more, resulting in substantial fluid and sodium loss.

#### MINOR HEAT DISORDERS

Heat cramps are painful muscle contractions following exercise. They begin an hour or more after stopping exercise and most often involve heavily used muscles in the calves, thighs, and abdomen. Rest and passive stretching of the muscle, supplemented by commercial rehydration solutions or water and salt, rapidly relieve symptoms. Water with a salty snack is usually sufficient. Travelers can make a simple oral salt solution by adding one-fourth to one-half teaspoon of table salt (or two 1-g salt tablets) to 1 L of water. To improve taste, a few teaspoons of sugar or orange or lemon juice may be added to the mixture.

Heat syncope—sudden fainting caused by vasodilation—occurs in unacclimatized people standing in the heat or after 15–20 minutes of exercise. Consciousness rapidly returns when the patient is supine. Rest, relief from heat, and oral rehydration are adequate treatment.

Heat edema, another minor heat disorder, occurs more frequently in women than in men. Characterized by mild swelling of the hands and feet during the first few days of heat exposure, this condition typically resolves spontaneously. Travelers should not treat heat edema with diuretics, which can both delay heat acclimatization and cause dehydration.

Prickly heat (miliaria or heat rash) manifests as small, red, raised itchy bumps on the skin caused by obstruction of the sweat ducts. It resolves spontaneously, aided by relief from heat and avoiding continued sweating. Travelers can best prevent prickly heat by wearing light, loose clothing and avoiding heavy, continuous sweating.

## MAJOR HEAT DISORDERS

### HEAT EXHAUSTION

Most people who experience acute collapse or other symptoms associated with exercise in the heat are suffering from heat exhaustion—the inability to continue exertion in the heat. The presumed cause of heat exhaustion is loss of fluid and electrolytes, but there are no objective markers to define the syndrome, which is a spectrum ranging from minor complaints to a vague boundary shared with heat stroke. Transient mental changes, such as irritability, confusion, or irrational behavior, may be present in heat exhaustion, but major neurologic signs such as seizures or coma indicate heat stroke or profound hyponatremia. Body temperature may be normal or mildly to moderately elevated.

Most cases of heat exhaustion can be treated with supine rest in the shade or other cool place and oral water or fluids containing glucose and salt; subsequently, spontaneous cooling occurs, and patients recover within hours. As previously described, travelers can prepare a simple oral salt solution by adding one-fourth to one-half teaspoon of table salt (or two 1-g salt tablets) to 1 L of water. Adding 4–6 teaspoons of sugar, one-quarter cup of orange juice, or 2 teaspoons of lemon juice can improve the taste. Commercial sports-electrolyte drinks are also effective. Plain water plus salty snacks may be more palatable and equally effective. Subacute heat exhaustion may develop over several days and is often misdiagnosed as "summer flu" because of findings of weakness, fatigue, headache, dizziness, anorexia, nausea, vomiting, and diarrhea. Treatment is as described for acute heat exhaustion.

### EXERCISE-ASSOCIATED HYPONATREMIA

Symptoms of heat exhaustion and early exercise-associated hyponatremia are similar. Hyponatremia can be distinguished from heat illnesses by persistent alteration of mental status without elevated body temperature, delayed onset of major neurologic symptoms (confusion, seizures, or coma), or deterioration up to 24 hours after cessation of exercise and removal from heat. Where medical care and clinical laboratory resources are available, measure serum sodium to diagnose hyponatremia and guide treatment.

Hyponatremia occurs in both endurance athletes and recreational hikers, due in some measure to physiologic mechanisms that result in failure of the kidneys to correct salt and fluid imbalances properly. Excess fluid retention occurs when antidiuretic hormone (secreted inappropriately) influences the kidneys to both retain water and excrete sodium. Sodium losses through sweat also contribute to hyponatremia. In the field setting, altered mental status in a patient with normal body temperature and a history of taking in large volumes of water suggests hyponatremia. The vague and nonspecific symptoms are the same as those described for hyponatremia in other settings, including anorexia, nausea, emesis, headache, muscle weakness, lethargy, confusion, and seizures.

The recommendation to force fluid intake during prolonged exercise and the attitude that "you can't drink too much" are major contributors to exercise-associated hyponatremia. Prevention includes drinking only enough to relieve thirst. During prolonged exercise (>12 hours) or heat exposure, supplemental sodium should be taken. Most sports-electrolyte drinks do not contain sufficient amounts of sodium to prevent hyponatremia; on the other hand, salt tablets often cause nausea and vomiting. For hikers, food is the most efficient vehicle for salt replacement. Snacks should include not just sweets, but salty foods such as trail mix, crackers, and pretzels.

Restrict fluid if hyponatremia is suspected (neurologic symptoms in the absence of hyperthermia or other diagnoses). In conscious patients who can tolerate oral intake, give salty snacks with sips of water or a solution of concentrated broth (2–4 bouillon cubes in 1/2 cup of water). Obtunded patients may require hypertonic saline.

3

## HEAT STROKE

Heat stroke is an extreme medical emergency requiring aggressive cooling measures and hospitalization for support. Heat stroke is the only form of heat illness in which the mechanisms for thermal homeostasis have failed, and the body does not spontaneously restore the temperature to normal. Uncontrolled fever and circulatory collapse cause organ damage to the brain, liver, kidneys, and heart. Damage is related to duration as well as peak elevation of body temperature.

The onset of heat stroke may be acute or gradual. Acute (also known as exertional) heat stroke is characterized by collapse while exercising in the heat, usually with profuse sweating. It can affect healthy, physically fit people. By contrast, gradual or nonexertional (referred to sometimes as classic or epidemic) heat stroke occurs in chronically ill people experiencing passive exposure to heat. Sufferers of nonexertional heat stroke tend not to perspire. Victims of both exertional and nonexertional heat stroke demonstrate altered mental status and markedly elevated body temperature.

Early symptoms are similar to those of heat exhaustion, with confusion or change in personality, loss of coordination, dizziness, headache, and nausea that progress to more severe symptoms. A presumptive diagnosis of heat stroke is made in the field when people have elevation of body temperature (hyperpyrexia) and marked alteration of mental status, including delirium, convulsions, and coma. Body temperatures in excess of 106°F (41°C) can occur in heat stroke; even without a thermometer, people will feel hot to the touch. If a thermometer is available, a rectal temperature is the safest and most reliable way to check the temperature of someone with suspected heat stroke; an axillary temperature may give a reasonable estimation.

In the field, immediately institute cooling measures by these methods:

- Maintain the airway if victim is unconscious.

- Move the victim to the shade or some cool place out of the sun.

- Use evaporative cooling: remove excess clothing to maximize skin exposure, spray tepid water on the skin, and maintain air movement over the body by fanning. Alternatively, place cool or cold wet towels over the body and fan to promote evaporation.

- Apply ice or cold packs to the neck, axillas, groin, and as much of the body as possible. Vigorously massage the skin to limit constriction of blood vessels and to prevent shivering, which will increase body temperature.

- Immerse the victim in cool or cold water, such as a nearby pool or natural body of water or bath—an ice bath cools fastest. Always attend and hold the person while in the water.

- Encourage rehydration for those able to take oral fluids.

Heat stroke is life threatening, and many complications occur in the first 24–48 hours, including liver or kidney damage and abnormal bleeding. Most victims have significant dehydration and many require hospital intensive care management to replace fluid losses. If evacuation to a hospital is delayed, monitor closely for several hours for temperature swings.

## Prevention of Heat Disorders

### HEAT ACCLIMATIZATION

Heat acclimatization is a process of physiologic adaptation that occurs in residents of and visitors to hot environments. Increased sweating with less salt content, and decreased energy expenditure with lower rise in body temperature for a given workload, is the result. Only partial adaptation occurs from passive exposure to heat. Full acclimatization, especially cardiovascular, requires 1–2 hours of exercise in the heat each day. With a suitable amount of daily exercise, most acclimatization changes occur within 10 days. Decay of acclimatization occurs within days to weeks if there is no heat exposure.

### PHYSICAL CONDITIONING AND ACCLIMATIZATION

If possible, all travelers should acclimatize before departing for hot climates by exercising ≥1 hour daily in the heat. Physically fit travelers have improved exercise tolerance and capacity but still benefit from acclimatization. If this is not possible, advise travelers to limit exercise intensity and duration during their first week of travel. It is a good idea to conform to the local practice in most hot regions and avoid strenuous activity during the hottest part of the day.

## CLOTHING

Clothing should be lightweight, loose, and light colored to allow maximum air circulation for evaporation yet give protection from the sun (see Sun Exposure in this chapter). A wide-brimmed hat markedly reduces radiant heat exposure.

## FLUID AND ELECTROLYTE REPLACEMENT

During exertion, fluid intake improves performance and decreases the likelihood of illness. Reliance on thirst alone is not sufficient to prevent mild dehydration, but forcing a person who is not thirsty to drink water creates the potential danger of hyponatremia. During mild to moderate exertion, electrolyte replacement offers no advantage over plain water. For those exercising many hours in the heat, however, salt replacement is recommended. Eating salty snacks or lightly salting mealtime food or fluids is the most efficient way to replace salt losses. Salt tablets swallowed whole may cause gastrointestinal irritation and vomiting; they may be better tolerated if dissolved in 1 L of water. Urine volume and color are a reasonable means to monitor fluid needs.

## PROBLEMS ASSOCIATED WITH A COLD CLIMATE

### Risk for Travelers

Travelers do not have to be in an arctic or high-elevation environment to encounter problems with cold. Humidity, rain, and wind can produce hypothermia with temperatures around 50°F (10°C). Even in temperate climates, people can rapidly become hypothermic in the water. Although reports of severe hypothermia in international travelers are rare, those planning trips to wilderness areas should be familiar with the major mechanisms of heat loss (convection, conduction, radiation) and how to mitigate them (by taking shelter from the wind, getting and staying dry, and keeping warm by building a fire).

Being caught without shelter in a wilderness environment represents a significant risk for accidental hypothermia. Many high-elevation travel destinations, however, are not wilderness areas. Local inhabitants and villages offer shelter and protection from extreme cold weather. In Nepal, for example, trekkers almost never experience hypothermia except in rare instances in which they get lost in a storm.

## Clinical Presentations

### HYPOTHERMIA

Hypothermia is defined as a core body temperature below 95°F (35°C). When people are faced with an environment in which they cannot keep warm, they first feel chilled. They then shiver, and eventually stop shivering as their metabolic reserves are exhausted. Body temperature continues to decrease, depending on ambient temperatures. As core body temperature falls, neurologic function decreases; almost all hypothermic people with a core temperature of 86°F (30°C) or lower are comatose. The record low core body temperature in an adult who survived is 56°F (13°C).

Travelers headed to cold climates should ask questions and research clothing and equipment. Modern clothing, gloves, and particularly footwear have greatly decreased the chances of suffering cold injury in extreme climates. Cold injuries occur more often after accidents, such as avalanches or unexpected nights outside, than during normal recreational activities.

Those engaging in recreational activities or working around cold water face a different sort of risk. Within 15 minutes, immersion hypothermia can render a person unable to swim or float. In these cases, a personal flotation device is critical, as is knowledge about self-rescue and righting a capsized boat.

Other medical conditions associated with cold affect mainly the skin and the extremities. These can be divided into nonfreezing cold injuries and freezing injuries (frostbite).

## NONFREEZING COLD INJURY

Nonfreezing cold injuries include trench foot (immersion foot), pernio (chilblains), and cold urticaria. Trench foot is caused by prolonged immersion of the feet in cold water (32°F–59°F; 0°C–15°C). The damage is mainly to nerves and blood vessels, and the result is pain aggravated by heat and a dependent position of the limb. Severe cases can take months to resolve. Unlike frostbite, avoid rapid rewarming of immersion foot, which can make the damage much worse.

Pernio are localized, inflammatory lesions occurring mainly on the hands after exposure to only moderately cold weather. The bluish-red lesions are thought to be caused by prolonged, cold-induced vasoconstriction. Rapid rewarming makes the pain worse; slow rewarming is preferred. Nifedipine may be an effective treatment.

Cold urticaria are localized or general wheals with itching. It is not the absolute temperature but the rate of change of temperature that induces this form of skin lesion.

## FREEZING COLD INJURY

Frostbite describes tissue damage caused by direct freezing of the skin. Once severe tissue damage occurs, little can be done. Fortunately, modern equipment and clothing are available to protect adventure tourists from frostbite. The condition now occurs mainly as the result of accidents, severe unexpected weather, or failure to plan appropriately.

Frostbite is usually graded like burns. First-degree frostbite involves reddening of the skin without deeper damage. The prognosis for complete healing is virtually 100%. Second-degree frostbite involves blister formation. Blisters filled with clear fluid have a better prognosis than blood-tinged blisters. Third-degree frostbite represents full-thickness injury to the skin and possibly the underlying tissues. No blisters form, the skin darkens over time and may turn black. If the tissue is completely devascularized, amputation will be necessary.

Severely frostbitten skin is numb and appears whitish or waxy. The generally accepted method for treating a frozen digit or limb is rapid rewarming in water heated to 104°F–108°F (40°C–42°C). Immerse the frozen area completely in the heated water. Use a thermometer to ensure the water is kept at the correct temperature. Rewarming can be associated with severe pain, so analgesics should be given if needed. Once rewarmed, protect frostbitten skin against freezing again. It is better to keep digits frozen a little longer and rapidly rewarm them than to allow them to thaw out slowly or to thaw and refreeze. A cycle of freeze-thaw-refreeze is devastating to tissue, often resulting in amputation.

Once the area has rewarmed, examine for blisters and note whether they extend to the end of the digit. Proximal blisters usually mean that the tissue distal to the blister has suffered full-thickness damage. For treatment, avoid further mechanical trauma to the area and prevent infection. In the field, wash the area thoroughly with a disinfectant such as povidone iodine, put dressings between the toes or fingers to prevent maceration, use fluffs (expanded gauze sponges) for padding, and cover with a roller gauze bandage. These dressings can be left on safely for up to 3 days at a time. By leaving the dressings on longer, travelers can preserve what may be limited supplies of bandages. Prophylactic antibiotics are not needed in most situations.

In the rare situation in which a foreign traveler suffers frostbite and can be evacuated to an advanced medical setting within 24–72 hours, there may be a role for thrombolytic agents, such as prostacyclin and recombinant tissue plasminogen activator. Clinicians managing a case of frostbite within the first 72 hours should carefully consider the risks and benefits of using these drugs; consultation with an expert is strongly recommended. Beyond 72 hours after thawing, these interventions are probably not beneficial.

Once a frostbite patient has reached a definitive medical setting, there should be no rush to do surgery. The usual time from injury to surgery is 4–5 weeks. Technetium (Tc)-99 scintigraphy and magnetic resonance imaging can be used to define the extent of the damage. Once the delineation between dead and viable tissue becomes clear, surgery that preserves the remaining digits can be planned.

**3**

## BIBLIOGRAPHY

1. Aleeban M, Mackey TK. Global Health and Visa Policy Reform to address dangers of Hajj during summer seasons. Front Public Health. 2016 Dec 22;4:280.

2. Armstrong LE, Casa DJ, Millard-Stafford M, Moran DS, Pyne SW, Roberts WO. American College of Sports Medicine position stand. Exertional heat illness during training and competition. Med Sci Sports Exerc. 2007 Mar; 39(3):556–72.

3. Bennett BL, Hew-Butler T, Hoffman MD, Roger sIR, Rosner MH, Wilderness Medical Society. Wilderness Medical Society practice guidelines for treatment of exercise-associated hyponatremia: 2014 update. Wilderness Environ Med. 2014 Dec; 25(4 Suppl):S30–42.

4. Cauchy E, Cheguillaume B, Chetaille E. A controlled trial of a prostacyclin and rt-PA in the treatment of severe frostbite. N Engl J Med. 2011 Jan 13; 364(2):189–90.

5. Epstein Y, Moran DS. Extremes of temperature and hydration. In: Keystone JS, Kozarsky PE, Connor BA, Nothdurft HD, editors. Travel Medicine. Philadelphia: Saunders Elsevier; 2013. pp. 381–90.

6. Freer L, Imray CHE. Frostbite. In: Auerbach PS, editor. Wilderness Medicine. 6th ed. Philadelphia: Mosby Elsevier; 2012. pp. 181–201.

7. Hadad E, Rav-Acha M, Heled Y, Epstein Y, Moran DS. Heat stroke: a review of cooling methods. Sports Med. 2004; 34(8):501–11.

8. Lipman GS, Eifling KP, Ellis MA, Gaudio FG, Otten EM, Grissom CK, et al. Wilderness Medical Society practice guidelines for the prevention and treatment of heat-related illness: 2014 update. Wilderness Environ Med. 2014 Dec; 25(4 Suppl):S55–65.

9. Noweir MH, Bafail AO, Jomoah IM. Study of heat exposure during Hajj (pilgrimage). Environ Monit Assess. 2008 Dec;147(1–3):279–95.

10. O'Brien KK, Leon LR, Kenefick RW. Clinical management of heat-related illnesses. In: Auerbach PS, editor. Wilderness Medicine. 6th ed. Philadelphia: Mosby Elsevier; 2012. pp. 232–8.

11. Porter AM. Collapse from exertional heat illness: implications and subsequent decisions. Mil Med. 2003 Jan;168(1):76–81.

12. Rogers IR, Hew-Butler T. Exercise-associated hyponatremia: overzealous fluid consumption. Wilderness Environ Med. 2009 Summer; 20(2):139–43.

**3**

# AIR QUALITY & IONIZING RADIATION

Armin Ansari, Suzanne Beavers

## AIR QUALITY

Although air pollution has decreased in many parts of the world, it represents a significant and growing health problem for the residents of some cities in certain industrializing countries. Polluted air can be difficult or impossible for travelers to avoid, and the risk to otherwise healthy people who have only limited exposure is generally low. Conversely, those with preexisting heart and lung disease, children, and older adults have an increased risk of adverse health effects from even short-term exposure to air pollution.

Travelers, particularly those with underlying cardiorespiratory disease, should be familiar with the air quality at their destination. The AirNow website (http://airnow.gov) provides basic information about local air quality using the Air Quality Index (AQI) (Table 3-1). The World Air Quality Index project shows real-time air quality/air pollution data for more than 10,000 air stations in more than 80 countries around the world (https://waqi.info/) and the World Health Organization posts historical data on outdoor air pollution in urban areas at http://gamapserver.who.int/gho/interactive_charts/phe/oap_exposure/atlas.html.

Travelers should be mindful of, and limit exposures to, indoor air pollution and carbon monoxide (Table 3-2). Secondhand smoke from smoking tobacco is an important contributor to indoor air pollution. Other potential sources of indoor air pollutants include cooking or combustion

## Table 3-1. Air quality index

| AIR QUALITY INDEX LEVELS OF HEALTH CONCERN | AIR QUALITY INDEX VALUES | MEANING |
| --- | --- | --- |
| Good | 0 to 50 | Satisfactory air quality<br>Air pollution poses little or no risk |
| Moderate | 51 to 100 | Acceptable air quality<br>Some pollutants may represent a moderate health concern for highly sensitive people |
| Unhealthy for Sensitive Groups | 101 to 150 | Members of sensitive groups may experience health effects<br>General public not likely to be affected |
| Unhealthy | 151 to 200 | Everyone may begin to experience health effects<br>Sensitive groups may experience more serious health effects |
| Very Unhealthy | 201 to 300 | Health alert: everyone may experience more serious health effects |
| Hazardous | 301 to 500 | Health warnings of emergency conditions<br>Entire population is more likely to be affected |

Air Quality Index Basics. [cited 2018 Jan 22]. Available from: www.airnow.gov/index.cfm?action=aqibasics.aqi.

## Table 3-2. Strategies to mitigate adverse health effects of air pollution

| ENVIRONMENTAL SOURCE | POLLUTANTS | TRAVELER CATEGORY | MITIGATION STRATEGIES |
| --- | --- | --- | --- |
| Outdoor air | Poor air quality (high levels of air pollution) or areas potentially affected by wildland fires | Travelers with preexisting asthma, chronic obstructive pulmonary disease, heart disease | Limit strenuous or prolonged outdoor activity |
| | | All travelers | Facemasks (decision to wear should be left to the traveler)[1] |
| Indoor air | High levels of smoke (for example, from cooking and combustion sources, tobacco, incense, and candles) | Long-term travelers and expatriates | Consider purchasing indoor air filtration system |
| | | All travelers | Avoidance |

[1] CDC has no recommendations regarding facemask use for travelers. One small study in Beijing showed that wearing a dust respirator with valves appeared to mitigate the negative health effects of air pollution on blood pressure and heart rate. However, the respirators used in the study had better filtration than the surgical or nuisance dust masks commonly worn in some countries.

sources, such as kerosene, coal, wood, or animal dung. Major sources of indoor carbon monoxide include gas ranges and ovens, unvented gas or kerosene space heaters, and coal- or wood-burning stoves. Ceremonial incense and candles are often unrecognized asthma triggers.

## MOLD

Travelers may visit flooded areas as part of emergency, medical, or humanitarian relief missions. Water damage to buildings can lead to mold contamination. Mold is a more serious health hazard for the immunocompromised or for people who have respiratory problems such as asthma. To prevent exposures that could result in adverse health effects, travelers should adhere to the following recommendations:

- Avoid areas where mold contamination is obvious.

- When working in moldy environments, use personal protective equipment (PPE), such as gloves, goggles, and a NIOSH-approved N95 respirator or higher. To learn more about mold and respirators, visit www.cdc.gov/disasters/disease/respiratory.html. Travelers should anticipate needing to bring sufficient quantities of PPE with them, as supplies may be scarce or not available in the countries visited.

- Keep hands, skin, and eyes clean and free from mold-contaminated dust.

- Review recommendations for dealing with mold: www.cdc.gov/mold/cleanup.htm.

## RADIATION

Background radiation levels can vary substantially from region to region, but these variations are natural and do not represent a health concern. In addition, several regions in the world have high natural background radiation. Examples of these areas include Guarapari (Brazil), Kerala (India), Ramsar (Iran), and Yangjiang (China), and traveling to these areas does not pose a threat to health. By contrast, travelers should be aware of (and avoid) regions known to be contaminated with radioactive materials. Areas surrounding the Chernobyl nuclear power plant in Ukraine and the Fukushima Daiichi nuclear power plant in Japan, for example, have radiation levels that greatly exceed background and represent a significant risk to health and safety.

The Chernobyl plant is located 100 km (62 miles) northwest of Kiev. The 1986 accident contaminated regions in 3 republics—Ukraine, Belarus, and Russia—but the highest radioactive ground contamination is within 30 km (19 miles) of Chernobyl.

The Fukushima Daiichi plant is located 240 km (150 miles) north of Tokyo. After the accident in 2011, the area within a 20-km (32-mile) radius of the plant was evacuated; Japanese authorities also advised evacuation from locations farther away to the northwest of the plant. As Japanese authorities continue to clean the affected areas and monitor the situation, access requirements and travel advisories change. The Department of State recommends against all unnecessary travel to areas designated by the Japanese government as restricted because of radioactive contamination. For up-to-date safety information or current travel advisories for any country, see the Department of State's website (https://travel.state.gov/content/travel/en/traveladvisories/traveladvisories.html) or check with the US mission in that country.

In most countries, areas of known radioactive contamination are fenced or marked with signs. Any traveler seeking long-term (more than a few months) residence near a known or suspected contaminated area should consult with staff of the nearest US embassy and inquire about any advisories regarding drinking water quality or purchase of meat, fruit, and vegetables from local farmers.

Radiation emergencies are rare events. In case of such an emergency, travelers should follow instructions provided by local authorities. If such information is not forthcoming, US travelers should seek advice from the nearest US embassy or consulate.

Natural disasters (such as floods) may displace industrial or clinical radioactive sources. In all circumstances, travelers should exercise caution when they encounter unknown objects or equipment, especially if they bear the basic radiation trefoil symbol or other radiation signs (see www.remm.nlm.gov/radsign.htm for examples).

Travelers who encounter a questionable object should avoid touching or moving it, and notify local authorities as quickly as possible.

## BIBLIOGRAPHY

1. Ansari A. Radiation threats and your safety: a guide to preparation and response for professionals and community. Boca Raton (FL): Chapman & Hall/CRC; 2009.
2. Brandt M, Brown C, Burkhart J, Burton N, Cox-Ganser J, Damon S, et al. Mold prevention strategies and possible health effects in the aftermath of hurricanes and major floods. MMWR Recomm Rep. 2006 Jun 9; 55(RR-8):1–27.
3. Brook RD, Rajagopalan S, Pope CA 3rd, Brook JR, Bhatnagar A, Diez-Roux AV, et al. Particulate matter air pollution and cardiovascular disease: An update to the scientific statement from the American Heart Association. Circulation. 2010 Jun 1; 121(21):2331–78.
4. Eisenbud M, Gesell TF. Environmental Radioactivity: from Natural, Industrial, and Military Sources. 4th ed. San Diego Academic Press; 1997.
5. Guarnieri M, Balmes JR. Outdoor air pollution and asthma. Lancet. 2014; 383(9928):1581–92.
6. Langrish JP, Mills NL, Chan JK, Leseman DL, Aitken RJ, Fokkens PH, et al. Beneficial cardiovascular effects of reducing exposure to particulate air pollution with a simple facemask. Part Fibre Toxicol. 2009; 6:8.
7. Nuclear Emergency Response Headquarters, Government of Japan. Report of Japanese Government to IAEA Ministerial Conference on Nuclear Safety: the accident at TEPCO's Fukushima nuclear power stations. 2011 [cited 2016 Sep. 19]. Available from: http://japan.kantei.go.jp/kan/topics/201106/iaea_houkokusho_e.html.
8. Shofer S, Chen TM, Gokhale J, Kuschner WG. Outdoor air pollution: counseling and exposure risk reduction. Am J Med Sci. 2007 Apr; 333(4):257–60.
9. United Nations Scientific Committee on the Effects of Atomic Radiation. Annex B: Exposures from natural radiation sources. In: Sources and Effects of Ionizing Radiation, Volume I. New York: United Nations; 2000. p 121.
10. United Nations Scientific Committee on the Effects of Atomic Radiation. Annex J: Exposure and effects of the Chernobyl accident. In: Sources and Effects of Ionizing Radiation, Volume II. New York: United Nations; 2000. p. 451–556.
11. US Department of Health and Human Services. The health consequences of involuntary exposure to tobacco smoke: a report of the Surgeon General. Atlanta, GA: US Department of Health and Human Services, Centers for Disease Control and Prevention, Coordinating Center for Health Promotion, National Center for Chronic Disease Prevention and Health Promotion, Office on Smoking and Health; 2006 [cited 2016 Sep. 22]. Available from: www.ncbi.nlm.nih.gov/books/NBK44324/.

# ANIMAL BITES & STINGS (ZOONOTIC EXPOSURES)

Kendra Stauffer, Ryan M. Wallace, G. Gale Galland, Nina Marano

## HUMAN INTERACTION WITH ANIMALS: A RISK FACTOR FOR INJURY & ILLNESS

Animals do not have to be sick to be a risk to humans. Animals such as poultry, reptiles, and goats, carry human pathogens as normal flora. Other animals, such as rodents, bats, and nonhuman primates, can be subclinical carriers of pathogens. Animals, even those in close association with humans, such as dogs or animals in petting zoos, can attack if they feel threatened, are protecting their young or territory, or are injured or ill.

Travelers should be aware that attacks by domestic animals are far more common than attacks by wildlife, and secondary infections of wounds may result in serious illness or death.

This section will cover the most common routes of transmission of illness and injury from animals and will highlight those animals that are common reservoirs of zoonotic diseases (Table 3-3). See the respective disease sections in Chapter 4 for more detailed information on specific diseases.

## ROUTES OF TRANSMISSION

### Bites and Scratches

Bites from certain mammals encountered during foreign travel (monkeys, dogs, bats, and rodents) present a risk for serious infection. Saliva from these animals can be contaminated so heavily with pathogens that a bite may not be required to cause human infection; contact with a preexisting cut or scratch or mucous membrane can represent sufficient exposure.

### PREVENTION

Before departure, travelers should have a current tetanus vaccination or documentation of a booster vaccination in the previous 5–10 years (see Chapter 4, Tetanus). Travel health providers should also assess a traveler's need for preexposure rabies immunization (see Chapter 4, Rabies). During travel, people should never try to pet, handle, or feed unfamiliar animals (domestic or wild, even in captive settings such as game ranches or petting zoos), particularly in areas where rabies is enzootic. Avoiding unfamiliar animals can help mitigate the risk of exposure to rabies, and travelers should avoid the

## Table 3-3. Common reservoirs of zoonotic diseases and mechanisms/routes of human infection

| ANIMAL RESERVOIR | DISEASES TRANSMITTED BY MECHANISM/ROUTE OF INFECTION | | RECOMMENDATIONS FOR TRAVELERS |
| --- | --- | --- | --- |
| | BITES & SCRATCHES | INHALATION & INGESTION | |
| Dogs & Cats | Globally, dogs pose the highest risk for rabies transmission. | Dogs and cats carry bacteria, viruses, and parasites in their saliva, feces, and urine that can cause severe disease in humans (e.g., *Pasteurella* spp. or *Bartonella* spp.). | Avoid unfamiliar dog and cats (even if they appear tame). Clean bite and scratch wounds promptly and seek medical care. |
| Bats | Globally, bats pose a high risk for rabies transmission. Tiny teeth and lack of apparent wound/trauma may lead people to trivialize a bite or scratch and not seek care. | Bats carry numerous pathogens including *Histoplasma* spp. and hemorrhagic fever viruses Exposure can occur during adventure activities such as caving[1] and can include mucosal or cutaneous exposure to bat saliva or droppings. | Seek medical advice even in the absence of an obvious bite wound, including: waking up to find a bat in the room or finding a bat in the room of an unattended small child or other person unable to reliably report a bite. |
| Monkeys | Monkeys carry serious, often fatal zoonotic viruses. Macaque bites can transmit B virus, a virus related to the herpes simplex viruses. | | Avoid interacting with monkeys, even if they appear tame. |

(continued)

## Table 3-3. Common reservoirs of zoonotic diseases and mechanisms/routes of human infection (continued)

| ANIMAL RESERVOIR | DISEASES TRANSMITTED BY MECHANISM/ROUTE OF INFECTION | | RECOMMENDATIONS FOR TRAVELERS |
| --- | --- | --- | --- |
| | BITES & SCRATCHES | INHALATION & INGESTION | |
| Rodents | Rodent bites and scratches can transmit rat-bite fever, lymphocytic choriomeningitis virus, viral hemorrhagic fevers, monkeypox, and many other zoonotic pathogens. | Rodents carry 85 unique zoonotic pathogens<br>Fleas, ticks, and mites on rodents can spread:<br>• Plague<br>• Rickettsial infections<br>• Lyme disease<br>• Tickborne encephalitis<br>• Tularemia<br>• Bartonellosis<br>Diseases transmitted through contact with rodent feces and urine:<br>• Lymphocytic choriomeningitis virus<br>• Viral hemorrhagic fevers<br>• Salmonellosis<br>• Leptospirosis<br>• Hantavirus<br>Disease spread through direct contact with rodents: monkeypox | Avoid places with evidence of rodent infestation. |
| Birds | | Associated with cases of highly pathogenic avian influenza in humans<br>Diseases transmitted though bird feces or aerosol exposure:<br>• Histoplasmosis<br>• Salmonellosis<br>• Psittacosis<br>• Avian mycobacteriosis | Do not eat uncooked or undercooked poultry or poultry products.<br>Avoid contact with live poultry or wild birds. |

[1] A recent example of an indirect exposure is an imported case of Marburg fever in a tourist who had visited a cave inhabited by bats (Python Cave in western Uganda). This case illustrates the risk of acquiring diseases from indirect contact with cave-dwelling bats. This same cave was the source of a fatal case of Marburg hemorrhagic fever in a Dutch tourist in 2008.

temptation to adopt stray animals from abroad. Advise parents traveling with young children to watch them carefully around unfamiliar animals, as they are more likely to be bitten or scratched and to sustain more severe injuries.

## MANAGEMENT

Travelers should clean all bite and scratch wounds quickly with soap and water to prevent infection. Wounds contaminated by necrotic tissue, dirt, or other foreign materials should be debrided promptly by health care professionals, if present.

Often, a course of antibiotics is appropriate after dog or cat bites or scratches, as these can lead to local or systemic infections.

Wound care is especially important for exposures where rabies or tetanus is a concern. Health care professionals should evaluate travelers bitten or scratched by any animal, but particularly if the attack was unprovoked, to assess the need for rabies postexposure prophylaxis (PEP). In many countries dogs, terrestrial carnivores, and bats are the most commonly reported rabid animals; a health care professional should treat high-risk exposure immediately.

Rabies is comparatively rare in primates and rodents. Nevertheless, travelers should seek evaluation from a health care professional, especially if an attack was unprovoked or the animal appeared ill. Additionally, if bitten or scratched by a monkey, travelers should be evaluated for B virus PEP (see Chapter 4, B Virus).

Travelers with high-risk exposures (including animal bites and scratches) not vaccinated for tetanus will require a dose of tetanus toxoid–containing vaccine (Tdap, Td, or DTaP). This applies to those who received their most recent tetanus toxoid–containing vaccine >5 years before their exposure and those who have not received ≥3 doses of tetanus toxoid–containing vaccines.

## Stings and Envenomations

Snakes, insects, and marine fish and invertebrates are hazards in many locations. Snakebites usually occur in areas where dense human populations coexist with dense snake populations, such as Southeast Asia, sub-Saharan Africa, and tropical areas in the Americas; 25%–40% of venomous snakebites result in negligible or trivial envenomation.

Bites and stings from spiders and scorpions can be painful and can result in illness and death, particularly among infants and children. Other insects and arthropods, such as mosquitoes and ticks, can transmit infections (see the Mosquitoes, Ticks & Other Arthropods section in this chapter).

Most injuries from marine fish and invertebrates occur from chance encounters or defensive maneuvers. Resulting wounds have many common characteristics: bacterial contamination, foreign bodies, and occasionally venom. The incidence of venomous injuries from marine fish and invertebrates is rising as the popularity of surfing, scuba diving, and snorkeling increases. Most species responsible for human injuries, including stingrays, jellyfish, stonefish, sea urchins, and scorpionfish, live in tropical coastal waters.

Avoiding stinging and venomous animals is a traveler's best precaution. Most stings and envenomation result from startling, stepping on, handling, attempting to feed, or otherwise harassing the animal.

- Before engaging in recreational activities, travelers should try to learn about the animals they may encounter, including their characteristics and habitats.

- Travelers should be aware of their surroundings:
  - > Especially at night and during warm weather when snakes tend to be more active
  - > When water conditions create poor visibility, rough water, currents, or confined areas
- Travelers should wear protective clothing:
  - > Heavy, ankle-high or higher boots and long sleeves and pants when walking outdoors in areas possibly inhabited by venomous snakes and biting insects
  - > Rash guards, swim boots, or other protective footwear in water where these animals are present
- See Mosquitoes, Ticks & Other Arthropods section in this chapter for information on proper insect repellent use.

### MANAGEMENT

Advise travelers to seek immediate medical attention any time a sting or envenomation occurs. In case of injury, species identification can help direct the best course of treatment. Photographs of the animal can aid medical personnel. Immobilization of affected limbs and application of pressure bandages that do not restrict blood flow are recommended first aid measures during victim transport to a medical facility.

Incision at bite sites and use of tourniquets to restrict blood flow to affected extremities should not be used as therapeutic options. Snakebite care is controversial and should be left to local emergency medical personnel. Specific antivenoms are available for some snakes in some areas; knowing the species of snake involved may prove critical to management. Consultation with a herpetologist can be beneficial.

If the traveler does not see or recognize the animal, health care providers will need to base treatment on the nature of the injury and the clinical effects. Bear in mind that—in some cases, at least—signs and symptoms may not appear for hours after contact. Symptoms can range from localized mild swelling and redness to more severe findings, such as difficulty breathing or swallowing, chest pain, or intense pain at the sting or bite site. Management will vary according to the severity of symptoms; therapy may include diphenhydramine, steroids, pain medication, and antibiotics.

## Inhalation and Ingestion

The normal flora in the saliva, urine, and feces of many animals are pathogenic for humans. However, exposure to animal body fluids is not always obvious or recognized. For example, water contaminated with animal urine or feces may be used to wash food items.

## PREVENTION

Discourage travelers from going into caves, tunnels, or mines housing large populations of animals. Travelers planning to enter densely populated animal habitats (such as bat caves) should don protective equipment (face shield, respirator, gloves) and clothing. Upon leaving, they should then doff dirty equipment and clothing and wash or bathe as soon as possible. Travelers should not eat or drink anything potentially contaminated by animal feces or urine. Avoiding dusty animal enclosures or housing can help prevent the inhaling of aerosolized urine and/or feces.

## MANAGEMENT

Illness related to animal excreta may not appear for hours or even weeks after exposure. Health care providers must take highly detailed travel histories that include all activities resulting in exposure to or contact with animals and their habitats. Base treatment of illness on signs, symptoms, and the specific pathogen.

## BIBLIOGRAPHY

1. Callahan M. Bites, stings and envenoming injuries. In: Keystone JS, Freedman DO, Kozarsky PE, Connor BA, Nothdurft HD, editors. Travel Medicine. 3rd ed. Philadelphia: Saunders Elsevier; 2013. pp. 413–24.

2. Cohen JI, Davenport DS, Stewart JA, et al. Recommendations for prevention of and therapy for exposure to B virus (cercopithecine herpesvirus 1). Clin Infect Dis. 2002 Nov 15; 35(10):1191–203.

3. Daly RF, House J, Stanek D, Stobierski MG. Compendium of measures to prevent disease associated with animals in public settings. J Am Vet Med Assoc. 2017; 251(11):1268–92.

4. Diaz JH. The global epidemiology, syndromic classification, management, and prevention of spider bites. Am J Trop Med Hyg. 2004; 71(2):239–50.

5. Gibbons RV. Cryptogenic rabies, bats, and the question of aerosol transmission. Ann Emerg Med. 2002; 39(5):528–36.

6. Han BA, Kramer AM, Drake JM. Global patterns of zoonotic disease in mammals. Trends Parasitol. 2016; 32(7):565–77.

7. Hifumi T, Sakai A, Kondo Y, Yamamoto A, Morine N, Ato M, et al. Venomous snake bites: clinical diagnosis and treatment. J Intensive Care. 2015; 3(16):1–9.

8. Lankau EW, Cohen NJ, Jentes ES, Adams LE, Bell TR, Blanton JD, et al. Prevention and control of rabies in an age of global travel: a review of travel- and trade-associated rabies events—United States, 1986–2012. Zoonoses Public Health. 2014; 61(5):305–16.

9. Meerburg BG, Singleton GR, Kijlstra A. Rodent-borne diseases and their risks for public health. Crit Rev Microbiol. 2009; 35(3):221–70.

10. World Health Organization. WHO Expert Consultation on rabies, Second report. World Health Organ Tech Rep Ser. 2013; 982:1–139.

# SCUBA DIVING: DECOMPRESSION ILLNESS & OTHER DIVE-RELATED INJURIES

Daniel A. Nord, Gregory A. Raczniak, James M. Chimiak

Published estimates report anywhere from 0.5 million to 4 million people in the United States participate in recreational diving; many travel to tropical areas of the world to dive. Divers face a variety of medical challenges, but because dive injuries are generally rare, few clinicians are trained in their prevention, diagnosis, and treatment. The onus, then, is on the recreational diver to assess potential risks before diving, recognize signs of injury, and seek qualified dive medicine help when needed.

## PREPARING FOR DIVE TRAVEL

Planning for dive-related travel should take into account chronic health conditions, any recent changes in health (including pregnancy, injuries, and surgeries), and medication use. Underlying respiratory conditions, such as asthma, chronic obstructive pulmonary disease, or a history of spontaneous pneumothorax, can challenge the breathing capacity required of divers. Mental health disorders (such as anxiety, claustrophobia, or substance abuse) and disorders affecting central nervous system higher function and consciousness (such as seizures) raise special concerns about diving fitness. Although medications should be reviewed for their compatibility with diving, it is usually the underlying condition for which the medication is taken that is of concern.

People with known risk factors for coronary artery disease, including but not limited to an abnormal lipid profile, elevated blood pressure, diabetes, and smoking history, who wish to either begin a dive program or continue diving, should undergo a physical examination to assess their cardiovascular fitness. This may include an electrocardiogram or exercise treadmill test. Diving is a potentially strenuous activity that can put substantial demands on the cardiovascular system. Serious injury and death are associated with poor physical conditioning; regular aerobic exercise should already be part of a diver's routine before arriving for their dive physical.

Health care workers providing travel medicine examinations for divers should also remind their patients of actions they can take in advance to reduce or eliminate risks. Identifying and assessing potential hazards (such as weather, water conditions, planned depth, bottom time, and environment) better enables divers to make decisions about acceptable risk. Preparing for a safe dive also includes having an up-to-date emergency action plan, on-hand first aid supplies (with ample oxygen), and reliable communication devices. Using correct and well-maintained protective equipment, diving with supervision, and ensuring that medical care is available in the event of an emergency are other controls that can be implemented. Finally, a diver should never feel compelled to make a dive.

## DIVING DISORDERS

### Barotrauma

Barotrauma is an injury to soft tissues resulting from a pressure differential between an airspace in the body and the ambient pressure. The resultant expansion or contraction of that space can cause injury.

#### EAR AND SINUS

The most common injury in divers is ear barotrauma (Box 3-3). On descent, failure to equalize pressure changes within the middle ear space creates a pressure gradient across the eardrum. As the middle ear tissues swell with edema—a consequence of the increased pressure—the

## BOX 3-3. Symptoms of ear barotrauma

- Pain
- Tinnitus (ringing in the ears)
- Vertigo (dizziness or sensation of spinning)
- Sensation of fullness
- Sense of "water" in the ear (serous fluid/blood accumulation in the middle ear)
- Decreased hearing

pressure difference across the eardrum pushes it into the middle ear space causing it to bleed and possibly rupture.

Forceful equalization under these conditions can increase the pressure differential between the inner ear and the middle ear, resulting in round window rupture with perilymph leakage and inner ear damage. To avoid these pathologic processes, divers must learn proper equalization techniques. The physician can coach this effort by observing movement of the tympanic membrane using simple otoscopy.

Paranasal sinuses, because of their relatively narrow connecting passageways, are especially susceptible to barotrauma, generally on descent. With small changes in pressure (depth), symptoms are usually mild and subacute but can be exacerbated by continued diving. Larger pressure changes can be more injurious, especially with forceful attempts at equilibration (such as the Valsalva maneuver).

Additional risk factors for ear and sinus barotrauma include:

- Use of solid earplugs
- Medication (such as overuse or prolonged use of decongestants leading to rebound congestion)
- Ear or sinus surgery
- Nasal deformity or polyps
- Chronic nasal and sinus disease that interferes with equilibration during the large barometric pressure changes encountered while diving

Divers who suspect they may have ear or sinus barotrauma should discontinue diving and seek medical attention.

## PULMONARY

A scuba diver reduces the risk of lung overpressure problems by breathing normally and ascending slowly when breathing compressed gas. Overexpansion of the lungs can result if a scuba diver ascends toward the surface without proper exhalation, which may happen, for example, when a novice diver panics. During ascent, compressed gas trapped in the lung increases in volume until the expansion exceeds the elastic limit of lung tissue, causing damage and allowing gas bubbles to escape into 3 possible locations:

- **Pleural space.** Gas entering the pleural space can cause lung collapse or pneumothorax.

- **Mediastinum.** Gas entering the space around the heart, trachea, and esophagus causes mediastinal emphysema and frequently tracks under the skin (subcutaneous emphysema) or into the tissue around the larynx, sometimes precipitating a change in voice characteristics.

- **Pulmonary vasculature.** Gas rupturing the alveolar walls can enter the pulmonary capillaries and pass via the pulmonary veins to the left side of the heart, resulting in arterial gas embolism (AGE).

While mediastinal or subcutaneous emphysema may resolve spontaneously, pneumothorax generally requires specific treatment to remove the air and reinflate the lung. AGE is a medical emergency, requiring urgent intervention with hyperbaric oxygen therapy (recompression treatment).

Lung overinflation injuries from scuba diving can range from mild to dramatic and life threatening. Although pulmonary barotrauma is uncommon in divers, prompt medical evaluation is necessary, and clinicians must rule out this condition in patients presenting with post-dive respiratory or neurologic symptoms.

## Decompression Illness

Decompression illness (DCI) describes the dysbaric injuries (such as AGE) and decompression sickness (DCS). Because scientists consider the two diseases to result from separate causes, they are described here separately. However, from a clinical and practical standpoint, distinguishing between them in the field may be impossible and unnecessary, since the initial treatment is the same for both (Box 3-4). DCI can occur even in divers who have carefully followed the standard decompression tables and the principles of "safe" diving. Serious permanent injury or death may result from AGE or DCS.

### ARTERIAL GAS EMBOLISM

Gas entering the arterial blood through ruptured pulmonary vessels can distribute bubbles into the body tissues, including the heart and brain, where they can disrupt circulation or damage vessel walls. The presentation of AGE ranges from minimal neurologic findings to dramatic symptoms requiring urgent and aggressive treatment.

In general, a clinician should suspect AGE in any scuba diver who surfaces unconscious or loses consciousness within 10 minutes after surfacing. Initiate basic life support, including administration of the highest fraction of oxygen. Since relapses can and do occur, evacuate rapidly to a hyperbaric oxygen treatment facility even if the diver appears to have recovered fully.

### DECOMPRESSION SICKNESS

Breathing air under pressure causes excess inert gas (usually nitrogen) to dissolve in and saturate body tissues. The amount of gas dissolved is proportional to—and increases with—the total depth and time a diver is below the surface. As the diver ascends, the excess dissolved gas must be cleared through respiration. Depending on the amount of gas dissolved and the rate of ascent, some can supersaturate tissues, where it separates from

## BOX 3-4. Decompression illness syndromes—clinical findings

| ARTERIAL GAS EMBOLISM | DECOMPRESSION SICKNESS |
|---|---|
| Chest pain or bloody sputum | Coughing spasms or shortness of breath |
| Loss of consciousness | Collapse or unconsciousness |
| Personality change, difficulty thinking, or confusion | Personality changes |
| Muscular weakness | Weakness |
| Paralysis | Paralysis |
| Numbness or paresthesias | Numbness or tingling |
| Dizziness | Dizziness |
| Ataxia | Staggering, loss of coordination, or tremors |
| Blurred vision | Mottling or marbling of skin |
| Convulsions | Loss of bowel or bladder function |
| | Itching |
| | Joint aches or pain |
| | Unusual fatigue |

solution to form bubbles, interfering with blood flow and tissue oxygenation.

## Other Conditions Related to Diving

**Drowning:** Any incapacitation while underwater can result in drowning (see Injury & Trauma in this chapter).

**Nitrogen narcosis:** At increasing depths, the partial pressure of nitrogen increases, causing narcosis in all divers. The impairment can be life threatening. This narcosis quickly clears on ascent and is *not* seen on the surface after a dive, which helps differentiate this condition from AGE.

**Oxygen toxicity:** At increasing partial pressures of oxygen, levels in the blood become high enough to cause seizures. This is not seen when diving on air at recreational depth limits.

**Immersion (induced) pulmonary edema (IPE):** The hemodynamic effects of water immersion account for a shift of fluid from peripheral to central circulation that can result in higher pressures within the pulmonary capillary bed, forcing excess fluid into the lungs. Symptoms and signs of IPE generally begin on descent or at depth and include chest pain, dyspnea, wheezing, and productive cough with frothy sputum. Although not entirely well understood, age, overhydration, overexertion, negative inspiratory pressure, and left ventricular hypertrophy are believed to increase IPE risk in otherwise healthy divers. Anyone experiencing acute pulmonary edema while diving requires a workup to rule out myocardial ischemia, evaluation of left ventricular function, hypertrophy, and valvular integrity.

**Hazardous marine life:** Oceans and waterways are filled with marine animals, most of which are generally harmless unless threatened. Most injuries are the result of chance encounters or defensive maneuvers. Resulting wounds have many common characteristics: bacterial contamination, foreign bodies, and occasionally venom. See Animal Bites & Stings (Zoonotic Exposures) in this chapter for prevention and injury management recommendations.

## FLYING AFTER DIVING

The risk of developing decompression sickness increases when divers go to increased altitude too soon after a dive. The cabin pressure of commercial aircraft may be the equivalent of 6,000–8,000 ft (1,829–2,438 m). Thus, divers should wait before flying at an altitude >2,000 ft (610 m) for:

- ≥12 hours after surfacing from a single no-decompression dive
- ≥18 hours after multiple dives or multiple days of diving
- 24–48 hours after a dive that required decompression stops

These recommended preflight surface intervals reduce, but do not eliminate, risk of DCS. Longer surface intervals further reduce this risk.

## DIVING AFTER FLYING

There are no guidelines for diving after flying. Divers should wait a sufficient period of time to acclimate mentally and physically to their new location in order to focus solely on the dive.

## PREVENTING DIVING DISORDERS

Recreational divers should dive conservatively and well within the no-decompression limits of their dive tables or computers. Risk factors for DCI are primarily dive depth, dive time, and rate of ascent. Additional factors such as repetitive dives, strenuous exercise, overhead situations (such as caves or wrecks), dives to depths >60 ft. (18 m), altitude exposure soon after a dive, difficult diving conditions (for example, decreased visibility, currents, wave action) and certain physiologic variables also increase risk. Caution divers to stay well hydrated and rested and dive within the limits of their training. Diving is a skill that requires training and certification and should be done with a companion (or buddy).

# TREATMENT OF DIVING DISORDERS

Definitive treatment of DCI begins with early recognition of symptoms, followed by recompression with hyperbaric oxygen. Any unusual symptoms occurring soon after a dive should be suspect and properly evaluated. Breathing a high concentration (100%) of supplemental oxygen is recommended. Surface-level oxygen given for first aid may relieve the signs and symptoms of DCI and should be administered as soon as possible.

Because of either incidental causes, immersion, or DCI itself, which can cause capillary leakage, divers are often dehydrated. Administration of isotonic glucose-free intravenous fluid is recommended in most cases. Oral rehydration fluids may also be helpful, provided they can be administered safely ( for example, if the diver is conscious and can maintain his or her airway).

The definitive treatment of DCI is recompression and oxygen administration in a hyperbaric chamber. It is worth noting that stable or remitting symptoms of mild DCI (such as limb pain, constitutional symptoms, some cutaneous sensory changes, or rash) in divers reporting from remote locations without a hyperbaric facility may not require recompression. Such conditions involve reasonable decision making with a qualified dive medicine physician and should take into account the prevailing circumstances, complicated logistics, the hazardous nature of evacuation, and the likelihood of disadvantaging the patient by failing to recompress.

Divers Alert Network (DAN) maintains 24-hour emergency consultation and evacuation assistance at 919-684-9111 (collect calls are accepted). DAN can help with the medical management of injured divers, deciding if recompression is needed, providing the location of the closest recompression facility, and arranging patient transport. Divers and health care providers can also contact DAN for routine, nonemergency consultation by telephone at 919-684-2948, extension 6222, or by accessing the DAN website (www.diversalertnetwork.org).

Travelers who plan to scuba dive may want to ascertain whether recompression facilities are available at their destination before embarking on their trip.

## BIBLIOGRAPHY

1. Brubakk AO, Neuman TS, Bennett PB, Elliott DH. Bennett and Elliott's Physiology and Medicine of Diving. 5th ed. London: Saunders; 2003.

2. Dear G, Pollock NW. DAN America Dive and Travel Medical Guide. 5th ed. Durham, NC: Divers Alert Network; 2009.

3. Mitchell SJ, Doolette DJ, Wachholz, CJ, Vann RD, editors. Management of Mild or Marginal Decompression Illness in Remote Locations. Sydney, Australia: Undersea and Hyperbaric Medical Society; 2004.

4. Moon RE. Treatment of decompression illness. In: Bove AA, Davis JC, editors. Bove and Davis' Diving Medicine. 4th ed. Philadelphia: WB Saunders; 2004. pp. 195–223.

5. Neuman TS, Thom SR. Physiology and medicine of hyperbaric oxygen therapy. Philadelphia, PA: Saunders; 2008.

6. Sheffield P, Vann RD. Flying after recreational diving, workshop proceedings of the Divers Alert Network 2002 May 2. Durham, NC: Divers Alert Network; 2004 [cited 2016 Sep. 22]. Available from: www. diversalertnetwork.org/research/projects/fad/workshop/FADWorkshopProceedings.pdf.

7. The heart and diving: immersion pulmonary edema. Durham, NC: Divers Alert Network; 2017 [cited 2018 Mar. 23]. Available from: www.diversalertnetwork.org/health/heart/immersion-pulmonary-edema.

8. US Navy Diving Manual Revision 6 Change A. Publication Number SS521-AG-PRO-010 0910-LP-106-0957. 2011 [cited 2016 Mar, 16]. Available from: http://www.usu.edu/scuba/navy_manual6.pdf.

# ZOONOSES: THE ONE HEALTH APPROACH

Ria R. Ghai, Casey Barton Behravesh

**3**

The One Health approach to zoonotic illnesses is predicated on the connection that exists between people, animals, and the environment. As a discipline, One Health includes specialists from multiple health sectors: human medicine and public health, veterinary medicine, and environmental health; its areas of interest cover zoonotic diseases, antimicrobial resistance, food safety and food security, vectorborne diseases, and other shared health threats at the human–animal–environment interface.

No single sector can address challenges at the human–animal–environment interface alone, but coordinated efforts to identify and manage animal or environmental sources of infection can prevent, detect, and respond to infectious disease threats. For example, programs that use a One Health approach between medical and veterinary professionals have controlled rabies in animals; annual or biannual mass dog vaccination campaigns prevent human rabies deaths.

## ZOONOTIC DISEASES

Diseases addressed by the One Health approach are typically zoonotic. Approximately 60% of all known human infectious disease agents originate in animals, including brucellosis, anthrax, and salmonellosis. Most new or emerging infectious diseases in humans are zoonotic, such as Ebola, Middle East respiratory syndrome, and highly pathogenic avian influenza. Further, 80% of disease agents identified with bioterrorism potential are zoonotic.

## ONE HEALTH AND TRAVEL MEDICINE

International travelers may be at risk of zoonotic diseases through a variety of exposures not limited to wild or domestic animal contact or insect vectors. Contaminated environmental surfaces, freshwater sources (such as ponds and rivers), and food and beverages have also been implicated as sources of zoonotic illness in humans. Failure to identify sources of exposure associated with a traveler's destination, itinerary, and activities can delay correct diagnosis and treatment and potentially increase the risk for further transmission of disease.

Patients benefit when health care providers employ the One Health approach. In the pretravel consultation, providers should make travelers aware of zoonotic and other infectious disease risks in the areas where they are traveling, encouraging them to take measures to reduce those risks (for example, through vaccinations or prophylactic medications). In the posttravel setting, providers should ask questions about interactions with animals (such as pets, free-roaming animals, livestock, and wildlife), including the apparent health of these animals, and animal habitats encountered during travel. Occasionally, health care providers and veterinarians may need to consult together on a patient with a suspected zoonotic disease.

## Zoonotic Transmission: Direct and Indirect Animal Contact

Travelers must remain aware of the risks associated with animal contact. Direct contact with the saliva, blood, urine, mucus, feces, or other body fluids of an infected animal increases the risk of exposure to zoonotic pathogens; common routes of contact include petting or handling animals and being bitten or scratched (for details see Animal Bites & Stings [Zoonotic Exposures] in this chapter). Additionally, ecotourism ventures that involve riding animals such as horses, camels, or elephants pose a potential risk for injury or zoonotic diseases. However, it is difficult to know which animals could be carrying pathogenic organisms, especially since animal carriers can appear healthy. Contact with environmental surfaces where animals have been can also pose a risk of zoonotic disease transmission. Travelers should avoid contact with animals and their secretions, and if animal contact cannot be avoided, travelers should ensure they are up-to-date with recommended vaccinations and seek medical care if bitten or scratched.

## Zoonotic Transmission: Exposure to Disease Vectors

Rickettsial diseases, plague (*Yersinia pestis* infection), and yellow fever are all examples of zoonotic diseases transmitted by insect vectors. Travelers can minimize exposure to vectors by adhering to insect precautions and regularly performing tick checks on people and any traveling pets (for details see Mosquitoes, Ticks & Other Arthropods in this chapter).

## Zoonotic Transmission: Foodborne Exposure

Because many foodborne pathogens have an animal reservoir, consuming raw or undercooked animal parts or products exposes travelers to zoonotic pathogens. In many developing countries, for example, unpasteurized milk or dairy products (cheese, for example) made from unpasteurized milk carries the risk of *Brucella*, *Campylobacter*, *Cryptosporidium*, *Listeria*, and others. Travelers should avoid eating bushmeat— raw, smoked, or partially processed meat from bats, nonhuman primates, rodents, or other wild animals. Advise travelers to eat only fully cooked meat, fish, shellfish, eggs, and other foods, and to drink only pasteurized milk and dairy products, to reduce the risk of foodborne illness while traveling (see Chapter 2, Food & Water Precautions, for more details).

### BIBLIOGRAPHY

1. Angelo KM, Barbre K, Shieh WJ, Kozarsky PE, Blau DM, Sotir MJ, Zaki SR. International travelers with infectious diseases determined by pathology results, Centers for Disease Control and Prevention—United States, 1995–2015. Trav Med Infect Dis. 2017;19:8–15.

2. Centers for Disease Control and Prevention. One Health. [cited 2018 Mar 19–21]. Available from: www.cdc.gov/onehealth/index.html.

3. Centers for Disease Control and Prevention. Healthy Pets, Healthy People. [cited 2018 Mar 19–21]. Available from: www.cdc.gov/healthypets/.

4. Daly RF, House J, Stanek D, Stobierski MG. Compendium of measures to prevent disease associated with animals in public settings, 2017. J Am Vet Med Assoc. 2017; 251(11):1269–92.

5. Day M. Human-animal health interactions: the role of One Health. Am Fam Phys. 2016;93(5):344–6.

6. Hurley JW, Friend M. Zoonoses and travel. In: Friend M, editor. Disease emergence and resurgence: the wildlife-human connection. Reston (VA): US Geological Survey; 2006. p. 191–206.

3

*Perspectives* sections are written as editorial discussions aiming to add depth and clinical perspective to the official recommendations contained in the book. The views and opinions expressed in this section are those of the author and do not necessarily represent the official position of CDC.

# HIGH-ALTITUDE TRAVEL & ALTITUDE ILLNESS

Peter H. Hackett, David R. Shlim

Environments significantly above sea level expose travelers to cold, low humidity, increased ultraviolet radiation, and decreased air pressure, all of which can cause problems. The biggest concern, however, is hypoxia. At an elevation of 10,000 ft (3,000 m) above sea level, for example, the inspired $PO_2$ is a little more than two-thirds (69%) what it is at sea level. The magnitude of hypoxic stress depends on elevation, rate of ascent, and duration of exposure. Sleeping at high elevation produces the most hypoxemia; day trips to high elevations with return to low elevation are much less stressful on the body. Typical high-elevation destinations include Cusco (11,000 ft; 3,300 m), La Paz (12,000 ft; 3,640 m), Lhasa (12,100 ft; 3,650 m), Everest Base Camp (17,700 ft; 5,400 m), and Kilimanjaro (19,341 ft; 5,895 m; see Chapter 10, Tanzania: Kilimanjaro).

The human body adjusts very well to moderate hypoxia, but requires time to do so (Box 3-5). The process of acute acclimatization to high elevation takes 3–5 days; therefore, acclimatizing for a few days at 8,000–9,000 ft (2,500–2,750 m) before proceeding to a higher elevation is ideal. Acclimatization prevents altitude illness, improves sleep and cognition, and increases comfort and well-being, although exercise performance will always be reduced compared to what it would be at lower elevations. Increase in ventilation is the most important factor in acute acclimatization; therefore, respiratory depressants must be avoided. Expanded red-cell production does not play a role in acute acclimatization, although hemoglobin concentration is increased within 48 hours because of diuresis and decreased plasma volume.

## RISK FOR TRAVELERS

Inadequate acclimatization may lead to altitude illness in any traveler going to 8,000 ft (2,500 m) or higher, and sometimes even at lower elevations. Susceptibility and resistance to altitude illness are genetic traits, and no simple screening tests are available to predict risk. Training or physical fitness do not affect risk. Children are equally susceptible as adults; people aged >50 years slightly so. How a traveler has responded to high elevations previously is the most reliable guide for future trips if the elevation and rate of ascent are similar, although this is not an infallible predictor. Given a baseline susceptibility, 3 factors largely influence the risk of a traveler developing altitude illness: elevation at destination, rate of ascent, and

---

BOX 3-5.   ## Tips for acclimatization

- Ascend gradually, if possible. Avoid going directly from low elevation to more than 9,000 ft (2,750 m) sleeping elevation in 1 day. Once above 9,000 ft (2,750 m), move sleeping elevation no higher than 1,600 ft (500 m) per day, and plan an extra day for acclimatization every 3,300 ft (1,000 m).
- Consider using acetazolamide to speed acclimatization if abrupt ascent is unavoidable.
- Avoid alcohol for the first 48 hours; continue caffeine if a regular user.
- Participate in only mild exercise for the first 48 hours.
- Having a high-elevation exposure (greater than 9,000 ft [2,750 m]) for 2 nights or more, within 30 days before the trip, is useful, but closer to the trip departure is better.

## Table 3-4. Risk categories for acute mountain sickness

| RISK CATEGORY | DESCRIPTION | PROPHYLAXIS RECOMMENDATIONS |
|---|---|---|
| Low | • People with no prior history of altitude illness and ascending to less than 9,000 ft (2,750 m)<br>• People taking ≥2 days to arrive at 8,200–9,800 ft (2,500–3,000 m), with subsequent increases in sleeping elevation less than 1,600 ft (500 m) per day, and an extra day for acclimatization every 3,300 ft (1,000 m) | Acetazolamide prophylaxis generally not indicated. |
| Moderate | • People with prior history of AMS and ascending to 8,200–9,200 ft (2,500–2,800 m) or higher in 1 day<br>• No history of AMS and ascending to more than 9,200 ft (2,800 m) in 1 day<br>• All people ascending more than 1,600 ft (500 m) per day (increase in sleeping elevation) at elevations above 9,900 ft (3,000 m), but with an extra day for acclimatization every 3,300 ft (1,000 m) | Acetazolamide prophylaxis would be beneficial and should be considered. |
| High | • History of AMS and ascending to more than 9,200 ft (2,800 m) in 1 day<br>• All people with a prior history of HAPE or HACE<br>• All people ascending to more than 11,400 ft (3,500 m) in 1 day<br>• All people ascending more than 1,600 ft (500 m) per day (increase in sleeping elevation) above 9,800 ft (3,000 m), without extra days for acclimatization<br>• Very rapid ascents (such as less than 7-day ascents of Mount Kilimanjaro) | Acetazolamide prophylaxis strongly recommended. |

Abbreviations: AMS, acute mountain sickness; HACE, high-altitude cerebral edema; HAPE, high-altitude pulmonary edema.

exertion (Table 3-4). Creating an itinerary to avoid any occurrence of altitude illness is difficult because of variations in individual susceptibility, as well as in starting points and terrain. The goal for the traveler may not be to avoid all symptoms of altitude illness but to have no more than mild illness.

Some common destinations (such as the ones mentioned above) require rapid ascent by airplane to >3,400 meters, placing travelers in the high-risk category (Table 3-4). Chemoprophylaxis may be necessary for these travelers, in addition to 2–4 days of acclimatization before going higher. In some cases, such as Cusco and La Paz, the traveler can descend to elevations much lower than the airport to sleep.

## CLINICAL PRESENTATION

Altitude illness is divided into 3 syndromes: acute mountain sickness (AMS), high-altitude cerebral edema (HACE), and high-altitude pulmonary edema (HAPE).

## Acute Mountain Sickness

AMS is the most common form of altitude illness, affecting, for example, 25% of all visitors sleeping above 8,000 ft (2,500 m) in Colorado. Symptoms are similar to those of an alcohol hangover: headache is the cardinal symptom, sometimes accompanied by fatigue, loss of appetite, nausea, and occasionally vomiting. Headache onset is usually 2–12 hours after arrival at a higher elevation and often during or after the first night. Preverbal children may develop loss of appetite, irritability, and pallor. AMS generally resolves with 12–48 hours of acclimatization.

## High-Altitude Cerebral Edema

HACE is a severe progression of AMS and is rare; it is most often associated with HAPE. In addition to AMS symptoms, lethargy becomes profound, with drowsiness, confusion, and ataxia on tandem gait test, similar to alcohol intoxication. A person with HACE requires immediate descent; if the person fails to descend, death can occur within 24 hours of developing ataxia.

## High-Altitude Pulmonary Edema

HAPE can occur by itself or in conjunction with AMS and HACE; incidence is 1 per 10,000 skiers in Colorado and up to 1 per 100 climbers at more than 14,000 ft (4,270 m). Initial symptoms are increased breathlessness with exertion, and eventually increased breathlessness at rest, associated with weakness and cough. Oxygen or descent is lifesaving. HAPE can be more rapidly fatal than HACE.

## Preexisting Medical Problems

Travelers with medical conditions such as heart failure, myocardial ischemia (angina), sickle cell disease, any form of pulmonary insufficiency or preexisting hypoxemia, or obstructive sleep apnea (OSA) should consult a physician familiar with high-altitude medical issues before undertaking such travel (Table 3-5).

Travel to high elevations does not appear to increase the risk for new events due to ischemic heart disease in previously healthy persons. Patients with well-controlled asthma, hypertension, atrial arrhythmia, and seizure disorders at low elevations generally do well at high elevations. All patients with OSA should receive acetazolamide; those with mild to moderate OSA may do well without their CPAP machines, while those with severe OSA should avoid high elevation travel unless given supplemental oxygen in addition to their CPAP. People with diabetes can travel safely to high elevations, but they must be accustomed to exercise and carefully monitor their blood glucose. Altitude illness can trigger diabetic ketoacidosis, which may be more difficult to treat in those taking

## Table 3-5. Ascent risk associated with various underlying medical conditions

| LIKELY NO EXTRA RISK | CAUTION REQUIRED[1] | ASCENT CONTRAINDICATED |
|---|---|---|
| Children and adolescents | Infants <6 weeks old | Sickle cell anemia |
| Elderly people | Compensated heart failure | Severe chronic obstructive |
| Sedentary people | Morbid obesity | pulmonary disease |
| Mild obesity | Cystic fibrosis (FEV$_1$ 30%–50% | Pulmonary hypertension with |
| Well-controlled asthma | predicted) | pulmonary artery systolic |
| Diabetes mellitus | Poorly controlled arrhythmia | pressure >60 mm Hg |
| Coronary artery disease | Poorly controlled asthma | Unstable angina |
| following revascularization | Poorly controlled hypertension | Decompensated heart failure |
| Mild chronic obstructive | Moderate chronic obstructive | High-risk pregnancy |
| pulmonary disease | pulmonary disease | Cystic fibrosis (FEV$_1$ <30% predicted) |
| Low-risk pregnancy | Severe obstructive sleep apnea | Recent myocardial infarction or |
| Mild–moderate obstructive | Stable angina | stroke (<90 days) |
| sleep apnea | Nonrevascularized coronary artery | Untreated cerebral vascular |
| Controlled hypertension | disease | aneurysms or arteriovenous |
| Controlled seizure disorder | Sickle cell trait | malformations |
| Psychiatric disorders | Poorly controlled seizure disorder | Cerebral space-occupying lesions |
| Neoplastic diseases | Cirrhosis | |
| | Mild pulmonary hypertension | |
| | Radial keratotomy surgery | |

Abbreviations: FEV$_1$, forced expiratory volume in 1 s.
[1] Patients with these conditions most often require consultation with a physician experienced in high-altitude medicine and a comprehensive management plan.

acetazolamide. Not all glucose meters read accurately at high elevations.

Most people do not have visual problems at high elevations. However, at very high elevations some people who have had radial keratotomy may develop acute farsightedness and be unable to care for themselves. LASIK and other newer procedures may produce only minor visual disturbances at high elevations.

Travel to high elevations during pregnancy warrants confirmation of good maternal health and verification of a low-risk gestation. A discussion with the traveler of the dangers of having a pregnancy complication in remote, mountainous terrain is also appropriate. That said, there are no studies or case reports of harm to a fetus if the mother travels briefly to high elevations during her pregnancy. It may nevertheless be prudent to recommend that pregnant women do not stay at sleeping elevations above 10,000 ft (3,048 m).

## DIAGNOSIS AND TREATMENT

### Acute Mountain Sickness/ High-Altitude Cerebral Edema

The differential diagnosis of AMS/HACE is broad and includes dehydration, exhaustion, hypoglycemia, hypothermia, hyponatremia, carbon monoxide poisoning, infections, drug effects, and neurologic problems including migraine. Focal neurologic symptoms and seizures are rare in HACE and should lead to suspicion of an intracranial lesion or seizure disorder. Descending ≥300 m in elevation relieves HACE symptoms rapidly. Alternatively, supplemental oxygen at 2 L per minute relieves headache quickly and helps resolve AMS over hours, but it is rarely available. People with AMS can also safely remain at their current elevation and treat symptoms with nonopiate analgesics and antiemetics, such as ondansetron. They may also take acetazolamide, which speeds acclimatization and effectively treats AMS but is better for prophylaxis than treatment. Dexamethasone is more effective than acetazolamide at rapidly relieving the symptoms of moderate to severe AMS. If symptoms are getting worse while the traveler is resting at the same elevation, or in spite of medication, he or she must descend.

HACE is an extension of AMS characterized by neurologic findings, particularly ataxia, confusion, or altered mental status. HACE may also occur in the presence of HAPE. Initiate descent in any person suspected of having HACE. If descent is not feasible because of logistical issues, supplemental oxygen or a portable hyperbaric chamber in addition to dexamethasone can be lifesaving.

## High-Altitude Pulmonary Edema

Although the progression of decreased exercise tolerance, increased breathlessness, and breathlessness at rest is almost always recognizable as HAPE, the differential diagnosis includes pneumonia, bronchospasm, myocardial infarction, or pulmonary embolism. Descent in this situation is urgent and mandatory, accomplished with as little exertion as is feasible for the patient. If descent is not immediately possible, supplemental oxygen or a portable hyperbaric chamber is critical. Patients with HAPE who have access to oxygen (at a hospital or high-altitude medical clinic, for example) may not need to descend to lower elevation and can be treated with oxygen at the current elevation. In the field setting, where resources are limited and there is a lower margin for error, nifedipine can be used as an adjunct to descent, oxygen, or portable hyperbaric therapy. A phosphodiesterase inhibitor may be used if nifedipine is not available, but concurrent use of multiple pulmonary vasodilators is not recommended.

## MEDICATIONS

In addition to the discussion below, recommendations for the usage and dosing of medications to prevent and treat altitude illness are outlined in Table 3-6.

### Acetazolamide

Acetazolamide prevents AMS when taken before ascent; it can also help speed recovery if taken after symptoms have developed. The drug works by acidifying the blood and reducing the respiratory alkalosis associated with high elevations, thus increasing respiration and arterial oxygenation and speeding acclimatization. An effective dose that minimizes the

## Table 3-6. Recommended medication dosing to prevent and treat altitude illness

| MEDICATION | USE | ROUTE | DOSE |
|---|---|---|---|
| Acetazolamide | AMS, HACE prevention | Oral | 125 mg twice a day; 250 mg twice a day if >100 kg<br>Pediatrics: 2.5 mg/kg every 12 h, up to 125 mg |
| | AMS treatment[1] | Oral | 250 mg twice a day |
| Dexamethasone | AMS, HACE prevention | Oral | 2 mg every 6 h or 4 mg every 12 h<br>Pediatrics: should not be used for prophylaxis |
| | AMS, HACE treatment | Oral, IV, IM | AMS: 4 mg every 6 h<br>HACE: 8 mg once, then 4 mg every 6 h<br>Pediatrics: 0.15 mg/kg/dose every 6 h up to 4 mg |
| Nifedipine | HAPE prevention | Oral | 30 mg SR version every 12 h, or 20 mg SR version every 8 h |
| | HAPE treatment | Oral | 30 mg SR version every 12 h, or 20 mg SR version every 8 h |
| Tadalafil | HAPE prevention | Oral | 10 mg twice a day |
| Sildenafil | HAPE prevention | Oral | 50 mg every 8 h |

Abbreviations: AMS, acute mountain sickness; HACE, high-altitude cerebral edema; HAPE, high-altitude pulmonary edema; IM, intramuscular; IV, intravenous; SR, sustained release.
[1] Acetazolamide can also be used at this dose as an *adjunct* to dexamethasone in HACE treatment, but dexamethasone remains the primary treatment for that disorder.

common side effects of increased urination and paresthesias of the fingers and toes is 125 mg every 12 hours, beginning the day before ascent and continuing the first 2 days at elevation, or longer if ascent continues.

Allergic reactions to acetazolamide are uncommon. As a nonantimicrobial sulfonamide, it does not cross-react with antimicrobial sulfonamides. However, it is best avoided by people with history of anaphylaxis to any sulfa. People with history of severe penicillin allergy have occasionally had allergic reactions to acetazolamide. The pediatric dose is 5 mg/kg/day in divided doses, up to 125 mg twice a day.

### Dexamethasone

Dexamethasone is effective for preventing and treating AMS and HACE and prevents HAPE as well. Unlike acetazolamide, if the drug is discontinued at elevation before acclimatization, mild rebound can occur. Acetazolamide is preferable to prevent AMS while ascending, with dexamethasone reserved as an adjunct treatment for descent. The adult dose is 4 mg every 6 hours. An increasing trend is to use dexamethasone for "summit day" on high peaks such as Kilimanjaro and Aconcagua, in order to prevent abrupt altitude illness.

### Nifedipine

Nifedipine both prevents and ameliorates HAPE. For prevention, it is generally reserved for people who are particularly susceptible to the condition. The adult dose for prevention or treatment is 30 mg of extended release every 12 hours or 20 mg every 8 hours.

## OTHER MEDICATIONS

Phosphodiesterase-5 inhibitors can also selectively lower pulmonary artery pressure, with less effect on systemic blood pressure. Tadalafil, 10 mg twice a day during ascent, can prevent HAPE; it may also have use as a treatment. Gingko biloba, 100–120 mg taken twice a day before ascent, reduced AMS in adults in some trials. It was not effective in other trials, though, possibly due to variation in ingredients (see Chapter 2, Complementary and Integrative Health Approaches). Recent studies have shown ibuprofen 600 mg every 8 hours to be noninferior to acetazolamide in preventing AMS, although ibuprofen does not improve acclimatization or reduce periodic breathing. It is, however, over-the-counter, inexpensive, and well tolerated.

## PREVENTION OF SEVERE ALTITUDE ILLNESS OR DEATH

The main point of instructing travelers about altitude illness is not to eliminate the possibility of mild illness but to prevent death or evacuation. Since the onset of symptoms and the clinical course are sufficiently slow and predictable, there is no reason for anyone to die from altitude illness unless trapped by weather or geography in a situation in which descent is impossible. Travelers who adhere to 3 principles can prevent death or serious consequences from altitude illness:

- Know the early symptoms of altitude illness and be willing to acknowledge when they are present.

- Never ascend to sleep at a higher elevation when experiencing symptoms of altitude illness, no matter how minor they seem.

- Descend if the symptoms become worse while resting at the same elevation.

For trekking groups and expeditions going into remote high-elevation areas, where descent to a lower elevation could be problematic, a pressurization bag (such as the Gamow bag) can be beneficial. A foot pump produces an increased pressure of 2 lb/in², mimicking a descent of 5,000–6,000 ft (1,500–1,800 m) depending on the starting elevation. The total packed weight of bag and pump is about 14 lb (6.5 kg). Oxygen is an excellent option for emergency use but is often impractical.

### BIBLIOGRAPHY

1. Bartsch P, Swenson ER. Acute high-altitude illnesses. N Engl J Med. 2013 Oct 24; 369(17):1666–7.

2. Hackett P. High altitude and common medical conditions. In: Hornbein TF, Schoene RB, editors. High Altitude: an Exploration of Human Adaptation. New York: Marcel Dekker; 2001. pp. 839–85.

3. Hackett PH, Roach RC. High altitude cerebral edema. High Alt Med Biol. 2004 Summer; 5(2):136–46.

4. Hackett PH, Roach RC. High-altitude medicine and physiology. In: Auerbach PS, editor. Wilderness Medicine. 6th ed. Philadelphia: Mosby Elsevier; 2012. pp. 2–32.

5. Johnson TS, Rock PB, Fulco CS, Trad LA, Spark RF, Maher JT. Prevention of acute mountain sickness by dexamethasone. N Engl J Med. 1984 Mar 15; 310(11):683–6.

6. Luks AM, McIntosh SE, Grissom CK, Auerbach PS, Rodway GW, Schoene RB, et al. Wilderness Medical Society consensus guidelines for the prevention and treatment of acute altitude illness. Wilderness Environ Med. 2010 Jun; 21(2):146–55.

7. Luks AM, Swenson ER. Medication and dosage considerations in the prophylaxis and treatment of high-altitude illness. Chest. 2008 Mar; 133(3):744–55.

8. Maggiorini M, Brunner-La Rocca HP, Peth S, Fischler M, Bohm T, Bernheim A, et al. Both tadalafil and dexamethasone may reduce the incidence of high-altitude pulmonary edema: a randomized trial. Ann Intern Med. 2006 Oct 3; 145(7):497–506.

9. Pollard AJ, Murdoch DR. The High Altitude Medicine Handbook. 3rd ed. Abingdon, UK: Radcliffe Medical Press; 2003.

10. Pollard AJ, Niermeyer S, Barry P, Bartsch P, Berghold F, Bishop RA, et al. Children at high altitude: an international consensus statement by an ad hoc committee of the International Society for Mountain Medicine, March 12, 2001. High Alt Med Biol. 2001 Fall; 2(3):389–403.

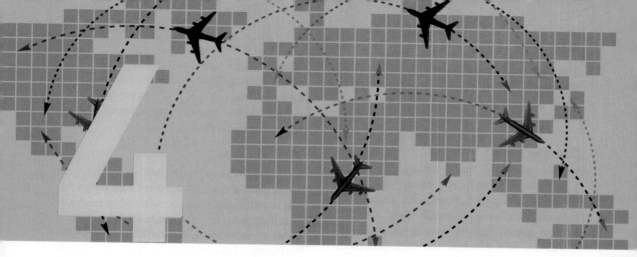

# Travel-Related Infectious Diseases

## AMEBIASIS

Jennifer R. Cope, Ibne K. Ali

### INFECTIOUS AGENT

The protozoan parasite *Entamoeba histolytica*, possibly other *Entamoeba* spp.

### TRANSMISSION

Fecal–oral route, either by eating or drinking fecally contaminated food or water or person-to-person contact (such as by diaper changing or sexual activity).

### EPIDEMIOLOGY

Amebiasis is distributed worldwide, particularly in the tropics, most commonly in areas of poor sanitation. Long-term travelers (duration >6 months) are significantly more likely than short-term travelers (duration <1 month) to develop *E. histolytica* infection. Recent immigrants and refugees from these areas are also at risk. Outbreaks among men who have sex with men have been reported. People at higher risk for severe disease are those who are pregnant, immunocompromised, or receiving corticosteroids; associations with diabetes and alcohol use have also been reported.

### CLINICAL PRESENTATION

Most patients have a gradual illness onset days or weeks after infection. Symptoms include cramps, watery or bloody diarrhea, and weight loss, and may last several weeks. Occasionally, the parasite may spread to other organs (extraintestinal amebiasis), most commonly the liver. Amebic liver abscesses may be asymptomatic, but most patients present with fever, right upper quadrant abdominal pain, and weight loss, usually in the absence of diarrhea. Men are at higher risk of developing amebic liver abscess than are women for reasons not fully understood.

## DIAGNOSIS

Microscopy does not distinguish between *E. histolytica* (known to be pathogenic), *E. bangladeshi*, *E. dispar*, and *E. moshkovskii*. *E. dispar* and *E. moshkovskii* have historically been considered nonpathogenic, but evidence is mounting that *E. moshkovskii* can cause illness; *E. bangladeshi* has only recently been identified, so its pathogenic potential is not well understood. More specific tests such as enzyme immunoassay or PCR are needed to confirm the diagnosis of *E. histolytica*. Additionally, serologic tests can help diagnose extraintestinal amebiasis.

CDC's Free-Living and Intestinal Amebas laboratory can make a specific diagnosis by using a duplex real-time PCR capable of detecting and distinguishing *E. histolytica* and *E. dispar* in stool and liver aspirate samples. More information about this testing and the CDC point of contact can be found at www.cdc.gov/laboratory/specimen-submission/detail.html?CDCTestCode=CDC-10478.

## TREATMENT

For symptomatic intestinal infection and extraintestinal disease, treatment with metronidazole or tinidazole should be followed by treatment with iodoquinol or paromomycin. Asymptomatic patients infected with *E. histolytica* should also be treated with iodoquinol or paromomycin, because they can infect others and because 4%–10% develop disease within a year if left untreated.

## PREVENTION

Food and water precautions (see Chapter 2, Food & Water Precautions) and hand hygiene. Avoid fecal exposure during sexual activity.

**CDC website:** www.cdc.gov/parasites/amebiasis

### BIBLIOGRAPHY

1. Choudhuri G, Rangan M. Amebic infection in humans. Indian J Gastroenterol. 2012 Jul;31(4):153–62.
2. Escolà-Vergé L, Arando M, Vall M, Rovira R, Espasa M, Sulleiro E, et al. Outbreak of intestinal amoebiasis among men who have sex with men, Barcelona (Spain), October 2017 and January 2017. Euro Surveill. 2017 Jul 27;22(30):pii:30581.
3. Heredia RD, Fonseca JA, Lopez MC. Entamoeba moshkovskii perspectives of a new agent to be considered in the diagnosis of amebiasis. Acta Trop. 2012 Sep;123(3):139–45.
4. Lachish T, Wieder-Finesod A, Schwartz E. Amebic liver abscess in Israeli travelers: a retrospective study. Am J Trop Med Hyg. 2016 May 4;94(5):1015–19.
5. Shimokawa C, Kabir M, Taniuchi M, Mondal D, Kobayashi S, Ali IK, et al. Entamoeba moshkovskii is associated with diarrhea in infants and causes diarrhea and colitis in mice. J Infect Dis. 2012 Sep 1;206(5):744–51.
6. Shirley D, Moonah S. Fulminant amebic colitis after corticosteroid therapy: a systematic review. PLoS Negl Trop Dis. 2016 Jul 28;10(7):e0004879.
7. Ximenez C, Moran P, Rojas L, Valadez A, Gomez A, Ramiro M, et al. Novelties on amoebiasis: a neglected tropical disease. J Glob Infect Dis. 2011 Apr;3(2):166–74.

# ANGIOSTRONGYLIASIS, NEUROLOGIC

Anne Straily, Barbara L. Herwaldt

## INFECTIOUS AGENT

*Angiostrongylus cantonensis*, rat lungworm, a nematode parasite.

## TRANSMISSION

Various species of rats are the definitive hosts of the parasite, known as the rat lungworm.

Parasites from rats only infect snails and slugs, which are the intermediate hosts. Infective larvae have also been found in paratenic (transport) hosts, such as freshwater shrimp, crabs, and frogs, which become infected by consuming infected snails and slugs. Transmission to humans occurs by ingesting infected intermediate or paratenic hosts or by consuming contaminated raw produce or vegetable juices.

## EPIDEMIOLOGY

Most described cases have occurred in Asia and the Pacific Basin (such as in parts of Thailand, Taiwan, mainland China, Australia, the Hawaiian Islands, and other Pacific Islands); however, cases have been reported in many areas of the world, including the Caribbean.

## CLINICAL PRESENTATION

Incubation period is typically 1–3 weeks but ranges from 1 day to >6 weeks. *A. cantonensis* is considered the most common infectious cause of eosinophilic meningitis in humans. Common manifestations include headache, photophobia, stiff neck, abnormal skin sensations (such as tingling or painful feelings), nausea, vomiting, fatigue, and body aches. A low-grade fever may occur. Symptoms are usually self-limited but may persist for weeks or months. Severe cases can be associated with paralysis, blindness, or death.

## DIAGNOSIS

Typically presumptive, on the basis of clinical and epidemiologic criteria in people with otherwise unexplained eosinophilic meningitis. PCR testing of cerebrospinal fluid is available at CDC (www.cdc.gov/dpdx; 404-718-4745; parasites@cdc.gov). Immunodiagnostic tests have been developed (for example, in research settings) but are not approved or licensed for clinical use in the United States.

## TREATMENT

The larvae die spontaneously and supportive care usually suffices, including analgesics for pain and corticosteroids to limit inflammation. No antihelminthic drugs have been proven to be effective in treatment.

## PREVENTION

Food and water precautions, particularly:

- Avoid eating raw or undercooked snails, slugs, and other possible hosts.

- Eat raw produce, such as lettuce, only if it has been thoroughly washed or treated with bleach. Such measures might provide some protection but may not eliminate the risk.

- If a catchment tank is used as a source of water, ensure that it is covered to prevent intrusion by slugs and snails. Also keep drink containers covered.

- Wear gloves (and wash hands) if snails or slugs are handled.

**CDC website**: www.cdc.gov/parasites/angiostrongylus

BIBLIOGRAPHY

1. Barratt J, Chan D, Sandaradura I, Malik R, Spielman D, Lee R, et al. Angiostrongylus cantonensis: a review of its distribution, molecular biology and clinical significance as a human pathogen. Parasitol. 2016 May;143:1087–118.

2. Eamsobhana P. Eosinophilic meningitis caused by Angiostrongylus cantonensis—a neglected disease with escalating importance. Trop Biomed. 2014 Apr;31(4):569–78.

3. Hochberg NS, Blackburn BG, Park SY, Sejvar JJ, Effler PV, Herwaldt BL. Eosinophilic meningitis attributable to Angiostrongylus cantonensis infection in Hawaii: clinical characteristics and potential exposures. Am J Trop Med Hyg. 2011 Oct;85(4):685–90.

4. Qvarnstrom Y, Xayavong M, da Silva AC, Park SY, Whelen AC, Calimlim PS, et al. Real-time polymerase chain reaction detection of Angiostrongylus cantonensis DNA in cerebrospinal fluid from patients with eosinophilic meningitis. Am J Trop Med Hyg. 2016 Jan;94(1):176–81.

5. Wang Q-P, Wu Z-D, Wei J, Owen RL, Lun Z-R. Human Angiostrongylus cantonensis: an update. Eur J Clin Microbiol Infect Dis. 2012 Jul;31:389–95.

# ANTHRAX

Kate Hendricks, Antonio R. Vieira, Chung K. Marston

## INFECTIOUS AGENT

Aerobic, gram-positive, encapsulated, spore-forming, nonmotile, nonhemolytic, rod-shaped bacterium *Bacillus anthracis*.

## TRANSMISSION

Most human infections with *B. anthracis* result from handling *B. anthracis*–infected animals, their carcasses, or their meat, hides, or wool. Products derived from infected animals, such as drumheads and wool clothing, are additional, documented sources of human infection.

Anthrax has 4 main clinical presentations—cutaneous, ingestion, injection, and inhalation. Anthrax meningitis can complicate any of the 4 main clinical presentations. It can also occur with no obvious portal of entry, in which case it is called primary anthrax meningitis.

Spores introduced through the skin can result in cutaneous anthrax; abrasion of the skin increases susceptibility. Eating meat from infected animals can result in ingestion (also called gastrointestinal) anthrax. Reports since 2000 document *B. anthracis* soft-tissue infections in intravenous heroin users in northern Europe. Aerosolized spores from contaminated hides or wool can cause inhalation anthrax. Anthrax in humans generally is not considered contagious; person-to-person transmission of cutaneous anthrax has been reported only rarely.

## EPIDEMIOLOGY

Anthrax is a zoonotic disease primarily affecting ruminant herbivores such as cattle, sheep, goats, antelope, and deer that become infected by ingesting contaminated vegetation, water, or soil; humans are generally incidental hosts. Anthrax is most common in agricultural regions in Central and South America, sub-Saharan Africa, central and southwestern Asia, and southern and eastern Europe. Although outbreaks still occur in livestock and wild herbivores in the United States, Canada, and Western Europe, human anthrax in these areas is now rare.

Worldwide, the most commonly reported form of anthrax in humans is cutaneous anthrax (95%–99%). Anthrax can occur after playing or handling drums made from contaminated goatskins. Although the risk of acquiring anthrax from drums imported from anthrax-endemic countries appears low, life-threatening or fatal disease is possible. Cases of cutaneous (4), ingestion (1), and inhalation (3) anthrax have been reported in people who have handled, played, or made drums; others who have been in the same place as people who participated in these activities have also been infected.

In 2006, a case of travel-associated anthrax (the cutaneous form of the disease) was reported in a woman who traveled with a small group of tourists to Namibia, Botswana, and South Africa. Outbreaks of cutaneous and ingestion anthrax have been associated with handling infected animals and butchering and eating meat from those animals. Most of these outbreaks have occurred in endemic areas in Asia and Africa.

Severe soft-tissue infections, including cases complicated by sepsis and systemic infection, are suspected to be due to recreational use of heroin contaminated with *B. anthracis* spores. No associated cases have been identified in people who have not taken heroin.

Inhalation exposure was historically associated with the industrial processing of hides or wool (hence, "woolsorters' disease"). More recently, bioterrorist activities were implicated as a source of inhalation exposure. Occasional anthrax cases have occurred, in the United States and elsewhere, in which the exposure source remains unidentified.

# CLINICAL PRESENTATION

## Cutaneous Anthrax

Cutaneous anthrax usually develops 1–7 days after exposure, but incubation periods as long as 17 days have been reported. Before antimicrobial therapy, almost a quarter of patients with cutaneous anthrax died. The case-fatality ratio is <2% with antimicrobial therapy.

Localized itching, followed by the development of a painless papule, heralds cutaneous anthrax. The papule then turns into a vesicle that enlarges and ulcerates, ultimately becoming a depressed black eschar, 7–10 days after the appearance of the initial lesion. Edema around lesions is characteristic, sometimes with secondary vesicles, hyperemia, and regional lymphadenopathy. Head, neck, forearms, and hands are the most commonly affected sites. Patients may have malaise and headache; about one-third are febrile.

## Ingestion Anthrax

Ingestion anthrax usually develops 1–7 days after eating contaminated meat; however, incubations as long as 16 days have been reported. Left untreated, more than half of cases will die; with treatment, the case-fatality ratio decreases slightly, to <40%. There are 2 main types of ingestion anthrax: oropharyngeal and intestinal. Fever and chills are usual with either. The oropharyngeal type is characterized by severe sore throat, difficulty swallowing, swelling of the neck, and regional lymphadenopathy; airway compromise and death can occur. Nausea, vomiting, and diarrhea (which may be bloody) are more typical of intestinal anthrax; marked ascites may also develop. Later symptoms can include shortness of breath and altered mental status with shock and death occurring 2–5 days after disease onset.

## Injection Anthrax

Anthrax in injection drug users usually develops within 1–4 days of exposure; death occurs in more than a quarter of confirmed cases. Cases present with severe soft-tissue infection manifested by swelling, erythema, and excessive bruising at the injection site; pain may be less than anticipated for the degree of swelling. In approximately one-third of cases, patients become septic.

## Inhalation Anthrax

Inhalation anthrax usually develops within a week after exposure, but the incubation period may be prolonged (up to 2 months). Before 2001, fatality ratios for inhalation anthrax were 90%; since then, they have fallen to 45%. During the first few days of illness, most patients exhibit fever, chills, and fatigue. These symptoms may be accompanied by cough, shortness of breath, chest pain, and nausea or vomiting, making inhalation anthrax difficult to distinguish from influenza and community-acquired pneumonia. This is often described as the prodromal period.

Over the next day or so, shortness of breath, cough, and chest pain become more common, and nonthoracic complaints such as nausea, vomiting, altered mental status, diaphoresis, and headache develop in one-third or more of patients. Upper respiratory tract symptoms occur in only a quarter of patients, and myalgias are rare. Altered mental status or shortness of breath generally brings patients to the attention of the medical establishment and heralds the fulminant phase of illness.

## Anthrax Meningitis

Anthrax meningitis may develop from hematogenous spread of any of the clinical forms of anthrax, or it may occur alone; half of all reported cases are sequelae of cutaneous anthrax. The condition should be suspected in patients with anthrax who have severe headache, altered mental status (including confusion), meningeal signs, or neurologic deficits of any kind. Most, but not all, cases of anthrax meningitis are fatal.

## DIAGNOSIS

Include anthrax in the differential diagnosis of returning travelers with unexplained fevers or new skin lesions. Ask about recent travel to anthrax-endemic areas (www.cdc.gov/anthrax/specificgroups/travelers.html). Inquire about activities (such as drumming) and souvenir purchases, including animal-hide drums and woolen clothing.

Clinicians can use any of several methods to make a laboratory diagnosis of anthrax infection: bacterial culture and isolation of *B. anthracis*;

detection of bacterial DNA, antigens, or toxins; or detection of a host immune response to *B. anthracis*. Anthrax lethal toxin can be detected in acute-phase serum, although serologic testing of host antibody responses requires acute- and convalescent-phase sera for diagnosis.

In the United States, anthrax is a nationally notifiable disease. Laboratory Response Network reference laboratories can perform confirmatory testing, such as isolate identification, and CDC laboratories—in addition to performing isolate identification—are capable of conducting other complex tests such as mass spectrometry for toxin, quantitative serology, and antigen detection in tissues. Internationally, relevant national reference laboratories should perform testing. CDC provides specimen collection and submission guidelines and algorithms for laboratory diagnosis at www.cdc.gov/anthrax/lab-testing/index.html. Collect specimens for culture before initiating antimicrobial therapy.

Diagnostic procedures for inhalation anthrax include thoracic imaging studies to detect a widened mediastinum or pleural effusion. Drainage of pleural effusions can be useful for diagnosis and can increase survival, as it removes a nidus for toxin. Unless contraindicated, lumbar puncture should be performed to rule out meningitis in all patients with systemic illness.

## TREATMENT

Treat naturally occurring localized or uncomplicated cutaneous anthrax with 7–10 days of a single oral antibiotic. First-line agents include ciprofloxacin (or an equivalent fluoroquinolone) or doxycycline; clindamycin is an alternative, as are penicillins if the isolate is penicillin susceptible. Treat systemic anthrax with combination broad-spectrum intravenous antibiotics pending the results of confirmatory testing; delays in initiating therapy may prove fatal.

Online recommendations for the treatment and prevention of anthrax are available:

- Adults: wwwnc.cdc.gov/eid/article/20/2/13-0687_article

- Pregnant, postpartum, and lactating women: wwwnc.cdc.gov/eid/article/20/2/13-0611_article

- Children: http://pediatrics.aappublications.org/content/133/5/e1411

## PREVENTION

In 2010, CDC published updated recommendations from the Advisory Committee on Immunization Practices for preexposure use of anthrax vaccine and for postexposure management of previously unvaccinated people (www.cdc.gov/mmwr/preview/mmwrhtml/rr5906a1.htm). Vaccination against anthrax is not recommended for the majority of travelers.

To prevent anthrax exposures while visiting anthrax-endemic countries, travelers should avoid direct and indirect contact with animal carcasses and should not eat meat from animals butchered after having been found dead or ill. No tests are available to determine if animal products are free from *B. anthracis* spore contamination; travelers should be aware of regulations concerning (and restrictions against) the importation of prohibited animal products, trophies, and souvenirs.

Additional information regarding import regulations may be found in the following references:

- Yellow Book 2020, Appendix E, Taking Animals & Animal Products Across International Borders (www.cdc.gov/importation/animal-products.html)

- US Department of Agriculture, Animal and Plant Health Inspection Service, import-export regulations (www.aphis.usda.gov/aphis/ourfocus/importexport)

- World Organisation for Animal Health, Terrestrial Animal Health Code, Anthrax (www.oie.int/en/animal-health-in-the-world/animal-diseases/anthrax)

A map of anthrax-endemic countries and guidance for travelers visiting those countries can be found at www.cdc.gov/anthrax/specificgroups/travelers.html.

**CDC website:** www.cdc.gov/anthrax

## BIBLIOGRAPHY

1. Bales ME, Dannenberg AL, Brachman PS, Kaufmann AF, Klatsky PC, Ashford DA. Epidemiologic response to anthrax outbreaks: field investigations, 1950–2001. Emerg Infect Dis. 2002 Oct;8(10):1163–74.

2. Beatty ME, Ashford DA, Griffin PM, Tauxe RV, Sobel J. Gastrointestinal anthrax. Arch Int Med. 2003 Nov;163:2527–31.

3. Bradley JS, Peacock G, Krug S, et al. Pediatric anthrax clinical management. Pediatrics. 2014 May;133(5):e1411–36.

4. CDC. Gastrointestinal anthrax after an animal-hide drumming event—New Hampshire and Massachusetts, 2009. MMWR Morb Mortal Wkly Rep. 2010 Jul 23;59(28):872–7.

5. Hendricks KA, Wright ME, Shadomy SV, Bradley JS, Morrow MG, Pavia AT, et al. Centers for disease control and prevention expert panel meetings on prevention and treatment of anthrax in adults. Emerg Infect Dis. 2014 Feb;20(2). Available from: wwwnc.cdc.gov/eid/article/20/2/13-0687_article.

6. Holty JEC, Bravata DM, Liu H, Olshen RA, McDonald KM, Owens DK. Systematic review: a century of inhalational anthrax cases from 1900 to 2005. Ann Intern Med. 2006;144:270–80.

7. Katharios-Lanwermeyer S, Holty JE, Person M, et al. Identifying meningitis during an anthrax mass casualty incident: systematic review of systemic anthrax since 1880. Clin Infect Dis. 2016 June;62:1537–45.

8. Meaney-Delman D, Zotti ME, Creanga AA, Misegades LK, Wako E, Treadwell TA, et al. Special considerations for prophylaxis for and treatment of anthrax in pregnant and postpartum women. Emerg Infect Dis. 2014 Feb;20(2). Available from: wwwnc.cdc.gov/eid/article/20/2/13-0611_article.

9. National Anthrax Outbreak Control Team. An outbreak of anthrax among drug users in Scotland, December 2009 to December 2010. Health Protection Scotland, 2011.

10. Van den Enden E, Van Gompel A, Van Esbroeck M. Cutaneous anthrax, Belgian traveler. Emerg Infect Dis. 2006 Mar;12(3):523–5.

**4**

# B VIRUS (MACACINE HERPESVIRUS 1)

D. Scott Schmid

## INFECTIOUS AGENT

*Macacine herpesvirus 1*, or B virus, is an enveloped, double-stranded DNA virus in the family Herpesviridae, genus *Simplexvirus*. B virus is also commonly referred to as herpes B, monkey B virus, herpesvirus simiae, and herpesvirus B. B virus is commonly found among macaques, a genus of Old World monkeys.

## TRANSMISSION

Transmission is typically caused by bites or scratches from an infected macaque but may also occur through contact with body fluids or tissues of an infected macaque. A single case of human-to-human spread has been documented, in which a woman became infected through direct contact with the lesions of her infected spouse.

## EPIDEMIOLOGY

Macaques are the natural reservoir for B virus infection. No other primates are known to carry B virus infection unless they have become infected by contact with infected macaques. Although B virus infections in macaques are usually asymptomatic or cause only mild disease, approximately 70% of untreated infections in humans are fatal. People at risk for B virus infection are veterinarians, laboratory workers, and others who have close contact with macaques or macaque cell cultures, but infections in humans are rare. Since B virus was identified in 1932, fewer than 50 cases of human infection have been documented.

## CLINICAL PRESENTATION

Disease onset typically occurs within 1 month of exposure, although the actual incubation period can be as short as 3–7 days. The first signs of disease typically include influenzalike symptoms (fever, headache, myalgia) and sometimes vesicular lesions near the exposure site. Localized neurologic symptoms such as pain, numbness, or itching may occur near the wound site. Lymphadenitis, lymphangitis, nausea, vomiting, and abdominal pain may also occur. Spread of the infection to the central nervous system (CNS) causes acute ascending encephalomyelitis. Most patients with CNS involvement die despite antiviral therapy and supportive care, and those who survive usually suffer serious neurologic sequelae. Respiratory failure associated with ascending paralysis is the most common cause of death.

## DIAGNOSIS

In the United States, diagnostic testing of human specimens is performed only at the National B Virus Resource Center at Georgia State University. Detection of viral DNA by B virus PCR from clinical specimens is the standard for diagnosis of infection. Detection of B virus-specific antibodies in serum is also diagnostic. Culture is generally unsuccessful, as the virus is unlikely to remain viable during transit or after being frozen and thawed. For more information, see www2.gsu.edu/~wwwvir/.

## FIRST AID AND TREATMENT

For any suspected exposure, immediate first aid is crucial. The wound should be cleansed by thoroughly washing and scrubbing the area with soap, concentrated detergent solution, povidone iodine, or chlorhexidine and water. The wound should then be irrigated with running water for 15–20 minutes. For urine splashes to the eyes, repeated eye flushes should be performed for several minutes. **Specimens for testing should not be obtained from wound sites before washing because this may force virus more deeply into the wound.**

Antiviral therapy is recommended as postexposure prophylaxis in high-risk exposures (see www.cdc.gov/herpesbvirus/firstaid-treatment.html). When recommended, the drug of choice is valacyclovir, and an alternative is acyclovir. If B virus infection is diagnosed, treatment consists of intravenous acyclovir or ganciclovir, depending on whether CNS symptoms are present.

## PREVENTION

Adhering to laboratory and animal facility protocols will reduce the risk of B virus transmission among laboratory workers. Visitors to parks and other tourist destinations (such as certain religious temples) with free-roaming macaques should avoid contact with these animals (including feeding or petting them).

**CDC website:** www.cdc.gov/herpesbvirus/index.html

BIBLIOGRAPHY

1. CDC. Notice to readers: Occupational safety and health in the care and use of nonhuman primates. MMWR. 2003;52(38);920. Available from: www.cdc.gov/mmwr/preview/mmwrhtml/mm5238a8.htm.

2. Closewood LC WD. Section VIII—Agent summary statements. In: Closwood LC WD, editor. Biosafety in microbiological and biomedical laboratories. 5th ed. Washington, DC: US Department of Health and Human Services; 2009. pp. 205–8.

3. Cohen JI, Davenport DS, Stewart JA, Deitchman S, Hilliard JK, Chapman LE, B virus Working Group. Recommendations for prevention of and therapy for exposure to B virus (cercopithicine Herpesvirus 1). Clin Infect Dis. 2002;35:1191–203.

4. National Institute for Occupational Safety and Health (NIOSH). Hazard ID 5—Cercopithicine herpesvirus 1 (B virus) infection resulting from ocular exposure. Atlanta: CDC; 1999 [cited 2016 Sep 21]. Available from: www.cdc.gov/niosh/docs/99-100/.

5. National Association of State Public Health Veterinarians, Inc. (NASPHV). Compendium of measures to prevent disease associated with animals in public settings, 2009. MMWR Recomm Rep. 2009;58(RR-05):1–15.

# *BARTONELLA* INFECTIONS

Christina A. Nelson

## INFECTIOUS AGENT

Gram-negative bacteria in the genus *Bartonella*. Human illness is primarily caused by *Bartonella henselae* (cat-scratch disease [CSD]), *B. quintana* (trench fever), and *B. bacilliformis* (Carrión disease). A variety of *Bartonella* spp. can cause culture-negative endocarditis; other clinical syndromes due to *Bartonella* spp. such as ocular disease, osteomyelitis, and encephalitis have been reported. Additional *Bartonella* spp. that cause human illness have been described recently.

## TRANSMISSION

*B. henselae* is contracted through scratches from domestic or feral cats, particularly kittens. Direct transmission to humans by the bite of infected cat fleas is likely to occur but has not yet been proven. *B. quintana* is transmitted by the human body louse. *B. bacilliformis* is transmitted by infected sand flies (genus *Lutzomyia*).

## EPIDEMIOLOGY

CSD and trench fever are distributed worldwide. In the United States, CSD is more common in children, southern states, and during the months of August through January. Trench fever typically occurs in populations that do not have access to proper hygiene, such as refugees and the homeless. Carrión disease has limited geographic distribution; transmission occurs in the Andes Mountains at 1,000–3,000 m (3,281–9,843 ft) elevation in Peru, Colombia, and Ecuador; sporadic cases have also been reported in Bolivia, Chile, and possibly Guatemala. Most cases are reported in Peru. Short-term travelers to endemic areas are likely at low risk.

## CLINICAL PRESENTATION

CSD typically manifests as a papule or pustule at the inoculation site and enlarged, tender lymph nodes that develop proximal to the inoculation site 1–3 weeks after exposure. *B. henselae* infection may also cause prolonged fever, follicular conjunctivitis, neuroretinitis, or encephalitis. Trench fever symptoms include fever, headache, transient rash, and bone pain (mainly in the shins, neck, and back).

Some *Bartonella* spp. can cause subacute endocarditis, which is often culture-negative. Bacillary angiomatosis may present as skin, subcutaneous, or bone lesions and is caused by *B. henselae* or *B. quintana*; peliosis hepatis manifests as liver lesions and is caused by *B. henselae*. Both occur primarily in people infected with HIV.

Carrión disease has 2 distinct phases: an acute phase (Oroya fever) characterized by fever, myalgia, headache, and anemia and an eruptive phase (verruga peruana) characterized by red-to-purple nodular skin lesions.

## DIAGNOSIS

CSD can be diagnosed clinically in patients with typical presentation and a compatible exposure history. Serology can confirm the diagnosis, although cross-reactivity may limit interpretation in some circumstances. Serology is available from some commercial laboratories, however, consultation is available from the CDC. *B. henselae* may also be detected by PCR or culture of lymph node aspirates by using special techniques.

Trench fever can be diagnosed by serology or blood culture for *B. quintana*. PCR may also aid the diagnosis of disseminated *Bartonella* infections when performed by clinical laboratories using validated methods. Endocarditis caused by *Bartonella* spp. can be diagnosed by elevated serology of the patient and by PCR or culture of excised heart valve tissue.

Oroya fever is typically diagnosed via blood culture or direct observation of the bacilli in peripheral blood smears, though sensitivity of these methods is low. PCR and serologic testing may also aid diagnosis.

## TREATMENT

Most cases of typical CSD eventually resolve without treatment, however antibiotics may shorten the course of disease. Azithromycin has been shown to speed the decrease in lymph node volume. A small percentage of people will develop disseminated disease with severe complications; however, it is unknown whether antibiotic treatment reduces the risk of progression to atypical disease.

Various antibiotics are effective against *Bartonella* infections, and regimens including agents such as tetracyclines, fluoroquinolones, trimethoprim-sulfamethoxazole, rifampin, and aminoglycosides have been used. Recommended regimens and duration of treatment vary by clinical disease.

## PREVENTION

Avoid rough play with cats, particularly strays and kittens, to prevent scratches. This is especially important for immunocompromised people. Flea control for cats and limiting outdoor roaming of cats also decrease the risk that they carry *B. henselae*. Wash hands promptly after handling cats. Protect against bites of sand flies and body lice (see Chapter 3, Mosquitoes, Ticks & Other Arthropods).

**CDC website:** www.cdc.gov/bartonella

### BIBLIOGRAPHY

1. Angelakis E, Raoult D. Pathogenicity and treatment of Bartonella infections. Int J Antimicrob Agents. 2014 Jul;44(1):16–25.

2. Eremeeva ME, Gerns HL, Lydy SL, Goo JS, Ryan ET, Mathew SS, et al. Bacteremia, fever, and splenomegaly caused by a newly recognized *Bartonella* species. N Engl J Med. 2007 Jun 7;356(23):2381–7.

3. Florin TA, Zaoutis TE, Zaoutis LB. Beyond cat scratch disease: widening spectrum of Bartonella henselae infection. Pediatrics. 2008 May;121(5):e1413–25.

4. Fournier PE, Thuny F, Richet H, Lepidi H, Casalta JP, Arzouni JP, et al. Comprehensive diagnostic strategy for blood culture-negative endocarditis: a prospective study of 819 new cases. Clin Infect Dis. 2010 Jul 15;51(2):131–40.

5. Nelson CA, Saha S, Mead PS. Cat-scratch disease in the United States, 2005–2013. Emerg Infect Dis. 2016 Oct;22(10):1741–6.

# BRUCELLOSIS

María E. Negrón, Rebekah Tiller, Grishma Kharod

## INFECTIOUS AGENT

*Brucella* spp., the causative agents for brucellosis, are facultative, intracellular, gram-negative coccobacilli. The main *Brucella* spp. known to cause human disease are *Brucella abortus* (including the livestock vaccine strain *Brucella abortus* RB51), *B. melitensis*, *B. suis*, and *B. canis*.

## TRANSMISSION

Brucellosis is a classical bacterial zoonosis since animals are the only source of infection. Humans most commonly acquire the infection through consumption of unpasteurized dairy products (such as raw milk, soft cheese, butter, and ice cream). The bacteria can also enter the body via skin wounds, mucous membranes, or inhalation, so direct contact with infected animal tissues or fluids can be a risk for exposure. Particularly important is direct contact with birthing tissues from infected animals or blood while dressing a carcass during hunting activities. Infection through eating undercooked meat from infected animals can occur, although this is less likely because of lower bacterial loads in muscle. Person-to-person transmission has been reported but is rare.

# EPIDEMIOLOGY

More than 500,000 new human cases of brucellosis are reported worldwide each year. However, this number is likely an underestimate as brucellosis cases are underreported and often misdiagnosed because symptoms are nonspecific, physicians may lack awareness, and laboratory capacity for diagnosis is limited. *B. melitensis* is the most frequently reported cause of human illness worldwide, while the most widespread potential source of infection is *B. abortus*. Human infections occur most frequently among people who have traveled to or who live in areas where the disease is endemic in animals (mainly cattle, sheep, and goats) along the Mediterranean Basin, South and Central America, Eastern Europe, Asia, Africa, and the Middle East. Although not commonly reported in travelers, clinicians should also be aware of the possibility of *B. suis* or *B. canis* infection, as these *Brucella* species are present in animal populations (such as *B. suis* in feral swine and caribou/reindeer and *B. canis* in canines) that certain travelers may contact.

# CLINICAL PRESENTATION

The incubation period is usually 2–4 weeks (range, 5 days to 6 months). Initial presentation is nonspecific and includes fever, malaise, arthralgia, myalgia, fatigue, headache, and night sweats. Focal infections are common and can affect most organs in the body. Osteoarticular involvement is the most common brucellosis complication, and reproductive system involvement is the second most common. Although rare, endocarditis can occur and is the principal cause of death among brucellosis patients.

# DIAGNOSIS

Blood culture is considered the diagnostic gold standard, but isolation rates may vary considerably (25%–80%) depending on stage of infection, previous use of antibiotics, type and volume of clinical specimen, and culture method used. Bacterial growth can be observed within 3–5 days in culture but may take longer; therefore, cultures should be held for ≥10 days before considering the sample culture-negative. To increase recovery of the organism when focal disease is suspected, samples for culture should be collected from the affected area (for example, cerebrospinal fluid, joint aspirate, or urine). Inform the laboratory if brucellosis is suspected when submitting blood, bone marrow, or other clinical specimen for culture, as the bacteria take longer to grow, and laboratory personnel require additional personal protective equipment when handling.

Serologic testing is the most common method for diagnosis. The serum agglutination test (SAT) is the standard method for serologic diagnosis and detects IgM, IgG, and IgA. In general, ELISA tests have good sensitivity and specificity and can detect IgM and IgG. Some limitations to the use of serologic tests must be taken into consideration when diagnosing *Brucella* infections, as most serologic assays for brucellosis show variable levels of cross-reactivity with other gram-negative bacteria (for example, *E. coli* O:157, *Francisella tularensis*, and *Yersinia enterocolitica*). *Brucella* antibodies can persist for more than a year despite successful antibiotic treatment. Last, no validated serologic assays are available to detect antibodies produced against infections caused by *B. canis* and *B. abortus* RB51 strain. If infection by either of these organisms is possible or suspected, culture should be performed.

# TREATMENT

A combined regimen of doxycycline (or oral tetracycline) and rifampin for ≥6 weeks is the recommended treatment for uncomplicated infection. For complicated brucellosis (endocarditis, meningitis, osteomyelitis) an aminoglycoside in combination with tetracycline should be considered, and duration of therapy is often extended for 4–6 months. *B. abortus* RB51 is resistant to rifampin, so treatment for brucellosis due to this strain should be altered accordingly (for example, doxycycline in combination with trimethoprim-sulfamethoxazole, unless contraindicated). Other agents have been used in various combinations; treatment should be guided by someone with expertise in infectious diseases. Late diagnosis or incorrect therapy can result in relapse.

# PREVENTION

Avoid unpasteurized dairy products and undercooked meat, especially when traveling to countries where brucellosis is endemic.

Wear protective equipment (rubber gloves, goggles or face shields, and gowns or aprons) when dressing or butchering wild animals or when handling birthing products from animals potentially infected with *Brucella* spp. Clinicians should inform clinical microbiology laboratories when submitting specimens from patients with suspected brucellosis to ensure proper biosafety precautions in the laboratory when handling specimens and specimen derivatives.

For questions on laboratory diagnostics, postexposure guidance, or treatment, please contact the CDC Bacterial Special Pathogens Branch (bspb@cdc.gov).

**CDC website**: www.cdc.gov/brucellosis

## BIBLIOGRAPHY

1. Al Dahouk S, Nockler K. Implications of laboratory diagnosis on brucellosis therapy. Expert Rev Anti Infect Ther. 2011 Jul;9(7):833–45.
2. Ariza J, Bosilkovski M, Cascio A, Colmenero JD, Corbel MJ, Falagas ME, et al. Perspectives for the treatment of brucellosis in the 21st century: the Ioannina recommendations. PLoS Med. 2007 Dec;4(12):e317.
3. Centers for Disease Control and Prevention. Brucellosis reference guide: exposures, testing, and prevention. Atlanta, GA: US Department of Health and Human Services, CDC; 2017. Available from: www.cdc.gov/brucellosis/pdf/brucellosi-reference-guide.pdf.
4. Corbel M. Brucellosis in Humans and Animals: FAO, OIE, WHO; 2006 [cited 2018 Mar]. Available from: www.who.int/csr/resources/publications/Brucellosis.pdf.
5. Cossaboom CM, Kharod GA, Salzer JS, et al. *Notes from the Field: Brucella abortus* Vaccine Strain RB51 Infection and Exposures Associated with Raw Milk Consumption—Wise County, Texas, 2017. MMWR Morb Mortal Wkly Rep 2018;67:286. Available from: http://dx.doi.org/10.15585/mmwr.mm6709a4.
6. Memish ZA, Balkhy HH. Brucellosis and international travel. J Travel Med. 2004 Jan–Feb;11(1):49–55.
7. Organization WH. Brucellosis. Geneva: World Health Organization; 2012 [cited 2016 Sep 21]. Available from: www.who.int/zoonoses/diseases/brucellosis/en/.
8. Rhodes HM, Williams DN, Hansen GT. Invasive human brucellosis infection in travelers to and immigrants from the Horn of Africa related to the consumption of raw camel milk. Travel Med Infect Dis. 2016 May–Jun;14(3):255–60.
9. World Health Organization. Brucellosis. Geneva: World Health Organization; 2012 [cited 2016 Sep 21]. Available from: www.who.int/zoonoses/diseases/brucellosis/en/.
10. Yousefi-Nooraie R, Mortaz-Hejri S, Mehrani M, Sadeghipour P. Antibiotics for treating human brucellosis. Cochrane Database Syst Rev. 2012;10:Cd007179.

# CAMPYLOBACTERIOSIS

Mark E. Laughlin, Kevin Chatham-Stephens, Aimee L. Geissler

## INFECTIOUS AGENT

Infection is caused by gram-negative, spiral-shaped microaerophilic bacteria of the family Campylobacteraceae. Most infections are caused by *Campylobacter jejuni*; at least 18 other species, including *C. coli*, also cause infection. *C. jejuni* and *C. coli* are carried normally in the intestinal tracts of many domestic and wild animals.

## TRANSMISSION

The major modes of transmission include eating contaminated foods (especially undercooked chicken and foods contaminated by raw chicken), drinking contaminated water or milk (unpasteurized milk, most commonly), and having contact with animals, particularly farm animals such as cows and chickens, as well as domestic cats and dogs. *Campylobacter* can also be transmitted from person to person by the fecal–oral route.

## EPIDEMIOLOGY

*Campylobacter* is a leading cause of bacterial diarrheal disease worldwide and caused

96 million cases in 2010; in the United States, it is estimated to cause 1.3 million human illnesses every year. The risk of infection is highest in travelers to Africa and South America, especially to areas with poor restaurant hygiene and inadequate sanitation. The infectious dose is small; <500 organisms can cause disease.

## CLINICAL PRESENTATION

Incubation period is typically 2–4 days but can range from 1 to 10 days. Campylobacteriosis is characterized by diarrhea (frequently bloody), abdominal pain, fever, and occasionally nausea and vomiting. More severe illness can occur, including dehydration, bloodstream infection, and symptoms mimicking acute appendicitis or ulcerative colitis. People with campylobacteriosis are at increased risk for postinfectious complications, including reactive arthritis (2%–5% of patients), irritable bowel syndrome (9%–13%), and Guillain-Barré syndrome (GBS) (0.1%). *C. jejuni* is the most frequently observed antecedent bacterial infection in cases of GBS; symptoms usually begin 1–3 weeks after the onset of *Campylobacter* enteritis.

## DIAGNOSIS

Diagnosis is traditionally based on isolation of the organism from stool specimens or rectal swabs by using selective media incubated under reduced oxygen tension at 42°C (107.6°F) for 72 hours. A stool specimen should be collected as early after symptom onset as possible and before antibiotic treatment is initiated. Because the organism is fastidious, a delay in transporting the specimen to the laboratory will affect the viability of *Campylobacter* spp. A laboratory may reject stool samples without preservative that are in transit for more than 2 hours. If transport and processing are not possible within 2 hours of stool sample collection, specimens should be placed in transport medium according to standard guidelines. Only through culture can *Campylobacter* be subtyped and tested for antimicrobial susceptibility. Rapid culture-independent diagnostic tests, including both antigen tests and nucleic acid–based tests, are becoming widely available and more commonly used. The sensitivity and specificity of stool antigen tests are variable, and in settings of low prevalence, the positive predictive value is likely to be low. Therefore, laboratories should confirm positive results of stool antigen tests by culture. Nucleic acid–based tests have recently been approved and appear to have higher sensitivity and specificity than the antigen tests. Campylobacteriosis is a nationally notifiable disease.

## TREATMENT

The disease is generally self-limited, lasting a week or less. Antibiotic therapy decreases the duration of symptoms and bacterial shedding if administered early in the course of disease. Because campylobacteriosis generally cannot be distinguished from other causes of travelers' diarrhea without a diagnostic test, the use of empiric antibiotics in travelers should follow the guidelines for travelers' diarrhea.

Rates of antibiotic resistance, especially fluoroquinolone resistance, have risen sharply in the past 20 years, and high rates of resistance are now seen in many regions. Travel abroad is a risk factor for infection with resistant *Campylobacter*. Clinicians should suspect resistant infection in returning travelers with campylobacteriosis in whom empiric fluoroquinolone treatment has failed. When fluoroquinolone resistance is proven or suspected, azithromycin is usually the next choice of treatment, although resistance to macrolides has also been reported.

## PREVENTION

No vaccine is available. Prevention is best achieved by adhering to standard food and water safety precautions (see Chapter 2, Food & Water Precautions) and thorough handwashing after contact with animals or environments that may be contaminated with animal feces. Antibiotic prophylaxis is not recommended.

**CDC website:** www.cdc.gov/foodsafety/ diseases/campylobacter

## BIBLIOGRAPHY

1. Fitzgerald C, Nachamkin I. Campylobacter and Arcobacter. In: Jorgensen JH, Pfaller MA, Carroll KC, Funke G, Landry ML, Richter SS, et al., editors. Manual of Clinical Microbiology. 11th ed. Washington, D.C.: American Society for Microbiology Press; 2015. pp. 998–1012.

2. Geissler AL, Bustos Carrillo F, Swanson K, Patrick ME, Fullerton KE, Bennett C, et al. Increasing Campylobacter infections, outbreaks, and antimicrobial resistance in the United States, 2004–2012. Clin Infect Dis. 2017 Jul;65(10):1624–31.

3. Humphrey T, O'Brien S, Madsen M. Campylobacters as zoonotic pathogens: a food production perspective. Int J Food Microbiol. 2007 Jul 15;117(3):237–57.

4. Kaakoush NO, Castaño-Rodríguiz N, Mitchell HA, Man SM. Global epidemiology of Campylobacter infection. Clin Microbiol Rev. 2015 July;28(3):687–720.

5. Kendall ME, Crim S, Fullerton K, Han PV, Cronquist AB, Shiferaw B, et al. Travel-associated enteric infections diagnosed after return to the United States, Foodborne Diseases Active Surveillance Network (FoodNet), 2004–2009. Clin Infect Dis. 2012 Jun;54 Suppl 5:S480–7.

6. Tribble DR. Resistant pathogens as causes of traveller's diarrhea globally and impact(s) on treatment failure and recommendations. J. Travel Med. 2017 Apr 1;24(Suppl 1):S6–12.

7. World Health Organization. The global view of campylobacteriosis: report of an expert consultation. Geneva: World Health Organization; 2012 [cited 2016 Sep 21]. Available from: http://apps.who.int/ iris/bitstr eam/10665/80751/1/9789241564601_eng. pdf?ua=1.

# CHIKUNGUNYA

J. Erin Staples, Susan L. Hills, Ann M. Powers, Kristina M. Angelo

## INFECTIOUS AGENT

Chikungunya virus is a single-stranded RNA virus that belongs to the family Togaviridae, genus *Alphavirus.*

## TRANSMISSION

Chikungunya virus is transmitted to humans via the bite of an infected mosquito of the *Aedes* spp., predominantly *Aedes aegypti* and *Ae. albopictus.* Mosquitoes become infected when they feed on viremic nonhuman or human primates, which are likely the main amplifying reservoirs of the virus. Humans are typically viremic shortly before and in the first 2–6 days of illness. Bloodborne transmission is possible; 1 case has been documented in a health care worker who was stuck with a needle after drawing blood from an infected patient. Furthermore, chikungunya virus has been identified in donated blood products undergoing screening, though no transfusion-associated cases been identified to date. Cases have also been documented among laboratory personnel handling infected blood and through aerosol exposure in the laboratory. Maternal–fetal transmission has been documented during pregnancy; the highest risk occurs in the perinatal period when a woman is viremic at the time of delivery. Studies have not found virus in breast milk.

## EPIDEMIOLOGY

Chikungunya virus often causes large outbreaks with high attack rates, affecting one-third to three-quarters of the population in areas where the virus is circulating. Outbreaks of chikungunya have occurred in Africa, Asia, Europe, the Americas, and islands in the Indian and Pacific Oceans. In late 2013, the first locally acquired cases of chikungunya were reported in the Americas on islands in the Caribbean. By the end of 2017, more than 2.6 million suspect cases of chikungunya had been reported in the Americas. Since then, the virus has continued to circulate and cause sporadic disease cases and periodic outbreaks in many areas of the world.

Risk to travelers is highest in areas experiencing ongoing epidemics of the disease. Most epidemics occur during the tropical rainy season and abate during the dry season. However, outbreaks in Africa have occurred after periods of drought, where open water containers near human habitation served as vector-breeding sites. Risk of infection exists primarily during the day, as the primary vector, *Ae. aegypti*, aggressively bites during the daytime. *Ae. aegypti* mosquitoes bite indoors or outdoors near dwellings. They lay their eggs in domestic containers that hold water, including buckets and flowerpots.

Both adults and children can become infected and symptomatic with the disease. From 2010 through 2013, 110 cases of chikungunya were identified or reported among US travelers, who predominantly traveled to areas with known ongoing outbreaks. However, following the outbreaks in the Americas, from 2014–2017, >4,000 chikungunya cases were reported among US travelers, and 13 locally acquired cases were reported in the continental United States. In addition, US territories (Puerto Rico, US Virgin Islands, and American Samoa) reported locally acquired cases during 2014–2015, with Puerto Rico also reporting sporadic cases since 2016.

Characteristics of chikungunya and other arboviral diseases are shown in Box 4-1.

## CLINICAL PRESENTATION

Approximately 3%–28% of people infected with chikungunya virus will remain asymptomatic. For people who develop symptomatic illness, the incubation period is typically 3–7 days (range, 1–12 days). Disease is most often characterized by sudden onset of high fever (temperature typically >102°F [39°C]) and joint pains. Other symptoms may include headache, myalgia, arthritis, conjunctivitis, nausea, vomiting, or a maculopapular rash. Fevers typically last from several days up to 1 week; the fever can be biphasic. Joint symptoms are typically severe and can be debilitating. They usually involve multiple joints, typically bilateral and symmetric. The joint pains occur most commonly in hands and feet, but they can affect more proximal joints. Rash usually occurs after onset of fever. It typically involves the trunk and extremities but also can include the palms, soles, and face.

Abnormal laboratory findings can include thrombocytopenia, lymphopenia, and elevated creatinine and liver function tests. Rare but serious complications of the disease can occur, including myocarditis, ocular disease (uveitis, retinitis), hepatitis, acute renal disease, severe bullous lesions, and neurologic disease, such as meningoencephalitis, Guillain-Barré syndrome, myelitis, or cranial nerve palsies. Groups identified as having increased risk for more severe disease include neonates exposed intrapartum, adults >65 years of age, and people with underlying medical conditions, such as hypertension, diabetes, or heart disease.

Acute symptoms of chikungunya typically resolve in 7–10 days. Fatalities associated with infection occur but are rare and most commonly reported in older adults and those with comorbidities. Some patients will have a relapse of rheumatologic symptoms such as polyarthralgia, polyarthritis, tenosynovitis, or Raynaud syndrome in the months after acute illness. Studies have reported variable proportions, ranging from 5% to 80%, of patients with persistent joint pains, as well as prolonged fatigue, for months or years after their illness.

Pregnant women have symptoms and outcomes similar to those of other people, and most infections that occur during pregnancy will not result in the virus being transmitted to the fetus. However, intrapartum transmission can result in neonatal complications, including neurologic disease, hemorrhagic symptoms, and myocardial disease. There are also rare reports of spontaneous abortions after maternal infection during the first trimester.

## DIAGNOSIS

The differential diagnosis of chikungunya virus infection depends on the clinical signs and symptoms as well as where the person was suspected of being infected. Diseases that should be considered in the differential diagnosis include dengue, Zika, malaria, leptospirosis, parvovirus, enterovirus, group A *Streptococcus*, rubella, measles, adenovirus, postinfectious arthritis, rheumatologic conditions, or alphavirus infections (including Mayaro, Ross River, Barmah Forest, o'nyong'nyong, and Sindbis viruses).

Preliminary diagnosis is based on the patient's clinical features, places and dates of travel, and exposures. Laboratory diagnosis is generally accomplished by testing serum to detect virus, viral

4

BOX 4-1.

# Arboviral diseases

*What are arboviruses?*

Viruses that are spread to humans by an infected arthropod vector, such as ticks, mosquitoes, and sandflies.

*What are the general characteristics of arboviral diseases?*

- Include a number of emerging and reemerging infectious diseases.
- Vary by geographic distribution and clinical syndrome.
- Classified into 7 main families: Flaviviridae, Togaviridae, Peribunyaviridae, Phenuiviridae, Nairoviridae, Orthoviridae, and Reoviridae.

| FAMILY | VIRUS | GEOGRAPHIC DISTRIBUTION | VECTOR | TYPICAL CLINICAL SYNDROME |
|---|---|---|---|---|
| Flaviviridae | Alkhurma virus | Egypt, Saudi Arabia | Tick | Hemorrhagic fever |
| | Dengue viruses | Americas, Caribbean, Africa, Asia, Middle East | Mosquito | Febrile illness, arthralgia, rash, hemorrhagic fever, rarely shock |
| | Japanese encephalitis virus | Asia, Western Pacific | Mosquito | Encephalitis |
| | Kyasanur Forest disease virus | India | Tick | Hemorrhagic fever |
| | Louping ill virus | Europe | Tick | Encephalitis |
| | Murray Valley encephalitis virus | Australia, Papua New Guinea | Mosquito | Encephalitis |
| | Omsk hemorrhagic fever virus | Siberia | Tick | Hemorrhagic fever |
| | Powassan virus | North America | Tick | Encephalitis |
| | Rocio virus | South America | Mosquito | Encephalitis |
| | Saint Louis encephalitis virus | North America | Mosquito | Encephalitis |
| | Tickborne encephalitis virus | Europe, Asia (Russia) | Tick | Encephalitis |
| | West Nile virus | Africa, Europe, Middle East, North America, West Asia, SE Asia | Mosquito | Febrile illness, neuroinvasive disease (rare) |
| | Yellow fever virus | Africa, South America | Mosquito | Hemorrhagic fever, hepatitis |
| | Zika virus | Americas, Caribbean, Africa, Asia, Western Pacific | Mosquito | Febrile illness, arthralgia, rash |

BOX 4-1. Arboviral diseases (continued)

| FAMILY | VIRUS | GEOGRAPHIC DISTRIBUTION | VECTOR | TYPICAL CLINICAL SYNDROME |
|---|---|---|---|---|
| Togaviridae | Barmah Forest virus | Australia | Mosquito | Febrile illness, arthralgia, rash |
| | Chikungunya virus | Americas, Caribbean, Africa, Asia, Europe, Western Pacific | Mosquito | Febrile illness, arthralgia, rash |
| | Eastern equine encephalitis virus | North America, Caribbean | Mosquito | Encephalitis |
| | Mayaro virus | Americas, Caribbean | Mosquito | Febrile illness, arthralgia, rash |
| | Madariaga virus | Central and South America | Mosquito | Febrile illness, encephalitis |
| | O'nyong-nyong virus | Africa | Mosquito | Febrile illness, arthralgia, rash |
| | Ross River virus | Australia, South Pacific | Mosquito | Febrile illness, arthralgia, rash |
| | Semliki Forest virus | Africa | Mosquito | Febrile illness, rare encephalitis |
| | Sindbis virus | Northern Europe, Asia, Africa, Australia | Mosquito | Febrile illness, arthralgia, rash |
| | Venezuelan equine encephalitis virus | Americas | Mosquito | Encephalitis |
| | Western equine encephalitis virus | Americas | Mosquito | Encephalitis |
| Peribunyaviridae | Bunyamwera virus | Africa | Mosquito | Febrile illness, arthralgia, rash |
| | Bwamba virus | Africa | Mosquito | Febrile illness, arthralgia, rash |
| | California encephalitis virus | North America | Mosquito | Encephalitis |
| | Jamestown Canyon virus | North America | Mosquito | Encephalitis |
| | La Crosse encephalitis virus | North America | Mosquito | Encephalitis |
| | Oropouche virus | Americas, Caribbean | Mosquito | Febrile illness, arthralgia, rash |
| | Rift Valley fever virus | Africa, Middle East | Mosquito | Febrile illness, myalgia, rare encephalitis, rare hemorrhage |
| | Toscana virus | Mediterranean | Sandfly | Encephalitis |

(continued)

BOX 4-1.

# Arboviral diseases (continued)

| FAMILY | VIRUS | GEOGRAPHIC DISTRIBUTION | VECTOR | TYPICAL CLINICAL SYNDROME |
|--------|-------|-------------------------|--------|---------------------------|
| Phenuiviridae | Heartland virus | North America | Tick | Febrile illness, arthralgia |
| | Rift Valley fever virus | Africa, Middle East | Mosquito | Febrile illness, myalgia, rare |
| | Sandfly fever viruses | North Africa, Mediterranean, Middle East | Sandfly | Febrile illness, myalgia |
| | Severe fever with thrombocytopenia syndrome virus | East Asia | Tick | Hemorrhagic fever |
| | Toscana virus | Mediterranean | Sandfly | Encephalitis |
| Nairoviridae | Crimean Congo hemorrhagic fever virus | Africa, Middle East, Asia, Eastern Europe | Tick | Hemorrhagic fever |
| Reoviridae | Banna virus | Asia | Mosquito | Febrile illness, rare encephalitis |
| | Colorado tick fever virus | North America | Tick | Febrile illness, arthralgia, rash |
| Orthomyxoviridae | Bourbon virus | North America | Tick | Fever, acute respiratory distress, multiorgan failure |
| | Thogoto virus | Africa, Europe | Tick | Meningoencephalitis |

nucleic acid, or virus-specific IgM and neutralizing antibodies. During the first week after onset of symptoms, chikungunya can often be diagnosed by performing viral culture or nucleic acid amplification on serum. Virus-specific IgM and neutralizing antibodies normally develop toward the end of the first week of illness. Therefore, to definitively rule out the diagnosis, convalescent-phase samples should be obtained from patients whose acute-phase samples test negative.

Testing for chikungunya virus is performed at several state health department laboratories and commercial laboratories. Confirmatory testing for virus-specific neutralizing antibodies is available through CDC (Division of Vector-borne Diseases, 970-221-6400). Health care providers should report suspected chikungunya cases to their state or local health departments to facilitate diagnosis and mitigate the risk of local transmission. Because chikungunya is a nationally notifiable disease, state health departments should report laboratory-confirmed cases to CDC through ArboNET, the national surveillance system for arboviral diseases.

## TREATMENT

No specific antiviral treatment is available for chikungunya; however, a number of therapeutic options are being investigated. Treatment for symptoms can include rest, fluids, and use of analgesics and antipyretics. Nonsteroidal anti-inflammatory drugs can be used to help with acute fever and pain. In dengue-endemic areas, however, acetaminophen is the preferred first-line treatment for fever and joint pain until dengue can be ruled out, to reduce the risk of hemorrhage. For patients with persistent joint pain, use of nonsteroidal anti-inflammatory drugs, corticosteroids including topical preparations, and physical therapy may help lessen the symptoms.

## PREVENTION

Currently, no vaccine or preventive drug is available. However, several candidate vaccines are in various stages of development. The best way to prevent infection is to avoid mosquito bites (see Chapter 3, Mosquitoes, Ticks & Other Arthropods). Travelers at increased risk for more severe disease, including travelers with underlying medical conditions and women who are late in their pregnancy (as their fetuses are at increased risk), may consider avoiding travel to areas with ongoing outbreaks. If travel is unavoidable, emphasize the need for protective measures against mosquito bites.

**CDC website:** www.cdc.gov/chikungunya

### BIBLIOGRAPHY

1. CDC. Chikungunya virus in the United States. Atlanta: CDC; 2017 [cited 2018 Mar 23]. Available from: www.cdc.gov/chikungunya/geo/united-states.html.

2. Duvignaud A, Fianu A, Bertolotti A, Jaubert J, Michault A, Poubeau P, et al. Rheumatism and chronic fatigue, the two facets of post-chikungunya disease: the TELECHIK cohort study on Reunion Island. Epidemiol Infect. 2018 Apr;146(5):633–41.

3. Lindsey NP, Staples JE, Fischer M. Chikungunya virus disease among travelers—United States, 2014–2016. Am J Trop Med Hyg. 2018 Jan;98(1):192–7.

4. Mehta R, Soares CN, Medialdea-Carrera R, Ellul M, da Silva MTT, Rosala-Hallas A, et al. The spectrum of neurological disease associated with Zika and chikungunya viruses in adults in Rio de Janeiro, Brazil: a case series. PLoS Negl Trop Dis. 2018 Feb 12;12(2):e0006212.

5. Pan American Health Organization. Chikungunya: Data, Maps and Statistics. Washington, DC: Pan American Health Organization; 2018 [cited 2018 Mar 23]. Available from: www.paho.org/hq/index.php?option=com_topics&view=readall&cid=5927&Itemid=40931&lang=en.

6. Powers AM. Vaccine and therapeutic options to control chikungunya virus. Clin Microbiol Rev. 2017 Dec;31(1):e00104–16.

7. Simon F, Javelle E, Cabie A, Bouquillard E, Troisgros O, Gentile G, et al. French guidelines for the management of chikungunya (acute and persistent presentations). November 2014. Med Mal Infect. 2015 Jul;45(7):243–63.

8. Tomashek KM, Lorenzi OD, Andújar-Pérez DA, Torres-Velásquez BC, Hunsperger EA, et al. Clinical and epidemiologic characteristics of dengue and other etiologic agents among patients with acute febrile illness, Puerto Rico, 2012–2015. PLoS Negl Trop Dis. 2017 Sep;11(9):e0005859.

9. World Health Organization. Chikungunya: case definitions for acute, atypical and chronic cases. Conclusions of an expert consultation, Managua, Nicaragua, 20–21 May 2015. Wkly Epidemiol Rec. 2015 Aug 14;90(33):410–14.

# CHOLERA

Hammad S. N'cho, Karen K. Wong, Eric D. Mintz

## INFECTIOUS AGENT

Cholera is an acute bacterial intestinal infection caused by toxigenic *Vibrio cholerae* O-group 1 or O-group 139. Many other serogroups of *V. cholerae*, with or without the cholera toxin gene (including the nontoxigenic strains of the O1 and O139 serogroups), can cause a choleralike illness. Only toxigenic strains of serogroups O1 and O139 have caused widespread epidemics and are reportable to the World Health Organization (WHO) as "cholera." *V. cholerae* O1 is the source of an ongoing global pandemic, while the O139 serogroup remains localized to a few areas in Asia.

*V. cholerae* O1 has 2 biotypes, classical and El Tor, and each biotype has 2 distinct serotypes, Inaba and Ogawa. The symptoms of infection are indistinguishable, although more people infected with the El Tor biotype remain asymptomatic or have only a mild illness. Globally, most cases of cholera are caused by O1 El Tor organisms. In recent years, an El Tor variant that has characteristics of both classical and El Tor biotypes and may be more virulent than older El Tor strains has emerged in Asia and spread to Africa and the Caribbean. This strain is responsible for the epidemic on Hispaniola and appears to cause a higher proportion of severe episodes of cholera with the potential for higher death rates.

## TRANSMISSION

Toxigenic *V. cholerae* O1 and O139 are free-living bacterial organisms found in fresh and brackish water, often in association with copepods or other zooplankton, shellfish, and aquatic plants. Cholera infections are most commonly acquired from drinking water in which *V. cholerae* is found naturally or into which it has been introduced from the feces of an infected person. Other common vehicles include fish and shellfish. Other foods, including produce, are less commonly implicated. Direct transmission from person to person, even to health care workers during epidemics, has been reported but is infrequent.

## EPIDEMIOLOGY

Cholera is endemic in approximately 50 countries, primarily in Africa and South and Southeast Asia, and can emerge in dramatic epidemics, although most cases go unreported. In October 2010, a large cholera epidemic began in Haiti and spread to the Dominican Republic and Cuba; it is now endemic at much lower levels in Haiti and the Dominican Republic, though small outbreaks still occur. Sporadic cases associated with travel to or from cholera-affected countries in Asia and Africa continue to occur.

From 2010 through 2016, 107 cases of cholera were confirmed in the United States among people who had traveled internationally in the week before illness. Of these, approximately 75% were associated with travel to the Caribbean, and 10% were associated with travel to India or Pakistan; other travel destinations reported included countries in Southeast Asia and both East and West Africa. There is a risk of cholera infection for travelers to areas where cholera is endemic or where there is an active epidemic. This risk is increased for those who drink untreated water, do not follow handwashing recommendations, do not use latrines or other sanitation systems, or eat raw or undercooked food, especially seafood. Health care and response workers in cholera-affected areas, such as in an outbreak or after a disaster, may also be at increased risk of cholera. People who have low gastric acidity or those with blood type O are at higher risk of severe cholera illness. **Travelers who consistently observe safe food, water, sanitation, and handwashing recommendations while in countries affected by cholera have virtually no risk of acquiring cholera.**

## CLINICAL PRESENTATION

Cholera most commonly manifests as acute watery diarrhea in an afebrile person. Infection is often mild or asymptomatic, but it can be severe. Severe cholera is characterized by profuse watery diarrhea, described as "rice-water stools," often accompanied by nausea and vomiting, that can rapidly lead to severe volume depletion. Signs and symptoms include tachycardia, loss of skin turgor, dry mucous membranes, hypotension, and thirst. Additional symptoms, including muscle cramps, are secondary to the resulting electrolyte imbalances. If untreated, rapid loss of body fluids can lead to severe dehydration, hypovolemic shock, and death within hours. With adequate and timely rehydration, the case-fatality ratio is <1%.

## DIAGNOSIS

Cholera is confirmed through culture of a stool specimen or rectal swab. Cary-Blair medium can be used for transport, and selective media such as taurocholate-tellurite-gelatin agar and thiosulfate-citrate-bile salts agar may be used for isolation and identification. Reagents for serogrouping *V. cholerae* isolates are available in state health department laboratories. Culture-independent diagnostic tests (CIDT) do not yield an isolate for antimicrobial susceptibility testing and subtyping. Reflex culture to recover an isolate should be performed when a diagnosis of *V. cholerae* is derived from a CIDT, and the isolate should be forwarded to a public health laboratory for additional characterization. All isolates obtained in the United States should be sent to CDC via state health department laboratories for identification and virulence testing. Cholera is a nationally notifiable disease.

## TREATMENT

Rehydration is the cornerstone of cholera treatment. Oral rehydration solution and, when necessary, intravenous fluids and electrolytes, if administered in a timely manner and in adequate volumes, will reduce case-fatality ratios to <1%. Antibiotics reduce fluid requirements and duration of illness and are indicated in conjunction with aggressive hydration for severe cases and for those with moderate dehydration and ongoing fluid losses. Whenever possible, antimicrobial susceptibility testing should inform treatment choices. In most countries, doxycycline is recommended as the first-line antibiotic treatment for adults, and azithromycin is recommended for children and pregnant women. Multidrug-resistant isolates are emerging, particularly in South Asia, with resistance to quinolones, trimethoprim-sulfamethoxazole, and tetracycline. The strain from Hispaniola is also multidrug resistant; however, it is still sensitive to doxycycline and tetracycline. Zinc supplementation reduces the severity and duration of cholera and other diarrheal diseases in children living in resource-limited areas.

## PREVENTION

### Food and Water

Safe food and water precautions and frequent handwashing are critical in preventing cholera (see Chapter 2, Food & Water Precautions). Chemoprophylaxis is not indicated.

### Vaccine

No country or territory requires vaccination against cholera as a condition for entry. CVD 103-HgR, a single-dose oral cholera vaccine (Vaxchora, PaxVax), is licensed and available in the United

States. The vaccine was previously marketed under the names Orochol and Mutacol in other countries. Vaxchora was approved in June 2016 for use in adults ≥18 years of age.

### INDICATIONS

The Advisory Committee on Immunization Practices (ACIP) recommends CVD 103-HgR vaccine for adult travelers (age 18–64 years) to an area of active cholera transmission. An area of active cholera transmission is defined as a province, state, or other administrative subdivision within a country with endemic or epidemic cholera caused by toxigenic *V. cholerae* O1 and includes areas with cholera activity within the last year that are prone to recurrence of cholera epidemics; it does not include areas where rare sporadic cases have been reported. A list of countries where cholera vaccine can be considered for travelers is found at wwwnc.cdc.gov/travel/diseases/cholera. However, cholera activity may be found only in certain parts of a country or in certain settings, and information about places with cholera activity may be incomplete because of variations in surveillance and reporting. Additional country-specific information may be found on the country-specific travel pages.

The vaccine is not routinely recommended for most travelers from the United States, as most do not visit areas with active cholera transmission.

### VACCINE EFFICACY

Adults aged 18–45 years who received Vaxchora were protected against severe diarrhea after oral *V. cholerae* O1 challenge at 10 days and at 3 months after vaccination (vaccine efficacy 90% and 80%, respectively). In adults aged 46–64 years, vibriocidal antibody seroconversion rates, the best available marker for protection against cholera, were noninferior to the response seen in adults aged 18–45 years.

### VACCINE ADMINISTRATION

Vaxchora is administered in a single oral dose, which consists of ingestion of the entire contents of 1 double-chambered sachet. Vaxchora should be taken at least 10 days before potential cholera exposure. Eating or drinking should be avoided for 60 minutes before and after oral ingestion of Vaxchora. Prepare and administer Vaxchora in a health care setting equipped to dispose of medical waste.

## BOOSTER DOSES

The safety and efficacy of revaccination with CVD 103-HgR have not been established.

## VACCINE SAFETY AND ADVERSE REACTIONS

Serious adverse events were rare among recipients of Orochol and Mutacol, the previously marketed formulation of the CVD 103-HgR vaccine. Systemic adverse events, which may include diarrhea and headache, occur at similar rates in Vaxchora recipients and nonrecipients.

## PRECAUTIONS AND CONTRAINDICATIONS

Vaxchora is contraindicated in people with a history of severe allergic reaction to any ingredient of Vaxchora or to a previous dose of any cholera vaccine. A study with the older formulation of CVD 103-HgR showed that concomitant use of chloroquine decreased the immune response to the vaccine; therefore, antimalarial prophylaxis with chloroquine should begin no sooner than 10 days after administration of Vaxchora. Coadministration of mefloquine and proguanil with CVD 103-HgR did not diminish the vaccine's immunogenicity. Antibiotics may decrease the immune response to CVD 103-HgR, so vaccine should not be administered to patients who have received antibiotics in the previous 14 days.

Vaxchora is not currently licensed for use in children <18 years of age. No information is available on the use of Vaxchora during pregnancy or lactation. The safety and effectiveness of Vaxchora have not been established in immunocompromised people. There was no difference in adverse events reported among HIV-positive recipients of an older formulation of the CVD 103-HgR vaccine and those who received placebo.

Vaxchora may be shed in the stool for at least 7 days, and the vaccine strain may be transmitted to nonvaccinated close contacts. Clinicians and travelers should use caution when considering whether to use the vaccine in people with immunocompromised close contacts.

**CDC website:** www.cdc.gov/cholera

## BIBLIOGRAPHY

1. Chen WH, Cohen MB, Kirkpatrick BD, Brady RC, Galloway D, Gurwith M, et al. Single-dose live oral cholera vaccine CVD 103-HgR protects against human experimental infection with Vibrio cholerae O1 El Tor. Clin Infect Dis. 2016 Jun 1;62(11):1329–35.

2. Danzig L, editor. Vaxchora™ clinical data summary. Meeting of the Advisory Committee on Immunization Practices; 2016 Feb 24; Atlanta, GA.

3. Freedman DO. Re-born in the USA: Another cholera vaccine for travelers. 2016. Travel Med Infect Dis. July–Aug; 14(4):295–6.

4. Harris JB, LaRocque RC, Qadri F, Ryan ET, Calderwood SB. Cholera. Lancet. 2012 Jun 30;379(9835):2466–76.

5. Kollaritsch H, Que JU, Kunz C, Wiedermann G, Herzog C, Cryz SJ, Jr. Safety and immunogenicity of live oral cholera and typhoid vaccines administered alone or in combination with antimalarial drugs, oral polio vaccine, or yellow fever vaccine. J Infect Dis. 1997 Apr;175(4):871–5.

6. Loharikar A, Newton AE, Stroika S, Freeman M, Greene KD, Parsons MB, et al. Cholera in the United States, 2001–2011: a reflection of patterns of global epidemiology and travel. Epidemiol Infect. 2015 March;143(4):695–703.

7. Schilling KA, Cartwright EJ, Stamper J, Locke M, Esposito DH, Balaban V, et al. Diarrheal illness among US residents providing medical services in Haiti during the cholera epidemic, 2010–2011. J Travel Med. 2014 Jan–Feb;21(1):55–7.

8. Wong KK, Burdette E, Mahon BE, Mintz ED, Ryan ET, Reingold RL. Recommendations of the Advisory Committee on Immunization Practices for use of cholera vaccine. MMWR Morb Mortal Wkly Rep. 2017 May;66(18):482–485.

9. Wong KK, Mahon BE, Reingold A. CVD 103-HgR vaccine for travelers. Travel Med Infect Dis. 2016 Nov—Dec;14(6):632–633.

10. World Health Organization. Cholera, 2016. Wkly Epidemiol Rec. 2017 Sep 8;92(36):521–536.

# COCCIDIOIDOMYCOSIS (VALLEY FEVER)

Orion Z. McCotter, Tom M. Chiller

## INFECTIOUS AGENT

The fungi *Coccidioides immitis* and *C. posadasii*.

## TRANSMISSION

Through inhalation of fungal conidia from the environment. Not transmitted from person to person.

## EPIDEMIOLOGY

Endemic in the western United States, particularly Arizona and Southern California, and parts of Mexico and Central and South America. Travelers are at increased risk if they participate in activities that expose them to soil disruption and outdoor dust. Outbreaks have been associated with activities such as construction, archaeological excavation, and military training exercises.

## CLINICAL PRESENTATION

The incubation period is 7–21 days. Most infections (60%) are asymptomatic. Symptomatic infection ranges from primary pulmonary illness to severe disseminated disease. Primary pulmonary coccidioidomycosis is characterized by fatigue, cough, fever, shortness of breath, headache, night sweats, muscle aches, joint pain, and rash. These infections are often self-limited, and symptoms typically resolve in a few weeks to months. However, 5%–10% of people go on to develop serious or chronic lung disease, such as cavitary pneumonia, fibrosis, and bronchiectasis. In rare instances (approximately 1% of infections), dissemination to the central nervous system, joints, bones, or skin may occur.

Older people (≥65 years), people with diabetes, and people who smoke are at increased risk of developing severe pulmonary complications. People with depressed cellular immune function, pregnant women, and people of African American or Filipino descent are at increased risk of developing disseminated disease.

## DIAGNOSIS

The methods most commonly used to diagnose coccidioidomycosis are serology, culture, histopathology, and molecular techniques. EIA is a sensitive serologic method to detect IgM and IgG. Immunodiffusion and complement fixation can also detect antibodies and are often used to confirm diagnosis. Lateral flow assays to detect any antibodies in serum became available in 2018. Isolation of *Coccidioides* from fungal culture of respiratory specimens or tissue provides a definitive diagnosis. Microscopy of sputum or tissue can identify *Coccidioides* spherules but has low sensitivity. Molecular techniques include DNA probe for confirmation of cultures, as well as PCR for direct detection from clinical specimens, which became available in early 2018. Coccidioidomycosis is a nationally notifiable disease in the United States.

## TREATMENT

Expert opinions differ on the proper management of patients with uncomplicated primary pulmonary disease in the absence of risk factors for severe or disseminated disease. Some experts recommend no therapy since most illnesses are self-limited, whereas others advise treatment to reduce the intensity or duration of symptoms. Treatment with antifungal agents has not been proven to prevent dissemination. People at high risk for dissemination and people with the following clinical manifestations should receive antifungal therapy:

- Severe acute pulmonary disease
- Chronic pulmonary disease
- Disseminated disease

Depending on the clinical situation, a variety of antifungal agents may be used.

## PREVENTION

Limit exposure to outdoor dust in endemic areas.

### BIBLIOGRAPHY

1. Ampel NM. Coccidioidomycosis. In: Kauffman CA, Pappas PG, Sobel JD, Dismukes WE, editors. Essentials of Clinical Mycology. New York: Springer Science+Business Media, LLC; 2011. pp. 349–66.

2. Ampel NM. Coccidioidomycosis: a review of recent advances. Clin Chest Med. 2009 Jun;30(2):241–51.

3. CDC. Coccidioidomycosis in travelers returning from Mexico–Pennsylvania, 2000. MMWR. 2000;49(44):1004–6.

4. Chiller TM, Galgiani JN, Stevens DA. Coccidioidomycosis. Infect Dis Clin North Am. 2003 Mar;17(1):41–57, viii.

5. Crum NF, Lederman ER, Stafford CM, Parrish JS, Wallace MR. Coccidioidomycosis: a descriptive survey of a reemerging disease. Clinical characteristics and current controversies. Medicine (Baltimore). 2004 May;83(3):149–75.

6. Freedman M, Jackson BR, McCotter O, Benedict K. Coccidioidomycosis outbreaks, United States and worldwide, 1940–2015. Emerg Infect Dis. 2018;24(3):417–423.

7. Galgiani JN, Ampel NM, Blair JE, Catanzaro A, Geertsma F, Hoover SE, et al. 2016 Infectious Diseases Society of America (IDSA) clinical practice guideline for the treatment of coccidioidomycosis. Clin Infect Dis. 2016 Jul 27;63(6):e112–46.

8. Rosenstein NE, Emery KW, Werner SB, Kao A, Johnson R, Rogers D, et al. Risk factors for severe pulmonary and disseminated coccidioidomycosis: Kern County, California, 1995–1996. Clin Infect Dis. 2001 Mar 1;32(5):708–15.

9. Thompson GR, 3rd. Pulmonary coccidioidomycosis. Semin Respir Crit Care Med. 2011 Dec;32(6):754–63.

10. Twarog, Meryl, George R. Thompson III. Coccidioidomycosis: recent updates. Seminars in respiratory and critical care medicine. Thieme Medical Publishers, 2015. Vol. 36. No. 05.

**CDC website:** www.cdc.gov/fungal/diseases/ coccidioidomycosis

# CRYPTOSPORIDIOSIS

Michele C. Hlavsa, Dawn M. Roellig

## INFECTIOUS AGENT

Among the many protozoan parasites in the genus *Cryptosporidium*, *Cryptosporidium hominis* and *C. parvum* cause >90% of human infections.

## TRANSMISSION

*Cryptosporidium* is transmitted via the fecal–oral route. Its low infectious dose, prolonged survival in moist environments, protracted communicability, and extreme chlorine tolerance make *Cryptosporidium* ideally suited for transmission through contaminated drinking or recreational water (such as swimming pools). Transmission can also occur through eating contaminated food, through contact with infected animals (particularly preweaned bovine calves) or people (for example, when providing direct care or during oral-anal sex), or through contact with fecally contaminated surfaces.

## EPIDEMIOLOGY

Cryptosporidiosis is endemic worldwide, and the highest rates are found in developing countries. International travel is a risk factor for sporadic cryptosporidiosis in the United States and other industrialized nations; however, few studies have assessed the prevalence of cryptosporidiosis in travelers. One study found a 3% prevalence of *Cryptosporidium* infection among those with travelers' diarrhea; cryptosporidiosis was associated with travel to Latin America and to Asia, India in particular.

Another report identified a 6% prevalence of *Cryptosporidium* infection among North American travelers to Mexico. The authors of this study reported associations between duration of stay (longer visits associated with an increased risk of *Cryptosporidium* vs. bacterial diarrhea) and specific destination (travel to 2 cities in Mexico, in particular, increased the likelihood of *Cryptosporidium* infection).

## CLINICAL PRESENTATION

Symptoms (most commonly, profuse, watery diarrhea) begin within 2 weeks (typically 5–7 days) after infection and are generally self-limited. Other symptoms can include abdominal pain, flatulence, urgency, nausea, vomiting, and low-grade fever. In immunocompetent people, symptoms typically resolve within 2–3 weeks; patients may experience a recurrence of symptoms after a brief period of recovery and before complete symptom resolution.

Clinical presentation of cryptosporidiosis in immunocompromised patients varies with level of immunosuppression, ranging from no symptoms or transient disease to relapsing or chronic diarrhea or even choleralike diarrhea, which can lead to dehydration and life-threatening wasting and malabsorption. Extraintestinal cryptosporidiosis (in the biliary or respiratory tract and rarely the pancreas) has been documented in children and immunocompromised hosts.

## DIAGNOSIS

Routine ova and parasite testing does not typically include *Cryptosporidium*; clinicians should specifically request testing for this organism when *Cryptosporidium* infection is suspected. New molecular enteric panel assays generally include *Cryptosporidium* as a target pathogen. Intermittent excretion of *Cryptosporidium* in the stool necessitates collection of multiple samples (specimens collected on 3 separate days) to increase test sensitivity.

Other diagnostic techniques include microscopy with direct fluorescent antibody (DFA; considered the gold standard), enzyme immunoassay (EIA) kits, molecular assays, microscopy with modified acid-fast staining, and rapid immunochromatographic cartridge assays. Rapid immunochromatographic cartridge assays can generate false-positive results; consider confirmation microscopy for specimens identified as positive by this method.

Infections caused by the different *Cryptosporidium* species and subtypes can differ clinically. However, despite all the variations in clinical presentation caused by this protozoan, most *Cryptosporidium* species, all with multiple subtypes, are indistinguishable by traditional diagnostic tests. To better understand cryptosporidiosis epidemiology and track infection sources, CDC has launched CryptoNet (www.cdc.gov/parasites/crypto/cryptonet.html), which provides *Cryptosporidium* genotyping and subtyping services in collaboration with state public health agencies. CryptoNet recommends not using formalin to preserve stool for *Cryptosporidium* testing because formalin impedes reliable genotyping and subtyping. Cryptosporidiosis is a nationally notifiable disease.

## TREATMENT

Most immunocompetent people recover without treatment. The US Food and Drug Administration has approved nitazoxanide as a treatment for cryptosporidiosis in immunocompetent people aged ≥1 year. Nitazoxanide has not been shown to be an effective treatment of cryptosporidiosis in immunocompromised patients. However, dramatic clinical and parasitologic responses without specific treatment have been reported in these patients following reconstitution of the immune system. Protease inhibitors might have direct anti-*Cryptosporidium* activity. Oral rehydration is the most effective supportive therapy in both immunocompetent and immunocompromised patients.

## PREVENTION

Careful adherence to food and water precautions (see Chapter 2, Food & Water Precautions) and proper handwashing techniques (www.cdc.gov/handwashing/when-how-handwashing.html) can decrease the risk of infection. Alcohol-based hand sanitizers are not effective against the parasite. Treat water for drinking by filtering with an absolute 1-µm filter or heating to a rolling boil for 1 minute. *Cryptosporidium* is extremely tolerant of halogens (such as chlorine or iodine). To protect themselves, swimmers should avoid ingestion of recreational water. To protect others, cryptosporidiosis patients should not enter recreational water while ill with diarrhea and for the first 2 weeks after symptoms have completely resolved because of prolonged excretion of infectious oocysts.

**CDC website:** www.cdc.gov/parasites/crypto/index.html

## BIBLIOGRAPHY

1. Adamu H, Petros B, Zhang G, Kassa H, Amer S, Ye J, et al. Distribution and clinical manifestations of Cryptosporidium species and subtypes in HIV/AIDS patients in Ethiopia. PLoS Negl Trop Dis. 2014;8(4):e2831.

2. Garcia LS, Arrowood M, Kokoskin E, Paltridge GP, Pillai DR, Procop GW, et al. Laboratory diagnosis of parasites from the gastrointestinal tract. Clin Microbiol Rev. 2017 Nov 15;31(1). pii:e00025–17.

3. Kotloff KL, Nataro JP, Blackwelder WC, Nasrin D, Farag TH, Panchalingam S, et al. Burden and aetiology of diarrhoeal disease in infants and young children in developing countries (the Global Enteric Multicenter Study, GEMS): a prospective, case-control study. Lancet. 2013 Jul 20;382(9888):209–22.

4. Nair P, Mohamed JA, DuPont HL, Figueroa JF, Carlin LG, Jiang ZD, et al. Epidemiology of cryptosporidiosis in North American travelers to Mexico. Am J Trop Med Hyg. 2008 Aug;79(2):210–14.

5. Pantenburg B, Cabada MM, White AC, Jr. Treatment of cryptosporidiosis. Expert Rev Anti Infect Ther. 2009 May;7(4):385–91.

6. Roy SL, DeLong SM, Stenzel SA, Shiferaw B, Roberts JM, Khalakdina A, et al. Risk factors for sporadic cryptosporidiosis among immunocompetent persons in the United States from 1999–2001. J Clin Microbiol. 2004 Jul;42(7):2944–51.

7. Weitzel T, Wichmann O, Muhlberger N, Reuter B, Hoof HD, Jelinek T. Epidemiological and clinical features of travel-associated cryptosporidiosis. Clin Microbiol Infect. 2006 Sep;12(9):921–4.

# CUTANEOUS LARVA MIGRANS

Susan Montgomery

## INFECTIOUS AGENT

Larval stages of dog and cat hookworms (usually *Ancylostoma* spp.).

## TRANSMISSION

Skin contact with contaminated soil or sand.

## EPIDEMIOLOGY

Most cases are reported in travelers to the Caribbean, Africa, Asia, and South America. Beaches (and sandboxes) where domestic animals may roam are a common source of infection. Infection occurs in short-term as well as long-term travelers.

## CLINICAL PRESENTATION

Creeping eruption usually appears 1–5 days after skin penetration, but the incubation period may be ≥1 month. Typically, a serpiginous, erythematous track appears in the skin and is associated with intense itchiness and mild swelling. Usual locations are the foot and buttocks, although any skin surface coming in contact with contaminated soil can be affected.

## DIAGNOSIS

Diagnosed on the basis of characteristic skin lesions. Biopsy is not recommended.

## TREATMENT

Cutaneous larva migrans is self-limiting; migrating larvae usually die after 5–6 weeks. Albendazole is very effective for treatment. Ivermectin is effective but not approved for this indication. Symptomatic treatment for frequent severe itching may be helpful.

## PREVENTION

Reduce contact with contaminated soil by wearing shoes and protective clothing and using barriers such as towels when seated on the ground.

### BIBLIOGRAPHY

1. Caumes E. Treatment of cutaneous larva migrans. Clin Infect Dis. 2000 May;30(5):811–14.
2. Heukelbach J, Feldmeier H. Epidemiological and clinical characteristics of hookworm-related cutaneous larva migrans. Lancet Infect Dis. 2008 May;8(5):302–9.
3. Hochedez P, Caumes E. Hookworm-related cutaneous larva migrans. J Travel Med. 2007 Sep–Oct;14(5):326–33.
4. Lederman ER, Weld LH, Elyazar IR, von Sonnenburg F, Loutan L, Schwartz E, et al. Dermatologic conditions of the ill returned traveler: an analysis from the GeoSentinel Surveillance Network. Int J Infect Dis. 2008 Nov;12(6):593–602.
5. Vanhaecke C, Perignon A, Monsel G, Regnier S, Bricaire F, Caumes E. The efficacy of single dose ivermectin in the treatment of hookworm related cutaneous larva migrans varies depending on the clinical presentation. J Eur Acad Dermatol Venereol. 2014 May;28(5):655–7.

**CDC website:** www.cdc.gov/parasites/zoonotichookworm

**4**

# CYCLOSPORIASIS

Barbara L. Herwaldt

## INFECTIOUS AGENT

*Cyclospora cayetanensis*, a coccidian protozoan parasite.

## TRANSMISSION

Ingestion of infective *Cyclospora* oocysts, such as in contaminated food or water.

## EPIDEMIOLOGY

Most common in tropical and subtropical regions, where outbreaks are frequently seasonal (such as during summers and rainy season in Nepal); even short-term travelers can become infected. Outbreaks in the United States and Canada have been linked to imported fresh produce.

## CLINICAL PRESENTATION

Incubation period averages 1 week (range, 2 days to ≥2 weeks). Onset of symptoms is often abrupt but can be gradual; some people have an influenzalike prodrome. The most common symptom is watery diarrhea, which can be profuse. Other symptoms can include anorexia, weight loss, abdominal cramps, bloating, nausea, body aches, vomiting, and low-grade fever. If untreated, the illness can last for several weeks or months, with a remitting-relapsing course.

## DIAGNOSIS

Diagnosed by detecting *Cyclospora* oocysts or DNA in stool specimens. Stool examinations for ova and parasites usually do not include methods for detecting *Cyclospora* unless testing for this parasite is specifically requested. Diagnostic assistance for *Cyclospora* and other parasitic diseases is also available from CDC (www.cdc.gov/dpdx; 404-718-4745; parasites@cdc.gov). Cyclosporiasis is a nationally notifiable disease.

## TREATMENT

Trimethoprim-sulfamethoxazole; no highly effective alternatives have been identified.

## PREVENTION

Food and water precautions (see Chapter 2, Food & Water Precautions); disinfection with chlorine or iodine is unlikely to be effective.

**CDC website:** www.cdc.gov/parasites/cyclosporiasis

## BIBLIOGRAPHY

1. Abanyie F, Harvey RR, Harris JR, Wiegand RE, Gaul L, Desvignes-Kendrick M, et al. 2013 multistate outbreaks of Cyclospora cayetanensis infections associated with fresh produce: focus on the Texas investigations. Epidemiol Infect. 2015 Dec;143(16):3451–8.

2. Cama VA, Mathison BA. Infections by intestinal occidian and Giardia duodenalis. Clin Lab Med. 2015 Jun;35(2):423–44.

3. Hall RL, Jones JL, Herwaldt BL. Surveillance for laboratory-confirmed sporadic cases of cyclosporiasis—United States, 1997–2008. MMWR Surveill Summ. 2011 Apr 8;60(2):1–11.

4. Herwaldt BL. Cyclospora cayetanensis: a review, focusing on the outbreaks of cyclosporiasis in the 1990s. Clin Infect Dis. 2000 Oct;31(4):1040–57.

5. Marques DFP, Alexander CL, Chalmers RM, Chiodini P, Elson R, Freedman J, et al. Cyclosporiasis in travelers returning to the United Kingdom from Mexico in summer 2017: lessons from the recent past to inform the future. Euro Surveill. 2017 Aug 3;22(32). Pii: 30592.

6. Ortega YR, Sanchez R. Update on Cyclospora cayetanensis, a food-borne and waterborne parasite. Clin Microbiol Rev. 2010 Jan;23(1):218–34.

**4**

# CYSTICERCOSIS

Susan Montgomery, Barbara L. Herwaldt, Sharon L. Roy

## INFECTIOUS AGENT

*Taenia solium,* a cestode parasite.

## TRANSMISSION

Ingestion of eggs, excreted by a human carrier of the adult *T. solium* tapeworm, via fecally contaminated food or through close contact with the carrier. Autoinfection is also possible. Larval cysts of *T. solium* infect brain, muscle, or other tissues. Eating undercooked pork with cysticerci results in tapeworm infection (taeniasis), not human cysticercosis.

## EPIDEMIOLOGY

Common where sanitary conditions are poor and where pigs have access to human feces. Occurs globally; endemic areas include Latin America, sub-Saharan Africa, India, and East Asia. Uncommon in travelers. Seen in immigrants from endemic regions.

## CLINICAL PRESENTATION

The latent period ranges from months to decades. Symptoms depend on the number, location, and stage of cysts. The most important clinical manifestations are caused by cysts in the brain, where cysts can be parenchymal or extraparenchymal (ventricular, subarachnoid).

The 2 most common presentations are seizures and increased intracranial pressure. Other presentations include encephalitis, symptoms of space-occupying lesions, and hydrocephalus. Cysticercosis should be excluded in any adult with new-onset seizures who comes from an endemic area or has had potential exposure to a tapeworm carrier.

## DIAGNOSIS

Neuroimaging studies (CT and MRI) and confirmatory serologic testing. The most specific serologic test is the enzyme-linked immunotransfer blot, but the test results may be negative in up to 30% of patients with a single parenchymal lesion.

## TREATMENT

Control of symptoms is the cornerstone of therapy. Anticonvulsants, corticosteroids, or both may be indicated. For some lesions, surgical intervention may be the treatment of choice. Antiparasitic treatment (albendazole, praziquantel) is not indicated for all presentations of neurocysticercosis. In complicated cases, the priority is neurologic management (for example, corticosteroids, mannitol), neurosurgical management, or both. In 2018, guidelines for the clinical management of neurocysticercosis were published by the Infectious Diseases Society of America and the American Society of Tropical Medicine and Hygiene. Clinicians can consult CDC to obtain more information about diagnosis and treatment (CDC Parasitic Diseases Inquiries: 404-718-4745 or parasites@cdc.gov).

## BIBLIOGRAPHY

1. Del Brutto OH. Neurocysticercosis among international travelers to disease-endemic areas. J Travel Med. 2012 Mar–Apr;19(2):112–17.

2. Garcia HH, Gonzales I, Lescano AG, Bustos JA, Pretell EJ, Saavedra H, et al. Enhanced steroid dosing reduces seizures during antiparasitic treatment for cysticercosis and early after. Epilepsia. 2014 Sep;55(9):1452–9.

3. Garcia HH, Gonzales I, Lescano AG, Bustos JA, Zimic M, Escalante D, et al. Efficacy of combined antiparasitic therapy with praziquantel and albendazole for neurocysticercosis: a double-blind, andomized controlled trial. Lancet Infect Dis. 2014 Aug;14(8):687–95.

4. White AC, Coyle CM, Rajshekhar V, Singh G, Hauser WA, Mohanty A, et al. Diagnosis and treatment of neurocysticercosis: 2017 clinical practice guidelines by the Infectious Diseases Society of America (IDSA) and the American Society of Tropical Medicine and Hygiene (ASTMH). Clin Infect Dis. 2018 Feb; https://doi.org/10.1093/cid/cix1084.

## PREVENTION

Food and water precautions (see Chapter 2, Food & Water Precautions).

**CDC website:** www.cdc.gov/parasites/cysticercosis

# DENGUE

Tyler M. Sharp, Janice Perez-Padilla, Stephen H. Waterman

## INFECTIOUS AGENT

Dengue, an acute febrile illness, is caused by infection with any of 4 related positive-sense, single-stranded RNA viruses of the genus *Flavivirus*, dengue viruses 1, 2, 3, or 4.

## TRANSMISSION

Almost all transmission occurs through the bite of infected *Aedes* mosquitoes, primarily *Aedes aegypti* and *Ae. albopictus*. Because of the approximately 7-day viremia in humans, bloodborne transmission is possible through exposure to infected blood, organs, or other tissues (such as bone marrow). In addition, perinatal dengue transmission occurs when the mother is infected near the time of birth, in which infection occurs via microtransfusions when the placenta is detached or through mucosal contact with mother's blood during birth. Congenital transmission has not been documented. Dengue viruses may also be transmitted through breast milk. There is no evidence of sexual transmission.

## EPIDEMIOLOGY

Dengue is endemic throughout the tropics and subtropics and is a leading cause of febrile illness among travelers returning from Latin America, the Caribbean, and Southeast Asia. Dengue occurs in >100 countries worldwide (Maps 4-1 through 4-3), including Puerto Rico, the US Virgin Islands, and US-affiliated Pacific Islands. Sporadic outbreaks with local transmission have occurred in Florida, Hawaii, and Texas along the border with Mexico. Although the geographic distribution of dengue is similar to that of malaria, dengue is more of a risk in urban and residential areas than is malaria. DengueMap (www.healthmap.org/dengue/index.php) shows up-to-date information on areas of ongoing transmission.

## CLINICAL PRESENTATION

An estimated 40%–80% of infections are asymptomatic. Symptomatic infection (dengue) most commonly presents as a mild to moderate, non-specific, acute febrile illness. However, as many

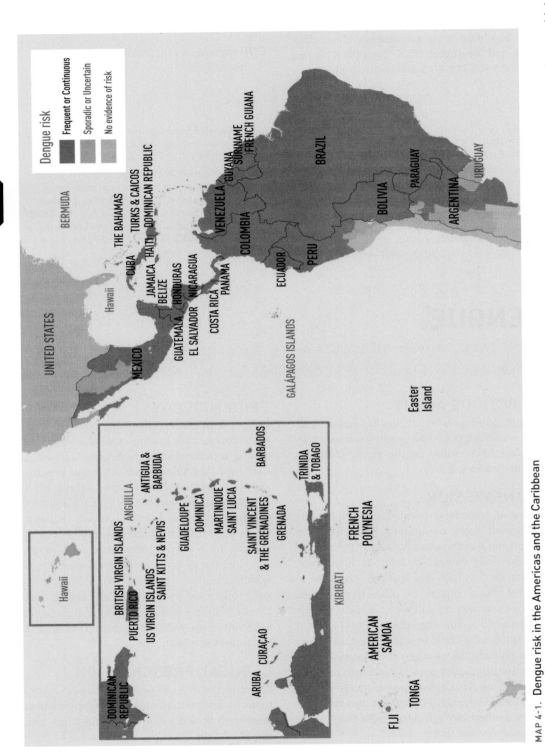

**MAP 4-1. Dengue risk in the Americas and the Caribbean**

Risk areas are shown on a national level except for where evidence exists of different risk levels at subnational regions. Areas that are too small to be seen on the regional maps are labeled in dark blue or light blue depending on their risk categorization.

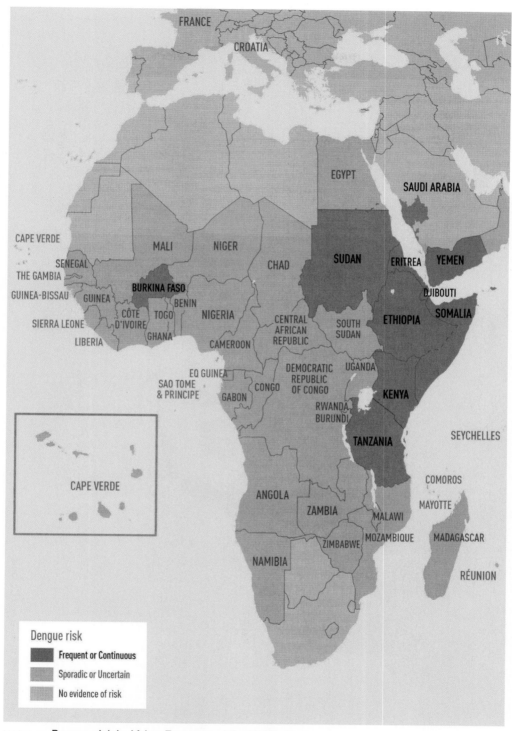

**MAP 4-2. Dengue risk in Africa, Europe, and the Middle East**

Risk areas are shown on a national level except for where evidence exists of different risk levels at subnational regions. Areas that are too small to be seen on the regional maps are labeled in dark blue or light blue depending on their risk categorization.

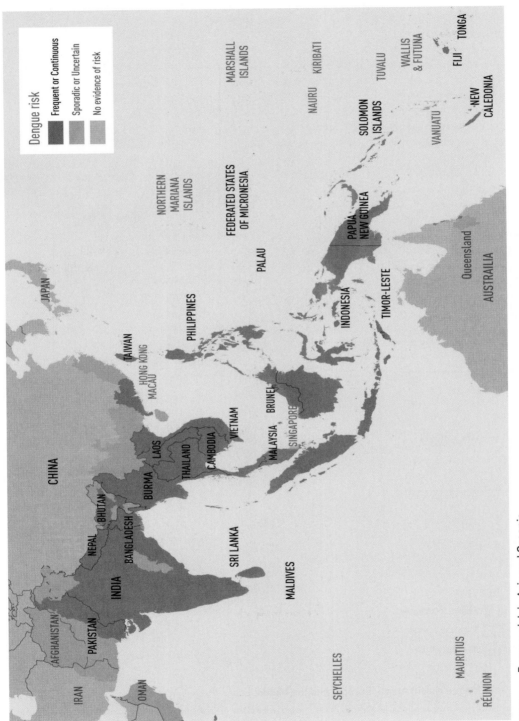

**Dengue risk**

Frequent or Continuous
Sporadic or Uncertain
No evidence of risk

IRAN

AFGHANISTAN

PAKISTAN

OMAN

CHINA

NEPAL

BHUTAN

BANGLADESH

INDIA

BURMA

LAOS

THAILAND

CAMBODIA

VIETNAM

SRI LANKA

MALDIVES

JAPAN

TAIWAN

HONG KONG

MACAU

PHILIPPINES

MALAYSIA

BRUNEI

SINGAPORE

NORTHERN
MARIANA
ISLANDS

FEDERATED STATES
OF MICRONESIA

PALAU

INDONESIA

TIMOR-LESTE

MARSHALL
ISLANDS

NAURU

KIRIBATI

PAPUA
NEW GUINEA

SOLOMON
ISLANDS

VANUATU

TUVALU

WALLIS
& FUTUNA

NEW
CALEDONIA

FIJI

TONGA

Queensland

AUSTRAILIA

SEYCHELLES

MAURITIUS

RÉUNION

**MAP 4-3. Dengue risk in Asia and Oceania**

as 5% of all dengue patients develop severe, life-threatening disease. Early clinical findings are nonspecific but require a high index of suspicion, because recognizing early signs of shock and promptly initiating intensive supportive therapy can reduce risk of death among patients with severe dengue by at least 20-fold to <0.5%. See Box 4-2 for information regarding the World Health Organization guidelines for classifying dengue.

Dengue begins abruptly after an incubation period of 5–7 days (range, 3–10 days), and the course follows 3 phases: febrile, critical, and convalescent. Fever typically lasts 2–7 days and can be biphasic. Other signs and symptoms may include severe headache; retroorbital pain; muscle, joint, and bone pain; macular or maculopapular rash; and minor hemorrhagic manifestations, including petechiae, ecchymosis, purpura, epistaxis, bleeding gums, hematuria, or a positive tourniquet test result. Some patients have an injected oropharynx and facial erythema in the first 24–48 hours after onset. Warning signs of progression to severe dengue occur in the late febrile phase around the time of defervescence and include persistent vomiting, severe abdominal pain, fluid accumulation, mucosal bleeding, difficulty breathing, lethargy/restlessness, postural hypotension, liver enlargement, and progressive increase in hematocrit (hemoconcentration).

The critical phase of dengue begins at defervescence and typically lasts 24–48 hours. Most patients clinically improve during this phase, but those with substantial plasma leakage develop severe dengue as a result of a marked increase in vascular permeability. Initially, physiologic compensatory mechanisms maintain adequate circulation, which narrows pulse pressure as diastolic blood pressure increases. Patients with severe plasma leakage have pleural effusions or ascites, hypoproteinemia, and hemoconcentration. Patients may appear well despite early signs of shock. However, once hypotension develops, systolic blood pressure rapidly declines, and irreversible shock and death may ensue despite resuscitation efforts. Patients can also develop severe hemorrhagic manifestations, including hematemesis, bloody stool, melena, or menorrhagia, especially if they have prolonged shock. Uncommon manifestations include hepatitis, myocarditis, pancreatitis, and encephalitis.

As plasma leakage subsides, the patient enters the convalescent phase and begins to reabsorb

## BOX 4-2. Guidelines for classifying dengue

In November 2009, the World Health Organization (WHO) issued a new guideline that classifies symptomatic cases as dengue or severe dengue.

**Dengue** is defined by a combination of ≥2 clinical findings in a febrile person who traveled to or lives in a dengue-endemic area. Clinical findings include nausea, vomiting, rash, aches and pains, a positive tourniquet test, leukopenia, and the following warning signs: abdominal pain or tenderness, persistent vomiting, clinical fluid accumulation, mucosal bleeding, lethargy, restlessness, liver enlargement, and postural hypotension. The presence of a warning sign may predict severe dengue in a patient.

**Severe dengue** is defined by dengue with any of the following symptoms: severe plasma leakage leading to shock or fluid accumulation with respiratory distress; severe bleeding; or severe organ impairment such as elevated transaminases ≥1,000 IU/L, impaired consciousness, or heart impairment.

From 1975 through 2009, symptomatic dengue virus infections were classified according to the WHO guidelines as dengue fever, dengue hemorrhagic fever (DHF), and dengue shock syndrome (the most severe form of DHF). The case definition was changed to the 2009 clinical classification after reports that the case definition of DHF was both too difficult to apply in resource-limited settings and too specific, as it failed to identify a substantial proportion of severe dengue cases, including cases of hepatic failure and encephalitis. The 2009 clinical classification has been criticized for being overly inclusive, as it allows several different ways to qualify for severe dengue, and nonspecific warning signs are used as diagnostic criteria for dengue.

extravasated intravenous fluids and pleural and abdominal effusions. As a patient's well-being improves, hemodynamic status stabilizes (although he or she may manifest bradycardia), and diuresis ensues. The patient's hematocrit stabilizes or may fall because of the dilutional effect of the reabsorbed fluid, and the white cell count usually starts to rise, followed by a recovery of the platelet count. The convalescent-phase rash may desquamate and be pruritic.

Laboratory findings commonly include thrombocytopenia, hyponatremia, elevated aspartate aminotransferase and alanine aminotransferase, and a normal erythrocyte sedimentation rate.

Data are limited on health outcomes of dengue in pregnancy and effects of maternal infection on the developing fetus. Perinatal transmission can occur, and peripartum maternal infection may increase the likelihood of symptomatic infection in the newborn. Of 41 perinatal transmission cases described in the literature, all developed thrombocytopenia, most had evidence of plasma leakage evidenced by ascites or pleural effusions, and fever was absent in only 2. Nearly 40% had a hemorrhagic manifestation, and one-fourth had hypotension. Symptoms in perinatally infected neonates typically present during the first week of life. Placental transfer of maternal IgG against dengue virus (from a previous maternal infection) may increase risk for severe dengue among infants infected at 6–12 months of age when the protective effect of these antibodies wanes.

## DIAGNOSIS

Clinicians should consider dengue in a patient who was in an endemic area within 2 weeks of symptom onset. Because dengue is a nationally notifiable disease, all suspected cases should be reported to the state or local health department. Laboratory confirmation can be made from a single acute-phase serum specimen obtained early (≤7 days after fever onset) in the illness by detecting viral genomic sequences with RT-PCR or dengue nonstructural protein 1 (NS1) antigen by immunoassay. Later in the illness (≥4 days after fever onset), IgM against dengue virus can be detected with ELISA. For patients presenting during the first week after fever onset, diagnostic testing should include a test for dengue virus (RT-PCR or NS1) and IgM (Figure 4-1). For

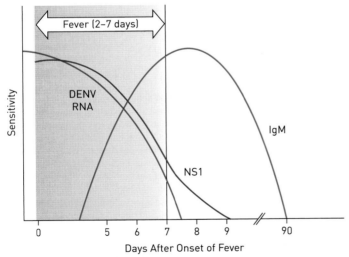

FIGURE 4-1. **Relative sensitivity of detection of dengue virus nucleic acid, antigen, and IgM**[1]

Abbreviations: DENV, dengue virus; NS1, nonstructural protein 1.
[1] DENV RNA and NS1 are detectable during the first week of illness. Anti-DENV IgM is detectable starting approximately 5 days after illness onset. Although most cases only have detectable IgM anti-DENV for 14–20 days after illness onset, in some cases it may be detectable for up to 90 days. Routine testing of anti-DENV IgG with a single sample is not useful in identifying patients with dengue.

patients presenting >1 week after fever onset, an IgM test is most useful. In the United States, both IgM ELISA and real-time RT-PCR are approved as in vitro diagnostic tests.

Presence of virus by RT-PCR or NS1 antigen in a single diagnostic specimen is considered laboratory confirmation of dengue in patients with a compatible clinical and travel history. IgM in a single serum sample suggests a probable recent dengue infection and should be considered diagnostic for dengue if the infection most likely occurred in a place where other potentially cross-reactive flaviviruses (such as Zika, West Nile, yellow fever, and Japanese encephalitis viruses) are not a risk. If infection is likely to have occurred in a place where other potentially cross-reactive flaviviruses circulate, both molecular and serologic diagnostic testing should be performed to detect evidence of infection with dengue and the other flaviviruses.

IgG by ELISA in a single serum sample is not useful for routine diagnostic testing because it remains detectable for life after infection. In addition, people infected with or vaccinated against other flaviviruses (such as yellow fever or Japanese encephalitis) may produce cross-reactive flavivirus antibodies, yielding false-positive serologic dengue diagnostic test results.

Dengue diagnostic testing (molecular and serologic) is available from several commercial reference diagnostic laboratories, state public health laboratories, and CDC (www.cdc.gov/Dengue/clinicalLab/index.html). Consultation on dengue diagnostic testing can be obtained from CDC at 787-706-2399.

## TREATMENT

No specific antiviral agents exist for dengue. Patients should be advised to stay well hydrated and to avoid aspirin (acetylsalicylic acid), aspirin-containing drugs, and other nonsteroidal anti-inflammatory drugs (such as ibuprofen) because of their anticoagulant properties. Fever should be controlled with acetaminophen and tepid sponge baths. Febrile patients should avoid mosquito bites to reduce risk of further transmission. For those who develop severe dengue, close observation and frequent monitoring in an intensive care unit setting may be required. Prophylactic platelet transfusions in dengue patients are not beneficial and may contribute to fluid overload. Similarly, administration of corticosteroids has no demonstrated benefit and is potentially harmful to patients; corticosteroids should not be used except in the case of autoimmune-related complications.

## PREVENTION

A vaccine to prevent dengue (Dengvaxia) has been licensed in almost 20 countries and approved for commercial use in 11 countries. However, in late 2017, the vaccine manufacturer, Sanofi Pasteur, announced that people who receive the vaccine and have not been previously infected with a dengue virus may be at risk of developing more severe manifestations of dengue. The Philippines suspended its dengue vaccine program, and other countries have specified that only people who have been infected with a dengue virus should receive the vaccine. Two other dengue vaccines are currently in phase 3 clinical trials, for which completion is expected in 2018 and 2019.

No prophylaxis is available to prevent dengue. Risk increases with duration of travel and disease incidence in the travel destination (such as during the rainy season and during epidemics). Travelers going to the tropics for any length of time should avoid mosquito bites by taking the following preventive measures:

- Select accommodations with well-screened windows and doors or air conditioning when possible. *Aedes* mosquitoes typically live indoors and are often found in dark, cool places, such as in closets, under beds, behind curtains, in bathrooms, and on porches.

- Wear clothing that covers the arms and legs, especially during the early morning and late afternoon, when risk of being bitten is the highest.

- Use insect repellent (see Chapter 3, Mosquitoes, Ticks & Other Arthropods).

- For longer-term travelers, empty and clean or cover any standing water that can be mosquito-breeding sites in the local residence (such as water storage tanks or flowerpots).

**CDC website:** www.cdc.gov/dengue

## BIBLIOGRAPHY

1. Arragain L, Dupont-Rouzeyrol M, O'Connor O, Sigur N, Grangeon JP, Huguon E, et al. Vertical transmission of dengue virus in the peripartum period and viral kinetics in newborns and breast milk: new data. J Pediatric Infect Dis. 2017 Nov 24;6(4):324–31.

2. Clapham HE, Cummings DAT, Johansson MA. Immune status alters the probability of apparent illness due to dengue virus infection: evidence from a pooled analysis across multiple cohort and cluster studies. PLoS Negl Trop Dis. 2017 Sep 27;11(9):e0005926.

3. Guzman MG, Halstead SB, Artsob H, Buchy P, Farrar J, Gubler DJ, et al. Dengue: a continuing global threat. Nat Rev Microbiol. 2010 Dec;8(12 Suppl):S7–16.

4. Lam PK, Tam DT, Diet TV, Tam CT, Tien NT, Kieu NT, et al. Clinical characteristics of dengue shock syndrome in Vietnamese children: a 10-year prospective study in a single hospital. Clin Infect Dis. 2013 Dec;57(11):1577–86.

5. Leder K, Torresi J, Libman MD, Cramer JP, Castelli F, Schlagenhauf P, et al. GeoSentinel surveillance of illness in returned travelers, 2007–2011. Ann Intern Med. 2013 Mar 19;158(6):456–68.

6. Schwartz E, Weld LH, Wilder-Smith A, von Sonnenburg F, Keystone JS, Kain KC, et al. Seasonality, annual trends, and characteristics of dengue among ill returned travelers, 1997–2006. Emerg Infect Dis. 2008 Jul;14(7):1081–8.

7. Simmons CP, Farrar JJ, van Vinh Chau N, Wills B. Dengue. N Engl J Med. 2012 Apr 12;366(15):1423–32.

8. Srikiatkhachorn A, Rothman AL, Gibbons RV, Sittisombut N, Malasit P, Ennis FA, et al. Dengue—how best to classify it. Clin Infect Dis. 2011 Sep;53(6):563–7.

9. Stanaway JD, Shepard DS, Undurraqa EA, Halasa YA, Coffeng LE, Brady OJ. The global burden of dengue: an analysis from the Global Burden of Disease Study 2013. Lancet Infect Dis. 2016 Jun;16(6):712–23.

10. Tomashek KM, Margolis HS. Dengue: a potential transfusion-transmitted disease. Transfusion. 2011 Aug;51(8):1654–60.

11. World Health Organization. Dengue guidelines for diagnosis, treatment, prevention and control: new edition. Geneva: World Health Organization; 2009. [cited 2019 Apr 1]. Available from: www.who.int/rpc/guidelines/9789241547871/en/.

# DIPHTHERIA

Tejpratap S. P. Tiwari, Anna Acosta

## INFECTIOUS AGENT

Toxigenic strains of *Corynebacterium diphtheriae* biotype *mitis, gravis, intermedius*, or *belfanti*.

## TRANSMISSION

Person-to-person through oral or respiratory droplets, close physical contact, and rarely, by fomites. Cutaneous diphtheria can be transmitted by contact with discharge from skin lesions.

## EPIDEMIOLOGY

Endemic in many countries in Asia, the South Pacific, the Middle East, Eastern Europe and in Haiti and the Dominican Republic. Since 2016, respiratory diphtheria outbreaks have occurred in Indonesia, Bangladesh, Myanmar, Vietnam, Venezuela, Haiti, South Africa, and Yemen. Cutaneous diphtheria is common in tropical countries. Respiratory and cutaneous diphtheria have been reported in travelers, though rarely. Diphtheria can affect any age group.

## CLINICAL PRESENTATION

The incubation period is 2–5 days (range, 1–10 days). Affected anatomic sites include the mucous membranes of the upper respiratory tract (nose, pharynx, tonsils, larynx, and trachea [respiratory diphtheria]), skin (cutaneous diphtheria), or rarely, mucous membranes at other sites (eye, ear, vulva). Nasal diphtheria can be asymptomatic or mild, with a blood-tinged discharge.

Respiratory diphtheria has a gradual onset and is characterized by a mild fever (rarely >101°F [38.3°C]), sore throat, difficulty swallowing, malaise, loss of appetite, and if the larynx is involved, hoarseness. The hallmark of respiratory diphtheria is a pseudomembrane that appears within 2–3 days of illness over the mucous lining of the tonsils, pharynx, larynx, or nares and that can extend into the trachea. The pseudomembrane is firm, fleshy, grey, and adherent; it typically will bleed after attempts to remove or dislodge it. Fatal airway obstruction can result if the pseudomembrane extends into the larynx or trachea or if a piece of it becomes dislodged. Case-fatality ratio is 5%–10%.

## DIAGNOSIS

A presumptive diagnosis is usually based on clinical features. Diagnosis is confirmed by isolating *C. diphtheriae* from culture of nasal or throat swabs or membrane tissue and testing for toxin production by the Elek test. Diphtheria is a nationally notifiable disease.

## TREATMENT

Patients with respiratory diphtheria require hospitalization to monitor response to treatment and manage complications. Equine diphtheria antitoxin (DAT) is the mainstay of treatment and can be administered without waiting for laboratory confirmation. In the United States, DAT is available to physicians under an investigational new drug protocol by contacting their state health departments and then CDC at 770-488-7100.

In addition to DAT, an antibiotic (erythromycin or penicillin) should be used to eliminate the causative organisms, stop exotoxin production, and reduce communicability. Supportive care (airway, cardiac monitoring) is required. Antimicrobial prophylaxis (erythromycin or penicillin) is recommended for close contacts of patients.

## PREVENTION

All travelers should be up-to-date with diphtheria toxoid vaccine before departure. After a primary series and childhood and adolescent boosters, booster doses with a diphtheria toxoid–containing vaccine at 10-year intervals given either as Td (tetanus-diphtheria) or Tdap (tetanus-diphtheria-acellular pertussis if not previously given) should be given to all adults. This booster is particularly important for travelers who will live or work with local populations in countries where diphtheria is endemic.

**CDC website:** www.cdc.gov/diphtheria

BIBLIOGRAPHY

1. CDC. Fatal respiratory diphtheria in a US traveler to Haiti—Pennsylvania, 2003. MMWR Morb Mortal Wkly Rep. 2004 Jan 9;52(53):1285–6.
2. CDC. Updated recommendations for use of tetanus toxoid, reduced diphtheria toxoid and acellular pertussis (Tdap) vaccine in adults aged 65 years and older—Advisory Committee on Immunization Practices (ACIP), 2012. MMWR Morb Mortal Wkly Rep. 2012 June 29;61(25):468–70.
3. Pan American Health Organization/World Health Organization. Epidemiological Update: Diphtheria. 15 December 2017, Washington, DC: PAHO/WHO; 2017
4. World Health Organization. Diphtheria vaccine: WHO position paper—August 2017. Wkly Epidemiol Rec. 2017 August 4;92(31):417–36.
5. World Health Organization. Review of the epidemiology of diphtheria—2000–2016. [cited 2018 Feb 20]. Available from: www.who.int/immunization/sage/meetings/2017/april/presentations_background_docs/en.

# ECHINOCOCCOSIS

Barbara L. Herwaldt, Susan Montgomery, Sharon L. Roy

## INFECTIOUS AGENT

Cestode parasites of the genus *Echinococcus*, including *E. granulosus*, *E. multilocularis*, and others.

## TRANSMISSION

Ingestion of *Echinococcus* eggs shed in the feces of infected definitive hosts (dogs and other canids for *E. granulosus*; foxes and other canids for *E. multilocularis*), such as by hand-to-mouth transfer of eggs and by consumption of fecally contaminated food, water, or soil.

## EPIDEMIOLOGY

The two main forms of echinococcosis in humans are cystic echinococcosis (CE), which is caused by *E. granulosus* (also other species), and alveolar echinococcosis (AE), which is caused by *E. multilocularis*. CE is found in parts of the Americas (including in South American foci, such as in Peru), Eurasia, Africa, and Australia—including in pastoral and rangeland areas, where transmission often is maintained by dog–sheep–dog cycles. AE is found in the northern hemisphere, in parts of Eurasia and North America. Although indigenous human cases of CE and AE have been reported in the United States, most US cases of echinococcosis have been imported.

## CLINICAL PRESENTATION

People with CE and AE may remain asymptomatic for years. The nature and severity of the clinical manifestations depend in part on the location, size, and other characteristics of the lesions that develop and the associated complications. In CE, the lesions are cystic (referred to as hydatid cysts) and most commonly develop in the liver; the next most common site is the lungs, but cysts may develop in other organ systems. AE usually affects the liver; direct extension to (and destruction) of contiguous tissues may occur, as may metastatic lesions.

## DIAGNOSIS

A presumptive diagnosis can be based on a combination of the person's exposure history and imaging studies, such as an ultrasound or CT scan. Lesions may be found incidentally in asymptomatic people. Serologic testing also may be helpful. Additional information and diagnostic assistance (serologic, parasitologic, and molecular) are available through CDC (www.cdc.gov/dpdx; 404-718-4745; parasites@cdc.gov).

## TREATMENT

For CE, WHO has developed an image-based staging system that facilitates selecting among potential case-management strategies, including observation without treatment, percutaneous approaches, surgical resection, and benzimidazole therapy (albendazole [drug of choice] or mebendazole). For AE, treatment strategies include complete surgical removal of infected tissue (if resectable) and long-term benzimidazole therapy; untreated AE progresses and ultimately leads to death.

## PREVENTION

Advise travelers to avoid contact with dogs and wild canids in endemic areas. Also advise travelers not to drink untreated water from streams, canals, lakes, or rivers, and to observe food and water precautions (see Chapter 2, Food & Water Precautions).

**CDC website:** www.cdc.gov/parasites/echinococcosis

BIBLIOGRAPHY

1. Brunetti E, Kern P, Vuitton DA; Writing Panel for the WHO-IWGE. Expert consensus for the diagnosis and treatment of cystic and alveolar echinococcosis in humans. Acta Trop. 2010 Apr;114(1):1–16.

2. Deplazes P, Rinaldi L, Alvarez Rojas CA, Torgerson PR, Harandi MF, Romig T, et al. Global distribution of alveolar and cystic echinococcosis. Adv Parasitol. 2017;95:315–493.

3. Kern P, Menezes da Silva A, Akhan O, Müllhaupt B, Vizcaychipi KA, Budke C, et al. The echinococcoses: diagnosis, clinical management and burden of disease. Adv Parasitol. 2017;96:259–369.

4. Mandal S, Mandal MD. Human cystic echinococcosis: epidemiologic, zoonotic, clinical, diagnostic and therapeutic aspects. Asian Pac J Trop Med. 2012 Apr;5(4):253–60.

5. Stojkovic M, Rosenberger K, Kauczor HU, Junghanss T, Hosch W. Diagnosing and staging of cystic echinococcosis: how do CT and MRI perform in comparison to ultrasound? PLoS Negl Trop Dis. 2012;6(10):e1880.

# *ESCHERICHIA COLI*, DIARRHEAGENIC

Alison Winstead, Jennifer C. Hunter, Patricia M. Griffin

## INFECTIOUS AGENT

*Escherichia coli* are gram-negative bacteria that inhabit the gastrointestinal tract. Most strains do not cause illness. Pathogenic *E. coli* are categorized into pathotypes on the basis of their virulence genes. Six pathotypes are associated with diarrhea (diarrheagenic): enterotoxigenic *E. coli* (ETEC), Shiga toxin–producing *E. coli* (STEC), enteropathogenic *E. coli* (EPEC), enteroaggregative *E. coli* (EAEC), enteroinvasive *E. coli* (EIEC), and possibly diffusely adherent *E. coli* (DAEC). Other pathotypes that are common causes of urinary tract infections, bloodstream infections, and meningitis are not covered here. Serotypes of *E. coli* are determined by surface antigens (O and H), and specific serotypes tend to cluster within specific pathotypes. Some *E. coli* have virulence factors of more than 1 pathotype, and new strains of *E. coli* continue to be recognized as causes of foodborne disease. An example is the O104:H4 strain that caused an outbreak in Germany in 2011; it produced Shiga toxin and had adherence properties typical of EAEC.

STEC are also called verotoxigenic *E. coli* (VTEC), and the term enterohemorrhagic *E. coli* (EHEC) is commonly used to specify STEC strains capable of causing human illness, especially bloody diarrhea and hemolytic uremic syndrome (HUS).

## TRANSMISSION

Diarrheagenic pathotypes can be passed in the feces of humans and other animals. Transmission occurs through the fecal–oral route, primarily via consumption of contaminated food or water, and also through person-to-person contact, contact with animals or their environment, and swimming in untreated water. Humans constitute the main reservoir for non-STEC pathotypes that cause diarrhea in humans. The intestinal tracts of animals, especially cattle and other ruminants, are the primary reservoirs of STEC.

## EPIDEMIOLOGY

Travel to less-developed countries is associated with a higher risk for travelers' diarrhea, including some types of *E. coli* infection. Travel-associated infections caused by *E. coli* are likely underrecognized because illness may occur during travel, health care is often not sought or illness is treated empirically, and most clinical laboratories do not use methods that can detect non-STEC diarrheagenic *E. coli*. The WHO Global Burden of Foodborne Diseases report estimates that >300 million illnesses and nearly 200,000 deaths are caused by diarrheagenic *E. coli* globally each year. Rates of infection vary by region. ETEC is the most common pathotype that causes diarrhea among travelers returning from most regions. Risk of non-STEC diarrheagenic *E. coli* infections (primarily ETEC) can be divided into 3 grades, according to the destination country:

- Low-risk countries include the United States, Canada, Australia, New Zealand, Japan, and countries in Northern and Western Europe.

- Intermediate-risk countries include those in Eastern Europe, South Africa, and some of the Caribbean islands.

- High-risk areas include most of Asia, the Middle East, Africa, Mexico, and Central and South America.

STEC infections are more commonly reported in industrialized countries than in less-developed countries. Among international travelers, about 75% of STEC infections are caused by non-O157 serotypes. Additional information about travelers' diarrhea is available in Chapter 2, Travelers' Diarrhea.

## CLINICAL PRESENTATION

Non-STEC diarrheagenic *E. coli* infections have an incubation period ranging from 8 hours to 3 days. The median incubation period of STEC infections is 3–4 days, with a range of 1–10 days. The clinical manifestations of diarrheagenic *E. coli* vary by pathotype (Table 4-1).

## Table 4-1. Mechanism of pathogenesis and typical clinical syndrome of *Escherichia coli* pathotypes

| PATHOTYPE | MECHANISM OF PATHOGENESIS | INCUBATION PERIOD | DURATION OF ILLNESS | TYPICAL CLINICAL SYNDROME |
|---|---|---|---|---|
| ETEC | Small bowel adherence via various adhesions that confer host specificity; heat-stable or heat-labile enterotoxin production | 10–72 hours | 1–5 days | Acute watery diarrhea, afebrile, occasionally severe |
| EAEC | Small and large bowel adherence mediated via various adhesions and accessory proteins; enterotoxin and cytotoxin production | 8–48 hours | 3–14 days; persistent diarrhea (>14 days) has been reported | Watery diarrhea with mucous, occasionally bloody; can cause prolonged or persistent diarrhea in children |
| EPEC | Small bowel adherence and epithelial cell effacement mediated by intimin | 9–12 hours | 12 days | Severe acute watery diarrhea; may be persistent; common cause of infant diarrhea in developing countries |
| EIEC | Mucosal invasion and inflammation of large bowel | 10–18 hours | 4–7 days | Watery diarrhea that may progress to bloody diarrhea (dysentery-like syndrome), fever |
| DAEC | Diffuse adherence to epithelial cells | Unknown | Unknown | Watery diarrhea but pathogenicity not conclusively demonstrated |
| STEC | Large bowel adherence mediated via intimin (or less commonly by other adhesions); Shiga toxin 1, Shiga toxin 2 production; Shiga toxin production is linked to induction of the bacteriophages carrying the Shiga toxin genes; some antibiotics induce these bacteriophages | 1–10 days (usually 3–4 days) | Typically 5–7 days; persistent diarrhea (>14 days) has been reported | Watery diarrhea that progresses (often for STEC O157, less often for non-O157) to bloody diarrhea in 1–3 days; abdominal cramps and tenderness; if fever present, low-grade; hemolytic uremic syndrome complicates approximately 6% of diagnosed STEC O157 infections (15% among children aged <5 years) and 1% of non-O157 STEC infections |

Abbreviations: ETEC, enterotoxigenic *E. coli*; EAEC, enteroaggregative *E. coli*; EPEC, enteropathogenic *E. coli*; EIEC, enteroinvasive *E. coli*; DAEC, diffusely adherent *E. coli*; STEC, Shiga toxin–producing *E. coli*.

4

## DIAGNOSIS

Many patients with travel-associated *E. coli* infections, especially those with nonbloody diarrhea, as commonly occurs with ETEC infection, are likely to be managed symptomatically and are unlikely to have the diagnosis confirmed by a laboratory. Most US clinical laboratories do not routinely use tests that can detect diarrheagenic *E. coli* other than STEC. Recently approved nucleic acid amplification tests that detect genes encoding putative virulence factors associated with non-STEC *E. coli* pathotypes (ETEC, EPEC, EAEC, EIEC) are now available in some clinical laboratories. However, the combination of virulence factors necessary for an *E. coli* strain to be a pathogen has not been determined for all pathotypes. For example, one PCR-based test relies on the *eae* gene that encodes the adhesion factor intimin to produce an EPEC result. However, many case-control studies have detected this gene with similar frequency in *E. coli* isolated from healthy people as from those with acute diarrhea. Therefore, EPEC might not be the etiology of illness for a person with diarrhea and a PCR-based EPEC result. The state public health and CDC laboratories can assist in the investigation of outbreaks for which an etiology has not been identified by testing for non-STEC *E. coli* pathotypes using PCR or whole genome sequence analysis; this is one way particular *E. coli* strains are recognized as pathogens.

When a decision is made to identify a cause of an acute diarrheal illness, in addition to routine culture for *Salmonella, Shigella*, and *Campylobacter*, the stool sample should be cultured for *E. coli* O157:H7 and simultaneously assayed for Shiga toxin with a test that detects the toxins or the genes that encode them. For more information, see www.cdc.gov/mmwr/preview/mmwrhtml/rr5812a1.htm. All presumptive *E. coli* O157 isolates and Shiga toxin–positive specimens should be sent to a public health laboratory for further characterization and for outbreak detection. Rapid, accurate diagnosis of STEC infection is important, because early clinical management decisions can affect patient outcomes, and early detection can help prevent secondary spread.

## TREATMENT

Patients with profuse diarrhea or vomiting should be rehydrated. Evidence from studies of children with STEC O157 infection indicates that early use of intravenous fluids (within the first 4 days of diarrhea onset) may decrease the risk of oligoanuric renal failure. Antibiotics to treat non-STEC diarrheagenic *E. coli* include fluoroquinolones such as ciprofloxacin, macrolides such as azithromycin, and rifaximin. Clinicians treating a patient whose clinical syndrome suggests STEC infection (Table 4-1) should be aware that administering certain antimicrobial agents may increase the risk of HUS. Resistance to antibiotics is increasing worldwide. The decision to use an antibiotic should be weighed carefully against the severity of illness, the possibility that the pathogen is resistant, and the risk of adverse reactions such as rash, antibiotic-associated colitis, and vaginal yeast infection. Antimotility agents should be avoided in patients with bloody diarrhea and patients with STEC infection, because these agents may increase the risk of complications, including toxic megacolon and HUS. (See Chapter 2, Travelers' Diarrhea and Chapter 7, Traveling Safely with Infants & Children for information about managing travelers' diarrhea in children.)

## PREVENTION

No vaccine is available for *E. coli* infection, nor are any medications recommended for prevention. Taking antibiotics can adversely affect the intestinal microbiota and increase susceptibility to gut infections. Food and water are primary sources of *E. coli* infection, so travelers should be reminded of the importance of adhering to food and water precautions (see Chapter 2, Food & Water Precautions). People who may be exposed to livestock, especially ruminants, should be instructed about the importance of handwashing in preventing infection. Because soap and water may not be readily available in at-risk areas, travelers should consider taking hand sanitizer that contains ≥60% alcohol. During *E. coli* outbreaks, clinicians should alert people traveling to affected areas and should be cognizant of possible infections among returning travelers.

**CDC website:** www.cdc.gov/ecoli

## BIBLIOGRAPHY

1. Frank C, Werber D, Cramer JP, Askar M, Faber M, an der Heiden M, et al. Epidemic profile of Shiga-toxin–producing Escherichia coli O104: H4 outbreak in Germany. New Engl J Med. 2011 Nov 10;365(19):1771–80.

2. Havelaar AH, Kirk MD, Torgerson PR, Gibb HJ, Hald T, Lake RJ, et al. World Health Organization global estimates and regional comparisons of the burden of foodborne disease in 2010. PLoS Med. 2015;12(12):e1001923.

3. Kaper JB, Nataro JP, Mobley HL. Pathogenic Escherichia coli. Nat Rev Microbiol. 2004 Feb;2(2):123–40.

4. Kotloff KL, Nataro JP, Blackwelder WC, Nasrin D, Farag TH, Panchalingam S, et al. Burden and aetiology of diarrhoeal disease in infants and young children in developing countries (the Global Enteric Multicenter Study, GEMS): a prospective, case-control study. Lancet. 2013;382(9888):209–22.

5. Mintz ED. Enterotoxigenic Escherichia coli: outbreak surveillance and molecular testing. Clin Infect Dis. 2006 Jun 1;42(11):1518–20.

6. Mody RK, Griffin PM. Editorial commentary: increasing evidence that certain antibiotics should be avoided for Shiga toxin-producing Escherichia coli infections: more data needed. Clin Infect Dis. 2016 May;62(10):1259–61.

7. Shane AL, Mody RK, Crump JA, Tarr PI, Steiner TS, Kotloff K, et al. 2017 Infectious Diseases Society of America clinical practice guidelines for the diagnosis and management of infectious diarrhea. Clin Infect Dis. 2017 Oct 19;65(12):e45–80.

# FASCIOLIASIS

Barbara L. Herwaldt, Sharon L. Roy

## INFECTIOUS AGENT

Trematode flatworms *Fasciola hepatica* and *F. gigantica*.

## TRANSMISSION

Consumption of watercress or other aquatic plants contaminated with infective metacercariae; potentially in other ways, such as by ingestion of contaminated water.

## EPIDEMIOLOGY

*F. hepatica* is found in parts of the Americas, Europe, the Middle East, Africa, Asia, and Oceania, especially in areas where sheep or cattle are reared. *F. gigantica* has a more limited distribution (parts of Africa and Asia).

## CLINICAL PRESENTATION

The acute phase of the infection (also known as the migratory, invasive, or hepatic phase) can last up to approximately 3–4 months. Although most infected people are asymptomatic during the acute phase, the clinical manifestations can include marked eosinophilia, fever, abdominal pain, other gastrointestinal symptoms, respiratory symptoms (such as cough), and urticaria. The chronic (biliary) phase begins when immature worms (larval flukes) reach the bile ducts; mature into adult worms, which may live up to a decade or longer; and start to produce eggs. The clinical manifestations, if any, during the chronic phase may reflect biliary tract disease (such as cholangitis, biliary tract obstruction, cholecystitis); pancreatitis also may occur.

## DIAGNOSIS

Detection of eggs in stool or duodenal or biliary aspirates. Serologic testing may be useful during the acute phase (egg production does not start until at least 3–4 months after exposure, whereas parasite antibodies may become detectable within 2–4 weeks) and the chronic phase (particularly if egg production is intermittent or at low levels). Serologic testing is available through CDC (www.cdc.gov/dpdx; 404-718-4745; parasites@cdc.gov). Imaging studies, such as ultrasonogram and CT of the hepatobiliary tract, may be helpful.

## TREATMENT

First-line treatment is with triclabendazole, which is not commercially available in the United States; it is available to US-licensed physicians through the CDC Drug Service, under a special protocol, which requires both CDC and FDA to agree that the drug is indicated for treatment of a particular patient (404-718-4745; parasites@cdc.gov). Nitazoxanide therapy might be helpful in some patients. In some patients with biliary tract obstruction, removal of adult flukes (such as via endoscopic retrograde cholangiopancreatography) may be indicated.

## PREVENTION

Avoid eating uncooked aquatic plants, including watercress, especially from *Fasciola*-endemic grazing areas. See Chapter 2, Food & Water Precautions.

**CDC website:** www.cdc.gov/parasites/fasciola

### BIBLIOGRAPHY

1. Ashrafi K, Bargues MD, O'Neill S, Mas-Coma S. Fascioliasis: a worldwide parasitic disease of importance in travel medicine. Travel Med Infect Dis. 2014 Nov–Dec;12(6 Pt A):636–49.

2. Fürst T, Keiser J, Utzinger J. Global burden of human food-borne trematodiasis: a systematic review and meta-analysis. Lancet Infect Dis. 2012 Mar;12(3):210–21.

3. Mas-Coma S, Bargues MD, Valero MA. Human fascioliasis infection sources, their diversity, incidence factors, analytical methods and prevention measures. Parasitology. 2018;1–35. https://doi.org/10.1017/S0031182018000914

4. Mas-Coma S, Valero MA, Bargues MD. Fascioliasis. Adv Exp Med Biol. 2014;766:77–114.

5. Rowan SE, Levi ME, Youngwerth JM, Brauer B, Everson GT, Johnson SC. The variable presentations and broadening geographic distribution of hepatic fascioliasis. Clin Gastroenterol Hepatol. 2012 Jun;10(6):598–602.

**4**

# FILARIASIS, LYMPHATIC

Christine Dubray, Sharon L. Roy

## INFECTIOUS AGENT

Filarial nematodes *Wuchereria bancrofti*, *Brugia malayi*, and *B. timori*.

## TRANSMISSION

Through the bite of infected *Aedes*, *Culex*, *Anopheles*, or *Mansonia* mosquitoes.

## EPIDEMIOLOGY

Found in sub-Saharan Africa, Egypt, southern Asia, the western Pacific Islands, the northeastern coast of Brazil, Guyana, Haiti, and the Dominican Republic. Travelers are at low risk, although infection has been documented in long-term travelers. Most infections in the United States are seen in immigrants and refugees.

## CLINICAL PRESENTATION

Most infections are asymptomatic, but lymphatic dysfunction may lead to lymphedema of the leg, scrotum, penis, arm, or breast years after infection. Acute episodes of recurrent secondary infections in people with lymphatic dysfunction characterized by painful swelling of an affected limb, fever, or chills hasten the progression of lymphedema to its advanced stage, known as elephantiasis. Tropical pulmonary eosinophilia (TPE) syndrome is a potentially serious progressive lung disease that presents with nocturnal cough, wheezing, and fever, resulting from immune hyperresponsiveness to microfilariae in the pulmonary capillaries. Most cases of TPE have been reported in long-term residents from Asia. Men aged 20–40 years are most commonly affected.

## DIAGNOSIS

Microscopic detection of microfilariae on an appropriately timed thick blood film. Determination of serum antifilarial IgG is also a diagnostically useful test, especially when microfilariae are not identifiable. This assay is available through the National Institutes of Health (301-496-5398) or through CDC (www.cdc.gov/dpdx; 404-718-4745; parasites@cdc.gov). Microfilariae are usually not detected in patients with tropical pulmonary eosinophilia. Diagnosis requires epidemiologic risk and filarial antibody testing.

## TREATMENT

The drug of choice, diethylcarbamazine (DEC), can be obtained from CDC under an investigational new drug protocol. DEC is contraindicated in patients who may also have onchocerciasis. Before DEC treatment for lymphatic filariasis, onchocerciasis should be excluded in all patients with a consistent exposure history because of the possibility of severe exacerbations of skin and eye involvement (Mazzotti reaction). In addition, DEC should be used with extreme caution in patients with circulating *Loa loa* microfilaria because of the potential for life-threatening side effects.

Patients with lymphedema and hydrocele can benefit from lymphedema management and, in the case of hydrocele, surgical repair. There is evidence that a 4–8-week course of doxycycline (200 mg daily) can both sterilize adult worms and improve lymphatic pathologic features.

## PREVENTION

Mosquito precautions (see Chapter 3, Mosquitoes, Ticks & Other Arthropods).

**CDC website:** www.cdc.gov/parasites/ lymphaticfilariasis

### BIBLIOGRAPHY

1. Debrah AY, Mand S, Specht S, Marfo-Debrekyei Y, Batsa L, Pfarr K, et al. Doxycycline reduces plasma VEGF-C/ sVEGFR-3 and improves pathology in lymphatic filariasis. PLoS Pathogens. 2006 Sep;2(9):e92.

2. Eberhard ML, Lammie PJ. Laboratory diagnosis of filariasis. Clin Lab Med. 1991 Dec;11(4):977–1010.

3. Hoerauf A, Pfarr K, Mand S, Bebrah AY, Specht S. Filariasis in Africa—treatment challenges and prospects. Clin Microbiol Infect. 2011 Jul;17(7):977–85.

4. Lipner EM, Law MA, Barnett E, Keystone JS, von Sonnenburg F, Loutan L, et al. Filariasis in travelers presenting to the GeoSentinel Surveillance Network. PLoS Negl Trop Dis. 2007;1(3):e88.

5. Magill AJ, Ryan ET, Hill DR, Solomon T. Hunter's Tropical Medicine and Emerging Infectious Diseases. 9th ed. New York: Elsevier; 2013.

6. WHO. Global programme to eliminate lymphatic filariasis: progress report, 2016. Wkly Epidemiol Rec. 2017;92(40):594–607.

# FLUKES, LUNG

Kristina M. Angelo

## INFECTIOUS AGENTS

*Paragonimus westermani* (and other species).

## TRANSMISSION

Lung fluke infections are transmitted by eating raw, partially cooked, pickled, or salted crab or crawfish that are infected with the immature form of the parasite. Ingested larval stages of the parasite are released when the infected crustacean is digested and then migrates from the intestines to other parts of the body. Most end up in the lungs, where they develop into adults and produce eggs. Human infections can persist for 20 years.

## EPIDEMIOLOGY

Human disease is caused by at least 15 species of *Paragonimus*, which vary by geographic area and definitive host. *Paragonimus* species are found in the Americas, western Africa, and Asia. *Paragonimus westermani*, the most common cause of human disease, occurs predominantly in eastern and southern Asia.

## CLINICAL PRESENTATION

Patients with *Paragonimus* infection can present with an acute syndrome within 2 days to 2 weeks after ingestion. Infections of longer duration can present with signs and symptoms similar to tuberculosis, with cough, shortness of breath, and hemoptysis. Extrapulmonary infections may occur and cause serious disease when there is central nervous system involvement. Infections are usually associated with eosinophilia, especially during the larval migration stage.

## DIAGNOSIS AND TREATMENT

If there is clinical suspicion of a lung fluke infection, travelers should be referred to an infectious disease specialist. Diagnosis is usually made by identifying eggs in stool or sputum. Serologic testing for *P. westermani*–specific antibodies can be helpful, especially for diagnosis of extrapulmonary infection; depending on the serologic assay, this testing can detect infections with other *Paragonimus* species because of differing levels of cross-reactivity among species. Treatment is with praziquantel. Clinicians can consult CDC to obtain more information about diagnosis and treatment (CDC Parasitic Diseases Inquiries: 404-718-4745 or parasites@cdc.gov).

## PREVENTION

Avoid eating raw or undercooked freshwater snails, crab, or crawfish.

**CDC website:** www.cdc.gov/parasites/ paragonimus/

### BIBLIOGRAPHY

1. Fischer PU, Weil GJ. North American paragonimiasis: epidemiology and diagnostic strategies. Exp Rev Anti-Infect Ther 2015;13(6):779–786.
2. World Health Organization. Paragonimiasis. Geneva: World Health Organization; 2018.
[cited 2018 Aug 3]. Available from: www.who.int/ foodborne_trematode_infections/paragonimiasis/en.
3. Xia Y, Ju Y, Chen J, You C. Hemorrhagic stroke and cerebral paragonimiasis. Stroke. 2014 Nov;45(11):3420–2.

**4**

# GIARDIASIS

Katharine M. Benedict, Dawn M. Roellig

## INFECTIOUS AGENT

The anaerobic protozoan parasite *Giardia duodenalis* (formerly known as *G. lamblia* or *G. intestinalis*).

## TRANSMISSION

*Giardia* is transmitted via the fecal–oral route. Its low infectious dose, protracted communicability, and moderate chlorine tolerance make *Giardia* ideally suited for transmission through drinking and recreational water. Transmission also occurs through contact with feces (for example, when providing direct patient care or during sexual activity), eating contaminated food, or contact with fecally contaminated surfaces.

## EPIDEMIOLOGY

*Giardia* is endemic worldwide, including in the United States. *Giardia*-related acute diarrhea was a top 10 diagnosis in ill US travelers returning from the Caribbean, Middle East, Eastern Europe, Central America, South America, North Africa, sub-Saharan Africa, and South-Central Asia. The risk of infection increases with duration of travel. Backpackers or campers who drink untreated water from lakes or rivers are also more likely to be infected. *Giardia* is commonly identified in routine screening of refugees and internationally adopted children, although many are asymptomatic.

## CLINICAL PRESENTATION

Many infected people are asymptomatic, though if symptoms develop, they typically develop 1–2 weeks after exposure and generally resolve within 2–4 weeks. Symptoms include diarrhea (often with foul-smelling, greasy stools), abdominal cramps, bloating, flatulence, fatigue, anorexia, and nausea. Usually, a patient presents with the gradual onset of 2–5 loose stools per day and gradually increasing fatigue. Sometimes upper gastrointestinal symptoms are prominent. Weight loss may occur over time. Fever and vomiting are uncommon. Reactive arthritis, irritable bowel syndrome, and other chronic symptoms sometimes occur after infection with *Giardia* (see Chapter 11, Travelers' Diarrhea in Returned Travelers).

## DIAGNOSIS

*Giardia* cysts or trophozoites are not consistently seen in the stools of infected patients. Diagnostic sensitivity can be increased by examining up to 3 stool specimens over several days. New molecular enteric panel assays generally include *Giardia* as a target pathogen. Diagnostic techniques include microscopy with direct fluorescent antibody testing (considered the gold standard), rapid immunochromatographic cartridge assays, enzyme immunoassay kits, microscopy with trichrome staining, and molecular assays. Only molecular testing (such as PCR) can be used to identify the genotypes and subtypes of *Giardia*. Retesting is recommended only if symptoms persist after treatment. In the United States, giardiasis is a nationally notifiable disease.

### BIBLIOGRAPHY

1. Abramowicz M, editor. Drugs for Parasitic Infections. New Rochelle (NY): The Medical Letter; 2013.

2. Adam EA, Yoder JS, Gould LH, Hlavsa MC, Gargano JW. Giardiasis outbreaks in the United States, 1971–2011. Epidemiol Infect. 2016 Oct;144(13):2790–801.

3. Escobedo AA, Lalle M, Hrastnik NI, Rodriguez-Morales AJ, Castro-Sanchez E, Cimerman S, et al. Combination therapy in the management of giardiasis: what laboratory and clinical studies tell us, so far. Acta Trop. 2016 Oct;162:196–205.

4. Halliez, MC, Buret AG. Extra-intestinal and long term consequences of *Giardia duodenalis* infections. World J Gastroenterol. 2013 Dec 21;19(47):8974–85.

5. Soares R, Tasca T. Giardiasis: an update review on sensitivity and specificity of methods for laboratorial diagnosis. J Microbiol Methods. 2016 Oct;129:98–102.

6. Swirski AL, Pearl DL, Peregrine AS, Pintar K. A comparison of exposure to risk factors for giardiasis in non-travellers, domestic travellers and international travellers in a Canadian community, 2006–2012. Epidemiol Infect. 2016;144(5):980–99.

## TREATMENT

Effective treatments include metronidazole, tinidazole, and nitazoxanide. An alternative is paromomycin. Because making a definitive diagnosis is difficult, empiric treatment can be used in patients with the appropriate history and typical symptoms.

## PREVENTION

The best defense against giardiasis is thorough frequent handwashing, strict adherence to standard food and water precautions (see Chapter 2, Food & Water Precautions), and minimizing fecal–oral exposures during sexual activity.

**CDC website:** www.cdc.gov/parasites/giardia

# HAND, FOOT & MOUTH DISEASE

Holly M. Biggs

## INFECTIOUS AGENT

In the United States, coxsackievirus A16 is an important cause of hand, foot, and mouth disease (HFMD). More recently, coxsackievirus A6 has been implicated as the cause of outbreaks and sporadic cases in the United States and internationally. In the Asia-Pacific region, enterovirus 71 is a common etiologic agent.

## TRANSMISSION

Direct person-to-person contact with the saliva, nose and throat secretions, vesicle fluid, or stool of an infected person.

## EPIDEMIOLOGY

A common illness in young children, HFMD has a worldwide distribution. Outbreaks often occur during summer and early fall in the United States. Large outbreaks in Cambodia, China, Japan, Korea, Malaysia, Singapore, Thailand, Taiwan, and Vietnam have been reported in the past 2 decades. Seasonal patterns in Asia vary between climatic zones. In temperate Asia, including mainland China, cases tend to peak during the early summer.

## CLINICAL PRESENTATION

Incubation period is 3–6 days. Patients usually present with fever and malaise, followed by sore throat and the appearance of vesicles in the mouth (typically anterior, involving the buccal mucosa, tongue, or hard palate) and a peripheral rash, often papulovesicular, on the hands (palms) and feet (soles). In some cases, particularly with coxsackievirus A6 infection, rash may be more widespread, the lesions enlarging and coalescing to form bullae. Lesions usually resolve within about a week. Onychomadesis (shedding of the nails) and desquamation of the palms or soles can occur during convalescence. Rare complications include aseptic meningitis and encephalitis. In a small proportion of children with enterovirus 71 infection in Asia, severe manifestations, including central nervous system disease and death, have occurred.

## DIAGNOSIS

Diagnosis is usually clinical. Confirmatory laboratory testing using RT-PCR assays is available and performed for atypical or severe cases. Preferred samples for testing include vesicle fluid, throat or buccal swabs, or stool. RT-PCR assays to detect enterovirus RNA are available at many commercial or reference laboratories. The CDC Picornavirus Laboratory performs enterovirus testing and typing in consultation with state or local health departments: www.cdc.gov/non-polio-enterovirus/lab-testing/index.html.

## TREATMENT
Supportive care.

## PREVENTION
Avoiding close contact with infected people, maintaining good hand hygiene, and disinfecting potentially contaminated surfaces, including toys.

**CDC website:** www.cdc.gov/hand-foot-mouth

### BIBLIOGRAPHY

1. American Academy of Pediatrics. Enterovirus (nonpoliovirus). In: Kimberlin DW, Brady MT, Jackson MA, Long SS, editors. Red Book: 2015 Report of the Committee on Infectious Diseases. American Academy of Pediatrics; 2015. pp. 333–6.

2. Buttery VW, Kenyon C, Grunewald S, Oberste MS, Nix WA. Atypical presentations of hand, foot, and mouth disease caused by coxsackievirus A6—Minnesota, 2014. MMWR Morb Mortal Wkly Rep. 2015;64(29):805.

3. Koh WM, Bogich T, Siegel K, et al. The epidemiology of hand, foot and mouth disease in Asia: a systematic review and analysis. Pediatr Infect Dis J. 2016;35(10):e285–300.

4. World Health Organization. A guide to clinical management and public health response for hand, foot and mouth disease (HFMD). Geneva: World Health Organization; 2011 [cited 2018 Mar 123]. Available from: www.wpro.who.int/publications/docs/GuidancefortheclinicalmanagementofHFMD.pdf.

5. World Health Organization. Emerging disease surveillance and response: hand, foot and mouth disease. [cited 2018 Mar 13]. Available from: www.wpro.who.int/emerging_diseases/HFMD/en.

# HELICOBACTER PYLORI

Bradley A. Connor

## INFECTIOUS AGENT
*Helicobacter pylori* is a small, curved, microaerophilic, gram-negative, rod-shaped bacterium.

## TRANSMISSION
Believed to be mainly fecal–oral or possibly oral–oral.

## EPIDEMIOLOGY
About two-thirds of the world's population is infected, but it is more common in developing countries. Short-term travelers do not appear to be at significant risk of acquiring *H. pylori* through travel, but expatriates and long-stay travelers may be at higher risk.

## CLINICAL PRESENTATION
Usually asymptomatic, but *H. pylori* is the major cause of peptic ulcer disease and gastritis worldwide, which often present as gnawing or burning epigastric pain. Less commonly, symptoms

include nausea, vomiting, or loss of appetite. Infected people have a 2-fold to 6-fold increased risk of developing gastric cancer and mucosal associated-lymphoid-type (MALT) lymphoma compared with their uninfected counterparts.

## DIAGNOSIS

Fecal antigen assay, urea breath test, rapid urease test, or histology of biopsy specimen. A positive serology indicates present or past infection.

## TREATMENT

Asymptomatic infections do not need to be treated. Patients with active duodenal or gastric ulcers should be treated if they are infected. Treatment should be determined on an individual basis. Standard treatment is bismuth quadruple therapy (PPI or $H_2$-blocker + bismuth + metronidazole + tetracycline). Clarithromycin triple therapy (proton pump inhibitor [PPI] + clarithromycin + amoxicillin or metronidazole) can be used in regions where *H. pylori* clarithromycin resistance is known to be <15% and in patients with no previous history of macrolide exposure. See http://gi.org/guideline/treatment-of-helicobacter-pylori-infection.

## PREVENTION

No specific recommendations.

### BIBLIOGRAPHY

1. Chey WD, Leontiadis GI, Howden CW, Moss SF. ACG clinical guideline: treatment of Helicobacter pylori infection. Am J Gastroenterol. 2017;112:212–38.

2. Lindkvist P, Wadstrom T, Giesecke J. Helicobacter pylori infection and foreign travel. J Infect Dis. 1995 Oct;172(4):1135–6.

3. Potasman, I, Yitzhak A. Helicobacter pylori serostatus in backpackers following travel to tropical countries. Am J Trop Med Hyg. 1998;58(3):305–8.

# HELMINTHS, SOIL-TRANSMITTED

Christine Dubray, Sharon Roy

## INFECTIOUS AGENTS

*Ascaris lumbricoides* (roundworm), *Ancylostoma duodenale* (hookworm), *Necator americanus* (hookworm), and *Trichuris trichiura* (whipworm) are helminths (parasitic worms) that infect the intestine and are transmitted via contaminated soil.

## TRANSMISSION

Eggs are passed in feces from an infected person. Hookworm eggs are not infective—the eggs must hatch and release larvae that need to mature in the soil before they become infective. Infection with roundworm and whipworm occurs when eggs in soil have become infective and are ingested. Hookworm infection (see the Cutaneous Larva Migrans section in this chapter) usually occurs when larvae penetrate the skin of people walking barefoot on contaminated soil. However, the hookworm *Ancylostoma duodenale* can also be transmitted when larvae are ingested.

## EPIDEMIOLOGY

A large part of the world's population is infected with 1 or more of these helminths, and the prevalence is highest in tropical and subtropical countries where water supplies and sanitation are poor. Travelers to these countries should be at low risk of infection if preventive measures are taken. Infections in the United States are typically seen in immigrant and refugee populations. Since these worms do not multiply in hosts, reinfection occurs only as a result of additional contacts with the infective stages.

## CLINICAL PRESENTATION

Most infections are asymptomatic, especially when few worms are present. Pulmonary symptoms (Löffler syndrome) occur in a small percentage of patients when roundworm larvae pass through the lungs. Löffler syndrome is associated with fever and marked eosinophilia. Roundworms can also cause intestinal discomfort, obstruction, and impaired nutritional status. Hookworm infection can lead to anemia due to blood loss and chronic protein deficiency. Whipworm infection can cause chronic abdominal pain, diarrhea, blood loss, dysentery, and rectal prolapse. However, travelers are rarely at risk, because these more severe manifestations are generally associated with high worm burdens seen in indigenous populations.

### BIBLIOGRAPHY

1. Bethony J, Brooker S, Albonico M, Geiger SM, Loukas A, Diemert D, et al. Soil-transmitted helminth infections: ascariasis, trichuriasis, and hookworm. Lancet. 2006 May 6;367(9521):1521–32.

2. Brooker S, Bundy DAP. Soil-transmitted helminths (geohelminths). In: Cook GC, Zumla A, editors.

Manson's Tropical Diseases. 22nd ed. London: Saunders; 2009. pp. 1515–48.

3. Brooker S, Clements AC, Bundy DA. Global epidemiology, ecology and control of soil-transmitted helminth infections. Adv Parasitol. 2006;62:221–61.

## DIAGNOSIS

The standard method for diagnosing soil-transmitted helminths is by identifying eggs in a stool specimen using a microscope.

## TREATMENT

The drugs most commonly used are albendazole and mebendazole.

## PREVENTION

Food and water precautions (see Chapter 2, Food & Water Precautions). To avoid hookworm infection, travelers should not walk barefoot in areas where hookworm is common and where there may be human fecal contamination of the soil. In general, avoid ingesting soil that may be contaminated with human feces, including where human fecal matter or wastewater is used to fertilize crops.

**CDC website:** www.cdc.gov/parasites/sth

# HENIPAVIRUSES

Trevor Shoemaker, Mary Joung Choi

## INFECTIOUS AGENT

Enveloped, single-stranded RNA viruses in the genus *Henipavirus*, family Paramyxovirus. Of the 5 identified *Henipavirus* spp., Hendra virus and Nipah virus are highly virulent emerging pathogens that cause outbreaks in humans and are associated with high case-fatality ratios. Three additional species—Cedar virus, Ghanaian bat virus, and Mojiang virus—are not known to cause human disease.

## TRANSMISSION

Pteropid fruit bats (flying foxes) are the reservoir hosts. Hendra virus is transmitted through direct contact with infected horses or body fluids or tissues of infected horses; horses are infected through exposure to bat urine. Hendra virus is not transmitted person to person or directly from bats to humans. Nipah virus is transmitted through contact with infected pigs or bats (a common exposure is consumption of date palm sap contaminated with bat excretions). Person-to-person transmission of Nipah virus has been reported through close contact (including respiratory droplets) with infected people; transmission is facilitated by cultural and health care practices in which friends and family members care for ill patients.

## EPIDEMIOLOGY

Henipavirus outbreaks in humans have occurred in northern Australia and Southeast Asia; Nipah virus outbreaks in humans were reported in 1999 in Malaysia and Singapore and are reported almost annually in India and Bangladesh. However, pteropid bats can be found throughout the tropics and subtropics, and henipaviruses have been isolated from these bats in Central and South America, Asia, Oceania, and East Africa. Hendra virus has been reported nearly annually since 1994 in the eastern states of Australia.

## CLINICAL PRESENTATION

Incubation period is approximately 5–16 days (and rarely up to 2 months). Both Hendra and Nipah virus infections can cause a severe influenzalike illness with fever, myalgia, headache, and dizziness. This may progress to severe encephalitis with confusion, abnormal reflexes, seizures, and coma; respiratory symptoms may also be present. Relapsing or late-onset encephalitis can occur months or years after acute illness. The case-fatality ratio of Hendra virus is 57% (among 7 known human cases, 4 were fatal). Case-fatality ratios for Nipah virus infection are 40%–70% but have been 100% in some human outbreaks.

## DIAGNOSIS

Laboratory diagnosis is made by using a combination of tests, including ELISA of serum or cerebrospinal fluid (CSF); RT-PCR of serum, CSF, or throat swabs; and virus isolation from CSF or throat swabs.

## TREATMENT

There is no specific antiviral treatment for henipavirus infections; therapy consists of supportive care and management of complications. Ribavirin has shown in vitro effectiveness but its clinical usefulness is unknown. A monoclonal serotherapy has been proposed for Hendra in Australia.

## PREVENTION

Travelers should avoid contact with sick horses, pigs, bats, or their excretions. Travelers should not consume raw date palm sap or products made from raw sap. A Hendra virus vaccine for horses has been licensed in Australia and has potential future benefit to prevent henipavirus infection in humans.

**CDC website:** www.cdc.gov/vhf/hendra/index. html and www.cdc.gov/vhf/nipah/index.html

BIBLIOGRAPHY

1. Ang BSP, Lim TCC, Wang L. Nipah virus infection. J Clin Microbiol. 2018;56(6):e01875–17.
2. Croser EL, Marsh GA. The changing face of the henipaviruses. Veterinary Microbiol. 2013;167(1–2):151–8.
3. Weatherman S, Feldmann H, de Wit E. Transmission of henipaviruses. Curr Opin Virol. 2018;28:7–11.

# HEPATITIS A

Noele P. Nelson

## INFECTIOUS AGENT

Hepatitis A virus (HAV) is a nonenveloped RNA virus classified as a picornavirus.

## TRANSMISSION

HAV is transmitted through direct person-to-person contact (fecal–oral transmission) or through ingestion of contaminated food or water. HAV can survive in the environment for prolonged periods at low pH. Freezing does not inactivate HAV, and it can be transmitted through ice and frozen foods. Heat inactivation must occur at high temperatures (>185°F [>85°C] for 1 minute). HAV can be transmitted from contaminated raw or inadequately cooked foods and through handling foods after cooking. Recent large-scale outbreaks have been caused by contaminated food (such as frozen berries, seafood, and fresh fruit and vegetables) and through person-to-person spread among injection and noninjection drug users and homeless people.

HAV is shed in the feces of infected people. People are most infectious 1–2 weeks before the onset of clinical signs and symptoms (jaundice or elevation of liver enzymes), when the concentration of virus is highest in the stool and blood. Viral excretion and the risk of transmission diminish rapidly after liver dysfunction or symptoms appear, which is concurrent with the appearance of circulating antibodies to HAV. Infants and children can shed virus for up to 6 months after infection.

## EPIDEMIOLOGY

HAV is common in areas with inadequate sanitation and limited access to clean water. In highly endemic areas (such as parts of Africa and Asia), a large proportion of adults in the population are immune to HAV, and epidemics of hepatitis A are uncommon. In areas of intermediate endemicity (such as Central and South America, Eastern Europe, and parts of Asia), childhood transmission is less frequent, more adolescents and adults are susceptible to infection, and outbreaks are more likely. In areas of low endemicity (such as the United States and Western Europe), infection is less common, but disease occurs among people in high-risk groups and as communitywide outbreaks.

In the United States, the most frequently identified risk factors for hepatitis A infection vary from year to year. Risk groups recommended to receive the hepatitis A vaccine by the Advisory Committee for Immunization Practices (ACIP), include international travelers, users of injection and noninjection drugs, men who have sex with men (MSM), people with chronic liver disease, people with clotting-factor disorders, people who work with nonhuman primates, and people who anticipate close personal contact with an international adoptee. In addition, homelessness was approved as an indication for hepatitis A vaccination by ACIP at the October 2018 meeting.

Hepatitis A is among the most common vaccine-preventable infections acquired during travel. Cases of travel-related hepatitis A can occur in travelers to developed countries and developing countries, who have "standard" tourist itineraries, accommodations, and eating behaviors. Risk is highest for those who live in or visit rural areas, trek in backcountry areas, or frequently eat or drink in settings of poor sanitation. Common-source food exposures are increasingly recognized as a risk for hepatitis A, and sporadic outbreaks have been reported in Europe, Australia, North America, and other regions with low levels of endemic transmission. Multinational HAV outbreaks among MSM have been described, including since 2016 among MSM who have traveled to areas with ongoing HAV transmission among MSM in European Union countries. In the United States, outbreaks of hepatitis A in multiple states have been identified among homeless people and people who use injection and noninjection drugs. The homeless population has emerged as a high-risk group for hepatitis A infection in these recent US outbreaks.

## CLINICAL PRESENTATION

The incubation period averages 28 days (range, 15–50 days). Infection can be asymptomatic or range in severity from a mild illness lasting 1–2 weeks to a severely disabling disease lasting several months. Clinical manifestations include the abrupt onset of fever, malaise, anorexia, nausea, and abdominal discomfort, followed within a few days by jaundice. The likelihood of having symptoms with HAV infection is related to the age of the infected person. In children aged <6 years, most (70%) infections are asymptomatic; jaundice is uncommon in symptomatic young children. Among older children and adults, the illness usually lasts <2 months, although approximately 10%–15% of infected people have prolonged or relapsing symptoms over a 6- to 9-month period. Severe hepatic and extrahepatic complications, including fulminant hepatitis and liver failure, are rare but more common in older adults and people with underlying liver disease. Chronic infection does not occur. The overall case-fatality ratio varies according to the population affected.

## DIAGNOSIS

HAV cannot be differentiated from other types of viral hepatitis on the basis of clinical or epidemiologic features. Diagnosis requires a positive test for antibody to HAV (anti-HAV) IgM in serum, detectable from 2 weeks before the onset of symptoms to approximately 6 months afterward.

Serologic tests for total anti-HAV (IgG and IgM) are available commercially. A positive total anti-HAV result and a negative IgM anti-HAV result indicate past infection or vaccination and immunity. The presence of serum IgM anti-HAV usually indicates current or recent infection and does not distinguish between immunity from infection and vaccination. Acute hepatitis A is a nationally notifiable disease.

## TREATMENT

Supportive care.

## PREVENTION

Vaccination or immune globulin (IG), food and water precautions, maintaining standards of hygiene and sanitation.

## Vaccine

Two monovalent hepatitis A vaccines, Vaqta (Merck & Co, Inc., Whitehouse Station, NJ) and Havrix (GlaxoSmithKline Beecham Biologicals, Rixensart, Belgium), are approved for people ≥12 months of age in a 2-dose series. A combined hepatitis A and hepatitis B (Twinrix, GlaxoSmithKline) vaccine is approved for people ≥18 years of age in the United States (Table 4-2). The immunogenicity of the combination vaccine is equivalent to that of the monovalent hepatitis A and hepatitis B vaccines when tested after completion of the recommended schedule.

### INDICATIONS FOR USE

All susceptible people traveling for any purpose, frequency, or duration to countries with high or intermediate HAV endemicity should be vaccinated or receive IG before departure. Many travel health clinicians feel that all travelers should be educated about hepatitis A and be given the opportunity for immunization. Prevalence patterns of HAV infection vary among regions within a country,

## Table 4-2. Vaccines to prevent hepatitis A

| VACCINE | TRADE NAME (MANUFACTURER) | AGE (Y) | DOSE | ROUTE | SCHEDULE | BOOSTER |
|---|---|---|---|---|---|---|
| Hepatitis A vaccine, inactivated | Havrix (GlaxoSmithKline) | 1–18 | 0.5 mL (720 ELU) | IM | 0, 6–12 mo | None |
| | | ≥19 | 1.0 mL (1,440 ELU) | IM | 0, 6–12 mo | None |
| Hepatitis A vaccine, inactivated | Vaqta (Merck & Co., Inc.) | 1–18 | 0.5 mL (25 U) | IM | 0, 6–18 mo | None |
| | | ≥19 | 1.0 mL (50 U) | IM | 0, 6–18 mo | None |
| Combined hepatitis A and B vaccine | Twinrix (GlaxoSmithKline) | ≥18 (primary) | 1.0 mL (720 ELU HAV + 20 µg HBsAg) | IM | 0, 1, 6 mo | None |
| | | ≥18 (accelerated) | same as above | IM | 0, 7, 21–30 d | 12 mo |

Abbreviations: ELU, ELISA units of inactivated HAV; IM, intramuscular; U, units HAV antigen; HAV, hepatitis A virus; HBsAg, hepatitis B surface antigen.

and in some areas limited data result in uncertainty in endemicity maps, especially in low- and middle-income countries. Countries where the prevalence of HAV infection is decreasing have growing numbers of susceptible people and are at risk for outbreaks of hepatitis A. In recent years, large outbreaks of hepatitis A were reported in developed countries among people who had been exposed to imported food contaminated with HAV, MSM, drug users, and the homeless. Taking into account the complexity of interpreting hepatitis A risk maps and potential risk of foodborne hepatitis A in countries with low endemicity, some experts advise people traveling outside the United States to consider hepatitis A vaccination regardless of destination.

Vaccination is recommended for unvaccinated household members and other people who anticipate close personal contact (such as household contacts or regular babysitters) with an international adoptee from a country of high or intermediate endemicity during the 60 days after arrival of the child in the United States. The first dose of the 2-dose hepatitis A vaccine series should be administered as soon as adoption is planned, ideally ≥2 weeks before the arrival of the child (see Chapter 7, International Adoption).

## VACCINE ADMINISTRATION

One dose of single-antigen hepatitis A vaccine administered at any time before departure can provide adequate protection for most healthy travelers. However, single-dose, long-term protection data are limited. The monovalent vaccine series should be completed according to the licensed schedule for long-term protection.

Hepatitis A vaccine should be administered to infants aged 6–11 months traveling outside the United States when protection against hepatitis A is recommended. Although hepatitis A vaccine is considered safe and immunogenic in infants, hepatitis A vaccine doses administered before 12 months of age might result in a suboptimal immune response, particularly in infants with passively acquired maternal antibody. Therefore, hepatitis A vaccine doses administered at <12 months of age are not considered for long-term protection, and the 2-dose hepatitis A vaccine series should be initiated at

age 12 months according to the routine, age-appropriate vaccine schedule. Adults aged >40 years, immunocompromised people, people with chronic liver disease, and people with other chronic medical conditions planning travel in <2 weeks may receive IG (0.1 mL/kg) in addition to vaccine at a separate injection site based on provider risk assessment, including considerations of the traveler's age, immune status and underlying conditions, risk of exposure, and availability of IG.

Infants aged <6 months and travelers who are allergic to a vaccine component or elect not to receive vaccine should receive a single dose of IG (0.1 mL/kg), which provides effective protection against HAV infection for up to 1 month. Those who do not receive vaccination and plan to travel for 1–2 months should receive an IG dose of 0.2 mL/kg, which can be repeated every 2 months thereafter if the traveler remains in a high-risk setting, though hepatitis A vaccination should be encouraged if not contraindicated.

No data on single-dose hepatitis A vaccine efficacy are available for Twinrix. An alternate, accelerated 4-dose schedule is available for Twinrix; doses can be administered at 0, 7, and 21–30 days, followed by a dose at 12 months. (For more information, see www.cdc.gov/mmwr/volumes/66/wr/mm6636a5.htm?s_cid=mm6636a5_e.) Although vaccinating an immune traveler is not contraindicated and does not increase the risk for adverse effects, screening for total anti-HAV before travel can be useful in some circumstances to determine susceptibility and eliminate unnecessary vaccination. Postvaccination testing for serologic response is not indicated.

## OTHER VACCINE CONSIDERATIONS

Using vaccine according to the licensed schedule is preferable. An interrupted series does not need to be restarted. More than 95% of vaccinated people develop levels of anti-HAV that correlate with protection 1 month after the first dose. Given their similar immunogenicity, a series that has been started with one brand of hepatitis A monovalent vaccine may be completed with another brand of monovalent vaccine. For children and adults who complete the primary series, booster doses of vaccine are not recommended.

## VACCINE SAFETY AND ADVERSE REACTIONS

Among adults, the most frequently reported side effects after hepatitis A vaccination are tenderness or pain at the injection site (56%–67%) and headache (14%–16%). Among children (11–25 months of age), the most common reported side effects are pain or tenderness at the injection site (32%–37%) and redness (21%–29%). No serious adverse events in children or adults have been reported that could be attributed definitively to the vaccine; no increase in serious adverse events has been identified among vaccinated people compared with baseline rates.

## PRECAUTIONS AND CONTRAINDICATIONS

Hepatitis A–containing vaccines should not be administered to travelers with a history of hypersensitivity to any vaccine component, including neomycin. Twinrix should not be administered to people with a history of hypersensitivity to yeast. The tip caps of prefilled syringes of Havrix and Twinrix and the vial stopper, syringe plunger stopper, and tip caps of Vaqta may contain dry natural rubber, which may cause allergic reactions in latex-sensitive people. Because hepatitis A vaccine consists of inactivated virus, and hepatitis B vaccine consists of a recombinant protein, no special precautions are needed for vaccination of immunocompromised travelers. Providers should check precautions and contraindications before administering IG.

## PREGNANCY

Hepatitis A vaccine is considered safe for pregnant women. A recent review of the Vaccine Adverse Event Reporting System did not identify any concerning patterns of adverse events in pregnant women or their infants after hepatitis A vaccination (Havrix, Vaqta) or hepatitis A and B combined vaccination (Twinrix) during pregnancy. Hepatitis A vaccine should be administered to pregnant women who are at high risk of exposure and to pregnant women who want protection according to the adult immunization schedule.

## POSTEXPOSURE PROPHYLAXIS

Travelers who are exposed to HAV but not symptomatic and who have not received hepatitis A vaccine previously should be administered 1 dose of monovalent hepatitis A vaccine or IG (0.1 mL/kg) as soon as possible, ideally within 2 weeks of exposure. The efficacy of IG or vaccine when administered >2 weeks after exposure has not been established.

Hepatitis A vaccines should be administered for postexposure prophylaxis for all people aged ≥12 months. In addition to hepatitis A vaccine, IG (0.1 mL/kg) should be administered to people who are immunocompromised or who have chronic liver disease and may be administered to people aged >40 years depending on the provider's risk assessment, which should include consideration of the exposed person's age, immune status and underlying conditions, exposure type (risk of transmission), and availability of IG. People aged <12 months and people who are allergic to a vaccine component or elect not to receive vaccine should receive a single dose of IG (0.1 mL/kg) only. Twinrix should not be used for postexposure prophylaxis, because no data are available on the efficacy of combination vaccine for prophylaxis after exposure to HAV.

More detailed information can be found in the Advisory Committee on Immunization Practices recommendations at www.cdc.gov/mmwr/volumes/67/wr/mm6743a5.htm?s_cid=mm6743a5_w.

**CDC website:** www.cdc.gov/hepatitis/HAV

## BIBLIOGRAPHY

1. Averhoff FM, Khudyakov Y, Nelson NP. Vaccines. 7th ed. Philadelphia: Saunders Elsevier; 2016.

2. CDC. Viral hepatitis surveillance—United States, 2016 [cited 2018 Mar 15]. Available from: www.cdc.gov/hepatitis/statistics/2016surveillance/pdfs/2016HepSurveillanceRpt.pdf.

3. Collier MG, Khudyakov YE, Selvage D, Adams-Cameron M, Epson E, Cronquist A, et al. Outbreak of hepatitis A in the USA associated with frozen pomegranate arils imported from Turkey: an epidemiological case study. Lancet Infect Dis. 2014 Oct;14(10):976–81.

4. Fiore AE, Wasley A, Bell BP. Prevention of hepatitis A through active or passive immunization: recommendations of the Advisory Committee on Immunization Practices (ACIP). MMWR Recomm Rep. 2006 May 19;55(RR-7):1–23.

5. Foster M. Ramachandran S, Myatt K, Donovan D, Bohm S, Fielder J, et al. Hepatitis A outbreaks associated with

4

drug use and homelessness—California, Kentucky, Michigan, and Utah, 2017. MMWR Morb Mortal Wkly Rep. 2018 Nov 2;67(43):1208–10.

6. Jacobsen KH. Globalization and the changing epidemiology of hepatitis A virus. Cold Spring Harb Perspect Med. 2018 Oct 1;8(10). pii: a031716. doi: 10.1101/cshperspect.a031716.

7. Latash J, Dorsinville M, Del Rosso P, Antwi M, Reddy V, Waechter H, et al. Notes from the field: increase in reported hepatitis A infections among men who have sex with men—New York City, January–August 2017. MMWR Morb Mortal Wkly Rep. 2017 Sep 22;66(37):999–1000.

8. Moro PL, Museru OI, Niu M, Lewis P, Broder K. Reports to the Vaccine Adverse Event Reporting System after hepatitis A and hepatitis AB vaccines in pregnant women. Am J Obstet Gynecol. 2014 Jun;210(6):561.e1–6.

9. Nelson NP, Link-Gelles R, Hofmeister MG, Romero JR, Moore KL, Ward JW, et al. Update: recommendations of the Advisory Committee on Immunization Practices for use of hepatitis A vaccine for postexposure prophylaxis and for preexposure prophylaxis for international travel. MMWR Morb Mortal Wkly Rep. 2018 Nov 2;67(43):1216–20.

# HEPATITIS B

Aaron M. Harris

**4**

## INFECTIOUS AGENT

Hepatitis B virus (HBV), a small, circular, partially double-stranded DNA virus in the family Hepadnaviridae

## TRANSMISSION

HBV is transmitted by contact with contaminated blood, blood products, and other body fluids (such as semen). Examples of exposures associated with transmission that travelers may encounter include poor infection control during medical or dental procedures, receipt of blood products, injection drug use, tattooing or acupuncture, and unprotected sex.

## EPIDEMIOLOGY

HBV is a leading cause of chronic hepatitis, liver cirrhosis, and hepatocellular carcinoma worldwide, resulting in an estimated 887,000 deaths per year. An estimated 257 million people have chronic HBV infection globally. Although accurate data are lacking from many countries, Map 4-4 shows the estimated prevalence of chronic HBV infection by country. No data are available to show the specific risk to travelers; however, published reports of travelers acquiring hepatitis B are rare, and the risk for travelers who do not have high-risk behaviors or exposures is low. The risk for HBV infection may be higher in countries where the prevalence of chronic HBV infection is ≥2%, such as in the western Pacific

and African regions; expatriates, missionaries, and long-term development workers may be at increased risk for HBV infection in such countries. All travelers should be aware of how HBV is transmitted and take measures to minimize their exposures.

## CLINICAL PRESENTATION

HBV infection primarily affects the liver. Typically, the incubation period for hepatitis B is 90 days (range, 60–150 days). Newly acquired acute HBV infections only cause symptoms some of the time. The presence of signs and symptoms varies by age. Most children under age 5 years and newly infected immunosuppressed adults are generally asymptomatic, whereas 30%–50% of people aged ≥5 years have signs and symptoms. When present, the typical signs and symptoms of acute infection include malaise, fatigue, poor appetite, nausea, vomiting, abdominal pain, fever, dark urine, light color (clay-colored) stool, joint pain, and jaundice. The overall case-fatality ratio of acute hepatitis B is approximately 1%.

Some acute HBV infections will resolve on their own, but some will develop into chronic infection. The risk of acute hepatitis B progressing to chronic HBV infection depends on the age at the time of initial infection as follows: >90% of neonates and infants, 25%–50% of children aged 1–5 years, and <5% of older children and adults. Most people with chronic HBV infection are asymptomatic and have

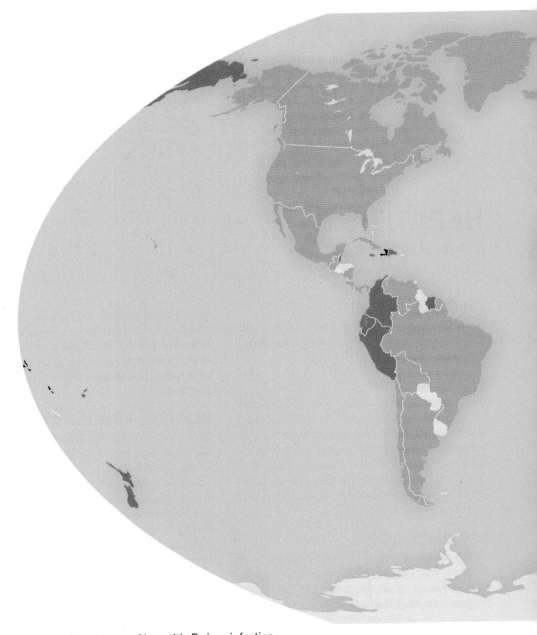

**MAP 4-4.** Prevalence of hepatitis B virus infection

Disease data source: Schweitzer A, Horn J, Mikolajczyk R, Krause G, Ott J. Estimations of worldwide prevalence of chronic hepatitis B virus infection: a systematic review of data published between 1965 and 2013. Lancet. 2015 Jul 28;386(10003):1546–55.

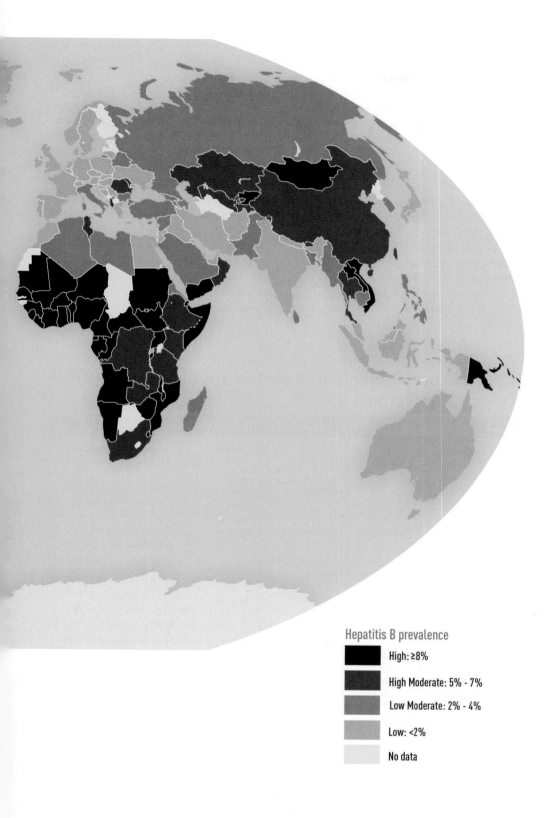

Hepatitis B prevalence

- High: ≥8%
- High Moderate: 5% - 7%
- Low Moderate: 2% - 4%
- Low: <2%
- No data

4

no evidence of liver disease. However, 15%–40% of people with chronic HBV infection will develop liver cirrhosis, hepatocellular carcinoma, or liver failure, and 25% die prematurely of these complications. People infected with HBV are susceptible to infection with hepatitis D virus; coinfection increases the risk of fulminant hepatitis and rapidly progressive liver disease.

## DIAGNOSIS

The clinical diagnosis of acute HBV infection is based on signs or symptoms consistent with viral hepatitis and elevated hepatic transaminases but cannot be distinguished from other causes of acute hepatitis. Serologic markers specific for hepatitis B are necessary to diagnose HBV infection and for appropriate clinical management (Table 4-3). These markers can differentiate between acute, resolving, and chronic infection. Hepatitis B is a nationally notifiable disease.

## TREATMENT

There are no medications available to treat acute HBV; treatment is supportive. There are several antiviral medications for people with chronic HBV infection. People with chronic HBV should be under the care of a health professional and receive a thorough physical examination and laboratory testing to determine the need for antiviral therapy and ongoing monitoring for hepatocellular carcinoma and liver damage related to chronic HBV infection. American Association for the Study of Liver Diseases (AASLD) practice guidelines are available for the treatment of chronic HBV infection and can be found at www.aasld.org/publications/practice-guidelines-0.

## Table 4-3. Interpretation of serologic test results for hepatitis B virus infection

| CLINICAL STATE | HBSAG | TOTAL ANTI-HBS | TOTAL ANTI-HBC | ACTION |
|---|---|---|---|---|
| Chronic infection | Positive | Negative | Positive | Link to hepatitis B-directed care |
| Acute | Positive | Negative | Positive (IgM anti-HBc) | Link to hepatitis B-directed care |
| Resolved infection | Negative | Positive | Positive | Counseling, reassurance |
| Immune (immunization) | Negative | Positive | Negative | Reassurance |
| Susceptible (never infected and no evidence of immunization) | Negative | Negative | Negative | Vaccinate |
| Isolated core antibody[1] | Negative | Negative | Positive | Depends on situation |

Abbreviations: HBsAg, hepatitis B surface antigen; anti-HBc, antibody to hepatitis B core antigen; anti-HBs, antibody to hepatitis B surface antigen; hepatitis B-directed care, physical exam and laboratory evaluation for liver transaminase, HBV DNA, and hepatitis B e antigen.
From: Abara WE, Qaseem A, Schillie S, McMahon BJ, Harris AM. Hepatitis B vaccination, screening, and linkage to care: best practice advice from the American College of Physicians and the Centers for Disease Control and Prevention. Ann Intern Med. 2017;167(11):794-804.
[1] Can be a result of:
- False positive, repeat testing required.
- Past infection, no action needed.
- Occult HBV infection, needs to be known if patient ever becomes immunosuppressed or given chemotherapy or treated with antiviral therapy for hepatitis C virus infection. Consider monitoring HBV DNA.
- Passive transfer to infant born to HBsAg-positive mother; no specific action needed.

# PREVENTION

## Vaccine

### INDICATIONS FOR USE

Hepatitis B vaccination should be administered to all unvaccinated people traveling to areas with intermediate to high prevalence of chronic HBV infection (HBV surface antigen prevalence ≥2%). Complete vaccination information and recommendations for the United States are available at www.cdc.gov/vaccines/hcp/acip-recs/vacc-specific/hepb.html. Vaccination to prevent hepatitis B should be considered for all international travelers, regardless of destination.

### VACCINE ADMINISTRATION

Multiple hepatitis B vaccines are available (Table 4-4). The vaccine is administered either as a 2-dose series on a 0- and 1-month schedule (for Heplisav-B) or a 3-dose series on a 0-, 1-, and 6-month schedule (for Engerix-B, Recombivax HB, and Twinrix). For the 2-dose vaccine, the second dose should be given ≥1 month after the first dose. For 3-dose vaccines, the third dose should be given ≥2 months after the second dose and ≥4 months after the first dose. The third dose of Engerix-B should not be administered before age 24 weeks. Four doses of hepatitis B vaccine can be administered when a combination vaccine containing hepatitis B is administered after the birth dose. Postexposure prophylaxis with hepatitis B immune globulin (HBIG) administered in conjunction with hepatitis B vaccine is effective in preventing transmission after exposure to HBV; hepatitis B vaccine alone may also be used if HBIG is not available.

Heplisav-B (Dynavax Technologies Corporation) is licensed for a 2-dose schedule for adults aged ≥18 years; Recombivax HB (Merck & Co.) is licensed for a 2-dose schedule for children aged 11–15 years; and Engerix-B (GlaxoSmithKline) is licensed for a 4-dose schedule, with the first 3 doses within 2 months and a booster at 12 months (doses at 0, 1, 2, and 12 months). A combined hepatitis A and hepatitis B vaccine (Twinrix) can also be used on a 3-dose schedule (0, 7, and 21–30 days), with a booster at 12 months. The prescribing information should always be consulted when administering alternate schedules and formulations. Whenever feasible, the same manufacturer's vaccines should be used to complete the series; however, vaccination should not be deferred when the manufacturer of previously administered doses is unknown or when the vaccine from the same manufacturer is unavailable. The 2-dose Heplisav-B vaccine series only applies when both doses in the series consist of Heplisav-B. Series consisting of a combination of 1 dose of Heplisav-B and a vaccine from a different manufacturer should adhere to the 3-dose schedule. Protection from the primary vaccination series is robust, and >95% of healthy people achieve immunity after completion of the vaccine series. Serologic testing and booster vaccination are not recommended before travel for immunocompetent adults who have been previously vaccinated.

### SPECIAL SITUATIONS

Ideally, vaccination with Heplisav-B should begin ≥1 month before travel so the full vaccine series can be completed before departure. When vaccines other than Heplisav-B are used, vaccination should begin ≥6 months before travel. Because some protection is provided by 1 or 2 doses, the vaccine series should be initiated, if indicated, even if it cannot be completed before departure. Optimal protection, however, is not conferred until after the vaccine series is completed, and travelers should be advised to complete the vaccine series. An approved accelerated vaccination schedule can be used for people traveling on short notice who face imminent exposure or for emergency responders to disaster areas. The accelerated vaccination schedule for the combined hepatitis A and hepatitis B vaccine, Twinrix, calls for vaccine doses administered at days 0, 7, and 21–30; a booster should be administered at 12 months to promote long-term immunity. Alternatively, Heplisav-B may be used as a 2-dose series at 0 and 4 weeks to protect against hepatitis B alone.

### VACCINE SAFETY AND ADVERSE REACTIONS

There are safe hepatitis B vaccines available for people of all ages, and adverse reactions are rare. The most common adverse reactions are soreness

# Table 4-4. Vaccines to prevent hepatitis B

| VACCINE | TRADE NAME (MANUFACTURER) | AGE (Y) | DOSE | ROUTE | SCHEDULE | BOOSTER |
|---|---|---|---|---|---|---|
| Hepatitis B vaccine, recombinant with novel adjuvant (1018) | Heplisav-B (Dynavax Technologies) | >18 | 0.5 mL (20 µg HBsAg and 3000 µg of 1018) | IM | 0, 1 mo | None |
| Hepatitis B vaccine, recombinant[1] | Engerix-B (GlaxoSmithKline) | 0–19 (primary) | 0.5 mL (10 µg HBsAg) | IM | 0, 1, 6 mo | None |
| | | 0–10 (accelerated) | 0.5 mL (10 µg HBsAg) | IM | 0, 1, 2 mo | 12 mo |
| | | 11–19 (accelerated) | 1 mL (20 µg HBsAg) | IM | 0, 1, 2 mo | 12 mo |
| | | ≥20 (primary) | 1 mL (20 µg HBsAg) | IM | 0, 1, 6 mo | None |
| | | ≥20 (accelerated) | 1 mL (20 µg HBsAg) | IM | 0, 1, 2 mo | 12 mo |
| Hepatitis B vaccine, recombinant[1] | Recombivax HB (Merck & Co., Inc.) | 0–19 (primary) | 0.5 mL (5 µg HBsAg) | IM | 0, 1, 6 mo | None |
| | | 11–15 (adolescent accelerated) | 1 mL (10 µg HBsAg) | IM | 0, 4–6 mo | None |
| | | ≥20 (primary) | 1 mL (10 µg HBsAg) | IM | 0, 1, 6 mo | None |
| Combined hepatitis A and B vaccine | Twinrix (GlaxoSmithKline) | ≥18 (primary) | 1 mL (720 ELU HAV + 20 µg HBsAg) | IM | 0, 1, 6 mo | None |
| | | ≥18 (accelerated) | 1 mL (720 ELU HAV + 20 µg HBsAg) | IM | 0, 7, 21–30 d | 12 mo |

Abbreviations: HBsAg, hepatitis B surface antigen; IM, intramuscular; ELU, ELISA units of inactivated HAV; HAV, hepatitis A virus.
[1] Consult the prescribing information for differences in dosing for hemodialysis and other immunocompromised patients.

at the injection site (3%–29%) and low-grade fever (temperature >99.9°F [37.7°C]; 1%–6%). Hepatitis B vaccines should not be administered to people with a history of hypersensitivity to any vaccine component, including yeast. The vaccine contains a recombinant protein (hepatitis B surface antigen) that is noninfectious and contains an adjuvant (either aluminum [for Engerix-B, Recombivax HB, Twinrix] or 1018 [small synthetic immunostimulatory cytidine-phosphate-guanosine oligodeoxynucleotide motif for Heplisav-B]).

Limited data indicate no apparent risk of adverse events to the mother or the developing fetus when licensed 3-dose series hepatitis B vaccine is administered to pregnant women. There are no data on use of 2-dose series vaccines (Heplisav-B) in pregnant women. HBV infection affecting a pregnant woman can result in serious disease for the mother and chronic infection for the newborn. Neither pregnancy nor lactation should be considered a contraindication for use of licensed 3-dose series hepatitis B vaccines.

## Personal Protection Measures

As part of the pretravel education process, all travelers should be counseled and given information about the risks for hepatitis B and other bloodborne pathogens from contaminated equipment or items used during medical, dental, or cosmetic procedures; blood products; injection drug use; any activities or procedures that involve piercing the skin or mucosa; or unprotected sexual activity. When seeking medical or dental care or cosmetic procedures (such as tattooing or piercing), travelers should be advised against the use of equipment that has not been adequately sterilized or disinfected, reuse of contaminated equipment, and unsafe injecting practices (such as reuse of disposable needles and syringes). HBV and other bloodborne pathogens can be transmitted if tools are not sterile or if personnel do not follow proper infection-control procedures. Travelers should consider the health risks when receiving medical or dental care overseas; information may be available from the US embassy. The health risks should be strongly considered when deciding to obtain a tattoo or body piercing in areas where adequate sterilization or disinfection procedures might not be available or practiced.

**CDC website:** www.cdc.gov/hepatitis/HBV

BIBLIOGRAPHY

1. Abara WE, Qaseem A, Schillie S, McMahon BJ, Harris AM. Hepatitis B vaccination, screening, and linkage to care: best practice advice from the American College of Physicians and the Centers for Disease Control and Prevention. Ann Intern Med. 2017;167(11):794–804.

2. CDC. Updated US Public Health Service guidelines for the management of occupational exposures to HBV, HCV, and HIV and recommendations for post-exposure prophylaxis. MMWR Recomm Rep. 2001 Jun 29;50(RR-11):1–42.

3. Johnson DF, Leder K, Torresi J. Hepatitis B and C infection in international travelers. J of Trop Med. 2013 May–Jun;20(3):194–202.

4. Pepin J, Abou Chakra CN, Pepin E, Nault V, Valiquette L. Evolution of the global burden of viral infections from unsafe medical injections, 2000–2010. PLoS One. 2014;9(6):e99677.

5. Schillie S, Harris A, Link-Gelles R, Romero J, Ward J, Nelson N. Recommendations of the Advisory Committee on Immunization Practices for use of a hepatitis b vaccine with a novel adjuvant. MMWR Recomm Rep 2018;67(15);455–8.

6. Schillie S, Vellozzi C, Reingold A, Harris A, Haber P, Ward JW, et al. Prevention of hepatitis B virus infection in the United States: recommendations of the Advisory Committee on Immunization Practices. MMWR Recomm Rep 2018 Jan 12;67(RR-1):1–31.

7. Schweitzer A, Horn J, Mikolajczyk RT, Krause G, Ott JJ. Estimations of worldwide prevalence of chronic hepatitis B virus infection: a systematic review of data published between 1965 and 2013. Lancet. 2015 Oct 17;386(10003):1546–55.

8. Terrault NA, Bzowej NH, Chang KM, Hwang JP, Jonas MM, Murad MH. AASLD guidelines for treatment of chronic hepatitis B. Hepatology. 2016 Jan;63(1):261–83.

# HEPATITIS C

Philip Spradling

## INFECTIOUS AGENT

Hepatitis C virus (HCV) is a spherical, enveloped, positive-strand RNA virus. Seven distinct HCV genotypes and 67 subtypes have been identified, the distribution of which vary geographically worldwide.

## TRANSMISSION

Transmission of HCV is bloodborne and most often involves exposure to contaminated needles or syringes or receipt of blood or blood products that have not been screened for HCV. Although infrequent, HCV can be transmitted through other

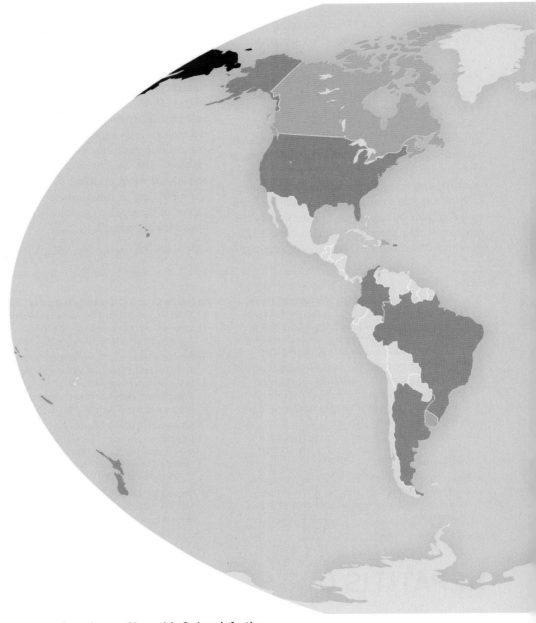

MAP 4-5. **Prevalence of hepatitis C virus infection**

The Polaris Observatory HCV Collaborators. Global prevalence and genotype distribution of hepatitis C virus infection in 2015: a modelling study. Lancet Gastroenterol Hepatol. 2017;2:161–76.

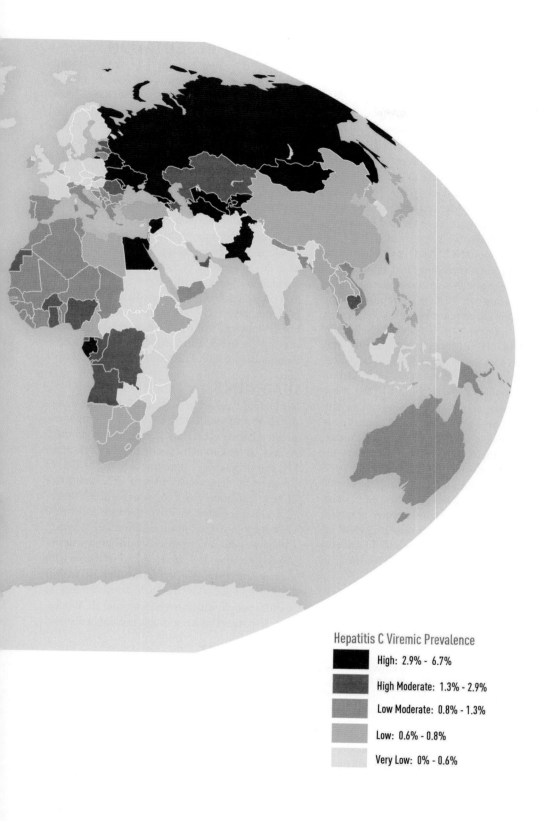

Hepatitis C Viremic Prevalence

High: 2.9% - 6.7%

High Moderate: 1.3% - 2.9%

Low Moderate: 0.8% - 1.3%

Low: 0.6% - 0.8%

Very Low: 0% - 0.6%

4

procedures that involve blood exposure, such as tattooing, during sexual contact, or perinatally from mother to child.

## EPIDEMIOLOGY

Globally, an estimated 71 million people are living with HCV infection (chronically infected), and approximately 400,000 were estimated to have died from HCV-related liver disease in 2013. Although the quality of epidemiologic data and prevalence estimates vary widely across countries and within regions, the most recent global estimates indicate that the viremic prevalence of HCV infection (prevalence of HCV RNA) is <1.0% in most developed countries, including the United States (Map 4-5). The prevalence is considerably higher in some countries in Eastern Europe (3.3% in Russia, 2.2% in Latvia) and certain countries in Africa (6.3% in Egypt, 7.0% in Gabon), the Middle East (3.0% in Syria), the South Caucasus and Central Asia (4.2% in Georgia, 4.3% in Uzbekistan) and southern and eastern Asia (3.8% in Pakistan, 6.4% in Mongolia, 2.1% in Taiwan). The most frequent current mode of transmission in the United States and most developed countries is through sharing of drug preparation and drug-injection equipment. In countries where HCV infection prevalence is higher relative to developed countries, the predominant mode of transmission is from unsafe injections and other health care exposures where infection-control practices are poor. Travelers' risk for contracting HCV infection is generally low, but they should exercise caution, as the following activities can result in blood exposure:

- Receiving blood transfusions that have not been screened for HCV

- Having medical or dental procedures

- Activities such as acupuncture, tattooing, being shaved, or injection drug use in which equipment has not been adequately sterilized or disinfected or in which contaminated equipment is reused

- Working in health care fields (medical, dental, or laboratory) that entail direct exposure to human blood

## CLINICAL PRESENTATION

HCV is a major cause of cirrhosis and hepatocellular cancer and is the leading reason for liver transplantation in the United States. Most people (80%) with acute HCV infection have no symptoms. If symptoms occur, they are indistinguishable from other forms of acute viral hepatitis and may include loss of appetite, abdominal pain, fatigue, nausea, dark urine, and jaundice. Of those infected, approximately 75%–85% will remain infected unless treated with antiviral medications. For people who develop chronic HCV infection, the most common symptom is fatigue. Cirrhosis develops in approximately 10%–20% of people after 20–30 years of chronic infection. This progression is often clinically silent, and evidence of liver disease may not occur until late in the course of the disease. HCV testing is required for diagnosis. However, testing is not routinely provided in many countries, and most HCV-infected people are unaware of their infection.

## DIAGNOSIS

Two major types of tests are available: IgG assays for HCV antibodies and nucleic acid amplification testing to detect HCV RNA in blood (viremia). Assays for IgM, to detect early or acute infection, are not available. Approximately 70%–75% of people who seroconvert to anti-HCV, indicative of acute infection, will progress to chronic infection and persistent viremia. Because a positive HCV antibody test cannot discriminate between someone who was previously infected but resolved or cleared the infection and someone with current infection, it is essential that HCV RNA testing follow a positive HCV antibody test to identify people with current (chronic) HCV infection. Hepatitis C is a nationally notifiable disease.

## TREATMENT

Since 2014, several new all-oral direct-acting antiviral agents have been approved for use in the United States and other countries. These new treatment regimens are of short duration (typically 12 weeks) with few side effects and cure rates exceeding 90% for those who complete treatment, regardless of HCV genotype, prior treatment status, and the presence of cirrhosis. Travelers who think they may have been exposed should be tested for HCV upon return and, if found to have current infection (HCV RNA-positive), be referred for care and evaluated for treatment. The most up-to-date treatment guidelines and information can be found at www.hcvguidelines.org.

## PREVENTION

No vaccine is available to prevent HCV infection, nor does immune globulin provide protection. Before traveling, people should check with their health care providers to understand the potential risk of infection and any precautions they should take. When seeking medical or dental care, travelers should be alert to the use of medical, surgical, or dental equipment that has not been adequately sterilized or disinfected; reuse of contaminated equipment; and unsafe injection practices (such as reuse of disposable needles and syringes). HCV and other bloodborne pathogens can be transmitted if instruments are not sterile or the clinician does not follow other proper infection-control procedures (washing hands, using latex gloves, and cleaning and disinfecting surfaces and instruments). In some parts of the world, such as parts of sub-Saharan Africa, blood donors may not be screened for HCV. Travelers should be advised to consider the health risks if they are considering a tattoo or body piercing or having a medical procedure in areas where adequate sterilization or disinfection procedures might not be practiced. Travelers should be advised to seek testing for HCV upon return if they received blood transfusions or sustained other blood exposures for which they could not assess the risks.

**CDC website:** www.cdc.gov/hepatitis/HCV

BIBLIOGRAPHY

1. American Association for Study of Liver Diseases (AASLD), Infectious Diseases Society of America (IDSA). Recommendations for testing, managing, and treating hepatitis C. [updated 2017 Sep 21]. Available from: www.hcvguidelines.org/.

2. CDC. Testing for HCV infection: an update of guidance for clinicians and laboratorians. MMWR Morb Mortal Wkly Rep. 2013 May 10;62(18):362–5.

3. GBD 2013 Mortality and Causes of Death Collaborators. Global, regional, and national age-sex specific all-cause and cause-specific mortality for 240 causes of death, 1990–2013: a systematic analysis for the Global Burden of Disease Study 2013. Lancet. 2015 Jan 10;385(9963):117–71.

4. Global Hepatitis Report 2017. Geneva: World Health Organization; 2017. Licence: CC BY-NC-SA 3.0 IGO. Available from: http://apps.who.int/iris/bitstr eam/10665/255016/1/9789241565455-eng.pdf?ua=1.

5. Messina JP, Humphreys I, Flaxman A, Brown A, Cooke GS, Pybus OG, et al. Global distribution and prevalence of hepatitis C virus genotypes. Hepatology. 2015 Jan;61(1):77–87.

6. Smith DB, Bukh J, Kuiken C, Muerhoff AS, Rice CM, Stapleton JT, et al. Expanded classification of hepatitis C virus into 7 genotypes and 67 subtypes: updated criteria and genotype assignment web resource. Hepatology. 2014 Jan;59(1):318–27.

7. Westbrook RH, Dusheiko G. Natural history of hepatitis C. J Hepatol. 2014 Nov;61(1 Suppl):S58–68.

# HEPATITIS E

Eyasu H. Teshale

## INFECTIOUS AGENT

Infection is caused by hepatitis E virus (HEV), a single-stranded, single-serotype, RNA virus belonging to the Herpesviridae family. Five HEV genotypes are known to cause human disease. HEV genotype 3 causes hepatitis E in developed countries, whereas genotypes 1, 2, 4, and 7 are associated with illness in developing countries. HEV genotype 1 and to some extent genotype 2 are associated with large waterborne outbreaks.

## TRANSMISSION

HEV genotypes 1 and 2 are transmitted primarily by the fecal–oral route. In regions with poor sanitation and limited access to safe drinking water, epidemics and interepidemic occurrences of hepatitis E are largely waterborne. In developing countries transmission to fetuses and neonates by women infected during pregnancy is common. In Japan and Europe, sporadic disease can be zoonotic and foodborne, associated with eating meat and offal (including liver) of deer, boars, and pigs and is mainly caused by HEV genotype 3. In France, disease can be acquired from eating *figatellu*, a sausage delicacy prepared from raw pig liver. A hepatitis E outbreak on a cruise ship was associated with consumption of shellfish. Transfusion-related hepatitis E is increasingly reported from countries in Europe. Rare domestically acquired symptomatic disease is observed in the United States, but its mode of transmission is generally unknown.

## EPIDEMIOLOGY

Every year HEV causes an estimated 20 million infections with 3.3 million symptomatic cases and 44,000 deaths, and the great majority of these occur in developing countries. Waterborne outbreaks (which can be large, often involving hundreds to thousands of people) have occurred in South and Central Asia, tropical East Asia, Africa, and Central America. In recent years, many large international outbreaks have occurred among refugees and internally displaced people living in camps. In outbreak-prone areas, interepidemic disease is sporadically encountered. Sporadic disease also occurs in regions that are not prone to outbreaks, such as the Middle East, temperate East Asia (including China), North and South America, and Europe.

During outbreaks of hepatitis E, clinical attack rates are highest in young adults aged 15–49 years. In HEV genotype 1–endemic areas, pregnant women—whether infected sporadically or during an outbreak—are at risk of their HEV infection progressing to liver failure and death. Miscarriages and neonatal deaths are common complications of HEV infection. In areas where infection is caused by HEV genotype 3, symptomatic disease is observed most frequently in adults aged >50 years. HEV genotype 3 infection acquired by people who are immunosuppressed, particularly recipients of solid-organ allografts, may progress to chronic infection.

People living in the United States are at highest risk of HEV infection when they travel to areas where epidemics have occurred, mainly from drinking contaminated water. When traveling in Japan and Europe, eating raw or inadequately cooked venison, boar meat, pig liver, pig meat, or food products derived from these is a risk factor for infection.

## CLINICAL PRESENTATION

The incubation period of HEV infection is 2–9 weeks (mean 6 weeks). Signs and symptoms of acute hepatitis E include jaundice, fever, loss of appetite, abdominal pain, and lethargy, and are indistinguishable from symptoms of other causes of viral hepatitis. Infection with HEV genotype 3, common in developed countries, can progress to chronic infection, whereas genotypes 1, 2, and 4 result only in acute infection. For most people, HEV infection and disease is self-limited. Pregnant women with HEV infection (especially those infected during the third trimester) may present with or progress to liver failure, and their fetuses are at risk of spontaneous abortion and premature delivery. To date, there is no evidence that HEV genotype 3 is associated with severe outcome in pregnant women. People with preexisting liver disease may undergo further hepatic decompensation with HEV infection. Recipients of solid organ transplants tend to have no symptoms associated with acute and chronic HEV infection, but progressive liver injury can result when infected with HEV genotype 3.

## DIAGNOSIS

The diagnosis of acute hepatitis E is established by detecting anti-HEV IgM in serum. Detecting HEV RNA in serum or stools further confirms the serologic diagnosis but is seldom required. Longer term, serial detection of HEV RNA in serum or stools, regardless of the HEV antibody serostatus, suggests chronic HEV infection. No diagnostic

4

test for HEV has been approved by the Food and Drug Administration.

## TREATMENT

Treatment is supportive. Oral ribavirin has been used to treat chronic hepatitis E in solid-organ transplant recipients.

## PREVENTION

Travelers should avoid drinking unboiled or unchlorinated water and beverages that contain unboiled water or ice. Travelers should eat only thoroughly cooked food, including seafood, meat, offal, and products derived from these (see Chapter 2, Food & Water Precautions). A safe and effective vaccine has been available in China since 2012; however it is not approved for use elsewhere.

**CDC website:** www.cdc.gov/hepatitis/HEV

### BIBLIOGRAPHY

1. Ankcorn MJ, Tedder RS. Hepatitis E: the current state of play. Tranfus Med. 2017 Apr;27(2):84–95.
2. Kamar N, Dalton HR, Abravanel F, Izopet J. Hepatitis E virus infection. Clin Microbiol Rev. 2014 Jan;27(1):116–38.
3. Kamar N, Izopet J, Tripon S, Bismuth M, Hillaire S, Dumortier J, et al. Ribavirin for chronic hepatitis E virus infection in transplant recipients. N Engl J Med. 2014 Mar 20;370(12):1111–20.
4. Khuroo MS, Khuroo MS. Hepatitis E: an emerging global disease—from discovery towards control and cure. J Viral Hepat. 2016 Feb;23(2):68–79.
5. Krawczynski K. Hepatitis E virus. Semin Liver Dis. 2013 Feb;33(1):1–93.
6. Riveiro-Barciela M, Minguez B, Girones R, Rodriguez-Frias F, Quer J, Buti M. Phylogenetic demonstration of hepatitis E infection transmitted by pork meat ingestion. J Clin Gastroenterol. 2015 Feb;49(2):165–8.

# HISTOPLASMOSIS

Brendan R. Jackson, Tom M. Chiller

## INFECTIOUS AGENT

*Histoplasma capsulatum,* a dimorphic fungus that grows as a mold in soil and as a yeast in animal and human hosts.

## TRANSMISSION

Through inhalation of spores (conidia) from soil (often soil contaminated with bat guano or bird droppings); not transmitted from person to person.

## EPIDEMIOLOGY

Distributed worldwide, except in Antarctica, but most often associated with river valleys. Activities that expose people to soil disruption or areas where bats live and birds roost, such as construction, excavation, demolition, farming, gardening, and caving, can increase risk of histoplasmosis. Outbreaks have been reported associated with travel to many countries in Central and South America, most often associated with visiting caves.

## CLINICAL PRESENTATION

Incubation period is typically 3–17 days for acute disease. Ninety percent of infections are asymptomatic or result in a mild influenzalike illness. Some infections may cause acute pulmonary histoplasmosis, manifested by high fever, headache, nonproductive cough, chills, weakness, pleuritic chest pain, and fatigue. Most people spontaneously recover 2–3 weeks after onset of symptoms, although fatigue may persist longer. High-dose exposure can lead to severe pulmonary disease. Dissemination, especially to the gastrointestinal tract and central nervous system, can occur in people who are immunocompromised.

## DIAGNOSIS

Several methods are available to diagnose histoplasmosis.

- Although the gold standards remain culture and histopathologic identification, antigen or antibody testing are commonly used.
  - > Rapid *Histoplasma* antigen testing by EIA on multiple specimen types (for example, urine, serum, plasma, bronchoalveolar lavage, or cerebrospinal fluid) is available at multiple US laboratories. Antigen testing is most sensitive in severely ill patients.
  - > Antibody testing by EIA, immunodiffusion (ID), and complement fixation (CF) can be used to detect subacute and chronic forms of histoplasmosis. Antibodies to *Histoplasma* typically become detectable in serum 4–8 weeks after infection. A small proportion (<5%) of people living in histoplasmosis-endemic areas have positive serology by CF or ID. Testing a single serum specimen can aid in diagnosis, but testing serial specimens offers greater specificity (detection of seroconversion and increases in antibody titer). An antibody response may be absent in immunocompromised people.
  - > Other endemic mycoses (such as blastomycosis, paracoccidioidomycosis, and talaromycosis [formerly penicilliosis]) can lead to false-positive antigen and antibody tests for *H. capsulatum*.

- Culture of *H. capsulatum* from bone marrow, blood, sputum, and tissue specimens is the definitive method but may take weeks to grow. DNA probe is sometimes used to confirm *H. capsulatum* in culture.

- Demonstration of the typical intracellular yeast forms in tissue by microscopic examination strongly supports the diagnosis of histoplasmosis when clinical, epidemiologic, and other laboratory studies are compatible. Molecular diagnostics, such as PCR on tissue specimens, are increasingly available to support microscopic findings, although the performance of these tests may vary.

## TREATMENT

Treatment is not usually indicated for immunocompetent people with acute, localized pulmonary infection. People with more extensive disease or persistent symptoms beyond 1 month are generally treated with an azole drug such as itraconazole for mild to moderate illness or amphotericin B for severe infection. Patients with acute respiratory distress may benefit from steroids as well as antifungal treatment.

## PREVENTION

People at increased risk for severe disease should avoid high-risk areas, such as bat-inhabited caves.

**CDC website:** www.cdc.gov/fungal/diseases/histoplasmosis

BIBLIOGRAPHY

1. Armstrong PA, Beard JD, Bonilla L, Arboleda N, Lindsley MD, Chae S, et al. Outbreak of severe histoplasmosis among tunnel workers—Dominican Republic, 2015. Clin Infect Dis. 2018 May 2;66(10):1550–1557. doi: 10.1093/cid/cix1067.

2. Azar MM, Hage CA. Laboratory diagnostics for histoplasmosis. J Clin Microbiol. 2017 Jun 1;55(6):1612–20.

3. CDC. Outbreak of histoplasmosis among travelers returning from El Salvador—Pennsylvania and Virginia, 2008. MMWR Morb Mortal Wkly Rep. 2008 Dec 19;57(50):1349–53.

4. Kauffman CA. Histoplasmosis: a clinical and laboratory update. Clin Microbiol Rev. 2007 Jan;20(1):115–32.

5. Morgan J, Cano MV, Feikin DR, Phelan M, Monroy OV, Morales PK, et al. A large outbreak of histoplasmosis among American travelers associated with a hotel in Acapulco, Mexico, spring 2001. Am J Trop Med Hyg. 2003 Dec;69(6):663–9.

6. Weinberg M, Weeks J, Lance-Parker S, Traeger M, Wiersma S, Phan Q, et al. Severe histoplasmosis in travelers to Nicaragua. Emerg Infect Dis. 2003 Oct;9(10):1322–5.

7. Wheat LJ, Freifeld AG, Kleiman MB, Baddley JW, McKinsey DS, Loyd JE, et al. Clinical practice guidelines for the management of patients with histoplasmosis: 2007 update by the Infectious Diseases Society of America. Clin Infect Dis. 2007 Oct 1;45(7):807–25.

# HIV INFECTION

Philip J. Peters, John T. Brooks

## INFECTIOUS AGENT

HIV, an enveloped positive-strand RNA virus in the Retroviridae family.

## TRANSMISSION

Transmitted through sexual contact, needle or syringe sharing, unsafe medical injection or blood transfusion, and organ or tissue transplantation. It can also be transmitted from mother to child during pregnancy, at birth, and postpartum through breastfeeding.

## EPIDEMIOLOGY

HIV infection occurs worldwide. As of June 2017, an estimated 36.7 million people were living with HIV infection. Sub-Saharan Africa is the most affected part of the world (25.5 million cases or 69% of all people living with HIV infection), and the Eastern Europe and central Asia region has experienced the largest increases in new HIV infections (60% increase from 2010 to 2016). Although the reported adult HIV prevalence in many regions of the world is low, certain populations are disproportionately affected, such as sex workers, people who inject drugs, men who have sex with men, transgender people, and prisoners. Sex workers are particularly vulnerable; the prevalence among sex workers is 12 times as high as in the general population.

The risk of HIV infection for international travelers is generally low. Travelers' risk of HIV exposure and infection is determined less by geographic destination and more by the behaviors in which they engage while traveling, such as unprotected sex and injection drug use. Travelers who might undergo scheduled or emergency medical procedures should be aware that HIV can be transmitted by unsafe nonsterile medical injection practices (reusing needles, syringes, or single-dose medication vials). This problem may be greater in low-income countries where the blood supply as well as organs and tissues used for transplantation may not be screened properly for HIV.

## CLINICAL PRESENTATION

As many as 90% of people will recall experiencing symptoms during the acute phase of HIV infection. Acute HIV infection can present as an infectious mononucleosis-like or influenzalike syndrome, but the clinical features are highly variable. Symptoms typically begin a median of 10 days after infection and can include fever, maculopapular rash, arthralgia, myalgia, malaise, lymphadenopathy, oral ulcers, pharyngitis, and weight loss. The presence of fever and rash have the best positive predictive value.

## DIAGNOSIS

HIV can be diagnosed with laboratory-based or point-of-care assays that detect anti-HIV antibodies, HIV p24 antigen, or HIV-1 RNA. In the United States, the recommended laboratory-based screening test for HIV is a combination antigen/antibody assay that detects antibodies against HIV, as well as p24 antigen. The combination antigen/antibody assay becomes reactive approximately 2–3 weeks after HIV infection. It is estimated that 99% of people will develop a reactive combination antigen/antibody result within 6 weeks of infection, but in rare cases, it can take up to 6 months to develop a reactive test result. Point-of-care HIV antibody tests performed on oral fluid (instead of blood) have been associated with a lower sensitivity during early HIV infection. The earliest time after exposure that HIV infection can be diagnosed is approximately 9 days, when HIV-1 RNA becomes detectable in blood. Travelers can find detailed information on HIV testing locations at gettested.cdc.gov.

## TREATMENT

Prompt medical care and effective treatment with antiretrovirals can partially reverse HIV-induced damage to the immune system, and prolong life. Effective treatment also substantially reduces the risk of HIV transmission to others. Detailed information on specific treatments is available from the Department of Health and Human Services AIDSinfo (www.aidsinfo.nih.gov). Travelers may contact AIDSinfo toll-free at 800-448-0440 (English or Spanish) or 888-480-3739 (TTY) for more information.

## PREVENTION

Travelers can reduce their risk of HIV infection in multiple ways. They can avoid sexual encounters with people whose HIV status is unknown, and use condoms consistently and correctly with all partners who are HIV infected or whose HIV status is unknown. They should also not inject drugs or share needles, and avoid exposure to blood or blood products and nonsterile invasive medical equipment. Travelers who do inject drugs should only use sterile, single-use syringes and needles that are safely disposed after every injection.

### Preexposure Prophylaxis

Preexposure prophylaxis (or PrEP) with tenofovir-emtricitabine is highly effective in preventing HIV infection and is recommended as a prevention option for adults at substantial risk of HIV acquisition (see www.cdc.gov/hiv/risk/prep). Travelers taking PrEP should carry proper documentation and be aware that some countries (see below for further information) may deny entry to people with evidence of HIV infection, which PrEP medications might mistakenly indicate to customs officials. Free, expert PrEP advice is available to health care professionals on the Clinician Consultation Center's PrEPline (855-448-7737; 11 AM–6 PM EST).

## Postexposure Prophylaxis

Postexposure prophylaxis (or PEP) with antiretroviral medications is another method to prevent HIV infection (see www.cdc.gov/hiv/risk/pep). PEP is recommended as a prevention option after a single high-risk exposure to HIV during sex, through sharing needles or syringes, or from a sexual assault. PEP must be started within 72 hours of a possible exposure. Travelers who will be working in a medical setting (such as a nurse volunteer drawing blood, or medical missionary performing surgeries) may have contact with HIV-infected or potentially infected biological materials. In certain settings, clinicians may prescribe PEP medications that a traveler could use in an emergency situation. Free, expert PEP advice is available to health care professionals on the Clinician Consultation Center's PEPline (888-448-4911; 11 AM–8 PM EST). Detailed advice regarding management of postexposure prophylaxis in the occupational setting is found in Chapter 9, Health Care Workers.

## HIV TESTING REQUIREMENTS FOR US TRAVELERS ENTERING FOREIGN COUNTRIES

International travelers should be advised that some countries screen incoming travelers (usually those with an extended stay) for HIV infection, and may deny entry to people with AIDS or evidence of HIV infection. People intending to visit a country for an extended stay should review that country's policies and requirements. This information is usually available from the consular officials of the individual nations. Information about entry and exit requirements compiled by the Department of State is found by country at http://travel.state.gov/content/passports/en/country.html.

**CDC website:** www.cdc.gov/hiv

BIBLIOGRAPHY

1. Brett-Major DM, Scott PT, Crowell TA, Polyak CS, Modjarrad K, Robb ML, et al. Are you PEPped and PrEPped for travel? Risk mitigation of HIV infection for travelers. Trop Dis Travel Med Vaccines. 2016 Nov 28;2:25.

2. CDC. Preexposure prophylaxis for the prevention of HIV in the United States: a clinical practice guideline. Atlanta 2014 [cited 2018 Feb 26]. Available from: www.cdc.gov/hiv/pdf/PrEPguidelines2014.pdf.

3. CDC. Preexposure prophylaxis for the prevention of HIV in the United States: clinical providers' supplement. Atlanta 2014 [cited 2018 Feb 26]. Available from: www.cdc.gov/hiv/pdf/PrEPProviderSupplement2014.pdf.

4. Joint United Nations Programme on HIV/ AIDS (UNAIDS). UNAIDS Data 2017. Geneva: UNAIDS; 2017 [cited 2018 Feb 26]. Available from: www.unaids.org/sites/default/files/ media_asset/20170720_Data_book_2017_en.pdf.

5. Kuhar DT, Henderson DK, Struble KA, Heneine W, Thomas V, Cheever LW, et al. Updated US Public Health Service guidelines for the management of occupational exposures to human immunodeficiency virus and recommendations for postexposure prophylaxis. Infect Control Hosp Epidemiol. 2013 Sep;34(9):875–92.

# INFLUENZA

Katherine Roguski, Alicia Fry

## INFECTIOUS AGENT

Influenza is caused by infection of the respiratory tract with influenza viruses, RNA viruses of the *Orthomyxovirus* genus. Influenza viruses are classified into 4 types: A, B, C, and D. Only virus types A and B commonly cause illness in humans. Influenza A viruses are further classified into subtypes based on 2 surface proteins, hemagglutinin (HA) and neuraminidase (NA). Although 4 types and subtypes of influenza virus cocirculate in humans worldwide (influenza A(H1N1), A(H3N2), and influenza B-Yamagata, B-Victoria viruses), the distribution of these viruses varies from year to year and between geographic areas and time of year. Information about circulating viruses in various regions can be found on the CDC website (www.cdc.gov/ flu/weekly) or the World Health Organization website (www.who.int/influenza/surveillance_ monitoring/updates/latest_update_GIP_sur- veillance/en/). Avian and swine influenza viruses can occasionally infect and cause disease in humans, usually associated with close exposure to infected animal populations. Notably, avian influenza A(H5N1) and A(H7N9) viruses, as well as swine-origin A(H1N1), A(H1N2), and A(H3N2) variant viruses, have led to sporadic human infections globally.

## TRANSMISSION

Influenza viruses spread from person to person, primarily through respiratory droplet transmission (such as when an infected person coughs or sneezes near a susceptible person). Transmission via large-particle droplets requires close proximity between the source and the recipient, because droplets generally travel only short distances (approximately 6 feet or less) through the air, before settling onto surfaces. Indirect (fomite) transmission can also occur, such as when a person touches a virus-contaminated surface and then touches his or her face. Airborne transmission via small-particle aerosols in the vicinity of the infectious person also occurs.

Most adults who are ill with influenza shed the virus in the upper respiratory tract and are infectious from the day before symptom onset to approximately 5–7 days after symptom onset. Infectiousness is highest within 3 days of illness onset and is correlated with fever. Children and those who are immunocompromised or severely ill may shed influenza virus for 10 days or more after the onset of symptoms. Seasonal influenza viruses have rarely been detected from non-respiratory sources such as stool or blood.

Although human infections due to avian or swine influenza viruses are rare, transmission of these viruses from birds or swine to humans is possible. Infected birds shed avian influenza virus in their saliva, mucus, and droppings, and transmission to humans can occur directly (through touching an infected animal or droplet spread) or indirectly (through inhalation of these viruses in the air or through fomite transmission on infected surfaces). See www.cdc.gov/flu/avianflu/ avian-in-humans.htm. Infected swine shed the virus in nasal secretions and can transmit viruses to humans in the same way seasonal influenza viruses spread among people (www.cdc. gov/flu/swineflu/people-raise-pigs-flu.htm).

Human-to-human transmission of swine or avian viruses is uncommon.

## EPIDEMIOLOGY

### Seasonal Influenza

Influenza circulation varies geographically. The risk of exposure to influenza during travel depends on the time of year and destination. In temperate regions, influenza typically circulates at higher levels during colder winter months: October to May in the Northern Hemisphere and April to September in the Southern Hemisphere. In many tropical or subtropical regions, influenza can occur throughout the year.

Influenza may be more common in children, especially in school-aged children. Rates of severe illness and death are typically highest among people aged ≥65 years, children <2 years, and people of any age who have underlying medical conditions that place them at increased risk for complications of influenza. CDC estimates that from 2010 through 2014, approximately 9.2–35.6 million symptomatic infections, 4.2–16.7 million outpatient visits, 139,000–708,000 hospitalizations, and 12,000–56,000 deaths associated with influenza viruses occurred each year in the United States (www.cdc.gov/flu/about/disease/burden.htm).

### Zoonotic Influenza

Influenza A viruses not only circulate among humans but also among many animal species populations, although influenza B viruses circulate widely only among humans. The primary reservoir for influenza A viruses is wild waterfowl and other wild birds, but viruses are common in domestic poultry and swine populations as well. Influenza A viruses can also infect other animal species, such as cats, dogs, horses, ferrets, sea lions, and bats.

Human infections with influenza A viruses from infected swine are uncommon and have been sporadically identified in the United States and other countries (www.cdc.gov/flu/swineflu/index.htm). When an influenza virus that normally circulates in swine (but not people) is detected in a person, it is called a "variant" influenza virus and denoted with the letter "v."

Human infections with influenza A(H1N1)v, A(H1N2)v, and A(H3N2)v have been identified. The largest outbreak in the United States occurred in 2012 when a total of 309 cases of human illnesses (1 of whom died) caused by A(H3N2) v viruses were identified. From 2013 through 2017, 119 human infections with variant viruses were identified in 16 states. Infrequent variant virus infections have also been identified and reported in other countries in Europe, the Americas, and Asia. Most people identified with variant influenza virus infections report contact with swine preceding their illness, suggesting swine-to-human spread. There have also been limited reports of human-to-human transmission of variant viruses. Seasonal human influenza viruses have also been known to infect swine, suggesting person-to-swine transmission. Agricultural fairs are a setting that can result in many human exposures to swine. Illnesses associated with variant virus infections have been mostly mild with symptoms similar to those of seasonal influenza; however, variant virus infections can also result in serious illness, causing hospitalization and death.

Avian influenza viruses do not commonly infect humans, although there have also been reports of sporadic disease resulting from these viruses (www.cdc.gov/flu/avianflu/index.htm). From 1997 through January 2018, 860 human illnesses caused by avian influenza A(H5N1) virus were reported globally, approximately 53% of which were fatal. Most disease from A(H5N1) has occurred after direct or close contact with sick or dead infected poultry. A(H5N1) virus is widespread among poultry in some countries in Asia and the Middle East (Map 4-6). Egypt and Indonesia have accounted for 65% of reported infections in humans globally. Instances of limited, nonsustained, human-to-human transmission of A(H5N1) virus have been reported. Since 2012, an increasing number of countries have reported detection of additional influenza H5 virus subtypes different from A(H5N1) among poultry and wild birds: A(H5N2), A(H5N3), A(H5N5), A(H5N6), A(H5N8), and A(H5N9) viruses. Of these virus subtypes, only A(H5N6) has been reported to cause illness in humans.

Avian influenza A(H7N9) virus emerged in China in 2013, and, as of January 2018, has caused

1,566 confirmed human illnesses. Most cases have been identified in mainland China, but several infections in people who reported exposure in mainland China and subsequent travel have been identified in Malaysia, Taiwan, Macao, and Hong Kong. In 2014, Canada reported the first imported A(H7N9) virus infection in North America in a traveler returning from China. Most of the people with infection caused by A(H7N9) had exposure to infected poultry or contaminated environments, such as live bird markets, and the virus has been found in poultry and environmental samples collected in China. A small proportion of human illnesses from A(H7N9) virus has been mild, but most patients have developed severe respiratory illness, and at least 39% have died.

In the United States, North American lineage avian influenza viruses are occasionally detected in wild, domestic, and commercial birds; these viruses are genetically different from those circulating in other regions of the world (www.aphis. usda.gov/aphis/ourfocus/animalhealth/animal-disease-information/avian-influenza-disease/defend-the-flock/defend-the-flock-ai-overview). From 2015 through 2017, H5 virus infections were identified in backyard and commercial poultry in 21 states. In 2016 and 2017, A(H7N8) and A(H7N9) viruses were identified in poultry flocks in 2 states. Although no human infections with H5, A(H7N8), or A(H7N9) viruses have been reported in the United States, surveillance in domestic birds and people exposed to infected birds is ongoing given the low but continued risk of transmission to humans.

Although rare, human infections with other avian influenza viruses, including A(H7N2) and A(H9N2), have been reported globally in recent years. In the United States, 3 infections with A(H7N2) virus were reported in humans in 2002, 2003, and 2016, all of whom recovered.

## CLINICAL PRESENTATION

Uncomplicated influenza illness is the most common presentation of influenza and is characterized by the abrupt onset of signs and symptoms that include fever, muscle aches, headache, malaise, nonproductive cough, sore throat, vomiting, and rhinitis. Less commonly, rashes have been associated with influenza infection.

Illness without fever can occur, especially in the elderly and infants. Children are more likely than adults to also experience nausea, vomiting, or diarrhea when ill with influenza. Physical findings are predominantly localized to the respiratory tract and include nasal discharge, pharyngeal inflammation without exudates, and occasionally rales on chest auscultation. The incubation period is usually 1–4 days after exposure. Influenza illness typically resolves within 1 week for most previously healthy children and adults who do not receive antiviral medication, although cough and malaise can persist for >2 weeks, especially in the elderly. Complications of influenza virus infection include primary influenza viral pneumonia, secondary bacterial pneumonia, parotitis, exacerbation of underlying medical conditions (such as pulmonary and cardiac disease), encephalopathy, myocarditis, myositis, coinfections with other viral or bacterial pathogens, and rarely, death.

Humans infected with variant influenza viruses have a clinical presentation similar to human influenza virus infections. Reported human infections with avian influenza A(H5N1) or A(H7N9) viruses often have severe pneumonia or respiratory failure and a high case-fatality ratio. However, it is uncommon for people with less severe illness to be tested for A(H5N1) or A(H7N9) viruses.

## DIAGNOSIS

Influenza can be difficult to distinguish from respiratory illnesses caused by other pathogens on the basis of signs and symptoms alone. The positive predictive value of clinical signs and symptoms for influenzalike illness (fever with either cough or sore throat) for laboratory-confirmed influenza virus infection is 30%–88%, depending on the level of influenza activity.

Diagnostic tests available for influenza include viral culture, rapid influenza diagnostic tests (RIDTs), immunofluorescence assays, and nucleic acid–based assays, such as RT-PCR (www.cdc.gov/flu/professionals/diagnosis/overview-testing-methods.htm). Most patients with clinical illness consistent with uncomplicated influenza in an area where influenza viruses are circulating do not require diagnostic testing for clinical management. Patients who

4

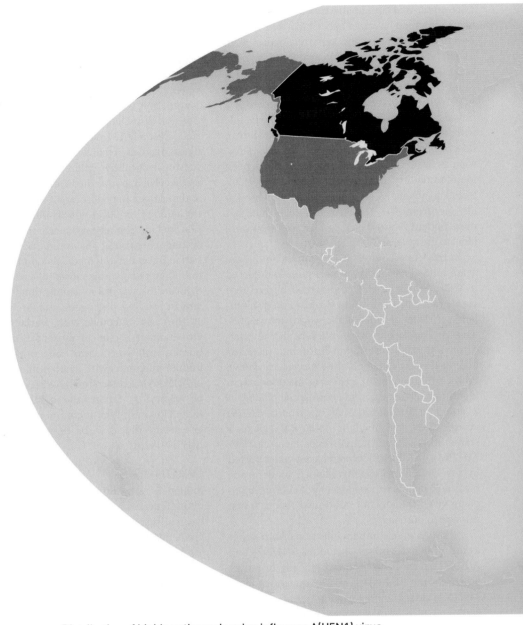

MAP 4-6. Distribution of highly pathogenic avian influenza A(H5N1) virus

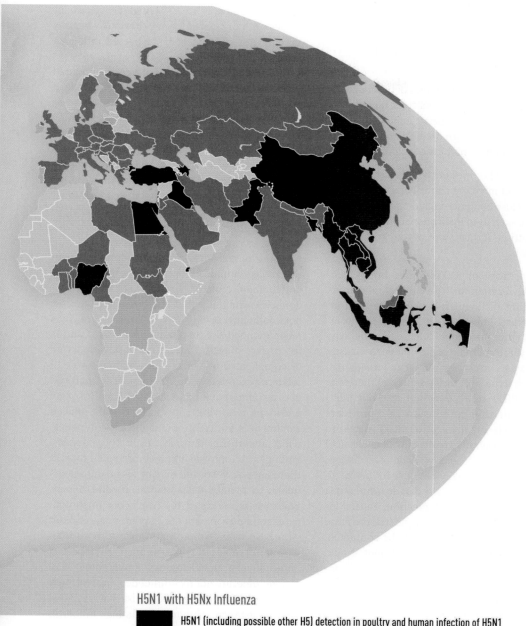

## H5N1 with H5Nx Influenza

■ H5N1 (including possible other H5) detection in poultry and human infection of H5N1

■ H5N1 (including possible other H5) detection in poultry since 2005

■ H5 detection in poultry (not H5N1) since 2005

■ No cases reported

should be considered for influenza diagnostic testing include the following:

- Hospitalized patients with suspected influenza

- Patients for whom a diagnosis of influenza will inform clinical care decisions, including patients who do not improve on antiviral therapy and those with medical conditions that place them at high risk of complications

- Patients for whom results of influenza testing would affect infection control or management of close contacts, including other patients, such as in institutional outbreaks or other settings (cruise ships or tour groups, for example)

The sensitivity of RIDTs varies but is substantially lower than for RT-PCR or viral culture. RIDTs cannot distinguish between seasonal influenza A virus infections and animal-origin influenza A virus infections, and their sensitivity to detect these animal-origin influenza viruses, including avian or variant influenza viruses, can vary by test type and virus subtype. Therefore, a negative RIDT result does not rule out influenza virus infection, and health care providers should not rely on a negative RIDT result to make decisions about treatment. Nucleic acid assays are the most sensitive diagnostic assays. However, no commercially available influenza diagnostic assay can specifically diagnose influenza variant virus or avian virus infection. Thus, if infection with these viruses is suspected, the state health department or CDC should be contacted. The decision to start antiviral treatment should not be delayed while waiting for results of confirmatory laboratory testing.

## Use of Antiviral Drugs

Early antiviral treatment can shorten the duration of fever and other symptoms and reduce the risk of complications from influenza. Antiviral treatment is recommended as early as possible for any patient with confirmed or suspected influenza who is hospitalized; has severe, complicated, or progressive illness; or is at a higher risk for influenza-associated complications (www.cdc.gov/flu/professionals/antivirals/

summary-clinicians.htm). Antiviral treatment can also be considered for any previously healthy patient with confirmed or suspected influenza not at high risk of complications.

Treatment is most effective if it can be initiated within 48 hours of illness onset. For hospitalized patients, those with severe illness, or those at higher risk of complications, antiviral therapy may still be beneficial if started >48 hours after illness onset. Four FDA-approved antiviral agents are recommended for the treatment and prophylaxis of influenza: oral oseltamivir (available as generic or Tamiflu, Genentech), inhaled zanamivir (Relenza, GlaxoSmithKline), intravenous (IV) peramivir (Rapivab, BioCryst Pharmaceuticals), and oral baloxavir (Xofluza, Genentech).

Three of the antiviral medications are neuraminidase inhibitors that have activity against both influenza A and B viruses; baloxavir is an endonuclease inhibitor that also has activity against both influenza A and B viruses. Oseltamivir is recommended for treatment for all ages and is the preferred agent to treat patients with severe or complicated influenza illness who are able to tolerate oral medications. Zanamivir is approved and recommended to treat those aged ≥7 years and for prophylaxis in those aged ≥5 years. Inhaled zanamivir is not recommended for use in people with underlying chronic respiratory disease. Peramivir is approved and recommended to treat those aged ≥2 years and may be useful in patients unable to tolerate or absorb oral antiviral therapy. Baloxavir is indicated to treat acute uncomplicated influenza in patients 12 years of age or older who have been symptomatic for no more than 48 hours (Table 4-5). Two other FDA-approved anti-influenza medications, amantadine and rimantadine, are not recommended for treatment or prophylaxis of influenza because of widespread viral resistance among circulating influenza A viruses. Amantadine and rimantadine are not active against influenza B viruses.

People at increased risk for complications of influenza should discuss antiviral treatment with their health care provider before travel to areas where influenza activity is occurring.

Antiviral drugs can also be used for prophylaxis, to prevent infection after close contact with a confirmed case; however, CDC does not recommend

## Table 4-5. Recommended dosage and duration of antiviral medications for treatment and prophylaxis of influenza A and B

| ANTIVIRAL AGENT | USE | CHILDREN | ADULTS |
|---|---|---|---|
| Oral oseltamivir | Treatment (5 days) | **If child is <1 year old[1]:** 3 mg/kg/dose twice daily.[2,3]<br>**If ≥1 year old, dose varies by child's weight:**<br>≤15 kg, the dose is 30 mg twice a day.<br>>15–23 kg, the dose is 45 mg twice a day.<br>>23–40 kg, the dose is 60 mg twice a day.<br>>40 kg, the dose is 75 mg twice a day. | 75 mg twice daily |
| | Prophylaxis (7 days) | **If child is <3 months old:** use of oseltamivir for prophylaxis is not recommended unless situation is judged critical because data in this age group are limited.<br>**If child is ≥3 months and <1 year old[1]:**<br>3 mg/kg/dose once daily.[2]<br>**If ≥1 year old, dose varies by child's weight:**<br>≤15 kg, the dose is 30 mg once a day.<br>>15–23 kg, the dose is 45 mg once a day.<br>>23–40 kg, the dose is 60 mg once a day.<br>>40 kg, the dose is 75 mg once a day. | 75 mg once daily |
| Inhaled zanamivir[4] | Treatment (5 days) | 10 mg (two 5-mg inhalations) twice daily<br>**(FDA approved and recommended for use in children ≥7 years)** | 10 mg (two 5-mg inhalations) twice daily |
| | Prophylaxis (7 days) | 10 mg (two 5-mg inhalations) once daily[4]<br>**(FDA approved for and recommended for use in children ≥5 years)** | 10 mg (two 5-mg inhalations) once daily |
| Intravenous peramivir[5] | Treatment (1 day) | (2–12 years of age) One 12-mg/kg dose, up to 600 mg maximum, via IV infusion for a minimum of 15 minutes[5]<br>**(FDA approved and recommended for use in children ≥2 years)** | (≥13 years) 600 mg dose via IV infusion for 15–30 minutes[5] |
| Oral baloxavir | Treatment (1 day) | **Weight 40 to <80 kg:** one 40 mg dose<br>**Weight ≥80 kg:** one 80 mg dose<br>**(FDA approved for use in children ≥12 years)** | |

[1] Oral oseltamivir is approved by the FDA for treatment of acute uncomplicated influenza within 2 days of illness onset with twice-daily dosing in people aged ≥14 days and for prophylaxis with once-daily dosing in people aged ≥1 year. Although not part of the FDA-approved indications, use of oral oseltamivir for treatment of influenza in infants <14 days old, and for prophylaxis in infants 3 months to 1 year of age, is recommended by CDC and the American Academy of Pediatrics (AAP).

[2] This is the FDA-approved oral oseltamivir treatment dose for infants aged ≥14 days and <1 year old and provides oseltamivir exposure in children similar to that achieved by the approved dose of 75 mg orally twice daily for adults, as shown in 2 studies of oseltamivir pharmacokinetics in children. The AAP recommended an oseltamivir treatment dose of 3.5 mg/kg orally twice daily for infants aged 9–11 months, on the basis of data that indicated that a higher dose of 3.5 mg/kg was needed to achieve the protocol-defined targeted exposure for this cohort as defined in the CASG 114 study. It is unknown whether this higher dose will improve efficacy or prevent the development of antiviral resistance. However, there is no evidence that the 3.5 mg/kg dose is harmful or causes more adverse events to infants in this age group.

[3] Current weight-based dosing recommendations are not appropriate for premature infants. Premature infants might have slower clearance of oral oseltamivir because of immature renal function, and doses recommended for full-term infants might lead to very high drug concentrations in this age group. CDC recommends dosing as also recommended by the American Academy of Pediatrics: 1.0 mg/kg/dose, orally, twice daily, for those <38 weeks postmenstrual age; 1.5 mg/kg/dose, orally, twice daily, for those 38–40 weeks postmenstrual age; 3.0 mg/kg/dose, orally, twice daily, for those >40 weeks postmenstrual age.

[4] Inhaled zanamivir is approved to treat acute uncomplicated influenza within 2 days of illness onset with twice-daily dosing in people aged ≥7 years and for prophylaxis with once-daily dosing in people aged ≥5 years.

[5] Intravenous peramivir is approved for treatment of acute uncomplicated influenza within 2 days of illness onset with a single dose in people aged ≥2 years. Daily dosing for a minimum of 5 days was used in clinical trials of hospitalized patients with influenza.

routine use of antiviral medications for prophylaxis except as one of multiple interventions to control institutional influenza outbreaks. Postexposure prophylaxis should be initiated within 48 hours of exposure and never later than 48 hours, because of the risk of treating infection with a subtherapeutic dose. Alternatively, exposed people can monitor for symptoms and initiate antiviral treatment early after symptoms begin.

CDC recommendations for antiviral use for variant virus infections are similar to seasonal influenza virus infection (www.cdc.gov/flu/professionals/antivirals/index.htm); however, CDC recommends antiviral treatment for all suspected cases of human infection with avian influenza viruses (www.cdc.gov/flu/avianflu/severe-potential.htm). Recommendations for exposure prophylaxis of close contacts of confirmed human infections of avian influenza A(H5N1) and A(H7N9) viruses are available at www.cdc.gov/flu/avianflu/novel-av-chemoprophylaxis-guidance.htm. Postexposure prophylaxis is not routinely recommended for people exposed to birds infected with A(H5N1) or A(H7N9). However, prophylaxis can be considered based on clinical judgment, with consideration given to the type of exposure and to whether the exposed person is at high risk for complications from influenza. If antiviral prophylaxis is initiated, twice daily treatment dosing for oseltamivir or zanamivir is recommended instead of once daily prophylaxis dosing (www.cdc.gov/flu/avianflu/guidance-exposed-persons.htm).

## VACCINES

### Available Vaccine Products and Indications for Use

In the United States, annual vaccination for seasonal influenza is recommended for those aged ≥6 months and is the most effective way to prevent influenza and its complications. Several influenza vaccines are approved for use in the United States (www.cdc.gov/flu/protect/vaccine/vaccines.htm) and can be grouped into categories: inactivated influenza vaccine (IIV), live attenuated influenza vaccine (LAIV), and recombinant influenza vaccine (RIV). For updates and the following season recommendations, providers should access www.cdc.gov/flu/professionals/acip/index.htm. For people for whom more than one type of vaccine is indicated, there is no preference for any particular category. During their first influenza season, children aged 6 months through 8 years require 2 doses of age-appropriate influenza vaccine (given ≥4 weeks apart) to induce sufficient immune response.

IIV can be administered by intramuscular injection, transdermally via needle-free jet injector, or intradermal injection depending on the product. IIVs are labeled for use in people aged ≥6 months, but specific age indications vary by manufacturer and product; label instructions should be followed. High-dose IIV and adjuvanted IIV vaccines, which may elicit higher levels of antibodies than standard-dose vaccines, are available for people aged ≥65 years. RIV is labeled for use in people aged ≥18 years. Cell-based inactivated vaccines are licensed for people aged ≥4 years. LAIV is administered as a nasal spray and is labeled for use in people aged 2–49 years.

Influenza vaccine composition can be trivalent, protecting against 3 different influenza viruses (2 influenza subtype A and 1 type influenza B), or quadrivalent, with protection against 4 different influenza viruses (2 influenza A subtypes and 2 influenza type B lineages). Quadrivalent vaccine includes a representative strain from 2 antigenically distinct influenza B lineages, B-Yamagata and B-Victoria.

CDC recommends that everyone aged ≥6 months get vaccinated yearly. Any traveler, including people at high risk for complications of influenza who did not receive the current seasonal influenza vaccine and who are traveling to parts of the world where influenza activity is ongoing, should consider influenza vaccination ≥2 weeks before departure.

No information is available about the benefits of revaccinating people before summer travel who were vaccinated during the preceding fall, and revaccination is not recommended. People at higher risk for influenza complications should consult with their health care provider to discuss the risk for influenza or other travel-related diseases before traveling during the summer.

Seasonal influenza vaccines are not expected to provide protection against human infection with animal-origin influenza viruses, including avian influenza A(H5N1 and H7N9) viruses. No commercially available influenza vaccines are available to protect against avian or swine influenza viruses.

## Vaccine Safety and Adverse Reactions

### INACTIVATED INFLUENZA VACCINE (IIV)

The most frequent side effects of vaccination with intramuscular and intradermal IIV in adults are soreness and redness at the vaccination site. These local injection-site reactions are slightly more common with vaccine administered intradermally, with needle-free jet injection and with high-dose IIV. They generally are mild and rarely interfere with the ability to conduct usual activities. Fever, malaise, myalgia, headache, and other systemic symptoms sometimes occur after vaccination; these may be more frequent in people with no previous exposure to the influenza virus antigens in the vaccine (such as young children) and are generally short-lived.

Guillain-Barré syndrome (GBS) was associated with the 1976 swine influenza vaccine, with an increased risk of 1 additional case of GBS per 100,000 people vaccinated. None of the studies of influenza vaccines other than the 1976 influenza vaccine has demonstrated a risk of GBS of similar magnitude. If there is an increased risk of GBS after seasonal influenza vaccines, it is small, approximately 1–2 additional cases per 1 million people vaccinated.

## Live Attenuated Influenza Vaccine (LAIV)

The most frequent side effects of LAIV reported in healthy adults include minor upper respiratory symptoms, runny nose, and sore throat, which are generally well tolerated. Some children and adolescents have reported fever, vomiting, myalgia, and wheezing. These symptoms, particularly fever, are more often associated with the first administered LAIV dose and are self-limited.

Children aged 2–4 years who have a history of wheezing in the past year or who have a diagnosis of asthma should not receive LAIV. Children and adults aged 2–49 years who have conditions that increase the risk of severe influenza, including pregnancy and immunocompromising conditions, should receive IIV or RIV and not LAIV. Caretakers of severely immunocompromised people should also not receive LAIV or should avoid contact with such people for 7 days after receipt of LAIV to decrease the risk of live virus transmission.

## Recombinant Influenza Vaccine (RIV)

The first RIV was licensed in the United States in January 2013. Limited postmarketing safety data are available, but prelicensure safety data indicate that the most common reactions were headache, fatigue, and myalgia. RIV is not indicated for people <18 years.

## Precautions and Contraindications

Influenza vaccine is contraindicated in people who have had a previous severe allergic reaction to influenza vaccine, regardless of which vaccine component was responsible for the reaction. Immediate hypersensitivity reactions (such as hives, angioedema, allergic asthma, and systemic anaphylaxis) rarely occur after influenza vaccination. These reactions likely result from hypersensitivity to vaccine components, one of which is residual egg protein. People with a history of egg allergy who have experienced only hives after exposure to eggs can receive any licensed and recommended influenza vaccine for their age and health status. Vaccine options are also available for people with a history of egg allergy with a history of severe reaction to egg; these are outlined at www.cdc.gov/flu/professionals/vaccination/vax-summary.htm#egg-allergy.

## PERSONAL PROTECTION MEASURES

Measures that may help prevent influenza virus infection and other infections during travel include avoiding close contact with sick people and washing hands often with soap and water (where soap and a safe source of water are not available, use of an alcohol-based hand sanitizer containing ≥60% alcohol is recommended). No recommendation can be made at this time for mask use by people without influenza illness symptoms outside the health care setting. If people are ill, they can help prevent the spread of illness to others by covering their nose and mouth when coughing and sneezing and avoiding close contact with others. If symptomatic people cannot avoid contact with others, consideration should be given to having them wear a mask when they are in close contact with others (www.cdc.gov/flu/professionals/infectioncontrol/maskguidance.htm).

The best way to prevent infection with animal-origin influenza viruses, including A(H5N1) and A(H7N9), is to follow standard travel safety precautions: follow good hand hygiene and food safety practices and avoid contact with sources of exposure. Most human infections with animal-origin influenza viruses have occurred after direct or close contact with infected poultry or swine. In countries where avian influenza virus outbreaks are occurring, travelers or those living abroad should avoid markets and farms where live animals are sold or raised, avoid contact with sick or dead animals, not eat undercooked or raw animal products (including eggs), and not eat or drink foods or beverages that contain animal blood.

**CDC website:** www.cdc.gov/flu

## BIBLIOGRAPHY

1. CDC. Prevention and control of seasonal influenza with vaccines: recommendations of the Advisory Committee on Immunization Practices, United States, 2017–18 influenza season. MMWR Morb Mortal Wkly Rep. 2017 Aug 25;66(2):1–20. Available from: www.cdc.gov/mmwr/volumes/66/rr/rr6602a1.htm.

2. Committee on Infectious Diseases. Recommendations for prevention and control of influenza in children, 2017–2018. Pediatrics. 2018 Jan;141(1):e20172550. Available from: http://pediatrics.aappublications.org/content/early/2017/09/01/peds.2017-2550

3. Donnelly CA, Finelli L, Cauchemez S, Olsen SJ, Doshi S, Jackson ML, et al. Serial intervals and the temporal distribution of secondary infections within households of 2009 pandemic influenza A(H1N1): implications for influenza control recommendations. Clin Infect Dis. 2011 Jan 1;52 Suppl 1:S123–30.

4. Lai S, Qin Y, Cowling BJ, Ren X, Wardrop NA, Gilbert M, et al. Global epidemiology of avian influenza A H5N1 virus infection in humans, 1997–2015: a systematic review of individual case data. Lancet Infect Dis. 2016 Jul;16(7):e108–18.

5. Merckx J, Wali R, Schiller I, Caya C, Gore GC, Chartrand C, et al. Diagnostic accuracy of novel and traditional rapid tests for influenza infection compared with reverse transcriptase polymerase chain reaction: a systematic review and meta-analysis. Ann Intern Med. 2017 Sep 19;167(6):394–409.

6. Muthuri SG, Venkatesan S, Myles PR, Leonardi-Bee J, Al Khuwaitir TSA, Al Mamun A, et al. Effectiveness of neuraminidase inhibitors in reducing mortality in patients admitted to hospital with influenza A H1N1pdm09 virus infection: a meta-analysis of individual participant data. 2014;2(5):395–404.

7. Rolfes MA, Foppa IM, Garg S, Flannery B, Brammer L, Singleton JA. Annual estimates of the burden of seasonal influenza in the United States: a tool for strengthening influenza surveillance and preparedness. Influenza Other Respir Viruses. 2018 Jan;12(1):132–7.

8. Su S, Gu M, Liu D, Cui J, Gao GF, Zhou J, et al. Epidemiology, evolution, and pathogenesis of H7N9 influenza viruses in five epidemic waves since 2013 in China. Trends Microbiol. 2017 Sep;25(9):713–28.

# JAPANESE ENCEPHALITIS

Susan L. Hills, Nicole P. Lindsey, Marc Fischer

## INFECTIOUS AGENT

Japanese encephalitis (JE) virus is a single-stranded RNA virus that belongs to the genus *Flavivirus* and is closely related to West Nile and Saint Louis encephalitis viruses.

## TRANSMISSION

JE virus is transmitted to humans through the bite of an infected mosquito, primarily *Culex* species. The virus is maintained in an enzootic cycle between mosquitoes and amplifying vertebrate hosts, primarily pigs and wading birds. Humans are incidental or dead-end hosts, because they usually do not develop a level or duration of viremia sufficient to infect mosquitoes.

## EPIDEMIOLOGY

JE virus is the most common vaccine-preventable cause of encephalitis in Asia, occurring throughout most of Asia and parts of the western Pacific (Map 4-7). Transmission principally occurs in rural agricultural areas, often associated with rice cultivation and flood irrigation. In some areas of Asia, these ecologic conditions may occur near, or occasionally within, urban centers. In temperate areas of Asia, transmission is seasonal, and human disease usually peaks in summer and fall. In the subtropics and tropics, seasonal transmission varies with monsoon rains and irrigation practices and may be prolonged or even occur year-round.

In endemic countries, where adults have acquired immunity through natural infection, JE is primarily a disease of children. However, travel-associated JE can occur among people of any age. For most travelers to Asia, the risk for JE is extremely low but varies based on destination, duration, season, and activities.

Before 1973, >300 cases of JE were reported among soldiers from the United States, the United Kingdom, Australia, and Russia. From 1973 through 2017, 84 JE cases among travelers or expatriates from nonendemic countries were published or reported to CDC. From the time a JE vaccine became available in the United States in 1993, through 2017, only 12 JE cases among US travelers were reported to CDC.

The overall incidence of JE among people from nonendemic countries traveling to Asia is estimated to be <1 case per 1 million travelers. However, expatriates and travelers who stay for prolonged periods in rural areas with active JE virus transmission might be at similar risk as the susceptible (pediatric) resident population (6–11 cases per 100,000 children per year). Travelers on even brief trips might be at increased risk if they have extensive outdoor or nighttime exposure in rural areas during periods of active transmission. Shorter-term (for example, <1 month) travelers whose visits are restricted to major urban areas are at minimal risk for JE. In some endemic areas, although there are few human cases among residents because of natural immunity among older people or vaccination, JE virus is still maintained locally in an enzootic cycle between animals and mosquitoes. Therefore, susceptible visitors may be at risk for infection.

## CLINICAL PRESENTATION

Most human infections with JE virus are asymptomatic; <1% of people infected with JE virus develop neurologic disease. Acute encephalitis is the most commonly recognized clinical manifestation of JE virus infection. Milder forms of disease, such as aseptic meningitis or undifferentiated febrile illness, also can occur. The incubation period is 5–15 days. Illness usually begins with sudden onset of fever, headache, and vomiting. Mental status changes, focal neurologic deficits, generalized weakness, and movement disorders may develop over the next few days. The classical description of JE includes a parkinsonian syndrome with mask-like facies, tremor, cogwheel rigidity, and choreoathetoid movements. Acute flaccid paralysis, with clinical and pathological features similar to those of poliomyelitis, has also been associated with JE virus infection. Seizures are common, especially among children. The case-fatality ratio is approximately 20%–30%. Among survivors, 30%–50% have serious neurologic, cognitive, or psychiatric sequelae.

Common clinical laboratory findings include moderate leukocytosis, mild anemia, and hyponatremia. Cerebrospinal fluid (CSF) typically has a mild to moderate pleocytosis with a lymphocytic predominance, slightly elevated protein, and normal ratio of CSF to plasma glucose.

## DIAGNOSIS

JE should be suspected in a patient with evidence of a neurologic infection (such as encephalitis, meningitis, or acute flaccid paralysis) who has recently traveled to or resided

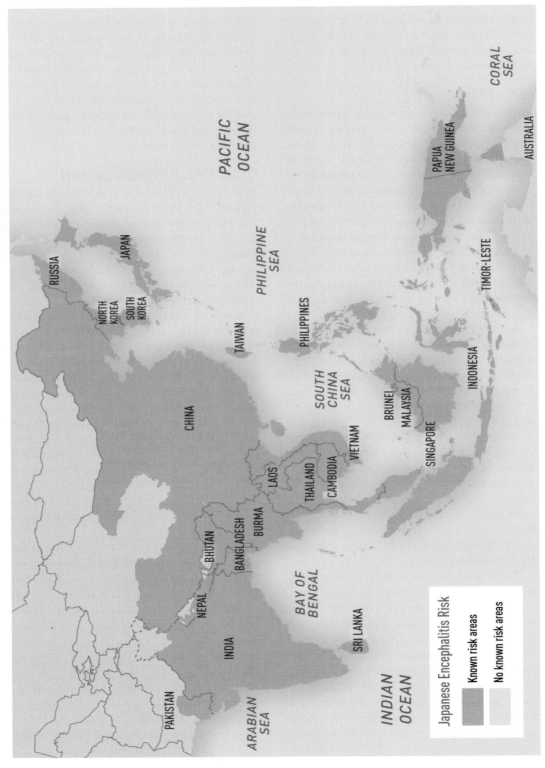

MAP 4-7. Distribution of Japanese encephalitis

**Japanese Encephalitis Risk**
Known risk areas
No known risk areas

in an endemic country in Asia or the western Pacific. Laboratory diagnosis of JE virus infection should be performed by using a JE virus-specific IgM-capture ELISA on CSF or serum. JE virus-specific IgM can be measured in the CSF of most patients by 4 days after onset of symptoms and in serum by 7 days after onset. Plaque reduction neutralization tests can be performed to confirm the presence of JE virus-specific neutralizing antibodies and discriminate between cross-reacting antibodies from closely related flaviviruses (such as dengue and West Nile viruses). A ≥4-fold rise in JE virus-specific neutralizing antibodies between acute- and convalescent-phase serum specimens may be used to confirm recent infection. Vaccination history, date of onset of symptoms, and information regarding other flaviviruses known to circulate in the geographic area that may cross-react in serologic assays need to be considered when interpreting results.

Humans have low levels of transient viremia and usually have neutralizing antibodies by the time distinctive clinical symptoms are recognized. Virus isolation and nucleic acid amplification tests are insensitive in detecting JE virus or viral RNA in blood or CSF and should not be used for ruling out a diagnosis of JE. Clinicians should contact their state or local health department or CDC at 970-221-6400 for assistance with diagnostic testing.

## TREATMENT

There is no specific antiviral treatment for JE; therapy consists of supportive care and management of complications.

## PREVENTION

### Personal Protection Measures

The best way to prevent mosquitoborne diseases, including JE, is to avoid mosquito bites (see Chapter 3, Mosquitoes, Ticks & Other Arthropods).

### Vaccine

One JE vaccine is licensed and available in the United States—an inactivated Vero cell culture–derived vaccine, Ixiaro (Table 4-6). Ixiaro is manufactured by Valneva Austria GmbH. It was approved in March 2009 for use in people aged ≥17 years and in May 2013 for use in children aged 2 months through 16 years. Other inactivated and live attenuated JE vaccines are manufactured and used

## Table 4-6. Vaccine to prevent Japanese encephalitis (JE)

| VACCINE | TRADE NAME (MANUFACTURER) | AGE | DOSE | ROUTE | SCHEDULE | BOOSTER[1] |
|---------|---------------------------|-----|------|-------|----------|------------|
| JE vaccine, inactivated | Ixiaro (Valneva) | 2 mo-2 y | 0.25 mL | IM | 0, 28 d | ≥1 y after primary series |
| | | 3-17 y | 0.5 mL | IM | 0, 28 d | ≥1 y after primary series |
| | | 18-65 y | 0.5 mL | IM | 0, 7-28 d | ≥1 year after primary series |
| | | >65 y | 0.5 mL | IM | 0, 28 d | ≥1 year after primary series |

Abbreviations: IM, intramuscular.
[1] If potential for JE virus exposure continues.

in other countries but are not licensed for use in the United States.

## INDICATIONS FOR USE OF JE VACCINE FOR TRAVELERS

Travelers to JE-endemic countries should be advised of the risks of JE disease and the importance of personal protective measures to reduce the risk for mosquito bites. When making recommendations regarding the use of JE vaccine for travelers, clinicians must consider the risks related to the specific travel itinerary, likelihood of future travel to JE-endemic countries, the high rate of death and disability when JE occurs, availability of an effective vaccine, the possibility but low probability of serious adverse events after immunization, and the traveler's personal perception and tolerance of risk. Evaluation of a traveler's risk should take into account travel location, duration, activities, accommodations, and seasonal patterns of disease in the areas to be visited (Table 4-7). The data in the table should be interpreted cautiously, because JE virus transmission activity varies within countries and from year to year, and surveillance data are often incomplete. Additional information on factors that increase risk is provided in "Japanese encephalitis vaccine: recommendations of the Advisory Committee on Immunization Practices (ACIP)" (www.cdc.gov/vaccines/hcp/acip-recs/vacc-specific/je.html).

The Advisory Committee on Immunization Practices recommends JE vaccine for people moving to a JE-endemic country, longer-term (for example, ≥1 month) travelers to JE-endemic arears, and frequent travelers to JE-endemic areas. Vaccine should also be considered for shorter-term (for example, <1 month) travelers with an increased risk of JE based on planned travel duration, season, location, activities, and accommodations. Vaccination should also be considered for travelers going to endemic areas, but who are uncertain of specific destinations, activities, or duration of travel.

JE vaccine is not recommended for travelers with very low-risk itineraries, such as shorter-term travel limited to urban areas or travel that occurs outside a well-defined JE virus transmission season.

## VACCINE EFFICACY AND IMMUNOGENICITY

There are no efficacy data for Ixiaro. The vaccine was licensed in the United States on the basis of its ability to induce JE virus–neutralizing antibodies as a surrogate for protection. In pivotal immunogenicity studies, 96% of adults and 100% of children aged 2 months through 17 years developed protective neutralizing antibodies at 28 days after receiving a primary immunization series of 2 doses administered 28 days apart. Among adults aged ≥65 years, 65% are seroprotected at 42 days after the 2-dose primary series.

A study in adults on persistence of protective neutralizing antibodies after a primary 2-dose series of Ixiaro showed that at 5 years postvaccination, 82% of subjects were seroprotected. However, the study was conducted in areas where tickborne encephalitis (TBE) vaccine is available. In a subgroup analysis, seroprotection rates at 24–60 months in the TBE vaccine group ranged from 94%–100%, compared with 64%–72% in the group in which TBE vaccine was not administered. TBE vaccine is not available in the United States; therefore, JE seroprotection rates for US travelers are likely to be most similar to the rates in the group not administered TBE vaccine.

One observational study investigated long-term protection following a booster dose of Ixiaro in adults. After a booster dose administered at 15 months, 96% of subjects were still seroprotected approximately 6 years later.

In a study conducted among children in a JE-endemic country, 90% of children were seroprotected at 36 months after the primary series. Seroprotection rates were variable by age group, but at least 81% of children in each age group were seroprotected. Among 150 children in this study who received a booster dose at 11 months after the primary series, 100% were seroprotected at 1 month, 12 months, and 24 months after the booster dose. In a study conducted among children from nonendemic countries, 89% were seroprotected at 3 years after a primary 2-dose series of Ixiaro.

## Table 4-7. Risk areas and transmission season for Japanese encephalitis (JE), by country[1,2,3]

| COUNTRY | RISK AREAS | TRANSMISSION SEASON | COMMENTS |
|---------|-----------|---------------------|----------|
| **Australia** | Outer Torres Strait Islands, northern Cape York | December–May; all human cases reported February–April | Rare cases reported from Outer Torres Strait Islands and 1 case previously reported from northern Queensland mainland Vaccine only recommended for Outer Torres Strait Islands |
| **Bangladesh** | Widespread | Year-round with most cases reported May–November | Cases reported from multiple areas, including Chittagong, Dhaka, Khulna, Rajshahi, Ranjpur, and Sylhet Divisions, so transmission likely countrywide |
| **Bhutan** | Presumed transmission in nonmountainous areas | Unknown | Rare cases reported but limited data Proximity to endemic areas of India and presence of vectors suggests transmission likely |
| **Brunei Darussalam** | Presumed widespread | Unknown | Limited data but outbreak reported in 2013 Proximity to Sarawak, Malaysia suggests ongoing transmission likely |
| **Burma (Myanmar)** | Presumed widespread | Year-round with most cases reported July–September | |
| **Cambodia** | Widespread | Year-round with peak season May–October | Cases reported from majority of provinces, so transmission likely countrywide |
| **China** | All provinces except Xinjiang and Qinghai | Peak season June–October | |
| **India** | Andhra Pradesh, Arunachal Pradesh, Assam, Bihar, Goa, Haryana, Jharkhand, Karnataka, Kerala, Maharashtra, Manipur, Meghalaya, Nagaland, Odisha, Punjab, Tamil Nadu, Telangana, Tripura, Uttar Pradesh, Uttarakhand, West Bengal | Peak season May–November, especially in northern India; the season may be extended or year-round in some areas, especially in southern India | |

(continued)

4

Table 4-7. Risk areas and transmission season for Japanese encephalitis (JE), by country[1,2,3] (continued)

| COUNTRY | RISK AREAS | TRANSMISSION SEASON | COMMENTS |
|---|---|---|---|
| Indonesia | Widespread | Year-round, with peak season varying by island | Cases reported from many islands, including Sumatra, Java, Kalimantan, Bali, Nusa Tenggara, and Papua, so transmission likely on all islands<br>Several traveler cases reported in recent years from Bali |
| Japan | All islands | June–October | Rare sporadic cases reported from all islands except Hokkaido<br>Enzootic transmission without reported human cases on Hokkaido |
| Lao People's Democratic Republic | Widespread | Year-round with peak season June–September | |
| Malaysia | Widespread | Year-round, with peak season in Sarawak from October–December | Much higher rates of disease reported from Sarawak than peninsular Malaysia |
| Nepal | Southern lowlands (Terai), some hill and mountain districts | Peak season June–October | Highest rates of disease reported from southern lowlands (Terai)<br>Vaccine not routinely recommended for those trekking in high-altitude areas |
| North Korea | Presumed widespread | Unknown<br>Proximity to South Korea suggests peak transmission May–November | |
| Pakistan | Unknown | Unknown | Very limited data<br>Rare cases reported from Sindh Province |
| Papua New Guinea | Widespread | Presumed year-round | Sporadic cases reported from Western Province, serologic evidence of disease from Gulf and Southern Highland Provinces, and 1 case reported from near Port Moresby, so transmission likely countrywide |

4

| | | | |
|---|---|---|---|
| **Philippines** | Widespread | Year-round with peak season April–August | Human, animal, and mosquito studies have indicated transmission in 32 provinces, so transmission likely on all islands |
| **Russia** | Primorsky Krai | June–September | Cases previously reported from Primorsky Krai<br>Vaccine not routinely recommended |
| **Singapore** | Presumed in focal areas | Year-round | Very rare sporadic cases reported<br>Vaccine not routinely recommended |
| **South Korea** | Widespread | May–November | |
| **Sri Lanka** | Widespread except in mountainous areas | Year-round with peak season November–February | |
| **Taiwan** | Widespread | Peak season May–October | |
| **Thailand** | Widespread | Year-round with peak season May–October, especially in northern Thailand | Highest rates of disease reported from Chiang Mai Valley<br>Several traveler cases reported in recent years from resort and coastal areas of southern Thailand |
| **Timor-Leste** | Presumed widespread | No data<br>Proximity to West Timor suggests year-round | |
| **Viet Nam** | Widespread | Year-round with peak season May–October, especially in northern Viet Nam | |

[1] Destination and transmission season information should be considered in association with travel duration and activities when making decisions on vaccination.
[2] Data are based on published and unpublished reports. Risk assessments should be performed cautiously, because risk can vary within areas and from year to year, and surveillance data regarding human cases and JE virus transmission are often incomplete. In some endemic areas, human cases among residents are limited because of vaccination or natural immunity among older people. However, because JE virus is maintained in an enzootic cycle between animals and mosquitoes, susceptible visitors to these areas still may be at risk for infection.
[3] Outbreaks previously occurred in the Western Pacific Islands of Guam (1947–1948) and Saipan (1990), but as they are no longer considered risk areas, they are not included in the table.

An accelerated primary series of 2 doses of Ixiaro administered 7 days apart has been studied in adults aged 18–65 years. In the accelerated schedule group, 99% of adults were seroprotected, compared with 100% of adults in the standard schedule group. The accelerated primary series was noninferior to the conventional dosing schedule.

## VACCINE ADMINISTRATION

The primary vaccination dose and schedule for Ixiaro varies by age (Table 4-6). To administer a 0.25-mL dose, health care providers must expel and discard half of the volume from the 0.5-mL prefilled syringe by pushing the plunger stopper up to the edge of the red line on the syringe barrel before injection. For all age groups, the 2-dose series should be completed ≥1 week before travel.

## BOOSTER DOSES

For adults and children, a booster dose (third dose) should be given at ≥1 year after completion of the primary Ixiaro series if ongoing exposure or reexposure to JE virus is expected.

There are limited data on the use of Ixiaro as a booster dose after a primary series with the mouse brain–derived inactivated JE vaccine. Three studies have been conducted, 2 in US military personnel and the other at 2 travel clinics in Europe. In 1 US military study and the European study, among adults who had previously received at least a primary series of mouse brain–derived inactivated JE vaccine, a single dose of Ixiaro adequately boosted neutralizing antibody levels and provided at least short-term protection. In 1 US military study investigating longer-term protection, the immunologic response at 12–23 months after 1 dose of Ixiaro in adults previously vaccinated with ≥3 doses of mouse brain–derived JE vaccine was

noninferior to the response after 2 doses of Ixiaro in JE vaccine-naïve adults. In addition, seroprotective titers against both vaccine virus strains persisted in all participants who could be followed up at 2 years in the European study (N = 18).

## VACCINE SAFETY AND ADVERSE REACTIONS

Ixiaro was licensed in the United States based on safety evaluations in almost 5,000 adults. Since licensure, >1 million doses of Ixiaro have been distributed in the United States. Local symptoms of pain and tenderness were the most commonly reported symptoms in a safety study with 1,993 adult participants who received 2 doses of Ixiaro. Headache, myalgia, fatigue, and an influenzalike illness were each reported at a rate of >10%. In children, fever was the most commonly reported systemic reaction in studies. Serious adverse events are reported only rarely.

## PRECAUTIONS AND CONTRAINDICATIONS

A severe allergic reaction after a previous dose of Ixiaro or any other JE vaccine, or to any component of Ixiaro, is a contraindication to administration of Ixiaro. Ixiaro contains protamine sulfate, a compound known to cause hypersensitivity reactions in some people. No studies of Ixiaro in pregnant women have been conducted. Pregnancy is a precaution for use of Ixiaro and in most instances, its administration to pregnant women should be deferred. However, pregnant women who must travel to an area where risk for JE virus infection is high should be vaccinated when the theoretical risk of immunization is outweighed by the risk of infection.

**CDC website:** www.cdc.gov/japaneseencephalitis

## BIBLIOGRAPHY

1. Dubischar KL, Kadlecek V, Sablan JB, Borja-Tabora CF, Gatchalian S, Eder-Lingelbach S, et al. Immunogenicity of the inactivated Japanese encephalitis virus vaccine Ixiaro in children from a Japanese encephalitis virus-endemic region. Pediatr Infect Dis J. 2017 Sep;36(9):898–904.

2. Dubischar KL, Kadlecek V, Sablan B Jr, Borja-Tabora CF, Gatchalian S, Eder-Lingelbach S, et al. Safety of the inactivated Japanese encephalitis virus vaccine Ixiaro in children: an open-label, randomized, active-controlled, phase 3 study. Pediatr Infect Dis J. 2017 Sep;36(9):889–97.

3. Hills SL, Walter EB, Atmar RL, Fischer M. Japanese encephalitis vaccine: recommendations of the Advisory Committee on Immunization Practices (ACIP). MMWR Recomm Rep. 2019. In press.

4. Jelinek T, Cromer MA, Cramer JP, Mills DJ, Lessans K, Gherardin AW, et al. Safety and immunogenicity of an inactivated Vero cell–derived Japanese encephalitis vaccine (Ixiaro, Jespect) in a pediatric population in JE nonendemic countries: an uncontrolled, open-label phase 3 study. Travel Med Infect Dis. 2018 Mar–Apr;22:18–24. doi: 10.1016/j.tmaid.2018.03.003.

5. Jelinek T, Burchard GD, Dieckmann S, Buhler S, Paulke-Korinek M, Nothdurft HD, et al. Short-term immunogenicity and safety of an accelerated

preexposure prophylaxis regimen with Japanese encephalitis vaccine in combination with a rabies vaccine: a phase III, multicenter, observer-blind study. J Travel Med. 2015 Jul-Aug;22(4):225–31.

6. Paulke-Korinek M, Kollaritsch H, Kundi M, Zwazl I, Seidl-Friedrich C, Jelinek T. Persistence of antibodies six years after booster vaccination with inactivated vaccine against Japanese encephalitis. Vaccine. 2015 Jul 9;33(30):3600–4.

7. Rabe IB, Miller ER, Fischer M, Hills SL. Adverse events following vaccination with an inactivated, Vero cell culture-derived Japanese encephalitis vaccine in the United States, 2009–2012. Vaccine. 2015 Jan 29;33(5):708–12.

**4**

# LEGIONELLOSIS (LEGIONNAIRES' DISEASE & PONTIAC FEVER)

Laura A. Cooley

## INFECTIOUS AGENT

Gram-negative bacteria of the genus *Legionella*. Most cases of Legionnaires' disease are caused by *Legionella pneumophila*, but all species of *Legionella* can cause disease.

## TRANSMISSION

The most common route of transmission is by inhalation of aerosolized water containing the bacteria, although transmission can sometimes occur through aspiration of water containing the bacteria. A single episode of possible person-to-person transmission of Legionnaires' disease has been reported.

*Legionella* is ubiquitous in freshwater sources worldwide, but quantities of *Legionella* in these environments are insufficient to cause disease. In the built environment, *Legionella* can amplify in water systems, depending on the conditions. Factors associated with amplification include warm water temperatures (77°F–108°F [25°C–42°C]); water stagnation; presence of scale, sediment, and biofilm in the pipes and fixtures; and absence of disinfectant. To cause disease,

*Legionella* spp. must then be aerosolized and inhaled by a susceptible host. The most common sources of transmission include potable water (via showerheads and faucets), cooling towers, hot tubs, and decorative fountains.

## EPIDEMIOLOGY

*Legionella* growth and transmission can occur anywhere in the world when the right conditions exist. However, capacity for diagnosing and reporting of cases of Legionnaires' disease are most well established in industrialized settings. In the United States, Legionnaires' disease is on the rise; the number of reported Legionnaires' disease cases has increased 350% from 2000 through 2016. Legionnaires' disease cases and outbreaks have been reported worldwide. Large outbreaks associated with cooling towers have been reported in Spain (449 confirmed cases, 2001) and Portugal (377 cases, 2014). In 2015, a cooling tower in Bronx, New York, was associated with 138 cases of Legionnaires' disease. Travel-associated outbreaks are commonly recognized. In 2016–2017, 51 confirmed cases of Legionnaires' disease were associated with travel to Dubai.

Despite the presence of *Legionella* spp. in many aquatic environments, the risk of developing Legionnaires' disease for most people is low. Travelers who are aged >50 years, are current or former smokers, have chronic lung conditions, or are immunocompromised are at increased risk for infection when exposed to aerosolized water containing *Legionella* spp. Travel-associated Legionnaires' disease outbreaks can occur in settings such as cruise ships, hotels, and resorts. Approximately 10%–15% of all reported cases of Legionnaires' disease in the United States occur in people who have traveled during the 10 days before symptom onset. Exposures among travelers can occur when a person is in or near a hot tub, showering in a hotel, standing near a decorative fountain, or touring in cities with buildings that have cooling towers. Patients with Legionnaires' disease often do not recall specific water exposures, as they frequently occur during normal activities.

## CLINICAL PRESENTATION

Legionellosis is composed of 2 clinically and epidemiologically distinct syndromes: Legionnaires' disease and Pontiac fever. Legionnaires' disease typically presents with severe pneumonia, which usually requires hospitalization and can be fatal in approximately 10% of cases. Symptom onset occurs 2–10 days (rarely, up to 19 days) after exposure. In outbreak settings, <5% of people exposed to the source of the outbreak develop Legionnaires' disease. Legionnaires' disease accounts for nearly all cases of legionellosis reported in the United States.

Pontiac fever is milder than Legionnaires' disease and presents as an influenzalike illness, with fever, headache, and muscle aches, but no signs of pneumonia. Pontiac fever can affect healthy people, as well as those with underlying illnesses, and symptoms occur within 72 hours of exposure. Nearly all patients fully recover without antibiotic therapy. Up to 95% of people exposed during outbreaks of Pontiac fever can develop symptoms of this disease.

## DIAGNOSIS

The preferred diagnostic tests for Legionnaires' disease are the *Legionella* urinary antigen test and culture of lower respiratory secretions (sputum, bronchoalveolar lavage) on media that supports growth of *Legionella* spp. The most commonly used diagnostic test, the urinary antigen test, only detects *L. pneumophila* serogroup 1; this serogroup accounts for 80%–90% of cases.

Isolation of *Legionella* by culture is important to detect non–*L. pneumophila* serogroup 1 species and serogroups and is necessary to compare clinical to environmental isolates during an outbreak investigation. Diagnosis by PCR of respiratory secretions is a newer, evolving technique. Because of differences in mechanism of disease, *Legionella* spp. cannot be isolated in people who have Pontiac fever. Legionnaires' disease and Pontiac fever are nationally notifiable diseases in the United States.

## TREATMENT

For travelers with suspected Legionnaires' disease, specific antibiotic treatment is necessary and should be administered promptly while diagnostic tests are being processed. Preferred agents include fluoroquinolones and macrolides. In severe cases, patients may have prolonged stays in intensive care units. Consultation with an infectious disease specialist is advised. Pontiac fever is a self-limited illness that requires supportive care only; antibiotics have no benefit.

## PREVENTION

There is no vaccine for Legionnaires' disease, and antibiotic prophylaxis is not effective. Water management programs for building water systems and devices at risk for *Legionella* growth and transmission can lower the potential for illnesses and outbreaks. Travelers at increased risk for infection, such as the elderly or those with immunocompromising conditions such as cancer or diabetes, may choose to avoid high-risk areas such as hot tubs. If exposure cannot be avoided, travelers should seek medical attention promptly if they develop symptoms of Legionnaires' disease or Pontiac fever.

**CDC website:** www.cdc.gov/legionella

## BIBLIOGRAPHY

1. CDC. Surveillance for travel-associated Legionnaires disease—United States, 2005–2006. MMWR Morb Mortal Wkly Rep. 2007 Dec 7;56(48):1261–3.

2. CDC. Vital signs: deficiencies in environmental control identified in outbreaks of Legionnaires' disease—North America, 2000–2014. MMWR Morb Mortal Wkly Rep. 2016 Jun 7;65(22):576–84.

3. Dabrera G, Brandsema P, Lofdahl M, Naik F, Cameron R, et al. Increase in Legionnaires' disease cases associated with travel to Dubai among travelers from the United Kingdom, Sweden, and the Netherlands, October 2016 to end August 2017. Euro Surveill. 2017 Sep;22(38):1–4.

4. de Jong B, Payne Hallstrom L, Robesyn E, Ursut D, Zucs P, Eldsnet. Travel-associated Legionnaires' disease in Europe, 2010. Euro Surveill. 2013;18(23):1–8.

5. George F, Shivaji T, Pinto CS, Serra LAO, Valente J, Albuquerque MJ, et al. A large outbreak of Legionnaires' disease in an industrial town in Portugal. Rev Port Saude Publica. 2016;34(3):199–208.

6. Mouchtouri VA, Rudge JW. Legionnaires' disease in hotels and passenger ships: a systematic review of evidence, sources, and contributing factors. J Travel Med. 2015 Sep–Oct;22(5):325–37.

**4**

# LEISHMANIASIS, CUTANEOUS

Barbara L. Herwaldt, Christine Dubray, Sharon L. Roy

Leishmaniasis is a parasitic disease found in parts of the tropics, subtropics, and southern Europe. Leishmaniasis has several different forms. This section focuses on cutaneous leishmaniasis (CL), the most common form, both in general and in travelers.

## INFECTIOUS AGENT

Leishmaniasis is caused by obligate intracellular protozoan parasites; >20 *Leishmania* species cause CL.

## TRANSMISSION

The parasites that cause CL are transmitted through the bites of infected female phlebotomine sand flies. CL also can occur after accidental occupational (laboratory) exposures to *Leishmania* parasites.

## EPIDEMIOLOGY

In the Old World (Eastern Hemisphere), CL is found in parts of the Middle East, Asia (particularly southwest and central Asia), Africa (particularly the tropical region and North Africa), and southern Europe. In the New World (Western Hemisphere), CL is found in parts of Mexico, Central America, and South America. Occasional cases have been reported in Texas and Oklahoma. CL is not found in Chile, Uruguay, or Canada. Overall, CL is found in focal areas of approximately 90 countries. More information is available at www.who.int/leishmaniasis/burden/endemic-priority-alphabetical/en.

The geographic distribution of cases of CL evaluated in countries such as the United States reflects travel and immigration patterns, such as travel to popular tourist destinations in Latin America (Costa Rica, for example). Cases of CL in US service personnel have reflected military activities (such as in Afghanistan and Iraq). CL is usually more common in rural than urban areas, but it is found in some periurban and urban areas (such as in Kabul, Afghanistan). The ecologic settings range from rainforests to arid regions.

The risk is highest from dusk to dawn because sand flies typically feed (bite) at night and during twilight hours. Although sand flies are less active during the hottest time of the day, they may bite if they are disturbed (for example, if people brush against tree trunks or other sites where sand flies are resting). Vector activity can easily be overlooked: sand flies do not make noise, they are small, and their bites might not be noticed.

Examples of types of travelers who might have an increased risk for CL include ecotourists, adventure travelers, bird watchers, Peace Corps volunteers, missionaries, military personnel, construction workers, and people who do research outdoors at night or twilight. However, even short-term travelers in leishmaniasis-endemic areas have developed CL.

## CLINICAL PRESENTATION

CL is characterized by skin lesions (open or closed sores), which typically develop within several weeks or months after exposure. In some people, the sores first appear months or years later, in the context of trauma (such as skin wounds or surgery). The sores can change in size and appearance over time. They typically progress from small papules to nodular plaques, and often lead to open sores with a raised border and central crater (ulcer), which can be covered with scales or crust. The lesions usually are painless but can be painful, particularly if open sores become infected with bacteria. Satellite lesions, regional lymphadenopathy, and nodular lymphangitis can be noted. The sores usually heal eventually, even without treatment. However, they can last for months or years and typically result in scarring.

A potential concern applies to some *Leishmania* species in South and Central America: some parasites might spread from the skin to the mucosal surfaces of the nose or mouth and cause sores there. This form of leishmaniasis, mucosal leishmaniasis (ML), might not be noticed until years after the original skin sores appear to have healed. Although ML is uncommon, it has occurred in travelers and expatriates, including in people whose cases of CL were not treated or were inadequately treated. The initial clinical manifestations typically involve the nose (chronic stuffiness, bleeding, and inflamed mucosa or sores) and less often the mouth; in advanced cases, ulcerative destruction of the nose, mouth, pharynx, and larynx can be noted (such as perforation of the nasal septum).

## DIAGNOSIS

Clinicians should consider CL in people with chronic (nonhealing) skin lesions who have been in areas where leishmaniasis is found. Laboratory confirmation of the diagnosis is achieved by detecting *Leishmania* parasites (or DNA) in infected tissue, through light-microscopic examination of stained specimens, culture techniques, or molecular methods.

CDC can assist in all aspects of the diagnostic evaluation. Identification of the *Leishmania* species can be important, particularly if >1 species is found where the patient traveled and if the species can have different clinical and prognostic implications. Serologic testing generally is not useful for CL but can provide supportive evidence for the diagnosis of ML.

For consultative services, contact CDC Parasitic Diseases Inquiries (404-718-4745; parasites@cdc.gov) or see www.cdc.gov/dpdx.

## TREATMENT

Decisions about whether and how to treat CL should be individualized, including whether to use a systemic (oral or parenteral) medication rather than a local or topical approach. All cases of ML should be treated with systemic therapy. Clinicians may consult with CDC staff about the relative merits of various approaches to treat CL and ML (see the Diagnosis section above for contact information). The response to a particular regimen may vary not only among *Leishmania* species but also for the same species in different geographic regions.

The oral agent miltefosine is FDA-approved to treat CL caused by 3 New World species in the *Viannia* subgenus [*Leishmania* (*V.*) *braziliensis*, *L.* (*V.*) *panamensis*, and *L.* (*V.*) *guyanensis*], as well as for ML caused by *L.* (*V.*) *braziliensis*, in adults and adolescents ≥12 years of age who weigh ≥30 kg and are not pregnant or breastfeeding during therapy or for 5 months thereafter. Miltefosine is available in the United States via www.profounda.com.

Various parenteral options (including liposomal amphotericin B) are commercially available, although not FDA-approved to treat CL or ML. The pentavalent antimonial compound sodium stibogluconate (Pentostam) is available to US-licensed physicians through the CDC Drug Service (404-639-3670) for intravenous or intramuscular administration under an investigational new drug protocol (see www.cdc.gov/laboratory/drugservice).

## PREVENTION

No vaccines or drugs to prevent infection are available. Preventive measures are aimed at reducing contact with sand flies by using personal protective measures (see Chapter 3, Mosquitoes, Ticks & Other Arthropods). Travelers should be advised to:

- Avoid outdoor activities, to the extent possible, especially from dusk to dawn, when sand flies generally are the most active.

- Wear protective clothing and apply insect repellent to exposed skin and under the edges of clothing, such as sleeves and pant legs, according to the manufacturer's instructions.

- Sleep in air-conditioned or well-screened areas. Spraying the quarters with insecticide might provide some protection. Fans or ventilators might inhibit the movement of sand flies, which are weak fliers.

Sand flies are so small (approximately 2–3 mm, less than one-eighth of an inch) that they can pass through the holes in ordinary bed nets. Although closely woven nets are available, they may be uncomfortable in hot climates. The effectiveness of bed nets can be enhanced by treatment with a pyrethroid-containing insecticide. The same treatment can be applied to window screens, curtains, bed sheets, and clothing.

**CDC website:** www.cdc.gov/parasites/ leishmaniasis

## BIBLIOGRAPHY

1. Aronson N, Herwaldt BL, Libman M, Pearson R, Lopez-Velez R, Weina P, et al. Diagnosis and treatment of leishmaniasis: clinical practice guidelines by the Infectious Diseases Society of America (IDSA) and the American Society of Tropical Medicine and Hygiene (ASTMH). Clin Infect Dis. 2016 Dec;63(12):e202–64.

2. Blum J, Buffet P, Visser L, Harms G, Bailey MS, Caumes E, et al. LeishMan recommendations for treatment of cutaneous and mucosal leishmaniasis in travelers, 2014. J Travel Med. 2014 Mar–Apr;21(2):116–29.

3. Blum J, Lockwood DN, Visser L, Harms G, Bailey MS, Caumes E, et al. Local or systemic treatment for New World cutaneous leishmaniasis? Re-evaluating the evidence for the risk of mucosal leishmaniasis. Int Health. 2012 Sep;4(3):153–63.

4. Hodiamont CJ, Kager PA, Bart A, de Vries HJ, van Thiel PP, Leenstra T, et al. Species-directed therapy for leishmaniasis in returning travellers: a comprehensive guide. PLoS Negl Trop Dis. 2014 May;8(5):e2832.

5. Karimkhani C, Wanga V, Coffeng LE, Naghavi P, Dellavalle RP, Naghavi M. Global burden of cutaneous leishmaniasis: a cross-sectional analysis from the Global Burden of Disease Study 2013. Lancet Infect Dis. 2016 May;16(5):584–91.

6. Murray HW. Leishmaniasis in the United States: treatment in 2012. Am J Trop Med Hyg. 2012 Mar;86(3):434–40.

7. World Health Organization. Control of the leishmaniases. Geneva: World Health Organization; 2010 [cited 2018 Mar 7]. Available from: http://apps.who.int/iris/bitstream/10665/44412/1/WHO_TRS_949_eng.pdf.

8. World Health Organization. Global leishmaniasis update, 2006–2015: a turning point in leishmaniasis surveillance. Wkly Epidemiol Rec. 2017 Sep;92(38):557–65.

# LEISHMANIASIS, VISCERAL

Barbara L. Herwaldt, Sharon L. Roy

Leishmaniasis is a parasitic disease found in parts of the tropics, subtropics, and southern Europe. Leishmaniasis has several different forms. This section focuses on visceral leishmaniasis (VL), which affects some of the internal organs of the body (such as the spleen, liver, and bone marrow).

## INFECTIOUS AGENT

VL is caused by obligate intracellular protozoan parasites, particularly by the species *Leishmania donovani* and *L. infantum* (considered synonymous with *L. chagasi*).

## TRANSMISSION

The parasites that cause VL are transmitted through the bite of infected female phlebotomine sand flies. Congenital and parenteral transmission (through blood transfusions and needle sharing) have been reported.

## EPIDEMIOLOGY

VL is usually more common in rural than urban areas, but it is found in some periurban areas (such as in northeastern Brazil). In the Old World (Eastern Hemisphere), VL is found in parts of Asia (particularly the Indian subcontinent and southwest and central Asia), the Middle East, Africa (particularly East Africa), and southern Europe. In the New World (Western Hemisphere), most cases occur in Brazil; some cases occur in scattered foci elsewhere in Latin America. Overall, VL is found in focal areas of >70 countries, with most (>90%) of the world's cases in the Indian subcontinent (India, Bangladesh, and Nepal), East Africa (Sudan, South Sudan, Ethiopia, Somalia, and Kenya), and Brazil. More information is available at www.who.int/leishmaniasis/burden/endemic-priority-alphabetical/en.

The geographic distribution of cases of VL evaluated in countries such as the United States reflects travel and immigration patterns. VL is uncommon in US travelers and expatriates. Occasional cases have been diagnosed in short-term travelers (tourists) to southern Europe and also in longer-term travelers (such as expatriates and deployed soldiers) to the Mediterranean region and other areas where VL is found.

## CLINICAL PRESENTATION

Among symptomatic people, the incubation period typically ranges from weeks to months. The onset of illness can be abrupt or gradual. Stereotypical manifestations of VL include fever, weight loss, hepatosplenomegaly (especially splenomegaly), and pancytopenia (anemia, leukopenia, and thrombocytopenia). If untreated, severe (advanced) cases of VL typically are fatal. Latent infection can become clinically manifest years to decades after exposure in people who become immunocompromised (such as HIV infection, immunosuppressive therapy, or biologic immunomodulatory therapy).

## DIAGNOSIS

Clinicians should consider VL in people with a relevant travel history (even in the distant past) and a persistent, unexplained febrile illness, especially if accompanied by other suggestive manifestations (such as splenomegaly and pancytopenia). Laboratory confirmation of the diagnosis is achieved by detecting *Leishmania* parasites (or DNA) in infected tissue (such as in bone marrow, liver, lymph node, or blood), through light-microscopic examination of stained specimens, culture techniques, or molecular methods. Serologic testing can provide supportive evidence for the diagnosis.

CDC can assist in all aspects of the diagnostic evaluation, including species identification. For consultative services, contact CDC Parasitic Diseases Inquiries (404-718-4745; parasites@cdc.gov) or see www.cdc.gov/dpdx.

## TREATMENT

Infected people should be advised to consult an infectious disease or tropical medicine specialist. Therapy for VL should be individualized with expert consultation. The relative merits of various approaches can be discussed with CDC staff (see the Diagnosis section above for contact information).

Liposomal amphotericin B (AmBisome) is approved by the Food and Drug Administration (FDA) to treat VL and generally constitutes the drug of choice for US patients. The oral agent miltefosine is FDA approved to treat VL in patients who are infected with *L. donovani*, are ≥12 years of age, weigh ≥30 kg, and are not pregnant or breastfeeding during therapy or for 5 months thereafter; the drug is available in the United States via www.profounda.com. The pentavalent antimonial compound sodium stibogluconate (Pentostam) is available to US-licensed physicians through the CDC Drug Service (404-639-3670) for parenteral administration under an investigational new drug protocol (see www.cdc.gov/laboratory/drugservice).

## PREVENTION

No vaccines or drugs to prevent infection are available. Preventive measures are aimed at reducing contact with sand flies (see Chapter 3, Mosquitoes, Ticks & Other Arthropods; and Prevention in the previous section, Cutaneous Leishmaniasis). Preventive measures include minimizing outdoor activities, to the extent possible, especially from dusk to dawn, when sand flies generally are the most active; wearing protective clothing; applying insect repellent to exposed skin; using bed nets treated with a pyrethroid-containing insecticide; and spraying dwellings with residual-action insecticides.

**CDC website:** www.cdc.gov/parasites/leishmaniasis

### BIBLIOGRAPHY

1. Aronson N, Herwaldt BL, Libman M, Pearson R, Lopez-Velez R, Weina P, et al. Diagnosis and treatment of leishmaniasis: clinical practice guidelines by the Infectious Diseases Society of America (IDSA) and the American Society of Tropical Medicine and Hygiene (ASTMH). Clin Infect Dis. 2016 Dec;63(12):e202–64.

2. Fletcher K, Issa R, Lockwood DN. Visceral leishmaniasis and immunocompromise as a risk factor for the development of visceral leishmaniasis: a changing pattern at the hospital for tropical diseases, London. PLoS One. 2015;10(4):e0121418.

3. Murray HW. Leishmaniasis in the United States: treatment in 2012. Am J Trop Med Hyg. 2012 Mar;86(3):434–40.

4. van Griensven J, Carrillo E, Lopez-Velez R, Lynen L, Moreno J. Leishmaniasis in immunosuppressed individuals. Clin Microbiol Infect. 2014 Apr;20(4):286–99.

5. World Health Organization. Control of the leishmaniases. Geneva: World Health Organization; 2010 [cited 2018 Mar 7]. Available from: http://apps.who.int/iris/bitstream/10665/44412/1/WHO_TRS_949_eng.pdf.

6. World Health Organization. Global leishmaniasis update, 2006–2015: a turning point in leishmaniasis surveillance. Wkly Epidemiol Rec. 2017 Sep;92(38):557–65.

# LEPTOSPIROSIS

Renee L. Galloway, Ilana J. Schafer, Robyn A. Stoddard

## INFECTIOUS AGENT

*Leptospira* spp., the causative agents of leptospirosis, are obligate aerobic, gram-negative spirochete bacteria.

## TRANSMISSION

The infection route is through abrasions or cuts in the skin, or through the conjunctiva and mucous membranes. Humans may be infected by direct contact with urine or reproductive fluids from infected animals, through contact with urine-contaminated water or soil, or by consuming contaminated food or water. Infection rarely occurs through animal bites or human-to-human contact.

## EPIDEMIOLOGY

Leptospirosis has worldwide distribution; incidence is higher in tropical climates. The estimated worldwide annual incidence is >1 million cases, including approximately 59,000 deaths. Regions with the estimated highest morbidity include South and Southeast Asia, Oceania, the Caribbean, parts of sub-Saharan Africa, and parts of Latin America. Outbreaks can occur after heavy rainfall or flooding in endemic areas, especially in urban areas of developing countries, where housing conditions and sanitation are poor. Outbreaks of leptospirosis have occurred in the United States after flooding in Hawaii, Florida, and Puerto Rico. Travelers participating in recreational freshwater activities, such as swimming or boating, are at increased risk, particularly after heavy rainfall or flooding. Prolonged exposure to contaminated water and activities that involve head immersion or swallowing water increase the risk of infection.

## CLINICAL PRESENTATION

The incubation period is 2–30 days, and illness usually occurs 5–14 days after exposure. While most infections are thought to be asymptomatic, clinical illness can present as a self-limiting acute febrile illness, estimated to occur in approximately 90% of clinical infections, or as a severe, potentially fatal illness with multiorgan dysfunction in 5%–10% of patients. In patients who progress to severe disease, the illness can be biphasic, with a temporary decrease in fever between phases. The acute, septicemic phase (approximately 7 days) presents as an acute febrile illness with symptoms including headache (can be severe and include retroorbital pain and photophobia), chills, myalgia (characteristically involving the calves and lower back), conjunctival suffusion (characteristic of leptospirosis but not occurring in all cases), nausea, vomiting, diarrhea, abdominal pain, cough, and rarely, a skin rash. The second or immune phase is characterized by antibody production and the presence of leptospires in the urine. In patients who progress to severe disease, symptoms can include jaundice, renal failure, hemorrhage, aseptic meningitis, cardiac arrhythmias, pulmonary insufficiency, and hemodynamic collapse. The classically described syndrome, Weil' disease, consists of renal and liver failure and has a case-fatality ratio of 5%–15%. Severe pulmonary hemorrhagic syndrome is a rare but severe form of leptospirosis that can have a case-fatality ratio >50%. Poor prognostic indicators include older age and development of altered mental status, respiratory insufficiency, or oliguria.

## DIAGNOSIS

Diagnosis of leptospirosis is usually based on serology; microscopic agglutination test (MAT), the reference standard, is best performed on paired acute and convalescent serum samples, and can only be performed at certain reference laboratories. Detection of the organism in blood or cerebrospinal fluid (for patients with meningitis) using real-time PCR can provide a more timely diagnosis during the acute, septicemic phase, and PCR can also be performed on urine after the first week of illness. Various serologic screening tests are available, including ELISA and multiple rapid diagnostic tests; the use of IgM-specific serologic screening tests is recommended, and positive screening tests should be confirmed with MAT. Culture is insensitive and slow and therefore not recommended as the sole diagnostic method. The Zoonoses and Select Agent Laboratory at CDC performs MAT and PCR for diagnosis of leptospirosis as well as culture identification and genotyping of isolates: www.cdc.gov/ncezid/dhcpp/bacterial_special/zoonoses_lab.html. Leptospirosis is a nationally notifiable disease—the Council for State and Territorial Epidemiologists' case definition can be found at wwwn.cdc.gov/nndss/conditions/leptospirosis/case-definition/2013.

## TREATMENT

Early antimicrobial therapy can be effective in decreasing the severity and duration of leptospirosis and should be initiated as soon as possible, without waiting for diagnostic test results, if leptospirosis is suspected. For patients with mild symptoms, doxycycline is a drug of choice (100 mg orally, twice daily), unless contraindicated; alternative options include ampicillin and amoxicillin. Intravenous penicillin (1.5 MU every 6 hours) is a drug of choice for patients with severe leptospirosis, and ceftriaxone was shown to be equally effective (1 g IV, once daily). As with other spirochetal diseases, antibiotic treatment of patients with leptospirosis may cause a Jarisch-Herxheimer reaction; however, this is rarely fatal. Patients with severe leptospirosis may require hospitalization and supportive therapy, including intravenous hydration and electrolyte supplementation, dialysis in the case of oliguric renal failure, and mechanical ventilation in the case of respiratory failure.

4

## PREVENTION

No vaccine is available in the United States. Travelers who might be at an increased risk for infection should be educated on exposure risks and advised to consider preventive measures such as chemoprophylaxis; wearing protective clothing, especially footwear; and covering cuts and abrasions with occlusive dressings. Limited studies have shown that chemoprophylaxis with doxycycline (200 mg orally, weekly), begun 1–2 days before and continuing through the period of exposure, might be effective in preventing clinical disease in adults and could be considered for people at high risk and with short-term exposures. The best way to prevent infection is to avoid exposure: travelers should avoid contact with potentially contaminated bodies of water, walking in flood waters, and contact with potentially infected animals or their body fluids.

**CDC website:** www.cdc.gov/leptospirosis

### BIBLIOGRAPHY

1. Barragan V, Olivas S, Keim P, Pearson T. Critical knowledge gaps in our understanding of environmental cycling and transmission of Leptospira spp. Appl Environ Microbiol. 2017 Sep 15;83(19).

2. Brett-Major DM, Coldren R. Antibiotics for leptospirosis. Cochrane Database Syst Rev. 2012 Feb 15;(2).

3. Brett-Major DM, Lipnick RJ Antibiotic prophylaxis for leptospirosis. Cochrane Database Syst Rev. 2009 Jul 8;(3):CD007342. doi: 10.1002/14651858.CD007342.pub2.

4. Costa F, Hagan JE, Calcagno J, Kane M, Torgerson P, Martinez-Silveira MS, et al. Global morbidity and mortality of leptospirosis: a systematic review. PLoS Negl Trop Dis. 2015;9(9):e0003898.

5. Galloway RL, Hoffmaster AR. Optimization of LipL32 PCR assay for increased sensitivity in diagnosing leptospirosis. Diagnostic microbiology and infectious disease. 2015 Jul;82(3):199–200.

6. Guerrier G, D'Ortenzio E. Jarisch-Herxheimer reaction among patients with leptospirosis: incidence and risk factors. Am J Trop Med Hyg. 2017 Apr;96(4):791–4.

7. Haake DA, Levett PN. Leptospira Species (Leptospirosis). In: Bennett JE, Dolin R, Blaser MJ, editors. Principles and Practice of Infectious Diseases. 8th ed. Philadelphia, PA: Saunders 2015. p. 2714–20.

8. Haake DA, Levett PN. Leptospirosis in humans. Curr Top Microbiol Immunol. 2015;387:65–97.

9. Jensenius M, Han PV, Schlagenhauf P, Schwartz E, Parola P, Castelli F, et al. Acute and potentially life-threatening tropical diseases in western travelers—a GeoSentinel multicenter study, 1996–2011. Am J Trop Med Hyg. 2013 Feb;88(2):397–404.

10. Picardeau M, Bertherat E, Jancloes M, Skouloudis AN, Durski K, Hartskeerl RA. Rapid tests for diagnosis of leptospirosis: current tools and emerging technologies. Diagn Microbiol Infect Dis. 2014 Jan;78(1):1–8.

# LYME DISEASE

Paul S. Mead

## INFECTIOUS AGENT

Spirochetes belonging to the *Borrelia burgdorferi* sensu lato complex, including *B. afzelii*, *B. burgdorferi* sensu stricto, and *B. garinii*.

## TRANSMISSION

Through the bite of *Ixodes* (blacklegged) ticks, typically, immature (nymphal) ticks. Nymphal ticks are small, about the size of a poppy seed, and elude easy detection. Patients with Lyme disease may be unaware that they had ever been bitten.

## EPIDEMIOLOGY

In Europe, Lyme is endemic from southern Scandinavia into the northern Mediterranean countries of Italy, Spain, and Greece and east from the British Isles into central Russia. Incidence is highest in central and Eastern European countries.

In Asia, infected ticks range from western Russia through Mongolia, northeastern China, and into Japan; however, human infection appears to be uncommon in most of these areas. In North America, highly endemic areas are the northeastern and north-central United States. Transmission has not been documented in the tropics. Lyme disease is occasionally reported in travelers to the United States returning to their home countries; it should be considered in the differential diagnosis of those with consistent symptoms and a history of hiking or camping.

## CLINICAL PRESENTATION

Incubation period is typically 3–30 days. Approximately 80% of people infected with *B. burgdorferi* develop a characteristic rash, erythema migrans (EM), within 30 days of exposure. EM is a red, expanding rash, with or without central clearing, often accompanied by symptoms of fatigue, fever, headache, mild stiff neck, arthralgia, or myalgia. Within days or weeks, infection can spread to other parts of the body, causing more serious neurologic conditions (meningitis, radiculopathy, and facial palsy) or cardiac abnormalities (myocarditis with atrioventricular heart block).

Untreated, infection can progress over a period of months to cause monoarticular or oligoarticular arthritis, peripheral neuropathy, or encephalopathy. These long-term sequelae can be observed to occur over variable periods of time, ranging from 1 week to a few years.

## DIAGNOSIS

Observation of an EM rash with a history of recent travel to an endemic area (with or without history of tick bite) is sufficient. For patients with evidence of disseminated infection (musculoskeletal, neurologic, or cardiac manifestations), 2-tiered serologic testing, consisting of an ELISA/IFA and confirmatory Western blot, is recommended. Patients suspected of becoming infected with Lyme disease while traveling overseas should be tested by using a C6-based ELISA, as other serologic tests may not detect infection with European species of *Borrelia*. Lyme disease is nationally notifiable.

## TREATMENT

Most patients can be treated with oral doxycycline, amoxicillin, or cefuroxime axetil or with intravenous ceftriaxone (see www.cdc.gov/lyme). Diagnosis and management of disseminated infection can be complicated and usually requires referral to an infectious disease, rheumatologist, or other specialist.

## PREVENTION

Avoid tick habitats, use insect repellent on exposed skin and clothing, and carefully check every day for attached ticks. Minimize areas of exposed skin by wearing long-sleeved shirts, long pants, and closed shoes; tucking shirts in and tucking pants into socks can help reduce risk (see Chapter 3, Mosquitoes, Ticks & Other Arthropods).

**CDC website:** www.cdc.gov/lyme

### BIBLIOGRAPHY

1. Hu LT. Lyme disease. Ann Intern Med. 2016 Nov 1;165(9):677.

2. Sanchez E, Vannier E, Wormser GP, Hu LT. Diagnosis, treatment, and prevention of Lyme disease, human granulocytic anaplasmosis, and babesiosis: A review. JAMA. 2016 Apr 26;315(16):1767–77.

3. Steere AC, Strle F, Wormser GP, Hu LT, Branda JA, Hovius JW, Li X, Mead PS. Lyme borreliosis. Nat Rev Dis Primers. 2016 Dec 15;2:16090.

# MALARIA

Kathrine R. Tan, Paul M. Arguin

## INFECTIOUS AGENT

Malaria in humans is caused by protozoan parasites of the genus *Plasmodium*: *Plasmodium falciparum, P. vivax, P. ovale*, or *P. malariae*. In addition, *P. knowlesi*, a parasite of Old World (Eastern Hemisphere) monkeys, has been documented as a cause of human infections and some deaths in Southeast Asia.

## TRANSMISSION

*Plasmodium* species are transmitted by the bite of an infective female *Anopheles* mosquito. Occasionally, transmission occurs by blood transfusion, organ transplantation, needle sharing, nosocomially, or from mother to fetus.

## EPIDEMIOLOGY

Malaria is a major international public health problem; 91 countries reported an estimated 216 million infections and 445,000 deaths in 2016, according to the World Health Organization (WHO) World Malaria Report 2017. Travelers going to malaria-endemic countries are at risk for contracting the disease, and almost all of the approximately 1,700 cases per year of malaria in the United States are imported.

Information about malaria transmission in specific countries is derived from various sources, including WHO (see Chapter 2, Yellow Fever Vaccine & Malaria Prophylaxis Information, by Country). The information presented here was accurate at the time of publication; however, the risk of malaria can change rapidly and from year to year (because of changes in local weather conditions, mosquito vector density, and prevalence of infection). Updated information can be found on the CDC website at www.cdc.gov/malaria.

Malaria transmission occurs in large areas of Africa, Latin America, parts of the Caribbean, Asia (including South Asia, Southeast Asia, and the Middle East), Eastern Europe, and the South Pacific (Maps 4-8 and 4-9).

The risk for acquiring malaria differs substantially from traveler to traveler and from region to region, even within a single country. This variability is a function of the intensity of transmission within the various regions and the itinerary, duration, season, and type of travel. Risk also varies by travelers' adherence to mosquito precautions and prophylaxis recommendations. In 2015, 1,513 cases of malaria (including 11 deaths) were diagnosed in the United States and its territories and were reported to CDC. Of these cases for which country of acquisition was known, 85% were acquired in Africa, 9% in Asia, 5% in the Caribbean and the Americas, and 1% in Oceania or the Middle East.

## CLINICAL PRESENTATION

Malaria is characterized by fever and influenzalike symptoms, including chills, headache, myalgias, and malaise; these symptoms can occur intermittently. In severe disease, seizures, mental confusion, kidney failure, acute respiratory distress syndrome, coma, and death may occur. Malaria symptoms can develop as early as 7 days after being bitten by an infectious mosquito in a malaria-endemic area and as late as several months or more after exposure. Suspected or confirmed malaria, especially *P. falciparum*, is a medical emergency requiring urgent intervention, as clinical deterioration can occur rapidly and unpredictably. See Box 4-3 for frequently asked clinical questions.

## DIAGNOSIS

Travelers who have symptoms of malaria should seek medical evaluation as soon as possible. Consider malaria in any patient with a febrile illness who has recently returned from a malaria-endemic country.

Blood smear microscopy remains the most important method for malaria diagnosis. Microscopy can provide immediate information about the presence of parasites, allow quantification

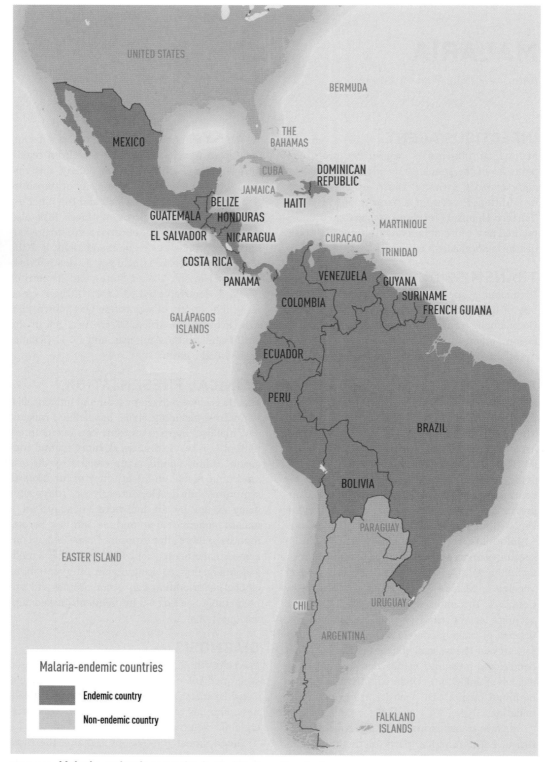

MAP 4-8. **Malaria-endemic countries in the Western Hemisphere**

In this map, countries with areas endemic for malaria are shaded completely even if transmission occurs only in a small part of the country. For more specific within-country malaria transmission information, see Chapter 2, Yellow Fever Vaccine & Malaria Prophylaxis Information, by Country.

# BOX 4-3. Clinician frequently asked questions

**How do I address concerns about side effects from prophylaxis?**

- Prophylaxis can be started earlier if there are concerns about tolerating a particular medication. For example, mefloquine can be started 3–4 weeks in advance to allow potential adverse events to occur before travel. If unacceptable side effects develop, there would be time to change the medication before the traveler's departure.
- The drugs used for antimalarial prophylaxis are generally well tolerated. However, side effects can occur. Minor side effects usually do not require stopping the drug. Clinicians should determine if symptoms are related to the medicine and make a medication change if needed.

**What should be done if a dose of prophylaxis is missed?**

- In comparison with drugs with short half-lives, which are taken daily, drugs with longer half-lives, which are taken weekly, offer the advantage of a wider margin of error if the traveler is late with a dose.
- For a weekly drug, prophylactic blood levels can remain adequate if they are only 1–2 days late. If this is the case, the traveler can take a dose as soon as possible, then resume weekly doses on the originally scheduled day. If the traveler is >2 days late, blood levels may not be adequate. The traveler should take a dose as soon as possible. The weekly doses should resume at this new day of the week (the next dose is 1 week later, then weekly thereafter).
- For a daily drug, if the traveler is 1–2 days late, protective blood levels are less likely to be maintained. They should take a dose as soon as possible and resume the daily schedule at the new time of day.

**What happens if too high a dose of prophylaxis is taken?**

- Overdose of antimalarials, particularly chloroquine, can be fatal. Medications should be stored in childproof containers out of reach of infants and children.

**Isn't malaria a treatable disease? Why not carry a treatment dose of antimalarials instead of taking malaria prophylaxis?**

- Malaria could be fatal even when treated, which is why it is always preferable to prevent malaria cases rather than rely on treating infections after they occur.

**What should be done if fever develops while traveling in a malaria-endemic area?**

- Malaria could be fatal if treatment is delayed. Medical help should be sought promptly if malaria is suspected. Travelers should continue to take malaria prophylaxis while in the malaria-endemic area.

**What should be done if a traveler who took malaria prophylaxis develops fever after returning from their trip?**

- Malaria prophylaxis, while highly effective, is not 100% effective. Travelers should be advised that they should seek medical care immediately if fever develops, report their travel history, get tested for malaria, and get treated promptly if infection is confirmed.
- Malaria smear results or a rapid diagnostic test must be done immediately (within a few hours). These tests should not be sent out to reference laboratories with results available only days to weeks later. Empiric treatment with antimalarials is not recommended as the malaria smear provides critical information for appropriate treatment. If a patient has an illness suggestive of severe malaria, a compatible travel history in an area where malaria transmission occurs, and malaria testing is not immediately available, it is advisable to start treatment as soon as possible, even before the diagnosis is established. CDC recommendations for malaria treatment can be found at www.cdc.gov/malaria/diagnosis_treatment/index.html.

of the density of the infection, and allow determination of the species of the malaria parasite—all of which are necessary for providing the most appropriate treatment. Microscopy results should ideally be available within a few hours. These tests should be performed immediately when ordered by a health care provider. They should not be saved for the most qualified staff to perform or batched for convenience. In addition, these tests should not be sent out to reference laboratories with results available only days to weeks later. Assistance with speciation of

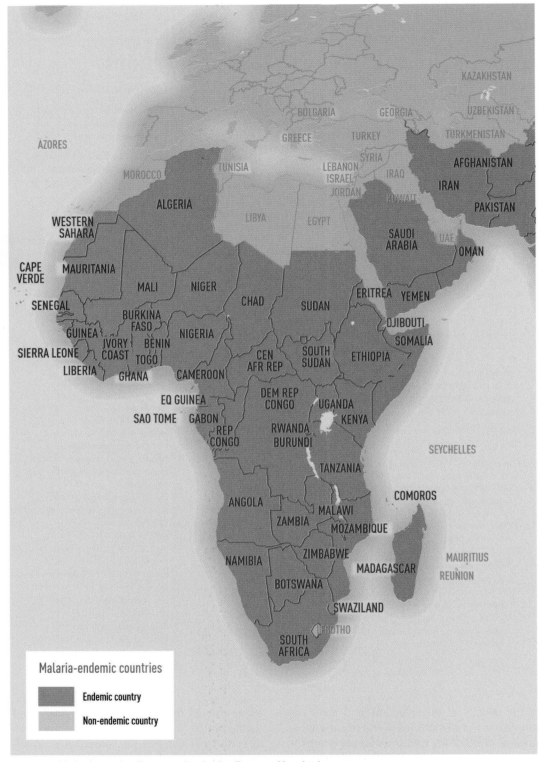

Malaria-endemic countries

- Endemic country
- Non-endemic country

MAP 4-9. **Malaria-endemic countries in the Eastern Hemisphere**

In this map, countries with areas endemic for malaria are shaded completely even if transmission occurs only in a small part of the country. For more specific within-country malaria transmission information, see Chapter 2, Yellow Fever Vaccine & Malaria Prophylaxis Information, by Country.

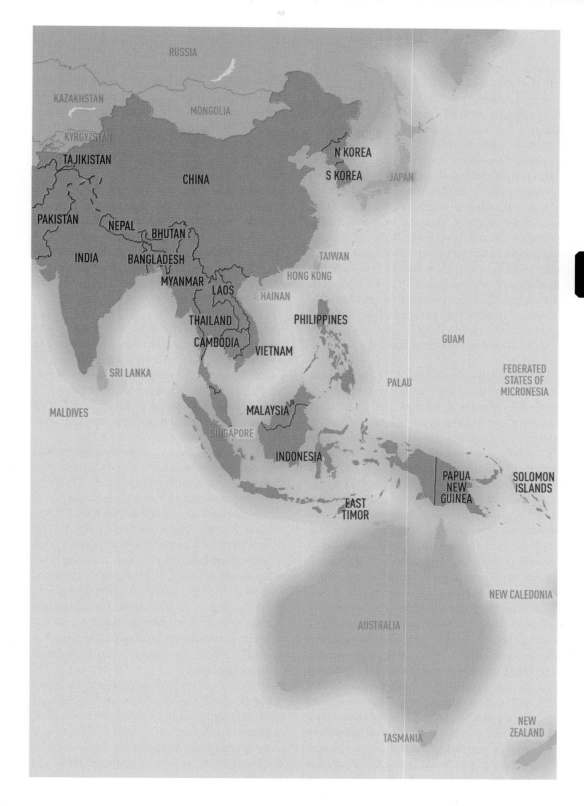

4

malaria on smears is available from CDC (www.cdc.gov/dpdx).

Rapid diagnostic tests (RDTs) for malaria detect antigens derived from malaria parasites. Malaria RDTs are immunochromatographic tests that most often use a dipstick or cassette format and provide results in 2–15 minutes. RDTs offer a useful alternative to microscopy in situations where reliable microscopic diagnosis is not immediately available. Although RDTs can detect malaria antigens within minutes, they have several limitations. RDTs cannot distinguish between all of the *Plasmodium* species that affect humans, they may be less sensitive than expert microscopy or PCR for diagnosis, they cannot quantify parasitemia, and an RDT-positive test result may persist for days or weeks after an infection has been treated and cleared. Thus, RDTs are not useful for assessing response to therapy.

Both positive and negative RDT results must always be confirmed by microscopy. Microscopy confirmation of the RDT result should occur as soon as possible because the information on the presence, density, and parasite species is critical for optimal management of malaria. The Food and Drug Administration (FDA) has approved an RDT (the BinaxNOW Malaria test) for hospital and commercial laboratory use; the test is not approved for use by individual clinicians or patients. Laboratories that do not provide in-house, on-the-spot microscopy services should maintain a stock of malaria RDTs so that they will be able to perform immediate malaria diagnostic testing when needed.

PCR tests are also available to detect malaria parasites. Although these tests are more sensitive than routine microscopy, results are not usually available as quickly as microscopy results, thus limiting the utility of this test for acute diagnosis and initial clinical management. Use of PCR testing is encouraged to confirm the species of malaria parasite and detect mixed infections. As noted above, the CDC malaria laboratory can assist in speciating malaria by microscopy. It also provides PCR-based species confirmation. And, the CDC laboratory can assess malaria parasites for mutations that confer resistance to medications (www.cdc.gov/dpdx).

In resource-limited settings, and particularly in sub-Saharan Africa, overdiagnosis and the rate of false-positive microscopy for malaria may be high. Warn travelers that a local diagnosis of malaria may be incorrect. In such cases, acutely ill travelers should seek the best available medical services, and continue their prophylaxis regimen until they have a definitive diagnosis.

In the United States, reporting malaria disease is mandatory. Health care providers must report laboratory-diagnosed cases of malaria occurring in the United States and its territories to local or state health departments. More information on reporting malaria can be found at www.cdc.gov/malaria/report.html.

## TREATMENT

Malaria can be treated effectively early in the course of the disease, but delay of therapy can have serious or even fatal consequences. Specific treatment options depend on the species of malaria, the severity of infection, the likelihood of drug resistance (based on where the infection was acquired), and the patient's age and pregnancy status.

Detailed CDC recommendations for malaria treatment can be found at www.cdc.gov/malaria/diagnosis_treatment/treatment.html. Clinicians who require assistance with the diagnosis or treatment of malaria should call the CDC Malaria Hotline (770-488-7788 or toll-free at 855-856-4713) from 9 AM to 5 PM Eastern Time. After hours or on weekends and holidays, clinicians requiring assistance should call the CDC Emergency Operations Center at 770-488-7100 and ask the operator to page the subject matter expert on call for the Malaria Branch. In addition, it is advisable to consult with a clinician who has specialized travel or tropical medicine expertise or with an infectious disease physician.

Travelers who reject the advice to take prophylaxis, who choose a suboptimal drug regimen (such as chloroquine in an area with chloroquine-resistant *P. falciparum*), or who require a less-than-optimal drug regimen for medical reasons, are at increased risk for acquiring malaria and then needing prompt treatment while overseas.

In addition, some travelers who are taking effective prophylaxis but who will be in remote

What is a reliable supply?

| A reliable supply is a complete course of an approved malaria treatment regimen obtained in the United States before travel. | A reliable supply:<br><br>• Is not counterfeit or substandard | • Will not interact adversely with the patient's other medicines, including prophylaxis<br>• Will not deplete local resources in the destination country |
|---|---|---|

areas may decide, in consultation with their travel health provider, to take along a reliable supply of a full course of an approved malaria treatment regimen (see Box 4-4 for the definition of reliable supply). In the event that a traveler carrying a reliable supply is diagnosed with malaria, he or she will have immediate access to treatment. CDC recommends that the reliable supply be acquired in the United States to allow the traveler's doctor to consider the traveler's other medical conditions or medications when selecting an antimalarial, to avoid the possibility of obtaining counterfeit drugs in the local pharmacy or market, and to avoid depleting local resources. In rare instances when access to medical care is not available and the traveler develops a febrile illness consistent with malaria, the reliable supply medication can be self-administered presumptively. Advise travelers that this self-treatment of a possible malarial infection is only a temporary measure and that prompt medical evaluation is imperative.

Two malaria treatment regimens available in the United States can be prescribed as a reliable supply: atovaquone-proguanil and artemether-lumefantrine. The use of the same or related drugs that have been taken for prophylaxis is not recommended to treat malaria. For example, atovaquone-proguanil may be used as a reliable supply medication by travelers not taking atovaquone-proguanil for prophylaxis. See Table 4-8 for the dosing recommendation.

Medications that are not used in the United States to treat malaria, such as halofantrine or sulfadoxine-pyrimethamine, are widely available overseas. CDC does not recommend halofantrine for treatment because of documented adverse cardiac events, including deaths. These adverse events have occurred in people with and without preexisting cardiac problems and both in the presence and absence of other antimalarial drugs. Sulfadoxine-pyrimethamine is not recommended because of widespread resistance to this drug.

## PREVENTION

Malaria prevention consists of a combination of mosquito avoidance measures and chemoprophylaxis. Prevention measures must address all malaria species in the area of travel and apply to both short-term and long-term travelers. Although highly efficacious, the recommended interventions are not 100% effective.

Preventing malaria involves striking a balance between effectiveness and safety: ensuring that all people at risk for infection use the recommended prevention measures and preventing rare occurrences of adverse effects. An individual risk assessment should be conducted for every traveler, taking into account not only the destination country but also the detailed itinerary, including specific cities, types of accommodation, season, and style of travel. Traveler characteristics (such as pregnancy or underlying health conditions) and malaria characteristics at the destination (such as intensity of transmission and local parasite resistance to drugs) may modify the risk assessment. Depending on the level of risk, it may be appropriate to recommend no specific interventions, mosquito avoidance measures only, or mosquito avoidance measures plus prophylaxis.

Several factors increase a traveler's risk for malaria. Travel—even for short periods of time—to areas with intense malaria transmission can result in infection. Malaria transmission is not distributed homogeneously throughout a country, so it will be important to review the

## Table 4-8. Reliable supply regimens for malaria treatment

| DRUG[1] | ADULT DOSE | PEDIATRIC DOSE | COMMENTS |
|---|---|---|---|
| ATOVAQUONE-PROGUANIL The adult tablet contains 250 mg atovaquone and 100 mg proguanil. The pediatric tablet contains 62.5 mg atovaquone and 25 mg proguanil. | 4 adult tablets, orally as a single daily dose for 3 consecutive days | Daily dose to be taken for 3 consecutive days: 5–8 kg: 2 pediatric tablets 9–10 kg: 3 pediatric tablets 11–20 kg: 1 adult tablet 21–30 kg: 2 adult tablets 31–40 kg: 3 adult tablets >41 kg: 4 adult tablets | Contraindicated in people with severe renal impairment (creatinine clearance <30 mL/min). Not recommended for people on atovaquone-proguanil prophylaxis. Not recommended for children weighing <5 kg, pregnant women, and women breastfeeding infants weighing <5 kg. |
| ARTEMETHER-LUMEFANTRINE One tablet contains 20 mg artemether and 120 mg lumefantrine. | A 3-day treatment schedule with a total of 6 oral doses is recommended for both adult and pediatric patients based on weight. The patient should receive the initial dose, followed by the second dose 8 hours later, then 1 dose twice per day for the following 2 days. 5 to <15 kg: 1 tablet per dose 15 to <25 kg: 2 tablets per dose 25 to <35 kg: 3 tablets per dose ≥35 kg: 4 tablets per dose | | Not for people on mefloquine prophylaxis. Not recommended for children weighing <5 kg, and women breastfeeding infants weighing <5 kg. |

[1] If used for presumptive self-treatment, medical care should be sought as soon as possible.

exact itinerary to determine if travel will occur in highly endemic areas. In countries where malaria is seasonal, travel during peak transmission season also increases risk. Travelers going to rural areas or staying in accommodations without screens or air conditioning will also be at higher risk. The highest risk for malaria is associated with first- and second-generation immigrants living in nonendemic countries who return to their countries of origin to visit friends and relatives (VFRs). VFR travelers often perceive themselves to be at no risk because they grew up in a malarious country and consider themselves immune. However, acquired immunity is lost quickly, and VFRs should be considered to have the same risk as other nonimmune travelers (see Chapter 9, Visiting Friends & Relatives: VFR Travel). Travelers should also be reminded that even if a person has had malaria before, he or she can get it again, and preventive measures are still necessary.

## Mosquito Avoidance Measures

Because of the nocturnal feeding habits of *Anopheles* mosquitoes, malaria transmission occurs primarily between dusk and dawn. Contact with mosquitoes can be reduced by remaining in well-screened areas, sleeping under mosquito nets (preferably insecticide-treated nets), using an effective insecticide spray in living and sleeping areas during evening and nighttime hours, and wearing clothes that cover most of the body.

All travelers should use an effective mosquito repellent, such as those that contain DEET (see Chapter 3, Mosquitoes, Ticks & Other Arthropods). Repellents should be applied to exposed parts of the skin when mosquitoes are likely to be present. If travelers are also wearing sunscreen, sunscreen should be applied first and insect repellent second. In addition to using a topical insect repellent, a permethrin-containing product may be applied to bed nets and clothing for additional protection against mosquitoes.

## Chemoprophylaxis

All recommended primary prophylaxis regimens involve taking a medicine before, during, and after travel to an area with malaria. Beginning the drug before travel allows the antimalarial agent to be in the blood before the traveler is exposed to malaria parasites. In choosing a prophylaxis regimen before travel, the traveler and the travel health provider should consider several factors. These include the presence of antimalarial drug resistance in the area of travel (see Chapter 2, Yellow Fever Vaccine & Malaria Prophylaxis Information, by Country), length of travel, the patient's other medical conditions, allergy history, medications being taken (to assess potential drug interactions), and potential side effects. Long-term travelers, defined as people who travel for ≥6 months, have additional considerations, listed in Box 4-5. Table 4-9 lists some of the benefits and limitations of medicines used for malaria prophylaxis; additional information about choosing a malaria prophylaxis regimen can be found at www.cdc.gov/malaria/travelers/drugs.html.

In addition to primary prophylaxis, presumptive antirelapse therapy (also known as terminal prophylaxis) uses a medication toward the end of the exposure period (or immediately thereafter) to prevent relapses or delayed-onset clinical presentations of malaria caused by hypnozoites (dormant liver stages) of *P. vivax* or *P. ovale*. Because most malarious areas of the world (except the Caribbean) have at least 1 species of relapsing malaria, travelers to these areas have some risk for acquiring either *P. vivax* or *P. ovale*, although the actual risk for an individual traveler is difficult to define. Presumptive antirelapse therapy is generally indicated only for people who have had prolonged exposure in malaria-endemic areas (for example, missionaries, military personnel, or Peace Corps volunteers).

### OBTAINING MEDICATIONS OVERSEAS

The medications recommended for prophylaxis of malaria may be available at overseas destinations. However, combinations of these medications and additional drugs that are not recommended may be commonly prescribed and used in other countries. Travelers should be strongly discouraged from obtaining prophylaxis medications while abroad. The quality of these products is not known; they may have been produced by substandard manufacturing practices, may be counterfeit, may contain contaminants, may not be protective, and could be dangerous. Additional information on this topic can be found in Chapter 6, *Perspectives*: Avoiding Poorly

---

**BOX 4-5.** Malaria considerations for the long-term traveler (travel >6 months)

**Considerations**

- Malaria preventive measures are the same for both short- and long-term travelers
- Increased risk of acquiring malaria—longer stay means increased duration of exposure
- Laxity in attention to mosquito avoidance over time
- Poor adherence to a lengthy course of malaria prophylaxis due to forgetfulness, fear of side effects, and the possible waning of a sense of risk and need
- Travel between highly endemic or low-endemic areas within a country or region
- Decreased sense of risk and concern about malaria after engaging in local conversations and lore (particularly regarding malaria immunity over time)
- Becoming ill with malaria in countries with limited access and quality of health care

**Additional advice for long-term travelers**

- Emphasize continued adherence to and safety of malaria prophylaxis drugs
- Develop a plan for seeking immediate care when ill with fever, including where to get promptly tested and treated for malaria
- Advise traveler to purchase travel insurance, including contingencies for medical evacuation
- Consider having a reliable supply of a treatment dose of antimalarials available in case malaria is diagnosed

# Table 4-9. Considerations when choosing a drug for malaria prophylaxis

| DRUG | REASONS TO CONSIDER USE OF THIS DRUG | REASONS TO CONSIDER AVOIDING USE OF THIS DRUG |
|---|---|---|
| Atovaquone-proguanil | • Good for last-minute travelers because the drug is started 1–2 days before travel.<br>• Some people prefer to take a daily medicine.<br>• Good choice for shorter trips because the traveler takes the medicine for only 7 days after traveling rather than 4 weeks.<br>• Well tolerated—side effects uncommon.<br>• Pediatric tablets are available and may be more convenient. | • Cannot be used by women who are pregnant or breastfeeding a child that weighs <5 kg.<br>• Cannot be taken by people with severe renal impairment.<br>• Tends to be more expensive than some of the other options (especially for long trips).<br>• Some people (including children) would rather not take a medicine every day. |
| Chloroquine | • Some people would rather take medicine weekly.<br>• Good choice for long trips because it is taken only weekly.<br>• Some people are already taking hydroxychloroquine chronically for rheumatologic conditions; in those instances, they may not have to take an additional medicine.<br>• Can be used in all trimesters of pregnancy. | • Cannot be used in areas with chloroquine or mefloquine resistance.<br>• May exacerbate psoriasis.<br>• Some people would rather not take a weekly medication.<br>• For short trips, some people would rather not take medication for 4 weeks after travel.<br>• Not a good choice for last-minute travelers, because drug needs to be started 1–2 weeks before travel. |
| Doxycycline | • Some people prefer to take a daily medicine.<br>• Good for last-minute travelers because the drug is started 1–2 days before travel.<br>• Tends to be the least expensive antimalarial.<br>• People already taking doxycycline chronically to prevent acne do not have to take an additional medicine.<br>• Doxycycline also can prevent some additional infections (such as rickettsial infections and leptospirosis), so it may be preferred by people planning to hike, camp, and swim in fresh water. | • Cannot be used by pregnant women and children aged <8 years.<br>• Some people would rather not take a medicine every day.<br>• For short trips, some people would rather not take medication for 4 weeks after travel.<br>• Women prone to getting vaginal yeast infections when taking antibiotics may prefer taking a different medicine.<br>• People may want to avoid the increased risk of sun sensitivity.<br>• Some people are concerned about the potential of getting an upset stomach from doxycycline. |
| Mefloquine | • Some people would rather take medicine weekly.<br>• Good choice for long trips because it is taken only weekly.<br>• Can be used in all trimesters of pregnancy. | • Cannot be used in areas with mefloquine resistance.<br>• Cannot be used in patients with certain psychiatric conditions.<br>• Cannot be used in patients with a seizure disorder.<br>• Not recommended for people with cardiac conduction abnormalities.<br>• Not a good choice for last-minute travelers because drug needs to be started ≥2 weeks before travel.<br>• Some people would rather not take a weekly medication.<br>• For short trips, some people would rather not take medication for 4 weeks after travel. |

# Table 4-9. Considerations when choosing a drug for malaria prophylaxis (continued)

| DRUG | REASONS TO CONSIDER USE OF THIS DRUG | REASONS TO CONSIDER AVOIDING USE OF THIS DRUG |
|---|---|---|
| Primaquine | • One of the most effective drugs for prevention of *P. vivax*, so it is a good choice for travel to places with >90% *P. vivax*.<br>• Good choice for shorter trips because the traveler takes the medicine for 7 days after traveling rather than 4 weeks.<br>• Good for last-minute travelers because the drug is started 1–2 days before travel.<br>• Some people prefer to take a daily medicine. | • Cannot be used in patients with G6PD deficiency.<br>• Cannot be used in patients who have not been tested for G6PD deficiency.<br>• There are costs and delays associated with getting a G6PD test; however, it only has to be done once. Once a normal G6PD level is verified and documented, the test does not have to be repeated the next time primaquine or tafenoquine is considered.<br>• Cannot be used by pregnant women.<br>• Cannot be used by women who are breastfeeding, unless the infant has also been tested for G6PD deficiency.<br>• Some people (including children) would rather not take a medicine every day.<br>• Some people are concerned about the potential of getting an upset stomach from primaquine. |
| Tafenoquine | • One of the most effective drugs for prevention of *P. vivax* malaria but also prevents *P. falciparum*.<br>• Good choice for shorter trips because the traveler takes the medicine once, 1 week after traveling rather than 4 weeks.<br>• Good for last-minute travelers because the drug is started 3 days before travel. | • Cannot be used in people with G6PD deficiency.<br>• Cannot be used in patients who have not been tested for G6PD deficiency.<br>• There are costs and delays associated with getting a G6PD test; however, it only has to be done once. Once a normal G6PD level is verified and documented, the test does not have to be repeated the next time tafenoquine or primaquine is considered.<br>• Cannot be used by children<br>• Cannot be used by pregnant women.<br>• Cannot be used by women who are breastfeeding.<br>• Not recommended in those with psychotic disorders |

Regulated Medicines and Medical Products during Travel, and on the FDA website (www.fda.gov/Drugs/ResourcesForYou/Consumers/BuyingUsingMedicineSafely/BuyingMedicinefromOutsidetheUnitedStates/default.htm).

## MEDICATIONS USED FOR PROPHYLAXIS

### ATOVAQUONE-PROGUANIL

Atovaquone-proguanil (Malarone) is a fixed combination of the drugs atovaquone and proguanil. Prophylaxis should begin 1–2 days before travel to malarious areas and should be taken daily, at the same time each day, while in the malarious areas, and daily for 7 days after leaving the areas (see Table 4-10 for recommended dosages). Atovaquone-proguanil is well tolerated, and side effects are rare. The most common adverse effects reported in people using atovaquone-proguanil for prophylaxis or treatment are abdominal pain, nausea, vomiting, and headache. Atovaquone-proguanil is not recommended for prophylaxis in children weighing <5 kg (11 lb), pregnant women,

## Table 4-10.  Drugs used in the prophylaxis of malaria

| DRUG | USAGE | ADULT DOSE | PEDIATRIC DOSE | COMMENTS |
|------|-------|-----------|----------------|----------|
| Atovaquone-proguanil | Prophylaxis in all areas | Adult tablets contain 250 mg atovaquone and 100 mg proguanil hydrochloride. 1 adult tablet orally, daily | Pediatric tablets contain 62.5 mg atovaquone and 25 mg proguanil hydrochloride.<br>• 5–8 kg: 1/2 pediatric tablet daily<br>• 8–10 kg: 3/4 pediatric tablet daily<br>• 10–20 kg: 1 pediatric tablet daily<br>• 20–30 kg: 2 pediatric tablets daily<br>• 30–40 kg: 3 pediatric tablets daily<br>• >40 kg: 1 adult tablet daily | Begin 1–2 days before travel to malarious areas. Take daily at the same time each day while in the malarious area and for 7 days after leaving such areas. Contraindicated in people with severe renal impairment (creatinine clearance <30 mL/min). Atovaquone-proguanil should be taken with food or a milky drink. Not recommended for prophylaxis for children weighing <5 kg, pregnant women, and women breastfeeding infants weighing <5 kg. Partial tablet doses may need to be prepared by a pharmacist and dispensed in individual capsules, as described in the text. |
| Chloroquine | Prophylaxis only in areas with chloroquine-sensitive malaria | 300 mg base (500 mg salt) orally, once/week | 5 mg/kg base (8.3 mg/kg salt) orally, once/week, up to a maximum adult dose of 300 mg base | Begin 1–2 weeks before travel to malarious areas. Take weekly on the same day of the week while in the malarious area and for 4 weeks after leaving such areas. May exacerbate psoriasis. |
| Doxycycline | Prophylaxis in all areas | 100 mg orally, daily | ≥8 years of age: 2.2 mg/kg up to adult dose of 100 mg/day | Begin 1–2 days before travel to malarious areas. Take daily at the same time each day while in the malarious area and for 4 weeks after leaving such areas. Contraindicated in children aged <8 years and pregnant women. |
| Hydroxychloroquine | An alternative to chloroquine for prophylaxis only in areas with chloroquine-sensitive malaria | 310 mg base (400 mg salt) orally, once/week | 5 mg/kg base (6.5 mg/kg salt) orally, once/week, up to a maximum adult dose of 310 mg base | Begin 1–2 weeks before travel to malarious areas. Take weekly on the same day of the week while in the malarious area and for 4 weeks after leaving such areas. |

4

| Medication | Use | Dose | Pediatric dose | Comments |
|---|---|---|---|---|
| Mefloquine | Prophylaxis in areas with mefloquine-sensitive malaria | 228 mg base (250 mg salt) orally, once/week | ≤9 kg: 4.6 mg/kg base (5 mg/kg salt) orally, once/week<br>>9–19 kg: 1/4 tablet once/week<br>>19–30 kg: 1/2 tablet once/week<br>>30–45 kg: 3/4 tablet once/week<br>>45 kg: 1 tablet once/week | Begin ≥2 weeks before travel to malarious areas. Take weekly on the same day of the week while in the malarious area and for 4 weeks after leaving such areas. Contraindicated in people allergic to mefloquine or related compounds (quinine, quinidine) and in people with active depression, a recent history of depression, generalized anxiety disorder, psychosis, schizophrenia, other major psychiatric disorders, or seizures. Use with caution in people with psychiatric disturbances or a previous history of depression. Not recommended for people with cardiac conduction abnormalities. |
| Primaquine [1] | Prophylaxis for short-duration travel to areas with principally P. vivax | 30 mg base (52.6 mg salt) orally, daily | 0.5 mg/kg base (0.8 mg/kg salt) up to adult dose orally, daily | Begin 1–2 days before travel to malarious areas. Take daily at the same time each day while in the malarious area and for 7 days after leaving such areas. |
|  | Presumptive antirelapse therapy (PART or terminal prophylaxis) to decrease the risk for relapses of P. vivax and P. ovale | 30 mg base (52.6 mg salt) orally, daily | 0.5 mg/kg base (0.8 mg/kg salt) up to adult dose orally, daily | PART indicated for people with prolonged exposure to P. vivax, P. ovale, or both: daily for 14 days after departure from the malarious area. Contraindicated in people with G6PD deficiency. Also contraindicated during pregnancy and lactation, unless the infant being breastfed has a documented normal G6PD level. |
| Tafenoquine [1] | Prophylaxis in all areas | 200 mg orally | Not indicated in children <16 years old | Begin taking daily for 3 days prior to travel to malarious areas. Then, take weekly while at the malarious area, and for 1 week after leaving the malarious area. |
|  | Presumptive antirelapse therapy (PART or terminal prophylaxis) to decrease the risk for relapses of P. vivax and P. ovale | 300mg orally | 300 mg orally | PART indicated for people who had prolonged exposure to P. vivax, P. ovale or both: Administered as a single dose. Contraindicated in people with G6PD deficiency. Also contraindicated during pregnancy and lactation unless the infant being breastfed has a documented normal G6PD level |

Abbreviation: PART, presumptive antirelapse therapy.
[1] All people who take primaquine or tafenoquine should have a documented normal G6PD level before starting the medication.

4

or patients with severe renal impairment (creatinine clearance <30 mL/min). Proguanil may increase the effect of warfarin, so international normalized ratio monitoring or adjustment of warfarin dosage may be needed. However, there are no data regarding the clinical impact of the administration of atovaquone-proguanil and warfarin at the same time.

## CHLOROQUINE AND HYDROXYCHLOROQUINE

Chloroquine phosphate or hydroxychloroquine sulfate (Plaquenil) can be used for prevention of malaria only in destinations where chloroquine resistance is not present (see Chapter 2, Yellow Fever Vaccine & Malaria Prophylaxis Information, by Country). Prophylaxis should begin 1–2 weeks before travel to malarious areas. It should be continued by taking the drug once a week, on the same day of the week, during travel in malarious areas and for 4 weeks after a traveler leaves these areas (see Table 4-10 for recommended dosages).

Reported side effects include gastrointestinal disturbance, headache, dizziness, blurred vision, insomnia, and pruritus, but generally, these effects do not require that the drug be discontinued. High doses of chloroquine, such as those used to treat rheumatoid arthritis, have been associated with retinopathy; this serious side effect appears to be extremely unlikely when chloroquine is used for routine weekly malaria prophylaxis. Chloroquine and related compounds have been reported to exacerbate psoriasis. People who experience uncomfortable side effects after taking chloroquine may tolerate the drug better by taking it with meals. As an alternative, the related compound hydroxychloroquine sulfate may be better tolerated.

## DOXYCYCLINE

Doxycycline prophylaxis should begin 1–2 days before travel to malarious areas. It should be continued once a day, at the same time each day, during travel in malarious areas and daily for 4 weeks after the traveler leaves such areas. Insufficient data exist on the antimalarial prophylactic efficacy of related compounds such as minocycline (commonly prescribed for the treatment of acne). People on a long-term regimen of minocycline who need malaria prophylaxis should stop taking minocycline 1–2 days before travel and start doxycycline instead. Minocycline can be restarted after the full course of doxycycline is completed (see Table 4-10 for recommended dosages).

Doxycycline can cause photosensitivity, usually manifested as an exaggerated sunburn reaction. The risk for such a reaction can be minimized by avoiding prolonged, direct exposure to the sun and by using sunscreen. In addition, doxycycline use is associated with an increased frequency of vaginal yeast infections. Gastrointestinal side effects (nausea or vomiting) may be minimized by taking the drug with a meal or by specifically prescribing doxycycline monohydrate or the enteric-coated doxycycline hyclate, rather than the generic doxycycline hyclate, which is often less expensive. To reduce the risk for esophagitis, travelers should be advised to swallow the medicine with sufficient fluids and not to take doxycycline shortly before going to bed. Doxycycline is contraindicated in people with an allergy to tetracyclines, during pregnancy, and in infants and children aged <8 years. Vaccination with the oral typhoid vaccine Ty21a should be delayed for ≥24 hours after taking a dose of doxycycline.

## MEFLOQUINE

Mefloquine prophylaxis should begin ≥2 weeks before travel to malarious areas. It should be continued once a week, on the same day of the week, during travel in malarious areas and for 4 weeks after a traveler leaves such areas (see Table 4-10 for recommended dosages).

Mefloquine has been associated with rare but serious adverse reactions (such as psychoses or seizures) at prophylactic doses; these reactions are more frequent with the higher doses used for treatment. Other side effects that have occurred in prophylaxis studies include gastrointestinal disturbance, headache, insomnia, abnormal dreams, visual disturbances, depression, anxiety disorder, and dizziness. Other more severe neuropsychiatric disorders have been occasionally reported and include sensory and motor neuropathies (such as paresthesia, tremor, and ataxia), agitation or restlessness, mood changes, panic attacks, forgetfulness, confusion, hallucinations, aggression, paranoia, and encephalopathy. On occasion, psychiatric symptoms have been reported to continue long after mefloquine has been stopped.

FDA also includes a boxed warning about rare reports of persistent dizziness after mefloquine use. Mefloquine is contraindicated for use by travelers with a known hypersensitivity to mefloquine or related compounds (such as quinine or quinidine) and in people with active depression, a recent history of depression, generalized anxiety disorder, psychosis, schizophrenia, other major psychiatric disorders, or seizures. Mefloquine should be avoided in people with psychiatric disturbances or a history of depression.

A review of available data suggests that mefloquine may be used safely in people concurrently on β-blockers, if they have no underlying arrhythmia. However, mefloquine is not recommended for people with cardiac conduction abnormalities. Any traveler receiving a prescription for mefloquine must also receive a copy of the FDA medication guide, which can be found at www.accessdata.fda.gov/drugsatfda_docs/label/2008/019591s023lbl.pdf.

### PRIMAQUINE

Primaquine phosphate has 2 distinct uses for malaria prevention in people with normal G6PD levels (see cautionary note below): primary prophylaxis in areas with primarily *P. vivax* and presumptive antirelapse therapy (terminal prophylaxis). When taken for primary prophylaxis, primaquine should be taken 1–2 days before travel to malarious areas, daily, at the same time each day, while in the malarious area, and daily for 7 days after leaving the area (see Table 4-10 for recommended dosages).

When used for presumptive antirelapse therapy, primaquine is administered for 14 days after the traveler has left a malarious area. When chloroquine, doxycycline, or mefloquine is used for primary prophylaxis, primaquine is usually taken during the last 2 weeks of postexposure prophylaxis. When atovaquone-proguanil is used for prophylaxis, primaquine may be taken during the final 7 days of atovaquone-proguanil, and then for an additional 7 days. Primaquine should be given concurrently with the primary prophylaxis medication. However, if that is not feasible, the primaquine course should still be administered after the primary prophylaxis medication has been completed. Primary prophylaxis with primaquine or tafenoquine (see below) obviates the need for presumptive antirelapse therapy.

The most common adverse event in people with normal G6PD levels is gastrointestinal upset if primaquine is taken on an empty stomach. This problem is minimized or eliminated if primaquine is taken with food.

In G6PD-deficient people, primaquine can cause fatal hemolysis. **Before primaquine is used, G6PD deficiency MUST be ruled out by laboratory testing.**

### TAFENOQUINE

Tafenoquine (Arakoda 100-mg tablets, Krintafel 150-mg tablets) can be used to prevent malaria in adults and as presumptive antirelapse therapy for people >16 years of age (see Table 4-10 for recommended dosages).

When used for prophylaxis, a loading dose of tafenoquine is taken daily for 3 days before leaving for a malaria-endemic area. Maintenance doses are taken weekly while in the malarious area (start 7 days after loading dose is complete) and a final dose in the week after leaving the area. Doses should be taken on the same day each week.

For presumptive antirelapse therapy, one 300-mg dose of tafenoquine is administered after leaving the malarious area. Ideally, this single dose should overlap with the last dose of the antimalarial used for prophylaxis, but if that approach is not feasible, tafenoquine can be taken after primary prophylaxis has been completed. As with primaquine, presumptive antirelapse therapy is not needed if tafenoquine is taken for primary prophylaxis.

Like primaquine, tafenoquine can cause fatal hemolysis in people with G6PD deficiency. **Before tafenoquine is used, G6PD deficiency MUST be ruled out by laboratory testing.** Tafenoquine is also contraindicated in pregnancy and during breastfeeding. Rare psychiatric adverse events have been observed in people with a history of psychotic disorder using tafenoquine at higher doses. Therefore, tafenoquine should not be used as prophylaxis in people with a history of psychotic disorder, but can be administered for presumptive antirelapse therapy, which is likely to be associated with a very small risk of psychiatric adverse reactions. The most common adverse events reported with use of tafenoquine are gastrointestinal disturbances, dizziness, headache, and clinically nonsignificant decreases in hemoglobin. Tafenoquine should be taken with food.

## TRAVEL TO AREAS WITH LIMITED MALARIA TRANSMISSION

For destinations where malaria cases occur sporadically and risk for infection to travelers is assessed as being low, CDC recommends that travelers use mosquito avoidance measures only, and no prophylaxis should be prescribed (see Chapter 2, Yellow Fever Vaccine & Malaria Prophylaxis Information, by Country).

## TRAVEL TO AREAS WITH CHLOROQUINE-SENSITIVE MALARIA

Areas with chloroquine-sensitive malaria include many Latin American countries where there is predominantly *P. vivax* malaria. Chloroquine-sensitive *P. falciparum* is present in the Caribbean and Central American countries west of the Panama Canal. For destinations where chloroquine-sensitive malaria is present, in addition to mosquito avoidance measures, the many effective prophylaxis options include chloroquine, atovaquone-proguanil, doxycycline, mefloquine, and tafenoquine. In countries where there is predominantly *P. vivax*, primaquine is an additional option.

## TRAVEL TO AREAS WITH CHLOROQUINE-RESISTANT MALARIA

Chloroquine-resistant *P. falciparum* is found in all parts of the world except the Caribbean and countries west of the Panama Canal. Although chloroquine-resistant *P. falciparum* predominates in Africa, it is found in combination with chloroquine-sensitive *P. vivax* malaria in South America and Asia. Resistance of *P. vivax* to chloroquine has been confirmed only in Papua New Guinea and Indonesia. For destinations where any chloroquine-resistant malaria is present, in addition to mosquito avoidance measures,

prophylaxis options are atovaquone-proguanil, doxycycline, mefloquine, and tafenoquine.

## TRAVEL TO AREAS WITH MEFLOQUINE-RESISTANT MALARIA

Mefloquine-resistant *P. falciparum* has been confirmed in Southeast Asia on the borders of Thailand with Burma (Myanmar) and Cambodia, in the western provinces of Cambodia, in the eastern states of Burma on the border between Burma and China, along the borders of Laos and Burma, the adjacent parts of the Thailand-Cambodia border, and in southern Vietnam. For destinations where mefloquine-resistant malaria is present, in addition to mosquito avoidance measures, prophylaxis options are atovaquone-proguanil, doxycycline, and tafenoquine.

## PROPHYLAXIS FOR INFANTS, CHILDREN, AND ADOLESCENTS

All children traveling to malaria-endemic areas should use recommended prevention measures, which often include taking an antimalarial drug. In the United States, antimalarial drugs are available only in oral formulations and may taste bitter. Pediatric doses should be calculated carefully according to body weight but should never exceed the adult dose. Pharmacists can pulverize tablets and prepare gelatin capsules for each measured dose. If the child is unable to swallow the capsules or tablets, parents should prepare the child's dose of medication by breaking open the gelatin capsule or crushing the pill and mixing the drug with a small amount of something sweet, such as applesauce, chocolate syrup, or jelly, to ensure the entire dose is delivered to the child. Giving the dose on a full stomach may minimize stomach upset and vomiting.

Chloroquine and mefloquine are options for infants and children of all ages and weights, depending on drug resistance at their destination. Primaquine can be used for children who are not G6PD deficient traveling to areas with principally *P. vivax*. Doxycycline may be used for children aged ≥8 years. Atovaquone-proguanil may be used as prophylaxis for infants and children weighing ≥5 kg (11 lb). Prophylactic dosing for children weighing <11 kg (24 lb) constitutes off-label use in the United States. Pediatric dosing regimens are included in Table 4-10.

## PROPHYLAXIS DURING PREGNANCY AND BREASTFEEDING

Malaria infection in pregnant women can be more severe than in nonpregnant women. Malaria increases the risk for adverse pregnancy outcomes, including prematurity, spontaneous abortion, and stillbirth. For these reasons, and because no prophylaxis regimen is completely effective, women who are pregnant or likely to become pregnant should be advised to avoid travel to areas with malaria transmission if possible (see Chapter 7, Pregnant Travelers). If travel to a malarious area cannot be deferred, use of an effective prophylaxis regimen is essential (along with mosquito avoidance measures).

Pregnant women traveling to areas where chloroquine-resistant *P. falciparum* has not been reported may take chloroquine prophylaxis. Chloroquine has not been found to have harmful effects on the fetus when used in the recommended doses for malaria prophylaxis; therefore, pregnancy is not a contraindication for malaria prophylaxis with chloroquine or hydroxychloroquine.

For travel to areas where chloroquine resistance is present, mefloquine is the only medication recommended for malaria prophylaxis during pregnancy. Studies of mefloquine use during pregnancy have found no indication of adverse effects on the fetus.

Experts are evaluating the safety of atovaquone-proguanil use during pregnancy. Proguanil has been used for decades in pregnant women; however, until such time as these data are fully evaluated, atovaquone-proguanil is not recommended for use during pregnancy. Doxycycline is contraindicated for malaria prophylaxis during pregnancy because of the risk for adverse effects seen with tetracycline, a related drug, on the fetus. These adverse effects include discoloration and dysplasia of the teeth and inhibition of bone growth. Primaquine and tafenoquine should not be used during pregnancy because the drug may be passed transplacentally to a G6PD-deficient fetus and cause hemolytic anemia in utero.

Women planning to become pregnant may use the same medications that are recommended for use during pregnancy. CDC does not make recommendations about delaying pregnancy after the use of malaria prophylaxis medicines. However, if women or their health care providers wish to decrease the amount of antimalarial drug in the body before conception, Table 4-11 provides information on the half-lives of the recommended

## Table 4-11. Half-lives of malaria prophylaxis drugs

| DRUG | HALF-LIFE |
|---|---|
| Atovaquone | 2–3 days |
| Chloroquine | 1–2 months |
| Doxycycline | 15–24 hours |
| Hydroxychloroquine | 1–2 months |
| Mefloquine | 2–4 weeks |
| Primaquine | 4–7 hours |
| Proguanil | 12–25 hours |
| Tafenoquine | 14–28 days |

malaria prophylaxis medicines. After 2, 4, and 6 half-lives, approximately 25%, 6%, and 2%, respectively, of the drug remains in the body.

Very small amounts of antimalarial drugs are excreted in the breast milk of lactating women. Because the quantity of antimalarial drugs transferred in breast milk is insufficient to provide adequate protection against malaria, infants who require prophylaxis must receive the recommended dosages of antimalarial drugs listed in Table 4-10. Because chloroquine and mefloquine may be prescribed safely to infants, it is also safe for infants to be exposed to the small amounts excreted in breast milk. Data about the use of doxycycline in lactating women are very limited; most experts, however, consider the theoretical possibility of adverse events to the infant to be remote.

Although no information is available on the amount of primaquine that enters human breast milk, both the mother and infant should be tested for G6PD deficiency before primaquine is given to a woman who is breastfeeding. Because data are not yet available on the safety of atovaquone-proguanil prophylaxis in infants weighing <5 kg (11 lb), CDC does not recommend this drug to prevent malaria in women breastfeeding infants weighing <5 kg. However, it can be used to treat women who are breastfeeding infants of any weight when the potential benefit outweighs the potential risk to the infant (such as treating a breastfeeding woman who has acquired *P. falciparum* malaria in an area of multidrug-resistant strains and who cannot tolerate other treatment options). No data are available on the safety of tafenoquine in infants, so tafenoquine is not recommended in women who are breastfeeding.

## CHOOSING A DRUG TO PREVENT MALARIA

Recommendations for drugs to prevent malaria differ by country of travel and can be found in Chapter 2, Yellow Fever Vaccine & Malaria Prophylaxis Information, by Country. Recommended drugs for each country are listed in alphabetical order and have comparable efficacy in that country. No antimalarial drug is 100% protective; therefore, prophylaxis must be combined with mosquito avoidance and personal protective measures (such as insect repellent, long sleeves, long pants, sleeping in a mosquito-free setting or using an insecticide-treated bed net). When several different drugs are recommended for an area, Table 4-9 may help in the decision-making process.

## CHANGING MEDICATIONS AS A RESULT OF SIDE EFFECTS DURING PROPHYLAXIS

Medications recommended for prophylaxis against malaria have different modes of action that affect the parasites at different stages of the life cycle. Thus, if the medication needs to be changed because of side effects before a full course has been completed, there are some special considerations (see Table 4-12).

# BLOOD DONATION AFTER TRAVEL TO MALARIOUS AREAS

People who have been in an area where malaria transmission occurs should defer donating blood for a period of time after returning from the malarious area to prevent transmission of malaria through blood transfusion (Table 4-13).

Risk assessments may differ between travel health providers and blood banks. A travel health provider advising a traveler going to a country with relatively low malaria transmission for a short period of time and engaging in low-risk behaviors may choose insect avoidance only and no prophylaxis for the traveler. However, upon the traveler's return, a blood bank may still choose to defer that traveler for 1 year because of the travel to an area where transmission occurs.

**CDC website:** www.cdc.gov/malaria

## Table 4-12. Changing medications as a result of side effects during malaria chemoprophylaxis

| DRUG BEING STOPPED | DRUG BEING STARTED | COMMENTS |
|---|---|---|
| Mefloquine | Doxycycline | Begin doxycycline, continue daily while in malaria-endemic area, and continue for 4 weeks after leaving malaria-endemic area. |
| | Atovaquone-proguanil | If the switch occurs ≥3 weeks before departure from the endemic area, atovaquone-proguanil should be taken daily for the rest of the stay in the endemic area and for 1 week thereafter.<br>If the switch occurs <3 weeks before departure from the endemic area, atovaquone-proguanil should be taken daily for 4 weeks after the switch.<br>If the switch occurs after departure from the endemic area, atovaquone-proguanil should be taken daily until 4 weeks after the date of departure. |
| | Chloroquine | Not recommended. |
| | Primaquine | This switch would be unlikely as primaquine is recommended only for primary prophylaxis in areas with mainly *P. vivax* for people with normal G6PD activity. Should that be the case, begin primaquine, continue daily while in malaria-endemic area, and continue for 7 days after leaving malaria-endemic area. |
| | Tafenoquine | For people with normal G6PD activity, begin tafenoquine as soon as possible after the last dose of mefloquine while in the malarious area. Take daily for 3 days, weekly while in the malarious area and a final dose in the week after leaving the malarious area. |
| Doxycycline | Mefloquine | Not recommended. |
| | Atovaquone-proguanil | If the switch occurs ≥3 weeks before departure from the endemic area, atovaquone-proguanil should be taken daily for the rest of the stay in the endemic area and for 1 week thereafter.<br>If the switch occurs <3 weeks before departure from the endemic area, atovaquone-proguanil should be taken daily for 4 weeks after the switch.<br>If the switch occurs after departure from the endemic area, atovaquone-proguanil should be taken daily until 4 weeks after the date of departure. |
| | Chloroquine | Not recommended. |
| | Primaquine | This switch would be unlikely as primaquine is recommended only for primary prophylaxis in areas with mainly *P. vivax* for people with normal G6PD activity. Should that be the case, begin primaquine, continue daily while in malaria-endemic area, and continue for 7 days after leaving malaria-endemic area. |
| | Tafenoquine | Not recommended. |

(continued)

## Table 4-12. Changing medications as a result of side effects during malaria chemoprophylaxis (continued)

| DRUG BEING STOPPED | DRUG BEING STARTED | COMMENTS |
|---|---|---|
| Atovaquone-proguanil | Doxycycline | Begin doxycycline, continue daily while in malaria-endemic area, and continue for 4 weeks after leaving malaria-endemic area. |
| | Mefloquine | Not recommended. |
| | Chloroquine | Not recommended. |
| | Primaquine | This switch would be unlikely as primaquine is recommended only for primary prophylaxis in areas with mainly *P. vivax* for people with normal G6PD activity. Should that be the case, begin primaquine, continue daily while in malaria-endemic area, and continue for 7 days after leaving malaria-endemic area. |
| | Tafenoquine | Not recommended. |
| Chloroquine | Doxycycline | Begin doxycycline, continue daily while in malaria-endemic area, and continue for 4 weeks after leaving malaria-endemic area. |
| | Atovaquone-proguanil | If the switch occurs ≥3 weeks before departure from the endemic area, atovaquone-proguanil should be taken daily for the rest of the stay in the endemic area and for 1 week thereafter. If the switch occurs <3 weeks before departure from the endemic area, atovaquone-proguanil should be taken daily for 4 weeks after the switch. If the switch occurs following departure from the endemic area, atovaquone-proguanil should be taken daily until 4 weeks after the date of departure. |
| | Mefloquine | Not recommended. |
| | Primaquine | Primaquine is recommended only for primary prophylaxis in areas with mainly *P. vivax* for people with normal G6PD activity. Should that be the case, begin primaquine, continue daily while in malaria-endemic area, and continue for 7 days after leaving malaria-endemic area. |
| | Tafenoquine | For people with normal G6PD activity, begin tafenoquine as soon as possible after the last dose of chloroquine while in the malarious area. Take daily for 3 days, weekly while in the malarious area, and a final dose in the week after leaving the malarious area. |
| Primaquine | Doxycycline | Begin doxycycline, continue daily while in malaria-endemic area, and continue for 4 weeks after leaving malaria-endemic area. |
| | Atovaquone-proguanil | Begin atovaquone-proguanil, continue daily while in malaria-endemic area, and continue for 7 days after leaving malaria-endemic area. |
| | Chloroquine | Not recommended. |
| | Mefloquine | Not recommended. |
| | Tafenoquine | Not recommended. |

## Table 4-13. Food and Drug Administration recommendations for deferring blood donation in people returning from malarious areas

| GROUP | BLOOD DONATION DEFERRAL |
|---|---|
| Travelers to malaria-endemic areas | May not donate blood for 1 year after travel. |
| Former residents of malaria-endemic areas | May not donate blood for 3 years after departing. If they return to a malaria-endemic area within that 3-year period, they are deferred for an additional 3 years. |
| People diagnosed with malaria | May not donate for 3 years after treatment. |

### BIBLIOGRAPHY

1. Angelo KM, Libman M, Caumes E, Hamer DH, Kain KC, Leder K, et al. Malaria after international travel: a GeoSentinel analysis, 2003–2016. Malar J. 2017 Jul 20;16(1):293.

2. Boggild AK, Parise ME, Lewis LS, Kain KC. Atovaquone-proguanil: report from the CDC expert meeting on malaria chemoprophylaxis (II). Am J Trop Med Hyg. 2007 Feb;76(2):208–23.

3. Davlantes EA, Tan KR, Arguin PM. Quantifying malaria risk in travelers: a quixotic pursuit. J Travel Med. 2017 Sep 1;24(6).

4. Hill DR, Baird JK, Parise ME, Lewis LS, Ryan ET, Magill AJ. Primaquine: report from CDC expert meeting on malaria chemoprophylaxis I. Am J Trop Med Hyg. 2006 Sep;75(3):402–15.

5. Hwang J, Cullen KA, Kachur SP, Arguin PM, Baird JK. Severe morbidity and mortality risk from malaria in the United States, 1985–2011. Open Forum Infect Dis. 2014 Jun 30;1(1).

6. Lupi E, Hatz C, Schlagenhauf P. The efficacy of repellents against Aedes, Anopheles, Culex and Ixodes spp.—a literature review. Travel Med Infect Dis. 2013 Nov–Dec;11(6):374–411.

7. Mace KE, Arguin PM, Tan KR. Malaria Surveillance—United States, 2015. MMWR Surveill Summ 2018;67 (No. SS-7):1–28. doi: http://dx.doi.org/10.15585/mmwr.ss6707a1

8. Novitt-Moreno A, Ransom J, Dow, G, Smith B, Read LT, Toovey S. Tafenoquine for malaria prophylaxis in adults: an integrated safety analysis. Travel Med Infect Dis. 2017 May–Jun;17:19–27.

9. Tan KR, Magill AJ, Parise ME, Arguin PM. Doxycycline for malaria chemoprophylaxis and treatment: report from the CDC expert meeting on malaria chemoprophylaxis. Am J Trop Med Hyg. 2011 Apr;84(4):517–31.

# MEASLES (RUBEOLA)

Paul A. Gastañaduy, James L. Goodson

## INFECTIOUS AGENT

Measles virus is a member of the genus *Morbillivirus* of the family Paramyxoviridae.

## TRANSMISSION

Measles is transmitted from person to person primarily by the airborne route as aerosolized droplet nuclei. Infected people are usually contagious from 4 days before until 4 days after rash onset. Measles is among the most contagious viral diseases known; secondary attack rates are ≥90% in susceptible household and institutional contacts. Humans are the only natural host for sustaining measles virus transmission, which makes global eradication of measles feasible.

## EPIDEMIOLOGY

The number of reported measles cases in the United States has declined from nearly 500,000 annually in the decade before the measles vaccine program to 37–667 cases annually from 2001 through 2017. As a result of high vaccination coverage and implementation of measles elimination strategies in the Americas, measles in the United States was declared eliminated (defined as the absence of endemic measles virus transmission in a defined geographic area for ≥12 months in the presence of a well-performing surveillance system) in 2000. In September 2016, the Americas became the first region in the world to be certified as having verified elimination of endemic measles virus transmission. However, measles virus continues to be imported into the region from other parts of the world, and recent prolonged outbreaks resulting from measles virus importations highlight the challenges faced in maintaining elimination.

Globally, in 2016, the annual reported measles incidence was 19 cases per million population. Given the large global incidence and high communicability of the disease, travelers may be exposed to the virus in almost any country they visit where measles is endemic or where large outbreaks are occurring, particularly those outside the Western Hemisphere. Most measles cases imported into the United States have come from unvaccinated US residents who became infected while traveling abroad, became symptomatic after returning to the United States, and in some cases infected others in their communities, causing outbreaks.

Humanitarian emergencies following natural disasters, famine, war, large-scale population movements, and disease outbreaks can disrupt immunization services and create persistent reservoirs for vaccine-preventable diseases and for measles virus, in particular. Protracted armed conflict and absence of a centralized government can cripple efforts to provide basic public health services to local civilian populations, including the delivery of vaccinations to children. Aid workers and volunteers in humanitarian emergencies are thus also at an increased risk of being exposed to measles.

Additional information on global measles elimination efforts is available on the Measles & Rubella Initiative website at www.measlesrubellainitiative.org.

## CLINICAL PRESENTATION

The incubation period ranges from 7 to 21 days from exposure to onset of fever; rash usually appears about 14 days after exposure. Symptoms include prodromal fever that can rise as high as 105°F (40.6°C), conjunctivitis, coryza (runny nose), cough, and small spots with white or bluish-white centers on an erythematous base on the buccal mucosa (Koplik spots). A characteristic red, blotchy (maculopapular) rash appears on the third to seventh day after the onset of prodromal symptoms. The rash begins on the face, becomes generalized, and lasts 4–7 days. Common complications include diarrhea (8%), middle ear infection (7%–9%), and pneumonia (1%–6%). Encephalitis, which can result in permanent brain damage, occurs in approximately 1 per 1,000–2,000 cases of measles. The risk of serious complications and death is highest for children aged ≤5 years and adults aged ≥20 years. It is also higher in populations with poor nutritional status.

Subacute sclerosing panencephalitis (SSPE) is a progressive neurologic disorder caused by measles virus that usually presents 5–10 years after recovery from the initial primary measles virus infection. SSPE is manifested by mental and motor deterioration, progressing to coma and death and occurs in approximately 1–2 in 10,000 reported measles cases, with a higher rate among children <5 years of age.

## DIAGNOSIS

Laboratory criteria for diagnosis include any of the following: a positive serologic test for measles-specific IgM, IgG seroconversion or a significant rise in measles IgG level by any standard serologic assay, isolation of measles virus, or detection of measles virus RNA by RT-PCR.

A clinical case of measles illness is characterized by all of the following:

- Generalized maculopapular rash lasting ≥3 days

- Temperature of ≥101°F (38.3°C)

- Cough, coryza, or conjunctivitis

A confirmed case is one with an acute febrile rash illness with laboratory confirmation or direct epidemiologic linkage to a laboratory-confirmed case. In a laboratory-confirmed case or epidemiologically linked case, the temperature does not need to reach ≥101°F (38.3°C) and the rash does not need to last ≥3 days.

Measles is a nationally notifiable disease.

## TREATMENT

Treatment is supportive. The World Health Organization recommends vitamin A for all children with acute measles, regardless of their country of residence, to reduce the risk of complications. Vitamin A is administered once a day for 2 days at the following doses:

- 50,000 IU for infants aged <6 months

- 100,000 IU for infants aged 6–11 months

- 200,000 IU for children aged ≥12 months

An additional (third) age-specific dose of vitamin A should be given 2–4 weeks later to children with clinical signs and symptoms of vitamin A deficiency. Parenteral and oral formulations of vitamin A are available in the United States.

## PREVENTION

Measles has been preventable since 1963 through vaccination. People who do not have evidence of measles immunity should be considered at risk for measles, particularly during international travel. Acceptable presumptive evidence of immunity to measles for international travelers includes meeting any of the following criteria:

- Written documentation of age-appropriate vaccination with a live* measles-containing vaccine (MMR or MMRV):
  > For infants aged 6–11 months, documented administration of 1 dose of MMR

  > For people aged ≥12 months, 2 doses of MMR or MMRV (the first dose should be administered at age ≥12 months; the second dose should be administered no earlier than 28 days after the first dose)

- Laboratory evidence of immunity

- Laboratory confirmation of disease

- Birth before 1957

Verbal or self-reported history of vaccination is not considered valid presumptive evidence of immunity.

### Vaccine

Measles vaccine contains live, attenuated measles virus. In the United States, it is available only in combination formulations, such as measles-mumps-rubella (MMR) and measles-mumps-rubella-varicella (MMRV) vaccines. MMRV vaccine is licensed for children aged 12 months through 12 years and may be used in place of MMR vaccine if vaccination for measles, mumps, rubella, and varicella is needed.

International travelers, including people traveling to industrialized countries, who do not have presumptive evidence of measles immunity and who have no contraindications to MMR or MMRV, should receive MMR or MMRV before travel according to the following guidelines:

- Infants aged 6–11 months should receive 1 MMR dose. Infants vaccinated before age 12 months must be revaccinated on or after the first birthday with 2 doses of MMR or MMRV separated by ≥28 days. MMRV is not licensed for children aged <12 months.

- Preschool and school-age children (aged ≥12 months) should be given 2 MMR or MMRV doses separated by ≥28 days.

- Adults born in or after 1957 should be given 2 MMR doses separated by ≥28 days.

* From 1963 through 1967, a formalin-inactivated measles vaccine was available in the United States and was administered to an estimated 600,000–900,000 people. It was discontinued when it became apparent that the immunity it produced was short-lived. People who received this vaccine should be considered unvaccinated.

One dose of MMR is approximately 85% effective when administered at age 9 months; MMR and MMRV are 93% effective when administered at age ≥1 year. Vaccine effectiveness of 2 doses is 97%.

Measles-containing vaccine and immune globulin (IG) may be effective as postexposure prophylaxis. MMR or MMRV, if administered within 72 hours after initial exposure to measles virus, may provide some protection. If the exposure does not result in infection, the vaccine should induce protection against subsequent measles virus infection. IG can be used to prevent or mitigate measles in a susceptible person when administered within 6 days of exposure. However, any immunity conferred is temporary unless modified or typical measles occurs, and the person should receive MMR or MMRV 6 months after intramuscularly administered IG or 8 months after intravenously administered IG, provided the person is then aged ≥12 months and the vaccine is not otherwise contraindicated.

## VACCINE SAFETY AND ADVERSE REACTIONS

In rare circumstances, MMR vaccination has been associated with the following adverse events:

- Anaphylaxis (approximately 3.5–10 occurrences per million doses administered)

- Thrombocytopenia (approximately 1 occurrence per 30,000–40,000 doses during the 6 weeks after immunization)

- Febrile seizures (approximately 1 occurrence per 3,000 doses administered, but overall, the rate of febrile seizures after measles-containing vaccine is much lower than the rate with measles disease)

- Joint symptoms (Arthralgia develops among approximately 25% of nonimmune postpubertal women from the rubella component of the MMR vaccination. Approximately 10% have acute arthritislike signs and symptoms that generally persist for 1 day to 3 weeks and rarely recur. Chronic joint symptoms are rare, if they occur at all.)

There is no evidence to support a causal link between MMR vaccination and hearing loss, retinopathy, optic neuritis, ocular palsies, Guillain-Barré syndrome, cerebellar ataxia, Crohn's disease, or autism.

## CONTRAINDICATIONS AND PRECAUTIONS
### CONTRAINDICATIONS
*Allergy*—People with severe allergy (hives, swelling of the mouth or throat, difficulty breathing, hypotension, and shock) to gelatin or neomycin, or who have had a severe allergic reaction to a prior dose of MMR or MMRV vaccine, should not be vaccinated or revaccinated. MMR or MMRV vaccine may be administered to people who are allergic to eggs without prior routine skin testing or the use of special protocols.

*Pregnancy*—MMR vaccines should not be administered to pregnant women or to those attempting to become pregnant. Because of the theoretical risk to the fetus when the mother receives a live-virus vaccine, women should be counseled to avoid becoming pregnant for 28 days after receipt of MMR vaccine.

*Immunosuppression*—Enhanced replication of live vaccine viruses can occur in people who have immune deficiency disorders. Death related to vaccine-associated measles virus infection has been reported among severely immunocompromised people. Therefore, severely immunosuppressed people should not be vaccinated with MMR or MMRV vaccine. For a thorough discussion of recommendations for immunocompromised travelers, see Chapter 5, Immunocompromised Travelers.

- People with leukemia in remission, and off chemotherapy, who were not immune to measles when diagnosed with leukemia, may receive MMR vaccine. At least 3 months should elapse after termination of chemotherapy before administration of the first dose.

- MMR vaccination is recommended for all people aged ≥12 months with HIV infection who do not have evidence of measles, rubella, and mumps immunity or evidence of severe immunosuppression. The assessment of severe immunosuppression can be on the basis of CD4 values (count or percentage); absence of severe immunosuppression is defined as CD4 percentages ≥15% for ≥6 months at any age or CD4 count ≥200 cells/mm$^3$ for ≥6 months for people aged >5 years.

- People who have received high-dose corticosteroid therapy (in general, considered to be ≥20 mg prednisone or equivalent daily for a duration of ≥14 days) should avoid vaccination with MMR or MMRV for ≥1 month after cessation of steroid therapy. Corticosteroid therapy usually is not a contraindication when administration is short-term (<14 days) or a low to moderate dose (<20 mg of prednisone or equivalent per day).

- In general, MMR or MMRV vaccine should be withheld for ≥3 months after cessation of other immunosuppressive therapies and remission of the underlying disease. This interval is based on the assumptions that the immune response will have been restored in 3 months and the underlying disease for which the therapy was given remains in remission.

## PRECAUTIONS

*Thrombocytopenia*—The benefits of primary immunization are usually greater than the potential risks of thrombocytopenia. However, avoiding a subsequent dose of MMR or MMRV vaccine may be prudent if an episode of thrombocytopenia occurred within approximately 6 weeks after a previous dose of vaccine.

*Personal or family history of seizures of any etiology*—Compared with administration of separate MMR and varicella vaccines at the same visit, use of MMRV vaccine is associated with a higher risk for fever and febrile seizures 5–12 days after the first dose among children aged 12–23 months. Approximately 1 additional febrile seizure occurs for every 2,300–2,600 MMRV vaccine doses administered. Use of separate MMR and varicella vaccines avoids this increased risk for fever and febrile seizures.

**CDC website:** www.cdc.gov/measles

## BIBLIOGRAPHY

1. American Academy of Pediatrics. Measles. In: Pickering LK, editor. Red Book: 2015 Report of the Committee on Infectious Diseases. 30th ed. Elk Grove Village, IL: American Academy of Pediatrics; 2015. pp. 535–47.

2. Bellini WJ, Rota JS, Lowe LE, Katz RS, Dyken PR, Zaki SR, et al. Subacute sclerosing panencephalitis: more cases of this fatal disease are prevented by measles immunization than was previously recognized. J Infect Dis. 2005 Nov 15;192(10):1686–93.

3. CDC. General recommendations on immunization—recommendations of the Advisory Committee on Immunization Practices (ACIP). MMWR Recomm Rep. 2011;60(RR-02):1–60.

4. CDC. Prevention of measles, rubella, congenital rubella syndrome, and mumps, 2013: summary recommendations of the Advisory Committee on Immunization Practices (ACIP). MMWR Recomm Rep. 2013 Jun 14;62(RR-04):1–34.

5. Dabbagh A, Patel MK, Dumolard L, Gacic-Dobo M, Mulders MN, Okwo-Bele JM, et al. Progress toward regional measles elimination—worldwide, 2000–2016. MMWR Morb Mortal Wkly Rep. 2017;66(42):1148–53.

6. Measles & Rubella Initiative [Internet]. Washington, DC: American Red Cross; 2014 [cited 2016 Sep 25]. Available from: www.measlesrubellainitiative.org.

7. National Notifiable Diseases Surveillance System. Measles (rubeola): 2013 case definition. Atlanta: CDC; 2013 [cited 2019 Jan 10]. Available from: wwwn.cdc.gov/NNDSS/script/casedef.aspx?CondYrID=908&-DatePub=1/1/2013.

8. Perry RT, Halsey NA. The clinical significance of measles: a review. J Infect Dis. 2004 May 1;189 Suppl 1:S4–16.

9. Rota PA, Moss WJ, Takeda M, de Swart RL, Thompson KM, Goodson JL. Measles. Nat Rev Dis Primers. 2016;2:16049.

10. Strebel PM, Papania MJ, Gastañaduy PA, Goodson JL. Measles vaccines. In: Vaccines. 7th ed. Elsevier; 2017.

11. World Health Organization. Measles [fact sheet no. 286]. Geneva: World Health Organization; 2014 [cited 2016 Sep 25]. Available from: www.who.int/mediacentre/factsheets/fs286/en/.

12. World Health Organization. Information sheet: Observed rate of vaccine reactions: Measles, mumps, and rubella vaccines. Geneva: World Health Organization; 2014 [cited 2018 Apr 25]. Available from: www.who.int/vaccine_safety/initiative/tools/vaccinfosheets/en/.

13. World Health Organization. Measles vaccines: WHO position paper—April 2017. Wkly Epidemiol Rec. 2017;92(17): 205–27.

4

# MELIOIDOSIS

David D. Blaney, Jay E. Gee

## INFECTIOUS AGENT

*Burkholderia pseudomallei*, a saprophytic gram-negative bacillus, is the causative agent of melioidosis. The bacteria are found in soil and water, widely distributed in tropical and sub-tropical countries.

## TRANSMISSION

Transmission can occur through subcutaneous inoculation, ingestion, or inhalation; person-to-person transmission is extremely rare but may occur through contact with the blood or body fluids of an infected person.

## EPIDEMIOLOGY

Melioidosis is endemic to Southeast Asia, Papua New Guinea, much of the Indian subcontinent, southern China, Hong Kong, and Taiwan and is considered highly endemic to northeast Thailand, Malaysia, Singapore, and northern Australia. Sporadic cases have been reported among residents of or travelers to Aruba, Colombia, Costa Rica, El Salvador, Guatemala, Guadeloupe, Honduras, Martinique, Mexico, Panama, Venezuela, and many other countries in the Americas, as well as Puerto Rico. In northeastern Brazil, clusters of melioidosis have been reported. The true extent of the distribution of the bacteria remains unknown and is considered underreported or unrecognized in many tropical and subtropical areas, and more than 165,000 cases are estimated to occur annually.

The risk is highest for adventure travelers, ecotourists, military personnel, construction and resource extraction workers, and other people whose contact with contaminated soil or water may expose them to the bacteria; infections have been reported in people who have spent less than a week in an endemic area. Cases, especially presenting as pneumonias, are often associated with periods of high rainfall such as during typhoons or the monsoon season. Risk factors for invasive melioidosis include diabetes, excessive alcohol use, chronic renal disease, chronic lung disease (such as cystic fibrosis or chronic obstructive pulmonary disease), thalassemia, and malignancy or other non-HIV-related immune suppression.

## CLINICAL PRESENTATION

Incubation period is generally 1–21 days; with a high inoculum, symptoms can develop in a few hours. Melioidosis may also remain latent for months or years before symptoms develop. Melioidosis may occur as a subclinical infection, localized infection (such as cutaneous abscess), pneumonia, meningoencephalitis, sepsis, or chronic suppurative infection. The latter may mimic tuberculosis, with fever, weight loss, productive cough, and upper lobe infiltrate, with or without cavitation. More than 50% of cases present with pneumonia.

## DIAGNOSIS

Culture of *B. pseudomallei* from blood, sputum, pus, urine, synovial fluid, peritoneal fluid, or pericardial fluid is diagnostic. Indirect hemagglutination assay is a widely used serologic test but is not considered confirmatory. Diagnostic assistance is available through CDC (www.cdc.gov/ncezid/dhcpp/bacterial_special/zoonoses_lab.html).

## TREATMENT

Intravenous ceftazidime, or meropenem for severe cases with sepsis, is typically used for initial treatment, for a minimum of 14 days; depending on response to therapy, this initial treatment may be extended for up to 8 weeks. This is usually followed by 3–6 months of eradication treatment with an oral agent such as trimethoprim-sulfamethoxazole. Relapse may be seen, especially in patients who received a shorter-than-recommended course of therapy.

## PREVENTION

Travelers should use personal protective equipment such as waterproof boots and gloves to protect against contact with soil and water in endemic areas and thoroughly clean skin lacerations, abrasions, or burns contaminated with soil or surface water.

**CDC website:** www.cdc.gov/melioidosis

## BIBLIOGRAPHY

1. Benoit TJ, Blaney DD, Doker TJ, Gee JE, Elrod MG, Rolim DB, et al. A review of melioidosis cases in the Americas. Am J Trop Med Hyg. 2015 Dec;93(6):1134–9.

2. Cheng JW, Hayden MK, Singh K, Heimler I, Gee JE, Proia L, Sha BE. *Burkholderia pseudomallei* Infection in US Traveler Returning from Mexico, 2014. Emerg Infect Dis. 2015 Oct;21(10):1884–5.

3. Currie BJ. Melioidosis: evolving concepts in epidemiology, pathogenesis, and treatment. Semin Respir Crit Care Med. 2015 Feb;36(1):111–25.

4. Doker TJ, Sharp TM, Rivera-Garcia B, Perez-Padilla J, Benoit TJ, Ellis EM, et al. Contact investigation of melioidosis cases reveals regional endemicity in Puerto Rico. Clin Infect Dis. 2015 Jan 15;60(2):243–50.

5. Limmathurotsakul D, Golding N, Dance DA, Messina JP, Pigott DM, Moyes CL, et al. Predicted global distribution of Burkholderia pseudomallei and burden of melioidosis. Nat Microbiol. 2016;1:15008.

6. Limmathurotsakul D, Kanoksil M, Wuthiekanun V, Kitphati R, deStavola B, Day NP, et al. Activities of daily living associated with acquisition of melioidosis in northeast Thailand: a matched case-control study. PLoS Negl Trop Dis. 2013;7(2):e2072.

7. Wiersinga WJ, Virk HS, Torres AG, Currie BJ, Peacock SJ, Dance DAB, Limmathurotsakul D. Melioidosis. Nat Rev Dis Primers. 2018 Feb 1;4:17107.

**4**

# MENINGOCOCCAL DISEASE

Sarah A. Mbaeyi, Lucy A. McNamara

## INFECTIOUS AGENT

*Neisseria meningitidis* is a gram-negative diplococcus. Meningococci are classified into serogroups on the basis of the composition of the capsular polysaccharide. The 6 major meningococcal serogroups associated with disease are A, B, C, W, X, and Y.

## TRANSMISSION

Spread through respiratory secretions; requires close contact. Both asymptomatic carriers and people with overt meningococcal disease can serve as sources of infection. Asymptomatic carriage is transient and typically affects approximately 5%–10% of the population at any given time.

## EPIDEMIOLOGY

*N. meningitidis* is found worldwide, but the highest incidence occurs in the "meningitis belt" of sub-Saharan Africa (Map 4-10). Meningococcal disease is hyperendemic to this region, and periodic epidemics during the dry season (December–June) reach up to 1,000 cases per 100,000 population. By contrast, rates of disease in the United States, Europe, Australia, and South America range from 0.12 to 3 cases per 100,000 population per year.

Although meningococcal outbreaks can occur anywhere in the world, they are most common in the African meningitis belt, and large-scale epidemics occur every 5–12 years. Historically, outbreaks in the meningitis belt were primarily due to serogroup A. However, with the introduction of a monovalent serogroup A meningococcal conjugate vaccine (MenAfriVac) in the region starting in 2010, recent meningococcal outbreaks in the meningitis belt have primarily been due to serogroups C and W, although serogroup X outbreaks are also reported.

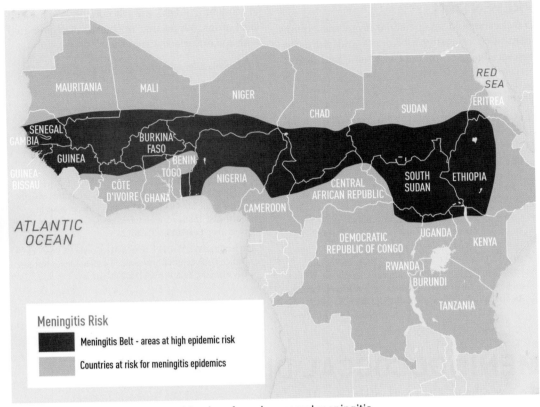

**MAP 4-10. Areas with frequent epidemics of meningococcal meningitis**

Disease data source: World Health Organization. International Travel and Health. Geneva, Switzerland: 2015.

Outside the meningitis belt, infants and adolescents have the highest rates of disease. In meningitis belt countries, high rates of disease are seen in people up to age 30 years, and the highest rates are in children and adolescents aged 5– 14 years. Risk for travelers is highest in people visiting meningitis belt countries who have prolonged contact with local populations during an epidemic. The Hajj pilgrimage to Saudi Arabia has also been associated with outbreaks of meningococcal disease in returning pilgrims and their contacts.

## CLINICAL PRESENTATION

Meningococcal disease generally occurs 1–10 days after exposure and presents as meningitis in ≥50% of cases. Meningococcal meningitis is characterized by sudden onset of headache, fever, and stiffness of the neck, sometimes accompanied by nausea, vomiting, photophobia, or altered mental status. Approximately 40% of people with meningococcal disease present with meningococcal sepsis, known as meningococcemia. Symptoms of meningococcemia can include abrupt onset of fever, chills, vomiting, diarrhea, and a petechial or purpuric rash, which may progress to purpura fulminans. Meningococcemia often involves hypotension, acute adrenal hemorrhage, and multiorgan failure. Among infants and children aged <2 years, meningococcal disease may have nonspecific symptoms. Neck stiffness, usually seen in people with meningitis, may be absent in this age group. Meningococcal disease is rapidly progressive and has a case-fatality ratio of 10%–20%, even with antibiotic treatment. Without rapid treatment, fatality ratios can be much higher.

## DIAGNOSIS

Early diagnosis and treatment are critical. A lumbar puncture should be done to examine the cerebrospinal fluid (CSF) and perform a Gram stain. If possible, the lumbar puncture should be done before starting antibiotic therapy to ensure that bacteria, if present, can be cultured from CSF; however, lumbar puncture should not delay antibiotic treatment. In general, diagnosis is made by isolating *N. meningitidis* from a normally sterile body site (such as blood or CSF) through culture or by detection of *N. meningitidis*–specific nucleic acid by PCR.

The signs and symptoms of meningococcal meningitis are similar to those of other causes of bacterial meningitis, such as *Haemophilus influenzae* and *Streptococcus pneumoniae*. The causative organism should be identified so that the correct antibiotics can be used for treatment and prophylaxis. Meningococcal disease is nationally notifiable in the United States and should be immediately reported to the state or local health department.

## TREATMENT

Meningococcal disease can be rapidly fatal and should always be viewed as a medical emergency. Antibiotic treatment must be started early in the course of the disease, and empirically when suspected and prior to the diagnostic test results. Several antibiotic choices are available, including third-generation cephalosporins.

## PREVENTION

### Vaccine

Four meningococcal vaccines are licensed and available in the United States. Refer to Table 4-14 for more information about available meningococcal vaccines. Approximately 7–10 days are required after vaccination for the development of protective antibody levels.

#### ROUTINE IMMUNIZATION

The Advisory Committee on Immunization Practices (ACIP) recommends routine administration of a quadrivalent meningococcal conjugate vaccine (MenACWY) for all people aged 11–18 years. A single dose of vaccine should be administered at age 11 or 12 years, and a booster dose should be administered at age 16 years. Routine immunization with MenACWY is not recommended for other age groups in the United States, with the exception of people at increased risk for meningococcal disease. Those at increased risk for meningococcal disease include people who have a persistent complement component deficiency (C3, C5-9, properdin, factor D, factor H, or people who are taking eculizumab [Soliris]), people who have functional or anatomic asplenia, or people with HIV. Vaccine, product, number of doses, and booster dose recommendations are based on age and risk factors and are described in detail for each risk group in the 2013 ACIP Meningococcal Disease Recommendations (www.cdc.gov/mmwr/preview/mmwrhtml/rr6202a1.htm) and additional ACIP policy notes (www.cdc.gov/vaccines/hcp/acip-recs/vacc-specific/mening.html).

Adolescents and young adults aged 16–23 years may also be vaccinated with a serogroup B meningococcal (MenB) vaccine series to provide short-term protection against most strains of serogroup B meningococcal disease. The preferred age for MenB vaccination is 16–18 years. ACIP also recommends routine use of MenB vaccine for people aged ≥10 years who are at increased risk for meningococcal disease, including people who have persistent complement component deficiency and people who have functional or anatomic asplenia. ACIP recommendations for MenB vaccines can be found at www.cdc.gov/vaccines/hcp/acip-recs/vacc-specific/mening.html.

#### IMMUNIZATION FOR TRAVELERS

ACIP recommends that travelers aged ≥2 months who visit or reside in parts of sub-Saharan Africa known as the "meningitis belt" (see Map 4-10) during the dry season (December–June) receive vaccination with a MenACWY vaccine before travel. Advisories for travelers to other countries are issued when outbreaks of meningococcal disease are recognized (see the CDC Travelers' Health website at www.cdc.gov/travel).

For infants aged <9 months, MenACWY-CRM (Menveo) is the only licensed and available

## Table 4-14. Meningococcal vaccines licensed and available in the United States

| VACCINE | TRADE NAME (MANUFACTURER) | AGE OF VACCINE INITIATION | DOSE | ROUTE | INTERVAL SINCE FIRST DOSE | BOOSTER |
|---|---|---|---|---|---|---|
| Meningococcal (serogroups A, C, W, and Y) oligosaccharide diphtheria CRM$_{197}$ conjugate vaccine (MenACWY-CRM)[1] | Menveo (GSK) | 2 mo<br>7–23 mo<br><br><br><br><br><br>≥ 2 y | 0.5 mL<br>0.5 mL<br><br><br><br><br><br>0.5 mL | IM<br>IM<br><br><br><br><br><br>IM | 0, 2, 4, 10 mo<br>0, 3 mo (2nd dose administered in 2nd year of life)<br>1 dose[2] | If at continued risk[3] |
| Meningococcal (serogroups A, C, W, and Y) polysaccharide diphtheria toxoid conjugate vaccine (MenACWY-D)[1] | Menactra (Sanofi Pasteur) | 9–23 mo<br>≥ 2 y | 0.5 mL<br>0.5 mL | IM<br>IM | 0, 3 mo<br>1 dose[2] | If at continued risk[3] |
| Meningococcal serogroup B vaccine (MenB-FHbp) | Trumenba (Pfizer) | 10–25 y | 0.5 mL | IM | 0, 1–2, 6 mo or 0, 6 mo (depending on indication)[4] | None |
| Meningococcal serogroup B vaccine (MenB-4C) | Bexsero (GSK) | 10–25 y | 0.5 mL | IM | 0, ≥1 mo | None |

Abbreviations: IM, intramuscular; SC, subcutaneous.
[1] If an infant is receiving the vaccine before travel, 2 doses may be administered as early as 8 weeks apart.
[2] For people with HIV, anatomic or functional asplenia, and people with persistent complement component deficiencies (C3, C5-9, properdin, factor D, factor H, or people taking eculizumab [Soliris]) should receive a 2-dose primary series 8–12 weeks apart.
[3] Revaccination with meningococcal conjugate vaccine (MenACWY-D or MenACWY-CRM) is recommended after 3 years for children who received their last dose at <7 years of age. Revaccination with meningococcal conjugate vaccine is recommended after 5 years for people who received their last dose at ≥7 years of age, and every 5 years thereafter for people who are at continued risk.
[4] In April 2016, FDA approved updates to the prescribing information for MenB-FHbp to allow for the administration of either a 3-dose schedule (0, 1–2, 6 months) or a 2-dose schedule (0, 6 months). The 3-dose schedule is preferred for groups at increased risk where more rapid protection is desired.

meningococcal vaccine. In children initiating vaccination at 2 months of age, MenACWY-CRM should be administered as a 4-dose series at 2, 4, 6, and 12 months of age. In children initiating vaccination at 7–23 months of age, MenACWY-CRM should be administered as a 2-dose series, with the second dose administered at ≥12 months of age and ≥3 months after the first dose, although it can be administered as early as 8 weeks after the first dose to precede travel.

For travelers initiating vaccination at ≥9 months (i.e., 9 months through 55 years), either MenACWY-CRM or MenACWY-D (Menactra) may be used. For travelers 9–23 months of age who receive MenACWY-D, 2 doses should be administered, with the second dose administered ≥3 months after the first dose, although it can be administered as early as 8 weeks after the first dose to precede travel. For most people aged ≥2 years, 1 dose of a MenACWY vaccine (MenACWY-CRM or MenACWY-D) is recommended before travel.

Additional dosing instructions for people with HIV, asplenia, or persistent complement component deficiencies are available in the 2013 ACIP Meningococcal Disease Recommendations (www.cdc.gov/mmwr/preview/mmwrhtml/rr6202a1.htm). Although not licensed for use in adults aged ≥56 years, MenACWY is the recommended vaccine for people in this age group, as the quadrivalent meningococcal polysaccharide vaccine (MPSV4) is no longer available in the United States.

Travelers to the Kingdom of Saudi Arabia (KSA) for Umrah or Hajj are required to provide documentation of quadrivalent vaccine at least 10 days and no more than 3 years before arrival for polysaccharide vaccine and no more than 5 years before arrival for conjugate vaccine (see www.moh.gov.sa/en/Hajj/Pages/HealthRegulations.aspx). Visa requirements should be confirmed with the KSA embassy. Although the KSA Ministry of Health currently advises against travel to Hajj for pregnant women or children, these groups should receive meningococcal vaccination according to licensed indications for their age if they travel.

International travelers at risk for meningococcal disease who were previously vaccinated with a quadrivalent vaccine should receive a booster dose. For children who completed the primary dose or series at <7 years of age, a booster dose of MenACWY should be administered after 3 years and repeated every 5 years thereafter if they live in or travel to a hyperendemic area. For people who received the primary dose or series at ≥7 years of age, a booster dose should be administered after 5 years and every 5 years thereafter if they live in or travel to a hyperendemic area.

MenB vaccine is not recommended for people who live in or travel to meningitis belt countries, as serogroup B disease is extremely rare in this region. MenB vaccine is not routinely recommended for travel to other regions of the world unless an outbreak of serogroup B disease has been reported.

A monovalent serogroup A meningococcal conjugate vaccine (MenAfriVac) has been introduced into meningitis belt countries since 2010 through mass vaccination campaigns and the routine childhood immunization schedule. This vaccine is not available in the United States for travelers and is not recommended in place of MenACWY vaccine for travelers who will be living in meningitis belt countries as it does not protect against serogroups C, W, and Y. In some countries outside the meningitis belt, meningococcal vaccination (such as monovalent conjugate C vaccine or MenB vaccine) may be recommended as part of the routine immunization program for infants. Infants residing in these countries may consider meningococcal vaccination according to the routine immunization recommendations of that country.

## VACCINE SAFETY AND ADVERSE REACTIONS

Low-grade fevers and local reactions, such as injection-site pain, arm swelling, and pain that limits movement of the injected arm, are side effects seen after MenACWY vaccine. Symptoms are generally mild to moderate and resolve within 48–72 hours. Severe adverse events, such as high fever, chills, joint pain, rash, or seizures are rare (<5% of vaccinees).

Although no clinical trials of meningococcal vaccines have been conducted in pregnant or lactating women, postlicensure safety data have not identified any serious safety concerns to the mother or fetus. Pregnancy or lactation should not preclude vaccination with MenACWY if indicated.

## PRECAUTIONS AND CONTRAINDICATIONS

People with moderate or severe acute illness should defer vaccination until their condition improves. Vaccination is contraindicated for people who have a severe allergic reaction to any component of the vaccines. All meningococcal vaccines are inactivated and may be given to immunosuppressed people.

## Antibiotic Chemoprophylaxis

In the United States and most industrialized countries, antibiotic chemoprophylaxis is recommended for close contacts of a patient with invasive meningococcal disease to prevent secondary cases. Chemoprophylaxis ideally should be initiated within 24 hours after the index patient is identified; prophylaxis given >2 weeks after exposure has little value. Antibiotics used for prophylaxis include ciprofloxacin, rifampin, and ceftriaxone. Ceftriaxone is recommended for pregnant women.

**CDC website:** www.cdc.gov/meningococcal

## BIBLIOGRAPHY

1. American Academy of Pediatrics. Meningococcal infections. In: Kimberlin DW, Brady MT, Jackson M, Long SS, editors. Red Book: 2015 Report of the Committee on Infectious Diseases. 30th ed. Elk Grove Village, IL: American Academy of Pediatrics; 2015. pp. 547–58.

2. CDC. Prevention and control of meningococcal disease: recommendations of the Advisory Committee on Immunization Practices (ACIP). MMWR Morb Mortal Wkly Rep. 2013;62(2):1–28.

3. Folaranmi T, Rubin L, Martin SW, Patel M, MacNeil JR. Use of serogroup B meningococcal vaccines in persons aged >/=10 years at increased risk for serogroup B meningococcal disease: recommendations of the Advisory Committee on Immunization Practices, 2015. MMWR Morb Mortal Wkly Rep. 2015 Jun 12;64(22):608–12.

4. Halperin SA, Bettinger JA, Greenwood B, Harrison LH, Jelfs J, Ladhani SN, et al. The changing and dynamic epidemiology of meningococcal disease. Vaccine. 2012 May 30;30 Suppl 2:B26–36.

5. MacNeil JR, Rubin L, Folaranmi T, Ortega-Sanchez IR, Patel M, Martin SW. Use of serogroup B meningococcal vaccines in adolescents and young adults: recommendations of the Advisory Committee on Immunization Practices, 2015. MMWR Morb Mortal Wkly Rep. 2015 Oct 23;64(41):1171–6.

6. Patton ME, Stephens D, Moore K, MacNeil JR. Updated recommendations for use of MenB-FHbp serogroup B meningococcal vaccine—Advisory Committee on Immunization Practices, 2016. MMWR Morb Mortal Wkly Rep. 2016 May 19;66(19):509–13.

7. Trotter CL, Lingani C, Fernandez K, Cooper LV, Bita A, Tevi-Benissan C, et al. Impact of MenAfriVac in nine countries of the African meningitis belt, 2010–2015: an analysis of surveillance data. Lancet Infect Dis. 2017 Aug;17(8):867–72.

8. World Health Organization. Epidemic meningitis control in countries of the African meningitis belt, 2016. Wkly Epidemiol Rec. 2017 Mar 31;92(13):145–54.

# MIDDLE EAST RESPIRATORY SYNDROME (MERS)

John T. Watson, Susan I. Gerber

## INFECTIOUS AGENT

The MERS coronavirus, a single-stranded, positive-sense RNA coronavirus that belongs to the family Coronaviridae, genus *Betacoronavirus*.

## TRANSMISSION

Transmission dynamics are not well understood. The MERS coronavirus is genetically similar to bat coronaviruses and has been detected in camels in North Africa and the Arabian Peninsula. Although exposure to dromedary camels is a risk factor for MERS, little is known about the specific exposures that result in primary human cases. Evidence suggests that the virus can be spread from person to person among close contacts, resulting in outbreaks in families and in health care settings. Sustained community transmission of MERS has not been shown.

## EPIDEMIOLOGY

MERS coronavirus is an emerging novel coronavirus that causes severe acute respiratory illness, and approximately 35% of confirmed cases have been fatal. MERS was first reported in September 2012, but illnesses with onsets as early as April 2012 were subsequently documented. Risk is ongoing in countries in or near the Arabian Peninsula. Index cases have lived in or recently traveled to Iran, Jordan, Kuwait, Lebanon, Oman, Qatar, Saudi Arabia, United Arab Emirates, or Yemen. MERS has also been identified in travelers from these countries returning to North America, Europe, Asia, and North Africa.

## CLINICAL PRESENTATION

MERS is associated with severe acute respiratory failure, multiple organ dysfunction, and high mortality, although the spectrum of illness and clinical course are not fully defined. Mild or asymptomatic cases have been documented among contacts of cases. For people who develop symptomatic illness, the incubation period is approximately 2–14 days; median incubation period is slightly more than 5 days. Disease is most often characterized by fever, cough, and shortness of breath. Other symptoms may include chills, sore throat, myalgias, arthralgias, diarrhea, and vomiting. Initial nonspecific symptoms can progress to pneumonia. Chest radiographs have shown variable pulmonary involvement.

In addition to acute and often severe respiratory compromise, serious complications of MERS include cardiovascular collapse and acute renal injury. Abnormal laboratory findings can include thrombocytopenia, lymphopenia, and elevated liver function tests. Older age and comorbidities are associated with poor outcomes.

## DIAGNOSIS

Several diagnostic assays have been developed to detect acute infection with MERS coronavirus, including real-time RT-PCR. Lower respiratory specimens (sputum, bronchoalveolar lavage, endotracheal aspirates) are the priority respiratory specimens for testing, although upper respiratory and serum specimens should also be collected, if possible. To increase the likelihood of detecting the virus, multiple specimens from these sites should be collected over the course of the illness. In the United States, most state laboratories are approved to test for MERS by using CDC's RT-PCR assay. Testing should be coordinated through state and local health departments and CDC.

In coordination with state and local health departments, health care providers should evaluate patients for MERS if they develop fever and pneumonia or acute respiratory distress syndrome within 14 days after traveling from countries in or near the Arabian Peninsula or have had close contact with a recent traveler from this area who has fever and acute respiratory illness.

## TREATMENT

No specific antiviral treatment is available. Treatment is limited to supportive care. Standard, contact, and airborne infection-control precautions are recommended for hospitalized patients with known or suspected MERS.

## PREVENTION

No vaccine or preventive drug is available. CDC recommends that travelers practice general hygiene precautions such as frequent handwashing; avoiding touching the eyes, nose, and mouth; and avoiding contact with sick people. The World Health Organization (WHO) considers certain groups to be at high risk for severe MERS, including people with diabetes, kidney failure, chronic lung disease, or immunocompromised people. WHO recommends that these groups take additional precautions: avoid contact with camels, do not drink raw camel milk or raw camel urine, and do not eat undercooked meat, particularly camel meat. For more information, see www.who.int/csr/disease/coronavirus_infections/faq/en.

**CDC website:** www.cdc.gov/coronavirus/mers

### BIBLIOGRAPHY

1. Arabi YM, Arifi AA, Balkhy HH, Najm H, Aldawood AS, Ghabashi A, et al. Clinical course and outcomes of critically ill patients with Middle East respiratory syndrome coronavirus infection. Ann Intern Med. 2014 Mar 18;160(6):389–97.

2. Arabi YM, Balkhy HH, Hayden FG, Bouchama A, Luke T, Baillie K, et al. Middle East respiratory syndrome. N Engl J Med. 2017 Feb 9;376:584–94.

3. CDC. Interim infection prevention and control recommendations for hospitalized patients with Middle East respiratory syndrome coronavirus (MERS-CoV). [updated 2015 June; cited 2018 Feb 26]. Available from: www.cdc.gov/coronavirus/mers/infection-prevention-control.html.

4. Memish ZA, Zumla AI, Al-Hakeem RF, Al-Rabeeah AA, Stephens GM. Family cluster of Middle East respiratory syndrome coronavirus infections. N Engl J Med. 2013 Jun 27;368(26):2487–94.

5. Oboho IK, Tomczyk SM, Al-Asmari AM, Banjar AA, Al-Mugti H, Aloraini MS, et al. 2014 MERS-CoV outbreak in Jeddah—a link to health care facilities. N Engl J Med. 2015 Feb 26;372(9):846–54.

6. World Health Organization. Coronavirus infections. [cited 2018 Feb 26]. Available from: www.who.int/csr/disease/coronavirus_infections/en/.

# MUMPS

Mariel A. Marlow, Nakia S. Clemmons

## INFECTIOUS AGENT

An enveloped, single-stranded, negative-sense RNA virus of the family Paramyxoviridae, genus *Rubulavirus*.

## TRANSMISSION

By respiratory droplets, saliva, or contact with contaminated fomites; requires close contact for spread. Transmission is most likely to occur 2 days before through 5 days after parotitis onset.

## EPIDEMIOLOGY

Endemic to many countries throughout the world. By the end of 2016, mumps-containing vaccine was being used routinely in 121 countries worldwide. Recently, there has been an increase in mumps outbreaks among highly vaccinated populations in industrialized nations. The risk of exposure among travelers is high in many countries.

## CLINICAL PRESENTATION

Average incubation period is 16–18 days (range, 12–25 days). Mumps is an acute systemic illness that classically presents with parotitis (acute onset of unilateral or bilateral tender, self-limited swelling of the parotid or other salivary glands), lasting 2–10 days. Nonspecific prodromal symptoms of low-grade fever, headache, malaise, myalgias, and anorexia may occur several days before parotitis onset. Infections may also be limited to nonspecific respiratory symptoms or asymptomatic. Complications, including orchitis, oophoritis, mastitis, hearing loss, aseptic meningitis, encephalitis, and pancreatitis may occur in the absence of parotitis.

## DIAGNOSIS

Usually clinically defined as acute parotitis or other salivary gland swelling lasting ≥2 days or orchitis or oophoritis, without other apparent cause. Laboratory confirmation of mumps involves detecting mumps virus by real-time RT-PCR or virus isolation by culture. Laboratory confirmation of mumps can be challenging; therefore, mumps cases should not be ruled out by negative laboratory results. For further information on laboratory testing, see www.cdc.gov/mumps/lab/index.html. Mumps is a nationally notifiable disease.

## TREATMENT

Supportive care is the mainstay of treatment.

## PREVENTION

Before departure from the United States, travelers aged ≥12 months who do not have acceptable evidence of mumps immunity (as documented by 2 doses of a mumps virus–containing vaccine, laboratory evidence of immunity, laboratory confirmation of disease, or birth before 1957) should be vaccinated with 2 doses of measles-mumps-rubella (MMR) vaccine ≥28 days apart (or 1 dose of MMR if previously administered 1 dose of MMR). Measles-mumps-rubella-varicella (MMRV) vaccine is licensed for children aged 12 months through 12 years and may be used if vaccination for measles, mumps, rubella, and varicella is indicated for this age group. There is no recommendation for vaccination against mumps for infants aged <12 months before international travel; however, infants aged 6–11 months should receive 1 dose of MMR vaccine before departure to protect against measles.

**CDC website:** www.cdc.gov/mumps

BIBLIOGRAPHY

1. CDC. Manual for the surveillance of vaccine-preventable diseases. Atlanta: CDC; 2018 [updated Dec 2017; cited 2018 Jan 29]. Available from: www.cdc.gov/vaccines/pubs/surv-manual/chpt09-mumps.pdf.

2. CDC. Prevention of measles, rubella, congenital rubella syndrome, and mumps, 2013: summary recommendations of the Advisory Committee on Immunization Practices (ACIP). MMWR Recomm Rep. 2013 Jun 14;62(RR-04):1–34.

3. Dayan GH, Quinlisk MP, Parker AA, Barskey AE, Harris ML, Schwartz JM, et al. Recent resurgence of mumps in the United States. N Engl J Med. 2008 Apr 10;358(15):1580–9.

4. Sabbe M & Vandermeulen. The resurgence of mumps and pertussis. Hum Vaccin Immunother. 2016 Jan 12:955–959.

5. Vygen S, Fischer A, Meurice L et al. Waning immunity against mumps in vaccinated young adults, France 2013. Euro Surveill. 2016;21:30156.

6. World Health Organization. Immunization, vaccines and biologicals: mumps. 2016 [updated August 9, 2017; cited 2018 Jan]. Available from: www.who.int/immunization/monitoring_surveillance/burden/vpd/surveillance_type/passive/mumps/en.

# NOROVIRUS

Cristina V. Cardemil, Aron J. Hall

## INFECTIOUS AGENT

Norovirus infection is caused by nonenveloped, single-stranded RNA viruses of the genus *Norovirus*, which have also been referred to as "Norwalk-like viruses," Norwalk viruses, and small round-structured viruses. Norovirus is a cause of viral gastroenteritis, sometimes referred to as "stomach flu"; however, there is no biologic association with influenza or influenza viruses.

## TRANSMISSION

Transmission occurs primarily through the fecal–oral route, either through direct person-to-person contact or indirectly via contaminated food or water. Norovirus is also spread through aerosols of vomitus and contaminated environmental surfaces and objects.

## EPIDEMIOLOGY

Norovirus infections are common throughout the world, and globally most children will have experienced ≥1 infection by the age of 5 years. Norovirus infections can occur year-round, but in temperate climates, norovirus activity peaks during the winter. Noroviruses are common in both developing and developed countries. Globally, norovirus is estimated to cause 18% of acute gastroenteritis cases and may be responsible for approximately 200,000 deaths annually. In the United States, norovirus is the leading cause of medically attended gastroenteritis in young children and of outbreaks of gastroenteritis; it is estimated to cause 19–21 million illnesses a year and approximately 50% of all foodborne disease outbreaks.

Norovirus outbreaks frequently occur in settings where people live in close quarters and can easily infect each other. Although most norovirus outbreaks occur in health care, school, and food-service settings, outbreaks also occur on cruise ships, and in hotels, camps, and dormitories. Norovirus is a well-known cause of travelers' diarrhea; prevalence in some settings is known to be greater than in others. Because coinfection and asymptomatic infection with norovirus are common, additional controlled studies are needed to determine exactly how frequently norovirus is the cause of disease.

Risk for infection is present anywhere food is prepared in an unsanitary manner and may become contaminated or where drinking water is inadequately treated. Of particular risk are "ready-to-eat" cold foods, such as sandwiches and salads. Raw shellfish, especially oysters, are also a frequent source of infection, because virus from contaminated water concentrates in the gut of these filter feeders. Contaminated ice has also been implicated in outbreaks.

Viral contamination of inanimate objects or environmental surfaces (fomites) may persist during and after outbreaks and be a source of infection. On cruise ships, for instance, environmental contamination has caused recurrent norovirus outbreaks on successive cruises with newly boarded passengers. Transmission of norovirus on airplanes has been reported during

4

both domestic and international flights and likely results from contamination of lavatories or from symptomatic passengers in the cabin.

## CLINICAL PRESENTATION

Infected people usually have an acute onset of vomiting with nonbloody diarrhea. The incubation period is 12–48 hours. Other symptoms include abdominal cramps, nausea, and sometimes a low-grade fever. Illness is generally self-limited, and full recovery can be expected in 1–3 days for most patients. In some cases, dehydration, especially in patients who are very young or elderly, may require medical attention.

## DIAGNOSIS

Norovirus infection is generally diagnosed based on symptoms. Norovirus diagnostic testing is not widely performed to guide clinical management of individual patients, but laboratory testing is used during outbreak investigations by public health agencies.

PCR-based multipathogen diagnostic panels are increasingly available for clinical and research purposes; these panels have good sensitivity and specificity to detect norovirus. The most common diagnostic test used at state public health laboratories and CDC is RT-PCR, which rapidly and reliably detects the virus in stool specimens. Several commercial enzyme immunoassays (EIAs) are also available to detect the virus in stool specimens. The specificity and sensitivity of EIAs are relatively poor compared with RT-PCR. For more information on laboratory diagnostic testing and specimen collection, see www.cdc.gov/norovirus/lab-testing/index.html.

## TREATMENT

Supportive care is the mainstay of treatment of norovirus disease, especially oral or intravenous rehydration. For routine management of acute gastroenteritis in children, antidiarrheals and antiemetics are not recommended because high-quality evidence for efficacy and their potential toxicity is lacking. For adults, antimotility, antisecretory, and antiemetic agents may be useful adjuncts to rehydration. Antibiotics are not useful in treating patients with norovirus disease.

## PREVENTION

No vaccine is currently available, although vaccine development efforts are advancing. Noroviruses are common and highly contagious, but the risk for infection can be minimized by frequent and proper handwashing and avoiding possibly contaminated food and water. Washing hands with soap and water for at least 20 seconds is considered the most effective way to reduce norovirus contamination; alcohol-based hand sanitizers might be useful between handwashings but should not be considered a substitute for soap and water.

In addition to handwashing, measures to prevent transmission of noroviruses between people traveling together include carefully cleaning up fecal material or vomit and disinfecting contaminated surfaces and toilet areas. Products should be approved by the Environmental Protection Agency for norovirus disinfection; alternatively, a dilute bleach solution (5–25 tablespoons bleach per gallon of water) may be used. Soiled articles of clothing should be washed at the maximum available cycle length and machine-dried at high heat.

To help prevent the spread of noroviruses, isolation may be considered for ill people on cruise ships and in institutional settings, including hospitals, long-term care facilities, and schools.

**CDC website:** www.cdc.gov/norovirus

BIBLIOGRAPHY

1. Ahmed SM, Hall AJ, Robinson AE et al. Global prevalence of norovirus in cases of gastroenteritis: a systematic review and meta-analysis. Lancet Infect Dis. 2014;14(8):725–30.

2. Ajami NJ, Kavanagh OV, Ramani S, Crawford SE, Atmar RL, Jiang ZD, et al. Seroepidemiology of norovirus-associated travelers' diarrhea. J Travel Med. 2014 Jan–Feb;21(1):6–11.

3. Aliabadi N, Lopman BA, Parashar UD, Hall AJ. Progress toward norovirus vaccines: considerations for further development and implementation in potential target populations. Expert Rev Vaccines. 2015;14(9):1241–53.

4. Cardemil CV, Parashar UD, Hall AJ. Norovirus Infection in older adults: epidemiology, risk factors, and opportunities for prevention and control. Infect Dis Clin North Am. 2017 Dec;31(4):839–70.

5. Hall AJ, Lopman BA, Payne DC, Patel MM, Gastañaduy PA, Vinje J, et al. Norovirus disease in the United States. Emerg Infect Dis. 2013 Aug;19(8):1198–205.

6. Hall AJ, Wikswo ME, Pringle K, Gould LH, Parashar UD. Vital signs: foodborne norovirus outbreaks—United States, 2009–2012. MMWR Morb Mortal Wkly Rep. 2014 Jun 6;63(22):491–5.

7. Kirk MD, Pires SM, Black RE et al. World Health Organization estimates of the global and regional disease burden of 22 foodborne bacterial, protozoal, and viral diseases, 2010: a data synthesis. PLoS Med. 2015;12(12):e1001921.

8. Simons MP, Pike BL, Hulseberg CE, Prouty MG, Swierczewski BE. Norovirus: new developments and implications for travelers' diarrhea. Trop Dis Travel Med Vaccines. 2016 Jan 12;2;1.

# ONCHOCERCIASIS (RIVER BLINDNESS)

Sharon L. Roy, Christine Dubray

## INFECTIOUS AGENT

*Onchocerca volvulus*, a filarial nematode.

## TRANSMISSION

Through female blackflies (genus *Simulium*), which typically bite during the day and breed near rapidly flowing rivers and streams.

## EPIDEMIOLOGY

Endemic to much of sub-Saharan Africa. Small endemic foci are also present in the Arabian Peninsula (Yemen) and in the Americas (Brazil and Venezuela). Foci center around blackfly breeding sites, which are located near rapidly flowing water. Most infections outside those in endemic populations occur in expatriate groups, such as missionaries, field scientists, and Peace Corps volunteers, though infection may sometimes occur in short-term travelers (<31 days).

## CLINICAL PRESENTATION

Highly pruritic, papular dermatitis; subcutaneous nodules; lymphadenitis; and ocular lesions, which can progress to visual loss and blindness. Symptoms begin after patent infections are established, which may take 18 months. Symptoms in travelers are primarily dermatologic (rash and pruritus) and may occur years after departure from endemic areas. Subcutaneous nodules are more common in endemic populations.

## DIAGNOSIS

Presence of microfilariae in superficial skin shavings or punch biopsy, adult worms in histologic sections of excised nodules, or characteristic eye lesions. Serologic testing is most useful for detecting infection when microfilariae are not identifiable. Determination of serum antifilarial antibody is available through the National Institutes of Health (301-496-5398) or CDC (www.cdc.gov/dpdx/; 404-718-4745; parasites@cdc.gov).

## TREATMENT

Ivermectin is the drug of choice. Repeated annual or semiannual doses may be required to control symptoms, as the drug kills the microfilariae but not the adult worms. Some experts recommend treating patients with 1 dose of ivermectin followed by 6 weeks of doxycycline to kill *Wolbachia*, an endosymbiotic rickettsialike bacterium that appears to be required for the survival of the *O. volvulus* adult worm and for embryo genesis. Diethylcarbamazine is contraindicated in onchocerciasis, because it has been associated with severe and fatal posttreatment reactions. An expert in tropical medicine should be consulted to help manage these patients.

## PREVENTION

Avoid blackfly habitats (fast-flowing rivers and streams) and use protection measures against biting insects (see Chapter 3, Mosquitoes, Ticks & Other Arthropods).

**CDC website:** www.cdc.gov/parasites/onchocerciasis/

### BIBLIOGRAPHY

1. Hoerauf A, Pfarr K, Mand S, Bebrah AY, Specht S. Filariasis in Africa—treatment challenges and prospects. Clin Microbiol Infect. 2011 Jul;17(7):977–85.

2. Klion AD. Filarial infections in travelers and immigrants. Curr Infect Dis Rep. 2008 Mar;10(1):50–7.

3. Lipner EM, Law MA, Barnett E, Keystone JS, von Sonnenburg F, Loutan L, et al. Filariasis in travelers presenting to the GeoSentinel Surveillance Network. PLoS Negl Trop Dis. 2007;1(3):e88.

4. McCarthy JS, Ottesen EA, Nutman TB. Onchocerciasis in endemic and nonendemic populations: differences in clinical presentation and immunologic findings. J Infect Dis. 1994 Sep;170(3):736–41.

5. Tielsch JM, Beeche A. Impact of ivermectin on illness and disability associated with onchocerciasis. Trop Med Int Health. 2004 Apr;9(4):A45–56.

6. WHO Department of Control of Neglected Tropical Diseases. Onchocerciasis—guidelines for stopping mass drug administration and verifying elimination of human onchocerciasis—criteria and procedures annexes. WHO Document Production Services, Geneva, Switzerland. WHO/HTM/NTD/PCT/2016. 1:1–36.

# PERTUSSIS

Tami H. Skoff, Anna Acosta

## INFECTIOUS AGENT

Fastidious gram-negative coccobacillus *Bordetella pertussis*.

## TRANSMISSION

Person-to-person transmission via aerosolized respiratory droplets or by direct contact with respiratory secretions.

## EPIDEMIOLOGY

Pertussis is endemic worldwide, even in areas with high vaccination rates. In recent years, pertussis has resurged in a number of countries with successful vaccination programs, especially countries that have transitioned from whole-cell pertussis vaccine formulations to acellular pertussis preparations, including the United States. In 2012, >48,000 cases of pertussis were reported nationally, the largest number in the United States since 1955. Disease rates are highest among young children in countries where vaccination coverage is low, primarily in the developing world. In developed countries, the reported incidence of pertussis is highest among infants too young to be vaccinated.

Immunity from childhood vaccination and natural disease wanes with time; therefore, adolescents and adults who have not received a tetanus-diphtheria-pertussis (Tdap) booster vaccination can become infected or reinfected with pertussis. US travelers are not at increased risk for disease specifically because of international travel, but they are at risk if they come in close contact with infected people. Infants, especially those who are too young to be protected by a complete vaccination series, are at highest risk for severe illness and death from pertussis.

## CLINICAL PRESENTATION

In classic disease, mild upper respiratory tract symptoms typically begin 7–10 days (range, 6–21 days) after exposure (catarrhal stage), followed by a cough that becomes paroxysmal (paroxysmal stage). Coughing paroxysms can vary in frequency and are often followed by vomiting. Fever is absent or minimal. The coughing paroxysms gradually resolve into milder and less frequent coughing, but paroxysms can recur with subsequent respiratory infections (convalescent stage). The clinical case definition for pertussis includes cough for ≥2 weeks with paroxysms, whoop, or posttussive vomiting.

Disease in infants aged <6 months can be atypical, with a short catarrhal stage, gagging, gasping, or apnea as early manifestations. Among infants aged <2 months, the case-fatality ratio is approximately 1%. Recently immunized children who develop disease may have mild cough illness; older children and adults may have prolonged cough with or without paroxysms. The cough gradually wanes over several weeks to months.

## DIAGNOSIS

Factors such as prior vaccination status, stage of disease, antibiotic use, specimen collection and transport conditions, and use of nonstandardized tests may affect the sensitivity, specificity, and interpretation of available diagnostic tests for *B. pertussis*. CDC guidelines for the laboratory confirmation of pertussis cases include culture and PCR (when the above clinical case definition is met); serology is not a confirmatory test included in the current case definition for reporting purposes. Direct fluorescent antibody (DFA) is no longer recommended as a diagnostic test for pertussis because of poor sensitivity and specificity. Pertussis is a nationally notifiable disease.

## TREATMENT

Macrolide antibiotics (azithromycin, clarithromycin, and erythromycin) are recommended to treat pertussis in people aged ≥1 month; for infants aged <1 month, azithromycin is the preferred antibiotic. Antimicrobial therapy with a macrolide antibiotic administered <3 weeks after

cough onset can limit transmission to others. Postexposure prophylaxis is recommended for all household contacts of cases and for people at high risk of developing severe disease (such as infants and women in the third trimester of pregnancy) or those who will have contact with a person at high risk of severe illness. The recommended agents and dosing regimens for prophylaxis are the same as for the treatment of pertussis.

## PREVENTION

### Vaccine

Travelers should be up-to-date with pertussis vaccinations before departure. Multiple pertussis vaccines are available in the United States for infants and children, and 2 vaccines are available for adolescents and adults. A complete listing of licensed vaccines can be found at www.fda.gov/BiologicsBloodVaccines/Vaccines/ApprovedProducts/ucm093833.htm.

#### INFANTS AND CHILDREN

In the United States, all infants and children should receive 5 doses of acellular pertussis vaccine in combination with diphtheria and tetanus toxoids (DTaP) at ages 2, 4, 6, and 15–18 months and 4–6 years. An accelerated schedule of doses may be used to complete the DTaP series.

Children aged 7–10 years who are not fully vaccinated against pertussis and for whom no contraindication to pertussis vaccine exists should receive a single dose of tetanus toxoid, reduced diphtheria toxoid, and acellular pertussis vaccine (Tdap) to provide protection against pertussis. If additional doses of tetanus and diphtheria toxoid-containing vaccines are needed, they should be given according to catch-up guidance, with Tdap preferred as the first dose (www.cdc.gov/vaccines/schedules/hcp/imz/catchup.html).

#### ADOLESCENTS AND ADULTS

Adolescents aged 11–18 years who have completed the recommended childhood DTwP/DTaP vaccination series and adults aged ≥19 years who have not previously received Tdap should receive a single dose of Tdap instead of tetanus and diphtheria toxoids (Td) vaccine for booster immunization against tetanus, diphtheria, and pertussis. To provide pertussis protection before travel, Tdap can be given regardless of the interval from the last Td, except to people for whom pertussis vaccination is contraindicated or for people who have previously received Tdap. Adolescents and adults who have never been immunized against pertussis, tetanus, or diphtheria; who have incomplete immunization; or whose immunity is uncertain should follow the catch-up schedule established for Td/Tdap.

## PREGNANT WOMEN

Women should have a dose of Tdap during *each* pregnancy, irrespective of their history of receiving Tdap. Although Tdap may be given at any time during pregnancy, to maximize the maternal antibody response and passive antibody transfer to the infant, optimal timing for Tdap administration is at 27–36 weeks' gestation, preferably during the earlier part of the period.

**CDC website:** www.cdc.gov/pertussis

## BIBLIOGRAPHY

1. Acosta AM, DeBolt C, Tasslimi A, Lewis M, Stewart LK, Misegades LK, et al. Tdap vaccine effectiveness in adolescents during the 2012 Washington State pertussis epidemic. Pediatrics. 2015 Jun;135(6):981–9.

2. American Academy of Pediatrics. Pertussis (whooping cough). In: Kimberlin DW, editor. Red Book: 2015 Report of the Committee on Infectious Diseases. 30th ed. Elk Grove Village, IL: American Academy of Pediatrics; 2015. pp. 608–21.

3. CDC. Pertussis (whooping cough) postexposure antimicrobial prophylaxis. [cited 2018 Jan. 1]. Available from: www.cdc.gov/pertussis/outbreaks/pep.html.

4. Edwards KM, Decker MD. Pertussis vaccines. In: Plotkin SA, Orenstein WA, Offit PA, editors. Vaccines. 6th ed. Philadelphia: Saunders Elsevier; 2012. p. 447–92.

5. Liang JL, Tiwari T, Moro P, Messonier NE, Reingold A, Sawyer M, et al. Prevention of pertussis, tetanus, and diphtheria with vaccines in the United States: recommendations of the Advisory Committee on Immunization Practices (ACIP). MMWR Recomm Rep. 2018 Apr 27;67(2):1–44.

6. Misegades LK, Winter K, Harriman K, Talarico J, Messonnier NE, Clark TA, et al. Association of childhood pertussis with receipt of 5 doses of pertussis vaccine by time since last vaccine dose, California, 2010. Jama. 2012 Nov 28;308(20):2126–32.

7. Skoff T, Blain A, Watt, J, Scherzinger K, McMahon M, Zansky S, et al. The impact of the U.S. maternal Tdap vaccination program on preventing pertussis in infants <2 months of age: a case-control evaluation. Clin Infect Dis. 2017 Nov 29;65(12):1977–1983. doi: 10.1093/cid/cix724.

8. Tan T, Dalby T, Forsyth K, Halperin SA, Heininger U, Hozbor D, et al. Pertussis across the globe: recent epidemiologic trends from 2000 to 2013. Pediatr Infect Dis J. 2015 Sep;34(9):e222–32.

9. Tiwari T, Murphy TV, Moran J. Recommended antimicrobial agents for the treatment and postexposure prophylaxis of pertussis: 2005 CDC Guidelines. MMWR Recomm Rep. 2005 Dec 9;54(RR-14):1–16.

# PINWORM (ENTEROBIASIS, OXYURIASIS, THREADWORM)

Christine Dubray

## INFECTIOUS AGENT

The intestinal nematode (roundworm) *Enterobius vermicularis*.

## TRANSMISSION

Egg transmission occurs by the fecal–oral route, either directly or indirectly via contaminated hands or objects such as clothes, toys, and bedding.

## EPIDEMIOLOGY

Pinworm is endemic worldwide and commonly clusters within families. Those most likely to be infected with pinworm are preschool- and school-age children, people who take care of infected children, and people who are institutionalized. Travelers are at risk if staying in crowded conditions with infected people.

## CLINICAL PRESENTATION

Incubation period is usually 1–2 months, but successive reinfections may be needed before symptoms appear. The most common symptom is an itchy anal region, which can disturb sleep; irritability and secondary infection of irritated skin can also occur. Adult worms can migrate from the anal area to other sites, including the vulva, vagina, and urethra. Appendicitis and enuresis have also been reported as possible associated conditions.

## DIAGNOSIS

The first option is to look for adult worms near the anus 2–3 hours after the infected person is asleep. The second option is microscopic identification of worm eggs collected by touching transparent tape to the anal area when the person first awakens in the morning. This method should be conducted on 3 consecutive mornings and before washing. The third option is microscopic examination of samples taken from under fingernails; samples should be taken before handwashing. Examining stool samples is not recommended because pinworm eggs are sparse.

## TREATMENT

Drugs of choice are mebendazole, albendazole, or pyrantel pamoate. Any of these drugs are given as 1 dose initially followed by another dose of the same drug 2 weeks later. The second dose is to eliminate possible reinfection since the first dose. Pyrantel pamoate is available without prescription in the United States. Mebendazole is available in the United States only through compounding pharmacies.

In households where >1 member is infected or where repeated, symptomatic infections occur, all household members should be treated at the same time. For children younger than 2 years of age, in whom experience with these drugs is limited, risks and benefits should be considered by a physician before drug administration. Infected people should also bathe (shower or stand-up baths) in the morning and change underwear and bedclothes frequently, preferably after bathing. Infected people should also practice personal hygiene measures such as washing hands before eating or preparing food, keeping fingernails short, not scratching the perianal region, and not biting nails.

## PREVENTION

Hand hygiene is the most effective method of prevention. Bed linen and underclothing of infected children should be changed first thing in the morning. They should not be shaken (to avoid contaminating the environment), and should be laundered promptly in hot water and dried in a hot dryer to kill any eggs that may be there.

**CDC website:** www.cdc.gov/parasites/pinworm

BIBLIOGRAPHY

1. American Academy of Pediatrics. Pinworm infection (Enterobius vermicularis). In: Kimberlin DW, editor. Red Book: 2015 Report of the Committee on Infectious Diseases. 30h ed. Elk Grove Village, IL: American Academy of Pediatrics; 2015. pp. 621–2.

2. American Public Health Association. Enterobiasis. In: Heyman DL, editor. Control of Communicable Diseases Manual. 20th ed. Washington, DC: American Public Health Association; 2014. pp. 187–8.

3. Kucik CJ, Martin GL, Sortor BV. Common intestinal parasites. Am Fam Physician. 2004 Mar 1;69(5):1161–9.

# PLAGUE (BUBONIC, PNEUMONIC, SEPTICEMIC)

Paul S. Mead

## INFECTIOUS AGENT

The gram-negative bacterium *Yersinia pestis*.

## TRANSMISSION

Usually through the bite of infected rodent fleas. Less common exposures include handling infected animal tissues (hunters, wildlife personnel), inhalation of infectious droplets from cats or dogs with plague, and, rarely, contact with a pneumonic plague patient.

## EPIDEMIOLOGY

Endemic to rural areas in central and southern Africa (especially eastern Democratic Republic of Congo, northwestern Uganda, and Madagascar), central Asia and the Indian subcontinent, the northeastern part of South America, and parts of the southwestern United States. Overall risk to travelers is low.

## CLINICAL PRESENTATION

Incubation period is typically 1–6 days. Symptoms and signs of the 3 clinical presentations of plague illness are as follows:

- Bubonic (most common)—rapid onset of fever; painful, swollen, and tender lymph nodes, usually inguinal, axillary, or cervical

- Pneumonic—high fever, overwhelming pneumonia, cough, bloody sputum, chills

- Septicemic—fever, prostration, hemorrhagic or thrombotic phenomena, progressing to acral gangrene

## DIAGNOSIS

*Y. pestis* can be isolated from bubo aspirates, blood cultures, or sputum culture if pneumonic. Diagnosis can be confirmed in public health laboratories by culture or serologic tests for the *Y. pestis* F1 antigen. Plague is a nationally notifiable disease.

## TREATMENT

There are a number of antibiotics used in the treatment of plague including gentamicin, doxycycline, ciprofloxacin, and levofloxacin. The parenteral antibiotic, moxifloxacin, may also be used. Parenteral streptomycin and chloramphenicol are alternatives.

## PREVENTION

Reduce contact with fleas and potentially infected rodents and other wildlife. No plague vaccine is available for commercial use in the United States. Antibiotics are used for postexposure prophylaxis.

**CDC website:** www.cdc.gov/plague

### BIBLIOGRAPHY

1. Bertherat E. Plague around the world, 2010–2015. WHO Wkly Epidemiol Rec. 2016;91:89–104.
2. Butler T. Plague gives surprises in the first decade of the 21st century in the United States and worldwide. Am J Trop Med Hyg. 2013;89:788–93.
3. Perry RD, Fetherston JD. Yersinia pestis—etiologic agent of plague. Clin Microbiol Rev. 1997 Jan;10(1):35–66.

# PNEUMOCOCCAL DISEASE

Fernanda C. Lessa

## INFECTIOUS AGENT

The gram-positive coccus *Streptococcus pneumoniae*.

## TRANSMISSION

Person to person through close contact via respiratory droplets.

## EPIDEMIOLOGY

*Streptococcus pneumoniae* is the most common bacterial cause of community-acquired pneumonia worldwide. Disease incidence is higher in developing than in industrialized countries. Risk is highest in young children, the elderly, and those with chronic illnesses or immune suppression.

## CLINICAL PRESENTATION

The major clinical syndromes of pneumococcal disease are pneumonia, bacteremia, and meningitis. Pneumococcal pneumonia classically presents with sudden onset of fever and malaise, pleuritic chest pain, cough with purulent or blood-tinged sputum, or dyspnea. In the elderly, fever, shortness of breath, or altered mental status may be the initial symptoms. Pneumococcal meningitis is less common than pneumonia, and symptoms may include headache, lethargy, vomiting, irritability, fever, stiff neck, and seizures. People with cochlear implants are at increased risk of pneumococcal meningitis.

## DIAGNOSIS

Isolation of *S. pneumoniae* from blood or other normally sterile body sites such as pleural fluid or cerebrospinal fluid (CSF). Tests are also available to detect pneumococcal antigen in body fluids.

A urinary antigen test for *S. pneumoniae* is commercially available, simple to use, and has reasonable specificity to detect pneumococcal infection in adults, making it a useful addition for diagnostic evaluation. A clinician should suspect pneumococcal pneumonia if a sputum specimen contains gram-positive diplococci, polymorphonuclear leukocytes, and few epithelial cells. Gram-positive diplococci on staining of CSF may indicate pneumococcal meningitis. High white blood cell counts should raise suspicion for bacterial infection.

## TREATMENT

Therapy depends on the syndrome, but patients who present with community-acquired pneumonia should be empirically treated for pneumococcal infection. Pneumococcal bacteria are resistant to ≥1 antibiotic in 30% of severe cases, although level and type of resistance varies among locations.

In outpatient settings, current clinical practice guidelines for pneumonia management recommend amoxicillin for children and macrolides (such as azithromycin) or doxycycline for previously healthy adults. For adults with chronic or immunosuppressing conditions, a respiratory fluoroquinolone (such as moxifloxacin or levofloxacin) or a β-lactam plus a macrolide is recommended. In inpatient settings, the initial treatment includes a broad-spectrum cephalosporin plus a macrolide or a respiratory fluoroquinolone alone. Vancomycin might be added until antibiotic susceptibility results are available.

Patients with presumptive pneumococcal meningitis by CSF staining should be treated with a broad-spectrum cephalosporin plus vancomycin until susceptibility results are available.

## PREVENTION

The 13-valent pneumococcal conjugate vaccine (PCV13) provides protection against the 13 serotypes responsible for most severe illness. PCV13 has been part of the US infant immunization schedule since 2010 and is also recommended for all adults aged ≥65 years and some adults aged 19–64 with immunocompromising conditions. A 23-valent pneumococcal polysaccharide vaccine (PPSV23) is recommended for all adults aged ≥65 years and people aged 2–64 years with

4

underlying medical conditions. The intervals between PCV13 and PPSV23 given in series differ by age and risk group (see www.cdc.gov/vaccines/vpd/pneumo/hcp/recommendations.html). PCV13 and PPSV23 should not be coadministered.

Adults aged ≥65 years who are immunocompetent should receive PPSV23 ≥1 year after PCV13, while those with immunocompromising conditions should receive PPSV23 ≥8 weeks after PCV13.

**CDC website:** www.cdc.gov/pneumococcal/

## BIBLIOGRAPHY

1. Bradley JS, Byington CL, Shah SS, Alverson B, Carter ER, Harrison C, et al. The management of community-acquired pneumonia in infants and children older than 3 months of age: clinical practice guidelines by the Pediatric Infectious Diseases Society and the Infectious Diseases Society of America. Clin Infect Dis. 2011 Oct;53(7):e25–76.

2. CDC. Intervals between PCV13 and PPSV23 vaccines: recommendations of the Advisory Committee on Immunization Practices (ACIP). MMWR Morb Mortal Wkly Rep. 2015 Sep 4;64(34):944–7.

3. CDC. Licensure of a 13-valent pneumococcal conjugate vaccine (PCV13) and recommendations for use among children—Advisory Committee on Immunization Practices (ACIP), 2010. MMWR Morb Mortal Wkly Rep. 2010 Mar 12;59(9):258–61.

4. CDC. Use of 13-valent pneumococcal conjugate vaccine and 23-valent pneumococcal polysaccharide vaccine among adults aged >/=65 years: recommendations of the Advisory Committee on Immunization Practices (ACIP).

MMWR Morb Mortal Wkly Rep. 2014 Sep 19;63(37):822–5.

5. CDC. Use of 13-valent pneumococcal conjugate vaccine and 23-valent pneumococcal polysaccharide vaccine among children aged 6–18 years with immunocompromising conditions: recommendations of the Advisory Committee on Immunization Practices (ACIP). MMWR Morb Mortal Wkly Rep. 2013 June 28, 2013;62(25):521–4.

6. Mandell LA, Wunderink RG, Anzueto A, Bartlett JG, Campbell GD, Dean NC, et al. Infectious Diseases Society of America/American Thoracic Society consensus guidelines on the management of community-acquired pneumonia in adults. Clin Infect Dis. 2007 Mar 1;44 Suppl 2:S27–72.

7. Rudan I, O'Brien KL, Nair H, Liu L, Theodoratou E, Qazi S, et al. Epidemiology and etiology of childhood pneumonia in 2010: estimates of incidence, severe morbidity, mortality, underlying risk factors and causative pathogens for 192 countries. J Glob Health. 2013 Jun;3(1):010401.

# POLIOMYELITIS

Concepción F. Estívariz, Janell Routh, Manisha Patel, Steven G. F. Wassilak

## INFECTIOUS AGENT

Polioviruses (genus *Enterovirus*) are small, nonenveloped viruses with a single-stranded RNA genome. Polioviruses are rapidly inactivated by heat, formaldehyde, chlorine, and ultraviolet light. There are 4 poliovirus serotypes, 1, 2 and 3, that have minimal heterotypic immunity between them.

## TRANSMISSION

The virus enters through the mouth and multiplies in the throat and gastrointestinal tract. Virus may be excreted in nasopharyngeal secretions for 1–2 weeks and in stools for 3–6 weeks, even in people who develop no symptoms after infection. Transmission occurs from person to person through the oral and fecal–oral routes.

## EPIDEMIOLOGY

Before a vaccine was available, infection with wild poliovirus (WPV) was common worldwide, with seasonal peaks and epidemics in the summer and fall in temperate areas. The incidence of poliomyelitis in the United States declined rapidly after the licensure of inactivated poliovirus vaccine (IPV) in 1955 and live oral polio vaccine (OPV) in the 1960s. The last cases of indigenously acquired polio in the United States occurred in 1979 and in the Americas in 1991.

Built upon the success in the Americas, the Global Polio Eradication Initiative (GPEI) was initiated in 1988 and has made great progress in interrupting WPV transmission globally, drastically reducing the number of countries where travelers are at risk for acquiring polio. WPV type 2 was last isolated in 1999 and declared eradicated in 2015; WPV type 3 has not been detected since November 2012. In 2018, WPV type 1 circulates in 3 countries: Afghanistan, Pakistan, and Nigeria.

In spite of progress made in eradicating WPVs globally, some polio-free countries with low vaccination coverage remain at risk for poliomyelitis outbreaks after importation of WPV type 1. Countries that have low OPV coverage in routine immunization are also at risk of experiencing poliomyelitis cases and outbreaks caused by circulating vaccine-derived poliovirus (cVDPVs). The live attenuated poliovirus strains contained in the Sabin OPV may circulate in areas with inadequate OPV coverage and revert to having wild-like characteristics. Rarely, OPV can cause paralytic polio in vaccine recipients or their close contacts (vaccine-associated paralytic poliomyelitis or VAPP).

From 2006 through 2015, more than 90% of cVDPV cases were type 2. Given the eradication of WPV type 2, experts recommended global withdrawal of OPV serotype 2. Approximately 155 OPV-using countries and territories switched from trivalent OPV (tOPV, containing serotypes 1, 2, and 3) to bivalent OPV (bOPV, containing serotypes 1 and 3) in April 2016. During 2017, WPV type 1 was responsible for 26 paralytic cases in Afghanistan and Pakistan, whereas cVDPV type 2 was responsible for 74 cases in Syria and 22 in the Democratic Republic of Congo. The cVDPV causing these large outbreaks emerged from OPV doses provided before April 2016.

Travelers to countries with current or recent WPV or cVDPV outbreaks may be at risk for exposure to poliovirus. The last documented case of WPV-associated paralysis in a US resident traveling abroad occurred in 1986 in a 29-year-old vaccinated adult who had been traveling in South and Southeast Asia. In 2005, an unvaccinated US adult traveling abroad acquired VAPP after contact with an infant recently vaccinated with OPV.

For additional information on the status of polio eradication efforts, countries or areas with active WPV or VDPV circulation, and vaccine recommendations, consult the travel notices on the CDC Travelers' Health website (www.cdc.gov/travel) and the GPEI website (www.polioeradication.org).

## CLINICAL PRESENTATION

Most poliovirus infections are asymptomatic; about 25% cause minor illness with total recovery. However, about 0.5% of unvaccinated people may develop acute flaccid paralysis. Paralysis may affect 1 or several limbs, and in severe cases it may result in quadriplegia, respiratory failure, and rarely, death. Many people partially recover muscle function, and some recover completely, but worsening of weakness or paralysis may occur 20–30 years later (postpolio syndrome). Adults with poliovirus paralysis have more severe disease and a worse prognosis than children.

## DIAGNOSIS

Poliovirus is identified in clinical specimens (usually stool) obtained from an acutely ill patient. Shedding in fecal specimens may be intermittent and declines over time, but poliovirus can be detected for up to 60 days after onset of paralysis. During the first 3–10 days following paralysis onset, poliovirus can also be detected from oropharyngeal specimens, but stool specimens are the preferred source for diagnosis. Poliovirus is rarely detected in the blood or cerebrospinal fluid.

Poliovirus is detected in specimens by cell culture, which is followed by PCR of isolates to identify the serotype and whether it is WPV, VDPV, or the vaccine (Sabin) strain. Genomic sequencing of poliovirus isolates determines the geographic origin of WPV and the estimated time of circulation since the original OPV dose for VDPV.

Paralytic polio is designated as "an immediately notifiable, extremely urgent" disease, which requires state and local health authorities to notify CDC within 4 hours of their notification. Because of new safety requirements in handling polioviruses, CDC is the only laboratory allowed to test specimens from a suspected case

4

of paralytic polio in the United States. CDC can be notified through the Emergency Operations Center (EOC, 770-488-7100) or through state health authorities. CDC's EOC will connect callers with polio SMEs who can provide consultation regarding the collection of clinical specimens and procedures.

## TREATMENT

Only symptomatic treatment is available.

## PREVENTION

### Vaccine

#### RECOMMENDATIONS FOR HEALTH PROTECTION

IPV is the only polio vaccine available in the United States since 2000, but bivalent OPV is used in most middle- and low-income countries and for global polio eradication activities. For complete information on recommendations for poliomyelitis vaccination, consult the Advisory Committee on Immunization Practices recommendations website (www.cdc.gov/vaccines/hcp/acip-recs/vacc-specific/polio.html) and the World Health Organization position paper on poliovirus vaccines (www.who.int/wer/2016/wer9112/en/).

Before traveling to areas that have WPV or VDPV circulation, travelers should ensure that they have completed the recommended age-appropriate polio vaccine series (see Infants and Children below). Adults who have completed a primary series should receive a single lifetime IPV booster dose if traveling to these areas. CDC also recommends a single lifetime IPV booster dose for adult travelers to some countries that border areas with WPV circulation based on evidence of historical cross-border transmission. These recommendations apply only to travelers to bordering countries with a high risk of exposure to someone with imported WPV infection, such as those working in health care settings, refugee camps, or other humanitarian aid settings.

Countries are considered to have WPV or VDPV circulation if they have evidence during the previous 12 months of poliovirus circulation (endemic WPV, active WPV or cVDPV outbreaks, or environmental isolation [sewage sampling]).

Since the situation is dynamic, refer to the CDC Travelers' Health website destination pages for the most up-to-date polio vaccine recommendations (wwwnc.cdc.gov/travel/destinations/list).

#### COUNTRY REQUIREMENTS

In May 2014, the Director General of the World Health Organization (WHO) declared the international spread of polio to be a public health emergency of international concern under the authority of the International Health Regulations (2005). To prevent further spread of disease, WHO issued temporary polio vaccine recommendations for long-term travelers (staying >4 weeks) and residents departing from countries with WPV transmission ("exporting WPV" or "infected with WPV"). The IHR emergency committee on polio meets every 3 months and updates these recommendations (available at www.who.int/mediacentre/news/statements). In November 2015, these recommendations were extended to long-term travelers (staying >4 weeks) and residents departing from countries with VDPV transmission ("infected with VDPV").

Clinicians should be aware that long-term travelers and residents may be required to show proof of polio vaccination when departing from these countries. All polio vaccination administration should be documented on an International Certificate of Vaccination or Prophylaxis (ICVP). The polio vaccine must be received between 4 weeks and 12 months before the date of departure from the polio-affected country. Country requirements may change, so clinicians should check for updates on the CDC Travelers' Health website (wwwnc.cdc.gov/travel/news-announcements/polio-guidance-new-requirements) for a list of affected countries, guidance on meeting the vaccination requirements, and instructions on how to order and fill out the ICVP.

#### INFANTS AND CHILDREN

In the United States, all infants and children should receive 4 doses of IPV, at ages 2, 4, and 6–18 months and 4–6 years. The final dose should be administered at age ≥4 years, regardless of the number of previous doses, and should

4

be given ≥6 months after the previous dose. A fourth dose in the routine IPV series is not necessary if the third dose was administered at age ≥4 years and ≥6 months after the previous dose. If the routine series cannot be administered within the recommended intervals before protection is needed, the following alternatives are recommended:

- The first dose should be given to infants at age ≥6 weeks.

- The second and third doses should be administered ≥4 weeks after the previous doses.

- The minimum interval between the third and fourth doses is 6 months.

If the age-appropriate series is not completed before departure, the remaining IPV doses to complete a full series should be administered when feasible, at the intervals recommended above.

### ADULTS

Adults who are traveling to areas where WPV or VDPV is actively circulating and who are unvaccinated, incompletely vaccinated, or whose vaccination status is unknown should receive a series of 3 doses: 2 doses of IPV administered at an interval of 4–8 weeks; a third dose should be administered 6–12 months after the second. If 3 doses of IPV cannot be administered within the recommended intervals before protection is needed, the alternatives are shown in Table 4-15.

### GUIDANCE FOR CHILDREN WHO HAVE RECEIVED POLIOVIRUS VACCINE OUTSIDE THE UNITED STATES

Vaccines administered outside the United States generally can be accepted as valid doses if the schedule is similar to that recommended in the United States. Vaccination against polio is also valid for children from countries that use an accelerated schedule. Only written, dated records are acceptable as evidence of previous vaccination. Please see www.cdc.gov/mmwr/volumes/66/wr/mm6601a6.htm and its erratum www.cdc.gov/mmwr/volumes/66/wr/mm6606a7.htm?s_cid=mm6606a7_w for information on interpreting international poliovirus vaccination documentation.

Children with full vaccination status, who have only received bOPV in the primary series because they were born after April 2016, or a combination of tOPV and bOPV, should be revaccinated with a full IPV series to ensure protection against all 3 poliovirus types. Children <18 years of age without adequate documentation of poliovirus vaccination should be vaccinated or revaccinated in accordance with the age-appropriate US IPV schedule.

The international adoption of children from countries or areas where WPV or VDPV is actively circulating is a special situation. International adoptees might not have completed a primary vaccination series against polio nor received a dose of polio vaccine before departure. Thus, there is a small risk that they could be infected with WPV or VDPV and remain infectious upon entry into the United States and potentially transmit to US household members and caregivers. As a

## Table 4-15. Alternative adult polio vaccine regimens

| TIME BEFORE TRAVEL | NUMBER OF DOSES[1] | INTERVAL BETWEEN DOSES |
|---|---|---|
| <4 weeks | 1 | Not Applicable |
| 4–8 weeks | 2 | 4 weeks |
| >8 weeks | 3 | 4 weeks |

[1] If <3 doses are administered, the remaining doses required to complete a 3-dose series should be administered when feasible, at the recommended intervals above, if the person remains at risk for poliovirus exposure.

measure of prudence, the polio vaccination status of all household members and caregivers of international adoptees whose origin is a country with active WPV or VDPV circulation should be assessed before the entry of the child into the United States. Those who are unvaccinated, incompletely vaccinated, or whose vaccination status is unknown should be brought up-to-date.

## VACCINE SAFETY AND ADVERSE REACTIONS

Minor local reactions (pain and redness) can occur after IPV administration. IPV should not be administered to people who have experienced a severe allergic reaction (such as anaphylaxis) after a previous dose of IPV. Because IPV contains trace amounts of streptomycin, polymyxin B, or neomycin, hypersensitivity reactions can occur after IPV administration among people allergic to these antibiotics.

## PREGNANCY AND BREASTFEEDING

If a pregnant woman is unvaccinated or incompletely vaccinated and requires immediate protection against polio because of planned travel to a country or area where WPV or VDPV is actively circulating, IPV can be administered as recommended for adults. Breastfeeding is not a contraindication to administration of polio vaccine to an infant or mother.

## PRECAUTIONS AND CONTRAINDICATIONS

IPV may be administered to people with diarrhea. Minor upper respiratory illnesses with or without fever, mild to moderate local reactions to a previous dose of IPV, current antimicrobial therapy, and the convalescent phase of acute illness are not contraindications to vaccination.

## IMMUNOSUPPRESSION

IPV may be administered safely to immunocompromised travelers and their household contacts. Although a protective immune response cannot be ensured, IPV might confer some protection to the immunocompromised person. People with certain primary immunodeficiency diseases should not be given OPV and should avoid contact with children vaccinated with OPV overseas in the previous 6 weeks.

**CDC website:** www.cdc.gov/polio

## BIBLIOGRAPHY

1. CDC. Updated recommendations of the Advisory Committee on Immunization Practices (ACIP) regarding routine poliovirus vaccination. MMWR Morb Mortal Wkly Rep. 2009 Aug 7;58(30):829–30.

2. Elhamidi Y, Mahamud A, Safdar M, Al Tamimi W, Jorba J, Mbaeyi C, et al. Progress toward poliomyelitis eradication—Pakistan, January 2016–September 2017. MMWR Morb Mortal Wkly Rep. 2017 Nov 24;66(46):1276–80.

3. Hampton LM, Farrell M, Ramirez-Gonzalez A, Menning L, Shendale S, Lewis I, et al. Cessation of trivalent oral poliovirus vaccine and introduction of inactivated poliovirus vaccine—worldwide, 2016. MMWR Morb Mortal Wkly Rep. 2016 Sep 9; 65(35): 934–8.

4. Jorba J, Diop OM, Iber J, Sutter RW, Wassilak SGF, Burns CC. Update on vaccine-derived polioviruses—worldwide, January 2016–June 2017. MMWR Morb Mortal Wkly Rep. 2017 Nov 3;66(43): 1185–91.

5. Marin M, Patel M, Oberste S, Pallansch MA. Guidance for assessment of poliovirus vaccination status and vaccination of children who have received poliovirus vaccine outside the United States. MMWR Morb Mortal Wkly Rep. 2017 Jan 13;66(01)23–5.

6. Martinez M, Shukla H, Nikulin J, Wadood MZ, Hadler S, Mbaeyi C, et al. Progress toward poliomyelitis eradication—Afghanistan, January 2016–June 2017. MMWR Morb Mortal Wkly Rep. 2017 Aug 18;66(32): 854–8.

7. Sutter RW, Kew OM, Cochi SL, Aylward RB. Poliovirus vaccine—live. In: Plotkin SA, Orenstein WA, Offit PA, editors. Vaccines. 6th ed. Philadelphia: Saunders Elsevier; 2012. pp. 598–645.

8. Vidor E, Plotkin SA. Poliovirus vaccine—inactivated. In: Plotkin SA, Orenstein WA, Offit PA, editors. Vaccines. 6th ed. Philadelphia: Saunders Elsevier; 2012. pp. 573–97.

9. Wallace GS, Seward JF, Pallansch MA. Interim CDC Guidance for polio vaccination for travel to and from countries affected by wild poliovirus. MMWR Morb Mortal Wkly Rep. 2014 July 11;63(27)591–594.

10. World Health Organization. Polio vaccines: WHO position paper—March, 2016. Wkly Epidemiol Rec. 2016 Mar 25;91(12):145–68.

# Q FEVER

Gilbert J. Kersh

## INFECTIOUS AGENT

The gram-negative intracellular bacterium *Coxiella burnetii*.

## TRANSMISSION

Most commonly through inhalation of aerosols or dust contaminated with dried birth fluids or excreta from infected animals (usually cattle, sheep, or goats). *C. burnetii* is highly infectious and persists in the environment. Infections via ingestion of contaminated, unpasteurized dairy products and human-to-human transmission via sexual contact have been rarely reported.

## EPIDEMIOLOGY

Distributed worldwide; the prevalence is highest in African and Middle Eastern countries. Reported rates of human infection are higher in France and Australia than in the United States. The largest known Q fever outbreak reported to date involved approximately 4,000 human cases and occurred during 2007–2010 in the Netherlands. Travelers who visit rural areas or farms with cattle, sheep, goats, or other livestock may be exposed to Q fever. Occupational exposure to infected animals (such as in farmers, veterinarians, butchers, meat packers, and seasonal or migrant farm workers), particularly during parturition, poses a high risk for disease transmission.

## CLINICAL PRESENTATION

It is estimated that more than half of acute infections are mild or asymptomatic. Incubation period is typically 2–3 weeks but may be shorter after exposure to large numbers of organisms. The most common presentation of acute infection is a self-limiting influenzalike illness, with pneumonia or hepatitis in more severe acute infections. Chronic infections occur primarily in patients with preexisting cardiac valvulopathies, vascular abnormalities, or immunosuppression. Women infected during pregnancy are at risk for adverse pregnancy outcomes unless treated. The most common manifestations of chronic disease are endocarditis and endovascular infections. Chronic infections may become apparent months or years after the initial exposure.

## DIAGNOSIS

Serologic evidence of a 4-fold rise in phase II IgG by indirect fluorescent antibody test between paired sera taken 3–4 weeks apart is the gold standard for diagnosis of acute infection. A single high serum phase II IgG titer (>1:128) in conjunction with clinical evidence of infection may be considered evidence of probable acute Q fever.

Chronic Q fever diagnosis requires a phase I IgG titer >1:512 and clinical evidence of persistent infection (for example, endocarditis, infected vascular aneurysm, osteomyelitis). Detection of *C. burnetii* in whole blood, serum, or tissue samples by PCR, immunohistochemical staining, or isolation can also be used to confirm chronic Q fever. Tests for direct detection of *C. burnetii* may not be widely available, but the Rickettsial Zoonoses Branch at CDC can provide assistance (www.cdc.gov/qfever/public-health/index.html). Q fever is a nationally notifiable disease.

## TREATMENT

Doxycycline has been used most frequently, although fluoroquinolones remain an alternative. Pregnant women, children aged <8 years with mild illness, and patients allergic to doxycycline may be treated with an antibiotic such as trimethoprim-sulfamethoxazole. Treatment for acute Q fever is not recommended for asymptomatic people or for those whose symptoms have resolved. Chronic *C. burnetii* infections require long-term combination therapy. The best outcomes are seen with the combination of doxycycline and hydroxychloroquine. Alternatives include trimethoprim-sulfamethoxazole, fluoroquinolones, and rifampin. Treatment of Q fever may also involve surgery.

## PREVENTION

Avoid areas where potentially infected animals are kept, and avoid consumption of unpasteurized dairy products. A human vaccine for Q fever has been developed and used in Australia, but it is not available in the United States.

**CDC website:** www.cdc.gov/qfever

### BIBLIOGRAPHY

1. Anderson A, Bijlmer H, Fournier PE, Graves S, Hartzell J, Kersh GJ, et al. Diagnosis and management of Q fever—United States, 2013: recommendations from CDC and the Q Fever Working Group. MMWR Recomm Rep. 2013 Mar 29;62(RR-03):1–30.

2. Delord M, Socolovschi C, Parola P. Rickettsioses and Q fever in travelers (2004–2013). Travel Med Infect Dis. 2014 Sep–Oct;12(5):443–58.

3. Million M, Thuny F, Richet H, Raoult D. Long-term outcome of Q fever endocarditis: a 26-year personal survey. Lancet Infect Dis. 2010 Aug;10(8):527–35.

4. Robyn MP, Newman AP, Amato M, Walawander M, Kothe C, Nerone JD, et al. Q fever outbreak among travelers to Germany who received live cell therapy—United States and Canada, 2014. MMWR Morb Mortal Wkly Rep. 2015 Oct 2;64(38):1071–3.

5. Roest HI, Tilburg JJ, van der Hoek W, Vellema P, van Zijderveld FG, Klaassen CH, et al. The Q fever epidemic in The Netherlands: history, onset, response and reflection. Epidemiol Infect. 2011 Jan;139(1):1–12.

# RABIES

Ryan M. Wallace, Brett W. Petersen, David R. Shlim

## INFECTIOUS AGENTS

Rabies is a fatal, acute, progressive encephalomyelitis caused by neurotropic viruses in the family Rhabdoviridae, genus *Lyssavirus*. Numerous and diverse variants of lyssaviruses are found in a wide variety of animal species throughout the world, all of which may cause fatal human rabies. Rabies virus is by far the most common lyssavirus infection of humans. Tens of millions of potential human exposures and tens of thousands of deaths from rabies virus occur each year.

## TRANSMISSION

The normal and most successful mode of transmission is inoculation of saliva from the bite of a rabid animal. Rabies virus is neurotropic and gains access to the peripheral nervous system by being taken up at a nerve synapse at the site of the bite. The virus travels through peripheral nerves to the central nervous system, where most viral replication occurs, before traveling back out through the peripheral nervous system. After reaching the salivary glands, virus can be secreted allowing the transmission cycle to repeat. Exposure of rabies virus to highly innervated tissue may increase the risk of successful infection. Exposure of rabies virus to anatomic sites nearer the central nervous system may reduce the incubation period. In addition to saliva, rabies virus may also be found in nervous tissues (central and peripheral) and tears. Infection from nonbite exposures, such as organ transplantation from infected humans, does occur. However, human-to-human transmission does not generally occur otherwise.

All mammals are believed to be susceptible to infection, but major rabies reservoirs are terrestrial carnivores and bats. Although dogs are the main reservoir in developing countries, the epidemiology of the disease differs from one region or country to another. All patients with mammal bites should be medically evaluated. **Bat bites anywhere in the world are a cause of concern and an indication to consider prophylaxis.**

## EPIDEMIOLOGY

Lyssaviruses, the causative agent for the disease rabies, have been found on all continents except Antarctica. Rabies virus is classified into 2 major genetic lineages: canine and New World bat. These 2 lineages can be further classified into rabies virus variants based on the reservoir species in which they circulate. Regionally, different viral variants are adapted to various mammalian hosts and perpetuate in dogs and wildlife, such as bats, foxes, jackals, mongooses, raccoons, and skunks. Canine rabies remains enzootic in many areas of the world, including Africa, Asia, and parts of Central and South America. In addition to rabies virus, the *Lyssavirus* genus includes 14 other viruses that all cause the disease rabies. Nonrabies lyssaviruses are found in Europe, Asia, Africa, and Australia; although they have caused human deaths, nonrabies lyssaviruses contribute relatively little to the global rabies burden compared to rabies virus.

Timely and specific information about the global occurrence of rabies is often difficult to find. Surveillance levels vary, and reporting status can change suddenly as a result of disease reintroduction or emergence. The rate of rabies exposures in travelers is at best an estimate and may range from 16 to 200 per 100,000 travelers.

## CLINICAL PRESENTATION

Clinical illness in humans begins following invasion of the peripheral and then central nervous system and culminates in acute fatal encephalitis. After infection, the asymptomatic incubation period is variable, but signs and symptoms most commonly develop within several weeks to several months after exposure. Pain and paresthesia at the site of exposure are often the first symptoms of disease. The disease then progresses rapidly from a nonspecific, prodromal phase with fever and vague symptoms to an acute, progressive encephalitis. The neurologic phase may be characterized by anxiety, paresis, paralysis, and other signs of encephalitis; spasms of swallowing muscles can be stimulated by the sight, sound, or perception of water (hydrophobia); and delirium and convulsions can develop, followed rapidly by coma and death. Once clinical signs manifest, patients die quickly in the absence of intensive supportive care.

## DIAGNOSIS

The diagnosis may be relatively simple in a patient with a compatible history and a classic clinical presentation (Box 4-6). However, clinical suspicion and prioritization of differential diagnoses may be complicated by variations in clinical presentation and a lack of exposure history. The exposure history can be difficult to elicit given that several weeks to months may have elapsed since the exposure occurred. Furthermore, the possibility of exposure to rabies virus may not be initially considered by

---

BOX 4-6. **World Health Organization, human rabies case definitions**

**Clinical case definition:** a person presenting with an acute neurologic syndrome (encephalitis) dominated by forms of hyperactivity (furious rabies) or paralytic syndromes (paralytic rabies) progressing toward coma and death, usually by cardiac or respiratory failure, typically within 7–10 days after the first symptom if no intensive care is instituted. Symptoms may include any of the following: aerophobia, hydrophobia, paresthesia or localized pain, dysphagia, localized weakness, nausea or vomiting.

**Suspected human rabies:** A case compatible with the clinical case definition.

**Probable human rabies:** A suspected case plus a reliable history of contact with a suspected, probable, or confirmed rabid animal.

**Confirmed human rabies:** A suspected or probable case confirmed in the laboratory.

clinicians and possible exposures might not be discussed with friends and family.

Definitive antemortem diagnosis requires high-complexity experimental test methods on multiple samples (serum, cerebrospinal fluid [CSF], saliva, and skin biopsy from the nape of the neck), which can be collected sequentially if initial testing is negative and clinical suspicion is high. Additional detailed information on diagnostic testing may be obtained from CDC (www.cdc.gov/rabies/specific_groups/doctors/ante_mortem.html). Rising levels of rabies virus– neutralizing antibodies, particularly in the CSF, is diagnostic in an unvaccinated, encephalitic patient. Rabies is a nationally notifiable disease.

CDC is designated as the national rabies reference laboratory for the United States, as well as a World Health Organization collaborating center for rabies and a World Organisation for Animal Health (OIE) rabies reference laboratory. As such, CDC performs public health testing for domestic and international health agencies, for both human and animal rabies diagnosis. Before submitting samples to CDC for rabies testing, the submitter must consult with program staff, obtain approval, and submit appropriate paperwork. Step-by-step instructions can be found at www.cdc.gov/rabies/resources/specimen-submission-guidelines.html.

## TREATMENT

There is not yet an evidence-based "best practices" medical approach to treating patients with rabies; most patients are managed with symptomatic and palliative supportive care. An experimental approach, known as the Milwaukee protocol, involves inducing coma and treating with antiviral drugs, but it remains controversial. Rabies is still considered universally fatal for practical purposes, and preventive measures ( for example, proper wound care, pre- and postexposure prophylaxis) are the only way to optimize survival if bitten by a rabid animal.

## PREVENTION

Rabies in travelers is best prevented by having a comprehensive strategy. This consists of 1) education about risks and the need to avoid bites from mammals, especially high-risk rabies reservoir species; 2) consultation with travel health professionals to determine if preexposure vaccination is recommended; 3) knowing how to prevent rabies after a bite; and 4) knowing how to obtain postexposure prophylaxis (PEP). The last may involve urgent importation of rabies biologics or travel to where PEP is available. A list of pretravel considerations in regards to rabies precautions can be found at www.cdc.gov/travel.

Not seeking PEP or receiving inadequate care is likely to result in death from rabies.

## Avoiding Animal Bites

Travelers to rabies-enzootic countries should be warned about the risk of rabies exposure and educated as to how to avoid animal bites. Travelers should avoid free-roaming mammals, avoid behaviors and actions that may provoke an animal to bite, and avoid contact with bats and other wildlife. Travelers who will spend time outdoors should be aware of dog-bite prevention techniques, such as avoidance of puppies when the mother is near, avoidance of dogs that are protecting a food source, and appropriate behavior around dogs.

Although nonhuman primates are rarely rabid, they are a common source of bites, mainly on the Indian subcontinent. In most instances these nonhuman primates cannot be followed up for rabies assessments, and the bite victims are recommended to receive PEP. Awareness of this risk and simple prevention is particularly effective. Travelers should be advised to not approach or otherwise interact with monkeys or carry food while monkeys are near, especially around monkeys that are habituated to tourists.

Travelers should be educated to not handle bats or other wildlife and consider the need for personal protective equipment before entering caves where bats may be found, given the risk for exposures to rabies virus, *Histoplasma* spp., viral hemorrhagic fever viruses, or other bat-associated pathogens. Many bats have tiny teeth, and wounds may not be readily apparent. Any suspected or documented bite or wound from a bat should be grounds for seeking PEP.

Children are at higher risk for rabies exposure and subsequent illness because of their inquisitive nature and inability to read behavioral cues from dogs and other animals. The smaller stature of children makes them more likely to experience severe bites to high-risk areas, such as the face and head. Also contributing to the higher risk is their attraction to animals and the possibility that they may not report an exposure.

## Preexposure Vaccination

Preexposure rabies vaccination may be recommended for certain international travelers based on the occurrence of animal rabies in the country of destination; the availability of antirabies biologics; the intended activities of the traveler, especially in remote areas; and the traveler's duration of stay. A decision to receive preexposure rabies immunization may also be based on the likelihood of repeat travel to at-risk destinations or long-term travel to a high-risk destination. Preexposure vaccination may be recommended for veterinarians, animal handlers, field biologists, cavers, missionaries, and certain laboratory workers. Table 4-16 provides criteria for preexposure vaccination. Regardless of whether preexposure vaccine is administered, travelers going to areas where the risk of rabies is high should be encouraged to purchase medical evacuation insurance (see Chapter 2, Travel Insurance,

## Table 4-16. Criteria for preexposure immunization for rabies

| RISK CATEGORY | NATURE OF RISK | TYPICAL POPULATIONS | PREEXPOSURE REGIMEN |
|---|---|---|---|
| Continuous | Virus present continuously, often in high concentrations Specific exposures (bite, nonbite, or aerosol) likely to go unrecognized | Rabies research laboratory workers[1] Rabies biologics production workers | Primary course; serologic testing every 6 months; booster vaccination if antibody titer is below acceptable level[2] |
| Frequent | Usually episodic exposure (bite, nonbite, or aerosol) with source recognized Possible unrecognized exposure | Rabies diagnostic laboratory workers[1] Cavers Veterinarians and staff Animal-control and wildlife workers in areas where rabies is enzootic All people who frequently handle bats | Primary course; serologic testing every 2 years; booster vaccination if antibody titer is below acceptable level[2] |
| Infrequent (greater than general population) | Exposure (bite or nonbite) nearly always episodic with source recognized | Veterinarians and animal control staff working with terrestrial carnivores in areas where rabies is uncommon to rare Veterinary students Travelers visiting areas where rabies is enzootic and immediate access to medical care, including biologics, is limited. | Primary course; no serologic testing or booster vaccination |
| Rare (general population) | Exposure (bite or nonbite) always episodic, with source recognized | US population at large, including people in rabies-epizootic areas | No preexposure immunization necessary |

[1] Judgment of relative risk and extra monitoring of vaccination status of laboratory workers are the responsibility of the laboratory supervisor (for more information, see: www.cdc.gov/biosafety/publications/bmbl5).
[2] Preexposure booster immunization consists of 1 dose of human diploid cell (rabies) vaccine or purified chick embryo cell vaccine, 1.0-mL dose, intramuscular (deltoid area). Per Advisory Committee on Immunization Practices recommendations, minimum acceptable antibody level is complete virus neutralization at a 1:5 serum dilution by the rapid fluorescent focus inhibition test, which is equivalent to approximately 0.1 IU/mL. A booster dose should be administered if titer falls below this level in populations that remain at risk.

## Table 4-17. Preexposure immunization for rabies[1]

| VACCINE | DOSE (ML) | NUMBER OF DOSES | SCHEDULE (DAYS)[2] | ROUTE |
|---------|-----------|-----------------|---------------------|-------|
| HDCV, Imovax (Sanofi) | 1.0 | 3 | 0, 7, and 21 or 28 | IM |
| PCEC, RabAvert (Novartis) | 1.0 | 3 | 0, 7, and 21 or 28 | IM |

Abbreviations: HDCV, human diploid cell vaccine; IM, intramuscular; PCEC, purified chick embryo cell.
[1] Patients who are immunosuppressed by disease or medications should postpone preexposure vaccinations and consider avoiding activities for which rabies preexposure prophylaxis is indicated during the period of expected immunosuppression. If this is not possible, immunosuppressed people who are at risk for rabies should have their antibody titers checked after vaccination.
[2] Every attempt should be made to adhere to recommended schedules; however, for most minor deviations (delays of a few days for individual doses), vaccination can be resumed as though the traveler were on schedule. If 3 doses of rabies vaccine cannot be completed before travel, the traveler should not start the series, as few data exist to guide PEP after a partial immunization series.

Travel Health Insurance & Medical Evacuation Insurance).

In the United States, preexposure vaccination consists of a series of 3 intramuscular injections given on days 0, 7, and 21 or 28 in the deltoid with human diploid cell rabies vaccine (HDCV) or purified chick embryo cell (PCEC) vaccine (Table 4-17). Travelers should receive all 3 preexposure immunizations before travel. If 3 doses of rabies vaccine cannot be completed before travel, the traveler should not start the series, as few data exist to guide PEP after a partial immunization series.

Preexposure vaccination does not eliminate the need for additional medical attention after a rabies exposure, but it simplifies PEP. Preexposure vaccination may also provide some protection when an exposure to rabies virus is unrecognized or PEP might be delayed. Travelers who have completed a 3-dose preexposure rabies immunization series or have received full PEP are considered previously vaccinated and do not require routine boosters. Routine testing for rabies virus-neutralizing antibody is not recommended for international travelers who are not otherwise in the frequent or continuous risk categories (Table 4-16).

## Wound Management

Any animal bite or scratch should be thoroughly cleaned with copious amounts of soap and water, povidone iodine, or other substances with virucidal activity. All travelers should be informed that immediately cleaning bite wounds as soon as possible substantially reduces the risk of rabies virus infection, especially when followed by timely administration of PEP. For unvaccinated patients, wounds that might require suturing should have the suturing delayed for a few days. If suturing is necessary to control bleeding or for functional or cosmetic reasons, rabies immune globulin (RIG) should be injected into all wounded tissues before suturing. The use of local anesthetic is not contraindicated in wound management.

## Postexposure Prophylaxis

### IN TRAVELERS WHO RECEIVED PREEXPOSURE VACCINATION

PEP for someone previously vaccinated consists of 2 doses of modern cell-culture vaccine given 3 days apart (days 0 and 3), ideally initiated shortly after the exposure. The booster doses do not have to be the same brand as the one in the original preexposure immunization series.

### IN TRAVELERS WHO DID NOT RECEIVE PREEXPOSURE VACCINATION

PEP for an unvaccinated patient consists of administration of RIG (20 IU/kg for human RIG or 40 IU/kg for equine RIG) and a series of 4 injections of rabies vaccine over 14 days, or 5 doses over a 1-month period in immunosuppressed patients (Table 4-18). After wound cleansing, as much of the dose-appropriate volume of RIG (Table 4-18) as is anatomically feasible should be injected at

## Table 4-18. Postexposure immunization for rabies[1]

| IMMUNIZATION STATUS | VACCINE/ PRODUCT | NUMBER OF DOSES | DOSE | SCHEDULE (DAYS)[2] | ROUTE |
|---|---|---|---|---|---|
| Not previously vaccinated | RIG plus | 20 IU/kg body weight | 1 | 0 | Infiltrated at bite site (if possible); remainder IM |
| Not previously vaccinated | HDCV or PCEC | 1.0 mL | 4[3] | 0, 3, 7, 14 (28 if immunocompromised[4]) | IM |
| Previously vaccinated[5,6] | HDCV or PCEC | 1.0 mL | 2 | 0, 3 | IM |

Abbreviations: RIG, rabies immune globulin; IM, intramuscular; HDCV, human diploid cell vaccine; PCEC, purified chick embryo cell.

[1] All postexposure prophylaxis should begin with immediate, thorough cleansing of all wounds with soap and water, povidone iodine, or other substances with virucidal activity.

[2] Every attempt should be made to adhere to recommended schedules; however, for most minor deviations (delays of a few days for individual doses), vaccination can be resumed as though the traveler were on schedule. When substantial deviations occur, immune status should be assessed by serologic testing 7–14 days after the final dose is administered.

[3] Five vaccine doses for the immunosuppressed patient. The first 4 vaccine doses are given on the same schedule as for an immunocompetent patient, and the fifth dose is given on day 28; patient follow-up should include monitoring antibody response. For more information, see: www.cdc.gov/mmwr/preview/mmwrhtml/rr5902a1.htm.

[4] CDC recommends 4 postexposure vaccine doses, on days 0, 3, 7, and 14, unless the patient is immunocompromised in some way, in which case a fifth dose is given at day 28.

[5] Preexposure immunization with HDCV or PCEC, prior postexposure prophylaxis with HDCV or PCEC, or people previously vaccinated with any other type of rabies vaccine and a documented history of positive rabies virus–neutralizing antibody response to the prior vaccination.

[6] RIG is not recommended.

the wound site. The intent is to put the RIG in the areas where saliva may have contaminated wounded tissue. If the wound is small and on a distal extremity such as a finger or toe, the health care provider must use clinical judgment to decide how much RIG to inject to avoid local tissue compression and complications. Any remaining dose should be administered intramuscularly at a site distant from the site of vaccine administration. If the wounds are extensive, the dose-appropriate volume of RIG must not be exceeded. If the volume is inadequate to inject all the wounds, the RIG may be diluted with normal saline to ensure sufficient volume to inject in all of the wounds. This is a particular issue in children whose body weight may be small in relation to the size and number of wounds.

RIG is difficult to access in many countries. If modern cell-culture vaccine is available but access to RIG is delayed, the vaccine series should be started as soon as possible, and RIG may be added to the regimen up to and including the seventh day after the first dose of vaccine was administered. After day 7, RIG is unlikely to provide benefit, as antibodies would be expected to be present from the patient's own vaccine-derived immune response.

Because rabies virus can persist in tissue for a long time before invading a peripheral nerve, a traveler who has sustained a bite that is suspicious for rabies should receive full PEP, including RIG, even if a considerable length of time has passed since the initial exposure. If there is a scar, or the patient remembers where the bite occurred, an appropriate amount of RIG should be injected in that area.

Human RIG is manufactured by plasmapheresis of blood from hyperimmunized volunteers. The total quantity of commercially produced human RIG falls short of worldwide demand, and it is not available in many developing countries. Equine RIG, purified fractions of equine RIG, and rabies monoclonal antibody products may be available in some countries where human RIG might not be available. Such products are preferable to no RIG.

The incidence of adverse events after the use of modern equine-derived RIG is low (0.8%–6.0%), and most reactions are minor. However, such products are not regulated by the Food and Drug Administration, and their use cannot be recommended unequivocally. In addition, unpurified antirabies serum of equine origin might still be used in some countries where neither human nor equine RIG is available.

Different PEP schedules, alternative routes of administration, and other rabies vaccines besides HDCV and PCEC may be used abroad. For example, commercially available purified Vero cell rabies vaccine and purified duck embryo cell vaccine are acceptable alternatives if available. However, other rabies vaccines or PEP regimens might require additional prophylaxis or confirmation of adequate rabies virus–neutralizing antibody titers. Assistance in managing complicated PEP scenarios can be obtained from experienced travel medicine professionals, health departments, and CDC (rabies@cdc.gov).

Rabies vaccine was once manufactured from viruses grown in animal brains, and some of these vaccines are still in use in developing countries. Typically, the brain-derived vaccines, also known as nerve tissue vaccines, can be identified if the traveler is offered a large-volume injection (5 mL) daily for approximately 14–21 days. Because of variability of potency in these preparations, which may limit effectiveness, and the risk of severe adverse reactions, the traveler should not accept these vaccines but travel to a location where acceptable vaccines and RIG are available.

## Rabies Vaccine

### VACCINE SAFETY AND ADVERSE REACTIONS

Travelers should be advised that they may experience local reactions after vaccination such as pain, erythema, swelling, or itching at the injection site, or mild systemic reactions such as headache, nausea, abdominal pain, muscle aches, and dizziness. Approximately 6% of people receiving booster vaccinations with HDCV may experience systemic hypersensitivity reactions characterized by urticaria, pruritus, and malaise. The likelihood of these reactions may be less with PCEC. Once initiated, rabies PEP should not be interrupted or discontinued because of local or mild systemic reactions to rabies vaccine. If an adverse event occurs with one of the vaccine types, consider switching to the alternative vaccine for the remainder of the series.

### PRECAUTIONS AND CONTRAINDICATIONS

Pregnancy is not a contraindication to PEP. In infants and children, the dose of HDCV or PCEC for preexposure or PEP is the same as that recommended for adults. The dose of RIG for PEP is based on body weight (Table 4-18).

**CDC website:** www.cdc.gov/rabies

## BIBLIOGRAPHY

1. Gautret P, Parola P. Rabies vaccination for international travelers. Vaccine. 2012 Jan 5;30(2):126–33.

2. Gautret P, Tantawichien T, Vu Hai V, Piyaphanee W. Determinants of pre-exposure rabies vaccination among foreign backpackers in Bangkok, Thailand. Vaccine. 2011 May 23;29(23):3931–4.

3. Malerczyk C, Detora L, Gniel D. Imported human rabies cases in Europe, the United States, and Japan, 1990 to 2010. J Travel Med. 2011 Nov–Dec; 18(6):402–7.

4. Mills DJ, Lau CL, Weinstein P. Animal bites and rabies exposure in Australian travellers. Med J Aust. 2011 Dec 19;195(11-12):673–5.

5. Rupprecht CE, Briggs D, Brown CM, Franka R, Katz SL, Kerr HD, et al. Use of a reduced (4-dose) vaccine schedule for postexposure prophylaxis to prevent human rabies: recommendations of the Advisory Committee on Immunization Practices. MMWR Recomm Rep. 2010 Mar 19;59(RR-2):1–9.

6. Rupprecht CE, Gibbons RV. Clinical practice. Prophylaxis against rabies. N Engl J Med. 2004 Dec 16;351(25):2626–35.

7. Smith A, Petrovic M, Solomon T, Fooks A. Death from rabies in a UK traveller returning from India. Euro Surveill. 2005 Jul;10(30):E050728 5.

8. van Thiel PP, de Bie RM, Eftimov F, Tepaske R, Zaaijer HL, van Doornum GJ, et al. Fatal human rabies due to Duvenhage virus from a bat in Kenya: failure of treatment with coma-induction, ketamine, and antiviral drugs. PLoS Negl Trop Dis. 2009;3(7):e428.

9. Warrell MJ, Warrell DA. Rabies and other lyssavirus diseases. Lancet. 2004 Mar 20;363(9413):959–69.

10. World Health Organization. WHO expert consultation on rabies. World Health Organ Tech Rep Ser. 2005;931:1–88.

# ALTERNATIVE APPROACHES TO RABIES IMMUNIZATION

David R. Shlim

Few topics in travel medicine prompt more concern and persistent questions than the prevention of rabies in travelers. Although we understand the basics of rabies prevention for travelers, the logistics of providing this care in a timely fashion remain a challenge. Unimmunized travelers who are exposed to rabies and other lyssaviruses require proper wound care, infiltration of human rabies immune globulin (RIG), and a series of 4 or 5 doses of rabies vaccine intramuscularly over a 2- to 4-week period. Travelers who receive 3 doses of rabies vaccine before travel need to receive 2 more doses of rabies vaccine, 3 days apart, after a viral exposure. Notably, human RIG and equine RIG are often unavailable in developing countries, although modern cell-culture rabies vaccines are increasingly available. Thus, preexposure rabies immunization can facilitate the traveler's access to adequate postexposure rabies prophylaxis.

Limiting the uptake of preexposure rabies immunization has been the cost of the vaccine in developed countries and the need for 3 clinic visits prior to travel. Three IM doses of rabies vaccine in the United States can now exceed $1,000 in cost. Even when modern cell-culture rabies vaccine was first introduced, at approximately $45 per dose in the early 1980s, many people already considered the vaccine too expensive. Thus, intradermal (ID) rabies immunization began almost as soon as the intramuscular (IM) human diploid cell vaccine (HDCV) was manufactured. By reconstituting the 1.0 mL of vaccine in the vial, practitioners could draw up approximately eight 0.1-mL doses. One problem was that the entire vial had to be used within a few hours of reconstituting, meaning that a provider had to either be in a busy clinic or line up groups of people, such as families, for rabies immunization at the same time.

Early studies of the immune response to ID rabies vaccine, using HDCV and later other rabies vaccines, were uniformly encouraging. Virtually 100% of vaccinees seroconverted. A 1982 statement by the US Advisory Committee on Immunization Practices (ACIP) reviewed data on >1,500 vaccinees and declared, "It appears that, with this vaccine, the 0.1-mL ID regimen is an acceptable alternative to the currently approved 1.0-mL IM regimen for preexposure prophylaxis." They called upon manufacturers to produce a product with appropriate packaging and labeling.

In 1986, the Mérieux Institute (now Sanofi Pasteur) received approval to market a 0.1-mL dose in an individual syringe. Sharing reconstituted vials of 1.0 mL between patients remained off-label. Although the new product solved the logistical problem of providing individual travelers with an ID dose, the cost of the prepackaged ID dose was 75% of the full 1.0-mL IM dose.

ACIP continued to endorse the concept of ID preexposure rabies immunization in a 1999 statement on rabies prevention. However, 3 lots of a prepackaged rabies ID vaccine were recalled in 2000 for having a potency that fell below the specification level before the expiration date. In 2001,

(continued)

# ALTERNATIVE APPROACHES TO RABIES IMMUNIZATION (CONTINUED)

the ID rabies vaccine was withdrawn from the market. Since then, authorities in the United States have not recommended sharing 1.0-mL vials for ID rabies immunization, as the manufacturer has not applied for the appropriate packaging and labeling to the Food and Drug Administration. This lack of endorsement of ID preexposure immunization has frustrated some travel medicine professionals.

With 2 decades more experience in using ID preexposure rabies immunization, the concept is fairly well accepted, but it remains off-label in the United States. Many clinics relying on preexposure ID dosing require the travelers to have a titer drawn after the series is completed to confirm seroconversion. This may save some money but requires a fourth clinic visit and even more time before travel.

Additional approaches have been taken to postexposure immunoprophylaxis, mainly driven by availability and cost of vaccine in resource-poor countries. Multi-dose ID and other abbreviated schedules have been used. From the point of view of the traveler, perhaps the best strategy would be to try to use postexposure regimens that are approved in the traveler's home country. This could create the most confidence and make it easier to complete regimens that have been started abroad in one's home country.

In late 2017, a World Health Organization (WHO) expert committee surprised many travel medicine practitioners by endorsing a 2-dose rabies preexposure immunization schedule. Although there have been some studies in limited numbers of subjects that support the notion that 2 doses may be adequate, the announcement seemed premature to some experts. In addition, WHO endorsed the use of wound-only administration of rabies immune globulin (RIG), an immunoglobulin-sparing technique in which RIG is injected around the wound (not to exceed the weight-calculated amount) but where the remaining calculated dose is not administered intramuscularly. This idea makes pathophysiologic sense, but there are many potential variables. Technique of the person injecting the RIG will be critical. With little written guidance available, some vaccine recipients may receive as little as 0.5 mL of RIG (in a small finger wound, for example), which may be <5% of historically recommended doses.

In the United States, practitioners should await ACIP and CDC guidance before adopting these new WHO recommendations. In the meantime, practitioners may face some challenging situations—treating people with a bite exposure who may have received the 2-dose preexposure regimen and having to decide how to proceed.

## BIBLIOGRAPHY

1. Bernard KW, Fishbein DB, Miller KD, Parker RA, Waterman S, Sumner JW, et al. Pre-exposure rabies immunization with human diploid cell vaccine: decreased antibody responses in persons immunized in developing countries. Am J Trop Med Hyg. 1985 May;34(3):633–47.

2. CDC. Recommendation of the Immunization Practices Advisory Committee (ACIP). Supplementary statement on pre-exposure rabies prophylaxis by the intradermal route. MMWR Morb Mortal Wkly Rep. 1982 Jun 4;31(21):279–80, 85.

3. Mills DJ, Lau CL, Fearnley EJ, Weinstein P. The immunogenicity of a modified intradermal pre-exposure rabies vaccination schedule--a case series of 420 travelers. J Travel Med. 2011 Sep–Oct;18(5):327–32.

4. Rabies vaccine and immunoglobulins: WHO position. [cited 2018 Mar 20]. Available from: http://apps.who.int/iris/bitstream/10665/259855/1/WHO-CDS-NTD-NZD-2018.04-eng.pdf?ua=1.

4

5. Soentjens P, Andries A, Aerssens A, Tsoumanis A, Ravinetto R, Heuninckx W, et al. Pre-exposure intradermal rabies vaccination: a non-inferiority trial in healthy adults on shortening the vaccination schedule from 28 to 7 days. Clin Infect Dis. 2019 Feb 1;68(4):607–14.

# RICKETTSIAL DISEASES (INCLUDING SPOTTED FEVER & TYPHUS FEVER RICKETTSIOSES, SCRUB TYPHUS, ANAPLASMOSIS, AND EHRLICHIOSES)

William L. Nicholson, Christopher D. Paddock

## INFECTIOUS AGENTS

Rickettsial infections are caused by multiple bacteria from the order Rickettsiales and genera *Rickettsia, Anaplasma, Ehrlichia, Neorickettsia, Neoehrlichia*, and *Orientia* (Table 4-19). *Rickettsia* spp. are classically divided into the spotted fever group (SFG) and the typhus group, although more recently these have been classified into as many as 4 groups. *Orientia* spp. make up the scrub typhus group. The rickettsial pathogens most likely to be encountered during travel outside the United States include *Rickettsia africae* (African tick-bite fever), *R. conorii* (Mediterranean spotted fever), *Anaplasma phagocytophilum* (anaplasmosis), *R. rickettsii* (known as both Rocky Mountain spotted fever and Brazilian spotted fever), *Orientia tsutsugamushi* (scrub typhus), and *R. typhi* (murine typhus).

## TRANSMISSION

Most rickettsial organisms are transmitted by the bites or infectious fluids (such as feces) inoculated into the skins from ectoparasites such as fleas, lice, mites, and ticks. Inhaling bacteria or inoculating conjunctiva with infectious material may also result in infection. The specific vectors that transmit each form of rickettsiae are listed in Table 4-19. Transmission of a few rickettsial diseases from transfusion of infected blood products or by organ transplantation is rare but has been reported.

## EPIDEMIOLOGY

All travelers are at risk of acquiring rickettsial infections during travel to endemic areas. Transmission occurs throughout the year but is increased during outdoor activities. Because of the 5- to 14-day incubation period for most rickettsial diseases, tourists may not experience symptoms during their trip, and onset may coincide with their return home or within a week after returning. Although the most commonly diagnosed rickettsial diseases in travelers are usually in the spotted fever or typhus groups, travelers may acquire a wide range of rickettsioses, including emerging and newly recognized species not well known by many health care providers (see Table 4-19).

## Table 4-19. Classification, primary arthropod vector, and host association of Rickettsiales known to cause disease in humans

| ANTIGENIC GROUP | DISEASE | SPECIES | VECTOR | ANIMAL HOST(S) | GEOGRAPHIC DISTRIBUTION |
|---|---|---|---|---|---|
| *Anaplasma* | Human anaplasmosis | *Anaplasma phagocytophilum* | Tick | Small mammals, rodents, deer | Primarily United States, worldwide |
| *Ehrlichia* | Human ehrlichiosis | *Ehrlichia chaffeensis* E. muris muris | Tick | Deer, wild and domestic dogs, domestic ruminants, rodents | United States, possibly elsewhere in world |
| | | *E. muris eauclairensis* *E. ewingii* *E. canis* | | Dogs | Worldwide; human cases in |
| | | | | Dogs | Venezuela, Costa Rica |
| *Neoehrlichia* | Human neoehrlichiosis | *Neoehrlichia mikurensis* | Tick | Rodents | Europe, Asia |
| *Neorickettsia* | Sennetsu fever | *Neorickettsia sennetsu* | Trematode | Fish | Japan, Malaysia, possibly other parts of Asia |
| Scrub typhus | Scrub typhus | *Orientia tsutsugamushi* | Larval mite (chigger) | Rodents | Asia–Pacific region from maritime Russia and China to Indonesia and North Australia to Afghanistan; recently recognized in Chile as well as some countries of Africa |
| | | *Orientia chuto* | Unknown | Unknown | United Arab Emirates |
| Spotted fever | Rickettsiosis | *Rickettsia aeschlimannii* | Tick | Unknown | South Africa, Morocco, Mediterranean littoral |
| | African tick-bite fever | *R. africae* | Tick | Ruminants | Sub-Saharan Africa, West Indies |
| | Rickettsialpox | *R. akari* | Mite | House mice, wild rodents | Countries of the former Soviet Union, South Africa, Korea, Turkey, Balkan countries, North and South America |

4

**326** TRAVEL-RELATED INFECTIOUS DISEASES

| Disease | Organism | Vector | Host | Distribution |
|---|---|---|---|---|
| Queensland tick typhus | R. australis | Tick | Rodents | Australia, Tasmania |
| Mediterranean spotted fever or Boutonneuse fever | R. conorii[1] | Tick | Dogs, rodents | Southern Europe, southern and western Asia, Africa, India |
| Cat flea rickettsiosis | R. felis | Flea | Domestic cats, rodents, opossums | Europe, North and South America, Africa, Asia |
| Far Eastern spotted fever | R. heilongjiangensis | Tick | Rodents | Far East of Russia, Northern China, eastern Asia |
| Aneruptive fever | R. Helvetica | Tick | Rodents | Central and northern Europe, Asia |
| Flinders Island spotted fever, Thai tick typhus | R. honei, including strain "marmionii" | Tick | Rodents, reptiles | Australia, Thailand |
| Japanese spotted fever | R. japonica | Tick | Rodents | Japan |
| Mediterranean spotted fever–like disease | R. massiliae | Tick | Unknown, possibly dogs | France, Greece, Spain, Portugal, Switzerland, Sicily, central Africa, Mali, United States |
| Mediterranean spotted fever–like illness | R. monacensis | Tick | Lizards, possibly birds | Europe, North Africa |
| Maculatum infection | R. parkeri | Tick | Rodents | North and South America |
| Tickborne lymphadenopathy (TIBOLA), Dermacentor–borne necrosis and lymphadenopathy (DEBONEL) | R. raoultii | Tick | Unknown | Europe, Asia |
| Rocky Mountain spotted fever, Brazilian spotted fever, febre maculosa, São Paulo exanthematic typhus, Minas Gerais exanthematic typhus | R. rickettsii | Tick | Rodents | North, Central, and South America |
| North Asian tick typhus, Siberian tick typhus | R. sibirica | Tick | Rodents | Russia, China, Mongolia |

(continued)

4

## Table 4-19. Classification, primary arthropod vector, and host association of Rickettsiales known to cause disease in humans (continued)

| ANTIGENIC GROUP | DISEASE | SPECIES | VECTOR | ANIMAL HOST(S) | GEOGRAPHIC DISTRIBUTION |
|---|---|---|---|---|---|
| | Lymphangitis-associated rickettsiosis | R. sibirica mongolotimonae | Tick | Rodents | Southern France, Portugal, China, Africa |
| | TIBOLA, DEBONEL | R. slovaca | Tick | Lagomorphs, rodents, European boar | Southern and eastern Europe, Asia; recently in US tick colony (unknown origin) |
| Typhus fever | Epidemic typhus, sylvatic typhus | R. prowazekii | Human body louse, flying squirrel ectoparasites | Humans, flying squirrels | Central Africa; Asia; North, Central and South America |
| | Murine typhus | R. typhi | Flea | Rodents | Temperate, tropical and subtropical areas worldwide |

[1] Includes 4 proposed subspecies that can be distinguished serologically and by PCR assay and that are the etiologic agents of Boutonneuse fever and Mediterranean tick fever in southern Europe and Africa (R. conorii subsp. conorii), Indian tick typhus in South Asia (R. conorii subsp. indica), Israeli tick typhus in southern Europe and Middle East (R. conorii subsp. israelensis), and Astrakhan spotted fever in the North Caspian region of Russia (R. conorii subsp. caspiae), respectively.

4

## Spotted Fever Group Rickettsioses

Tickborne spotted fever rickettsioses are the most frequently reported travel-associated rickettsial infections. Those who go on safari—especially those walking in the bush, game hunters, and ecotourists to southern Africa—are at risk for African tick-bite fever. This disease remains the most commonly reported rickettsial infection acquired during travel. Cases commonly occur as clusters among travel groups, and the diagnosis of African tick-bite fever in a member of a family or tourist group can alert other similarly exposed people to seek care if they develop symptoms. *R. africae* is also endemic to several Caribbean islands, and imported cases have been described from this region.

Travel-associated cases of Mediterranean spotted fever are less commonly reported but occur over an even larger region, including (but not limited to) much of Europe, Africa, India, and the Middle East. Rocky Mountain spotted fever (also known as Brazilian spotted fever, as well as other local names) occurs throughout much of the Western Hemisphere, and cases are reported from Canada, the United States, Mexico, and many countries of Central and South America, including Argentina, Brazil, Colombia, Costa Rica, and Panama. Clusters of illness may be reported in families or in geographic areas. Contact with dogs in rural and urban settings, and outdoor activities such as hiking, hunting, fishing, and camping increase the risk of infection.

The causative agent of rickettsialpox, *R. akari*, is transmitted by house mouse mites and circulates in mainly urban centers in Ukraine, South Africa, Korea, the Balkan states, and the United States. Outbreaks of rickettsialpox most often occur after contact with infected peridomestic rodents and their mites, especially during natural die-offs or exterminations of infected rodents that cause the mites to seek out new hosts, including humans.

## Typhus Group Rickettsioses

Flea-associated rickettsioses caused by *R. typhi* and *R. felis* are globally distributed, particularly in and around port cities and coastal regions with large rodent populations. Humans exposed to flea-infested cats, dogs, and peridomestic animals while traveling in endemic regions, or who enter or sleep in areas infested with rodents, are at most risk for fleaborne rickettsioses. Murine

typhus has been reported among travelers returning from Asia, Africa, and the Mediterranean Basin. Most cases acquired in the United States are reported from Hawaii, California, and Texas.

Epidemic typhus caused by *R. prowazekii* infection is reported rarely among tourists but can occur in communities and in refugee or incarcerated populations where body lice are prevalent. Outbreaks often occur during the colder months. Travelers at most risk for epidemic typhus include those who work with large homeless populations or who visit, impoverished areas, refugee camps, and regions that have recently experienced war or natural disasters. Active foci of epidemic typhus are known in the Andes regions of South America and some parts of Africa (including, but not limited to, Burundi, Ethiopia, and Rwanda). Louseborne epidemic typhus does not occur regularly in the United States, but a zoonotic reservoir exists in the southern flying squirrel, and sporadic sylvatic epidemic typhus cases are reported when they invade houses.

## Scrub Typhus Group Rickettsioses

Scrub typhus can be transmitted by many species of trombiculid mites encountered in high grass and brush and is endemic to northern Japan, Southeast Asia, Indonesia, eastern Australia, China, several parts of south-central Russia, India, and Sri Lanka; rare cases have been reported from the United Arab Emirates and Chile. More than 1 million cases occur annually, often in farmers or other occupationally exposed people. Most travel-acquired cases of scrub typhus are reported after visits to rural areas in countries where *O. tsutusgamushi* is endemic, but urban cases have also been described.

## Other Rickettsioses

Ehrlichiosis and anaplasmosis are tickborne infections most commonly reported in the United States, but pathogenic species can be found in many regions of the world. A variety of species are implicated in infection, but *E. chaffeensis* and *A. phagocytophilum* are most common. Infections with various *Ehrlichia* and *Anaplasma* spp. have also been reported in Europe, Africa, Asia, and South America.

*Neoehrlichia mikurensis* is a tickborne pathogen that occurs in many parts of Europe and Asia. It generally infects older or immunocompromised

4

people. Sennetsu fever, caused by *Neorickettsia sennetsu*, occurs in Japan, Malaysia, and possibly other parts of Asia. This disease can be contracted from eating raw fish infected with neorickettsiae-infected flukes.

## CLINICAL PRESENTATION

Rickettsial diseases are difficult to diagnose, even by health care providers experienced with these diseases. Most symptomatic rickettsial diseases cause moderate illness, but some Rocky Mountain and Brazilian spotted fevers, Mediterranean spotted fever, scrub typhus, and epidemic typhus may be fatal in 20%–60% of untreated cases. Prompt treatment is essential and results in improved outcomes.

Clinical presentations vary with the causative agent and patient; however, common symptoms that typically develop within 1–2 weeks of infection include fever, headache, malaise, rash, nausea, or vomiting. Many rickettsioses are accompanied by a maculopapular, vesicular, or petechial rash or sometimes an eschar at the site of the tick or mite bite.

African tick-bite fever is typically milder than some other rickettsioses, and recovery is improved with treatment. It should be suspected in a patient who presents with fever, headache, myalgia, and an eschar (tache noir) after recent travel to southern Africa. Mediterranean spotted fever is a potentially life-threatening rickettsial infection and should be suspected in patients with fever, rash, and eschar after recent travel to northern Africa or the Mediterranean basin. Rocky Mountain spotted fever is characterized by fever, headache, nausea, and abdominal pain. A rash is commonly reported but eschars are not.

Patients with murine or epidemic typhus usually present with a severe but nonspecific febrile illness, and approximately half present with a rash. Scrub typhus should be suspected in patients with a fever, headache, and myalgia after recent travel to Asia. Eschar, lymphadenopathy, cough, and encephalitis may be present.

Ehrlichiosis and anaplasmosis should be suspected in febrile patients with leukopenia with an exposure history. The clinical signs are similar to those of the rickettsioses.

## DIAGNOSIS

Diagnosis is usually based on clinical recognition, epidemiologic context, and serologic testing.

Serologic testing provides much stronger evidence when acute- and convalescent-phase serum samples are compared; a >4-fold rise in titer is diagnostic in indirect immunofluorescence antibody assays. Because of cross-reactivity of antigens, some antibodies may react in group-targeted serologic tests and provide evidence of exposure to the group level. PCR assays and immunohistochemical analyses may also be helpful, but useful results are highly dependent upon the type and timing of specimen submitted.

If an eschar is present, a swab or biopsy sample of the lesion can be evaluated by PCR and provides a species-specific diagnosis. If ehrlichiosis or anaplasmosis is suspected, PCR of a whole blood specimen provides the best diagnostic test. A buffy coat may provide presumptive evidence of infection if examined to identify characteristic intraleukocytic morulae. Ehrlichiosis, anaplasmosis, and spotted fever rickettsiosis are nationally notifiable diseases in the United States. Commercial laboratories offer rickettsial testing for rickettsioses, anaplasmosis, ehrlichiosis, and scrub typhus. However, some species-targeted serologic tests are not routinely available at commercial laboratories and are available only through the Rickettsial Branch at CDC (call 1-800-CDC-INFO).

## TREATMENT

Treatment of patients with possible rickettsioses should begin when the disease is suspected and while awaiting confirmatory testing, as certain infections can be rapidly progressive and fatal. Immediate empiric treatment with a tetracycline is recommended for all ages, most commonly doxycycline. Chloramphenicol may be an alternative in some cases, but its use is associated with increased risk of death, particularly from *R. rickettsii* infection, compared with use of a tetracycline. In some areas, tetracycline-resistant scrub typhus has been reported, and azithromycin may be an effective alternative. Limited clinical experience has shown that *A. phagocytophilum* and *R. africae* infections respond to treatment with rifampin, which may be an alternative drug for some pregnant or doxycycline-intolerant patients. Expert advice should be sought if alternative agents are being considered.

## PREVENTION

No vaccine is available for preventing rickettsial infections. Antibiotics are not recommended for prophylaxis of rickettsial diseases and should not be given to asymptomatic people.

Travelers should be instructed to minimize exposure to infectious arthropods during travel (including lice, fleas, ticks, mites) and to animal reservoirs (particularly dogs) when traveling in endemic areas. The proper use of insect or tick repellents on skin or clothing, self-examination after visits to vector-infested areas, and wearing protective clothing are ways to reduce risk. These precautions are especially important for people with underlying conditions that may compromise their immune systems, as these people may be more susceptible to severe disease. For more detailed information, see Chapter 3, Mosquitoes, Ticks & Other Arthropods.

**CDC website:** www.cdc.gov/ticks

### BIBLIOGRAPHY

1. Biggs, HM, Barton Behravesh C, Bradley KK, Dahlgren FS, Drexler NA, Dumler JS, et al. Diagnosis and management of tickborne rickettsial diseases: Rocky Mountain spotted fever and other spotted fever group rickettsioses, ehrlichiosis, and anaplasmosis—United States: A practical guide for health care and public health professionals. MMWR Recommendations and Reports 2016;65:1–44.

2. Cherry CC, Denison AM, Kato CY, Thornton K, CD Paddock. Diagnosis of spotted fever group rickettsioses in U.S. travelers returning from Africa, 2007–2016. Am J Trop Med Hyg. 2018 Jul;99(1):136–42.

3. Hendershot EF, Sexton DJ. Scrub typhus and rickettsial diseases in international travelers: a review. Curr Infect Dis Rep. 2009 Jan;11(1):66–72.

4. Jensenius M, Davis X, von Sonnenburg F, Schwartz E, Keystone JS, Leder K, et al. Multicenter GeoSentinel analysis of rickettsial diseases in international travelers, 1996–2008. Emerg Infect Dis. 2009 Nov;15(11):1791–8.

5. Leshem E, Meltzer E, Schwartz E. Travel-associated zoonotic bacterial diseases. Curr Opin Infect Dis. 2011 Oct;24(5):457–63.

6. Li H, Zheng YC, Ma L, Jia N, Jiang BG, Jiang RR, et al. Human infection with a novel tick-borne Anaplasma species in China: a surveillance study. Lancet Infect Dis. 2015 Jun; 15(6):663–70.

7. Nachega JB, Bottieau E, Zech F, Van Gompel A. Travel-acquired scrub typhus: emphasis on the differential diagnosis, treatment, and prevention strategies. J Travel Med. 2007 Sep–Oct;14(5):352–5.

8. Raoult D, Parola P, editors. Rickettsial Diseases. New York: Informa Healthcare USA; 2007.

9. Silaghi C, Beck R, Oteo JA, Pfeffer M, Sprong H. Neoehrlichiosis: an emerging tick-borne zoonosis caused by Candidatus Neoehrlichia mikurensis. Exp Appl Acarol 2016;68: 279–97.

10. Strand A, Paddock CD, Rinehart AR, Condit ME, Marus JR, Gillani S, et al. African tick bite fever treated successfully with rifampin in a patient with doxycycline intolerance. Clin Infect Dis 2017;65:1582–4.

4

# RUBELLA

Michelle Morales, Tatiana Lanzieri, Susan E. Reef

## INFECTIOUS AGENT

Rubella virus ( family Togaviridae, genus *Rubivirus*).

## TRANSMISSION

Person-to-person contact or droplets shed from the respiratory secretions of infected people. People may shed virus from 7 days before the onset of the rash to approximately 5–7 days after rash onset. Transmission from mother to fetus can also occur, with the highest risk of congenital rubella syndrome (CRS) if infection occurs in the first trimester. Infants with CRS can transmit virus for up to 1 year after birth.

## EPIDEMIOLOGY

Endemic rubella virus transmission was declared eliminated in the Americas in 2015; however, rubella virus continues to circulate widely, especially in Africa, the Middle East, and South and Southeast Asia. Globally, >100,000 infants are born each year with CRS, and >80% of those are born in Africa and some countries in South and Southeast Asia. In the United States, endemic rubella virus transmission was interrupted in 2001 and elimination was verified in 2004, but imported cases of both rubella and CRS continue to occur. From 2013 through 2015, a median of 6 (range, 5–9) imported cases were reported annually in the United States, and 3 CRS cases were reported during the same period.

## CLINICAL PRESENTATION

Average incubation period is 14 days (range, 12–23 days). Usually presents as a nonspecific, maculopapular, generalized rash that lasts ≤3 days with generalized lymphadenopathy. Rash may be preceded by low-grade fever, malaise, anorexia, mild conjunctivitis, runny nose, and sore throat. Adolescents and adults, especially women, can also present with transient arthritis. Asymptomatic rubella virus infections are common. Infection during early pregnancy can lead to miscarriage, fetal death, or infants born with severe birth defects known as CRS.

## DIAGNOSIS

Demonstration of specific rubella IgM or significant increase in rubella IgG in acute- and convalescent-phase specimens. RT-PCR can be used to detect virus infection; viral culture is also acceptable but is time-consuming and expensive. Rubella is a nationally notifiable disease.

## TREATMENT
Supportive care.

## PREVENTION
All travelers aged ≥12 months who do not have acceptable evidence of immunity to rubella (documented by ≥1 dose of rubella-containing vaccine on or after the first birthday, laboratory evidence of immunity, or birth before 1957) should be vaccinated with measles-mumps-rubella (MMR) vaccine. Before departure from the United States, infants aged 6–11 months should receive 1 dose of MMR vaccine (for measles protection), and children aged ≥12 months and adults should receive 2 doses of MMR vaccine ≥28 days apart.

MMR vaccine is contraindicated during pregnancy. Pregnant women who do not have acceptable evidence of rubella immunity should not travel to countries where rubella is endemic or areas with known rubella outbreaks, especially during the first 20 weeks of pregnancy, and should be vaccinated immediately postpartum. Health care providers should also ensure that all women of childbearing age and recent immigrants are up-to-date on their immunization against rubella or have evidence of immunity to rubella, because these groups are at the highest risk for maternal–fetal transmission of rubella virus, which can result in CRS.

**CDC website:** www.cdc.gov/rubella

### BIBLIOGRAPHY

1. Adams DA, Thomas KR, Jajosky RA, Foster L, Baroi G, Sharp P, et al. Summary of notifiable infectious diseases and conditions—United States, 2015. MMWR Morb Mortal Wkly Rep. 2017 Aug 11;64(53):1–143.

2. CDC. Rubella. In: Hamborsky J, Kroger A, Wolfe S, editors. Epidemiology and Prevention of Vaccine-Preventable Diseases. 13th ed. Washington, DC: Public Health Foundation; 2015. pp. 275–89.

3. Grant GB, Reef SE, Patel M, Knapp JK, Dabbagh A. Progress in rubella and congenital rubella syndrome control and elimination—worldwide, 2000–2016. MMWR Morb Mortal Wkly Rep. 2017 Nov 17;66(45):1256–60.

4. Reef SE, Plotkin SA. Rubella vaccines. In: Plotkin SA, Orenstein WA, Offit PA, Edwards KM, editors. Vaccines. 7th ed. Philadelphia: Elsevier; 2018. pp. 970–1000.

5. Vynnycky E, Adams EJ, Cutts FT, Reef SE, Navar AM, Simons E, et al. Using seroprevalence and immunisation coverage data to estimate the global burden of congenital rubella syndrome, 1996–2010: a systematic review. PLoS One. 2016;11(3):e0149160.

6. World Health Organization. Rubella vaccines: WHO position paper. Wkly Epidemiol Rec. 2011 July 15, 2011;86(29):301–16.

# SALMONELLOSIS (NONTYPHOIDAL)

Jessica M. Healy, Beau B. Bruce

## INFECTIOUS AGENT

*Salmonella enterica* subspecies *enterica* is a gram-negative, rod-shaped bacillus. More than 2,500 *Salmonella* serotypes have been identified, but only a small proportion are commonly associated with human illness. Nontyphoidal salmonellosis refers to illnesses caused by all serotypes of *Salmonella* except for Typhi, Paratyphi A, Paratyphi B (tartrate negative), and Paratyphi C.

## TRANSMISSION

Usually through the consumption of food or water contaminated with animal feces. Transmission can also occur through direct contact with infected animals or their environment and directly between humans.

## EPIDEMIOLOGY

Nontyphoidal salmonellae are one of the leading causes of bacterial diarrhea worldwide; they are estimated to cause approximately 153 million cases of gastroenteritis and 57,000 deaths globally each year. The risk of *Salmonella* infection among travelers returning to the United States varies by region of the world visited; the highest risk is among those who visited Africa (incidence of 25.8 cases per 100,000 air travelers), Latin America and the Caribbean (7.1 cases per 100,000), and Asia (5.8 cases per 100,000). A systematic review of travelers' diarrhea studies found that *Salmonella* (including typhoidal serotypes) was detected in <5% of patients who had traveled to Latin America, the Caribbean, and South Asia and in 5%–15% of patients who had traveled to Africa or Southeast Asia. *Salmonella* infection and carriage has been reported among internationally adopted children.

## CLINICAL PRESENTATION

Gastroenteritis is the most common clinical presentation of nontyphoidal *Salmonella* infection. The incubation period is typically 6–72 hours; although atypical, illness has been documented even 16 days after exposure. Illness is commonly manifested as acute diarrhea, abdominal pain, fever, and vomiting. The illness usually lasts 4–7 days, and most people recover without treatment.

Approximately 8% of people develop bacteremia or focal infection (such as meningitis, osteomyelitis, or septic arthritis). Serotypes more frequently associated with invasive infection include Dublin, Choleraesuis, and Typhimurium variant ST313 (currently only found in sub-Saharan Africa and Brazil). Rates of invasive infections and death are generally higher among infants, older adults, and people with immunosuppressive conditions (including HIV), hemoglobinopathies, and malignant neoplasms. Infection with antibiotic-resistant organisms has been associated with a higher risk of bloodstream infection and hospitalization.

## DIAGNOSIS

Culturing organisms continues to be the mainstay of clinical diagnostic testing for nontyphoidal *Salmonella* infection. Approximately 90% of isolates are obtained from routine stool culture, but isolates can also be obtained from other sites of infection if present, including blood, urine, abscesses, and cerebrospinal fluid. Although culture-independent diagnostic tests are used increasingly by clinical laboratories to diagnose *Salmonella* infection, isolates are necessary for serotyping and antimicrobial susceptibility testing. Serologic testing to detect infection with *Salmonella* is not advised.

Most states mandate that *Salmonella* isolates or clinical material be submitted to the local or state public health laboratory. To understand submission requirements in a particular state, clinical laboratories are advised to review the

**4**

disease reporting and mandatory isolate submission regulations of that state and to contact their local public health department with any questions. Salmonellosis is a nationally notifiable disease.

## TREATMENT

Current recommendations are to treat most patients with uncomplicated *Salmonella* infection with oral rehydration therapy but not with antimicrobial agents, as treatment can prolong bacterial shedding. Antimicrobial therapy should be considered for patients who are severely ill (those with severe diarrhea, high fever, or manifestations of extraintestinal infection) and for people at increased risk of invasive disease (infants, older adults, and the debilitated or immunosuppressed). When antimicrobial therapy is indicated, empiric treatment is usually required until susceptibility data are available. Resistance to antimicrobial agents varies by serotype and geographic region.

Fluoroquinolones are considered first-line treatment in adult travelers. However, resistance to fluoroquinolones among *Salmonella* strains is rising globally. In a study of international travelers diagnosed with *S. enterica* serotype Enteritidis infection in the United States, 24% of isolates showed decreased susceptibility to fluoroquinolones compared with only 3% of isolates from patients with no history of international travel. Azithromycin can be used for

children and is an alternative agent for adults returning from Latin America or Asia, where fluoroquinolone resistance in this organism may exceed 10%. Azithromycin resistance has been documented in multiple settings globally but is not commonly reported.

Invasive strains of nontyphoidal *Salmonella*, such as Typhimurium variant ST313, emerging in areas of sub-Saharan Africa, have shown resistance to chloramphenicol, ampicillin, trimethoprim-sulfamethoxazole, and cephalosporins. Resistance to older antimicrobial agents (chloramphenicol, ampicillin, and trimethoprim-sulfamethoxazole) has been present for many years among nontyphoidal *Salmonella* serotypes; these should not be considered first-line empiric agents in returning travelers (see Chapter 2, Travelers' Diarrhea).

## PREVENTION

No vaccine is available against nontyphoidal *Salmonella* infection. Preventive measures include food and water precautions (see Chapter 2, Food & Water Precautions), such as avoiding foods and drinks at high risk for contamination, and frequent handwashing, especially after contact with animals or their environment. Although rare, patients should be informed of the potential for continued bacterial shedding after symptoms have resolved.

**CDC website:** www.cdc.gov/salmonella

### BIBLIOGRAPHY

1. Almeida F, Aparecida Seribelli A, da Silva P, Inês Cazentini Medeiros M, dos Prazeres Rodrigues D, Gallina Moreira C, et al. Multilocus sequence typing of Salmonella Typhimurium reveals the presence of the highly invasive ST313 in Brazil. Infect Genet Evol. 2017 Jul;51:41–4.

2. American Public Health Association. Salmonellosis. In: Heymann DL, editor. Control of Communicable Diseases Manual. 20th ed. Washington, DC: American Public Health Association; 2015. pp. 532–35.

3. Association of Public Health Laboratories. State legal requirements for submission of isolates and other clinical materials by clinical laboratories: a review of state approaches 2015 [cited 2019 Jan 10]. Available from: www.aphl.org/aboutAPHL/publications/Documents/StateRequirements_Appendix_v6.pdf.

4. Crump JA, Sjölund-Karlssonb M, Gordonc MA, Parrye CM. Epidemiology, clinical presentation, laboratory diagnosis, antimicrobial resistance, and antimicrobial management of invasive salmonella infections. Clin Microbiol Rev. 2015 Oct 1;28(4):901–37.

5. Haselbeck AH, Panzner U, Im J, Baker S, Meyer CG, Marks F. Current perspectives on invasive nontyphoidal Salmonella disease. Curr Opin Infect Dis. 2017 Oct;30(5):498–503.

6. Jones TF, Ingram LA, Cieslak PR, Vugia DJ, Tobin-D'Angelo M, Hurd S, et al. Salmonellosis outcomes differ substantially by serotype. J Infect Dis. 2008 Jul 1;198(1):109–14.

7. Kendall ME, Crim S, Fullerton K, Han PV, Cronquist AB, Shiferaw B, et al. Travel-associated enteric infections diagnosed after return to the United States, Foodborne

Diseases Active Surveillance Network (FoodNet), 2004–2009. Clin Infect Dis. 2012 Jun;54 Suppl 5:S480–7.

8. Marzel A, Desai PT, Goren A, Schorr YI, Nissan I, Porwollik S, et al. Persistent infections by nontyphoidal salmonella in humans: epidemiology and genetics. Clin Infect Dis. 2016 Apr 1;62(7):879–86.

9. O'Donnell AT, Vieira AR, Huang JY, Whichard J, Cole D, Karp BE. Quinolone-resistant Salmonella enterica serotype Enteritidis infections associated with international travel. Clin Infect Dis. 2014 Nov 1;59(9):e139–41.

10. Steffen R, Hill DR, DuPont HL. Traveler's diarrhea: a clinical review. JAMA. 2015 Jan 6;313(1):71–80.

# SARCOCYSTOSIS

Douglas H. Esposito

## INFECTIOUS AGENT

Intracellular coccidian protozoan parasites in the genus *Sarcocystis*.

## TRANSMISSION

Humans are the natural definitive host for *Sarcocystis hominis, S. heydorni*, and *S. suihominis*, acquired by eating undercooked sarcocyst-containing beef or pork, resulting in intestinal sarcocystosis. Dead-end intermediate host infection can occur in humans with *S. nesbitti* and possibly other species when food, water, or soil contaminated with the feces from a reptilian sporocyst-shedding definitive host (likely snake) is ingested, resulting in muscular sarcocystosis.

## EPIDEMIOLOGY

Human intestinal sarcocystosis occurs worldwide, but the prevalence is poorly defined and may vary regionally. Outbreaks of symptomatic muscular sarcocystosis among tourists in Malaysia suggest that intermediate-host infection may be of public health significance. Most reported cases have been acquired in the tropics and subtropics, particularly in Southeast Asia.

## CLINICAL PRESENTATION

Most people with intestinal sarcocystosis are asymptomatic or experience mild gastroenteritis, though severe illness has been described. Differences in symptoms and illness severity and duration may reflect the number and species of the sarcocysts ingested. The disease is thought to be self-limited in immunocompetent hosts.

Intermediate-host infection may range from asymptomatic to severe and debilitating. In those with symptoms, onset occurs in the first 2 weeks after infection, and symptoms typically resolve in weeks to months. However, some patients may remain symptomatic for years. The most common symptoms are fever, fatigue, myalgia, headache, cough, and arthralgia. Less frequent are wheezing, nausea, vomiting, diarrhea, rash, lymphadenopathy, and symptoms reflecting cardiac involvement such as palpitations. Fever and muscle pain may be relapsing and can occur in 2 distinct phases: early (beginning during the second week after infection) and late (beginning during the sixth week after infection). Early-phase disease may reflect a generalized vasculitis, and late-phase disease may coincide with the onset of a diffuse focal myositis.

## DIAGNOSIS

Intestinal sarcocystosis should be considered in patients with gastroenteritis and a history of eating raw or undercooked meat. Oocysts or sporocysts can be confirmed in stool by light or fluorescence microscopy; PCR is not widely available, and no serologic assays have been validated for use in humans.

Muscular sarcocystosis should be considered in people presenting with myalgia, with or without fever, and a history of travel to a tropical or subtropical region, especially Malaysia. However, diagnosis during the early phase of infection is difficult because of the lack of specificity of symptoms and clinical and laboratory findings.

In the absence of an alternative diagnosis, serial investigations for evidence of myositis and eosinophilia should be considered. In those with myositis, trichinellosis should be excluded. Confirmation of muscular sarcocystosis requires biopsy and histologic observation of sarcocysts in muscle. Diagnostic assistance is available through CDC (www.cdc.gov/dpdx; dpdx@cdc.gov).

## TREATMENT
There are no proven medical treatments for sarcocystosis. Trimethoprim-sulfamethoxazole may have activity against schizonts in the early phase of muscular sarcocystosis, but data are scant. Glucocorticoids and nonsteroidal anti-inflammatories may improve the symptoms associated with myositis.

## PREVENTION
Intestinal sarcocystosis can be prevented by thoroughly cooking or freezing meat, which kills the infective bradyzoites. Muscular sarcocystosis can be prevented with standard food and water precautions (see Chapter 2, Food & Water Precautions).

**CDC website:** www.cdc.gov/parasites/ sarcocystosis/index.html

### BIBLIOGRAPHY

1. Dubey JP, van Wilpe E, Calero-Bernal R, Verma SK, Fayer R. *Sarcocystis heydorni*, n. sp. (Apicomplexa: Sarcocystidae) with cattle (Bos taurus) and human (Homo sapiens) cycle. Parasitol Res. 2015 Nov;114(11):4143–7.

2. Esposito DH, Stich A, Epelboin L, Malvy D, Han PV, Bottieau E, et al. Acute muscular sarcocystosis: an international investigation among ill travelers returning from Tioman Island, Malaysia, 2011–2012. Clin Infect Dis. 2014 Nov 15;59(10):1401–10.

3. Fayer R, Esposito DH, Dubey JP. Human infections with Sarcocystis species. Clin Microbiol Rev. 2015 Apr;28(2):295–311.

4. Italiano CM, Wong KT, AbuBakar S, Lau YL, Ramli N, Syed Omar SF, et al. Sarcocystis nesbitti causes acute, relapsing febrile myositis with a high attack rate: description of a large outbreak of muscular sarcocystosis in Pangkor Island, Malaysia, 2012. PLoS Negl Trop Dis. 2014 May;8(5):e2876.

5. Slesak G, Schafer J, Langeheinecke A, Tappe D. Prolonged clinical course of muscular sarcocystosis and effectiveness of cotrimoxazole among travelers to Tioman Island, Malaysia, 2011–2014. Clin Infect Dis. 2015 Jan 15;60(2):329.

6. Tappe D, Stich A, Langeheinecke A, von Sonnenburg F, Muntau B, Schafer J, et al. Suspected new wave of muscular sarcocystosis in travellers returning from Tioman Island, Malaysia, May 2014. Euro Surveill. 2014;19(21):pii=20816. https://doi.org/10.2807/1560-7917.ES2014.19.21.20816.

7. Wassermann M, Raisch L, Lyons JA, Natusch DJD, Richter S, Wirth M, et al. Examination of Sarcocystis spp. of giant snakes from Australia and Southeast Asia confirms presence of a known pathogen—Sarcocystis nesbitti. PLoS One. 2017 Nov 13;12(11):e0187984.

# SCABIES

Diana Martin

## INFECTIOUS AGENT
The human itch mite, *Sarcoptes scabiei* var. *hominis*.

## TRANSMISSION
Direct transmission of conventional scabies occurs after prolonged skin-to-skin contact with a person infested with the mite. Indirect transmission of conventional scabies through contact with contaminated objects is rare. Animals are not a source of scabies.

Crusted scabies, by contrast, is more highly contagious than conventional scabies. Although fewer than 20 mites typically are found on a host with conventional scabies, a person with crusted scabies (formerly called Norwegian scabies) may harbor thousands of mites in just a small area of skin. This large number greatly increases the chances that a person with crusted scabies will pass mites to others by both direct and indirect routes of transmission.

## EPIDEMIOLOGY

Scabies occurs worldwide and is transmitted most easily in settings where skin contact is common. Crusted scabies most commonly occurs among elderly, disabled, debilitated, or immuno-suppressed hosts, often in institutional settings. Scabies is more common in travelers with longer travel (>8 weeks) than in those who travel for shorter periods.

## CLINICAL PRESENTATION

Symptoms occur 2–6 weeks after an initial infestation. If someone has had scabies previously, symptoms appear much sooner (1–4 days after exposure). Conventional scabies is characterized by intense itching, particularly at night, and by a papular or papulovesicular erythematous rash. Characteristic features of crusted scabies include widespread crusting and scales containing large numbers of mites. Itching may be less prominent than in conventional scabies.

## DIAGNOSIS

Scabies is a clinical diagnosis. Telltale signs include burrows, typically found in skin folds and intertriginous areas in a patient with itching, and the characteristic rash. Although finding mites, mite eggs, or scybala (mite feces) under the microscope can confirm the diagnosis of scabies, microscopic identification of mites is far less sensitive than clinical diagnosis. Often misdiagnosed as psoriasis, crusted scabies can be diagnosed accurately by using skin scrapings because of the high number of mites in the sores.

## TREATMENT

Permethrin (5%) cream is the first-line treatment for conventional scabies. Apply the cream over the entire body (from the neck down), leaving it on for 8–12 hours or overnight. Then wash the cream off and reapply 1 week later. Treat household members and close contacts similarly.

Oral ivermectin is reported to be safe and effective to treat conventional scabies. Although not approved by the US Food and Drug Administration to treat scabies, consider off-label ivermectin use where topical treatment has failed or in patients who cannot tolerate other approved medications. The recommended oral dose is 200 µg/kg, repeated in 2 weeks.

Treat crusted scabies more aggressively by using a combination of permethrin and ivermectin. Daily full-body application of permethrin for 7 days and up to 7 doses of oral ivermectin may be required. Treatment of crusted scabies is best managed by a physician.

## PREVENTION

Avoidance is the best form of prevention. Prolonged skin-to-skin contact with people with conventional scabies and even brief skin-to-skin contact with people with crusted scabies are the primary routes of transmission. Do not share or handle clothing or bed linens used by an infested person, especially if the person has crusted scabies.

**CDC website:** www.cdc.gov/parasites/scabies

BIBLIOGRAPHY

1. Bouvresse S, Chosidow O. Scabies in healthcare settings. Curr Opin Infect Dis. 2010 Apr;23(2):111–18.

2. Currie BJ, McCarthy JS. Permethrin and ivermectin for scabies. N Engl J Med. 2010 Feb 25;362(8):717–25.

3. Davis JS, McGloughlin S, Tong SY, Walton SF, Currie BJ. A novel clinical grading scale to guide the management of crusted scabies. PLoS Negl Trop Dis. 2013;7(9):e2387.

4. Warkowski JA, Bolan GA. Sexually transmitted diseases treatment guidelines, 2015. MMWR Morb Mortal Wkly Rep. 2015 Jun 5;64(RR-03):1–137.

# SCHISTOSOMIASIS

Susan Montgomery

## INFECTIOUS AGENT

Schistosomiasis is caused by helminth parasites of the genus *Schistosoma*. Other helminth infections are discussed in the Helminths, Soil-Transmitted section earlier in this chapter.

## TRANSMISSION

Waterborne transmission occurs when larval cercariae, found in contaminated bodies of freshwater, penetrate the skin.

## EPIDEMIOLOGY

An estimated 85% of the world's cases of schistosomiasis are in Africa, where prevalence rates can exceed 50% in local populations. *Schistosoma mansoni* and *S. haematobium* are distributed throughout Africa; only *S. haematobium* is found in areas of the Middle East, and *S. japonicum* is found in Indonesia and parts of China and Southeast Asia (Map 4-11). Although schistosomiasis had been eliminated in Europe for decades, transmission of *S. haematobium* was reported in Corsica in 2014, where cases were identified among travelers who had bathed in the Cavu River. Two other species can infect humans: *S. mekongi*, found in Cambodia and Laos, and *S. intercalatum*, found in parts of Central and West Africa. These 2 species are rarely reported causes of human infection.

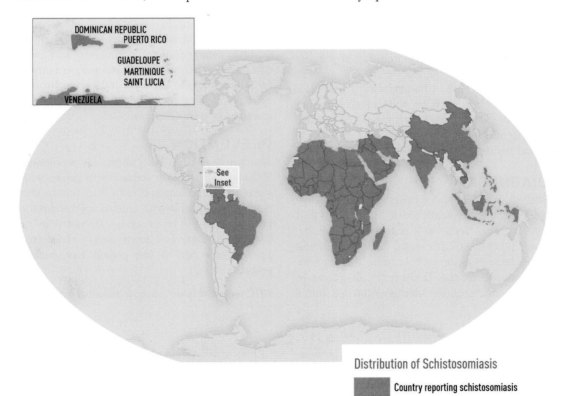

Distribution of Schistosomiasis

■ Country reporting schistosomiasis

MAP 4-11. **Distribution of schistosomiasis**

The distribution of schistosomiasis is highly focal; however, surveillance for schistosomiasis is limited in most countries. Therefore, this map shades entire countries where schistosomiasis transmission has been reported. The exception to this is France, where schistosomiasis has been reported on several islands, such as Guadeloupe, Martinique, and Corsica.

Many countries endemic for schistosomiasis have established control programs, but others do not. Countries where development has led to widespread improvements in sanitation and water safety, as well as successful schistosomiasis control programs, may have eliminated this disease. However, there are currently no international guidelines for verification of elimination.

Swimming, bathing, and wading in contaminated freshwater can result in infection; all ages are at risk. Human schistosomiasis is not acquired by contact with saltwater (oceans or seas). The distribution of schistosomiasis is very focal and determined by the presence of competent snail vectors, inadequate sanitation, and infected humans. The specific snail vectors can be difficult to identify, and whether snails are infected with human schistosome species can only be determined in the laboratory.

The geographic distribution of cases of schistosomiasis acquired by travelers reflects travel and immigration patterns. Most travel-associated cases of schistosomiasis are acquired in sub-Saharan Africa. Sites in Africa frequently visited by travelers are common sites of infection. These sites include rivers and water sources in the Banfora region (Burkina Faso) and areas populated by the Dogon people (Mali), Lake Malawi, Lake Tanganyika, Lake Victoria, the Omo River (Ethiopia), the Zambezi River, and the Nile River. However, as visitors travel to more remote sites, it is important to remember that most freshwater surface water sources in Africa are potentially contaminated and can be sources of infection. A local claim that there is no schistosomiasis in a body of freshwater is not necessarily reliable.

The types of travelers and expatriates potentially at increased risk for infection include adventure travelers, Peace Corps volunteers, missionaries, soldiers, and ecotourists. Outbreaks of schistosomiasis have occurred among adventure travelers on river trips in Africa.

## CLINICAL PRESENTATION

The incubation period is typically 14–84 days for acute schistosomiasis (Katayama syndrome), but chronic infection can remain asymptomatic for years. Penetration of cercariae can cause a rash that develops within hours or up to a week after contaminated water exposure. Acute schistosomiasis is characterized by fever, headache, myalgia, diarrhea, and respiratory symptoms. Eosinophilia is often present; painful hepatomegaly or splenomegaly may also occur.

The clinical manifestations of chronic schistosomiasis are the result of host immune responses to schistosome eggs. Eggs secreted by adult worm pairs living in the bloodstream become lodged in the capillaries of organs and cause granulomatous reactions. *S. mansoni* and *S. japonicum* eggs most commonly lodge in the blood vessels of the liver or intestine and can cause diarrhea, constipation, and blood in the stool. Chronic inflammation can lead to bowel wall ulceration, hyperplasia, and polyposis and, with heavy infections, to periportal liver fibrosis. *S. haematobium* eggs typically lodge in the urinary tract and can cause dysuria and hematuria. Calcifications in the bladder may appear late in the disease. *S. haematobium* infection can also cause genital symptoms and has been associated with increased risk of bladder cancer. As with acute schistosomiasis, eosinophilia may be present during chronic infection with any species.

Rarely, central nervous system manifestations of schistosomiasis may develop; this is thought to result from aberrant migration of adult worms or eggs depositing in the spinal cord or brain. Signs and symptoms are related to ectopic granulomas in the central nervous system and can present as transverse myelitis.

## DIAGNOSIS

Diagnosis is made by microscopic identification of parasite eggs in stool (*S. mansoni* or *S. japonicum*) or urine (*S. haematobium*). Serologic tests are useful to diagnose light infections because egg shedding may not be consistent in travelers and in others who have not had schistosomiasis previously. Antibody tests do not distinguish between past and current infection but are useful for identifying asymptomatic people who may have been exposed during travel and may benefit from treatment.

More detailed information and assistance with diagnosis may be obtained from CDC (www.cdc.gov/parasites/schistosomiasis or CDC Parasitic Diseases Inquiries, 404-718-4745).

4

## TREATMENT

Schistosomiasis is uncommon in the United States, and clinicians unfamiliar with management of the condition should consult an infectious disease or tropical medicine specialist for diagnosis and treatment. Praziquantel is used to treat schistosomiasis. Praziquantel is most effective against adult forms of the parasite and requires an immune response to the adult worm to be fully effective. Host immune response differences may affect individual response to treatment with praziquantel. Although a single course of treatment is usually curative, in lightly infected patients, the immune response may be less robust, and repeat treatment may be needed after 2–4 weeks to increase effectiveness.

## PREVENTION

No vaccine and no drugs are available for preventing infection. Preventive measures include avoiding wading, swimming, or other contact with freshwater in disease-endemic countries.

Untreated piped water coming directly from freshwater sources may contain cercariae, but filtering with fine-mesh filters, heating bathing water to 122°F (50°C) for 5 minutes, or allowing water to stand for ≥24 hours before exposure can prevent infection.

Swimming in adequately chlorinated swimming pools is safe, even in disease-endemic countries, although confirming adequate levels of chlorination is difficult. Vigorous towel-drying after accidental exposure to water has been suggested as a way to remove cercariae before they can penetrate, but this may only prevent some infections and should not be recommended as a preventive measure. Topical applications of insect repellents such as DEET can block penetrating cercariae, but the effect depends on the repellent formulation, may be short-lived, and does not provide adequate coverage to prevent infection reliably.

**CDC website:** www.cdc.gov/parasites/ schistosomiasis

### BIBLIOGRAPHY

1. Berry A, Mone H, Iriart X, Mouahid G, Aboo O, Boissier J, et al. Schistosomiasis haematobium, Corsica, France. Emerg Infect Dis. 2014 Sep;20(9):1595–7.

2. Campa P, Develoux M, Belkadi G, Magne D, Lame C, Carayon MJ, et al. Chronic Schistosoma mekongi in a traveler—case report and review of the literature. J Travel Med. 2014 Sep–Oct;21(5):361–3.

3. Clerinx J, Van Gompel A. Schistosomiasis in travellers and migrants. Travel Med Infect Dis. 2011 Jan;9(1):6–24.

4. Colley DG, Bustinduy A, Secor WE, King CH. Human schistosomiasis. Lancet. 2014 Jun;383(9936):2253–64.

5. Lingscheid T, Kurth F, Clerinx J, Marocco S, Trevino B, Schunk M, et al. Schistosomiasis in European travelers and migrants: analysis of 14 years TropNet surveillance data. Am J Trop Med Hyg. 2017 Aug;97(2):567–74.

6. Ross AG, Vickers D, Olds GR, Shah SM, McManus DP. Katayama syndrome. Lancet Infect Dis. 2007 Mar;7(3):218–24.

7. World Health Organization Expert Committee. Prevention and control of schistosomiasis and soil-transmitted helminthiasis. World Health Organ Tech Rep Ser. 2002;912:1–57.

# SHIGELLOSIS

Louise K. Francois Watkins, Grace D. Appiah

## INFECTIOUS AGENT

Shigellosis is an acute infection of the intestine caused by bacteria in the genus *Shigella*. There are 4 species of *Shigella*: *S. dysenteriae*, *S. flexneri*, *S. boydii*, and *S. sonnei* (also referred to as group A, B, C, and D, respectively). Several distinct serotypes are recognized within the first 3 species.

## TRANSMISSION

*Shigella*, which is host-adapted to humans and nonhuman primates, is transmitted via the fecal–oral route, including through direct person-to-person or sexual contact or indirectly through contaminated food, water, or fomites. Because as few as 10 organisms can cause infection, shigellosis is easily transmitted. It can be acquired even during short-term travel to settings with Western-style amenities.

In the United States, *S. sonnei* infection is usually transmitted through interpersonal contact, particularly among young children and their caregivers; however, outbreaks have also been linked to contaminated foods, infected food handlers, contaminated drinking water, swimming in contaminated water, and sexual activity.

## EPIDEMIOLOGY

Worldwide, *Shigella* is estimated to cause 80–165 million cases of disease and 600,000 deaths annually; of these, 20–119 million illnesses and 6,900–30,000 deaths are attributed to foodborne transmission. *Shigella* spp. are endemic in temperate and tropical climates. Transmission of *Shigella* spp. is most likely when hygiene and sanitation are insufficient. Shigellosis is caused predominantly by *S. sonnei* in industrialized countries, whereas *S. flexneri* prevails in the developing world. Infections caused by *S. boydii* and *S. dysenteriae* are less common globally but can make up a substantial proportion of *Shigella* spp. isolated in sub-Saharan Africa and South Asia.

*Shigella* spp. are detected in the stools of 5%–18% of patients with travelers' diarrhea, and studies in Australia and Canada found that 40%–50% of locally diagnosed shigellosis cases were associated with international travel. In a study of travel-associated enteric infections diagnosed after return to the United States, *Shigella* was the third most common bacterial pathogen isolated by clinical laboratories (of note, these laboratories did not test for enterotoxigenic *Escherichia coli*, a common cause of travelers' diarrhea). Many infections caused by *S. dysenteriae* (56%) and *S. boydii* (44%) were travel-associated, but infections caused by *S. flexneri* and *S. sonnei* were less often associated with travel (24% and 12%, respectively). In this study, the risk of infection caused by *Shigella* spp. was highest for people traveling to Africa, followed by Central America, South America, and Asia.

In 2014–2015, a large outbreak of *S. sonnei* occurred in the United States after travelers returned from India, Haiti, the Dominican Republic, and other countries with ciprofloxacin-resistant shigellosis. In 2015–2016, an outbreak of azithromycin-resistant *S. sonnei* infections occurred among men who have sex with men (MSM) and homeless people in Oregon. Outbreaks of infections caused by multidrug-resistant *Shigella*, including isolates resistant to azithromycin or ciprofloxacin, have been reported in Australia, Europe, Taiwan, Canada, and the United States among MSM. Infections caused by Shiga toxin–producing *S. flexneri* and *S. dysenteriae* have been reported repeatedly among travelers to Haiti and the Dominican Republic.

## CLINICAL PRESENTATION

Illness typically begins 1–2 days after exposure with symptoms lasting 5–7 days. Disease severity varies according to species: serotype *S. dysenteriae* serotype 1 (Sd1) is the agent of epidemic dysentery, whereas *S. sonnei* commonly causes milder, nondysenteric diarrheal illness. However, *Shigella* of any species can cause severe illness among people with compromised immune systems. Shigellosis is characterized by watery, bloody, or mucoid diarrhea; fever; stomach cramps; and nausea. Occasionally, patients experience vomiting, seizures (young children), or postinfectious manifestations, including reactive arthritis, glomerulonephritis, and intestinal perforation. Hemolytic uremic syndrome can occur after infection with Shiga toxin–producing strains, particularly Sd1.

## DIAGNOSIS

Rapid diagnostic tests for shigellosis are increasingly available in the United States; however, culture of a stool specimen or rectal swab should be conducted, including when a rapid test is positive, to obtain an isolate for species determination and antimicrobial susceptibility testing to guide treatment. Fecal specimens should be processed rapidly to optimize the chance of a positive culture. Shigellosis is a nationally notifiable disease in the United States.

## TREATMENT

Shigellosis can be mild and usually resolves within 5–7 days with supportive care alone; however, antimicrobial treatment given early in the course of illness can shorten the duration of symptoms and of carriage (asymptomatic shedding of the organism in the stool). Consider antimicrobial treatment for patients with severe disease or those with immune compromise.

When antimicrobial treatment is indicated for shigellosis associated with travel outside the United States, a fluoroquinolone, azithromycin, or ceftriaxone may be used empirically until antimicrobial susceptibility data are available, but clinicians should be aware that multidrug resistance among *Shigella* spp. is common. Shigellae acquired internationally are usually resistant to ampicillin and trimethoprim-sulfamethoxazole, and resistance to fluoroquinolones, azithromycin, and third- and fourth-generation cephalosporins occurs, particularly in South and East Asia. Additional information on antimicrobial resistance among US shigellosis cases is available at www.cdc.gov/narms/reports/index.html. Additional discussion of symptomatic management can be found in Chapter 2, Travelers' Diarrhea.

## PREVENTION

No vaccines are available for *Shigella*. The best defense against shigellosis is thorough, frequent handwashing, strict adherence to standard food and water safety precautions (see Chapter 2, Food & Water Precautions), and minimizing fecal-oral exposures during sexual activity. When soap and water are not available, alcohol-based hand sanitizers can be a useful adjunct to washing hands. General recommendations to prevent diarrhea while traveling are addressed in Chapter 2, Travelers' Diarrhea.

**CDC website:** www.cdc.gov/shigella

### BIBLIOGRAPHY

1. American Academy of Pediatrics. Shigella infections. In: Kimberlin DW, Brady MT, Jackson MA, Long SS, editors. Red Book: 2015 Report of the Committee on Infectious Diseases. 30th ed. Elk Grove Village, IL: American Academy of Pediatrics; 2015. pp. 706–9.

2. Baker KS, Dallman TJ, Ashton PM, Day M, Hughes G, Crook PD, et al. Intercontinental dissemination of azithromycin-resistant shigellosis through sexual transmission: a cross-sectional study. Lancet Infect Dis. 2015 Aug;15(8):913–21.

3. Bowen A, Grass J, Bicknese A, Campbell D, Hurd J, Kirkcaldy RD. Elevated risk for antimicrobial drug-resistant Shigella infection among men who have sex with men, United States, 2011–2015. Emerg Infect Dis. 2016 Sep;22(9):1613.

4. CDC. Importation and domestic transmission of Shigella sonnei resistant to ciprofloxacin—United States, May 2014–February 2015. MMWR Morb Mortal Wkly Rep. 2015 Apr 3;64(12):318–20.

5. Hines JZ, Pinsent T, Rees K, Vines J, Bowen A, Hurd J, et al. Notes from the field: Shigellosis outbreak mmong men who have sex with men and homeless persons—Oregon, 2015–2016. MMWR Morb Mortal Wkly Rep. 2016 Aug 12;65(31):812–13.

6. Kendall ME, Crim S, Fullerton K, Han PV, Cronquist AB, Shiferaw B, et al. Travel-associated enteric infections diagnosed after return to the United States, Foodborne Diseases Active Surveillance Network (FoodNet), 2004–2009. Clin Infect Dis. 2012 Jun;54 Suppl 5:S480–7.

7. Kirk MD, Pires SM, Black RE, Caipo M, Crump JA, Devleesschauwer B, et al. World Health Organization estimates of the global and regional disease burden of 22 foodborne bacterial, protozoal, and viral diseases, 2010: a data synthesis. PLoS Med. 2015 Dec 3;12(12):e1001921.

8. Li YL, Tewari D, Yealy CC, Fardig D, M'ikanatha NM. Surveillance for travel and domestically acquired multidrug-resistant human Shigella infections—Pennsylvania, 2006–2014. Health Secur. 2016 May–Jun;14(3):143–51.

9. McCrickard LS, Crim SM, Kim S, Bowen A. Disparities in severe shigellosis among adults—Foodborne diseases active surveillance network, 2002–2014. BMC Public Health. 2018 Feb 7;18(1):221.

10. Shane AL, Mody RK, Crump JA, Tarr PI, Steiner TS, Kotloff K, et al. 2017 Infectious Diseases Society of America clinical practice guidelines for the diagnosis and management of infectious diarrhea. Clin Infect Dis. 2017 Nov 29;65(12):1963–1973.

# SMALLPOX & OTHER ORTHOPOXVIRUS-ASSOCIATED INFECTIONS

Andrea M. McCollum

## INFECTIOUS AGENT

Smallpox is caused by variola virus, genus *Orthopoxvirus*. Other members of this genus that can infect humans are vaccinia virus, monkeypox virus, and cowpox virus. In 1980, the World Health Organization officially declared the worldwide eradication of smallpox.

## TRANSMISSION

### Smallpox & Vaccinia

Smallpox spread from person to person is principally respiratory; contact with infectious skin lesions or scabs is an uncommon mode of transmission.

Vaccinia virus is the live-virus component of contemporary smallpox vaccines. Rarely, infection can occur from touching the fluid or crust material from the inoculation lesion of someone recently vaccinated against smallpox. Human contact with animals infected with vaccinialike viruses has resulted in zoonotic infections in Colombia, Brazil, and India.

### Monkeypox

After zoonotic transmission, monkeypox spread from person to person is principally respiratory; contact with infectious skin lesions or scabs is another, albeit less common, means of person-to-person spread. African rodents and primates may harbor the virus and infect humans, but the reservoir host is unknown.

### Cowpox

Cowpox infection occurs after contact with infected animals; person-to-person transmission has not been observed.

## EPIDEMIOLOGY

### Smallpox & Vaccinia

The last documented case of naturally occurring (endemic) smallpox was in 1977. A single confirmed case of smallpox today could be the result of an intentional act (bioterrorism) and would be considered a global public health emergency.

Infections with wild vaccinialike viruses have been reported among cattle and buffalo herders in India and among dairy workers in southern Brazil and Colombia. Travelers touching affected bovines may acquire a localized, cutaneous infection. Immunosuppressed people or those with certain skin conditions are at an increased risk of developing systemic illness from handling infected animals.

### Monkeypox

Monkeypox is endemic to the tropical forested regions of West and Central Africa, notably the Congo Basin. Refugees and immigrants leaving the Democratic Republic of the Congo may be infected with monkeypox virus, but reports of this are rare. Recent literature documents the presence of this disease in other countries (Cameroon, Central African Republic, Côte d'Ivoire, Liberia, Nigeria, Republic of Congo, and Sierra Leone). Short-term travelers to monkeypox-endemic areas would not generally be at risk of infection. In 2018, however, both the United Kingdom and Israel reported imported cases of the disease in travelers returning home after visits to Nigeria. Rodents imported from West Africa were the source of a human monkeypox outbreak in the United States in 2003.

## Cowpox

Human infections with cowpox and cowpoxlike viruses have been reported in Europe and the Caucasus (cowpox and Akhmeta virus in Georgia). Travelers with direct, hands-on contact with affected bovines, felines, rodents, or captive exotics (zoo animals) may be at risk for cutaneous infection.

## CLINICAL PRESENTATION

Table 4-20 summarizes key clinical characteristics for orthopoxvirus infections in humans.

## Smallpox

Acute onset of fever >101°F (38.3°C), malaise, head and body aches, and sometimes vomiting is followed by development of a particular, characteristic rash: firm, deep-seated vesicles or pustules in the same stage of development. Clinically, the most common rash illness likely to be confused with smallpox is varicella (chickenpox).

## Monkeypox

As with smallpox, people experience a febrile prodrome followed by a widespread vesiculopustular rash involving the palms and soles. Marked lymphadenopathy is a distinguishing feature of monkeypox.

## Vaccinia and Cowpox

Human infections with vaccinia, wild vaccinialike viruses, cowpox, and cowpoxlike viruses are most often self-limited, characterized by localized vesicular-pustular (and in cowpox, occasionally ulcerative) lesions. Fever and other constitutional symptoms may occur briefly after lesions first appear. Lesions can be painful and can persist for weeks. Immunocompromised patients or those with exfoliative skin conditions (such as eczema or atopic dermatitis) are at higher risk of severe illness or death.

## DIAGNOSIS

PCR testing or virus isolation confirms orthopoxvirus infection. Health care providers can refer to the CDC smallpox website (www.cdc.gov/

## Table 4-20. Clinical characteristics of smallpox, monkeypox, cowpox, vaccinia (naturally occurring), and other similar orthopoxviruses

| CLINICAL CHARACTERISTIC | SMALLPOX | MONKEYPOX | COWPOX, VACCINIA, AND SIMILAR ORTHOPOXVIRUSES |
|---|---|---|---|
| Incubation period (days) | 7–19 | 5–17 | 2–4 |
| Fever | Yes, febrile prodrome present before the onset of lesions | Yes, febrile prodrome present before the onset of lesions | Yes, often with the onset of lesions |
| Malaise | Yes | Yes | Yes |
| Headache | Yes | Yes | Yes |
| Lymphadenopathy | No | Yes | Yes |
| Lesion distribution | Centrifugally disseminated rash; lesions often present on palms and soles | Centrifugally disseminated rash; lesions often present on palms and soles | Often localized lesions on the hands, face, and neck due to contact transmission |
| Lesion characteristics | Lesions are deep-seated and profound, well circumscribed, and often have a central point of umbilication. Lesions slowly progress from macule to papule to vesicle to pustule to crust, over a period of 2–4 weeks. | | |

smallpox/index.html) for guidance on the application of a clinical algorithm designed to aid in distinguishing orthopoxvirus infections from other disseminated rash illnesses, namely chickenpox (www.cdc.gov/smallpox/clinicians/algorithm-protocol.html). CDC (770-488-7100) can aid in clinical and laboratory diagnosis.

## TREATMENT

Treatment of orthopoxvirus infections is mainly supportive: hydration, nutritional supplementation, and prevention of secondary infections. Vaccinia and cowpox lesions should remain covered until the scab detaches to diminish chances of spreading virus to other parts of the body or to other people. Orthopoxvirus infections in patients at high risk for severe outcomes ( for example, immunocompromised or having an underlying skin condition) or with ocular infections represent significant management challenges. Clinicians should consult with CDC to explore treatment options including investigational use of antivirals.

## PREVENTION

Smallpox vaccine is not recommended for the average international traveler. It is recommended only for laboratory workers who handle variola virus (the agent of smallpox) or closely related orthopoxviruses and health care and public health officials who would be designated first responders in the event of an intentional release of variola virus. In addition, members of the US military may be required to receive the vaccine.

To reduce the chances of contracting other orthopoxvirus infections, travelers should avoid contact with rodents and sick or dead animals, including pets and domestic ruminants (cattle, buffalo), and direct contact with ill humans. For more information about orthopoxviruses, contact the CDC Poxvirus Inquiry Line (404-639-4129).

**CDC websites:** www.cdc.gov/poxvirus/index.html and www.cdc.gov/smallpox/index.html

4

### BIBLIOGRAPHY

1. Campe H, Zimmermann P, Glos K, Bayer M, Bergemann H, Dreweck C, et al. Cowpox virus transmission from pet rats to humans, Germany. Emerg Infect Dis. 2009 May;15(5):777–80.

2. Durski KN, McCollum AM, Nakazawa Y, Petersen BW, Reynolds MG, Briand S, et al. Emergence of monkeypox—West and Central Africa, 1970–2017. MMWR Morb Mortal Wkly Rep. 2018 Mar;67(10):306–10.

3. McCollum AM, Damon IK. Human monkeypox. Clin Infect Dis. 2014 Jun;58(2):260–7.

4. Petersen BW, Harms TJ, Reynolds MG, Harrison LH. Use of vaccinia virus smallpox vaccine in laboratory and health care personnel at risk for occupational exposure to orthopoxviruses—recommendations of the Advisory Committee on Immunization Practices (ACIP), 2015. MMWR Morb Mortal Wkly Rep. 2016 Mar;65(10);257–62.

5. Trindade GS, Guedes MI, Drumond BP, Mota BE, Abrahao JS, Lobato ZI, et al. Zoonotic vaccinia virus: clinical and immunological characteristics in a naturally infected patient. Clin Infect Dis. 2009 Feb 1; 48(3):e37–40.

# STRONGYLOIDIASIS

Anne Straily, Barbara L. Herwaldt, Susan Montgomery

## INFECTIOUS AGENT

An intestinal nematode, *Strongyloides stercoralis*.

## TRANSMISSION

Filariform larvae found in contaminated soil penetrate human skin. Person-to-person transmission is rare but documented.

## EPIDEMIOLOGY

Endemic to the tropics and subtropics; limited foci elsewhere, including Appalachia and the southeastern United States. Estimates of global prevalence range from 30 to 100 million. Most documented infections in the United States occur in immigrants, refugees, and military veterans who have lived in *Strongyloides*-endemic areas for long periods. Risk for short-term travelers is low, but infections can occur.

## CLINICAL PRESENTATION

Most infections are asymptomatic. With acute infections, a localized, pruritic, erythematous papular rash can develop at the site of skin penetration, followed by pulmonary symptoms (a Löffler-like pneumonitis), diarrhea, abdominal pain, and eosinophilia. Migrating larvae in the skin cause larva currens, a serpiginous urticarial rash.

Immunocompromised people, especially those receiving systemic corticosteroids, those infected with human T cell lymphotropic virus type 1 and those with hematologic malignancies or who have had hematopoietic stem cell or organ transplants, are at risk for hyperinfection or disseminated disease, characterized by abdominal pain, diffuse pulmonary infiltrates, and septicemia or meningitis from enteric bacteria. Untreated hyperinfection and disseminated strongyloidiasis are associated with high mortality rates.

## DIAGNOSIS

Peripheral blood eosinophilia is common in intestinal strongyloidiasis but often absent in hyperinfection and disseminated strongyloidiasis. Rhabditiform larvae can be visualized on microscopic examination of stool, either directly or by culture on agar plates. Repeated stool examinations or examination of duodenal contents may be necessary. Hyperinfection and disseminated strongyloidiasis are diagnosed by examining stool, sputum, cerebrospinal fluid, and other body fluids and tissues, which typically contain high numbers of filariform larvae. Serologic testing is available through commercial laboratories and through the National Institutes of Health and CDC (www.cdc.gov/dpdx; 404-718-4745; parasites@cdc.gov).

## TREATMENT

Treatment of choice for acute, chronic, and disseminated disease or hyperinfection is ivermectin. The alternative is albendazole, although it is associated with lower cure rates. Prolonged or repeated treatment may be necessary in patients with hyperinfection, disseminated disease, or coinfection with human T cell lymphotropic virus 1, as relapse can occur.

## PREVENTION

No vaccines or drugs to prevent infection are available. Protective measures include wearing shoes when walking in areas where humans may have defecated. It may be reasonable to perform serologic testing on patients at risk for *Strongyloides* infection who will be placed on corticosteroids or other immunosuppressive drug regimens, or who will undergo procedures such as transplantation that involve immunosuppression. If indicated, these patients should be treated before immunosuppression. Empiric treatment may be considered in people deemed at risk of strongyloidiasis in whom immediate immunosuppression is required.

**CDC website:** www.cdc.gov/parasites/strongyloides

### BIBLIOGRAPHY

1. Henriquez-Camacho C, Gotuzzo E, Echevarria J, White Jr AC, Terashima A, Samalvides F, et al. Ivermectin versus albendazole or thiabendazole for Strongyloides stercoralis infection. Cochrane Database Sys Rev. 2016 Jan;(1):CD007745.

2. Keiser PB, Nutman TB. Strongyloides stercoralis in the immunocompromised population. Clin Microbiol Rev. 2004 Jan;17(1):208–17.

3. Nutman TB. Human infection with Strongyloides stercoralis and other related Strongyloides species. Parasitology. 2017 Mar;144(3):263–73.

4. Puthiyakunnon S, Boddu S, Li Y, Zhou X, Wang C, Li J, et al. Strongyloidiasis—an insight into its global prevalence and management. PLoS Negl Trop Dis. 2014 Aug;8(8):e3018.

5. Requena-Mendez A, Buonfrate D, Gomez-Junyent J, Zammarchi L, Bisoffi A, Munoz J. Evidence-based guidelines for screening and management of strongyloidiasis in non-endemic countries. Am J Trop Med Hyg. 2017 Sep;97(3):645–52.

6. Seybolt LM, Christiansen D, Barnett ED. Diagnostic evaluation of newly arrived asymptomatic refugees with eosinophilia. Clin Infect Dis. 2006 Feb 1;42(3):363–7.

# TAENIASIS

Susan Montgomery

## INFECTIOUS AGENT

*Taenia solium* (pork tapeworm) and *T. saginata* or *T. asiatica* (beef tapeworm).

## TRANSMISSION

Eating raw or undercooked contaminated pork or beef.

## EPIDEMIOLOGY

The highest prevalences are in Latin America, Africa, and South and Southeast Asia. Taeniasis has been reported at lower rates in Eastern Europe, Spain, and Portugal. Tapeworm infections are unusual in travelers.

## CLINICAL PRESENTATION

The incubation period is 8–10 weeks for *T. solium* and 10–14 weeks for *T. saginata*. Symptoms may include abdominal discomfort, weight loss, anorexia, nausea, insomnia, weakness, perianal pruritus, and nervousness. Symptoms are less likely for *T. solium* infection than for *T. saginata* infection.

## DIAGNOSIS

Presence of eggs, proglottids (segments), or tapeworm antigens in the feces or on anal swabs. Differentiation of *T. solium* from *T. saginata* and *T. asiatica* is based on morphology of the scolex and gravid proglottids.

## TREATMENT

Praziquantel is the drug of choice, except in the setting of symptomatic neurocysticercosis (see Cysticercosis in this chapter). Niclosamide is an alternative but is not as widely available.

## PREVENTION

Avoid undercooked meat.

**CDC website:** www.cdc.gov/parasites/taeniasis

BIBLIOGRAPHY

1. Cantey PT, Coyle CM, Sorvillo FJ, Wilkins PP, Starr MC, Nash TE. Neglected parasitic infections in the United States: cysticercosis. Am J Trop Med Hyg. 2014 May;90(5):805–9.

2. Wittner M, White ACJ, Tanowitz HB. Taenia and other tapeworm infections. In: Guerrant RL, Walker DH, Weller PF, editors. Tropical Infectious Diseases: Principles, Pathogens and Practice. 3rd ed. Philadelphia: Saunders Elsevier; 2011. pp. 839–47.

3. Zammarchi L, Bonati M, Strohmeyer M, Albonico M, Requena-Mendez A, Bisoffi Z, et al. Screening, diagnosis and management of human cysticercosis and Taenia solium taeniasis: technical recommendations by the COHEMI project study group. Trop Med Int Health. 2017 Jul;22(7):881–94.

# TETANUS

Tejpratap S. P. Tiwari

## INFECTIOUS AGENT

*Clostridium tetani*, a spore-forming, anaerobic, gram-positive bacterium. Bacteria are ubiquitous in the environment.

## TRANSMISSION

Direct contamination of open wounds and non-intact skin. "Tetanus-prone" wounds include those contaminated with dirt, human or animal excreta, or saliva; punctures; burns; crush injuries; or injuries with necrotic tissue.

## EPIDEMIOLOGY

Distributed worldwide. More common in rural and agricultural regions, areas where contact with soil or animal excreta is likely, and areas where immunization is inadequate. Tetanus can affect any age group.

## CLINICAL PRESENTATION

Incubation period is 10 days (range, 3–21 days). Acute symptoms typically include muscle rigidity and spasms, often in the jaw (lockjaw) and neck. Tetanus is usually classified as local, cephalic, generalized, and neonatal. Symptoms of localized tetanus include muscle spasms confined to the injury site. Cephalic tetanus is characterized by head or face wound and flaccid cranial nerve palsies. Progression from these forms to generalized tetanus may occur. Generalized tetanus is characterized by lockjaw, generalized spasms, risus sardonicus, and opisthotonus. Neonatal tetanus occurs in newborns who have contaminated umbilical stumps and whose mothers are unimmunized or inadequately immunized. Severe tetanus can lead to respiratory failure and death. Case-fatality ratios are high even where modern intensive care is available.

## DIAGNOSIS

Diagnosis is clinical; no confirmatory laboratory tests are available. Tetanus is a nationally notifiable disease.

## TREATMENT

Tetanus requires hospitalization, treatment with human tetanus immune globulin (TIG), a tetanus toxoid booster, agents to control muscle spasm, aggressive wound care, and antibiotics. Metronidazole is the most appropriate antibiotic. The wound should be debrided widely and excised if possible.

## PREVENTION

All travelers should be up-to-date with tetanus toxoid vaccine before departure. Ensure adequate immunity to tetanus by completing the childhood primary vaccine series with tetanus toxoid, a booster dose during adolescence, and at 10-year intervals thereafter during adulthood. An age-appropriate tetanus toxoid–containing vaccine may be needed as early as 5 years since the last dose for high-risk wounds. In addition, for unvaccinated or inadequately vaccinated people or people with HIV infection or other severe immunodeficiency, a prophylactic dose of TIG may also be required. For detailed information regarding the tetanus vaccine, visit www.cdc.gov/vaccines/vpd-vac/tetanus.

**CDC website:** www.cdc.gov/tetanus

### BIBLIOGRAPHY

1. CDC. Updated recommendations for use of tetanus toxoid, reduced diphtheria toxoid and acellular pertussis (Tdap) vaccine in adults aged 65 years and older—Advisory Committee on Immunization Practices (ACIP), 2012. MMWR Morb Mortal Wkly Rep. 2012 June 29;61(25): 468–70.

2. Tiwari TSP. Tetanus. In: Kris Heggenhougen and Stella Quah, editors. International Encyclopedia of Public Health, Volume 2. San Diego: Academic Press; 2016.

3. World Health Organization. Tetanus vaccine: WHO position paper—February 2017. Wkly Epidemiol Rec. 2017;92(6):53–76.

# TICKBORNE ENCEPHALITIS

Marc Fischer, Carolyn V. Gould, Pierre E. Rollin

## INFECTIOUS AGENT

Tickborne encephalitis (TBE) virus is a single-stranded RNA virus that belongs to the genus *Flavivirus*. TBE virus has 3 subtypes: European, Siberian, and Far Eastern.

## TRANSMISSION

TBE virus is transmitted to humans through the bite of an infected tick of the *Ixodes* species, primarily *I. ricinus* (European subtype) or *I. persulcatus* (Siberian and Far Eastern subtypes). The virus is maintained in discrete areas of deciduous forests. Ticks act as both vector and virus reservoir, and small rodents are the primary amplifying host. TBE can also be acquired by ingesting unpasteurized dairy products (such as milk and cheese) from infected goats, sheep, or cows. TBE virus transmission has infrequently been reported through laboratory exposure and slaughtering viremic animals. Direct person-to-person spread of TBE virus occurs only rarely, through blood transfusion, solid organ transplantation, or breastfeeding.

## EPIDEMIOLOGY

TBE is endemic to focal areas of Europe and Asia, extending from eastern France to northern Japan and from northern Russia to Albania. Approximately 5,000–13,000 TBE cases are reported each year, with large annual fluctuations. Russia has the largest number of reported cases. The highest disease incidence has been reported from western Siberia, Slovenia, and the Baltic States (Estonia, Latvia, Lithuania). Other European countries with reported cases or known endemic areas include Albania, Austria, Belarus, Bosnia, Croatia, Czech Republic, Denmark, Finland, France, Germany, Hungary, Italy, Netherlands, Norway, Poland, Romania, Serbia, Slovakia, Sweden, Switzerland, and Ukraine. Asian countries with reported TBE cases or virus activity include China, Japan, Kazakhstan, Kyrgyzstan, Mongolia, and South Korea.

Most cases occur from April through November, with peaks in early and late summer when ticks are active. The incidence and severity of disease are highest in people aged ≥50 years. Most cases occur in areas <2,500 ft (750 m). In the last 30 years, the geographic range of TBE virus appears to have expanded to new areas, and the virus has been found at altitudes up to and above 5,000 ft (1,500 m). These trends are likely due to a complex combination of changes in diagnosis and surveillance, human activities and socioeconomic factors, and ecology and climate.

The overall risk of acquiring TBE for an unvaccinated visitor to a highly endemic area during the TBE virus transmission season has been estimated at 1 case per 10,000 person-months of exposure. Most TBE virus infections result from tick bites acquired in forested areas through activities such as camping; hiking; fishing; bicycling; collecting mushrooms, berries, or flowers; and outdoor occupations such as forestry or military training. The risk is negligible for people who remain in urban or unforested areas and who do not consume unpasteurized dairy products.

Vector tick population density and infection rates in TBE virus-endemic foci are highly variable. For example, TBE virus infection rates in *I. ricinus* in central Europe vary from <0.1% to approximately 5%, depending on geographic location and time of year, while rates of up to 40% have been reported in *I. persulcatus* in Siberia. The number of TBE cases reported from a country depends on the ecology and geographic distribution of TBE virus, the intensity of diagnosis and surveillance, and the vaccine coverage in the population. Therefore, the number of human TBE cases reported from an area may not be a reliable predictor of a traveler's risk for infection. The same ticks that transmit TBE virus can also transmit other pathogens, including *Borrelia burgdorferi* (the agent for Lyme disease), *Anaplasma phagocytophilum* (anaplasmosis), and *Babesia* spp. (babesiosis); simultaneous infection with multiple organisms has been described.

From 2000 through 2017, 8 cases of TBE among US travelers to Europe and China were reported. TBE is not a nationally notifiable disease in the United States.

## CLINICAL PRESENTATION

Approximately two-thirds of infections are asymptomatic. The median incubation period for TBE is 8 days (range, 4–28 days). The incubation period for milkborne exposure is usually shorter (3–4 days). Acute neuroinvasive disease is the most commonly recognized clinical manifestation of TBE virus infection. However, TBE disease often presents with milder forms of the disease or a biphasic course.

4

- First phase: nonspecific febrile illness with headache, myalgia, and fatigue. Usually lasts for several days and may be followed by an afebrile and relatively asymptomatic period. Up to two-thirds of patients recover without any further illness.

- Second phase: central nervous system involvement resulting in aseptic meningitis, encephalitis, or myelitis. Findings include meningeal signs, altered mental status, cognitive dysfunction, ataxia, rigidity, seizures, tremors, cranial nerve palsies, and limb paresis.

Disease severity increases with age. Although TBE tends to be less severe in children, residual symptoms and neurologic deficits have been described. Clinical course and long-term outcome also vary by TBE virus subtype, although some of the reported differences may be due to patient selection, access to medical care, or age-specific exposure. The European subtype is associated with milder disease, a case-fatality ratio of <2%, and neurologic sequelae in up to 30% of patients. The Far Eastern subtype is often associated with a more severe disease course, including a case-fatality ratio of 20%–40% and higher rates of severe neurologic sequelae. The Siberian subtype has a case-fatality ratio of 6%–8%, with rare reports of cases with slow or chronic progression over months.

## DIAGNOSIS

TBE should be suspected in travelers who develop a nonspecific febrile illness that progresses to neuroinvasive disease within 4 weeks of arriving from an endemic area. A history of tick bite may be a clue to this diagnosis; however, approximately 30% of TBE patients do not recall a tick bite.

Serology is typically used for laboratory diagnosis. IgM-capture ELISA performed on serum or cerebrospinal fluid is virtually always positive during the neuroinvasive phase of the illness. Vaccination history, date of onset of symptoms, and information regarding other flaviviruses known to circulate in the geographic area that may cross-react in serologic assays need to be considered when interpreting results. During the first phase of the illness, TBE virus or viral RNA can sometimes be detected in serum samples by virus isolation or RT-PCR. However, by the time neurologic symptoms are recognized, the virus or viral RNA is usually undetectable. Therefore, virus isolation and RT-PCR should not be used to rule out a diagnosis of TBE. Clinicians should contact their state or local health department, the CDC Viral Special Pathogens Branch (404-639-1115), or CDC Division of Vector-Borne Diseases (970-221-6400) for assistance with diagnostic testing.

## TREATMENT

There is no specific antiviral treatment for TBE; therapy consists of supportive care and management of complications.

## PREVENTION

### Personal Protection Measures

Travelers should avoid consuming unpasteurized dairy products and use all measures to avoid tick bites (see Chapter 3, Mosquitoes, Ticks & Other Arthropods).

### Vaccine

No TBE vaccines are licensed or available in the United States. Two inactivated cell culture-derived TBE vaccines are available in Europe, in adult and pediatric formulations: FSME-IMMUN (also marketed as TicoVac) (Pfizer, France) and Encepur (GSK, Germany). Two inactivated TBE vaccines are available in Russia: TBE-Moscow (Chumakov Institute) and EnceVir (Microgen). SenTaiBao (Changchun Institute of Biological Products in China) also manufactures an inactivated TBE vaccine. Immunogenicity studies suggest that the European and Russian vaccines provide cross-protection against all 3 TBE virus subtypes.

Although no formal efficacy trials of these vaccines have been conducted, immunogenicity data and postlicensure effectiveness studies suggest that their efficacy is >95%. Rare vaccine failures have been reported, particularly in people aged ≥50 years.

4

Because the routine primary vaccination series requires ≥6 months for completion, most travelers going to TBE-endemic areas will find avoiding tick bites to be more practical than vaccination. However, a rapid vaccination schedule has been evaluated for both European vaccines, and seroconversion rates are similar to those observed with the standard vaccination schedules. Travelers anticipating high-risk exposures, such as working or camping in forested areas or farmland, adventure travel, or living in TBE-endemic countries for extended periods, may wish to be vaccinated in Europe.

**CDC website:** www.cdc.gov/vhf/tbe

## BIBLIOGRAPHY

1. Bogovic P, Stupica D, Rojko T, Lotric-Furlan S, Vasic-Zupanc T, Kastrin A, et al. The long-term outcome of tick-borne encephalitis in Central Europe. Ticks Tick Borne Dis. 2018 Feb;9(2):369–78.

2. CDC. Tick-borne encephalitis among US travelers to Europe and Asia—2000–2009. MMWR Morb Mortal Wkly Rep. 2010 Mar 26;59(11):335–8.

3. Kollaritsch H, Paulke-Korinek M, Holzmann H, Hombach J, Bjorvatn B, Barrett A. Vaccines and vaccination against tick-borne encephalitis. Expert Rev Vaccines. 2012 Sep;11(9):1103–19.

4. Kunze U. Report of the 19th annual meeting of the International Scientific Working Group on Tick-Borne Encephalitis (ISW-TBE)—TBE in a changing world. Ticks Tick Borne Dis. 2018;9:146–50.

5. Lipowski D, Popiel M, Perlejewski K, Nakamura S, Bukowska-Osko I, Rzadkiewicz E, et al. A cluster of fatal tick-borne encephalitis virus infection in organ transplant setting. J Infect Dis. 2017;215:896–901.

6. McAuley AJ, Sawatsky B, Ksiazek T, Torres M, Korva M, Lotric-Furlan S, et al. Cross-neutralisation of viruses of the tick-borne encephalitis complex following tick-borne encephalitis vaccination and/or infection. NPJ Vaccines. 2017 Mar 13;2:5.

7. Steffen R. Epidemiology of tick-borne encephalitis (TBE) in international travellers to Western/Central Europe and conclusions on vaccination recommendations. J Travel Med. 2016 Apr;23(4):pii:taw018.

8. Suss J. Tick-borne encephalitis 2010: epidemiology, risk areas, and virus strains in Europe and Asia—an overview. Ticks Tick Borne Dis. 2011 Mar;2(1):2–15.

9. Taba P, Schmutzhard E, Forsberg P, Lutsar I, Ljostad U, Mygland A, et al. EAN consensus review on prevention, diagnosis, and management of tick-borne encephalitis. Eur J Neurol. 2017 Oct;24(10):1214-e61.

10. World Health Organization. Vaccines against tick-borne encephalitis: WHO position paper. Wkly Epidemiol Rec. 2011 Jun 10;86(24):241–56.

# TOXOPLASMOSIS

Anne Straily, Susan Montgomery

## INFECTIOUS AGENT

*Toxoplasma gondii,* an intracellular coccidian protozoan parasite.

## TRANSMISSION

Ingestion of soil, water, or food contaminated with cat feces, ingestion of undercooked meat or shellfish, congenital transmission from a woman infected during or shortly before pregnancy, and contaminated blood transfusion and organ transplantation.

## EPIDEMIOLOGY

*T. gondii* is endemic throughout most of the world. Risk is higher in developing and tropical countries, especially when people eat undercooked meat or shellfish, drink untreated water, or have extensive soil exposure. Congenital transmission can also occur if a woman is infected during pregnancy.

## CLINICAL PRESENTATION

Incubation period is 5–23 days. Symptoms may include influenzalike symptoms or a mononucleosis syndrome with prolonged fever, lymphadenopathy, elevated liver enzymes, lymphocytosis, and weakness. Rarely, chorioretinitis or disseminated disease can occur in immunocompetent people. In severely immunocompromised people, severe and even fatal encephalitis, pneumonitis, and other systemic illnesses can occur, most often from reactivation of a previous infection. Infants with congenital toxoplasmosis are often asymptomatic, but eye disease, neurologic disease, or other systemic symptoms can occur, and learning disabilities, cognitive deficits, or visual impairments may develop later in life.

## DIAGNOSIS

Serologic tests for *T. gondii* antibodies are available at commercial diagnostic laboratories; however, because of the inherent difficulty in diagnosing acute toxoplasmosis, physicians are advised to seek confirmatory testing through the reference laboratory at Sutter Health Palo Alto Medical Foundation Toxoplasma Serology Laboratory (www.pamf.org/serology). Eye disease is diagnosed by ocular examination. Diagnosis of toxoplasmic encephalitis in immunocompromised people (most often seen in people with AIDS) can be based on typical clinical course and identification of ≥1 mass lesion by CT or MRI. Biopsy may be needed to make a definitive diagnosis.

## TREATMENT

Treatment is reserved for acutely infected pregnant women and those with severe disease or who are immunocompromised. A number of regimens are available, but the recommended regimen includes pyrimethamine, sulfadiazine, and leucovorin (folinic acid). Alternative treatment regimens include clindamycin, atovaquone, and azithromycin, but these have not been extensively studied. The recommended treatment regimen for acutely infected pregnant women depends on the timing of infection during gestation; physicians are advised to seek consultation with a specialist before initiating therapy in these patients.

## PREVENTION

Food and water precautions (see Chapter 2, Food & Water Precautions). Avoid direct contact with soil or sand that may be contaminated with cat feces. If caring for a cat, change the litter box daily. If pregnant or immunocompromised, avoid changing cat litter, if possible, and do not adopt or handle stray cats. Wash hands with soap and water after gardening, contact with soil or sand, and after changing cat litter.

**CDC website:** www.cdc.gov/parasites/toxoplasmosis

### BIBLIOGRAPHY

1. Anand R, Jones CW, Ricks JH, Sofarelli TA, Hale DC. Acute primary toxoplasmosis in travelers returning from endemic countries. J Travel Med. 2012 Jan–Feb;19(1):57–60.

2. Montoya JG, Liesenfeld O. Toxoplasmosis. Lancet. 2004 Jun 12;363(9425):1965–76.

3. Maldonado YA, Read JS, AAP Committee on Infectious Diseases. Diagnosis, treatment, and prevention of congenital toxoplasmosis in the United States. Pediatrics. 2017;139(2):e20163860.

4. Panel on Opportunistic Infections in HIV-Infected Adults and Adolescents. Guidelines for the prevention and treatment of opportunistic infections in HIV-infected adults and adolescents: recommendations from the Centers for Disease Control and Prevention, the National Institutes of Health, and the HIV Medicine Association of the Infectious Diseases Society of America. [updated Nov 29 2018; cited 2019 Jan 10]. Available from: https://aidsinfo.nih.gov/contentfiles/lvguidelines/adult_oi.pdf.

5. Sepulveda-Arias JC, Gomez-Marin JE, Bobic B, Naranjo-Galvis CA, Djurkovic-Djakovic O. Toxoplasmosis as a travel risk. Travel Med Infect Dis. 2014 Nov–Dec;12(6 Pt A):592–601.

# TRYPANOSOMIASIS, AFRICAN (SLEEPING SICKNESS)

Sharon L. Roy, Barbara L. Herwaldt, Christine Dubray, Anne Straily

## INFECTIOUS AGENT

Two subspecies of the protozoan parasite *Trypanosoma brucei* (*T. b. rhodesiense* and *T. b. gambiense*).

## TRANSMISSION

The bite of an infected tsetse fly (*Glossina* spp.). Bloodborne and congenital transmission are rare.

## EPIDEMIOLOGY

Endemic to rural sub-Saharan Africa. *T. b. rhodesiense* is found in eastern and southeastern Africa, mainly Tanzania, Uganda, Malawi, Zambia, and Zimbabwe. *T. b. gambiense* is found in central Africa and in limited areas of West Africa, particularly in parts of Democratic Republic of the Congo, as well as Central African Republic, Angola, South Sudan, Guinea, Gabon, Congo, Chad, (northern) Uganda, and other countries. World Health Organization (WHO) maps of African trypanosomiasis cases, by country, are available at www.who.int/trypanosomiasis_african/country/foci_AFRO/en.

In 2016, the WHO received 2,184 reports of sleeping sickness cases; *T. b. gambiense* accounted for 98% of them. Many cases, however, are likely not recognized or reported. Tsetse flies inhabit rural, vegetated areas. Flies bite during the day, and <1% are infected. Risk for infection in travelers increases with the number of fly bites, which does not always correlate with duration of travel. Cases imported into the United States are rare; almost all are due to *T. b. rhodesiense*, typically during visits to national parks or game reserves.

## CLINICAL PRESENTATION

### T. b. rhodesiense

Clinical manifestations generally appear within 1–3 weeks after the infective bite and may include high fever, a chancre at the bite site (within a few days of the bite), skin rash, headache, myalgia, thrombocytopenia, and less commonly, splenomegaly, renal failure, or cardiac dysfunction. Central nervous system involvement can occur within a few weeks of the exposure and results in sleep cycle disturbance, mental deterioration, and (if not treated) death within months.

### T. b. gambiense

Clinical manifestations generally appear months to years after exposure, but the incubation period may be <1 month. Signs and symptoms are nonspecific and may include intermittent fever, headache, malaise, myalgia, arthralgia, facial edema, pruritus, lymphadenopathy, and weight loss. Central nervous system involvement occurs after several months to years of infection and is characterized by daytime somnolence and nighttime sleep disturbance, headache, and other neurologic manifestations (such as mood disorders, behavioral changes, and focal deficits). In residents of endemic areas, the clinical course of disease caused by *T. b. gambiense* generally progresses more slowly (with an estimated average total duration of 3 years) than that caused by *T. b. rhodesiense*, but both forms of African trypanosomiasis typically are fatal if not treated.

## DIAGNOSIS

Tsetse fly bites are characteristically painful, and a chancre may develop at the bite location. Diagnosis is made by identifying parasites in specimens of blood, chancre fluid or tissue, lymph node aspirate, or cerebrospinal fluid. Buffy-coat preparations concentrate the parasite, enabling easier visualization for diagnosis. All patients diagnosed with African trypanosomiasis must have their cerebrospinal fluid examined to determine whether there is involvement of the central nervous system, since the choice of treatment drugs depends on the disease stage. Diagnostic assistance is available through CDC (www.cdc.gov/dpdx; 404-718-4745; parasites@cdc.gov).

## TREATMENT

Infection can usually be cured by a course of antitrypanosomal therapy, although long-term sequelae, including permanent damage to the central nervous system, may occur. In the United States, particular treatment drugs (suramin, melarsoprol, eflornithine) are available through CDC under investigational protocols. Choice of treatment drug depends on species causing infection (*T. b. rhodesiense* or *T. b. gambiense*) and stage

of disease. Clinicians can consult with CDC for assistance with treatment.

## PREVENTION

Avoid tsetse fly bites. Travelers should wear wrist- and ankle-length clothing made of medium-weight fabric in neutral colors, as tsetse flies are attracted to bright or dark colors (especially blue and black) and can bite through lightweight clothing. Permethrin-impregnated clothing and use of DEET repellent might provide partial protection by reducing the number of bites—see Chapter 3, Mosquitoes, Ticks & Other Arthropods.

**CDC website:** www.cdc.gov/parasites/ sleepingsickness/

### BIBLIOGRAPHY

1. Büscher P, Cecchi G, Jamonneau V, Priotto G. Human African trypanosomiasis. Lancet. 2017;390(10110):2397–409.

2. Franco JR, Cecchi G, Priotto G, Paone M, Ciarra A, Grout L, et al. Monitoring the elimination of human African trypanosomiasis: Update to 2014. PLoS Negl Trop Dis. 2017;11(5):e0005585.

3. Franco JR, Simarro PP, Diarra A, Jannin JG. Epidemiology of human African trypanosomiasis. Clin Epidemiol. 2014;6:257–75.

4. Kennedy PGE. Clinical features, diagnosis, and treatment of human African trypanosomiasis (sleeping sickness). Lancet Neurol. 2013;12(2):186–94.

5. Neuberger A, Meltzer E, Leshem E, Dickstein Y, Stienlauf S, Schwartz E. The changing epidemiology of human African trypanosomiasis among patients from nonendemic countries—1902–2012. PLoS One. 2014;9:e88647.

6. World Health Organization. Control and surveillance of human African trypanosomiasis. World Health Organ Tech Rep Ser. 2013;984:1–237.

# TRYPANOSOMIASIS, AMERICAN (CHAGAS DISEASE)

Susan Montgomery, Sharon L. Roy, Christine Dubray

## INFECTIOUS AGENT

The protozoan parasite *Trypanosoma cruzi*.

## TRANSMISSION

Typically through feces of an infected triatomine insect (reduviid bug). Infection may occur when a bug bite is scratched, or by consuming food or beverages contaminated with infected bug feces; may also be transmitted through blood

transfusion, organ transplantation, or from mother to infant.

## EPIDEMIOLOGY

Endemic to many parts of Mexico and Central and South America; rare locally acquired cases reported in the southern United States. No vectorborne transmission has been documented in the Caribbean islands. In the United States,

Chagas disease is primarily a disease of immigrants from endemic areas of Latin America. The risk to travelers is extremely low, but they could be at risk if staying in poor-quality housing or from consuming contaminated food or beverages in endemic areas.

## CLINICAL PRESENTATION

Acute illness typically develops ≥1 week after exposure and lasts up to 60 days. A chagoma (indurated local swelling) may develop at the site of infection (such as the Romaña sign—edema of the eyelid and ocular tissues). Most infected people never develop symptoms but remain infected throughout their lives. Approximately 20%–30% of infected people develop chronic manifestations after a prolonged asymptomatic period. Chronic Chagas disease usually affects the heart; clinical signs include conduction system abnormalities, ventricular arrhythmias, and in late-stage disease, congestive cardiomyopathy. Chronic gastrointestinal problems (such as megaesophagus or megacolon) are less common and may develop with or without cardiac manifestations. Reactivation disease can occur in immunocompromised patients.

## DIAGNOSIS

During the acute phase, parasites may be detectable in fresh preparations of buffy coat or stained peripheral blood specimens; PCR testing may also help detect acute infection. After the acute phase, diagnosis requires 2 or more serologic tests (most commonly ELISA, immunoblot, and immunofluorescent antibody test) to detect *T. cruzi*–specific antibodies. PCR is not a useful diagnostic test for chronic-phase infections, since parasites are not detectable in the peripheral blood during this phase.

## TREATMENT

Antitrypanosomal drug treatment is always recommended for acute, early congenital, and reactivated *T. cruzi* infection, and for chronic *T. cruzi* infection in children aged <18 years old. In adults with chronic infection, treatment is usually recommended.

The 2 drugs used to treat Chagas disease are nifurtimox and benznidazole. Benznidazole is approved by FDA for use in children 2–12 years of age and is commercially available (see www.cdc.gov/parasites/chagas/health_professionals/tx.html for more information). Nifurtimox is not currently FDA approved. Nifurtimox is available under an investigational protocol from CDC. Side effects are common with both drugs and tend to be more frequent and more severe with increasing age. Contact CDC (chagas@cdc.gov; 404-718-4745) for assistance with clinical management.

## PREVENTION

Insect precautions (see Chapter 3, Mosquitoes, Ticks & Other Arthropods) and food and water precautions (see Chapter 2, Food & Water Precautions). Avoid sleeping in thatch, mud, and adobe housing in endemic areas; use insecticides in and around such homes. Insecticide-treated bed nets are helpful. Screening blood and organs for Chagas disease prevents transmission via transfusion or transplantation.

**CDC website:** www.cdc.gov/parasites/chagas

BIBLIOGRAPHY

1. Bern C. Antitrypanosomal therapy for chronic Chagas' disease. N Engl J Med. 2011 Jun 30;364(26):2527–34.

2. Bern C, Montgomery SP, Herwaldt BL, Rassi A Jr, Marin-Neto JA, Dantas RO, et al. Evaluation and treatment of Chagas disease in the United States: a systematic review. JAMA. 2007 Nov 14;298(18):2171–81.

3. Carter YL, Juliano JJ, Montgomery SP, Qvarnstrom Y. Acute Chagas disease in a returning traveler. Am J Trop Med Hyg. 2012 Dec;87(6):1038–40.

4. Edwards MS, Stimpert KK, Montgomery SP. Addressing the challenges of Chagas disease: an emerging health concern in the United States. Infect Dis Clin Pract. 2017 May;25(3):118–25.

5. Rassi A Jr, Rassi A, Marin-Neto JA. Chagas disease. Lancet. 2010 Apr 17;375(9723):1388–402.

# TUBERCULOSIS

Neela D. Goswami, Philip A. LoBue

## INFECTIOUS AGENT

*Mycobacterium tuberculosis* is a rod-shaped, nonmotile, slow-growing, acid-fast bacterium.

## TRANSMISSION

Tuberculosis (TB) transmission occurs when a contagious patient coughs, spreading bacilli through the air. Bovine TB (caused by the closely related *M. bovis*) can be transmitted by consuming unpasteurized dairy products from infected cattle.

## EPIDEMIOLOGY

Globally, 10.4 million new TB cases and 1.7 million TB-related deaths are estimated to occur each year. TB occurs throughout the world, but the incidence varies (see Map 4-12). In the United States, the annual incidence is <3 per 100,000 population, but in some countries in sub-Saharan Africa and Asia, the annual incidence is several hundred per 100,000.

Drug-resistant TB is of increasing concern. Multidrug-resistant (MDR) TB is resistant to the 2 most effective drugs, isoniazid and rifampin. Extensively drug-resistant (XDR) TB is resistant to isoniazid and rifampin, any fluoroquinolone, and ≥1 of 3 injectable second-line drugs (amikacin, kanamycin, or capreomycin). MDR TB is less common than drug-susceptible TB, but globally approximately 490,000 new cases of MDR TB are diagnosed each year, and some countries have proportions of MDR TB >25% (Table 4-21). MDR and XDR TB are of particular concern among HIV-infected or other immunocompromised people. As of 2016, XDR TB had been reported in 123 countries.

Before leaving the United States, travelers who anticipate possible prolonged exposure to TB (such as those spending time caring for patients or working in health care facilities, correctional facilities, or homeless shelters) or those who plan a prolonged stay in an endemic country should have a pretravel blood-based interferon-γ release assay (IGRA, such as QuantiFERON, T-SPOT. TB) or a 2-step tuberculin skin test (TST) (see *Perspectives*: Tuberculin Skin Testing of Travelers, later in this chapter).

If the predeparture test result is negative, the IGRA or single TST should be repeated 8–10 weeks after returning from travel. The predeparture test and follow-up test after traveler return should be the same test type to ensure accurate interpretation of results. Because people with HIV infection or other immunocompromising conditions are more likely to have an impaired response to either a skin or blood test, travelers should inform their clinicians about such conditions.

Although the risk of TB transmission on an airplane is low and dependent on infectiousness of the TB patient, seating proximity, flight duration and host factors, instances of transmission have occurred. To prevent TB transmission, people who have infectious TB (TB that can be spread to other people) should not travel by commercial airplanes or other commercial conveyances. Only TB of the lung or airway is infectious, and health department authorities determine whether a person is infectious based on the person's chest radiograph, sputum tests, symptoms, and treatment received. The World Health Organization (WHO) has issued guidelines for notifying passengers potentially exposed to TB aboard airplanes. Passengers concerned about possible exposure to TB should see their primary health care provider or visit their local health department clinic for evaluation.

Bovine TB (*M. bovis*) is a risk in travelers who consume unpasteurized dairy products in countries where *M. bovis* in cattle is common. Mexico is a common place of infection with *M. bovis* for US travelers.

## CLINICAL PRESENTATION

TB infection can be identified by a positive TST or IGRA result 8–10 weeks after exposure. Overall, only 5%–10% of otherwise healthy people have an infection that progresses to TB disease during their lifetime. Progression to disease can occur weeks to decades after initial infection. People with TB disease have symptoms or other manifestations of illness such as an abnormal chest radiograph. In the remainder, the infection remains in an inactive state (latent TB infection or LTBI) in which the infected person has no symptoms and cannot spread TB to others.

TB disease can affect any organ but most commonly the lungs (70%–80%). Typical TB symptoms include prolonged cough, fever, decreased appetite, weight loss, night sweats, and coughing up blood (hemoptysis). The most common sites for TB outside the lungs are the lymph nodes, pleura, bones and joints, brain and spinal cord lining (meningitis), kidneys, bladder, and genitalia.

The risk of progression to disease is much higher in immunosuppressed people (for example, 8%–10% per year in HIV-infected people not receiving antiretroviral therapy). People who are receiving tumor necrosis factor blockers to treat rheumatoid arthritis and other chronic inflammatory conditions are also at increased risk for disease progression.

## DIAGNOSIS

CDC/American Thoracic Society (ATS)/ Infectious Diseases Society of America (IDSA) have published diagnostic recommendations for both TB disease and LTBI. Sputum or other respiratory cultures and smears for acid-fast bacilli (AFB) should be collected for suspected cases of pulmonary TB, and for AFB smear-positive pulmonary cases, a nucleic acid amplification test (NAAT) positive for *M. tuberculosis* complex rapidly confirms the diagnosis. Similarly, diagnosis of extrapulmonary TB disease can be confirmed with a NAAT positive for *M. tuberculosis* complex or a culture positive for *M. tuberculosis* from affected body tissues or fluids. On average, it takes about 2 weeks to culture and identify *M. tuberculosis*, even with rapid culture techniques.

A preliminary diagnosis of TB can be made when AFB are seen by microscope on sputum smear or in other body tissues or fluids. However, microscopy cannot distinguish between *M. tuberculosis* and nontuberculous mycobacteria. This is particularly problematic in countries such as the United States where TB incidence is low. NAATs

are more rapid than culture and specific for *M. tuberculosis*. They are also more sensitive than the acid-fast bacillus smear but less sensitive than culture.

A diagnosis of TB disease can be made using clinical criteria in the absence of microbiologic confirmation. However, laboratory testing should be performed when feasible to confirm the diagnosis. Molecular tests for drug resistance can be performed directly on specimens and can guide initial treatment while culture results are pending. Culture-based susceptibility testing is recommended for all patients with a positive culture, regardless of the availability of molecular testing, to guide the final determination on the appropriate drug regimen.

LTBI is diagnosed by a positive IGRA or TST after further examinations (such as chest radiograph, symptom review) have excluded TB disease. TB is a nationally notifiable disease.

## TREATMENT

People with LTBI can be treated, and treatments are effective at preventing progression to TB disease. It is necessary to exclude TB disease before starting LTBI treatment. Current LTBI regimens in the United States for drug-susceptible TB include 3 months of once-weekly isoniazid and rifapentine (3HP), 4 months of daily rifampin, and 6–9 months of daily isoniazid. Given low completion rates of the 6- to 9-month isoniazid regimen, shorter-duration regimens are generally preferred. However, providers should choose the regimen on the basis of coexisting medical illness, potential for drug interactions, and drug-susceptibility results of the presumed source of exposure (if known). For example, rifampin has interactions with oral contraceptives and certain antiretroviral medications taken by people with HIV/AIDS.

For people who are at especially high risk for TB disease and may have difficulty adhering to treatment or are given an intermittent dosing regimen, directly observed therapy (DOT) for LTBI may be considered. Travelers who suspect that they have been exposed to TB should inform their health care provider of the possible exposure and receive a medical evaluation. Because drug resistance is relatively common in some parts of the world, travelers who have TST or IGRA conversion

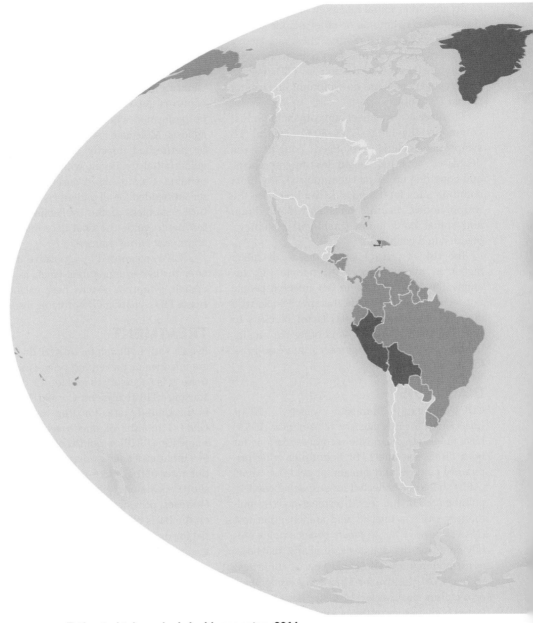

MAP 4-12. **Estimated tuberculosis incidence rates, 2016**

Data source: World Health Organization. Global Tuberculosis Report 2017 (www.who.int/tb/publications/global_report/gtbr2017_main_text.pdf) and http://gamapserver.who.int/mapLibrary/Files/Maps/gho_tb_incidence_2016.png Geneva: World Health Organization; 2017 [cited 2018 Feb 13].

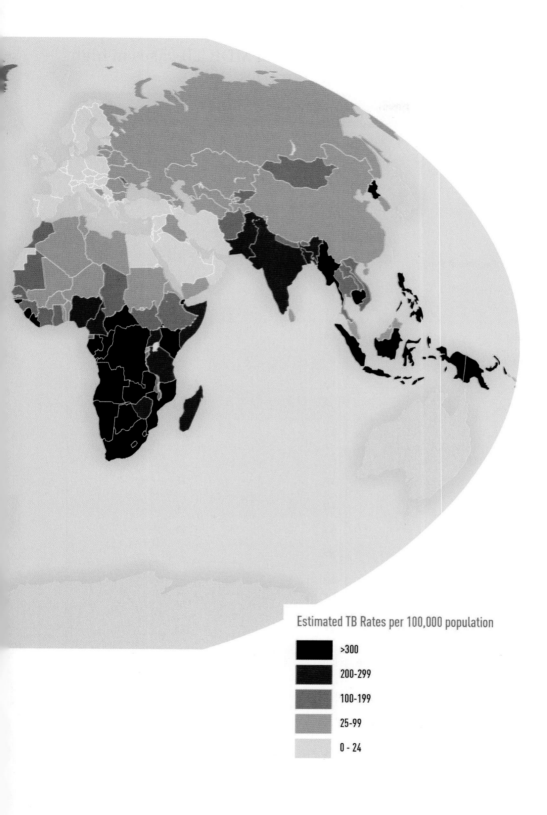

Estimated TB Rates per 100,000 population

■ >300
■ 200-299
■ 100-199
■ 25-99
□ 0 - 24

4

### Table 4-21.  Estimated proportion of MDR TB cases in high MDR TB burden countries, 2016

| COUNTRY | % OF NEW TB CASES THAT ARE MDR | % OF RETREATMENT TB CASES THAT ARE MDR |
|---|---|---|
| Angola | 2.6 | 18 |
| Azerbaijan | 13 | 39 |
| Bangladesh | 1.6 | 29 |
| Belarus | 38 | 72 |
| China | 7.1 | 24 |
| Democratic Republic of Congo | 2.2 | 17 |
| Ethiopia | 2.7 | 14 |
| India | 2.8 | 12 |
| Indonesia | 2.8 | 16 |
| Kazakhstan | 26 | 44 |
| Kenya | 1.3 | 9.4 |
| Kyrgyzstan | 27 | 60 |
| Mozambique | 3.7 | 20 |
| Myanmar (Burma) | 5.1 | 27 |
| Nigeria | 4.3 | 25 |
| Pakistan | 4.2 | 16 |
| Papua New Guinea | 3.4 | 26 |
| Peru | 6.3 | 24 |
| Philippines | 2.6 | 29 |
| Republic of Moldova | 26 | 56 |
| Russia | 27 | 65 |
| South Africa | 3.4 | 7.1 |
| Tajikistan | 22 | 45 |
| Thailand | 2.2 | 24 |
| Ukraine | 27 | 47 |
| Uzbekistan | 24 | 63 |
| Vietnam | 4.1 | 26 |
| Zimbabwe | 4.6 | 14 |

associated with international travel should consult experts in infectious diseases or pulmonary medicine.

Drug-susceptible TB disease is treated with a multiple-drug regimen administered by DOT for 6–9 months (usually isoniazid, rifampin, ethambutol, and pyrazinamide for 2 months, followed by isoniazid and rifampin for an additional 4 months). Patients with drug-resistant TB are more difficult to treat, requiring 4–6 drugs for 18–24 months, and should be managed by an expert in MDR/XDR TB. CDC/ATS/IDSA have published guidelines on treatment for drug-susceptible TB disease.

## PREVENTION

Travelers should avoid exposure to people with TB disease in crowded and enclosed environments (such as health care facilities, correctional facilities, or homeless shelters). Travelers who will be caring for patients or working in health care facilities where TB patients are likely to be encountered should be advised to consult infection control or occupational health experts about baseline LTBI screening and procedures for obtaining personal respiratory protective devices (such as N-95 respirators), along with respirator selection and training.

Based on WHO recommendations, bacillus Calmette-Guérin (BCG) vaccine is used once at birth in most developing countries to reduce the severe consequences of TB in infants and children. However, BCG vaccine has variable efficacy in preventing the adult forms of TB. Although not routinely recommended for use in the United States, some experts have advocated BCG vaccination for health care providers who are likely to be exposed to MDR or XDR TB patients in settings where the TB infection-control measures (such as those recommended in the United States) are not fully implemented. BCG may offer some protection in this circumstance; however, people who receive BCG vaccination must follow all recommended TB infection-control precautions to the greatest extent possible. Additionally, IGRA is preferred over the TST for pretravel and posttravel testing in people vaccinated with BCG, as BCG may result in false-positive TST results.

To prevent infections due to *M. bovis*, travelers should also avoid eating or drinking unpasteurized dairy products.

**CDC website:** www.cdc.gov/tb

## BIBLIOGRAPHY

1. American Thoracic Society, Infectious Diseases Society, CDC. Clinical practice guidelines: diagnosis of tuberculosis in adults and children. Clin Infect Dis. 2017 Jan;64(2):11–115.

2. American Thoracic Society, Infectious Diseases Society, CDC. Clinical practice guidelines: treatment of drug-susceptible tuberculosis. Clin Infect Dis. 2016 Oct;63(7):e147–95.

3. CDC. Availability of an assay for detecting Mycobacterium tuberculosis, including rifampin resistant strains, and considerations for its use—United States, 2013. MMWR Morb Mortal Wkly Rep. 2013 Oct 18;62(41):821–7.

4. Belknap R, Holland D, Feng PJ, Millet JP, Cayla JA, Martinson NA, et al. Self-administered versus directly observed once-weekly isoniazid and rifapentine treatment of latent tuberculosis infection: a randomized trial. Ann Intern Med. 2017 Nov 21;167(10):689–97.

5. Jensen PA, Lambert LA, Iademarco MF, Ridzon R. Guidelines for preventing the transmission of Mycobacterium tuberculosis in health-care settings, 2005. MMWR Recomm Rep. 2005 Dec 30;54(RR-17):1–141.

6. Lobue PA, Mermin JH. Latent tuberculosis infection: the final frontier of tuberculosis elimination in the USA. Lancet Infect Dis. 2017 Oct 17(10):e327–33.

7. Seaworth BJ, Armitge LY, Aronson NE, Hoft DF, Fleenor ME, Gardner AF, et al. Multidrugresistant tuberculosis. Recommendations for reducing risk during travel for healthcare and humanitarian work. Ann Am Thorac Soc. 2014 Mar;11(3):286–95.

8. World Health Organization. Global tuberculosis report 2017. Geneva: World Health Organization; 2017 [cited 2018 Mar 20]. Available from: www.who.int/tb/publications/global_report/gtbr2017_main_text.pdf.

9. World Health Organization. Tuberculosis and air travel: guidelines for prevention and control. 3rd ed. Geneva: World Health Organization; 2008 [cited 2018 Mar 20]. Available from: www.who.int/tb/publications/tb-airtravel-guidance/en/.

# TUBERCULIN SKIN TESTING OF TRAVELERS

Neela D. Goswami, Philip A. LoBue

Screening for asymptomatic tuberculosis (TB) infections should only be carried out for travelers at risk of acquiring TB at their destinations (see the preceding section on Tuberculosis). Screening with a tuberculin skin test (TST) or interferon-γ release assay (IGRA) in very low-risk travelers may result in false-positive test results, leading to unnecessary additional screening or unnecessary treatment. IGRAs, which require a blood draw, are approximately as specific as TST in people who have not been vaccinated with bacillus Calmette-Guérin (BCG) and are more specific in BCG-vaccinated populations. Using screening tests in very low-prevalence populations will likely produce more false positives than true positives.

Travelers at risk for TB infection include those going to live in a country with a high risk of TB or anyone intending to spend any length of time in routine contact with patients in health care facilities or populations living in congregate settings (such as homeless shelters, prisons, and refugee camps). The general recommendation is that people at low risk for exposure to TB, which includes most travelers, do not need to be screened before or after travel.

For travelers who anticipate a long stay or contact with a high-risk population, careful pretravel screening should be carried out with use of an IGRA or, when an IGRA is not available, 2-step pretravel TST screening. Guidelines recommend testing with an IGRA (over TST) for people aged ≥5 years in low-risk populations.

If an IGRA is used for pretravel testing and there is concern for a false positive in an otherwise low-risk traveler, a second test may be used, which confirms TB infection only if both tests are positive. If the IGRA result is negative, the traveler should have a repeat test 8–10 weeks after returning from the trip, but data are limited in supporting a recommendation for regular serial testing for a long-term traveler.

If the TST is used for pretravel testing, the 2-step TST should be used for any traveler undergoing TST testing for the first time. People whose baseline TSTs yield a negative result are retested 1–3 weeks after the initial test; if the second test result is negative, they are considered not infected. If the second test result is positive, they are classified as having had previous TB infection. The 2-step TST is recommended over single TST in this population for the following reasons:

- The use of 2-step testing can reduce the number of positive TSTs that would otherwise be misclassified as recent skin test conversions during future periodic screenings.

- Certain people who were infected with *Mycobacterium tuberculosis* years earlier exhibit waning delayed-type hypersensitivity to tuberculin. When they are skin tested years after infection, they might have a false-negative TST result (even though they are truly infected). However, the first TST might stimulate the ability to react to subsequent tests, resulting in a "booster" reaction. When the test is repeated, the reaction might be misinterpreted as a new infection (recent conversion) rather than a boosted reaction.

4

Two-step testing is important for travelers who will have potential prolonged or substantial TB exposure. Two-step testing before travel will detect boosting and potentially prevent "false conversions"—positive TST results that appear to indicate infection acquired during travel, but which are really the result of previous TB infection. This distinction is particularly important if the traveler is going to a country where multidrug-resistant (MDR) and extensively drug-resistant (XDR) TB are present: it would be critical to know whether the person's skin test had been positive before travel.

If the 2-step pretravel TST result is negative, the traveler should have a repeat TST 8–10 weeks after returning from the trip. During extended (>6 months) stays in or repeated travel to high-risk settings, a TST should be performed every 6–12 months, depending on the risk of exposure while traveling outside the United States, and 8–10 weeks after final return. Two-step testing should be considered for the baseline testing of people who report no history of a recent TST and who will receive repeated TSTs as part of ongoing monitoring.

People who have repeat TSTs must be tested with the same commercial antigen, since switching antigens can also lead to false TST

conversions. Two commercial TST antigens are approved by the Food and Drug Administration (FDA) and are commercially available in the United States: Aplisol (JHP Pharmaceuticals) and Tubersol (Sanofi Pasteur). For a traveler whose time before departure is short, a single-step TST would be an acceptable alternative if time is insufficient for the 2-step TST or the IGRAs are not available.

In general, it is best not to mix tests. There is up to 15% discordance between TST and IGRA, usually with the TST positive and the IGRA negative. There are multiple reasons for the discordance, and in any single person, it is often difficult to be confident about the reason for discordance. However, if the clinician decides to mix tests, it is better to go from TST to IGRA than the other way around, because the likelihood of having a discordant result with the TST negative and the IGRA positive is much lower. Such discordant results may become unavoidable as more medical establishments switch from TSTs to IGRAs.

The use of TSTs among travelers who are visiting friends and relatives in TB-endemic areas should take into account that the rate of TST positivity in people visiting their country of birth is often high. In a study among 53,000 adults in Tennessee, the prevalence of a positive TST among the

foreign born was 11 times that among the US born (34% vs 3%). Confirming TST status before travel would prevent the conclusion that a positive TST after travel was due to recent infection.

## BIBLIOGRAPHY

1. Brown ML, Henderson SJ, Ferguson RW, Jung P. Revisiting tuberculosis risk in Peace Corps Volunteers, 2006–13. J Travel Med. 2016 Jan;23(1).

2. Cobelens FG, van Deutekom H, Draayer-Jansen IW, Schepp-Beelen AC, van Gerven PJ, van Kessel RP, et al. Risk of infection with Mycobacterium tuberculosis in travelers to areas of high tuberculosis endemicity. Lancet. 2000 Aug 5;356(9228):461–5.

3. Denholm JT, Thevarajan I. Tuberculosis and the traveler: evaluating and reducing risk through travel consultation. J Travel Med. 2016 Mar 23(3).

4. Dorman SE, Belknap R, Graviss EA, Reeves R, Schluger N, Weinfurter P, et al. Interferon-gamma release assays and tuberculin skin testing for diagnosis of latent tuberculosis infection in healthcare workers in the United States. Am J Respir Crit Care Med. 2014 Jan 1;189(1):77–87.

5. Hagmann SH, Han PV, Stauffer WM, Miller AO, Connor BA, Hale DC. Travel-associated disease among US residents visiting US GeoSentinel clinics after return from international travel. Fam Pract. 2014 Dec;31(6):678–87.

6. Haley CA, Cain KP, Yu C, Garman KF, Wells CD, Laserson KF. Risk-based screening for latent tuberculosis infection. South Med J. 2008 Feb;101(2):142–9.

(continued)

## TUBERCULIN SKIN TESTING OF TRAVELERS (CONTINUED)

7. Kahwati LC, Feltner C, Halpern M, Woodell CL, Boland E, Amick HR, et al. Screening for latent tuberculosis infection in adults. Evidence Syntheses, No 142. AHRQ; 2016 Sep. Report No. 14-05212-EF-1. [cited 2018 Mar 20]. Available from: www.ncbi.nlm.nih.gov/pubmedhealth/PMH0089409.

8. Lewinsohn DM, Leonard MK, LoBue PA, Cohn DL, Daley CL, Desmond E, et al. American Thoracic Society/Infectious Diseases Society/Centers for Disease Control and Prevention clinical practice guidelines: diagnosis of tuberculosis in adults and children. Clin Infect Dis. 2017 Jan 15;64(2):111–5.

9. Mancuso JD, Tobler SK, Keep LW. Pseudoepidemics of tuberculin skin test conversions in the US Army after recent deployments. Am J Respir Crit Care Med. 2008 Jun 1;177(11):1285–9.

10. Marienau KJ, Cramer EH, Coleman MS, Marano N, Cetron MS. Flight related tuberculosis contact investigations in the United States: comparative risk and economic analysis of alternate protocols. Travel Med Infect Dis. 2014 Jan–Feb;12(1):54–62.

11. Seaworth BJ, Armitige LY, Aronson NE, Hoft DF, Fleenor ME, Gardner AF, et al. Multidrug-resistant tuberculosis. Recommendations for reducing risk during travel for healthcare and humanitarian work. Ann Am Thorac Soc. 2014 Mar;11(3):286–95.

12. US Preventive Services Task Force. Screening for latent TB infection in adults: US Preventive Services Task Force recommendation statement. JAMA. 2016 Sept 6;316(9):962–9.

# TYPHOID & PARATYPHOID FEVER

Grace D. Appiah, Michael J. Hughes, Kevin Chatham-Stephens

## INFECTIOUS AGENT

*Salmonella enterica* serotypes Typhi and Paratyphi A, Paratyphi B, and Paratyphi C cause potentially severe and occasionally life-threatening bacteremic illnesses referred to respectively as typhoid and paratyphoid fever, and collectively as enteric fever. Paratyphi B is differentiated into 2 distinct pathotypes on the basis of their ability to ferment tartrate—one is unable to ferment tartrate and is associated with paratyphoid fever (referred to as Paratyphi B), and the other ferments tartrate and is associated with uncomplicated gastroenteritis (referred to as Paratyphi B var. L(+) tartrate+).

## TRANSMISSION

Humans are the only source of these bacteria; no animal or environmental reservoirs have been identified. Typhoid and paratyphoid fever are acquired through consumption of water or food contaminated by feces of an acutely infected or convalescent person or a chronic, asymptomatic carrier. Risk for infection is high in low- and middle-income countries with endemic disease and poor access to safe food, water, and sanitation. Transmission through sexual contact, especially among men who have sex with men, has been documented rarely.

## EPIDEMIOLOGY

An estimated 26 million cases of typhoid fever and 5 million cases of paratyphoid fever occur worldwide each year, causing 215,000 deaths. In the United States during 2008–2015, approximately 350 culture-confirmed cases of typhoid fever and 90 cases of paratyphoid fever caused by Paratyphi A were reported each year. Cases of paratyphoid fever caused by Paratyphi B and Paratyphi C are rarely reported. Approximately 85% of typhoid fever and 92% of paratyphoid fever cases in the United States occur among international travelers; of those, 80% of typhoid and 91% of paratyphoid fever cases caused by Paratyphi A are acquired by travelers to southern Asia (primarily India, Pakistan, or Bangladesh). Other high-risk regions for typhoid and paratyphoid fever include Africa and Southeast Asia; lower-risk regions include East Asia, South America, and the Caribbean.

Travelers visiting friends and relatives are at increased risk, as they may be less careful with food and water while abroad and may not seek pretravel health consultation or typhoid vaccination (see Chapter 9, Visiting Friends and Relatives: VFR Travel). Although the risk of illness with typhoid or paratyphoid fever increases with the duration of stay, travelers have acquired typhoid fever even during visits of <1 week to countries where the disease is highly endemic (such as India, Pakistan, or Bangladesh).

## CLINICAL PRESENTATION

The incubation period of typhoid and paratyphoid infections is 6–30 days. The onset of illness is insidious, with gradually increasing fatigue and a fever that increases daily from low-grade to as high as 102°F–104°F (38°C–40°C) by the third to fourth day of illness. Fever is commonly lowest in the morning, peaking in the late afternoon or evening. Headache, malaise, and anorexia are nearly universal, and abdominal pain, diarrhea, or constipation are common. Vomiting and diarrhea are more common in children compared with adults. People can also have fatigue, myalgias, dry cough, and sore throat. Hepatosplenomegaly can often be detected. A transient, maculopapular rash of rose-colored spots can occasionally be seen on the trunk.

The clinical presentation is often confused with malaria, and typhoid fever should be suspected in a person with a history of travel to an endemic area who is not responding to antimalarial medication. Untreated, the disease can last for a month, and reported case-fatality ratios are 10%–30%. In comparison, the case-fatality ratio in disease treated early is usually <1%. The serious complications of typhoid fever occur in 10%–15%

of hospitalized patients, generally after 2–3 weeks of illness, and may include life-threatening gastrointestinal hemorrhage, intestinal perforation, and encephalopathy. Paratyphoid fever is usually described as less severe than typhoid fever; however, severe cases of Paratyphi A infection have been reported from Asia.

## DIAGNOSIS

Patients with typhoid or paratyphoid fever have bacteremia. Blood culture is the mainstay of diagnosis in typhoid and paratyphoid fever; however, a single culture is positive in only approximately 50% of cases. Multiple cultures increase the sensitivity and may be required to make the diagnosis. Bone marrow culture increases the diagnostic yield to approximately 80% of cases and is relatively unaffected by previous or concurrent antibiotic use. Stool culture is not usually positive during the first week of illness, so blood culture is preferred. Urine culture has a lower diagnostic yield than stool culture for acute cases.

The Widal test is unreliable but is widely used in developing countries because of its low cost. It measures elevated antibody titers in patients with recent typhoid or paratyphoid fever but may not accurately distinguish acute from past infection and lacks specificity, resulting in false-positive results. Serologic assays are not an adequate substitute for blood, stool, or bone marrow culture.

Because there are no definitive rapid diagnostic tests for typhoid or paratyphoid fever, the initial diagnosis often has to be made clinically. Typhoid and paratyphoid fever are clinically indistinguishable. The combination of a risk factor for infection and gradual onset of fever that increases in severity over several days should raise suspicion of typhoid or paratyphoid fever. Typhoid and paratyphoid fever are nationally notifiable diseases.

## TREATMENT

Antibiotic therapy shortens the clinical course of enteric fever and reduces the risk for death. Fluoroquinolones (such as ciprofloxacin) are often used for empiric treatment of enteric fever in adults and are considered the treatment of choice for fluoroquinolone-susceptible infections. However, most infections in the United States are acquired during travel abroad, particularly to regions where enteric fever is endemic and fluoroquinolone nonsusceptibility among Typhi and Paratyphi A isolates is common. Fluoroquinolone-nonsusceptible infections are also usually resistant to the synthetic quinolone, nalidixic acid, and have been associated with treatment failure or delayed clinical response.

In the United States, ≥90% of Typhi and Paratyphi A infections in travelers to South Asia were found to be fluoroquinolone-nonsusceptible or nalidixic acid–resistant, which suggests that treatment failures may occur among patients treated empirically with fluoroquinolones. Increasingly, azithromycin and ceftriaxone are being used to treat enteric fever. Through 2015, there was only 1 azithromycin-resistant Typhi isolate and no ceftriaxone-resistant Typhi or Paratyphi A isolates among isolates tested by CDC's National Antimicrobial Resistance Monitoring System. Additional data on antibiotic resistance among enteric fever cases in the United States can be found at www.cdc.gov/narmsnow. Emerging resistance to azithromycin and ceftriaxone among Typhi strains has been reported outside the United States.

Patients treated with an antibiotic may continue to have fever for 3–5 days, although the maximum temperature generally decreases each day. Patients may actually feel worse during the several days it takes for the fever to resolve. If fever in a person with a culture-confirmed typhoid or paratyphoid infection does not subside within 5 days, alternative antibiotics or persistent foci of infection such as an abscess, bone or joint infection, and other extraintestinal site of infection should be considered.

Relapse, reinfection, and chronic carriage can also occur. In up to 10% of patients, relapse occurs 1–3 weeks after clinical recovery, requiring additional antibiotic treatment. An estimated 1%–4% of treated patients become asymptomatic chronic carriers, excreting bacteria in stool for ≥12 months after acute infection and requiring a prolonged antibiotic course for eradication.

## PREVENTION

### Food and Water

Safe food and water precautions and frequent handwashing (especially before meals) are important in preventing typhoid and paratyphoid fever (see Chapter 2, Food & Water Precautions). Although vaccines are recommended to prevent typhoid fever, they are not 100% effective, and vaccine-induced immunity can be overwhelmed by a large bacterial inoculum; therefore, even vaccinated travelers should follow recommended food and water precautions. For paratyphoid fever, food and water precautions are the only prevention method, as no vaccines are available.

### Vaccine

#### INDICATIONS FOR USE

The Advisory Committee on Immunization Practices (ACIP) recommends typhoid vaccine for travelers to areas where there is a recognized risk for exposure to Typhi. Destination-specific vaccine recommendations are available at the CDC Travelers' Health website (www.cdc.gov/travel).

Two unconjugated typhoid vaccines are licensed and available in the United States:

- Vi capsular polysaccharide vaccine (ViCPS) (Typhim Vi, manufactured by Sanofi Pasteur) for intramuscular use

- Oral live attenuated vaccine (Vivotif, manufactured from the Ty21a strain of serotype Typhi by PaxVax)

Both typhoid vaccines protect 50%–80% of recipients; travelers should be reminded that typhoid immunization is not 100% effective, and typhoid fever could still occur. Neither licensed typhoid vaccine is indicated to prevent paratyphoid fever, although limited data from efficacy trials suggest that the live, oral typhoid Ty21a vaccine may provide some cross-protection against infection with Paratyphi B.

Newer, protein-conjugate Vi vaccines have been shown to have greater efficacy in children <2 years old and longer duration of protection than provided by Vi unconjugated polysaccharide vaccines. Two typhoid Vi conjugate vaccines (TCV) have been licensed in India (Typbar-TCV, manufactured by Bharat Biotech, and Peda Typh, manufactured by Biomed) for administration as a single 0.5-mL injection in children aged

≥6 months. Although neither vaccine is licensed or available in the United States currently, Tybar-TCV received WHO prequalification in 2018 and may be available in the future.

## VACCINE ADMINISTRATION

Table 4-22 provides information on vaccine dosage, administration, and revaccination. The time required for primary vaccination differs for the 2 vaccines, as do the lower age limits. Primary vaccination with ViCPS consists of one 0.5-mL (25-mg) dose administered intramuscularly. One dose should be given ≥2 weeks before travel. The manufacturer does not recommend the vaccine for infants or for children <2 years old. A booster dose is recommended every 2 years for people who remain at risk.

Primary vaccination with oral Ty21a vaccine consists of 4 capsules, 1 taken every other day. The capsules should be kept refrigerated (not frozen), and all 4 doses must be taken to achieve maximum efficacy. Each capsule should be taken with cool liquid no warmer than 98.6°F (37°C), approximately 1 hour before a meal and ≥2 hours after a previous meal. This regimen should be completed ≥1 week before potential exposure. What to do when a dose of the oral vaccine is missed or taken late is unclear. Some suggest that minor deviations in the dosing schedule, such as taking a dose 1 day late, may not have a large effect on how well the vaccine works. However, no studies have shown the effect of such deviations; thus, if 4 doses are not completed as directed, optimal immune response may not be achieved. The vaccine manufacturer recommends that the Ty21a vaccine not be administered to infants or to children aged <6 years. A booster dose is recommended every 5 years for people who remain at risk.

## VACCINE SAFETY AND ADVERSE REACTIONS

ViCPS vaccine is most often associated with headache (16%–20%) and injection-site reactions (7%). Adverse reactions to Ty21a vaccine are rare and mainly consist of abdominal discomfort, nausea, headache, fever, diarrhea, vomiting, and rash. Adverse reactions should be reported to the Vaccine Adverse Event Reporting System by visiting https://vaers.hhs.gov/index.html or calling 1-800-822-7967.

## PRECAUTIONS AND CONTRAINDICATIONS

Neither the ViCPS nor the Ty21a vaccine should be given to those with an acute febrile illness; in addition, Ty21a is not recommended for use in

## Table 4-22. Vaccines to prevent typhoid fever

| VACCINATION | AGE (Y) | DOSE, MODE OF ADMINISTRATION | NUMBER OF DOSES | DOSING INTERVAL | BOOSTING INTERVAL |
|---|---|---|---|---|---|
| **Oral, Live Attenuated Ty21a Vaccine (Vivotif)[1]** | | | | | |
| Primary series | ≥6 | 1 capsule,[2] oral | 4 | 48 hours | Not applicable |
| Booster | ≥6 | 1 capsule,[2] oral | 4 | 48 hours | Every 5 years |
| **Vi Capsular Polysaccharide Vaccine (Typhim Vi)** | | | | | |
| Primary series | ≥2 | 0.5 mL, intramuscular | 1 | Not applicable | Not applicable |
| Booster | ≥2 | 0.5 mL, intramuscular | 1 | Not applicable | Every 2 years |

[1] The vaccine must be kept refrigerated (35.6°F–46.4°F, 2°C–8°C).
[2] Administer with cool liquid no warmer than 98.6°F (37°C).

people with acute gastroenteritis. No information is available on the safety of either vaccine in pregnancy; it is prudent on theoretical grounds to avoid vaccinating pregnant women. However, the benefits of vaccinating pregnant women may outweigh potential risks when the likelihood of typhoid exposure is high; the inactivated vaccine (ViCPS) may be considered in these situations. Live attenuated Ty21a vaccine should not be given to pregnant women or immunocompromised travelers, including those infected with HIV.

The intramuscular vaccine presents a theoretically safer alternative for immunocompromised travelers. ACIP does not recommend against vaccinating household contacts of immunocompromised people with the Ty21a vaccine; although vaccine organisms can be shed transiently in the stool of vaccine recipients, secondary transmission of vaccine organisms has not been documented. The only contraindication to vaccination with ViCPS vaccine is a history of severe local or systemic reactions after a previous dose.

Theoretical concerns have been raised about the immunogenicity of live, attenuated Ty21a vaccine in people concurrently receiving antimicrobial agents, live vaccines, or immune globulin. The growth of the live Ty21a strain is inhibited in vitro by various antibacterial agents. The manufacturer advises that vaccination with the Ty21a vaccine should be delayed for >72 hours after the administration of any antibacterial agent, and antibiotics should not be given to a patient within 72 hours of the last dose of the Ty21a vaccine.

Available data do not suggest that simultaneous administration of yellow fever vaccine decreases the immunogenicity of the Ty21a vaccine. If typhoid vaccination is warranted, it should not be delayed because of administration of viral vaccines. No data are available on coadministration of the Ty21a vaccine and the oral cholera vaccine (lyophilized CVD 103-HgR [Vaxchora]); taking the first Ty21a vaccine dose ≥8 hours after oral cholera vaccine may decrease potential interference between the vaccines. Simultaneous administration of the Ty21a vaccine and immune globulin does not appear to pose a problem.

**CDC website:** www.cdc.gov/typhoid-fever

### BIBLIOGRAPHY

1. Buckle GC, Walker CL, Black RE. Typhoid fever and paratyphoid fever: systematic review to estimate global morbidity and mortality for 2010. J Glob Health. 2012 Jun;2(1):010401.

2. Crump JA, Mintz ED. Global trends in typhoid and paratyphoid fever. Clin Infect Dis. 2010 Jan 15;50(2):241–6.

3. Crump JA, Sjölund-Karlsson M, Gordon MA, Parry CM. Epidemiology, clinical presentation, laboratory diagnosis, antimicrobial resistance, and antimicrobial management of invasive Salmonella infections. Clin Microbiol Rev. 2015 Oct 1;28(4):90137.

4. Date KA, Bentsi-Enchill A, Marks F, Fox K. Typhoid fever vaccination strategies. Vaccine. 2015 Jun 19;33:C55–61.

5. Date KA, Newton AE, Medalla F, Blackstock A, Richardson L, McCullough A, et al. Changing patterns in enteric fever incidence and increasing antibiotic resistance of enteric fever isolates in the United States, 2008–2012. Clin Infect Dis. 2016 Aug 1;63(3):322–9.

6. Effa EE, Bukirwa H. Azithromycin for treating uncomplicated typhoid and paratyphoid fever (enteric fever). Cochrane Database Syst Rev. 2008(4):CD006083.

7. Gupta SK, Medalla F, Omondi MW, Whichard JM, Fields PI, Gerner-Smidt P, et al. Laboratory-based surveillance of paratyphoid fever in the United States: travel and antimicrobial resistance. Clin Infect Dis. 2008 Jun 1;46(11):1656–63.

8. Jackson BR, Iqbal S, Mahon B. Updated recommendations for the use of typhoid vaccine— Advisory Committee on Immunization Practices, United States, 2015. MMWR Morb Mortal Wkly Rep. 2015 Mar;64(11):305–8.

9. Klemm EJ, Shakoor S, Page AJ, Qamar FN, Judge K, Saeed DK, et al. Emergence of an extensively drug-resistant Salmonella enterica serovar Typhi clone harboring a promiscuous plasmid encoding resistance to fluoroquinolones and third-generation cephalosporins. mBio. 2018 Mar 7;9(1):e00105–18.

10. Lynch MF, Blanton EM, Bulens S, Polyak C, Vojdani J, Stevenson J, et al. Typhoid fever in the United States, 1999–2006. JAMA. 2009 Aug 26;302(8):859–65.

# VARICELLA (CHICKENPOX)

Mona Marin, Adriana S. Lopez

## INFECTIOUS AGENT

Varicella-zoster virus (VZV), a member of the herpesvirus family. Humans are the only reservoir of VZV, and disease occurs only in humans. After primary infection as varicella (chickenpox), VZV remains latent in the sensory-nerve ganglia and can reactivate later, causing herpes zoster (shingles).

## TRANSMISSION

Person to person—primarily via the respiratory route—by inhalation of aerosols from vesicular fluid of skin lesions of varicella or herpes zoster; VZV can also spread by direct contact with the vesicular fluid of skin lesions and possibly infected respiratory tract secretions. VZV enters the host through the upper respiratory tract or the conjunctiva. Varicella is a highly contagious viral disease with secondary attack ratios of approximately 85% (range, 61%–100%) in susceptible household contacts; contagiousness after community exposure is lower. Herpes zoster is approximately 20% as infectious as varicella; in susceptible people, contact with herpes zoster rash causes varicella, not herpes zoster.

The period of communicability of patients with varicella is estimated to begin 1–2 days before the onset of rash and ends when all lesions are crusted, typically 4–7 days after onset of rash in immunocompetent people. This period may be longer in immunocompromised people. Patients with herpes zoster are contagious while they have active, vesicular lesions (usually 7–10 days). In utero infection can also occur due to transplacental passage of the virus during maternal varicella infection.

## EPIDEMIOLOGY

Varicella occurs worldwide. In temperate climates, varicella tends to be a childhood disease, with peak incidence among preschool and school-aged children; <5% of adults are susceptible to varicella. Disease typically occurs during late winter and early spring. In tropical climates, by contrast, infection tends to be more common later in childhood, with higher susceptibility among adults than in temperate climates, especially in less densely populated areas. The highest incidence of disease in tropical climates occurs during the driest, coolest months.

With the implementation of the childhood varicella vaccination program in the United States in 1996, substantial declines have occurred in disease incidence. Although still endemic, the risk of exposure to VZV is now lower in the United States than in most other parts of the world. As of 2018, 18% of countries have introduced a routine varicella vaccination program, and an additional 6% have varicella vaccination programs for risk groups only.

Because varicella is endemic worldwide, all susceptible travelers are at risk of infection during travel. Additionally, exposure to herpes zoster poses a risk for varicella in susceptible travelers, although localized herpes zoster is much less contagious than varicella. Travelers at highest risk for severe varicella are infants, adults, and immunocompromised people without evidence of immunity (see criteria for evidence of immunity in "Prevention" below).

## CLINICAL PRESENTATION

Varicella is generally a mild disease in children, and most people recover without serious complications. The average incubation period is 14–16 days (range, 10–21 days). Infection is often characterized by a short (1- or 2-day) prodromal period (fever, malaise), although this may be absent in children, and a pruritic rash consisting of crops of macules, papules, and vesicles (typically 250–500 lesions), which appear in ≥3 successive waves and resolve by crusting. Characteristic for varicella is the presence of lesions in different stages of development at the same time.

Serious complications can occur, most commonly in infants, adults, and immunocompromised people. Complications include secondary bacterial infections of skin lesions, sometimes resulting in bacteremia/sepsis, pneumonia, cerebellar ataxia, encephalitis, and hemorrhagic conditions; rarely (about 1 in 40,000 varicella cases), these complications may result in death.

Modified varicella, also known as breakthrough varicella, can occur in vaccinated people. Breakthrough varicella is usually mild, with <50 lesions, low or no fever, and shorter duration of rash. The rash may be atypical in appearance with fewer vesicles and predominance of maculopapular lesions. Breakthrough varicella is contagious, although less so than varicella, in unvaccinated people.

## DIAGNOSIS

Often based on an appropriate exposure history and the presence of a generalized maculopapulovesicular rash, the clinical diagnosis of varicella in the United States has become increasingly challenging as a growing proportion of cases now occur in vaccinated people in whom disease is mild, and rash is atypical. Although not routinely recommended, laboratory diagnosis is likely to become increasingly useful.

For laboratory confirmation, skin lesions are the preferred specimen source. Vesicular swabs or scrapings and scabs from crusted lesions can be used to identify varicella-zoster virus DNA by PCR (preferred method, as it is the most sensitive and specific) or direct fluorescent antibody. In the absence of vesicles or scabs, scrapings of maculopapular lesions can be collected for testing.

Serologic tests may also be used to confirm disease but are less reliable than PCR or direct fluorescent antibody methods for virus identification. A significant rise in serum varicella IgG titers from acute- and convalescent-phase samples by any standard serologic assay can confirm a diagnosis retrospectively; these antibody tests may not be reliable in immunocompromised people.

Of note, testing for varicella-zoster IgM by using commercial kits is not recommended, because available methods lack sensitivity and specificity; false-positive IgM results are common in the presence of high IgG levels. Visit www.cdc.gov/chickenpox/lab-testing/collecting-specimens.html for additional information on specimen collection and testing for varicella. Varicella is a nationally notifiable disease in the United States.

## TREATMENT

Treatment with antivirals is not recommended routinely for otherwise healthy children with varicella. Consider treatment with oral acyclovir for people at increased risk for moderate to severe disease, such as people aged >12 years; people with chronic cutaneous or pulmonary disorders; people who are receiving long-term salicylate therapy; people who are receiving short, intermittent, or aerosolized courses of corticosteroids; and possibly secondary cases among household contacts. Intravenous acyclovir is recommended for immunocompromised people, including patients being treated with high-dose corticosteroids for ≥2 weeks and people with serious, virally mediated complications (such as pneumonia). Therapy initiated within 24 hours of onset maximizes efficacy.

## PREVENTION

### Vaccine

In the United States, all people, including those traveling or living abroad, should be assessed for varicella immunity, and those who do not have evidence of immunity or contraindications to vaccination should receive age-appropriate vaccination. Vaccination against varicella is not a requirement for entry into any country (including the United States), but people who do not have evidence of immunity should be considered at risk for varicella during international travel. Evidence of immunity to varicella includes any of the following:

- Documentation of age-appropriate vaccination
  - Preschool-aged children (≥12 months through 3 years of age): 1 dose
  - School-aged children (≥4 years of age), adolescents, and adults: 2 doses
- Laboratory evidence of immunity or laboratory confirmation of disease
- Birth in the United States before 1980 (not a criterion for health care personnel, pregnant women, and immunocompromised people)

4

- A health care provider's diagnosis of varicella or verification of a history of varicella

- A health care provider's diagnosis of herpes zoster or verification of a history of herpes zoster

Varicella vaccine contains live, attenuated VZV. Single-antigen varicella vaccine is licensed for people aged ≥12 months, and the combination measles-mumps-rubella-varicella (MMRV) vaccine is licensed only for children 1–12 years. CDC recommends varicella vaccine for all people aged ≥12 months without evidence of immunity to varicella who do not have contraindications to the vaccine. For children ≥12 months and <13 years: 2 doses of vaccine administered ≥3 months apart. Typically, the first dose is given at 12–15 months and the second at 4–6 years of age. The second dose may be given before age 4 however, provided it has been at least 3 months since the first dose. For people aged ≥13 years: 2 doses of vaccine administered at least 4 weeks apart.

Contraindications to vaccination include allergy to vaccine components, immune-compromising conditions or treatments, and pregnancy. When evidence of immunity is uncertain, a possible history of varicella is not a contraindication to varicella vaccination. Vaccine effectiveness is approximately 80% after 1 dose and 92%–95% after 2 doses.

## VACCINE SAFETY AND ADVERSE REACTIONS

The varicella vaccine is generally well tolerated. The most common adverse events after vaccination are self-limited injection-site reactions (pain, soreness, redness, and swelling). Fever or a varicellalike rash, usually consisting of a few lesions at the injection site or generalized rash with a small number of lesions, are reported less frequently.

Compared with use of separate MMR and varicella vaccines at the same visit, use of the combined MMRV vaccine is associated with a higher risk for fever and febrile seizures, approximately 1 additional febrile seizure for every 2,300–2,600 MMRV vaccine doses administered. Fever and febrile seizures

typically occur 5–12 days after the first dose of MMRV, with the greatest incidence among children aged 12–23 months. Use of separate MMR and varicella vaccines helps avoid this increased risk. For detailed information regarding the varicella vaccine, visit www.cdc.gov/chickenpox/vaccination.html.

## POSTEXPOSURE PROPHYLAXIS

### Vaccine

Varicella vaccine is recommended for postexposure administration to unvaccinated healthy people aged ≥12 months and without other evidence of immunity, to prevent or modify the disease. The vaccine should be administered as soon as possible within 5 days after exposure to rash, if there are no contraindications to use. Among children, protective efficacy was reported as ≥90% when vaccination occurred within 3 days of exposure. However, administration of a second dose is recommended for exposed people to bring them up-to-date on vaccination and for best protection against future exposures.

### Varicella Zoster Immune Globulin

People without evidence of immunity who have contraindications to vaccination and who are at risk for severe varicella and complications are recommended to receive postexposure prophylaxis with varicella zoster immune globulin. The varicella zoster immune globulin product licensed in the United States is VariZIG.

People who should receive VariZIG after exposure include immunocompromised people, pregnant women without evidence of immunity, and some neonates and infants. VariZIG provides maximum benefit when administered as soon as possible after exposure but may be effective if administered as late as 10 days after exposure. In the United States, VariZIG can be obtained from specialty distributors (available from https://varizig.com).

If VariZIG is not available, intravenous immune globulin (IVIG) can be considered (also within 10 days of exposure). In the absence of both VariZIG and IVIG, some experts recommend prophylaxis with acyclovir (80 mg/kg/day in 4 divided doses for 7 days; maximum dose,

800 mg, 4 times per day), beginning 7–10 days after exposure for people without evidence of immunity and with contraindications for varicella vaccination. Published data on the benefit of acyclovir as postexposure prophylaxis among immunocompromised people are limited.

**CDC website:** www.cdc.gov/chickenpox/

BIBLIOGRAPHY

1. American Academy of Pediatrics. Varicella-zoster infections. In: Kimberlin DW, Brady MT, Jackson MA, editors. Red Book: 2018 Report of the Committee on Infectious Diseases. 31st ed. Elk Grove Village, IL: American Academy of Pediatrics; 2018. pp. 869–82.

2. Bialek SR, Perella D, Zhang J, Mascola L, Viner K, Jackson C, et al. Impact of a routine two-dose varicella vaccination program on varicella epidemiology. Pediatrics. 2013 Nov;132(5):e1134–40.

3. CDC. Manual for the surveillance of vaccine-preventable diseases. Atlanta: CDC; 2018 [cited 2018 Mar 13]. Available from: www.cdc.gov/vaccines/pubs/surv-manual/chapters.html.

4. CDC. Updated recommendations for use of VariZIG—United States, 2013. MMWR Morb Mortal Wkly Rep. 2013 Jul 19;62(28):574–6.

5. Harpaz R, Ortega-Sanchez IR, Seward JF. Prevention of herpes zoster: recommendations of the Advisory Committee on Immunization Practices (ACIP). MMWR Recomm Rep. 2008 Jun 6;57(RR-5):1–30.

6. Marin M, Broder KR, Temte JL, Snider DE, Seward JF. Use of combination measles, mumps, rubella, and varicella vaccine: recommendations of the Advisory Committee on Immunization Practices (ACIP). MMWR Recomm Rep. 2010 May 7;59(RR-3):1–12.

7. Marin M, Guris D, Chaves SS, Schmid S, Seward JF. Prevention of varicella: recommendations of the Advisory Committee on Immunization Practices (ACIP). MMWR Recomm Rep. 2007 Jun 22;56(RR-4):1–40.

8. World Health Organization. WHO vaccine-preventable diseases: monitoring system. 2017 global summary 2017 [cited 2018 Mar 13]. Available from: http://apps.who.int/immunization_monitoring/globalsummary.

# VIRAL HEMORRHAGIC FEVERS

Trevor Shoemaker, Mary Choi

## INFECTIOUS AGENTS

Several families of enveloped RNA viruses cause viral hemorrhagic fevers (VHFs).

Filoviruses include the Ebola viruses, which cause Ebola virus disease (EVD), and Marburg virus, which causes Marburg virus disease (MVD). Arenaviruses include Lassa virus, lymphocytic choriomeningitis virus (LCMV), and Lujo, Guanarito, Machupo, Junin, Sabia, and Chapare viruses. Bunyaviruses include Rift Valley fever (RVF) virus, Crimean-Congo hemorrhagic fever (CCHF) virus, and hantavirus. The flaviviruses include dengue virus, yellow fever virus, Omsk hemorrhagic fever virus, Kyasanur Forest disease virus, and Alkhurma hemorrhagic fever virus (also see the Dengue and Yellow Fever sections in this chapter).

## TRANSMISSION

Some of the VHF viruses ( filoviruses, arenaviruses, CCHF virus) spread by direct contact with symptomatic patients, body fluids, or cadavers, or through inadequate infection control in health care settings. In community settings, disease transmission occurs when a person (without proper skin and mucous membrane protection) comes into direct physical contact with the blood or other infectious body fluids of patients in the acute phase of disease or who have died.

Zoonotic sources of VHF virus exposure include:

- Livestock, via slaughter or consumption of raw meat from infected animals or unpasteurized milk (CCHF, RVF, Alkhurma viruses)

- Rodents or insectivores, via direct contact with the animal or inhalation of, or contact with, materials contaminated with rodent excreta (arenaviruses, hantaviruses)

- The Egyptian fruit bat (*Rousettus aegyptiacus*), the natural reservoir for Marburg virus; bats are suspected reservoir species for the viruses within the genus *Ebolavirus*

- Mosquitoes (RVF virus) and ticks (CCHF, Omsk, Kyasanur Forest disease, Alkhurma viruses)

After recovery from acute EVD or MVD, the virus or its RNA persists in some specific body fluids of convalescent patients. Ebola virus RNA has been detected in breast milk up to 21 days after the onset of the disease and in vaginal secretions up to 33 days after onset. Ebola virus and Marburg virus have been cultured from ocular aqueous humor at 2 and 3 months after disease onset, respectively. Evidence suggests that Ebola and Marburg viruses can be sexually transmitted from a male survivor to his partner months after onset of disease. In pregnant women with EVD, there can be in utero transmission of Ebola virus to the fetus.

## EPIDEMIOLOGY

The viruses that cause VHF are distributed over much of the globe. Each virus is associated with one or more nonhuman host or vector species, restricting the virus and the initial contamination to the areas inhabited by these species. The diseases caused by these viruses are seen in people living in or having visited these areas. Humans are incidental hosts for these enzootic diseases; however, person-to-person transmission of some viruses can occur. Specific viruses are addressed below.

## Ebola and Marburg Virus Disease

People at greatest risk of EVD or MVD include family members, health care workers, or others who, without protective equipment, come into direct contact with infected patients or corpses; people who have come into contact or close proximity to bats (visiting bat caves); and people who have handled infected primates or carcasses. Additionally, sex partners of recent male EVD or MVD survivors may be at risk if they have had contact with virus-infected semen.

Countries where domestically acquired EVD cases have been reported and that should be considered areas where future epidemics could occur include Côte d'Ivoire, Democratic Republic of the Congo, Gabon, Guinea, Liberia, Republic of the Congo, Sierra Leone, South Sudan, and Uganda.

Typically, previous Ebola outbreaks had been limited in scope and geographic extent. However, in March of 2014, an outbreak of Ebola virus was detected in a rural area of Guinea near the border with Liberia and Sierra Leone. By June of 2014, cases were reported in all 3 countries and across many districts. The outbreak was the largest and most complex Ebola epidemic ever reported. Additional cases occurred in Nigeria, Senegal, Mali, Spain, the United Kingdom, Italy, and the United States, after infected people traveled from West Africa.

Countries with confirmed human cases of MVD include Angola, Democratic Republic of the Congo, Kenya, Uganda, and possibly Zimbabwe. Four cases of MVD have occurred in travelers visiting caves harboring bats, including Kitum Cave in Kenya and Python Cave in Maramagambo Forest, Uganda. Miners in the Democratic Republic of the Congo and Uganda have also acquired Marburg virus infection from working in underground mines harboring bats.

Reston virus is believed to be endemic to the Philippines but has not been shown to cause human disease.

## Lassa Fever and Other Arenaviral Diseases

Arenaviruses are maintained in rodents and transmitted to humans, except Tacaribe virus, which was found in bats but has not been reported to cause disease in humans. Most infections are mild, but some result in hemorrhagic fever with high death rates. Arenaviruses may be divided into 2 categories, Old World (eastern hemisphere) and New World (western hemisphere).

- Old World arenaviruses (and the diseases they cause) include Lassa virus (Lassa fever), Lujo virus, and LCMV (meningitis,

4

encephalitis, and congenital fetal infection in normal hosts; severe disease with multiple organ failure in organ transplant recipients). Lassa fever occurs across rural West Africa, with hyperendemic areas in parts of Sierra Leone, Guinea, Liberia, and Nigeria. Lujo virus has been described in Zambia and the Republic of South Africa during a health care-associated outbreak.

- New World arenaviruses (and the diseases they cause) include Junin (Argentine hemorrhagic fever), Machupo (Bolivian hemorrhagic fever), Guanarito (Venezuelan hemorrhagic fever), Sabia (Brazilian hemorrhagic fever), and Chapare virus (single case in Bolivia).

Reservoir host species are Old World rats and mice (family Muridae, subfamily Murinae) and New World rats and mice (family Muridae, subfamily Sigmodontinae). These rodent types are found worldwide, including Europe, Asia, Africa, and the Americas. Virus is transmitted through inhalation of rodent urine aerosols, ingestion of rodent-contaminated food, or by direct contact of broken skin or mucosa with rodent excreta. Risk of Lassa virus infection is associated with peridomestic rodent exposure, where inappropriate food storage increases the risk for exposure. Several cases of Lassa fever have been confirmed in international travelers staying in traditional dwellings in the countryside. Health care-associated transmission and close family member infection with Lassa, Lujo, and Machupo viruses occurs through droplet spread and direct contact.

## Rift Valley Fever and Other Bunyaviral Diseases

RVF primarily affects livestock, causing stillbirths and high mortality in neonatal cattle, sheep, and goats. In humans, RVF virus infection causes fever, hemorrhage, encephalitis, and retinitis. RVF virus is endemic to sub-Saharan Africa. Sporadic outbreaks have occurred in humans in Comoros, Egypt, Madagascar, Mali, Mauritania, Senegal, South Sudan, Sudan, and Uganda. Large epidemics occurred in Kenya, Somalia, and Tanzania in 1997–1998 and 2006–2007; Saudi Arabia and Yemen in 2000; Madagascar in 1990 and 2008; Botswana, Mauritania, Namibia, and South Africa in 2010; and Niger in 2016–2017. RVF virus is transmitted to livestock by mosquitoes, while people become infected more frequently through direct contact with clinically affected animals or their body fluids, including slaughter or consumption of infected animals.

CCHF is endemic to areas of Africa and Eurasia where ticks of the genus *Hyalomma* are found, including South Africa, the Balkans, the Middle East, Russia, and western China, and particularly to Turkey, Afghanistan, Iran, and Pakistan. The first human cases were reported in Spain in 2016. Primarily associated with livestock, *Hyalomma* ticks will also bite humans. Livestock and other hosts may develop CCHF viremia from tick bites but do not develop clinical disease. CCHF virus is transmitted to humans by infected ticks or by direct handling and preparation of fresh carcasses of infected animals, usually domestic livestock. Human-to-human transmission can occur through droplet or direct contact.

Hantaviruses cause hantavirus pulmonary syndrome (HPS) and hemorrhagic fever with renal syndrome (HFRS). The viruses that cause HPS are present in the New World; those that cause HFRS occur worldwide. The viruses that cause both HPS and HFRS are transmitted to humans through contact with urine, feces, or saliva of infected rodents. Travelers staying in rodent-infested dwellings are at risk for HPS and HFRS. Human-to-human transmission of hantavirus has been reported only with Andes virus in Chile and Argentina. The first reported case of imported Andes virus in the United States occurred in 2018 in a traveler returning from Chile and Argentina.

## CLINICAL PRESENTATION

Signs and symptoms vary by disease, but in general, patients with VHF present with abrupt onset of fever, myalgias, headache, and prostration, followed by coagulopathy with a petechial rash or ecchymoses and sometimes overt bleeding in severe forms. Gastrointestinal symptoms (diarrhea, vomiting, abdominal pain) are commonly observed. Vascular endothelial damage leads to shock and pulmonary edema, and liver injury is common.

Findings associated with specific viruses include renal failure (hantavirus); ecchymoses and bruises (CCHF virus); pharyngitis, retrosternal pain, hearing loss in adults and anasarca in newborns (Lassa virus); retinitis and partial blindness (RVF virus); and spontaneous abortion and birth defects (Lassa virus and LCMV). Laboratory abnormalities include elevations in liver enzymes, initial drop in leukocyte count, and thrombocytopenia. Because the incubation period may be as long as 21 days, patients may not develop illness until returning from travel; therefore, a thorough travel and exposure history is critical.

## DIAGNOSIS

US-based clinicians should notify local health authorities immediately of any suspected cases of VHF occurring in patients residing in the United States. For laboratory testing requests, notify the local or state health department. To notify the CDC directly regarding any patients requiring evacuation to the United States, contact the CDC Emergency Operations Center at 770-488-7100. Appropriate personal protective equipment is indicated for any patients where Lassa, Lujo, South American arenaviruses, or CCHF virus infection is suspected, and includes droplet and contact precautions.

Whole blood or serum may be tested for virologic (RT-PCR, antigen detection, virus isolation) and immunologic (IgM, IgG) evidence of infection. Tissue may be tested by immunohistochemistry, RT-PCR, and virus isolation. Postmortem skin biopsies fixed in formalin and blood collected by cardiac puncture within a few hours after death can be used for diagnosis. Consider collection of an oral swab from deceased cases when an alternative sample cannot be collected.

Special handling procedures are required when submitting blood and other body fluid specimens for diagnostic testing. Please contact the CDC Emergency Operations Center at 770-488-7100 for more information.

## TREATMENT

The mainstay of treatment for VHFs is early, aggressive, supportive care directed at maintaining effective intravascular volume and correcting electrolyte imbalances. Ribavirin is effective if given early in the course of disease for treating Lassa fever and other Old World arenaviruses, New World arenaviruses, and potentially CCHF, but it is not approved by the Food and Drug Administration (FDA) for these indications. Intravenous ribavirin can be obtained for compassionate use through FDA from Valeant Pharmaceuticals (Aliso Viejo, California). Requests should be initiated by the provider through FDA (301-796-1500 or after hours 866-300-4374), with simultaneous notification to Valeant Pharmaceuticals: 800-548-5100, extension 5 (domestic telephone). The process is explained on FDA's website (www.fda.gov/Drugs/ DevelopmentApprovalProcess/HowDrugsare DevelopedandApproved/ApprovalApplications/ InvestigationalNewDrugINDApplication/ ucm090039.htm).

There is no proven specific therapy for EVD. Several experimental immune therapy and antivirals treatments are under investigation. EVD patients may also have concomitant malaria infection. As such, empiric use of antimalarial therapy should be considered when rapid diagnostic testing is not immediately available. In general, NSAIDs such as ibuprofen and diclofenac are not recommended because of their antiplatelet activity.

There is no FDA-approved vaccine for any of the VHFs. Experimental Ebola vaccines are under development, including a recombinant vesicular stomatitis virus-based vaccine and a chimpanzee adenovirus-based vaccine. However, these investigational products are in the early stages of product development and are not yet available. Investigational vaccines exist for Argentine hemorrhagic fever and RVF; neither vaccine is approved by FDA or commercially available in the United States.

## PREVENTION

The risk of acquiring VHF is very low for international travelers. Travelers at increased risk for exposure include those engaging in animal research, and health care workers and others who, without adequate personal protection, provide care for patients in the community, particularly where outbreaks of VHF are occurring.

Prevention should focus on avoiding unprotected contact with sources of infection: people suspected of having VHF and hosts/vector species in endemic countries. Travelers should not visit locations where outbreaks are occurring, avoid contact with rodents and bats, and avoid blood or body fluids of livestock in RVF- and CCHF-endemic areas. To prevent vectorborne diseases, travelers should use insecticide-treated bed nets and wear insect repellent (see Chapter 3, Mosquitoes, Ticks & Other Arthropods).

For VHFs that can be transmitted person to person (EVD, MVD, Lassa Fever, CCHF), early identification and isolation of ill travelers, consistent implementation of basic infection control measures, and prompt notification of public health authorities are the keys to prevent secondary transmission. Early identification strategies include eliciting a travel history from all patients who present for care and posting signs and placards asking patients with recent international travel to self-identify. Those patients with recent international travel who have symptoms consistent with any VHF should be promptly isolated by placing them in a private room or a separate enclosed area with a private bathroom or covered bedside commode. To minimize disease transmission risk, only essential health care providers wearing personal protective equipment should evaluate a patient and provide care. Prompt notification of the facility's infection control program as well as state and local health departments is also key.

**CDC website:** www.cdc.gov/vhf.

## BIBLIOGRAPHY

1. Bah EI, Lamah MC, Fletcher T, Jacob ST, Brett-Major DM, Sall AA, et al. Clinical presentation of patients with Ebola virus disease in Conakry, Guinea. N Engl J Med. 2015 Jan 1;372(1):40–7.

2. CDC. Ebola virus disease—US healthcare workers and settings—personal protective equipment. 2016 [cited 2019 Jan 23]. Available from: www.cdc.gov/vhf/ebola/healthcare-us/ppe/index.html.

3. Ergonul O, Holbrook MR. Crimean-Congo hemorrhagic fever. In: Guerrant RL, Walker DH, Weller PF, editors. Tropical Infectious Diseases: Principles, Pathogens and Practice. 3rd ed. Philadelphia: Elsevier; 2011. pp. 466–9.

4. Ewer K, Rampling T, Venkatraman N, Bowyer G, Wright D, Lambe T, et al. A monovalent chimpanzee adenovirus Ebola vaccine boosted with MVA. N Engl J Med. 2016 Apr 28;374(17):1635–46.

5. Fowler RA, Fletcher T, Fischer WA, 2nd, Lamontagne F, Jacob S, Brett-Major D, et al. Caring for critically ill patients with Ebola virus disease. Perspectives from West Africa. Am J Respir Crit Care Med. 2014 Oct 1;190(7):733–7.

6. Osterholm MT, Moore KA, Kelley NS, Brosseau LM, Wong G, Murphy FA, et al. Transmission of Ebola viruses: what we know and what we do not know. mBio. 2015;6(2):e00137.

7. Peters CJ, Makino S, Morrill JC. Rift valley fever. In: Guerrant RL, Walker DH, Weller PF, editors. Tropical Infectious Diseases: Principles, Pathogens and Practice. 3rd ed. Philadelphia: Saunders Elsevier; 2011. pp. 462–5.

8. Peters CJ, Zaki SR. Overview of viral hemorrhagic fevers. In: Guerrant RL, Walker DH, Weller PF, editors. Tropical Infectious Diseases: Principles, Pathogens and Practice. 3rd ed. Philadelphia: Elsevier; 2011. pp. 441–8.

9. Regules JA, Beigel JH, Paolino KM, Voell J, Castellano AR, Munoz P, et al. A Recombinant vesicular stomatitis virus Ebola vaccine—preliminary report. N Engl J Med. 2015 Apr 1. doi: http://dx.doi.org/10.1056/NEJMoa1414216

10. Rollin PE, Nichol ST, Zaki S, Ksiazek TG. Arenaviruses and filoviruses. In: Jorgensen JH, Pfaller MA, Carroll KC, Funke G, Landry ML, Richter SS, et al., editors. Manual of Clinical Microbiology. 11th ed. Washington, DC: ASM Press; 2015. pp. 1669–86.

11. Uyeki TM, Mehta AK, Davey RT, Jr., Liddell AM, Wolf T, Vetter P, et al. Clinical management of Ebola virus disease in the United States and Europe. N Engl J Med. 2016 Feb 18;374(7):636–46.

12. Wahl-Jensen V, Peters CJ, Jahrling PB, Feldman H, Kuhn JH. Filovirus infections. In: Guerrant RL, Walker DH, Weller PF, editors. Tropical Infectious Diseases: Principles, Pathogens and Practice. 3rd ed. Philadelphia: Elsevier; 2011. pp. 483–91.

13. World Health Organization. Clinical care for survivors of Ebola virus disease. 2016 [cited 2019 Jan 23]. Available from: www.who.int/csr/resources/publications/ebola/guidance-survivors/en/.

# YELLOW FEVER

Mark D. Gershman, J. Erin Staples

## INFECTIOUS AGENT

Yellow fever (YF) virus is a single-stranded RNA virus that belongs to the genus *Flavivirus*.

## TRANSMISSION

Vectorborne transmission of YF virus occurs via the bite of an infected mosquito, primarily *Aedes* or *Haemagogus* spp. Nonhuman and human primates are the main reservoirs of the virus, with anthroponotic (human-to-vector-to-human) transmission occurring. There are 3 transmission cycles for YF virus: sylvatic (jungle), intermediate (savannah), and urban.

- The sylvatic (jungle) cycle involves transmission of virus between nonhuman primates and mosquito species found in forest canopy. Virus is transmitted via mosquitoes from monkeys to humans when occupational or recreational activities encroach into the jungle.

- In Africa, an intermediate (savannah) cycle involves transmission of YF virus from tree hole-breeding *Aedes* spp. to humans in jungle border areas. Virus may be transmitted from monkeys to humans or from human to human via these mosquitoes.

- The urban cycle involves transmission of virus between humans and peridomestic mosquitoes, primarily *Ae. aegypti*.

Humans infected with YF virus experience the highest levels of viremia shortly before onset of fever and for the first 3–5 days of illness, during which time they can transmit the virus to mosquitoes. Given the high level of viremia, bloodborne transmission theoretically can occur via transfusion or needlesticks. One case of perinatal transmission of wild-type YF virus has been documented from a woman who developed symptoms of YF, 3 days before giving birth. The infant tested positive for YF viral RNA and died of fulminant YF on the 12th day of life.

## EPIDEMIOLOGY

YF occurs in sub-Saharan Africa and tropical South America, where it is endemic and intermittently epidemic (see Tables 4-23 and 4-24 for a list of countries with risk of YF virus transmission). Most YF disease in humans is due to sylvatic or intermediate transmission cycles. However, urban YF occurs periodically in Africa and sporadically in the Americas. In areas of Africa with persistent circulation of YF virus, natural immunity accumulates with age; consequently, infants and children are at highest risk for disease. In South America, YF occurs most frequently in unimmunized young men exposed to mosquito vectors through their work in forested areas.

## RISK FOR TRAVELERS

A traveler's risk for acquiring YF is determined by various factors, including immunization status, location of travel, season, duration of exposure, occupational and recreational activities while traveling, and local rate of virus transmission at the time of travel. Although reported cases of human disease are the principal indicator of disease risk, case reports may be absent because of a low level of transmission, a high level of immunity in the population (because of vaccination, for example), or failure of local surveillance systems to detect cases. Since "epidemiologic silence" does not mean absence of risk, travelers should not go into endemic areas without taking protective measures.

YF virus transmission in rural West Africa is seasonal, with an elevated risk during the end of the rainy season and the beginning of the dry season (usually July–October). However, *Ae. aegypti* may transmit YF virus episodically, even during the dry season, in both rural and densely settled urban areas. The risk for infection by sylvatic vectors in South America is highest during the rainy season (January–May, with a peak incidence in February and March).

## Table 4-23. Countries with risk of yellow fever (YF) virus transmission[1]

| AFRICA | | | CENTRAL AND SOUTH AMERICA |
|---|---|---|---|
| Angola | Ethiopia[2] | Nigeria | Argentina[2] |
| Benin | Gabon | Senegal | Bolivia[2] |
| Burkina Faso | The Gambia | Sierra Leone | Brazil[2] |
| Burundi | Ghana | South Sudan | Colombia[2] |
| Cameroon | Guinea | Sudan[2] | Ecuador[2] |
| Central African Republic | Guinea-Bissau | Togo | French Guiana |
| Chad[2] | Kenya[2] | Uganda | Guyana |
| Congo, Republic of the | Liberia | | Panama[2] |
| Côte d'Ivoire | Mali[2] | | Paraguay |
| Democratic Republic of the Congo | Mauritania[2] | | Peru[2] |
| Equatorial Guinea | Niger[2] | | Suriname |
| | | | Trinidad and Tobago[2] |
| | | | Venezuela[2] |

[1] Defined by the World Health Organization as countries or areas where YF "has been reported currently or in the past and vectors and animal reservoirs currently exist." See current Annex 1 and country list on the WHO *International Travel and Health* webpage at www.who.int/ith/en.
[2] These countries are not holoendemic (only a portion of the country has risk of YF virus + transmission). See Maps 4-13 and 4-14 and YF vaccine recommendations (Yellow Fever Vaccine & Malaria Prophylaxis Information, by Country) for details.

From 1970 through 2015, 11 cases of YF were reported in travelers from the United States and Europe who traveled to West Africa (6 cases) or South America (5 cases). Eight of 11 travelers (73%) died. Only 1 traveler had a documented history of YF vaccination; that patient survived. Starting in 2016, the number of travel-associated YF cases increased substantially, primarily because of outbreaks in Angola and Brazil. From 2016 through mid-2018, more than 35 travel-associated cases were reported in unvaccinated travelers who were residents of nonendemic areas or countries, including at least 13 European travelers and 1 American traveler to Peru.

The risk of acquiring YF during travel is difficult to predict because of variations in ecologic determinants of virus transmission. For a 2-week stay, the estimated risks for illness and for death

## Table 4-24. Countries with low potential for exposure to yellow fever (YF) virus[1]

| AFRICA |
|---|
| Eritrea[2] |
| Rwanda |
| São Tomé and Príncipe |
| Somalia[2] |
| Tanzania |
| Zambia[2] |

[1] These countries are not on the World Health Organization list of countries with risk of YF virus transmission (Table 4-23). Therefore, proof of YF vaccination should not be required if traveling from any of these countries to another country with a vaccination entry requirement (unless that country requires proof of YF vaccination from all arriving travelers; see Table 4-27).
[2] These countries are classified as "low potential for exposure to YF virus" in only some areas; the remaining areas of these countries are classified as having no risk of exposure to YF virus.

due to YF for an unvaccinated traveler visiting an endemic area are as follows:

- In West Africa, 50 per 100,000 and 10 per 100,000, respectively

- In South America, 5 per 100,000 and 1 per 100,000, respectively

These estimates are based on the risk to indigenous populations, often during peak transmission season. They may not accurately reflect the risk to travelers who have a different immunity profile, take precautions against mosquito bites, and have less outdoor exposure. However, the risk of infection for travelers is likely higher during outbreaks, as demonstrated with recent outbreaks in Angola and Brazil.

## CLINICAL PRESENTATION

Most people infected with YF virus likely do not seek medical attention because they have minimal or no symptoms. For people who develop symptomatic illness, the incubation period is typically 3–6 days. The initial illness is nonspecific: fever, chills, headache, backache, myalgia, prostration, nausea, and vomiting. Most patients improve after the initial presentation. After a brief remission of up to 24 hours, approximately 12% of those infected progress to a more serious form of the disease, characterized by jaundice, hemorrhagic symptoms, and eventually shock and multisystem organ failure. The case-fatality ratio for severe cases is 30%–60%.

## DIAGNOSIS

The preliminary diagnosis is based on the patient's clinical features and exposure details. Laboratory diagnosis is best performed by:

- *Virus isolation or nucleic acid amplification tests performed early in the illness for YF virus or YF viral RNA.* By the time more overt symptoms are recognized, the virus or viral RNA may no longer be detectable. Therefore, virus isolation and nucleic acid amplification should not be used to rule out a diagnosis of YF.

- *Serologic assays to detect virus-specific IgM and IgG antibodies.* Because of cross-reactivity between antibodies raised against other flaviviruses, more specific antibody testing, such as a plaque reduction neutralization test, should be performed to confirm the infection.

Clinicians should contact their state or local health department or call the CDC Arboviral Diseases Branch at 970-221-6400 for assistance with diagnostic testing for YF virus infections. YF is a nationally notifiable disease.

## TREATMENT

There are no specific medications to treat YF virus infections; treatment is directed at symptomatic relief or life-saving interventions. Rest, fluids, and use of analgesics and antipyretics may relieve symptoms of aching and fever. Care should be taken to avoid medications such as aspirin or nonsteroidal anti-inflammatory drugs, which may increase the risk for bleeding. Infected people should be protected from further mosquito exposure (by staying indoors or under a mosquito net) during the first few days of illness, so they do not contribute to the transmission cycle.

## PREVENTION

### Personal Protection Measures

The best way to prevent mosquitoborne diseases, including YF, is to avoid mosquito bites (see Chapter 3, Mosquitoes, Ticks & Other Arthropods).

### Vaccine

YF is preventable by a relatively safe, effective vaccine. All YF vaccines currently manufactured are live attenuated viral vaccines. Only one YF vaccine (YF-VAX, Sanofi Pasteur) is licensed for use in the United States (Table 4-25). There have been periodic shortages of YF-VAX, including one that started in late 2015 that necessitated the importation and distribution of Stamaril, another YF vaccine produced by Sanofi Pasteur in France, under an expanded-access investigational new drug protocol.

There are no substantial differences in reactogenicity or immunogenicity of the different YF vaccine products, including those manufactured outside the United States. People who receive YF vaccines licensed in other countries but not approved by the US Food and Drug Administration (FDA) should be considered protected against YF. For the most up-to-date information

4

# Table 4-25. Vaccine to prevent yellow fever (YF)

| VACCINE | TRADE NAME (MANUFACTURER) | AGE | DOSE | ROUTE | SCHEDULE | BOOSTER |
|---|---|---|---|---|---|---|
| 17D | YF-VAX (Sanofi Pasteur) | ≥9 months[1] | 0.5mL[2] | SC | 1 dose | Not recommended for most[3] |

Abbreviation: SC, subcutaneous.

[1] Ages 6–8 months and ≥60 years are precautions and age <6 months is a contraindication to the use of YF vaccine.

[2] YF-VAX is available in single-dose and multiple-dose (5-dose) vials.

[3] For further details regarding revaccination see "Vaccine Administration" in this section.

on YF vaccine availability, providers should check the CDC Travelers' Health website at www.cdc.gov/travel.

## INDICATIONS FOR USE

YF vaccine is recommended for people aged ≥9 months who are traveling to or living in areas with risk for YF virus transmission in South America and Africa. In addition, some countries require proof of YF vaccination for entry. For country-specific YF vaccination recommendations and requirements, see Chapter 2, Yellow Fever Vaccine & Malaria Prophylaxis Information, by Country.

Because of the risk of serious adverse events after YF vaccination, clinicians should only vaccinate people who are at risk of exposure to YF virus or who require proof of vaccination to enter

a country. To minimize further the risk of serious adverse events, clinicians should carefully observe the contraindications and consider the precautions to vaccination before administering YF vaccine (Table 4-26). For additional information, refer to the YF vaccine recommendations of the Advisory Committee on Immunization Practices (ACIP) at www.cdc.gov/vaccines/hcp/acip-recs/vacc-specific/yf.html.

## VACCINE ADMINISTRATION

For all eligible people, a single 0.5-mL injection of reconstituted vaccine should be administered subcutaneously. Fractional dosing of yellow fever vaccine (administering a partial dose, usually 0.1 mL) has been used recently in several countries to control large yellow fever outbreaks during

# Table 4-26. Contraindications and precautions to yellow fever vaccine administration

| CONTRAINDICATIONS | PRECAUTIONS |
|---|---|
| • Allergy to vaccine component[1]<br>• Age <6 months<br>• Symptomatic HIV infection or CD4 T lymphocytes <200/mm³ (or <15% of total lymphocytes in children aged <6 years)[2]<br>• Thymus disorder associated with abnormal immune-cell function<br>• Primary immunodeficiencies<br>• Malignant neoplasms<br>• Transplantation<br>• Immunosuppressive and immunomodulatory therapies | • Age 6–8 months<br>• Age ≥60 years<br>• Asymptomatic HIV infection and CD4 T lymphocytes 200–499/mm³ (or 15%–24% of total lymphocytes in children aged <6 years)[2]<br>• Pregnancy<br>• Breastfeeding |

[1] If vaccination is considered, desensitization can be performed under direct supervision of a physician experienced in the management of anaphylaxis.

[2] Symptoms of HIV are classified in 1) Adults and Adolescents, Table 1. CDC. 1993 Revised classification system for HIV infection and expanded surveillance case definition for AIDS among adolescents and adults. MMWR Recomm Rep 1992;41(RR-17). Available from: www.cdc.gov/mmwr/preview/mmwrhtml/00018871.htm and 2) Panel on Antiretroviral Therapy and Medical Management of HIV-Infected Children. Guidelines for the use of antiretroviral agents in pediatric HIV infection. 2010. Available from http://aidsinfo.nih.gov/ContentFiles/PediatricGuidelines.pdf. pp. 20–2.

conditions of limited vaccine availability. **In the United States, FDA has not approved fractional dosing of yellow fever vaccine. Furthermore, the World Health Organization (WHO) notes that a fractional dose of yellow fever vaccine does not meet the requirements of a dose of vaccine according to the International Health Regulations (IHR); therefore, proof of vaccination may not be issued to a person who has received only a fractional dose.**

In 2014, the WHO Strategic Advisory Group of Experts on Immunization concluded that a single primary dose of YF vaccine provides sustained immunity and lifelong protection against YF disease and that a booster dose is not needed. In 2016, the IHR were officially amended to specify that a completed International Certificate of Vaccination or Prophylaxis (ICVP or "yellow card") is valid for the lifetime of the vaccinee, and countries cannot require proof of revaccination (booster) against YF as a condition of entry, even if the last vaccination was >10 years prior.

ACIP also stated that a single dose of YF vaccine provides long-lasting protection and is adequate for most travelers. However, these guidelines differ slightly from those of WHO. ACIP guidelines specify that additional doses of YF vaccine are recommended for the following groups of travelers:

- Women who were pregnant when they received their initial dose of vaccine should receive 1 additional dose before they are next at risk for YF.

- People who received a hematopoietic stem cell transplant after receiving a dose of YF vaccine should be revaccinated before they are next at risk for YF as long as they are sufficiently immunocompetent.

- People infected with HIV when they received their last dose of YF vaccine should receive a dose every 10 years if they continue to be at risk for YF.

Consider administering a booster dose for travelers who received their last dose of YF vaccine ≥10 years previously who will be going to higher-risk settings based on season, location, activities, and duration of travel. This includes travelers planning prolonged stays in endemic areas, those traveling to endemic areas such as rural West Africa during peak transmission season, or travelers visiting areas with ongoing outbreaks. Refer to the ACIP website (www.cdc.gov/vaccines/hcp/acip-recs/vacc-specific/yf.html) for all current ACIP YF vaccine recommendations.

Although booster doses of YF vaccine are not recommended for most travelers, and despite the recent changes to the IHR, clinicians and travelers should nonetheless review the entry requirements for destination countries. For more information on country-specific recommendations and requirements, see Chapter 2, Yellow Fever Vaccine & Malaria Prophylaxis Information, by Country.

## VACCINE SAFETY AND ADVERSE REACTIONS
### COMMON ADVERSE REACTIONS
Reactions to YF vaccine are generally mild; 10%–30% of vaccinees report mild systemic adverse events, including low-grade fever, headache, and myalgia that begin within days after vaccination and last 5–10 days.

### SEVERE ADVERSE REACTIONS
#### *HYPERSENSITIVITY*
Immediate hypersensitivity reactions, characterized by rash, urticaria, or bronchospasm are uncommon. Anaphylaxis after YF vaccine is reported to occur at a rate of 1.3 cases per 100,000 doses administered.

#### *YELLOW FEVER VACCINE–ASSOCIATED NEUROLOGIC DISEASE (YEL-AND)*
YEL-AND represents a conglomeration of clinical syndromes, including meningoencephalitis, Guillain-Barré syndrome, acute disseminated encephalomyelitis, and, rarely, cranial nerve palsies. Historically, YEL-AND was seen primarily among infants as encephalitis, but more recent reports have been among people of all ages. YEL-AND is rarely fatal.

Among all cases of YEL-AND reported globally, almost all occurred in first-time vaccine recipients. The onset of illness for documented cases in the United States is 2–56 days after vaccination. The incidence of YEL-AND in the United States is 0.8 per 100,000 doses administered but is higher (2.2 per 100,000 doses) in people aged ≥60 years.

### YELLOW FEVER VACCINE–ASSOCIATED VISCEROTROPIC DISEASE (YEL-AVD)

YEL-AVD is a severe illness similar to wild-type YF disease, with vaccine virus proliferating in multiple organs and often leading to multiorgan dysfunction or failure and occasionally death. Since the initial cases of YEL-AVD were published in 2001, >100 confirmed and suspected cases have been reported throughout the world.

YEL-AVD has been reported to occur only after the first dose of YF vaccine; there have been no laboratory-confirmed reports of YEL-AVD following booster doses. For YEL-AVD cases reported in the United States, the median time from YF vaccination until symptom onset is 4 days (range, 1–18 days). The case-fatality ratio is approximately 48% and the incidence is 0.3 cases per 100,000 doses of vaccine administered. The incidence of YEL-AVD is higher for people aged ≥60 years, 1.2 per 100,000 doses, and is even higher for people aged ≥70 years.

## CONTRAINDICATIONS

People who have a contraindication to YF vaccine should not be vaccinated. If travel to a YF-endemic area cannot be avoided, a medical waiver (Figure 4-3) should be provided, and protective measures against mosquito bites should be emphasized.

Contraindications to receiving YF vaccine include age <6 months, hypersensitivity to vaccine components, and various forms of altered immunity (including symptomatic HIV infection or HIV infection with severe immunosuppression).

### INFANTS YOUNGER THAN 6 MONTHS

YF vaccine is contraindicated in infants aged <6 months because the rate of YEL-AND is high (50–400 cases per 100,000 infants vaccinated). The mechanism of increased neurovirulence in infants is unknown but may be due to the immaturity of the blood–brain barrier, higher or more prolonged viremia, or immune system immaturity.

### HYPERSENSITIVITY

YF vaccine is contraindicated in people with a history of acute hypersensitivity reaction to a previous dose of the vaccine or to any of the vaccine components, including eggs, egg products, chicken proteins, or gelatin. The stopper used in

vials of vaccine also contains dry natural latex rubber, which may cause an allergic reaction. If vaccination of a person with a questionable history of hypersensitivity to a vaccine component is considered essential, skin testing and, if indicated, desensitization should be performed by an experienced clinician according to instructions provided by the manufacturer in the vaccine prescribing information.

### ALTERED IMMUNE STATUS
#### THYMUS DISORDER

YF vaccine is contraindicated in people with a thymus disorder associated with abnormal immune cell function, such as thymoma or myasthenia gravis. There is no evidence of immune dysfunction or increased risk of YF vaccine–associated serious adverse events in people who have undergone incidental thymectomy or who have had indirect radiation therapy in the distant past; these people can be vaccinated.

### HIV INFECTION

YF vaccine is contraindicated in people with AIDS or other clinical manifestations of HIV infection, including those with CD4 T lymphocyte values <200/mm³ or <15% of total lymphocytes for children aged <6 years. This recommendation is based on the potential increased risk of encephalitis in this population. See the following section ("Precautions") for guidance regarding other HIV-infected people not meeting the above criteria.

### IMMUNODEFICIENCIES (OTHER THAN THYMUS DISORDER OR HIV INFECTION)

YF vaccine is contraindicated in people who are immunodeficient or immunosuppressed, whether due to an underlying (primary) disorder or medical treatment. This includes organ transplant patients and those with malignant neoplasms. See Chapter 5, Immunocompromised Travelers.

### IMMUNOSUPPRESSIVE AND IMMUNOMODULATORY THERAPIES

YF vaccine is contraindicated in people whose immunologic response is either suppressed or modulated by current or recent radiation therapy or drugs. Drugs with known immunosuppressive or immunomodulatory properties include, but are not limited to, high-dose systemic corticosteroids, alkylating agents, antimetabolites, tumor necrosis factor-$\alpha$ inhibitors (such as etanercept), interleukin blocking agents (such as anakinra and tocilizumab), or other monoclonal antibodies targeting immune cells (such as rituximab or alemtuzumab). These people are presumed to be at increased risk for YF vaccine-associated serious adverse events, and the use of live attenuated vaccines is contraindicated in the package insert for most of these therapies (see Chapter 5, Immunocompromised Travelers). Live viral vaccines should be deferred in people who have discontinued these therapies until immune function has improved.

Family members of people with altered immune status, who themselves have no contraindications, can receive YF vaccine.

## PRECAUTIONS

If travel to a YF risk area is unavoidable for a person with a precaution to vaccination, the decision to vaccinate should balance the risks of YF virus exposure with the risk for an adverse event after vaccination. If international travel requirements, not risk of YF, are the only reason to vaccinate a person with a precaution to vaccination, the person should not be immunized and should be issued a medical waiver to fulfill health regulations.

Precautions to receiving YF vaccine include age 6–8 months, age ≥60 years, asymptomatic HIV infection with moderate immunosuppression, pregnancy, and breastfeeding.

### INFANTS AGED 6–8 MONTHS

Age 6–8 months is a precaution to receiving YF vaccine. Two cases of YEL-AND have been reported in infants aged 6–8 months. By 9 months of age, risk for YEL-AND is believed to be substantially lower. ACIP recommends that, whenever possible, travel to YF–endemic countries should be postponed or avoided for children aged 6–8 months.

### ADULTS 60 YEARS OF AGE OR OLDER

Age ≥60 years is a precaution to receiving YF vaccine, particularly a first ever dose. The rate of reported serious adverse events following YF vaccination in people aged ≥60 years is 7.7 per 100,000 doses distributed, compared with 3.8 per 100,000 for all YF vaccine recipients. The risks of YEL-AND and YEL-AVD are increased in this age group (see above). Given that YEL-AVD has been reported exclusively, and YEL-AND almost exclusively, in primary vaccine recipients, particular caution should be considered for older travelers receiving YF vaccine for the first time.

### HIV INFECTION

Asymptomatic HIV infection with CD4 T lymphocyte values 200–499/mm$^3$ or 15%–24% of total lymphocytes for children aged <6 years is a precaution to receiving YF vaccine (see also the previous discussion of HIV infection as a contraindication to YF vaccine administration). Combined studies of >500 HIV-infected people who had received YF vaccine reported no serious adverse events among patients considered moderately immunosuppressed based on their CD4 counts. However, HIV infection has been associated with a reduced immunologic response to a number of inactivated and live attenuated vaccines, including YF vaccine. The diminished immune response appears to be correlated with HIV RNA levels and CD4 T cell counts.

If an asymptomatic HIV-infected person has no evidence of immune suppression based on CD4 counts (CD4 T lymphocyte values ≥500/mm$^3$ or ≥25% of total lymphocytes for children aged <6 years), YF vaccine can be administered if recommended. Because vaccinating asymptomatic HIV-infected people might be less effective than vaccinating people not infected with HIV, measuring their neutralizing antibody response to vaccination should be considered before travel. Contact the state health department or the CDC Arboviral Diseases Branch (970-221-6400) to discuss serologic testing.

### PREGNANCY

Pregnancy is a precaution to receiving YF vaccine. The safety of YF vaccination during pregnancy has not been studied in any large prospective trials. A study of women vaccinated against YF early in their pregnancies detected no major malformations in their infants, although a slight increased risk for minor, mostly skin, malformations was noted. A higher rate of spontaneous abortions in pregnant women receiving the vaccine was reported but not substantiated by a subsequent study.

The proportion of women vaccinated during pregnancy who develop YF virus-specific IgG antibodies is variable depending on the study (39% or 98%) and may be correlated with the trimester in which they received the vaccine. Because pregnancy may affect immunologic function, serologic testing can be considered to document a protective immune response to the vaccine.

Although there are no specific data, ACIP recommends that a woman wait 4 weeks after receiving the YF vaccine before conceiving.

### BREASTFEEDING

Breastfeeding is a precaution to receiving YF vaccine. Three YEL-AND cases have been reported in exclusively breastfed infants whose mothers were vaccinated with YF vaccine. All 3 infants were diagnosed with encephalitis and aged <1 month at the time of exposure. Until specific research data are available, avoid vaccinating breastfeeding women against YF. However, when travel of nursing mothers to YF–endemic areas cannot be avoided or postponed, these women should be vaccinated. Although there are no data, some experts recommend that breastfeeding women who receive YF vaccine should temporarily suspend breastfeeding, pump, and discard pumped milk for at least 2 weeks after vaccination before resuming breastfeeding.

### OTHER CONSIDERATIONS

There are no data regarding possible increased adverse events or decreased vaccine efficacy after administration of YF vaccine to patients with other chronic medical conditions (such as renal disease, liver disease including hepatitis C virus infection, or diabetes mellitus). Limited data suggest that autoimmune disease, either by itself or in conjunction with other risk factors, including immunosuppressive medication, might increase the risk for YEL-AVD. Therefore, use caution if considering vaccination of such patients. Factors to consider in assessing patients' general level of immune competence include disease severity, duration, clinical stability, complications, comorbidities, and medications that the person is taking.

### SIMULTANEOUS ADMINISTRATION OF OTHER VACCINES AND DRUGS

No evidence exists that inactivated vaccines interfere with the immune response to YF vaccine. Therefore, inactivated vaccines can be administered either simultaneously or at any time before or after YF vaccination. ACIP recommends that YF vaccine be given at the same time as other live viral vaccines. Otherwise, the clinician should wait 30 days between vaccinations, as the immune response to a live viral vaccine might be impaired if administered within 30 days of another live viral vaccine.

Limited data suggest that coadministration of YF vaccine with measles-rubella (MR) or measles-mumps-rubella (MMR) vaccines might decrease the immune response. One study involving the simultaneous administration of YF and MMR vaccines and a second involving simultaneous administration of YF and MMR vaccines in children demonstrated a decreased immune response against all antigens except measles when the vaccines were given on the same day versus 30 days apart. Additional studies are needed to confirm these findings, but they suggest that if possible, YF and MMR should be given 30 days apart.

Data suggest oral Ty21a typhoid vaccine, a live bacterial vaccine, can be administered simultaneously or at any interval before or after YF vaccine. There are no data on the immune response to live attenuated oral cholera vaccine (Vaxchora) or nasally administered live attenuated influenza vaccine administered simultaneously with YF vaccine.

## INTERNATIONAL CERTIFICATE OF VACCINATION OR PROPHYLAXIS (ICVP)

The IHR allow countries to require proof of YF vaccination documented on an ICVP as a condition of entry for travelers arriving from certain countries, even if only in transit, to prevent importation and indigenous transmission of YF virus. Some countries require evidence of

## Table 4-27. Countries that require proof of yellow fever (YF) vaccination from all arriving travelers[1]

| | |
|---|---|
| Angola | Ghana |
| Burundi | Guinea-Bissau |
| Cameroon | Mali |
| Central African Republic | Niger |
| Chad | Sierra Leone |
| Congo, Republic of the | South Sudan |
| Côte d'Ivoire | Togo |
| Democratic Republic of the Congo | Uganda |
| Gabon | |

[1] Country requirements for YF vaccination are subject to change at any time; therefore, CDC encourages travelers to check with the destination country's embassy or consulate before departure.

vaccination from all entering travelers, which includes direct travel from the United States (Table 4-27). A traveler who has a specific contraindication to YF vaccine and who cannot avoid travel to a country requiring vaccination should request a waiver from a physician before embarking on travel (see the "Medical Waivers [Exemptions]" section below). Travelers arriving without proof of YF vaccination or a medical waiver to a country that has a YF vaccination entry requirement may be quarantined for up to 6 days, refused entry, or vaccinated on site.

## Authorization to Provide Vaccinations and to Validate the ICVP

People who received YF vaccination after December 15, 2007, must provide proof of vaccination on the new ICVP. If the person received the vaccine before December 15, 2007, their original International Certificate of Vaccination against Yellow Fever (ICV) card is still valid as proof of vaccination. Vaccinees should receive a completed ICVP (Figure 4-2), validated (stamped

and signed) with the stamp of the center where the vaccine was given (see below). Failure to secure validations can cause a traveler to be quarantined, denied entry, or possibly revaccinated at the point of entry to a country.

A properly filled out ICVP is valid beginning 10 days after the date of primary vaccination. As of July 2016, the YF vaccine booster requirement was eliminated in the IHR and a completed ICVP is considered valid for the lifetime of the vaccinee. Clinics may purchase ICVPs, CDC 731 (formerly PHS 731), from the US Government Publishing Office website (http://bookstore.gpo.gov) or by phone (866-512-1800).

## People Authorized to Sign the ICVP and Designated Yellow Fever Vaccination Centers

The ICVP must bear the signature of a licensed physician or a health care worker designated by the physician to supervise the administration of the vaccine (Figure 4-2). A signature stamp is not acceptable. YF vaccination must be given at an authorized center in possession of an official "uniform

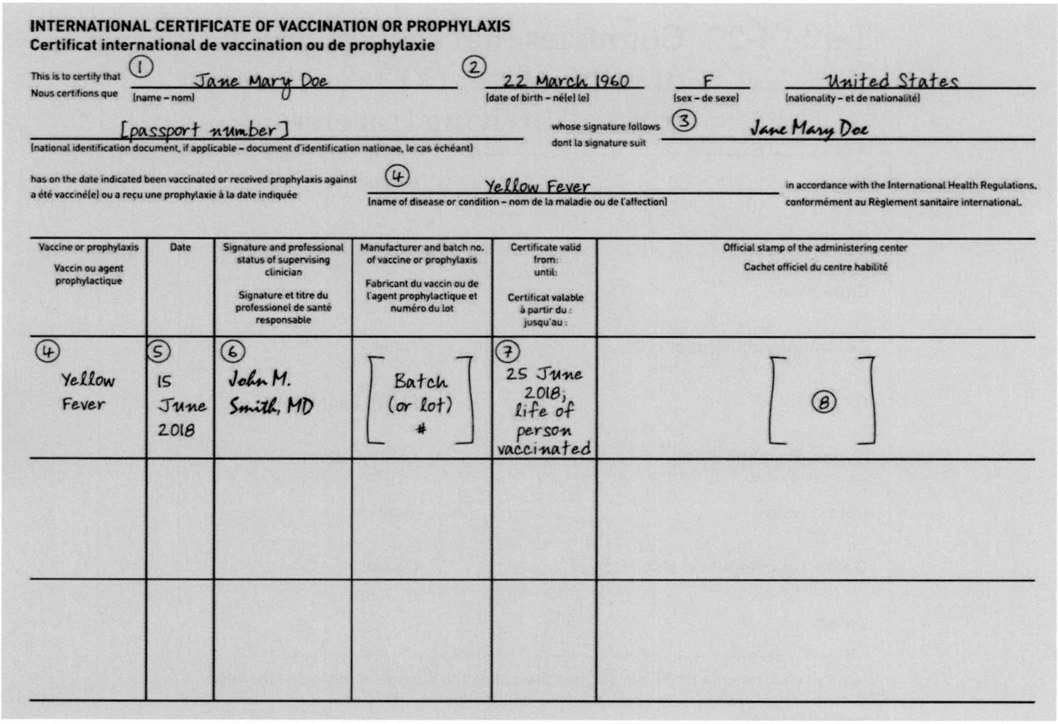

**INTERNATIONAL CERTIFICATE OF VACCINATION OR PROPHYLAXIS**
**Certificat international de vaccination ou de prophylaxie**

This is to certify that / Nous certifions que (1) Jane Mary Doe [name – nom] (2) 22 March 1960 [date of birth – né(e) le] F [sex – de sexe] United States [nationality – et de nationalité]

[passport number] [national identification document, if applicable – document d'identification nationae, le cas échéant] whose signature follows / dont la signature suit (3) Jane Mary Doe

has on the date indicated been vaccinated or received prophylaxis against / a été vacciné(e) ou a reçu une prophylaxie à la date indiquée (4) Yellow Fever [name of disease or condition – nom de la maladie ou de l'affection] in accordance with the International Health Regulations. / conformément au Règlement sanitaire international.

| Vaccine or prophylaxis<br>Vaccin ou agent prophylactique | Date | Signature and professional status of supervising clinician<br>Signature et titre du professionel de santé responsable | Manufacturer and batch no. of vaccine or prophylaxis<br>Fabricant du vaccin ou de l'agent prophylactique et numéro du lot | Certificate valid from: until:<br>Certificat valable à partir du : jusqu'au : | Official stamp of the administering center<br>Cachet officiel du centre habilité |
|---|---|---|---|---|---|
| (4) Yellow Fever | (5) 15 June 2018 | (6) John M. Smith, MD | [ Batch (or lot) # ] | (7) 25 June 2018; life of person vaccinated | [ (8) ] |
| | | | | | |
| | | | | | |

FIGURE 4-2. **Example International Certificate of Vaccination or Prophylaxis (ICVP)**

(1) Name should appear exactly as on the patient's passport.
(2, 5, 7) All dates should be entered with the day in numerals, followed by the month in letters, then the year. For example: in the above example, the patient's date of birth is 22 March 1960.
(3) This space is for the patient's signature.
(4) For a yellow fever (YF) vaccination, "Yellow Fever" should be written in both spaces. Should the ICVP be used for a required vaccination or prophylaxis against another disease or condition (following an amendment to the International Health Regulations or by recommendation of the World Health Organization), that disease or condition should be written in this space. Other vaccinations may be listed on the other side.
(5) The date on which the vaccination is given should be entered as shown above.
(6) A handwritten signature of the clinician—either the stamp holder or another health care provider authorized by the stamp holder—administering or supervising the administration of the vaccine (or prophylaxis) should appear in this box. A signature stamp is not acceptable.
(7) The certificate of YF vaccination (ICVP) is valid beginning 10 days after the date of primary vaccination, which should be noted in the box for "certificate valid from." As of July 2016, the YF vaccine booster requirement was eliminated in the IHR, and a completed ICVP is considered valid for the lifetime of the vaccinee. Suggested wording to write in the ICVP box for "certificate valid until" is "life of person vaccinated." For the most recent information on YF vaccination entry requirements by country, consult the destination pages of the CDC Travelers' Health website.
(8) The Uniform Stamp of the vaccinating center should appear in this box.

stamp," which can be used to validate the ICVP. In the United States, state health departments are responsible for designating nonfederal YF vaccination centers and issuing uniform stamps to clinicians. Information about the location and hours of YF vaccination centers may be obtained by visiting CDC's website at wwwnc.cdc.gov/travel/yellow-fever-vaccination-clinics-search.aspx.

## Medical Waivers (Exemptions)

A clinician issuing a waiver for YF vaccine should complete and sign the "Medical Contraindications to Vaccination" section of the ICVP (Figure 4-3). Reasons other than medical contraindications are not acceptable for exemption from vaccination. The clinician should also do the following:

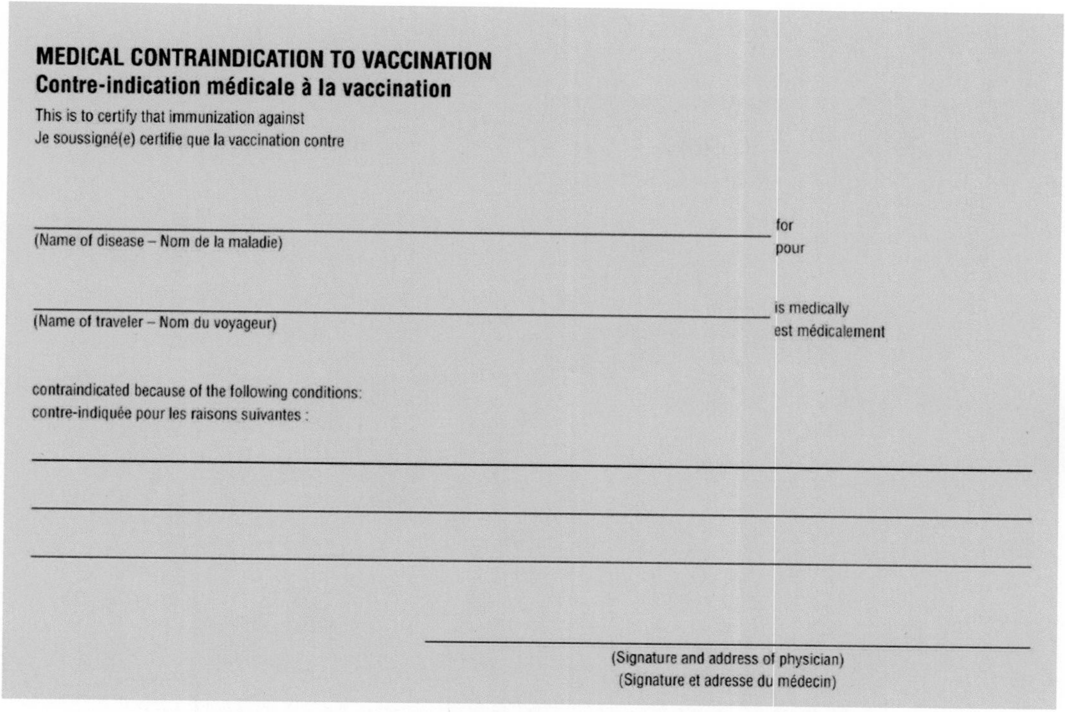

**MEDICAL CONTRAINDICATION TO VACCINATION**
**Contre-indication médicale à la vaccination**

This is to certify that immunization against
Je soussigné(e) certifie que la vaccination contre

_____ for
(Name of disease – Nom de la maladie)                pour

_____ is medically
(Name of traveler – Nom du voyageur)                 est médicalement

contraindicated because of the following conditions:
contre-indiquée pour les raisons suivantes :

_____

_____

_____

_____
                    (Signature and address of physician)
                    (Signature et adresse du médecin)

**4**

**FIGURE 4-3.** Medical Contraindication to Vaccination section of the International Certificate of Vaccination or Prophylaxis (ICVP)

- Provide the traveler with a signed and dated exemption letter on letterhead stationery, clearly stating the contraindications to vaccination and bearing the stamp used by the YF vaccination center to validate the ICVP.

- Advise the traveler that a medical waiver may not be accepted by the destination country.

- Inform the traveler of any increased risk for YF infection associated with lack of vaccination and how to minimize this risk by strictly adhering to mosquito bite prevention measures.

To improve the likelihood that the waiver will be accepted at the destination country, the clinician can suggest that the traveler take the following additional measures before beginning travel:

- Obtain specific and authoritative advice from the embassy or consulate of the destination country or countries.

- Request documentation of requirements for waivers from embassies or consulates and retain these, along with the completed Medical Contraindication to Vaccination section of the ICVP.

## REQUIREMENTS VERSUS RECOMMENDATIONS

Country entry _requirements_ for proof of YF vaccination under the IHR differ from CDC's _recommendations_. Countries may establish YF vaccine entry requirements to prevent the importation and transmission of YF virus. Travelers must comply with these requirements to enter the country, unless they have been issued a medical waiver. Certain countries require vaccination from travelers arriving from all countries (Table 4-27), while some countries require vaccination only for travelers above a certain age coming from countries with risk of YF virus transmission (see Chapter 2, Yellow Fever Vaccine & Malaria Prophylaxis Information, by Country).

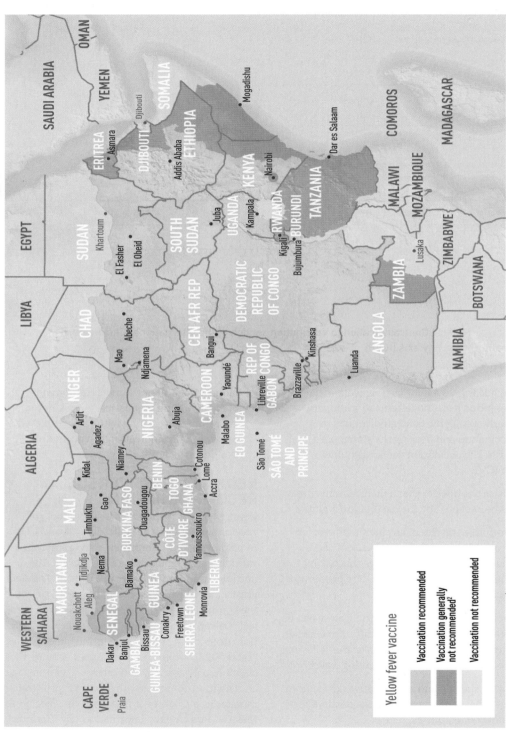

MAP 4-13. Yellow fever vaccine recommendations in Africa[1]

[1] Current as of August 2018. This map is an updated version of the 2010 map created by the Informal WHO Working Group on the Geographic Risk of Yellow Fever.

[2] Yellow fever (YF) vaccination is generally not recommended in areas where there is low potential for YF virus exposure. However, vaccination might be considered for a small subset of travelers to these areas who are at increased risk for exposure to YF virus because of prolonged travel, heavy exposure to mosquitoes, or inability to avoid mosquito bites. Consideration for vaccination of any traveler must take into account the traveler's risk of being infected with YF virus, country entry requirements, and individual risk factors for serious vaccine-associated adverse events (e.g, age, immune status).

**Yellow fever vaccine**

Vaccination recommended

Vaccination generally not recommended[2]

Vaccination not recommended

4

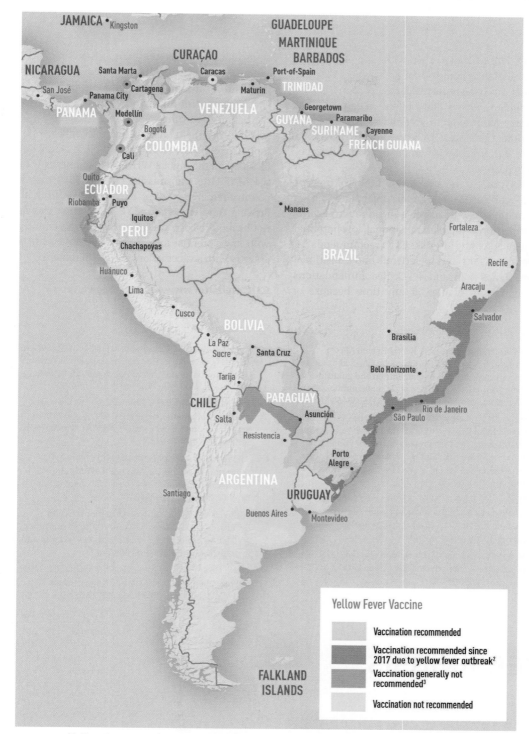

**Yellow Fever Vaccine**

Vaccination recommended

Vaccination recommended since 2017 due to yellow fever outbreak[2]

Vaccination generally not recommended[3]

Vaccination not recommended

MAP 4-14. **Yellow fever vaccine recommendations in the Americas**[1]

[1] Current as of August 2018. This map is an updated version of the 2010 map created by the Informal WHO Working Group on the Geographic Risk of Yellow Fever.

[2] In 2017, CDC expanded yellow fever vaccination recommendations for travelers to Brazil because of a large outbreak of yellow fever in multiple states in that country. Please refer to the CDC Travelers' Health website (www.cdc.gov/travel) for more information and updated recommendations.

[3] Yellow fever (YF) vaccination is generally not recommended in areas where there is low potential for YF virus exposure. However, vaccination might be considered for a small subset of travelers to these areas who are at increased risk for exposure to YF virus because of prolonged travel, heavy exposure to mosquitoes, or inability to avoid mosquito bites. Consideration for vaccination of any traveler must take into account the traveler's risk of being infected with YF virus, country entry requirements, and individual risk factors for serious vaccine-associated adverse events (such as age or immune status).

WHO defines those areas with risk of YF virus transmission as countries or areas where YF virus activity has been reported currently or in the past and where vectors and animal reservoirs exist. Country requirements are subject to change at any time; therefore, CDC encourages travelers to check with the relevant embassy or consulate before departure.

CDC bases its advice on how to prevent travel-associated YF virus infections on a destination-specific risk classification for YF virus transmission: endemic, transitional, low potential for exposure, and no risk. CDC recommends YF vaccination for travel to endemic and transitional areas (Maps 4-13 and 4-14). Recommendations are subject to change at any time because of

changes in YF virus circulation; therefore, CDC encourages travelers to check the destination pages for up-to-date vaccine information and to check for relevant travel notices on the CDC website before departure (www.cdc.gov/travel).

Countries that contain areas with only low potential for exposure to YF virus (Table 4-24) are not included on the official WHO list of countries with risk of YF virus transmission (Table 4-23). Unless a country requires proof of YF vaccination from all arriving travelers, proof of YF vaccination should not be required of travelers coming from a country with low potential for exposure to YF virus to a country with a vaccination entry requirement.

**CDC website:** www.cdc.gov/yellowfever

## BIBLIOGRAPHY

1. Gershman MD, Staples JE, Bentsi-Enchill AD, Breugelmans JG, Brito GS, Camacho LA, et al. Viscerotropic disease: case definition and guidelines for collection, analysis, and presentation of immunization safety data. Vaccine. 2012 Jul 13;30(33):5038–58.

2. Jentes ES, Poumerol G, Gershman MD, Hill DR, Lemarchand J, Lewis RF, et al. The revised global yellow fever risk map and recommendations for vaccination, 2010: consensus of the Informal WHO Working Group on Geographic Risk for Yellow Fever. Lancet Infect Dis. 2011 Aug;11(8):622–32.

3. Lindsey NP, Rabe IB, Miller ER, Fischer M, Staples JE. Adverse event reports following yellow fever vaccination, 2007–13. J Travel Med. 2016 Sep;23(5): doi.org/10.1093/jtm/taw045.

4. Monath TP, Cetron MS. Prevention of yellow fever in persons traveling to the tropics. Clin Infect Dis. 2002 May 15;34(10):1369–78.

5. Staples JE, Bocchini JA, Jr., Rubin L, Fischer M. Yellow fever vaccine booster doses: recommendations of the Advisory Committee on Immunization Practices, 2015. MMWR Morb Mortal Wkly Rep. 2015 Jun 19;64(23):647–50.

6. Staples JE, Gershman M, Fischer M. Yellow fever vaccine: recommendations of the Advisory Committee on Immunization Practices (ACIP). MMWR Recomm Rep. 2010 Jul 30;59(RR-7):1–27.

7. Staples JE, Monath TP, Gershman MD, Barrett ADT. Yellow fever vaccine. In: Plotkin SA, Orenstein WA, Offit PA, editors. Vaccines. 7th ed. Philadelphia: Elsevier; 2018. pp. 1181–1265.

8. World Health Organization. International Health Regulations, 2005. Geneva: World Health Organization; 2016 [cited 2018 Apr 23]. Available from: www.who.int/ihr/publications/9789241580496/en/.

9. World Health Organization. Vaccines and vaccination against yellow fever. WHO position paper—June 2013. Wkly Epidemiol Rec. 2013 Jul 5;88(27):269–83.

# YERSINIOSIS

Louise K. Francois Watkins, Cindy R. Friedman

## INFECTIOUS AGENT

*Yersinia* species are facultative anaerobic gram-negative coccobacilli. The most common species that cause yersiniosis are *Yersinia enterocolitica* (serogroups O:3, O:5,27, O:8,

and O:9), but disease is also caused by *Y. pseudotuberculosis. Yersinia pestis*, the causative agent of plague, is discussed in this chapter under the heading Plague (Bubonic, Pneumonic, Septicemic).

## TRANSMISSION

Transmission of *Yersinia* spp. may occur as a result of consuming or handling contaminated food (commonly raw or undercooked pork products, such as chitterlings); consuming milk that was not pasteurized, inadequately pasteurized, or contaminated after pasteurization; or being exposed to untreated water. *Yersinia* spp. may also be transmitted by direct or indirect contact with animals. Pigs are a major reservoir of pathogenic *Y. enterocolitica*, but a variety of other farm, wild, and domestic animals, such as cattle, deer, and dogs may harbor *Yersinia* spp. Transmission through blood product transfusions has been reported.

## EPIDEMIOLOGY

Yersiniosis is most commonly reported from northern Europe (particularly Scandinavia), Japan, and Canada; however, it is not a reportable condition in most countries, so infections in countries without surveillance programs may be underrepresented; it is not nationally reportable in the United States. In the United States, *Y. enterocolitica* causes about 92% of infections with known species information, accounting for an estimated 117,000 illnesses, 640 hospitalizations, and 35 deaths every year.

In temperate climates, the risk of infection is higher in cooler months. Children are infected more often than adults. People with diseases that cause high iron levels, such as hemochromatosis and thalassemia, including those on iron chelation treatment, are at higher risk for infection and severe disease. The incidence among travelers to developing countries is generally low. A US study found that approximately 6% of *Y. enterocolitica* infections were travel associated.

## CLINICAL PRESENTATION

The incubation period is 4–6 days (range, 1–14 days), and symptom onset may be more gradual compared with infections caused by other enteric pathogens. Enterocolitis is the most common clinical presentation; symptoms typically include fever, abdominal pain, and diarrhea, which may be bloody and can persist for several weeks. Sore throat may also occur, particularly in children. Mesenteric adenitis, which presents as pain mimicking appendicitis, has been well described. Necrotizing enterocolitis has been described in young infants. Reactive arthritis affecting the wrists, knees, and ankles can occur, usually 1 month after the initial diarrhea episode, resolving after 1–6 months. Erythema nodosum, manifesting as painful, raised red or purple lesions along the trunk and legs, can occur and usually resolves spontaneously within 1 month.

## DIAGNOSIS

Diagnosis is frequently made by isolating the organism from stool, blood, bile, wound, throat swab, mesenteric lymph node, cerebrospinal fluid, or peritoneal fluid. If yersiniosis is suspected, the clinical laboratory should be notified because cold enrichment, alkali treatment, or plating on CIN agar can be used to increase the likelihood of a positive culture. Several culture-independent diagnostic tests (CIDTs) are now available and have more than doubled the detection rate of *Yersinia* spp. in the United States. CIDT panels typically target only *Y. enterocolitica*, and the rarity of yersiniosis has precluded robust evaluation of the specificity and sensitivity of CIDT platforms through prospective studies. Culture is required to determine species and for antibiotic susceptibility testing.

## TREATMENT

Most infections are self-limited. Antibiotics should be given for moderate to severe cases. *Y. enterocolitica* isolates are usually susceptible to trimethoprim-sulfamethoxazole, aminoglycosides, third-generation cephalosporins, fluoroquinolones, and tetracyclines; they are typically resistant to first-generation cephalosporins and most penicillins. Antimicrobial therapy has no effect on postinfectious sequelae.

## PREVENTION

Travelers can reduce the risk of *Yersinia* spp. infection by avoiding consumption of raw or undercooked pork products, unpasteurized milk products, and untreated water (see Chapter 2, Food & Water Precautions). Washing hands with soap and water before eating and preparing food, after contact with animals, and after handling raw meat helps reduce risk.

**CDC website:** www.cdc.gov/yersinia

## BIBLIOGRAPHY

1. Chakraborty A, Komatsu K, Roberts M, Collins J, Beggs J, Turabelidze G, et al. The descriptive epidemiology of yersiniosis: a multistate study, 2005–2011. Public Health Rep. 2015 May–Jun;130(3):269–77.

2. Kendall ME, Crim S, Fullerton K, Han PV, Cronquist AB, Shiferaw B, et al. Travel-associated enteric infections diagnosed after return to the United States, Foodborne Diseases Active Surveillance Network (FoodNet), 2004–2009. Clin Infect Dis. 2012 Jun;54 Suppl 5:S480–7.

3. Long C, Jones TF, Vugia DJ, Scheftel J, Strockbine N, Ryan P, et al. Yersinia pseudotuberculosis and Y. enterocolitica infections, FoodNet, 1996–2007. Emerg Infect Dis. 2010 Mar;16(3):566–7.

4. Marder E, Griffin PM, Cieslak PR, Dunn J, Hurd S, Jervis R, et al. Preliminary incidence and trends of infections with pathogens transmitted commonly through food— Foodborne Diseases Active Surveillance Network, 10 U.S. Sites, 2006–2017. MMWR Morb Mortal Wkly Rep. 2018 Mar; 67(11);324–8.

5. Mead PS. Yersinia species, including plague. In: Bennett JE, Dolin R, Blaser MJ, editors. Mandell, Douglas, and Bennett's Principles and Practice of Infectious Diseases. 8th ed. Philadelphia: Saunders Elsevier; 2015. pp. 2615–17.

**4**

# ZIKA

J. Erin Staples, Stacey W. Martin, Marc Fischer

## INFECTIOUS AGENT

Zika virus is a single-stranded RNA virus of the Flaviviridae family, genus *Flavivirus*.

## TRANSMISSION

Transmission occurs through the bite of an infected *Aedes* species mosquito. Intrauterine, perinatal, sexual, laboratory, and possible transfusion-associated transmission have been reported. Zika virus has been detected in human milk, but the risk of transmission through breastfeeding is unknown.

## EPIDEMIOLOGY

Zika virus was first identified in Uganda in 1947. Before 2007, only sporadic human cases were reported from countries in Africa and Asia. In 2007, the first documented Zika virus disease outbreak was reported in the Federated States of Micronesia. Subsequent outbreaks of Zika virus disease occurred in countries in Southeast Asia and the Western Pacific.

Zika virus was identified for the first time in the Western hemisphere in 2015, with large outbreaks in Brazil. The virus then spread throughout much of the Americas, with 48 countries and territories reporting local transmission. In 2016, large outbreaks occurred in the Caribbean (Puerto Rico and the US Virgin Islands), and limited local transmission was identified in the mainland United States (parts of Florida and Texas). Since then, the number of reported Zika virus disease cases in the Americas has declined in all regions, though there have been occasional increases in reporting from some countries. Current information on Zika virus transmission and travel guidance can be found at wwwnc.cdc.gov/travel/page/zika-travel-information.

## CLINICAL PRESENTATION

Most Zika virus infections are asymptomatic. Symptomatic infections are generally mild. Commonly reported signs and symptoms include fever, maculopapular rash, arthralgia, and nonpurulent conjunctivitis. Other symptoms include myalgia, headache, edema, vomiting, retroorbital pain, and lymphadenopathy. Severe disease requiring hospitalization and deaths are uncommon. However, Guillain-Barré syndrome and rare reports of encephalopathy, meningoencephalitis, myelitis, uveitis, and severe thrombocytopenia have been associated with Zika virus infection.

Vertical transmission of the virus leads to congenital Zika virus infection; sequelae include microcephaly with brain anomalies (and other serious neurologic consequences) and fetal loss. The full range of functional disabilities caused by congenital Zika virus infection is not yet known. Short-term follow-up studies of young children with postnatal Zika virus infections have not identified neurodevelopmental problems; longer-term studies are needed, especially among infants infected during the neonatal period.

## DIAGNOSIS

Zika virus infection should be considered in patients with a clinically compatible illness who recently traveled to an area with ongoing transmission or who had sex with someone who lives in or traveled to those areas. Patients with suspected Zika virus infection should be evaluated and managed for possible dengue or chikungunya virus infection. Many other infectious diseases can appear similar to Zika virus infection, including malaria, dengue, rubella, measles, parvovirus, adenovirus, enterovirus, leptospirosis, rickettsiosis, and group A streptococcal infections.

Zika virus diagnostic testing can be accomplished using both molecular and serologic methods. Although false positives can occur, nucleic acid testing (NAT) provides confirmed evidence of recent infection and is the preferred test for people with suspected acute Zika virus disease. For returning nonpregnant travelers with suspected Zika virus disease, NAT should be performed on specimens collected <14 days after symptom onset.

Zika virus IgM antibodies typically develop within 3 days of symptom onset. However, IgM might be detectable for months after the initial infection, making it difficult to determine the timing of infection. In addition, false-positive IgM test results can occur because of nonspecific reactivity or cross-reactivity with other flaviviruses (such as dengue, West Nile, or yellow fever viruses). As incidence and risk of Zika virus infection decreases, a higher proportion of positive IgM tests will be falsely positive. Neutralizing antibody testing should be performed to confirm positive IgM test results and discriminate between cross-reacting antibodies. However, neutralizing antibodies might not distinguish Zika virus and cross-reacting antibodies in people previously infected with or vaccinated against a related flavivirus (secondary flavivirus infection).

Perform Zika virus IgM testing on NAT-negative specimens or serum collected ≥14 days after onset of symptoms. Pregnant women with recent possible Zika virus exposure and a clinically compatible illness should have concurrent NAT and IgM testing on specimens collected ≤12 weeks after symptom onset. For asymptomatic pregnant women, Zika virus testing is not routinely recommended unless there is ongoing Zika virus exposure. Additional information on diagnostic testing for Zika virus can be found at www.cdc.gov/zika/hc-providers/testing-for-zika-virus.html.

Most state health departments and many commercial laboratories perform Zika virus NAT and IgM testing. Confirmatory neutralizing antibody testing is available through several state health departments and CDC's Division of Vector-borne Diseases: 970-221-6400. Health care providers are encouraged to report suspected cases of Zika virus infection to their state or local health departments to facilitate diagnosis and mitigate the risk of local transmission in areas where *Aedes* species mosquitoes are active. Zika virus disease is a nationally notifiable condition. State health departments should report laboratory-confirmed cases to CDC according to the Council of State and Territorial Epidemiologists case definitions.

## TREATMENT

No specific antiviral treatment is available for Zika virus disease. Treatment is generally supportive and can include rest, fluids, and use of analgesics and antipyretics. Because aspirin and other nonsteroidal anti-inflammatory drugs (NSAIDs) can increase the risk of hemorrhage in patients with dengue, avoid use of these medications until dengue can be ruled out. People infected with Zika, dengue, or chikungunya virus should be protected from further mosquito exposure during the first week of illness to decrease the possibility of local transmission. Carefully evaluate pregnant women with laboratory evidence of Zika virus infection; closely manage these cases for possible adverse pregnancy outcomes. Guidance for the diagnosis, evaluation, and management of infants with possible congenital Zika virus infections is available at www.cdc.gov/pregnancy/zika/testing-follow-up/evaluation-testing.html.

## PREVENTION

No vaccine or preventive drug is available. However, several candidate vaccines are in various stages of development. All travelers to areas with Zika virus transmission should take steps to avoid mosquito bites to prevent the risk of Zika virus and other vectorborne infections (see Chapter 3, Mosquitoes, Ticks & Other Arthropods). Persons with possible Zika virus exposure who want to reduce their risk for sexual transmission of Zika virus to an uninfected partner should use condoms or abstain from sex. Blood donations in the United States are now routinely screened for Zika virus RNA to reduce the risk of transfusion-associated transmission.

Pregnant women should avoid travel to any area with risk of Zika virus transmission. Pregnant women who travel to one of these areas should talk to their health care provider before traveling and strictly follow steps to avoid mosquito bites or sexual transmission during travel. There is no restriction on the use of insect repellents by pregnant women if used in accordance with the instructions on the product label. Male partners of pregnant women who travel to areas with risk of Zika virus transmission should abstain from sex or use condoms for the duration of the pregnancy to avoid sexual transmission to their pregnant partners. Women and their partners who are trying to become—or who are interested in becoming—pregnant should take steps to protect themselves from Zika virus infection. Mothers are encouraged to breastfeed infants even after possible Zika virus exposure, as available evidence indicates the benefits of breastfeeding outweigh the theoretical risks associated with Zika virus infection transmission through breast milk.

**CDC website:** www.cdc.gov/zika

## BIBLIOGRAPHY

1. Adebanjo T, Godfred-Cato S, Viens L, Fischer M, Staples JE, Kuhnert-Tallman W, et al. Update: interim guidance for the diagnosis, evaluation, and management of infants with possible congenital Zika virus infection—United States, October 2017. MMWR Morb Mortal Wkly Rep. 2017;66(41):1089–99.

2. Duffy MR, Chen TH, Hancock WT, Powers AM, Kool JL, Lanciotti RS, et al. Zika virus outbreak on Yap Island, Federated States of Micronesia. N Engl J Med. 2009 Jun 11; 360(24):2536–43.

3. Gregory CJ, Oduyebo T, Brault AC, Brooks JT, Chung KW, Hills S, et al. Modes of transmission of Zika virus. J Infect Dis. 2017;216(10):S875–83.

4. Hall V, Walker WL, Lindsey NP, Lehman JA, Kolsin J, Landry K, et al. Update: noncongenital Zika virus disease cases—50 U.S. states and the District of Columbia, 2016. MMWR Morb Mortal Wkly Rep. 2018;67(9):265–9.

5. Hills SL, Fischer M, Petersen LR. Epidemiology of Zika virus infection. J Infect Disease. 2017;216(10):S868–74.

6. Krow-Lucal ER, de Andrade MR, Abath Cananéa JN, Staples JE, Coelho GE. Association and birth prevalence of microcephaly attributable to Zika virus infection among infants in Paraíba, Brazil, in 2015–16: a case-control study. Lancet Child Adol Health. 2018;2(3)205–13.

7. McArthur MA. Zika virus: Recent advances towards the development of vaccines and therapeutics. Viruses. 2017;9(6):143.

8. Oduyebo T, Polen KD, Walke HT, Reagan-Steiner S, Lathrop E, Rabe IB, et al. Update: interim guidance for health care providers caring for pregnant women with possible Zika virus exposure—United States (including U.S. territories), July 2017. MMWR Morb Mortal Wkly Rep. 2017;66(29):781–93.

9. Petersen LR, Jamieson DJ, Powers AM, Honein MA. Zika Virus. N Engl J Med. 2016 Apr 21; 374(16):1552–63.

10. Reynolds, MR, Jones AM, Petersen EE, Lee EH, Rice ME, Bingham A, et al. Vital signs: update on Zika virus–associated birth defects and evaluation of all U.S. infants with congenital Zika virus exposure—U.S. Zika Pregnancy Registry, 2016. MMWR Morb Mortal Wkly Rep. 2017;66(13):366–73.

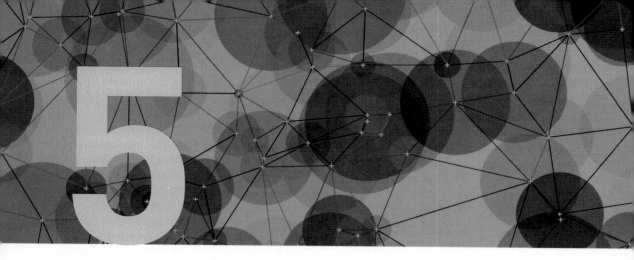

# 5

# Travelers with Additional Considerations

## IMMUNOCOMPROMISED TRAVELERS

Camille Nelson Kotton, Andrew T. Kroger, David O. Freedman

### APPROACH TO THE IMMUNOCOMPROMISED TRAVELER

Immunocompromised travelers make up 1%–2% of travelers seen in US travel clinics and pursue itineraries largely similar to those of immuno-competent travelers. The pretravel preparation of travelers with immune suppression due to any medical condition, drug, or treatment must take into consideration several issues:

- What is the cause of the immune suppression? Different conditions and medications produce widely varying degrees of immunocompromise, and there are many unknowns in this field. Guidance regarding vaccination of immuno-compromised travelers is less evidence-based than with other categories of travelers; this section provides recommendations based on the best available data and the practices of experienced clinicians.

- Is the traveler's underlying medical condition stable? The travel health care provider may need to contact the traveler's primary or specialty care providers (with the patient's permission) to discuss the traveler's fitness to travel, give specific medical advice for the proposed itinerary, verify the drugs and doses composing their usual maintenance regimen, and discuss whether any of the disease-prevention measures recommended for the proposed trip could destabilize the underlying medical condition, directly or through drug interactions.

- Do the conditions, medications, and treatments of the traveler constitute contraindications to, decrease the effectiveness of, or increase the risk for adverse events of any of the disease-prevention measures recommended for the proposed trip? Depending on the destination, such measures may include immunizations and drugs used for malaria chemoprophylaxis and management of travelers' diarrhea. Are there specific health hazards at the destination that would exacerbate the underlying condition or be more severe in an immunocompromised traveler? If so, can specific interventions be recommended to mitigate these risks?

- If an immunocompromised traveler were to become ill while traveling, what are the health care options (see Chapter 6, Obtaining Health Care Abroad)? What would the traveler do should medical evacuation be required? An immunocompromised traveler should have a plan for when and how to seek care overseas and how to pay for it.

The traveler's immune status is particularly relevant to immunizations. Overall considerations for vaccine recommendations, such as destination and the likely risk of exposure to disease, are the same for immunocompromised travelers as for other travelers. The risk of severe illness or death from a vaccine-preventable disease must be weighed against potential adverse events from administering a live vaccine to an immunocompromised patient. In some complex cases when travelers cannot tolerate recommended immunizations or prophylaxis, the traveler should consider changing the itinerary, altering the activities planned during travel, or deferring the trip.

For purposes of clinical assessment and approach to immunizations, immunocompromised travelers may be thought of as falling into 1 of 3 groups, based on mechanism and level of immune suppression. The 3 groups are people who have 1) medical conditions without significant immunologic compromise, 2) medical conditions and treatments associated with limited immune deficits, and 3) medical conditions or treatments associated with severe immune compromise. Vaccine recommendations for different categories of immunocompromised adults are shown in Table 5-1.

## MEDICAL CONDITIONS WITHOUT SIGNIFICANT IMMUNOLOGIC COMPROMISE

With regard to travel immunizations, travelers whose health status places them in any of the following groups are not considered significantly immunocompromised and should be prepared as any other traveler, although the nature of the underlying disease needs to be kept in mind.

1. Travelers receiving corticosteroid therapy under any of the following circumstances:
   > Short- or long-term daily or alternate-day therapy with <20 mg of prednisone or equivalent.
   > Maintenance steroids at physiologic doses (replacement therapy).
   > Steroid inhalers or topical steroids (skin, ears, or eyes).
   > Intraarticular, bursal, or tendon injection of steroids.
   > If >1 month has passed since high-dose steroids (≥20 mg per day of prednisone or equivalent for >2 weeks) have been used. After short-term (<2 weeks) therapy with daily or alternate-day dosing of ≥20 mg of prednisone or equivalent, some experts will still wait 2 weeks or more before administering live vaccines.

2. HIV patients without severe immunosuppression (for definitions of severe

# Table 5-1. Immunization of immunocompromised adults

| | HIV INFECTION, CD4 CELLS ≥200/MM³ | SEVERE IMMUNOSUPPRESSION (HIV/AIDS), CD4 CELLS <200/MM³ | SEVERE IMMUNOSUPPRESSION (NOT HIV-RELATED) | ASPLENIA | RENAL FAILURE |
|---|---|---|---|---|---|
| **Live Vaccines** | | | | | |
| Bacillus Calmette-Guérin (BCG) | X | X | X | U | U |
| Cholera | ND[1] | ND[1] | ND[1] | U | U |
| Influenza, live attenuated (LAIV) | X | X | X | X | P |
| Measles-mumps-rubella (MMR)[2] | R[2] | X[2] | X[2] | U | U |
| Typhoid, Ty21a | X | X | X | U | U |
| Varicella (adults)[3] | C[3] | X[3] | X[3] | U | U |
| Yellow fever[4] | P[4] | X[4] | X | U | OC[5] |
| Zoster-live (ZVL) | OC[6] | X[6] | X | U | U |
| **Inactivated Vaccines** | | | | | |
| DTaP | U | U | U | U | U |
| *Haemophilus influenzae* type b (Hib) | U | U | OC[7] | R[8] | U |
| Hepatitis A[9] | U | U | U | U | U |
| Hepatitis B[10] | R[10] | R[10] | U[10] | U[10] | R[11] |
| Human papillomavirus | U[12] | U[12] | U[12] | U | U |
| Influenza (inactivated) | R | R | R | R | R |
| Japanese encephalitis[13] | ND | ND | ND | ND | ND |
| Meningococcal conjugate (ACWY) | R[14] | R[14] | U | R[14] | U |
| Meningococcal group B | U | U | U | R | U |
| PCV13 followed by PPSV23[15] | R | R | R | R | R |
| Polio (IPV) | U | U | U | U | U |

(continued)

# Table 5-1. Immunization of immunocompromised adults (continued)

| | HIV INFECTION, CD4 CELLS ≥200/MM³ | SEVERE IMMUNOSUPPRESSION (HIV/AIDS), CD4 CELLS <200/MM³ | SEVERE IMMUNOSUPPRESSION (NOT HIV-RELATED) | ASPLENIA | RENAL FAILURE |
|---|---|---|---|---|---|
| Rabies | U | OC[16] | OC[16] | U | U |
| Td or Tdap | U | U | U | U | U |
| Typhoid, Vi | U | U | U | U | U |
| Zoster-recombinant (RZV) | OC | OC | OC | U | U |

Abbreviations: X, Contraindicated (per the Advisory Committee on Immunization Practices [ACIP]); U, Use as indicated for normal hosts; R, Recommended for all in this patient category; P, Precaution (per ACIP); OC, Other considerations; C, Consider; ND, No data; PCV13, 13-valent pneumococcal conjugate vaccine; PPSV23, 23-valent pneumococcal polysaccharide vaccine.

[1] No safety or efficacy data exist regarding use of the current formulation of CVD 103-HgR vaccine in HIV-positive adults or people with severe immunosuppression. Limited data from an older formulation of the CVD 103-HgR suggest no association between the vaccine and serious or systemic adverse events, and slightly lower immunogenicity of the vaccine in HIV-positive versus HIV-negative adults.

[2] MMR vaccination is recommended for all HIV-infected patients aged ≥12 months with (for patients aged <6 years) CD4 percentage ≥15% or (for patients aged ≥6 years) CD4 percentage ≥15% and CD4 counts ≥200/mm³ for ≥6 months if they are without evidence of measles immunity. Immune globulin may be administered for short-term protection of those facing high risk of measles and for whom MMR vaccine is contraindicated. Additional guidance is available at www.cdc.gov/mmwr/preview/mmwrhtml/rr6204a1.htm.

[3] Varicella vaccine should not be administered to people who have cellular immunodeficiencies, but people with impaired humoral immunity (including congenital or acquired hypoglobulinemia or dysglobulinemia) may be vaccinated. HIV-positive adults with CD4 counts ≥200 cells/mm³ may receive 2 doses of vaccine spaced at 3-month intervals. VariZIG (varicella zoster–specific immune globulin) is recommended for those exposed to varicella or herpes zoster if they do not have evidence of varicella immunity and have contraindications to vaccination.

[4] See details in Chapter 4, Yellow Fever. Yellow fever (YF) vaccination is a precaution for asymptomatic HIV-infected people with CD4 cell counts of 200–499/mm³. YF vaccination is not a precaution for people with asymptomatic HIV infection and CD4 cell counts ≥500/mm³. YF vaccine is also considered contraindicated by ACIP for symptomatic HIV patients without AIDS and with CD4 counts <200/mm³.

[5] No data suggest increased risk of serious adverse events after use of YF vaccine in people with these conditions; however, varying degrees of immune deficit might be present, and providers should carefully weigh vaccine risks and benefits before deciding to vaccinate people with these conditions.

[6] Also contraindicated by ACIP for symptomatic HIV patients without AIDS and with CD4 counts <200/mm³. No recommendation for asymptomatic HIV patients without AIDS and with CD4 counts ≥200/mm³. Recombinant zoster vaccine is the preferred agent.

[7] Recipients of a hematopoietic stem cell transplant should be vaccinated with a 3-dose regimen 6–12 months after a successful transplant, regardless of vaccination history; at least 4 weeks should separate doses.

[8] In adults, Hib is recommended for those with asplenia only if they have not previously received Hib vaccine.

[9] Routinely indicated for all men who have sex with men, hemophiliacs, patients with chronic hepatitis, injection drug users, and others.

[10] Hepatitis B vaccination is indicated for people at risk for infection by sexual exposure, including sex partners of hepatitis B surface antigen (HBsAg)-positive people, sexually active people who are not in a long-term mutually monogamous relationship, people seeking evaluation or treatment for a sexually transmitted disease, men who have sex with men, people at risk for infection by percutaneous or mucosal exposure to blood, current or recent injection drug users, household contacts of HBsAg-positive people, residents and staff of facilities for developmentally disabled people, health care and public safety workers with reasonably anticipated risk for exposure to blood or blood-contaminated body fluids, people with end-stage renal disease, international travelers to regions with high or intermediate levels (HBsAg prevalence >2%) of endemic HBV infection (see Map 4-4), people with chronic liver disease, and people with HIV infection.

[11] Adult patients ≥20 years old receiving hemodialysis or with other immunocompromising conditions should receive 1 dose of 40 µg/mL Recombivax HB administered on a 3-dose schedule at 0, 1, and 6 months or 2 doses of 20 µg/mL (Engerix-B) administered simultaneously on a 4-dose schedule at 0, 1, 2, and 6 months. Test for antibodies to hepatitis B virus surface antigen serum after vaccination and revaccinate if initial antibody response is absent or suboptimal (<10 mIU/mL). HIV-infected nonresponders may react to a subsequent vaccine course if CD4 cell counts rise to 500/mm³ after institution of highly active antiretroviral therapy. Heplisav-B (HepB-CpG) is an adjuvanted vaccine and should be administered as 2 doses, 1 month apart, in people ≥18 years of age, including hemodialysis and immunocompromised people. Postvaccination serologic testing is recommended. See text for discussion of other immunocompromised groups.

[12] HPV vaccine (3 dose schedule at 0, 1–2, and 6 months) is recommended through age 26 years. Should be administered as indicated for males and females but is additionally recommended for men 22–26 years of age in this patient category (otherwise male indication is through age 21 years). Female indication in each category is through 26 years of age.

[13] No safety or efficacy data exist regarding the use of Ixiaro in immunocompromised people. In general, inactivated vaccines can be administered safely to people with altered immunocompetence, using the usual doses and schedules, but the effectiveness might be suboptimal. The inactivated, Vero cell–derived Japanese encephalitis vaccine, Ixiaro, is the only Japanese encephalitis vaccine available in the United States; other types of Japanese encephalitis vaccines, including live vaccines, are available internationally but are not included here.

[14] Children aged 2–23 months should receive the vaccine in accordance with the age-appropriate, licensed, multidose schedule. For people aged ≥2 years, 2 doses ≥8 weeks apart are recommended. If the most recent dose was received at age <7 years, a booster dose should be administered 3 years after the primary series and every 5 years thereafter. If the most recent dose was received at age ≥7 years, a booster dose should be administered after 5 years, and every 5 years thereafter. See www.cdc.gov/mmwr/volumes/65/wr/pdfs/mm6543a3.pdf for more information.

[15] Previously unimmunized asplenic, HIV-infected, with chronic renal disease or nephrotic syndrome, or immunocompromised adults aged ≥5 years should receive 1 dose of 13-valent pneumococcal conjugate vaccine (PCV13) followed by 1 dose of pneumococcal polysaccharide vaccine (PPSV23) ≥8 weeks later. People with these conditions previously immunized with PPSV23 should follow catch-up guidelines per ACIP.

[16] For postexposure prophylaxis, both vaccine (5 doses at day 0, 3, 7, 14, 28) and immune globulin should be given to immunocompromised people, regardless of previous vaccination status.

immunosuppression, see www.cdc.gov/vaccines/hcp/acip-recs/general-recs/downloads/general-recs.pdf).

3. Travelers with a history of cancer who received their last chemotherapy treatment ≥3 months previously and whose malignancy is in remission. Those who have received immunotherapy with agents such as checkpoint inhibitors may need to wait longer; any vaccination should be discussed directly with their oncologist.

4. Hematopoietic stem cell transplant recipients or CAR-T cell recipients who are >2 years posttransplant, not on immunosuppressive drugs, with no evidence of ongoing malignancy, and without graft-versus-host disease.

5. Travelers with autoimmune disease (such as systemic lupus erythematosus, inflammatory bowel disease, or rheumatoid arthritis) who are not being treated with immunosuppressive or immunomodulatory drugs, although definitive data are lacking.

## MEDICAL CONDITIONS AND TREATMENTS ASSOCIATED WITH LIMITED IMMUNE DEFICITS

### Asymptomatic HIV Infection

Asymptomatic adults with HIV and CD4 cell counts of 200–499/mm³ are considered to have limited immune deficits and should be vaccinated according to the guidelines in Table 5-1. Meningococcal (MenACWY), pneumococcal, and

hepatitis B vaccines are recommended for HIV-positive patients regardless of travel plans. More specific recommendations are available for MMR (measles-mumps-rubella) vaccine (www.cdc.gov/mmwr/preview/mmwrhtml/rr6204a1.htm). CD4 counts while on antiretroviral drugs, rather than nadir counts, should be used to categorize people with HIV.

To achieve a maximal vaccine response with minimal risk, many clinicians advise a delay of 3 months after immune reconstitution (usually 6 months after initiation of antiretroviral therapy), if possible, before immunizations are administered; however, the optimal time to initiate vaccination after starting antiretroviral therapy has been identified as a gap in knowledge by the Infectious Diseases Society of America. For MMR vaccine, the recommendation is ≥6 months on antiretroviral therapy with the age- and CD4-based criteria. Although seroconversion rates and geometric mean titers of antibody in response to vaccines may be less than those measured in healthy controls, most vaccines can elicit protective levels of antibody in many HIV-infected patients in this category.

Single-antigen varicella vaccine should be considered for HIV-infected children aged 1–8 years who have CD4 percentages ≥15%. Vaccine may be considered, after weighing the risk for severe disease from wild virus and potential benefit of vaccination, for HIV-infected children aged >8 years with comparable levels of immune function (CD4 count ≥200 cells/mm³). Eligible children should receive 2 doses 3 months apart, with the first dose administered as soon as possible after the first birthday. Varicella vaccine is not recommended for HIV-infected children who have evidence of severe immunosuppression (CD4 percentage <15% for those 1–8 years of age and CD4 count <200 cells/mm$^3$ for those aged >8 years).

People with HIV may require vaccination with MMR or varicella vaccine. However, they also might receive periodic doses of intravenous immunoglobulin (IVIG), which may interfere with vaccine response. Varicella and MMR vaccines should be considered approximately 14 days before the next scheduled dose of IVIG. MMRV vaccine has not been studied in HIV-infected children and should not be substituted for single-antigen varicella vaccine.

Transient increases in HIV viral load, which return quickly to baseline, have been observed after administration of several different vaccines to asymptomatic HIV-infected people but does not occur in those well controlled on current antiretroviral therapies. The clinical significance of these increases is not known, but they do not preclude the use of any vaccine.

## Multiple Sclerosis (MS)

Inactivated vaccines, including influenza, hepatitis B, human papillomavirus, and tetanus vaccines, are generally considered safe for people with MS, although vaccination should be delayed during clinically significant relapses until patients have stabilized or begun to improve from the relapse, typically 4–6 weeks after it began. Published studies are lacking on the safety and efficacy of other vaccines, such as those against hepatitis A, meningococcal disease, pertussis, pneumococcal disease, polio, and typhoid. Inactivated vaccines are theoretically safe for people being treated with an interferon medication, glatiramer acetate, mitoxantrone, fingolimod, or natalizumab, although safety and efficacy data are lacking.

Modern MS therapy often includes aggressive and early immunomodulatory therapy for many MS patients, even those with stable disease. Live vaccines should not be given to people with MS during therapy with immunosuppressants such as mitoxantrone, azathioprine, methotrexate, or cyclophosphamide; during chronic corticosteroid therapy; or during therapy with any immunosuppressive biologic agents including nataluzimab

and alemtuzumab. Although definitive study of each medication is lacking, glatiramer acetate and interferon therapy are generally not classified by MS experts as immunosuppressive and do not preclude live vaccine administration.

Published studies suggest that mumps, measles, rubella, varicella, and zoster vaccines are safe in people with stable MS if administered 1 month before starting or at the appropriate interval (see Duration of Iatrogenic Immune Compromise below) after discontinuing immunosuppressive therapy. One study suggests yellow fever vaccine can exacerbate symptoms in MS patients; this risk together with the risk of yellow fever at the destination should be considered in consultation with the patient's neurologist before administering the vaccine to those at risk of yellow fever.

## Other Chronic Conditions

Chronic medical conditions that may be associated with varying degrees of immune deficit include asplenia and chronic renal disease. These patients should be vaccinated according to the guidelines in Table 5-1. Patients with complement deficiencies can receive any live or inactivated vaccine. Factors to consider in assessing the general level of immune competence of patients with chronic diseases include disease severity, duration, clinical stability, complications, comorbidities, and any potentially immune-suppressing treatment (see the next section in this chapter, Travelers with Chronic Illnesses).

Adults aged ≥19 years with most immunocompromising conditions who have not previously received the 13-valent pneumococcal conjugate vaccine (PCV13) or the 23-valent pneumococcal polysaccharide vaccine (PPSV23) should receive a single dose of PCV13 followed by a dose of PPSV23 ≥8 weeks later.

Those with anatomic or functional asplenia (including sickle cell disease), complement deficiency, or taking eculizumab are susceptible to overwhelming and rapidly progressive sepsis with certain bacterial pathogens despite indicated immunizations. Advise asplenic travelers to seek immediate medical advice if they develop a fever and be prepared to initiate self-treatment in the form of a broad-spectrum antibiotic; they should not travel to destinations where immediate access

5

to high standard medical care is not possible. People with asplenia generally are not considered immunocompromised for the purposes of vaccination, and live vaccines are not contraindicated.

Although response to vaccines may be diminished compared with people who have a functioning spleen, immunization against meningococcal (MenACWY and MenB), pneumococcal (see dosing above), and *Haemophilus influenzae* type b disease is recommended in these patients, regardless of travel plans. Age-appropriate dosing and schedules differ from competent hosts, and the recommended immunization schedules should be consulted (www.cdc.gov/vaccines/schedules/hcp/index.html).

People with terminal complement deficiencies, including anyone receiving the complement component inhibitor eculizumab, have increased susceptibility to meningococcal infections and should be immunized against meningococcal disease with both MenACWY and, if ≥10 years of age, MenB vaccine and could consider antimicrobial prophylaxis. The recommendations are the same as for patients with asplenia. Patients receiving eculizumab have increased risk of overwhelming meningococcal sepsis even after vaccination.

People with hypogammaglobulinemia or dysgammaglobulinemia may require vaccination with MMR or varicella vaccine. However, many people with these disorders also receive periodic doses of IVIG, which may interfere with vaccine response. Varicella and MMR vaccines should be considered approximately 14 days before the next scheduled dose of IVIG.

# MEDICAL CONDITIONS AND TREATMENTS ASSOCIATED WITH SEVERE IMMUNE COMPROMISE

## Severe Immune Compromise (Non-HIV)

Severely immunocompromised people include those who have active leukemia or lymphoma, generalized malignancy, aplastic anemia, graft-versus-host disease, or congenital immunodeficiency; others in this category include people who have received recent radiation therapy or checkpoint inhibitor treatment (therapy of autoimmune complications of treatment is immunosuppressive), those who have had solid-organ transplants and who are on active immunosuppression, and both CAR-T cell and hematopoietic stem cell transplant recipients (within 2 years of transplantation or still taking immunosuppressive drugs). The severely immunocompromised should generally not be given live vaccines, and inactivated vaccines are likely to be less effective; these patients should consider postponing travel until their immune function improves. For people likely to travel in the future, usual travel-related vaccines may be recommended before starting immunosuppressive therapies, if feasible. Administer inactivated vaccines ≥2 weeks and live vaccines ≥4 weeks before immunosuppression if possible (minimum 2 weeks before immunosuppression).

Special considerations apply for several common travel-related vaccines. Data indicate that immunocompromised people, notably those being treated with immunosuppressive drugs, may have inadequate seroconversion after a single dose of hepatitis A vaccine. For immunocompromised people (based on a provider guidance risk assessment) of any age who are traveling internationally, hepatitis A vaccine with additional immune globulin (IG) is recommended by the Advisory Committee on Immunization Practices (ACIP). The dose of IG, which varies according to planned duration of travel, is 0.1 mL/kg for travel up to one month; 0.2 mL/kg for travel up to 2 months; and for travel of more than 2 months, repeat doses of 0.2 mL/kg every 2 months. In general, IG should be administered immediately before travel. Immunocompromised travelers should make efforts to receive 2 doses of the hepatitis A vaccine over a 6-month period prior to their trip. Instead of concomitant IG, the approach of giving a second dose of vaccine ≥4 weeks after the first dose for time-constrained travelers who can get both doses before travel has been effective in select studies. For unvaccinated travelers who require postexposure prophylaxis during or after the trip, IG may be administered in addition to hepatitis A vaccine in people older than 40 years, depending on the providers' risk assessment (for example, patient age, immune status and underlying conditions, exposure type/risk of transmission, and availability of IG).

The humoral immune response to hepatitis B vaccine is reduced in children and adults who are immunocompromised. Limited data indicate that modified dosing regimens might increase response rates. Similar to dialysis patients, a 3-dose series of 40 µg Recombivax HB at 0, 1, and 6 months or a 4-dose series of 40 µg Engerix-B at 0, 1, 2, and 6 months should be used. Heplisav-B (HepB-CpG) is an adjuvanted vaccine and is recommended to be administered as 2 doses, 1 month apart in people ≥18 years of age. Postvaccination serologic testing following any hepatitis B vaccination series is recommended to confirm response to immunization in immunocompromised people.

Immunocompromised people deemed at risk for vaccine-preventable rabies should receive a full intramuscular vaccine course on days 0, 7, and 21 or 28. Abbreviated, low-dose, and intradermal series should not be used. Serologic postvaccination testing may be indicated. For postexposure rabies prophylaxis, all severely immunocompromised people should generally receive rabies vaccine at days 0, 3, 7, 14, and 28, plus human rabies immune globulin, irrespective of previous vaccination history.

Although no extra pretravel indication exists, many travel clinics administer zoster vaccines. Recombinant zoster vaccine (RZV), newly introduced in 2018 as preferential to zoster vaccine live (ZVL) in competent hosts, is not contraindicated in immunocompromised people, but no efficacy data in this population are available to inform a licensed indication by FDA.

People with chronic lymphocytic leukemia have poor humoral immunity, even early in the disease course, and rarely respond to vaccines. After hematopoietic stem cell transplant, complete revaccination with standard childhood vaccines should begin at 6 months, with the caveat that MMR and varicella vaccines should be administered 24 months after transplant and only if the recipient is assumed to be immunocompetent. Inactivated influenza vaccine should be administered beginning ≥6 months after hematopoietic stem cell transplant and annually thereafter; a dose of inactivated influenza vaccine can be given as early as 4 months after transplant if there is a community outbreak.

For solid-organ transplants, the risk of infection is highest in the first year after transplant, so travel to high-risk destinations should be postponed until after that time. For hematopoietic cell transplant (HCT), travel should ideally be delayed ≥2 years after transplant to allow for full revaccination.

Doses of inactivated vaccines received while concurrently receiving potent immunosuppressive therapy (see below) or during the 2 weeks before starting therapy should not be counted toward completing the primary vaccination series or relied upon to induce adequate immune responses. At least 3 months after potent immunosuppressive therapy is discontinued, patients should be revaccinated with all indicated inactivated vaccines.

People taking any of the following categories of medications are considered severely immunocompromised:

- **High-dose corticosteroids**—Most clinicians consider a dose of either >2 mg/kg of body weight or ≥20 mg per day of prednisone or equivalent in people who weigh >10 kg, when administered for ≥2 weeks, as sufficiently immunosuppressive to raise concern about the safety of vaccination with live vaccines. Furthermore, the immune response to vaccines may be impaired. Clinicians should wait ≥1 month after discontinuation of high-dose systemic corticosteroid therapy before administering a live-virus vaccine.

- **Alkylating agents** (such as cyclophosphamide).

- **Antimetabolites** (such as azathioprine, 6-mercaptopurine, methotrexate). However, low-dose monotherapy (methotrexate ≤0.4 mg/kg/week, azathioprine ≤3 mg/kg/day, or 6-mercaptopurine ≤1.5 mg/kg/day) with these drugs does not preclude administration of either zoster vaccine.

- **Transplant-related immunosuppressive drugs** (such as cyclosporine, tacrolimus, sirolimus, everolimus, azathioprine, and mycophenolate mofetil).

5

- **Cancer chemotherapeutic agents** are classified as severely immunosuppressive, as evidenced by increased rates of opportunistic infections and blunting of responses to certain vaccines among patient groups.[1] Vaccination following immunomodulatory therapies, such as checkpoint inhibitors, and CAR-T cell treatments have not been well studied, and until additional data are available, live attenuated vaccine should be avoided for many months after treatment.

- **Tumor necrosis factor (TNF) blockers** such as etanercept, adalimumab, certolizumab pegol, golimumab, and infliximab blunt the immune response to certain vaccines and certain chronic infections. When used alone or in combination regimens with other disease-modifying agents to treat rheumatoid disease, TNF blockers were associated with an impaired response to hepatitis A, influenza, and pneumococcal vaccines.
  - > Despite measurable impairment of the immune response, postvaccination antibody titers were often sufficient to provide protection for most people; therefore, treatment with TNF blockers does not preclude immunization against hepatitis A, influenza, and pneumococcal disease. When possible, all doses in the hepatitis A and pneumococcal series should be given before travel.
  - > The use of live vaccines is contraindicated according to the prescribing information for most of these therapies.

- **Other biologic agents** that are immunosuppressive or immunomodulatory may result in significant immunocompromise as outlined in Table 5-2. In particular, lymphocyte-depleting agents (thymoglobulin or alemtuzumab) and B cell–depleting agents (rituximab) are more significantly immunosuppressive. Consideration of the clinical context in which these were given is important, especially in hematologic malignancies.

The period of time clinicians should wait after discontinuation of immunosuppressive therapies before administering a live vaccine is not consistent across all live vaccines. For cancer chemotherapy, radiation therapy, and highly immunosuppressive medications (exclusive of lymphocyte-depleting agents and organ transplant immunosuppression), the waiting period is 3 months. For lymphocyte-depleting (alemtuzumab and rituximab) agents, the waiting period is ≥6 months, although some experts believe the waiting period should be ≥1 year.

For steroid regimens considered immunosuppressive (see above), wait 1 month. The live zoster vaccine (Zostavax) is exceptional and may be given 1 month after any highly immunosuppressive agent, although many experts advocate waiting ≥1 year for anti–B cell antibodies and other lymphocyte-depleting agents. The live zoster vaccine is now no longer preferred and should rarely, if ever, be used. People should instead receive the 2-dose recombinant shingles vaccine.

For agents not considered highly immunosuppressive (Table 5-2), consultation with the prescribing clinician (and possibly a hospital pharmacist) is recommended to manage individual patients and estimate degree of immunosuppression. No basis exists for interpreting laboratory studies of general immune parameters to predict vaccine safety or efficacy. Restarting immunosuppression after live vaccination has not been studied, but some experts would recommend waiting ≥1 month.

## Severe Immune Compromise Due to Symptomatic HIV/AIDS

Knowledge of the HIV-infected traveler's current CD4 T-lymphocyte count is necessary for optimal pretravel consultation. People with HIV and CD4 cell counts <200/mm³, history of an AIDS-defining illness without immune reconstitution,

---

[1] Some of these agents are less immunosuppressive than others, such as tamoxifen or trastuzumab given to breast cancer patients, but clinical data to support safety with live vaccines are lacking.

# Table 5-2. Immunosuppressive/immunomodulatory biologic agents that preclude use of live vaccines[1]

| GENERIC NAME | TRADE NAME | MECHANISM/TARGET OF ACTION |
|---|---|---|
| Abatacept | Orencia | Anti-CD28/CTLA-4 |
| Adalimumab | Humira | TNF blocker |
| Alemtuzumab | Campath | Anti-CD52 |
| Anakinra | Kineret | IL-1 antagonist |
| Atezolizumab | Tecentriq | PD-L1 |
| Avelumab | Bavencio | PD-L1 |
| Basiliximab | Simulect | IL-2R/CD25 |
| Belatacept | Nulojix | CTLA-4 |
| Bevacizumab | Avastin | VEGF |
| Certolizumab pegol | Cimzia | TNF blocker |
| Cetuximab | Erbitux | EGFR |
| Dasatinib | Sprycel | Bcr-Abl tyrosine kinase inhibitor |
| Dimethyl fumarate | Tecfidera | Activates the nuclear erythroid 2-related factor 2 transcriptional pathway |
| Etanercept | Enbrel | TNF blocker |
| Fingolimod | Gilenya | Sphingosine 1-phosphate receptor modulator |
| Glatiramer acetate | Copaxone | Immunomodulatory; target unknown |
| Golimumab | Simponi | TNF blocker |
| Ibritumomab tiuxetan | Zevalin | CD20 with radioisotope |
| Ibrutinib | Imbruvica | Tyrosine kinase inhibitor |
| Imatinib mesylate | Gleevec, STI 571 | Signal transduction inhibitor/protein-tyrosine kinase inhibitor |
| Infliximab | Remicade | TNF blocker |
| Interferon alfa | Pegasys, PegIntron | Block hepatitis C viral replication |
| Interferon beta-1a | Avonex, Rebif | Immunomodulatory; target unknown |
| Interferon beta-1b | Betaseron | Immunomodulatory; target unknown |
| Natalizumab | Tsabri | α4-integrin |

## Table 5-2. Immunosuppressive/immunomodulatory biologic agents that preclude use of live vaccines[1] (continued)

| GENERIC NAME | TRADE NAME | MECHANISM/TARGET OF ACTION |
|---|---|---|
| Nivolumab | Opdivo | PD-1 |
| Ofatumumab | Arzerra | CD20 |
| Panitumumab | Vectibix | EGFR |
| Pembrolizumab | Keytruda | PD-1 |
| Lenalidomide | Revlimid | Immunomodulatory |
| Rilonacept | Arcalyst | IL-1 |
| Rituximab | Rituxan | CD20 |
| Sarilumab | Kevzara | IL-6 |
| Secukinumab | Cosentyx | IL-17A |
| Sunitinib malate | Sutent | Multikinase inhibitor |
| Tocilizumab | Actemra | IL-6 |
| Tofacitinib | Xeljanz | JAK kinase inhibitor |
| Trastuzumab | Herceptin | Human EGFR 2 (HER2) |
| Ustekinumab | Stelara | IL-12, IL-23 |
| Vedolizumab | Entyvio | Binds integrin $\alpha_4\beta_7$ |

Abbreviations: CD, cluster of differentiation; CTLA, cytotoxic T-lymphocyte antigen; TNF, tumor necrosis factor; IL, interleukin; PD, programmed cell death protein; VEGF, vascular endothelial growth factor; EGFR, epidermal growth factor receptor.
[1] This table is based primarily on conservative expert opinion, given the lack of clinical data. Numerous agents are often given in combination with other agents (especially chemotherapy) and are immunosuppressive when given together. The list provides examples but is not inclusive of all biologic agents that suppress or modulate the immune system. Not all therapeutic monoclonal antibodies or other biologic agents result in immunosuppression; details of individual agents not listed here must be reviewed before determining whether live viral vaccines can be given. Interferon and glatiramer acetate given to multiple sclerosis patients are immunomodulators and are generally not classified by MS experts as immunosuppressive so do not preclude live vaccine administration (except perhaps YF vaccine), but clinical data to support safety with live vaccines are lacking.

or clinical manifestations of symptomatic HIV are considered to have severe immunosuppression (see Chapter 4, HIV Infection) and should not receive live viral or bacterial vaccines because of the risk that the vaccine could cause serious systemic disease.[2]

In newly diagnosed, treatment-naïve patients with CD4 cell counts <200/mm³, travel should be delayed pending reconstitution of CD4 cell counts with antiretroviral therapy and ideally complete suppression of detectable viral replication. Such postponement helps minimize risk of

[2] For MMR vaccine, severe immunosuppression is defined as CD4 percentages <15% at any age in addition to CD4 count <200/mm³ for people aged >5 years. See www.cdc.gov/mmwr/preview/mmwrhtml/rr6204a1.htm.

infection and avoid immune reconstitution illness during travel.

## SPECIAL CONSIDERATIONS FOR IMMUNOCOMPROMISED TRAVELERS

### Household Contacts

The live vaccines MMR, varicella, and rotavirus vaccines should be administered to susceptible household contacts and other close contacts of immunocompromised patients when indicated. Inactive influenza vaccine (IIV) is the preferred agent; however, household and other close contacts of mildly or moderately immunocompromised patients can safely receive LAIV if they are unable to receive IIV. LAIV is contraindicated in close contacts and caregivers of severely immunocompromised people who require a protected environment.

Zoster vaccine live and yellow fever vaccine may be administered when indicated. Smallpox vaccine (mostly for military personnel) is transmissible to immunocompromised household and intimate contacts; infection control measures among family members should be implemented. If a varicella vaccine recipient has a rash after vaccination, direct contact with susceptible household contacts with altered immunocompetence should be avoided until the rash resolves.

### Yellow Fever Vaccine

Unvaccinated travelers with severe immune compromise should be strongly discouraged from travel to destinations that present a true risk for yellow fever (YF). Significant immunosuppression is a contraindication to YF vaccination, as there is a risk of developing a serious adverse event, such as life-threatening yellow fever vaccine–associated viscerotropic disease and yellow fever vaccine–associated neurotropic disease. Additionally, YF vaccination is contraindicated in people with a history of a thymus disorder associated with abnormal immune cell function (e.g., thymoma or myasthenia gravis). This applies whether or not they have undergone therapeutic thymectomy (see "Altered Immune Status" under "Contraindications" in Chapter 4, Yellow Fever). There are no data to support IgA deficiency as a contraindication to YF vaccination.

If travel is unavoidable to an area where YF vaccine is recommended (see Maps 4-13 and 4-14) and the vaccine has not been given, these travelers should be informed of the risk of YF, carefully instructed in methods to avoid mosquito bites, and provided with a vaccination medical waiver (see Chapter 4, Yellow Fever). They may wish to travel during periods of lower disease activity. Travelers should be warned that vaccination waiver documents might not be accepted by some countries, and refusal of entry or quarantine is possible.

Patients with conditions that ACIP considers precautions (as opposed to contraindications) to administration of YF vaccine, such as asymptomatic HIV (see "Precautions" in Chapter 4, Yellow Fever) may be offered YF vaccine if travel to YF-endemic areas is unavoidable; recipients should be monitored closely for possible adverse effects. Studies show that higher CD4 cell counts and suppressed HIV viral loads seem to be the key determinants for development of protective neutralizing antibodies. Patients with undetectable viral loads respond well to YF vaccination regardless of CD4 count, although data are limited in those with CD4 counts <200 mm$^3$. As vaccine response may be suboptimal, such vaccinees are candidates for serologic testing 1 month after vaccination. For information about serologic testing, contact your state health department or CDC's Division of Vector-Borne Diseases at 970-221-6400. Data from clinical and epidemiologic studies are insufficient at this time to evaluate the actual risk of severe adverse effects associated with YF vaccine among recipients with limited immune deficits. If international travel requirements, and not true exposure risk, are the only reasons to vaccinate a traveler with asymptomatic HIV infection or a limited immune deficit, the physician should provide a waiver letter.

Booster doses of YF vaccine are no longer recommended for most travelers, because a single dose of yellow fever vaccine provides long-lasting protection. However, additional doses of yellow fever vaccine are recommended for certain populations (such as hematopoietic stem cell transplant recipients and people with HIV) who might not have as robust or sustained immune response to yellow fever vaccine compared with other recipients.

People who received a hematopoietic stem cell transplant after receiving a dose of yellow fever vaccine and who are sufficiently immunocompetent to be safely vaccinated should be revaccinated if travel puts them at risk of yellow fever. People who were infected with HIV when they received their last dose of yellow fever vaccine should receive a dose every 10 years if they continue to be at risk for yellow fever and if there are no precautions or contraindications based on their current CD4 cell counts. Recent data suggest that yellow fever vaccination before solid-organ transplant, even long before transplant, generally provides protective antibody levels after transplant.

## Response to Vaccination

Response to vaccination may be muted in severely immunocompromised hosts, and potential travelers should be informed about this. The immunosuppressive regimen does not predict the decrease in response to vaccination. Recent data in solid-organ transplant recipients vaccinated before transplant suggests that a prolonged phase of protective antibody titers can exist after transplant. In general, serologic testing for response to most travel-related vaccines is not clinically recommended.

## Malaria Prophylaxis

Immunocompromised travelers to malaria-endemic areas should be prescribed drugs for malaria prophylaxis and receive counseling about mosquito bite avoidance—the same as for immunocompetent travelers (see Chapter 4, Malaria). Special concerns for immunocompromised travelers include any of the following possibilities:

- Most current first-line regimens for HIV (integrase and entry inhibitors) have few drug interactions, but some older maintenance regimens for HIV may interact with drugs used for malaria prophylaxis. Notably, chloroquine, mefloquine, and primaquine may interact with older maintenance regimens for HIV, particularly those containing protease inhibitors.

- The underlying medical condition, notably splenectomy, or immunosuppressive regimen may predispose the immunocompromised traveler to more serious disease from malaria infection. Such travelers should be counseled to adhere conscientiously to mosquito avoidance techniques and the malaria prophylaxis.

- Malaria infection and the drugs used to treat it may exacerbate the underlying disease.

- The severity of malaria is increased in HIV-infected people; malaria infection increases HIV viral load and thus may exacerbate disease progression.

Commonly used integrase inhibitor (raltegravir, dolutegravir, elvitegravir)/NRTI combinations (brand names include Descovy-Tivicay, Truvada-Tivicay) have no known interactions with CDC-recommended prophylactic drugs, although the cobicistat booster coformulated with elvitegravir (Stribild, Genvoya) may theoretically increase mefloquine levels. The rilpivirine, emtricitabine, TAF/TDF combinations (Odefsey and Complera) similarly have no interactions with antimalarials.

Of older drugs, efavirenz lowers serum levels of both atovaquone and proguanil, but there is no evidence for clinical failure of these agents when used concurrently. Efavirenz could potentially increase the amount of hemotoxic metabolites of primaquine.

Antimalarial treatment regimens, including artemisinin derivatives, quinine/quinidine, lumefantrine (part of the artemether/lumefantrine combination, Coartem), and atovaquone and proguanil, may have potential interactions with many NNRTIs, PIs, and with the CCR5 receptor antagonist maraviroc. Advice from the CDC or another malaria expert should be sought when treating patients for malaria who are also on antiretrovirals.

Extra care must be taken in researching potential interactions in people with HIV who are receiving antiretroviral therapy. An interactive web-based resource for assessing possible drug interactions is found at the University of Liverpool website (www.hiv-druginteractions.org; a mobile application is available).

5

In organ transplant recipients, malaria prophylactic drugs may interact with calcineurin inhibitors and mTor inhibitors (tacrolimus, cyclosporine, sirolimus, everolimus). Mefloquine, chloroquine, primaquine, and doxycycline may cause elevated calcineurin inhibitor levels. Mefloquine, chloroquine, and calcineurin inhibitors may interact to prolong the QT interval. Some travel-related medications need to be dose-adjusted according to altered hepatic or renal function.

## ENTERIC INFECTIONS

Many foodborne and waterborne infections, such as those caused by *Salmonella*, *Shigella*, *Campylobacter*, *Giardia*, *Listeria*, and *Cryptosporidium*, can be severe or become chronic in immunocompromised people. All travelers should follow safe food and beverage precautions; travelers' diarrhea can nonetheless occur despite strict adherence. Meticulous hand hygiene, including frequent and thorough handwashing with soap, is the best prevention against gastroenteritis. Hands should be washed after contact with public surfaces, after any contact with animals or their living areas, and before preparing food or eating.

Because enteric pathogens, particularly *Shigella*, can also be acquired sexually, patients should be counseled about avoiding sex with people who have diarrhea; washing hands, genitals, and anus before and after sex; and using barriers during sex with partners who recently recovered from diarrhea.

To reduce the risk of cryptosporidiosis, giardiasis, and other waterborne infections, patients should avoid swallowing water during swimming and other water-based recreational activities and should not swim in water that might be contaminated (with sewage or animal waste, for example). Travelers with liver disease should avoid direct exposure to salt water that may contain *Vibrio* spp., and all immunocompromised hosts should avoid raw seafood. Patients and clinicians should be aware of the augmented risk of infection or colonization with multidrug-resistant organisms during travel, and should report recent travel to their doctors if ill afterwards.

Selecting antimicrobials to be used for self-treatment of travelers' diarrhea, if indicated, may require special consideration of potential drug interactions among patients already taking medications for chronic medical conditions. Fluoroquinolones, rifaximin, and rifamycin SV are active against several enteric bacterial pathogens and are not known to have significant interactions with highly active antiretroviral therapy (HAART) drugs. Macrolide antibiotics may have significant interactions with HAART drugs and sometimes with organ transplant–related immunosuppression. Fluoroquinolones as well as azithromycin in combination with calcineurin inhibitors and mTor inhibitors may cause a prolonged QT interval. Antibiotic prophylaxis for a limited duration may be considered for travelers with severe immune suppression, although it should be used with caution given the risk of selecting for multidrug-resistant organisms.

## REDUCING RISK FOR OTHER DISEASES

Geographically focal infections that pose an increased risk of severe outcome for immunocompromised people include visceral leishmaniasis and several fungal infections acquired by inhalation (such as *Talaromyces marneffei* [formerly *Penicillium marneffei*] infection in Southeast Asia and histoplasmosis and coccidioidomycosis in the Americas). Establishing the tuberculosis status of immunocompromised travelers going to regions endemic for tuberculosis may be helpful in the evaluation of subsequent illness. Depending on the traveler's degree of immune suppression, the baseline tuberculosis status may be assessed by obtaining a tuberculin skin test, *Mycobacterium tuberculosis* antigen–specific interferon-γ assay, or chest radiograph. The need for posttransplant testing (often 3 months after travel) depends on exposure risk during the trip, medical conditions, and other factors.

Patients with advanced HIV and transplant recipients frequently take either primary or secondary prophylaxis for opportunistic infections (such as *Pneumocystis*, *Mycobacterium*, and *Toxoplasma* spp.). Adherence to all indicated prophylactic regimens should be confirmed before travel (see Chapter 4, HIV Infection).

Key points to stress with immunocompromised travelers are summarized in Box 5-1.

## BOX 5-1. Key patient education points for the immunocompromised traveler

- Develop plan in case of illness at destination (clinic or hospital that would be able to care for immunocompromised host; how to use embassy resources and medical evacuation insurance).
- Bring extra medications in case of travel delays; ensure medications are labeled.
- Avoid taking medications purchased at destination (drug interactions or substandard, spurious, falsely labeled, falsified, and counterfeit medical products).
- Augmented risk of infection with multidrug-resistant organisms during and after travel; highlight such travel to clinicians if ill afterwards.
- Vigilant use of sun protection given dramatically elevated rates of skin cancer in immunocompromised hosts, also higher risk of photosensitivity from medications.
- Vigilant food and water precautions. Antibacterial hand wipes or an alcohol-based hand sanitizer containing at least 60% alcohol may be useful.
- Bring travel health/first aid kit.

## BIBLIOGRAPHY

1. Agarwal N, Ollington K, Kaneshiro M, Frenck R, Melmed GY. Are immunosuppressive medications associated with decreased responses to routine immunizations? A systematic review. Vaccine. 2012 Feb 14;30(8):1413–24.

2. Barte H, Horvath TH, Rutherford GW. Yellow fever vaccine for patients with HIV infection. Cochrane Database Syst Rev. 2014(1):Cd010929.

3. CDC. General recommendations on immunization—recommendations of the Advisory Committee on Immunization Practices (ACIP). MMWR Recomm Rep. 2011 Jan 28;60(2):1–64.

4. Dekkiche S, de Valliere S, D'Acremont V, Genton B. Travel-related health risks in moderately and severely immunocompromised patients: a case-control study. J Travel Med. 2016 Mar;23(3): pii: taw001. doi: 10.1093/jtm/taw001.

5. Farez MF, Correale J. Yellow fever vaccination and increased relapse rate in travelers with multiple sclerosis. Arch Neurol. 2011 Oct;68(10): 1267–71.

6. Garcia Garrido HM, Wieten RW, Grobusch MP, Goorhuis A. Response to hepatitis A vaccination in immunocompromised travelers. J Infect Dis. 2015 Aug 1;212(3):378–85.

7. Kotton CN, Hibberd PL. Travel medicine and transplant tourism in solid organ transplantation. Am J Transplant. 2013 Mar;13 Suppl 4:337–47.

8. Loebermann M, Winkelmann A, Hartung HP, Hengel H, Reisinger EC, Zettl UK. Vaccination against infection in patients with multiple sclerosis. Nat Rev Neurol. 2011;8(3):143–51.

9. Luks AM, Swenson ER. Evaluating the risks of high altitude travel in chronic liver disease patients. High Alt Med Biol. 2015 Jun;16(2):80–8.

10. Masur H, Brooks JT, Benson CA, Holmes KK, Pau AK, Kaplan JE. Prevention and treatment of opportunistic infections in HIV-infected adults and adolescents: updated guidelines from the Centers for Disease Control and Prevention, National Institutes of Health, and HIV Medicine Association of the Infectious Diseases Society of America. Clin Infect Dis. 2014 May;58(9):1308–11.

11. Pacanowski J, Lacombe K, Campa P, Dabrowska M, Poveda JD, Meynard JL, et al. Plasma HIV-RNA is the key determinant of long-term antibody persistence after yellow fever immunization in a cohort of 364 HIV-infected patients. J Acquir Immune Defic Syndr. 2012 Apr 1;59(4):360–7.

12. Perry RT, Plowe CV, Koumare B, Bougoudogo F, Kotloff KL, Losonsky GA, et al. A single dose of live oral cholera vaccine CVD 103-HgR is safe and immunogenic in HIV-infected and HIV-noninfected adults in Mali. Bull World Health Organ. 1998;76(1):63–71.

13. Rubin LG, Levin MJ, Ljungman P, Davies EG, Avery R, Tomblyn M, et al. 2013 IDSA clinical practice guideline for vaccination of the immunocompromised host. Clin Infect Dis. 2014 Feb;58(3):309–18.

14. Schwartz BS, Rosen J, Han PV, Hynes NA, Hagmann SH, Rao SR, et al. Immunocompromised travelers: demographic characteristics, travel destinations, and pretravel health care from the U.S. Global

5

TravEpiNet Consortium. Am J Trop Med Hyg. 2015 Nov;93(5):1110–16.

15. Visser LG. TNF-α antagonists and immunization. Curr Infect Dis Rep. 2011 Jun;13(3):243–7.

16. Wieten RW, Goorhuis A, Jonker EF, de Bree GJ, de Visser AW, van Genderen PJ, et al. 17D yellow fever vaccine elicits comparable long-term immune

responses in healthy individuals and immune-compromised patients. J Infect. 2016 Jun;72(6):713–22.

17. Wyplosz B, Burdet C, Francois H, Durrbach A, Duclos-Vallee JC, Mamzer-Bruneel MF, et al. Persistence of yellow fever vaccine-induced antibodies after solid organ transplantation. Am J Transplant. 2013 Sep;13(9):2458–61.

# TRAVELERS WITH DISABILITIES

Cynthia F. Hinton, John Eichwald

## OVERVIEW

According to the Americans with Disabilities Act, a person has a disability if he or she has a physical or mental impairment that substantially limits at least 1 major life activity. With proper preparation, many travelers with disabilities can travel internationally. Some travelers with disabilities, such as those with mobility limitations, vision or hearing loss, or cognitive disabilities may require special attention and adaptation of transportation services. The following recommendations may assist in ensuring safe, accessible travel for travelers with disabilities:

- Assess each international itinerary on an individual basis, in consultation with specialized travel agencies or tour operators.

- Consult travel health providers for additional recommendations.

- Plan ahead to ensure that necessary accommodations are available throughout the entire trip.

## BEFORE TRAVEL

Each country has its own standard of accessibility for people with disabilities. Several websites can help the traveler answer questions about accessibility. Visit https://travel.state.gov/content/travel/en/international-travel/International-Travel-Country-Information-Pages.html and enter a country or area to find information on accessibility for travelers with mobility limitations in the "Local Laws & Special Circumstances" section. Unlike the United States, many countries do not legally require

accommodations for people with disabilities. Read section 6 of the State Department's Human Rights Report for information of the human rights and social service framework protecting citizens with disabilities in the destination country (www.state.gov/j/drl/rls/hrrpt/index.htm).

- Consult with travel agents, hotels, airlines or cruise ship companies to learn about services during the trip and at the destination, including for service animals. Websites such as Mobility International USA (www.miusa.org) will have links to overseas disability organizations.

- Consult an organization that specializes in travel for people with intellectual disabilities (http://newdirectionstravel.org).

- Consider enrolling in the Smart Traveler Enrollment Program (STEP) to receive security messages and to make it easier for the US embassy or consulate to help in an emergency (https://step.state.gov/step/).

### Medical Considerations

- If the traveler's health insurance plan does not provide coverage overseas, the US State Department strongly recommends purchasing supplemental medical insurance and medical evacuation plans.

- Visit the web page "Your Health Abroad" for information about international travel (https://travel.state.gov/content/travel/en/international-travel/before-you-go/your-health-abroad.html).

- See the Travelers' Health page of the Centers for Disease Control website for health actions before, during, and after travel (www.cdc.gov/travel).

- Travelers should carry medical alert information and a letter from their health care provider describing medical conditions, medications, potential complications, and other pertinent medical information.

- Travelers should carry sufficient prescription medication to last the entire trip, including extra medicine in case of delay. Always carry prescriptions in their labeled containers, not in a pill pack.

- Some prescription medications that are legal in the United States are illegal in other countries. See https://travel.state.gov/content/travel/en/international-travel/International-Travel-Country-Information-Pages.html for the specific area where you will be traveling, and contact the foreign embassy or consulate for more information (www.usembassy.gov).

## Assistive Equipment

- Call the Transportation Security Administration's (TSA) helpline for travelers with disabilities and medical conditions at 855-787-2227 (toll-free), federal relay 711, or check TSA's website, (www.tsa.gov/travel/special-procedures) for answers to questions about screening policies, procedures, and the security checkpoints.

- Find out if there are specific policies for devices such as wheelchairs, portable machines, batteries, respirators, and oxygen.

- Consider renting wheelchairs and medical equipment at the destination. Research the availability of wheelchair and medical equipment providers. Websites such as Mobility International USA (www.miusa.org) or the European Network for Accessible Tourism (www.accessibletourism.org) will have links to overseas medical equipment providers.

- Consider the use of manual versus power wheelchairs. The country voltage, type of electrical plug, and reliability of the electrical infrastructure at the destination country may make one type of wheelchair preferable over another.

## Service Animals

- Contact the US embassy or consulate of the destination country for information on possible restrictions and cultural norms about service animals (www.usembassy.gov).

- Find out about any quarantine, vaccination, and documentation requirements.

- Consult veterinarians about tips for traveling with service animals.

- Contact destination hotels to make sure they will accommodate service animals.

## AIR TRAVEL

Many non-US airlines voluntarily adhere to codes of practice that are similar to US legislation based on guidelines from the International Civil Aviation Organization. However, these guidelines are not identical to those outlined in US legislation, and the degree of implementation may vary by airline and location. Travelers planning to fly between foreign countries or within a foreign country while abroad should check with the overseas airlines to ensure that the carriers adhere to accessibility standards adequate for their needs.

### Regulations and Codes

In 1986, Congress passed the Air Carrier Access Act (ACAA) to ensure that people with disabilities are treated without discrimination in a way consistent with the safe carriage of all air passengers. The regulations established by the Department of Transportation (DOT) apply to all flights of US airlines and flights to or from the United States by foreign carriers.

### Flight Information and Reservation Services

If an airline carrier provides telephone reservation and information service to the public, these services must be available to people who are deaf or hard-of-hearing through a telecommunications device for the deaf (TDD), telecommunications relay services, or other technology.

## Airports
As part of the ACAA, DOT rules require any airport terminal facility that receives federal financial assistance to enable or ensure high-contrast captioning. The captioning is required at all times on televisions and other audio-visual displays capable of displaying captions located in any common area of the terminal to which passengers have access, including the gate area, ticketing area, passenger lounges, and leased commercial shop and restaurant spaces.

## Security
The TSA has established a program for screening travelers with disabilities and their equipment, mobility aids, and devices. TSA permits prescriptions, liquid medications, and other liquids needed by people with disabilities and medical conditions. Travelers who have disabilities or medical conditions that may affect TSA screening may use notification cards to communicate with the officer. Travelers can learn more about the TSA guidelines for travelers with disabilities at www.tsa.gov/travel/special-procedures and print the card at www.tsa.gov/sites/default/files/disability_notification_card_508.pdf.

As with other people with disabilities or medical conditions, travelers who are deaf or hard-of-hearing can provide the TSA officer with a notification card or other medical documentation that describes their condition and informs the officer about the need for assistance with the screening process. Travelers are not required to remove any hearing aids or external cochlear implant devices. Additional screening, including a pat-down or device inspection, may be required if assistance devices alarm security technology.

## Ticket Counter, Gate, and Customer Service Desks
Current ACAA rules require people who are deaf or hard-of-hearing to self-identify in order to ensure the receipt of accessible information. Passenger information, including information about flight schedule changes, connections, gate assignments and baggage claim must be transmitted in a timely manner through an accessible method of communication to those who have identified themselves as having hearing impairment. Passengers with impaired hearing must identify themselves to carrier personnel at the gate area or the customer service desk even if they have already done so at the ticketing area. The rule does not require a sign language interpreter to ensure that a passenger who is deaf receives all pertinent information.

## In-Flight
All audio-visual displays played on aircraft for safety and informational purposes must use captioning or a sign language interpreter insert as part of the video presentation. The captioning must be in the predominant languages in which the carrier communicates with passengers on the flight. The current ACAA rule does not require the captioning of in-flight entertainment.

## Boarding and Deplaning
There may be no jetway with smaller airplanes, and travelers who use wheelchairs may need to be manually lifted up or down the stairs. Some airports have adapted hoists or lifts. An aisle chair is usually required to board and deplane. Travelers should be sure to mention they need an aisle chair, both when reserving tickets and when checking in at the airport (http://wheelchairtraveling.com/traveling-with-medical-equipment-or-a-wheelchair-handicap-limited-mobility-or-senior-at-airports-airplanes-and-all-aboutflying-faa-tsa-air-carriers-act).

## Assistance and Accommodations
Because of the ACAA, carriers may not refuse transportation on the basis of a disability. However, there are a few exceptions; for example, the carrier may refuse transportation if the person with a disability would endanger the health or safety of other passengers or if transporting the person would be a violation of Federal Aviation Administration safety rules. Travelers and their clinicians can learn more about these exceptions and other aspects of the ACAA at http://airconsumer.ost.dot.gov/publications/horizons.htm.

Air carriers are also obliged to accept a declaration by a passenger that he or she is self-reliant. A medical certificate (a written statement from the passenger's health care provider saying that the passenger is capable of completing the flight safely without requiring extraordinary medical care or endangering other passengers) can be required only in specific situations. If a person intends to travel with a possible communicable disease, will require a stretcher or oxygen, or if the person's medical condition can be reasonably expected to affect the operation of the flight, a medical certificate is typically required.

Under the guidelines of the ACAA, when a traveler with disability requests assistance, the airline is obliged to meet certain accessibility requirements. For example, carriers must provide access to the aircraft door (preferably by a level entry bridge), an aisle seat, and a seat with removable armrests. However, aircraft with <30 seats are generally exempt from these requirements. Any aircraft with >60 seats must have an onboard wheelchair (aisle chair), and personnel must help move the wheelchair from a seat to the lavatory area. Airline personnel are not required to transfer passengers from wheelchair to wheelchair, wheelchair to aircraft seat, or wheelchair to lavatory seat. In addition, airline personnel are not obliged to assist with feeding, visiting the lavatory, or dispensing medication to travelers. Only wide-body aircraft with ≥2 aisles are required to have fully accessible lavatories. Travelers with disabilities who require assistance should travel with a companion or attendant. Without reason, however, carriers may not require a person with a disability to travel with an attendant.

Airlines may not require advance notice of a passenger with a disability. They may, however, require up to 48 hours advance notice and 1-hour advance check-in for certain accommodations that require preparation time, such as the following services (if they are available on the flight):

- Medical oxygen for use on board the aircraft
- Carriage of an incubator
- Hook-up for a respirator to the aircraft electrical power supply

- Accommodation for a passenger who must travel in a stretcher
- Transportation of an electric wheelchair on an aircraft with <60 seats
- Provision by the airline of hazardous material packaging for batteries used in wheelchairs or other assistive devices
- Accommodation for a group of ≥10 people with disabilities who travel as a group
- Provision of an onboard wheelchair (aisle chair) for use on an aircraft that does not have an accessible lavatory

DOT maintains a toll-free hotline (800-778-4838 [voice] or 800-455-9880 [TTY], available 9 AM to 5 PM Eastern Time, Monday through Friday, except federal holidays) to provide general information to consumers about the rights of air travelers with disabilities and to assist air travelers with time-sensitive disability-related issues.

## CRUISE SHIPS

US companies or entities conducting programs or tours on cruise ships have obligations regarding access for travelers with disabilities, even if the ship itself is of foreign registry. However, all travelers with disabilities should check with individual cruise lines regarding availability of requested or needed items before booking. Cruise operators and travel agents that cater to travelers with special needs also exist.

## USEFUL LINKS

- Transportation Security Administration, Disabilities and Medical Conditions: www.tsa.gov/travel/special-procedures
- US Department of Transportation, Aviation Consumer Protection Division: www.transportation.gov/individuals/aviation-consumer-protection/service-animals-including-emotional-support-animals
- US Department of Transportation, Traveling with a Disability: www.transportation.gov/individuals/aviation-consumer-protection/traveling-disability

- US Department of State, Travel Health Website: https://travel.state.gov/content/travel/en/international-travel/before-you-go/your-health-abroad.html

- Aerospace Medical Association, medical publications for airline travel: www.asma.org/publications/medical-publications-for-airline-travel

- Mobility International USA: www.miusa.org

- Wheelchairtraveling.com: http://wheelchairtraveling.com

- New Directions Travel, Inc.: www.newdirectionstravel.org

- Society for Accessible Travel and Hospitality: www.sath.org

- National Association of the Deaf: www.nad.org/resources/transportation-and-travel/air-travel/air-carrier-access-act-acaa

- American Council of the Blind, Travel Resources: www.acb.org

- American Academy of Otolaryngology, Travel Tips for the Hearing Impaired: www.entnet.org/content/travel-tips-hearing-impaired

- European Network for Accessible Tourism: www.accessibletourism.org

## BIBLIOGRAPHY

1. Barnett, S. Communication with deaf and hard-of-hearing people: A guide for medical education. Academic Medicine. 2002; 77(7):694–700.

2. Bauer I. When travel is a challenge: travel medicine and the "dis-abled" traveler. Travel Medicine and Infectious Disease. 2018:22;66–72.

3. International Civil Aviation Organization. Manual on access to air transport by persons with disabilities. Montréal: International Civil Aviation Organization; 2013 [cited 2016 Sep 27]. Available

from: www.passepartouttraining.com/uploads/2013/03/ICAO-Manual-Doc-9984-1st-Edition-alltext-en_published_March-2013.pdf

4. National Association of the Deaf. Legal rights: The guide for deaf and hard of hearing people. Washington, DC: Gallaudet University Press; 2000.

5. Nondiscrimination on the basis of disability in air travel. 2003 [cited 2016 Sep 27]. Available from: http://airconsumer.dot.gov/rules/382short.pdf.

# TRAVELERS WITH CHRONIC ILLNESSES

Deborah Nicolls Barbeau, Gail A. Rosselot, Sue Ann McDevitt

## GENERAL TRAVEL PREPARATION: PRACTICAL CONSIDERATIONS

Although traveling abroad can be relaxing and rewarding, the physical demands of travel can be stressful, particularly for travelers with underlying chronic illnesses. With adequate preparation, however, such travelers can have safe and enjoyable trips. General recommendations

for advising patients with chronic illnesses include:

- Ensure that any chronic illnesses are well controlled. Patients with an underlying illness should see their health care providers to ensure that the management of their illness is optimized.

- Encourage patients to seek pretravel consultation ≥4–6 weeks before departure to ensure adequate time to respond to immunizations and, in some circumstances, to try medications before travel (see the Immunocompromised Travelers section in this chapter).

- Advise patients to consider a destination where they have access to quality care for their condition (see Chapter 6, Obtaining Health Care Abroad).

- Ask about previous health-related issues encountered during travel, such as complications during air travel.

- Advise the traveler about packing a health kit (see Chapter 6, Travel Health Kits).

- Advise travelers to pack medications and medical supplies (such as pouching for ostomies) in their original containers in carry-on luggage and to carry a copy of their prescriptions. Ensure the traveler has sufficient quantities of medications and proper storage conditions for the entire trip, plus extra in case of unexpected delays. Since medications should be taken based on elapsed time and not time of day, travelers may need guidance on scheduling when to take medications during and after crossing time zones.

- Advise travelers to check with the US embassy or consulate to clarify medication restrictions in the destination country. Some countries do not allow visitors to bring certain medications into the country, especially narcotics and psychotropic medications.

- Educate travelers regarding drug interactions (see Chapter 2, Interactions Among Travel Vaccines & Drugs). Medications (such as warfarin) used to treat chronic medical illnesses may interact with medications prescribed for self-treatment of travelers' diarrhea or malaria chemoprophylaxis. Discuss all medications used, either daily or on an as-needed basis.

- Provide a clinician's letter. The letter should be on office letterhead stationery and should outline existing medical conditions, medications prescribed (including generic names), and any equipment required to manage the condition.

- Discuss supplemental insurance. Three types of insurance policies can be considered: 1) trip cancellation in the event of illness; 2) supplemental insurance so that money paid for health care abroad may be reimbursed, since most medical insurance policies do not cover health care in other countries; and 3) medical evacuation insurance (see Chapter 6, Travel Insurance, Travel Health Insurance & Medical Evacuation Insurance). Travelers may need extra help in finding supplemental insurance, as some plans will not cover costs for preexisting conditions.

- Encourage travelers with underlying medical conditions to consider choosing a medical assistance company that allows them to store their medical history so it can be accessed worldwide (see Chapter 6, Obtaining Health Care Abroad).

- Help travelers devise a health plan. This plan should give instructions for managing minor problems or exacerbations of underlying illnesses and should include information about medical facilities available in the destination country (see Chapter 6, Obtaining Health Care Abroad).

- Advise travelers to wear a medical alert bracelet or carry medical information on his or her person (various brands of jewelry or tags, even electronic [through medical records apps], are available).

- Advise travelers to stay hydrated, wear loose-fitting clothing, and walk and stretch at regular intervals during long-distance travel (see Chapter 8, Deep Vein Thrombosis & Pulmonary Embolism).

## SPECIFIC CHRONIC ILLNESSES

Issues related to specific chronic medical illnesses are addressed in Table 5-3. These recommendations should be used in conjunction with

## Table 5-3. Special considerations for travelers with chronic medical illnesses

| CONDITION | ABSOLUTE AND RELATIVE CONTRAINDICATIONS TO AIRLINE TRAVEL | PRETRAVEL CONSIDERATIONS | IMMUNIZATION CONSIDERATIONS | MISCELLANEOUS |
|---|---|---|---|---|
| Cancer | Severe anemia (Hg <8.5 g/dL) Cerebral edema due to intracranial tumor ≤6 weeks since cranial surgery Cardiovascular, pulmonary, or gastrointestinal complications referred to below | Emphasize food and water precautions Plan for self-management of dehydration DVT precautions Supplemental oxygen Wear loose-fitting clothing to prevent worsening of lymphedema | Immunosuppressive medications may alter response to immunizations Live attenuated vaccines may be contraindicated Revaccination may be necessary following cancer treatment | Check for medication restrictions in the destination country, especially if controlled medications are required for pain management see the Immunocompromised Travelers section precedes this section in the chapter |
| Cardiovascular diseases | Following acute coronary syndrome: • those at very low risk and within 3 days after event • medium risk and within 10 days after event • high risk or awaiting further intervention or treatment—should defer air travel, until disease is stable Unstable angina CHF, severe, decompensated Uncontrolled hypertension CABG within 10 days CVA within 2 weeks Elective percutaneous coronary intervention within 2 days Uncontrolled arrhythmia Eisenmenger syndrome Severe symptomatic valvular heart disease | Supplemental oxygen plan for self-management of dehydration and volume overload; may include adjusting medications Bring copy of recent EKG Bring pacemaker or AICD card DVT precautions | Influenza Pneumococcal Hepatitis B | Have sublingual nitroglycerin available in carry-on bag Mefloquine not recommended for people with cardiac conduction abnormalities, particularly for those with ventricular arrhythmias Self-monitoring and management of INR should be tailored to the individual patient by the anticoagulant primary provider |

| Condition | Precautions | Counseling | Vaccines | Special considerations |
|---|---|---|---|---|
| Pulmonary diseases | Severe, labile asthma<br>Recent hospitalization for acute respiratory illness<br>Bullous lung disease<br>Active lower respiratory infection<br>Pneumothorax within 7 days (spontaneous pneumothorax) or 14 days (traumatic pneumothorax) | Supplemental oxygen<br>Discuss with airline need for other equipment on plane (such as nebulizer)<br>Plan for self-management of exacerbations (including COPD, asthma)<br>DVT precautions | Influenza<br>Pneumococcal<br>Hepatitis B | Consider carrying a short course of antibiotics and steroids for exacerbations<br>Consider advising an inhaler be available in carry-on bag, even if not routinely used |
| | Pleural effusion within 14 days<br>High supplemental oxygen requirements at baseline<br>Major chest surgery within 10days | | | |
| Gastrointestinal diseases | Major surgery, within 10–14 days<br>Uncomplicated appendectomy or laparoscopic surgery within 5 days<br>Gastrointestinal bleed within 24 hours<br>Colonoscopy within 24 hours<br>Partial bowel obstruction<br>Liver failure (especially cirrhosis or heavy alcohol use) | Emphasize food and water precautions<br>Consider prescribing prophylactic antibiotic for TD<br>Recommend avoiding undercooked seafood, if cirrhosis or heavy alcohol use (Vibrio vulnificus) | Influenza<br>Pneumococcal<br>Hepatitis A<br>Hepatitis B | May experience increased colostomy output during air travel<br>$H_2$ blockers and PPIs increase susceptibility to TD<br>Use mefloquine with caution in any chronic liver disease<br>For YF vaccine, see the Immunocompromised Travelers section precedes this section in the chapter |
| Renal failure and chronic renal insufficiency | None | Emphasize food and water precautions<br>Plan for self-management of dehydration, which can worsen renal function<br>Arrange dialysis abroad, if needed<br>Adjust medications for CrCl | Influenza<br>Pneumococcal<br>Hepatitis B | Know HIV, hepatitis C, and hepatitis B status<br>Atovaquone-proguanil contraindicated when CrCl <30 mL/min<br>AAKP and Global Dialysis websites can help with finding dialysis centers; check for accreditation<br>For YF vaccine, see the Immunocompromised Travelers section precedes this section in the chapter |

(continued)

# Table 5-3. Special considerations for travelers with chronic medical illnesses (continued)

| CONDITION | ABSOLUTE AND RELATIVE CONTRAINDICATIONS TO AIRLINE TRAVEL | PRETRAVEL CONSIDERATIONS | IMMUNIZATION CONSIDERATIONS | MISCELLANEOUS |
|---|---|---|---|---|
| Diabetes mellitus | None | Plan for self-management of dehydration, diabetic foot, and pressure sores<br>Insulin adjustments<br>Should check FSBG at 4- to 6-hour intervals during air travel<br>Discuss changes in insulin regimen or oral agent with diabetes specialist<br>Provide physician's letter stating need for all equipment, including syringes, glucose meter, and supplies | Influenza<br>Pneumococcal<br>Hepatitis B | Keep insulin and all glucose meter supplies in carry-on bag<br>Bring food and supplies needed to manage hypoglycemia during travel<br>Check feet daily for pressure sores<br>For YF vaccine, see the Immunocompromised Travelers section precedes this section in the chapter |
| Severe allergic reactions | None | Plan for managing allergic reactions while traveling and consider bringing a short course of steroids for possible allergic reactions<br>Should carry injectable epinephrine and antihistamines ($H_1$ and $H_2$ blockers)—always have on person | | Many airlines already have policies in place for dealing with peanut allergies<br>Make sure to carry injectable epinephrine in case of a severe reaction while in flight |
| Autoimmune and rheumatologic diseases | None | Should have a baseline TST or IGRA before starting TNF blockers | Immunosuppressive medications and TNF blockers may alter response to immunizations<br>Live attenuated vaccines may be contraindicated | Particular emphasis should be placed on food and water precautions and hand hygiene |

Abbreviations: DVT, deep vein thrombosis; CHF, congestive heart failure; CABG, coronary artery bypass graft; CVA, cerebrovascular accident; EKG, electrocardiogram; AICD, automatic implantable cardioverter defibrillators; Hg, hemoglobin; INR, international normalized ratio; COPD, chronic obstructive pulmonary disease; TD, travelers' diarrhea; PPIs, proton-pump inhibitors; YF, yellow fever; CrCl, creatinine clearance; AAKP, American Association of Kidney Patients; FSBG, fingerstick blood glucose; TST, tuberculin skin test; IGRA, interferon-γ release assay; TNF, tumor necrosis factor.

## BOX 5-2. Highly allergic travelers

Highly allergic travelers experience allergic reactions that can interrupt or alter planned activities or may require emergency medical care during travel. Language barriers, lack of emergency services, and unfamiliar environments and menus compound risk. Pretravel preparation and proactive communication can reduce the risk of severe allergic reactions (SARs), although travelers with a new severe allergy, recent SAR, or recurrent SARs warrant a specialist referral.

The travel medicine provider should assess and document the following:

- Date of allergy onset; specific and related triggers, last date of any allergy workup or specialist consult.
- Description of inhalation, ingested, contact, or injected (insects, snakes) allergy symptoms.
- History of anaphylaxis emergency, urgent care visits, or hospitalizations.
- Use of an epinephrine auto-injector, inhaler, inhaled or oral steroids; when and why last used.
- Additional recognized risk factors for SARs while traveling: younger age, adolescence, history of SAR hospitalization, history of >3 days use of corticosteroids, asthma and food allergy comorbidity, solo travel, multiple destinations, remote destinations, longer duration

of travel, outdoor activities (for inhalation and insect exposures), availability of specialist care at the destination, language barriers.

Providers should counsel travelers to:

- Bring several copies of a written plan for responding to SARs; always carry a copy, including one in destination languages, if possible.
- Research emergency services at destinations—where they are located and how to obtain them.
- *Never be too embarrassed to alert others about a severe allergy*; inform traveling companions, tour leaders, flight attendants, seat mates, restaurant and hotel staff; share customized care plan.
- Check expiration dates of prescriptions; carry extra supplies of all self-care therapies in carry-on luggage (antihistamines, inhalers, corticosteroids, epinephrine auto-injectors, nebulizers); medically necessary liquids and medications in excess of Transportation Security Administration limits are allowed in carry-on luggage; *do not purchase medications abroad*; bring a backpack or other bag to carry supplies at destination.
- Wear a medical identification bracelet; carry a card listing all medical conditions and medications; carry a medical

letter describing allergy, translated if possible.
- Recognize SAR signs and symptoms; know when and how to correctly use epinephrine auto-injectors.
- Purchase travel health insurance; confirm health insurance coverage for emergency services during travel.
- Anticipate dietary and environmental allergies for trains, airlines, and ships; bring along snacks or meals, if needed; ask to be seated away from pets.
- **Food allergies:** carry "chef cards" in English and destination languages (see www.foodallergy.org/life-food-allergies/managing-lifes-milestones/dining-out/food-allergy-chef-cards); bring a supply of nonperishable food in case safe food is not available; avoid "street food"; choose safe foods over exotic foods; consider eating at chain restaurants where ingredients may be more standardized; *always remember that dietary vigilance is critical; when in doubt, avoid a food item.*
- **Airborne allergies:** minimize outdoor activity when air quality is poor or pollen count is high; identify and reserve smoke-free (pet-free) accommodations and restaurants; even if asthma is stable, travel may exacerbate the condition; be sure to pack all equipment including spacers, nebulizers, and peak flow meters.

the other recommendations given throughout this book. Below is a noninclusive list of additional resources for information:

- American Association of Kidney Patients (www.aakp.org)
- American Diabetes Association (www.diabetes.org)
- American Heart Association (www.heart.org)
- American Lung Association (www.lung.org)
- American Society of Clinical Oncology (www.cancer.net)
- American Thoracic Society (www.thoracic.org)
- Anticoagulation Forum (www.acforum.org)
- British Thoracic Society (www.brit-thoracic.org.uk)
- Crohn's and Colitis Foundation of America (www.ccfa.org)
- Global Dialysis (www.globaldialysis.com)
- International Narcotics Control Board (www.incb.org)
- National Multiple Sclerosis Society (www.nationalmssociety.org)

- Transportation Security Administration (www.tsa.gov)
- Department of State (www.state.gov)
- Department of Transportation (www.transportation.gov)

Considerations for travelers with allergies are shown in Box 5-2.

Travelers may also want to investigate international health care accreditation agencies for centers that have been awarded recognition for high standards and good patient safety records. If travelers or their health care providers have concerns about fitness for air travel or the need to obtain a medical certificate before travel, the medical unit affiliated with the specific airline is a valuable source for information.

Travelers who require service animals, including emotional support animals, should check with the airline and the destination country to ensure the destination country permits the animal and that all required documentation is available. Remember to notify the airline well in advance if oxygen or other equipment is needed on the plane. The TSA Cares Helpline (toll-free at 855-787-2227) can also provide information on how to prepare for the airport security screening process with respect to a particular disability or medical condition.

## BIBLIOGRAPHY

1. Exemption from import/export requirements for personal medical use. 21 CFR Part 1301;2004. [cited 2016 Sep, 27]. Available from: www.deadiversion.usdoj.gov/21cfr/cfr/1301/1301_26.htm

2. Food allergy and anaphylaxis plan. FARE; 2018. [cited 2018 Apr 2]. Available from: www.foodallergy.org/life-with-food-allergies/food-allergy-anaphylaxis-emergency-care-plan.

3. IATA. Medical Manual. 11th Edition. June 2018 [cited 2018 Oct 23]. Available from: www.iata.org/publications/Documents/medical-manual.pdf.

4. Josephs LK, Coker RK, Thomas M, British Thoracic Society Air Travel Working Group. Managing patients with stable respiratory disease planning air travel: a primary care summary of the British Thoracic Society recommendations. Prim Care Respir J. 2013 Jun;22(2):234–8.

5. McCarthy AE, Burchard GD. The travelers with pre-existing disease. In: Keystone JS, Freedman DO,

Kozarsky PE, Connor BA, Nothdurft HD, editors. Travel Medicine. 3rd ed. Philadelphia: Saunders Elsevier; 2013. pp. 257–63.

6. Pinsker JE, Becker E, Mahnke CB, Ching M, Larson NS, Roy D. Extensive clinical experience: a simple guide to basal insulin adjustments for long-distance travel. J Diabetes Metab Disord. 2013;12(1):59.

7. Ringwald J, Strobel J, Eckstein R. Travel and oral anticoagulation. J Travel Med. 2009 Jul–Aug;16(4):276–83.

8. School tools: Allergy & asthma resources for families, clinicians and school nurses. AAAAI; 2018. [cited 2018 Apr 2]. Available from: www.aaaai.org/conditions-and-treatments/school-tools.

9. Smith D, Toff W, Joy M, Dowdall N, Johnston R, Clark L, et al. Fitness to fly for passengers with cardiovascular disease. Heart. 2010 Aug;96 Suppl 2:ii1–16.

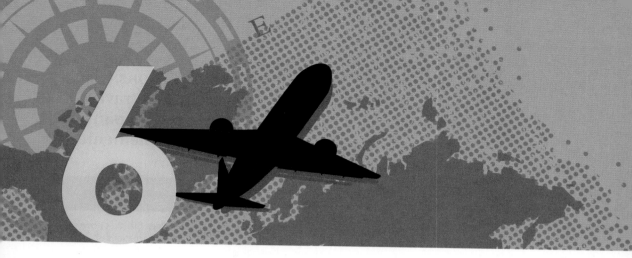

# Health Care Abroad

## TRAVEL INSURANCE, TRAVEL HEALTH INSURANCE & MEDICAL EVACUATION INSURANCE

Rhett J. Stoney

Severe illness or injury abroad may result in a financial burden to travelers. Travelers can substantially reduce their out-of-pocket costs for medical care received abroad by purchasing in advance specialized insurance policies for their trip, regardless of whether or not they have a domestic health insurance plan. The 3 types of policies are travel insurance, travel health insurance, and medical evacuation insurance. Each provides different types of coverage in the event of an illness or injury and may be of particular importance to travelers with preexisting medical conditions.

Basic accident or travel health insurance may be necessary for travelers with certain itineraries. For example, although cruise lines employ health care staff, the cost for medical treatment delivered on board a ship may not be included in the price of a passenger's ticket; travelers on cruise ships may wish to consider investing in specialized insurance policies.

### DOMESTIC HEALTH INSURANCE AND OVERSEAS TRAVEL

Some health insurance carriers in the United States cover medical emergencies that occur when policyholders travel internationally. Encourage patients to contact their insurer before traveling to learn what medical services, if any, their policies cover. Table 6-1 includes suggested questions travelers should ask their insurance company.

## Table 6-1. Coverage requirements, potential exclusions, and preexisting medical conditions: questions travelers should consider asking their insurance company when deciding whether to purchase supplemental insurance coverage

| COVERAGE REQUIREMENTS | POTENTIAL EXCLUSIONS | PREEXISTING MEDICAL CONDITIONS |
|---|---|---|
| Do I need preauthorization before receiving treatment, hospital admission, or other medical services? | Does this policy include/exclude coverage for treatment of injuries sustained while participating in high-risk activities (e.g., skydiving, scuba diving, and mountain climbing)? | Does this policy cover exacerbations of preexisting medical conditions? |
| Do I need a second opinion before I can receive emergency treatment? | Does this policy include/exclude coverage for psychiatric emergencies? | Does this policy cover complications of pregnancy and/or neonatal intensive care? |
| What are company policies regarding coverage of care received "out of network"? | Does this policy include/exclude coverage for treatment of injuries related to terrorist attacks, acts of war, or natural disasters? | |
| Does the company provide policyholders access to a 24/7/365 physician-backed support center? | | |

## PAYING FOR HEALTH SERVICES ABROAD

Include a discussion of insurance options as part of the pretravel consultation. Suggest that all travelers consider purchasing supplemental medical insurance coverage, particularly those going to remote destinations or places lacking high-quality medical facilities. Strongly encourage supplemental medical insurance coverage for any travelers planning extended international travel, those with underlying health conditions, and anyone who anticipates participating in high-risk activities overseas. In addition to covering costs of treatment or medical evacuation, travel health insurers can assist the international traveler by organizing and coordinating care and by keeping relatives informed in the event of a medical emergency. This is especially important when the traveler is severely ill or injured and requires a medical evacuation.

Even with a supplemental travel health insurance policy in force, receiving medical care abroad usually requires cash or credit card payment at the point of service. This can result in sizable expenditures of thousands of dollars. US citizens paying for health care received overseas are advised to obtain copies of all charges and receipts and, if necessary, to contact a US consular officer, who can assist them with transferring funds from the United States. The existence of nationalized health care services at a given destination does not ensure that health care costs of nonresidents are covered.

## TRAVEL INSURANCE

Travel insurance protects the financial investment in a trip, including lost baggage and trip cancellation. A traveler who becomes ill in advance of departure may be more likely to avoid or postpone travel if they know their financial investment in the trip is protected. Depending on the policy, travel insurance may or may not cover medical expenses abroad, so travelers need to research carefully the coverage offered to determine their need for additional travel health and medical evacuation insurance.

## SUPPLEMENTAL TRAVEL HEALTH AND MEDICAL EVACUATION INSURANCE

Travel health insurance and medical evacuation insurance are 2 types of short-term supplemental policies that cover health care costs incurred while abroad. Each is relatively inexpensive. Many commercial companies offer travel health insurance; travelers can purchase such policies separately or in conjunction with medical evacuation insurance. Frequent travelers can consider purchasing annual policies or even policies that provide coverage for repatriation to one's home country. Some recommended features to consider when purchasing supplemental travel health and medical evacuation insurance include the following:

- Arrangements made with hospitals to guarantee direct payment

- Assistance via a 24-hour physician-backed support center (critical for medical evacuation insurance)

- Emergency medical transport to facilities equivalent to those in the home country or to the home country itself (repatriation)

- Specific medical services, such as coverage of high-risk activities

Although travel health insurance covers some international health care costs, the quality of care may be inadequate, and medical evacuation (sometimes referred to as "medevac") from a resource-poor area to a hospital delivering definitive care may be necessary. The cost of medevac can exceed $100,000. In such cases, medevac insurance covers the cost of transportation, including transportation to another country if necessary. Some medical evacuation companies have more extensive experience working in some parts of the world than others do; travelers may want to ask about a company's resources in a given region, especially if planning trips to hard-to-reach locations in that region. Even if travelers select their insurance provider carefully, unexpected delays in care may still arise, especially in remote destinations. In special circumstances, therefore, if the health risks are too high, it may be advisable for a traveler to postpone or cancel their international trip.

## FINDING AN INSURANCE PROVIDER

The following organizations (not an all-inclusive list) provide information about purchasing travel health and medical evacuation insurance:

- Department of State (www.travel.state.gov)

- International Association for Medical Assistance to Travelers (www.iamat.org)

- US Travel Insurance Association (www.ustia.org)

- American Association of Retired Persons (www.aarp.org)

## SPECIAL CONSIDERATIONS FOR TRAVELERS WITH UNDERLYING MEDICAL CONDITIONS

Travelers with underlying medical conditions should discuss any concerns with the insurer before departure. In a study of international travelers with travel health insurance claims, insurance companies fully paid only two-thirds of claims. Preexisting illness and poor documentation were the main reasons for coverage refusal.

Beyond purchasing supplemental travel health insurance coverage, encourage travelers with medical conditions to take additional steps before departure. To facilitate ease of access to health records when overseas, travelers should store copies of those records with a medical assistance company. Instruct travelers to obtain letters from their health care providers listing all medical conditions and current medications (including their generic names), written in the local language, if possible. Transported medications should be in their original bottles and packed in carry-on luggage; to facilitate ease of entry through customs, travelers are advised to check beforehand with the destination country's embassy to ensure that none of the medications they are bringing with them is considered illegal there. Anyone with a known heart condition should carry a copy (paper or electronic) of his or her most recent electrocardiogram.

## SPECIAL CONSIDERATIONS FOR MEDICARE BENEFICIARIES

Except in limited circumstances, the Social Security Medicare program does not provide coverage for medical costs incurred outside the United States. **Medigap (Medicare supplement insurance) plans C, D, F, G, M, and N cover some emergency care outside the United States. After meeting the yearly $250 deductible, this benefit pays 80% of the cost of emergency care during the first 60 days of international travel. There is a $50,000 lifetime maximum.** International travelers can find more information on Medicare and Medigap options at www.medicare.gov/Pubs/pdf/11037-Medicare-Coverage-Outside-United-Stat.pdf. Medicare beneficiaries are no different from other travelers; they need to examine their coverage carefully and supplement it with additional travel health insurance, as required.

## CHECKLIST FOR DISCUSSING INSURANCE WITH TRAVELERS

Travel health providers can use the following points to guide the supplemental insurance discussion during the pretravel consultation:

- Determine travelers' health profile, including underlying medical conditions.

- Identify potential medical needs abroad, including health risks based on itinerary/destination, duration of travel, method of transportation (plane, ship, ground), lodgings/accommodations, and planned activities.

- Instruct travelers to review domestic health policies to identify gaps in coverage for identified potential medical needs.

- Discuss the differences between the 3 types of supplemental insurance (travel, travel health, and medical evacuation), and explain how to choose supplemental policies that cover potential medical needs abroad.

- Remind travelers of the steps to take should they require medical care abroad.

Traveler responsibilities regarding supplemental health insurance before and during travel include the following:

### Before Travel

- Carefully review domestic health insurance policies to determine what medical services are and are not covered overseas.

- Purchase supplemental travel health insurance coverage based on potential medical needs and health risks.

- Identify medical service providers at destination. (See www.iamat.org for a directory of English-speaking providers.)

- Check with insurance company/companies to confirm international health care providers accept the policy as payment for medical services rendered.

### During Travel

- Carry insurance policy identity cards (including supplemental travel health insurance) and insurance claim forms.

- Have contact information of medical providers at destination(s).

- Keep copies of all charges and receipts for medical care received.

### BIBLIOGRAPHY

1. American Association of Retired Persons, Education and Outreach. Overview of Medicare supplemental insurance. Washington, DC: American Association of Retired Persons; 2010 [cited 2018 Feb 21]. Available from: www.aarp.org/health/medicare-insurance/info-10-2008/overview_medicare_supplemental_insurance.html.

2. Centers for Medicare and Medicaid Services. Medicare coverage outside the United States. Baltimore: CMS; 2016 [cited 2018 Feb 21]. Available from: www.medicare.gov/Pubs/pdf/11037-Medicare-Coverage-Outside-United-Stat.pdf.

3. Flaherty G, De Freitas S. A heart for travel: travel health considerations for patients with heart disease and cardiac devices. Ir Med J. 2016 Dec 12;109(10):486.

4. Leggat PA, Carne J, Kedjarune U. Travel insurance and health. J Travel Med. 1999 Dec;6(4):243–8.

6

5. Leggat PA, Leggat FW. Travel insurance claims made by travelers from Australia. J Travel Med. 2002 Mar–Apr;9(2):59–65.

6. Teichman PG, Donchin Y, Kot RJ. International aeromedical evacuation. N Engl J Med. 2007 Jan 18;356(3):262–70.

7. US Department of State. Insurance providers for overseas coverage. Washington, DC: US Department of State; 2016 [cited 2018 Feb 21]. Available from: https://travel.state.gov/content/passports/en/go/health/insurance-providers.html.

# OBTAINING HEALTH CARE ABROAD

Carolina Uribe

While overseas, travelers may seek medical care ranging from treatment for self-limited minor infections to care for chronic conditions to sophisticated medical management of major illnesses or injuries. Because insurance plans may not cover emergency health care received abroad, travelers should check with their carriers before departure to confirm the limits of their coverage and to identify any additional coverage requirements. For example, travel health insurance alone does not usually pay for the cost of an emergency medical evacuation or an altered itinerary. Travelers may buy specific policies to cover these expenses, understanding that such policies often do not cover expenses related to preexisting conditions. Supplemental medical insurance plans purchased prior to traveling often furnish access to preselected local providers in many countries through a 24-hour emergency hotline (see Travel Insurance, Travel Health Insurance & Medical Evacuation Insurance in this chapter, for more details). At a minimum, travelers should be prepared to pay out-of-pocket at the time services are rendered (in some instances, even before care is received) and then afterward provide insurers with copies of bills and invoices to initiate reimbursement.

## LOCATING HEALTH CARE PROVIDERS AND FACILITIES ABROAD

The level and availability of medical care around the world varies from country to country and even within countries. Before going abroad, travelers should consider how they will access health care during their trip should a medical problem or emergency arise (Box 6-1). Encourage those likely to need health care to research thoroughly and identify potential health care providers and facilities at their destination. Dialysis patients, for example, need to arrange appointments in advance at a site with appropriate equipment. Pregnant travelers should know the names and locations of reliable obstetrical medical centers. More choices are generally available in urban areas than in rural or remote areas.

Travelers, particularly those with preexisting or complicated medical issues, should know the names of their condition(s), any allergies, their blood type, and current medications (including generic names), ideally in the local language. They should carry copies of prescriptions, including for glasses and contact lenses, and wear medical identification jewelry (such as a MedicAlert bracelet), as appropriate. Any number of mobile applications enable travelers to download their medical records, medications, electrocardiogram, and other information so that they are accessible when needed.

The following list of resources can help international travelers identify health care providers and facilities around the world. CDC does not endorse any particular provider or medical insurance company, and accreditation does not ensure a good outcome.

- The nearest US embassy or consulate (www.usembassy.gov) can help travelers locate medical services and notify friends, family, or employer of an emergency. They are available for emergencies 24 hours a day, 7 days a week,

## BOX 6-1. Patient checklist for obtaining health care abroad

- Consider travel health and evacuation insurance before travel.
- Evaluate health and avoid travel if feeling ill.
- Identify quality health care providers and facilities at destination.
- Download travel health mobile applications to input medical records, medications, and other health information so that it is accessible if needed.
- Pack adequate supply of medications and know how to get additional safe and effective medications while abroad.
- Request documentation of any medical care received abroad, including medications, and share with health care provider abroad and at home.
- If a blood transfusion is required while traveling, make every effort to ensure that the blood has been screened for transmissible diseases, including HIV.

overseas and in Washington, DC (888-407-4747 or 202-501-4444).

- The Department of State maintains a list of travel medical and evacuation insurance providers at https://travel.state.gov/content/passports/en/go/health/insurance-providers.html.

- The International Society of Travel Medicine maintains a directory of health care professionals with expertise in travel medicine in more than 80 countries. Search these clinics at www.istm.org.

- The International Association for Medical Assistance to Travelers maintains a network of physicians, hospitals, and clinics that have agreed to provide care to members. Membership is free, although donations are suggested. Search for clinics at www.iamat.org/doctors_clinics.cfm.

- Travel agencies, hotels, and credit card companies (especially those with special privileges) may also provide information.

- A number of countries or national travel medicine societies have websites related to travel medicine that provide access to clinicians, including the following:
  > Canada: Health Canada (www.phac-aspc.gc.ca and https://travel.gc.ca)
  > Great Britain: National Travel Health Network and Centre (www.nathnac.org)

and British Global and Travel Health Association (www.bgtha.org)
  > South Africa: South African Society of Travel Medicine (www.sastm.org.za)
  > Australia: Travel Medicine Alliance (www.travelmedicine.com.au)
  > China: International Travel Healthcare Association (http://en.itha.org.cn)

People who receive health care abroad may require ongoing care or experience complications afterward. They should request documentation of any medical care received, including a list of medications received, and share that information with any health care providers seen subsequently.

## AVOID TRAVEL WHEN ILL

Advise travelers to self-evaluate before leaving home to ensure they are healthy enough for their itinerary, and to self-monitor for illness during their trip. Traveling while ill increases the chances that a person will have to interact with an unfamiliar, and—in some locations, at least—inadequately equipped health care system. Moreover, ill travelers pose a risk not only to themselves but also, potentially, to other passengers and travel partners. For a variety of reasons, then, traveling while ill is best avoided.

People may be reluctant to postpone or cancel travel, however, due to loss of financial investment. Make travelers aware that some airlines conduct scans of people in the waiting area and during boarding; if a passenger appears visibly ill, they can be prohibited from boarding. Trip cancellation insurance can protect some or all of an investment in a trip, and may increase compliance with the recommendation not to travel when ill.

## DRUGS AND OTHER PHARMACEUTICALS

The quality of drugs and medical products purchased abroad may not meet the same regulated standards established by the US Food and Drug Administration. Worse yet, they could be counterfeit and contain no active (or even harmful) ingredients (see *Perspectives:* Avoiding Poorly Regulated Medicines and Medical Products during Travel, later in this chapter). If a traveler's original supply of medication is lost, stolen, or damaged, he or she should take steps to try to ensure that the replacement medicines they buy are safe and effective.

To minimize risks associated with substandard drugs and pharmaceuticals, travelers should:

- Bring with them the medicines they think they will need for the entire time they are away; include additional supply in case of trip delays. Hand carry all medications in carry-on luggage and not in checked baggage.

- Insist that health care providers use new needles and syringes when administering injections. Travelers who know they require injections can bring their own supplies along with a letter from their provider attesting to the need for this equipment.

- Carry an epinephrine autoinjector (epipen) in carry-on luggage, to treat known severe, potentially life-threatening allergies. Include a letter from the prescribing physician explaining the allergy and a copy of the prescription.

## BLOOD SAFETY

A medical emergency abroad, such as a motor vehicle crash or other trauma, could require a life-saving transfusion of blood or other blood components (e.g., platelets, fresh frozen plasma). Not all countries accurately, reliably, and systematically screen blood donations for infectious agents, putting recipients at increased risk of transfusion-related diseases. CDC recommends that travelers to developing countries receive transfusions of blood and blood products only when critically necessary. Although it can be difficult to ensure the safety of the blood supply, travelers can take a few measures to increase their chances of a safe blood transfusion, if needed:

- Ask about blood supply screening practices for transmissible diseases, including HIV. Although this is difficult to do at the point of service, travelers with known medical conditions that may require transfusions can increase their chances of obtaining higher-quality care by identifying medical services at their destination in advance of travel.

- Register with agencies that attempt to deliver reliable blood products rapidly to members at international locations. The Blood Care Foundation (www.bloodcare.org.uk/blood-transfusionsabroad.html) is one such organization.

All travelers should consider receiving hepatitis B virus immunization. This becomes especially important for travelers who frequently visit developing countries, longer-term travelers to developing countries, those with underlying medical conditions that increase their risk of requiring blood products while traveling, and travelers whose activities (such as adventure travel) put them at higher risk for serious injury.

6

## BIBLIOGRAPHY

1. Kolars JC. Rules of the road: a consumer's guide for travelers seeking health care in foreign lands. J Travel Med. 2002 Jul–Aug;9(4):198–201.

2. World Health Organization. Medicines: spurious/falsely-labelled/falsified/counterfeit (SFFC) medicines [fact sheet no. 275]. Geneva: World Health Organization; 2012 [updated January 2016, cited 2016 Sep 22]. Available from: www.who.int/mediacentre/factsheets/fs275/en/.

3. World Health Organization. Blood safety [fact sheet no. 279]. Geneva: World Health Organization; 2014 [updated July 2016, cited 2016 Sep 22]. Available from: www.who.int/mediacentre/factsheets/fs279/en/.

# AVOIDING POORLY REGULATED MEDICINES AND MEDICAL PRODUCTS DURING TRAVEL

Michael D. Green

In many low- to middle-income countries, national drug regulatory authorities lack the resources to monitor and enforce drug quality standards effectively and to keep poor-quality products (including drugs, vaccines, and medical devices) off the market. As a result, substandard and fake medicines are a public health concern in these locations. Many of these poor-quality products are also trafficked by pharmacy websites that appear to be reputable or located in countries with mature regulatory systems.

Poor regulatory oversight breeds poor-quality medicines, whether they are counterfeit, falsified, substandard, or degraded (Box 6-2). A recent report from the World Health Organization (WHO) states that 1 in 10 medical products circulating in low- and middle-income countries are either substandard or falsified. Another study found that 9%–41% of tested drugs failed quality specifications. In specific regions in Africa, Asia, and Latin America, the chance of purchasing a counterfeit drug may be >30%.

Since counterfeit drugs are not made by a legitimate manufacturer and are produced under unlawful circumstances, toxic contaminants or lack of proper ingredients may cause serious harm. For example, the active pharmaceutical ingredient may be completely lacking, present in small quantities, or substituted with a less effective compound. In addition, the wrong inactive ingredients (excipients) can contribute to poor drug dissolution, bioavailability, and toxicity. As a result, a patient may not respond to treatment or may have adverse reactions to unknown substituted or toxic ingredients.

Vaccines and other products, such as insecticide-treated mosquito nets, water purification devices, condoms, and disinfectants are also

---

## BOX 6-2. Definitions of poorly regulated medical products

**IMITATIONS**

*Counterfeit*: A counterfeit product bears the unauthorized representation of a registered trademark on a product identical or similar to one for which the trademark is registered.

*Falsified*: A falsified product falsely represents the product's identity, source, or both.

**AUTHENTICS**

*Substandard*: A substandard product fails to meet national specifications cited in an accepted pharmacopeia or in the manufacturer's approved dossier.

*Degraded*: A degraded product has undergone chemical or physical changes due to incorrect storage conditions.

subject to quality problems and counterfeiting. Vaccine integrity depends on a temperature-controlled supply chain, and, unlike medicines with stated amounts of active ingredients, the potency of vaccines is difficult to monitor and therefore easy to counterfeit. For example, WHO recently reported that falsified hepatitis B vaccines were circulating in Uganda. Insecticide-treated nets must meet standards to protect against diseases such as malaria; substandard nets were recently implicated as a cause of increased malaria incidence in Rwanda.

## HOW TO AVOID COUNTERFEIT DRUGS WHEN TRAVELING

The best way to avoid counterfeit drugs is to reduce the need to purchase medications abroad. Anticipated amounts of medications for chronic conditions (such as hypertension, diabetes, or arthritis), medications for travelers' diarrhea, and prophylactic medications for infectious diseases (such as malaria) should all be purchased before traveling. Purchasing these drugs online is not recommended, since the source of the medicines is always questionable. The traveler should also be aware that other health-related items such as medical

devices, mosquito nets, and insect repellents obtained abroad could also be counterfeit, falsified, or substandard.

Before departure, travelers should do the following:

- Obtain all medicines and other health-related items needed for the trip in advance. Prescriptions written in the United States usually cannot be filled overseas, and although many US prescription medications may be available for purchase over-the-counter in foreign countries, some may not be available at all. Checked baggage can get lost; therefore, travelers should pack medications and first aid items in a carry-on bag, and bring extra medicine in case of travel delays.

- Make sure medicines are in their original containers. If the drug is a prescription, the patient's name and dose regimen should appear on the container.

- Bring the "patient prescription information" sheet. This sheet provides information on common generic and brand names, use, side effects, precautions, and drug interactions.

- Because many countries have restrictions on medicines (including over-the-counter medications) entering their borders,

travelers should check with the embassies of their destination countries for prohibited items.

If travelers run out and require additional medications, they should take steps to ensure the medicines they buy are safe:

- Obtain medicines from a legitimate pharmacy. Patients should not buy from open markets, street vendors, or suspicious-looking pharmacies; they should request a receipt when making the purchase. The US embassy or consulate may be able to help locate legitimate local pharmacies.

- Do not buy medicines that are substantially cheaper than the typical price. Although generics are usually less expensive, many counterfeit brand names are sold at prices substantially lower than the normal.

- Make sure the medicines are in their original packages or containers. Travelers receiving medicines as loose tablets or capsules supplied in a plastic bag or envelope should ask the pharmacist to see the container from which the medicine was dispensed. The traveler should record the brand, batch number, and expiration date. Sometimes a wary consumer will prompt the seller into supplying quality medicine.

- Be familiar with medications. The size, shape, color, and taste of counterfeit medicines may be different from the authentic product. Discoloration, splits, cracks, spots, and stickiness of the tablets or capsules are indications of possible counterfeit. These defects may also indicate improper storage. Travelers should keep examples of authentic medications to compare if they purchase the same brand.

- Be familiar with the packaging. Different color inks, poor-quality printing or packaging materials, and misspelled words are clues to counterfeit drugs. Travelers should keep an example of packaging for comparison and observe the expiration date.

If the authentic packaging is unavailable or if the traveler is not familiar with the brand, he or she should compare the distinguishing features of the package with that of the insert or blister pack. For example, batch and lot numbers, manufacturing date, and expiration date should match.

## USEFUL WEBSITES

### General Information about Counterfeit Drugs

- CDC: wwwnc.cdc. gov/travel/page/ counterfeit-medicine

- World Health Organization: www. who.int/mediacentre/ factsheets/fs275/en

- Food and Drug Administration: www.fda. gov/drugs/drugsafety/ default.htm

- US Pharmacopeia: www. usp.org/global-public-health/medicines-quality-database

## Traveling and Customs Guidelines

Researching what travelers can pack, travel with, and bring back into the United States, is helpful in preparing for travel.

- Transportation Security Administration: www. tsa.gov/travel/ special-procedures

- Customs and Border Protection: www.cbp.gov/ travel/us-citizens/know-before-you-go/prohibited-and-restricted-item

- The International Society of Travel Medicine (ISTM) Pharmacist Professional

Group recently posted on the member section of the ISTM website a multi-country table of permissible medications based on information provided by the International Narcotics Control Board and embassies, though this information is subject to change

## BIBLIOGRAPHY

1. Institute of Medicine. Countering the problem of falsified and substandard drugs. Washington, DC: The National Academics Press; 2013 Feb.

2. Ministry of Health of Rwanda. MOH Reports. [cited 2018 Mar 30]. Available from: http://moh.gov.rw/index.php?id=99.

3. Nayyar GML, Bremen JG, Herrington JE. The global pandemic of falsified medicines: laboratory and field innovations and policy perspectives. Am J Trop Med Hyg 2015 Jun;92(6 suppl):2–7.

4. World Health Organization. Essential medicines and health products. Full list of Medical Products Alerts. 2018 [cited 2018 March 30]. Available from: www.who.int/medicines/publications/drugalerts/en/.

5. World Health Organization. Medicines: counterfeit medicines [fact sheet no. 275]. Geneva: World Health Organization; 2018 [cited 2018 Mar 30]. Available from: www.who.int/mediacentre/factsheets/fs275/en/.

# TRAVEL HEALTH KITS

Calvin Patimeteeporn

Regardless of their destination, international travelers should assemble and carry a travel health kit. Travelers should tailor the contents to their specific needs, the type and length of travel, and their destination(s). Kits can be assembled at home or purchased at a local store, pharmacy, or online. Travel health kits can help to ensure travelers have supplies they need to

- Manage preexisting medical conditions and treat any exacerbations of these conditions.

- Prevent illness and injury related to traveling.

- Take care of minor health problems as they occur.

By bringing medications from home, travelers can avoid having to purchase them at their destination. See *Perspectives:* Avoiding Poorly Regulated Medicines and Medical Products during Travel in this chapter for information about the risks associated with purchasing medications abroad. Even when the quality is reliable, the medications people are accustomed to taking at home may be sold under different names or with different ingredients and dosage units in other countries, presenting additional challenges.

## TRAVELING WITH MEDICATIONS

International travelers should carry all medications in their original containers with clear labels that easily identify the contents. Patient name and dosing regimen information should be included. Although travelers may prefer packing their medications into small bags, pillboxes, or daily-dose containers, officials at ports of entry may require a formal and proper identification of all medications.

Travelers should carry copies of all prescriptions, including their generic names, preferably translated into the local language of the destination. For controlled substances and injectable medications, travelers should carry a note on letterhead stationery from the prescribing clinician

or travel clinic. Translating the letter into the local language at the destination and attaching this translation to the original document may prove helpful if the document is needed during the trip. Some countries do not permit certain medications. If there is a question about these restrictions, particularly regarding controlled substances, travelers should contact the embassy or consulate of the destination country.

A travel health kit is useful only when easily accessible. It should be carried with the traveler at all times (such as in a carry-on bag), although sharp objects (like scissors and fine splinter tweezers) must remain in checked luggage. Travelers should make sure that any liquid or gel-based items packed in the carry-on bags do not exceed size limits. Exceptions are made for certain medical reasons; check the Transportation Security Administration for US outbound and inbound travel (call toll-free at 866-289-9673 Monday-Friday 8 AM to 11 PM, weekends and holidays 9 AM to 8 PM, or email TSA-ContactCenter@dhs.gov) and the embassy or consulate of the destination country for their restrictions.

## SUPPLIES FOR PREEXISTING MEDICAL CONDITIONS

Travelers with preexisting medical conditions should carry enough medication for the duration of their trip and an extra supply, in case the trip extends for any reason. If additional supplies or medications are needed to manage exacerbations of existing medical conditions, these should be carried as well. Consult with the clinician managing the traveler's preexisting medical conditions for the best plan of action (see Chapter 5, Travelers with Chronic Illnesses).

People with preexisting conditions, such as diabetes or allergies, should consider wearing an alert bracelet, making sure this information (in English and preferably translated into the local language of the destination) is also on a card in their wallet and with their other travel documents.

6

## GENERAL TRAVEL HEALTH KIT SUPPLIES

The following is a list of items that travelers should consider when assembling a basic travel health kit. See Chapters 5 and 9 for additional suggestions of contents for travelers with preexisting health conditions or specific reasons for travel.

### Prescription Medications and Supplies

- Medications taken on a regular basis at home

- Antibiotics for self-treatment of moderate to severe diarrhea[1]

- Medication to prevent malaria, if needed

- Medication to prevent or treat altitude illness, if needed

- Prescription glasses/contact lenses (consider packing an extra pair of each, in case lenses are damaged)

- Epinephrine auto-injectors[2] (such as an EpiPen 2-Pak), especially if history of severe allergic reaction or anaphylaxis; smaller-dose packages are available for children

- Diabetes testing supplies and insulin

- Needles or syringes, if needed for injectable medication. Needles and syringes can be difficult to purchase in some locations, so take more than what is needed for the length of the trip. These items will require a letter from the prescribing clinician on letterhead stationery.

- Medical alert bracelet or necklace

### Over-the-Counter Medications

- Medications taken on a regular basis at home

- Treatment for pain or fever (one or more of the following, or an alternative):
  - Acetaminophen
  - Aspirin
  - Ibuprofen

- Treatment for stomach upset or diarrhea:
  - Antidiarrheal medication (such as loperamide [Imodium] or bismuth subsalicylate [Pepto-Bismol])
  - Packets of oral rehydration salts for dehydration
  - Mild laxative
  - Antacid

- Treatment for mild upper respiratory tract conditions:
  - Antihistamine
  - Decongestant, alone or in combination with antihistamine
  - Cough suppressant or expectorant
  - Cough drops

- Anti–motion sickness medication

- Mild sedative or sleep aid

- Saline eye drops

- Saline nose drops or spray

### Basic First Aid Items

- Disposable latex-free gloves (≥2 pairs)

- Adhesive bandages, multiple sizes

- Gauze

- Adhesive tape

- Antiseptic wound cleanser

- Cotton swabs

- Antifungal and antibacterial spray or creams

- 1% hydrocortisone cream

- Anti-itch gel or cream for insect bites and stings

- Moleskin or molefoam for blister prevention and treatment

---

[1] For factors to consider when deciding whether to use an antibiotic for self-treatment of moderate to severe travelers' diarrhea, see Chapter 2, *Perspectives*: Antibiotics in Travelers' Diarrhea—Balancing the Risks & Benefits.

[2] Travelers with known, severe allergies should carry injectable epinephrine and antihistamines with them at all times, including during air, sea, and land travel. Travelers with a history of severe allergic reactions should consider bringing along a short course of oral steroid medication (prescription required from doctor) and antihistamines as additional treatment of a severe allergic reaction. For additional information, see Chapter 5, Travelers with Chronic Illnesses, Box 5-2, Highly allergic travelers.

- Digital thermometer
- Tweezers[3]
- Scissors[3]
- Safety pins
- Elastic/compression bandage wrap for sprains and strains
- Triangular bandage to wrap injuries and to make an arm or shoulder sling
- For travel in remote areas, consider a commercial suture kit
- First aid quick reference card

## Supplies to Prevent Illness or Injury

- Antibacterial hand wipes or an alcohol-based hand sanitizer, containing ≥60% alcohol
- Insect repellents for skin and clothing (see Chapter 3, Mosquitoes, Ticks & Other Arthropods for recommended types)
- Bed net (if needed, for protection against insect bites while sleeping)
- Sunscreen (≥15 SPF with UVA and UVB protection)
- Water purification tablets (if visiting remote areas, camping, or staying in areas where access to clean water is limited)
- Latex condoms
- Ear plugs
- Personal safety equipment (such as child safety seats and bicycle helmets)

## Documents

Travelers should both carry the following documents and leave copies with a family member or close contact who will remain in the United States, in case of an emergency.

- Proof of vaccination on an International Certificate of Vaccination or Prophylaxis (ICVP) card or medical waiver (if vaccinations are required)
- Copies of all prescriptions for medications, eye glasses/contacts, and other medical supplies (including generic names and preferably translated into the local language of the destination)
- Documentation of preexisting conditions, such as diabetes or allergies (in English and preferably translated into the local language of the destination)
- Health insurance, supplemental travel health insurance, medical evacuation insurance, and travel insurance information (carry contact information for all insurance providers and copies of claim forms)
- Contact card to be carried with the traveler at all times, including street addresses, phone numbers, and email addresses of the following:
  > Family member or close contact remaining in the United States
  > Health care provider(s) at home
  > Place(s) of lodging at the destination(s)
  > Hospitals or clinics (including emergency services) in your destination(s)
  > US embassy or consulate in the destination country or countries

See the Obtaining Health Care Abroad section in this chapter for information about how to locate local health care and embassy or consulate contacts.

## COMMERCIAL MEDICAL KITS

Commercial medical kits are available for a wide range of circumstances, from basic first aid to advanced emergency life support. A number of companies manufacture advanced medical kits for adventure travelers, customizing them based on specific travel needs. In addition, specialty kits are available for travelers managing diabetes, dealing with dental emergencies, and

---

[3] If traveling by air, travelers should pack these sharp items in checked baggage, since airport or airline security may confiscate them if packed in carry-on bags. Small bandage scissors with rounded tips may be available for purchase in certain stores or online.

participating in aquatic activities. Many pharmacy, grocery, retail, and outdoor sporting goods stores, as well as online retailers, sell their own basic first aid kits. Travelers who choose to purchase a preassembled kit should review the contents of the kit carefully to ensure that it has everything needed; any necessary additional items can be added.

## BIBLIOGRAPHY

1. Goodyer L. Travel medical kits. In: Keystone JS, Freedman DO, Kozarsky PE, Connor BA, Nothdurft HD, editors. Travel Medicine. 3rd ed. Philadelphia: Saunders Elsevier; 2013. pp. 63–6.

2. Harper LA, Bettinger J, Dismukes R, Kozarsky PE. Evaluation of the Coca-Cola company travel health kit. J Travel Med. 2002 Sep–Oct;9(5):244–6.

3. Rose SR, Keystone JS. Chapter 2, trip preparation. In: Rose SR, Keystone JS, editors. International Travel Health Guide. 2019 online ed. Northampton: Travel Medicine; 2019. Available from: www.travmed.com/pages/health-guide-chapter-2-trip-preparation.

**6**

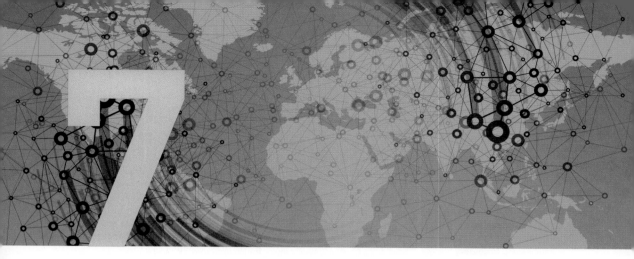

# Family Travel

## PREGNANT TRAVELERS

Diane F. Morof, I. Dale Carroll

Women experience physiologic changes in pregnancy that require special consideration when traveling. With careful preparation, however, most pregnant women are able to travel safely.

### PRETRAVEL EVALUATION

The pretravel evaluation of a pregnant traveler (Box 7-1) should begin with a careful medical and obstetric history, with particular attention paid to gestational age and evaluation for high-risk conditions. A visit with an obstetrician should be a part of the pretravel assessment, to ensure routine prenatal care as well as identify any potential problems. The traveler should be provided with a copy of her prenatal records and physician's contact information. Checking for immunity to various infectious diseases may obviate the need for some vaccines.

A review of the pregnant woman's travel itinerary, including destinations, accommodations, and activities, should guide pretravel health advice. Preparation includes educating the pregnant woman regarding avoidance of travel-associated risks, the management of minor pregnancy discomforts, and recognition of more serious complications. Bleeding, severe pelvic or abdominal pain, contractions or premature labor, premature rupture of the membranes, symptoms of preeclampsia (unusual swelling, severe headaches, nausea and vomiting, vision changes), severe vomiting, diarrhea, dehydration, and symptoms of deep vein thrombosis (unusual swelling of leg with pain in calf or thigh) or pulmonary embolism (unusual shortness of breath) require urgent medical attention.

Pregnant travelers should pack a health kit that includes items such as prescription medications, hemorrhoid cream, antiemetic drugs, antacids, prenatal vitamins, medication for vaginitis or yeast infection, and support hose, in addition to the items recommended for all travelers (see Chapter 6, Travel Health Kits).

## BOX 7-1. Pretravel consultation checklist for pregnant travelers

- Check for immunity to infectious diseases, for example, hepatitis A and B, rubella, varicella, measles, pertussis; update immunizations as needed (see text for contraindications during pregnancy)
- Policies and necessary paperwork
  - Supplemental travel insurance, travel health insurance, and medical evacuation insurance (research specific coverage information and limitations for pregnancy-related health issues)

- Check airline and cruise line policies for pregnant women
- Letter confirming due date and fitness to travel
- Copy of medical records
- Preparing for obstetric care at destination
  - Check medical insurance coverage
  - Arrange for obstetric care at destination, as needed
- Review signs and symptoms requiring immediate care
  - Pelvic or abdominal pain

- Bleeding
- Rupture of membranes
- Contractions or preterm labor
- Symptoms of preeclampsia (unusual swelling, severe headaches, nausea and vomiting, vision changes)
- Vomiting, diarrhea, dehydration
- Symptoms of potential deep vein thrombosis or pulmonary embolism (unusual swelling of leg with pain in calf or thigh, unusual shortness of breath)

Pregnant travelers should consider packing a blood pressure monitor if travel may limit access to a health center with blood pressure monitoring available.

## CONTRAINDICATIONS TO TRAVEL DURING PREGNANCY

Although travel is rarely contraindicated during a normal pregnancy, complicated pregnancies require extra consideration and may warrant a recommendation that travel be delayed (Box 7-2). Pregnant travelers should be advised that the risk of obstetric complications is highest in the first and third trimesters.

## PLANNING FOR EMERGENCY CARE

Obstetric emergencies are often sudden and life-threatening. Travel to areas where obstetric care may be less than the standard at home is inadvisable. For women traveling in the third trimester of pregnancy, it is recommended to identify international medical facilities capable of managing complications of pregnancy,

## BOX 7-2. Contraindications to travel during pregnancy

- **Absolute Contraindications**
  - Abruptio placentae
  - Active labor
  - Incompetent cervix
  - Premature labor
  - Premature rupture of membranes

  - Suspected ectopic pregnancy
  - Threatened abortion, vaginal bleeding
  - Toxemia, past or present
- **Relative Contraindications**
  - Abnormal presentation
  - Fetal growth restriction

  - History of infertility
  - History of miscarriage or ectopic pregnancy
  - Maternal age <15 or >35 years
  - Multiple gestation
  - Placenta previa or other placental abnormality

7

delivery, a cesarean section, and neonatal problems.

Many health insurance policies do not cover complications of pregnancy or the newborn overseas. Supplemental travel health insurance should be strongly considered to cover pregnancy-related problems and care of the neonate, as needed. Evacuation insurance that includes coverage of pregnancy-related complications is also highly encouraged.

## TRANSPORTATION CONSIDERATIONS

Pregnant women should be advised to wear seat belts, when available, on all forms of transport, including airplanes, cars, and buses. A diagonal shoulder strap with a lap belt provides the best protection. The shoulder belt should be worn between the breasts with the lap belt low across the upper thighs. When only a lap belt is available, it should be worn low, between the abdomen and the pelvis.

### Air Travel

Most commercial airlines allow pregnant travelers to fly until 36 weeks' gestation. Some limit international travel earlier in pregnancy, and some require documentation of gestational age. Pregnant travelers should check with the airline for specific requirements or guidance. Cabins of most commercial jetliners are pressurized to 6,000–8,000 ft (1,829–2,438 m) above sea level; the lower oxygen tension should not cause fetal problems in a normal pregnancy, but women with preexisting cardiovascular problems, sickle cell disease, or severe anemia (hemoglobin <8.0 g/dL) may experience the effects of low arterial oxygen saturation. Risks of air travel include potential exposure to communicable diseases, immobility, and the common discomforts of flying. Abdominal distention and pedal edema frequently occur. The pregnant traveler may benefit from an upgrade in airline seating and should seek convenient and practical accommodations (such as close proximity to the toilet) and aisle seating so she can move about frequently. Loose clothing and comfortable shoes are recommended.

Some experts report that the risk of deep vein thrombosis in pregnancy is 5–10 times higher than for nonpregnant women. Preventive measures include frequent stretching, walking and isometric leg exercises, and wearing graduated compression stockings (see Chapter 8, Deep Vein Thrombosis & Pulmonary Embolism).

Cosmic radiation during air travel poses little threat, but may be a consideration for pregnant travelers who are frequent fliers (such as aircrew). Older airport security machines are magnetometers and are not harmful to the fetus. Newer security machines use backscatter x-ray scanners, which emit low levels of radiation. Most experts agree that the risk of complications from radiation exposure from these scanners is extremely low.

### Cruise Ship Travel

Most cruise lines restrict travel beyond 28 weeks of pregnancy, and some as early as 24 weeks. Pregnant travelers may be required to carry a physician's note stating that they are fit to travel, including the estimated date of delivery. Pregnant women should check with the cruise line for specific requirements or guidance. The pregnant traveler planning a cruise should be advised regarding motion sickness, gastrointestinal and respiratory infections, and the risk of falls on a moving vessel.

## ENVIRONMENTAL CONSIDERATIONS

Air pollution may cause more health problems during pregnancy, as ciliary clearance of the bronchial tree is slowed and mucus more abundant. Body temperature regulation is not as efficient during pregnancy, and temperature extremes can cause more stress on the gravid woman. In addition, an increase in core temperature, such as with heat prostration or heat stroke, may harm the fetus. The vasodilatory effect of a hot environment might also cause fainting. For these reasons, accommodation should be sought in air-conditioned quarters and activities restricted in hot environments.

Pregnant women should avoid activities at high altitude unless trained for and accustomed to such activities; women unaccustomed to high altitudes may experience exaggerated breathlessness and palpitations. The common symptoms of acute mountain sickness (insomnia, headache, and nausea) are frequently also associated with pregnancy, and it may be difficult to distinguish the cause of the symptoms. Most experts recommend a slower ascent with adequate time for acclimatization. No studies or case reports show harm to a fetus if the mother travels briefly to high altitudes during pregnancy. However, it may be prudent to recommend that pregnant women not sleep at altitudes >12,000 ft (3,658 m), if possible. Probably the largest concern regarding high-altitude travel in pregnancy is that many such destinations are inaccessible and far from medical care (see Chapter 3, High-Altitude Travel & Altitude Sickness).

## ACTIVITIES

Pregnant travelers should be discouraged from undertaking unaccustomed vigorous activity. Swimming and snorkeling during pregnancy are generally safe, but waterskiing has resulted in falls that inject water into the birth canal. Most experts advise against scuba diving for pregnant women because of risk of fetal gas embolism during decompression. Riding bicycles, motorcycles, or animals presents risk of trauma to the abdomen.

## INFECTIOUS DISEASES

Respiratory and urinary infections and vaginitis are more likely to occur and to be more severe in pregnancy. Pregnant women who develop travelers' diarrhea or other gastrointestinal infections may be more vulnerable to dehydration than nonpregnant travelers. Strict hand hygiene and food and water precautions should be stressed (see Chapter 2, Food & Water Precautions). Bottled or boiled water is preferable to chemically treated or filtered water. Iodine-containing compounds should not be used to purify water for pregnant women because of potential effects on the fetal thyroid (see Chapter 2, Water Disinfection for Travelers). The treatment of choice for travelers' diarrhea is prompt and vigorous oral hydration; however, azithromycin may be given to pregnant women if clinically indicated. Use of bismuth subsalicylate is contraindicated because it is associated with intrauterine growth problems and premature fetal ductus arteriosus.

Hepatitis A and E are both spread by the fecal-oral route. Hepatitis A has been reported to increase the risk of placental abruption and premature delivery. Hepatitis E is more likely to cause severe disease during pregnancy and may result in a case-fatality ratio of 15%–30%; when acquired during the third trimester, it is also associated with fetal complications and fetal death. Some foodborne illnesses of particular concern during pregnancy include toxoplasmosis and listeriosis; the risk during pregnancy is that the infection will cross the placenta and cause spontaneous abortion, stillbirth, or congenital or neonatal infection. The pregnant traveler should be warned, therefore, to avoid unpasteurized cheeses and undercooked meat products. Risk of fetal infection increases with gestational age, but severity of infection is decreased.

Parasitic diseases are less common but may cause concern, particularly in women who are visiting friends and relatives in developing areas. In general, intestinal helminths rarely cause enough illness to warrant treatment during pregnancy. Most, in fact, can safely be addressed with symptomatic treatment until the pregnancy is over. On the other hand, protozoan intestinal infections, such as *Giardia*, *Entamoeba histolytica*, and *Cryptosporidium*, often do require treatment. These parasites may cause acute gastroenteritis, severe dehydration, chronic malabsorption resulting in fetal growth restriction, and in the case of *E. histolytica*, invasive disease, including amebic liver abscess and colitis. Pregnant women should avoid swimming or wading in freshwater lakes, streams, and rivers that may harbor schistosomes.

Pregnant women should avoid mosquito bites when traveling in areas where vectorborne diseases are endemic. Preventive measures include use of bed nets, insect repellents, and protective clothing (see Chapter 3, Mosquitoes, Ticks & Other Arthropods). A more recent concern for pregnant women is Zika virus infection. Zika virus is spread primarily through the bite of an infected *Aedes* mosquito (*Ae. aegypti* and *Ae. albopictus*) but can also be sexually transmitted. The illness associated with Zika may be asymptomatic or mild; however, some patients report acute onset of fever, rash, joint pain, and conjunctivitis that last for several days to a week after

7

infection. Birth defects that can be caused by Zika infection during pregnancy include microcephaly and brain abnormalities. Because of the risk of birth defects, CDC recommends pregnant women not travel to areas where Zika is a risk, and take precautions to avoid sexual transmission of the virus. If travel cannot be avoided, pregnant women should strictly follow steps to prevent mosquito bites. Additional information, including the most current list of countries and territories where Zika virus is a risk, is available at www.cdc.gov/travel. Guidance for pregnant women can be found at the CDC Zika website (www.cdc.gov/pregnancy/zika/index.html).

## MEDICATIONS

Various systems are used to classify drugs with regard to their safety in pregnancy. In most cases, it is preferable to refer to specific data regarding the effects of a given drug during pregnancy rather than simply to depend on a classification.

Analgesics that can be used during pregnancy include acetaminophen and some narcotics. Aspirin may increase the incidence of abruption, and other anti-inflammatory agents can cause premature closure of the ductus arteriosus. Constipation may require a mild bulk laxative. Several simple remedies are often effective in relieving the symptoms of morning sickness. Nonprescription remedies include ginger, which is available as a powder that can be mixed with food or drinks such as tea. It is also available in candy, such as lollipops. Similarly, pyridoxine (vitamin B6) is effective in reducing symptoms of morning sickness and is available in tablet form, as well as lozenges and lollipops. Antihistamines such as meclizine and dimenhydrinate are often used in pregnancy for morning sickness and motion sickness and appear to have a good safety record.

## VACCINES

In the best possible scenario, a woman should be up-to-date on routine vaccinations before she becomes pregnant. The most effective way of protecting the infant against many diseases is to immunize the mother. Tetanus, diphtheria, and pertussis (Tdap) vaccine should be given **during each pregnancy** irrespective of the woman's history of receiving Tdap. To maximize maternal antibody response and passive antibody transfer to the infant, **optimal timing for Tdap administration is between 27 and 36 weeks of gestation,** although it may be given at any time during pregnancy.

Annual influenza vaccine (inactivated) is recommended during any trimester for all women who are or will be pregnant during influenza season. For travelers, vaccination is recommended ≥2 weeks before departure if vaccine is available.

Certain vaccines, including meningococcal and hepatitis A and B vaccines that are considered safe during pregnancy, may be indicated based on risk. No adverse effects of inactivated polio vaccine (IPV) have been documented among pregnant women or their fetuses; however, vaccination of pregnant women should be avoided because of theoretical concerns. IPV can be administered in accordance with the recommended schedules for adults if a pregnant woman is at increased risk for infection and requires immediate protection against polio. Rabies postexposure prophylaxis with rabies immune globulin and vaccine should be administered after any moderate- or high-risk exposure to rabies; preexposure vaccine may be considered for travelers when the risk of exposure is substantial.

Most live-virus vaccines, including measles-mumps-rubella vaccine, varicella vaccine, and live attenuated influenza vaccine, are contraindicated during pregnancy; the exception is yellow fever vaccine, for which pregnancy is considered a precaution by the Advisory Committee on Immunization Practices (ACIP). If travel is unavoidable, and the risks for yellow fever virus exposure are felt to outweigh the risks of vaccination, a pregnant woman should be vaccinated. If the risks for vaccination are felt to outweigh the risks for yellow fever virus exposure, pregnant women should be issued a medical waiver to fulfill health regulations. Because pregnancy might affect immunologic function, serologic testing to document an immune response to yellow fever vaccine should be considered.

Postexposure prophylaxis of a nonimmune pregnant woman exposed to measles or varicella may be provided by administering immune globulin (IG) within 6 days for measles or varicella-zoster IG within 10 days for varicella.

Women planning to become pregnant should be advised to wait 4 weeks after receipt of a live-virus vaccine before conceiving. For certain travel-related vaccines, including Japanese encephalitis vaccine and typhoid vaccine, data are insufficient for a specific recommendation for use in pregnant women. A summary of current ACIP guidelines for vaccinating pregnant women is available at www.cdc.gov/vaccines/pregnancy/hcp/guidelines.html.

## MALARIA PROPHYLAXIS

Malaria may be much more serious in pregnant than in nonpregnant women and is associated with high risks of illness and death for both mother and child. Malaria in pregnancy may be characterized by heavy parasitemia, severe anemia, and sometimes profound hypoglycemia, and may be complicated by cerebral malaria and acute respiratory distress syndrome. Placental sequestration of parasites may result in fetal loss due to abruption, premature labor, or miscarriage. An infant born to an infected mother is apt to be of low birth weight, and, although rare, congenital malaria is a concern.

Because no prophylactic regimen provides complete protection, pregnant women should avoid or delay travel to malaria-endemic areas. However, if travel is unavoidable, pregnant women should take precautions to avoid mosquito bites, and use of an effective prophylactic regimen is essential.

Chloroquine and mefloquine are the drugs of choice for pregnant women for destinations with chloroquine-sensitive and chloroquine-resistant malaria, respectively. Doxycycline is contraindicated because of teratogenic effects on the fetus after the fourth month of pregnancy. Primaquine is contraindicated in pregnancy because the infant cannot be tested for G6PD deficiency, putting the infant at risk for hemolytic anemia. Atovaquone-proguanil is not recommended because of lack of available safety data. A list of the available antimalarial drugs and their uses and contraindications during pregnancy can be found in Table 4-10 and in Chapter 4, Malaria.

### BIBLIOGRAPHY

1. ACOG Committee on Obstetric Practice. ACOG Committee Opinion No. 443: Air travel during pregnancy. Obstet Gynecol. 2009 Oct;114(4):954–5.

2. Carroll ID, Williams DC. Pre-travel vaccination and medical prophylaxis in the pregnant traveler. Travel Med Infect Dis. 2008 Sep;6(5):259–75.

3. CDC. Guidelines for vaccinating pregnant women. Atlanta: CDC; 2014 [cited 2016 Sep 27]. Available from: www.cdc.gov/vaccines/pubs/preg-guide.html.

4. Dotters-Katz S, Kuller J, Heine RP. Parasitic infections in pregnancy. Obstet Gynecol Surv. 2011 Aug;66(8):515–25.

5. Hezelgrave NL, Whitty CJ, Shennan AH, Chappell LC. Advising on travel during pregnancy. BMJ. 2011;342:d2506.

6. Irvine MH, Einarson A, Bozzo P. Prophylactic use of antimalarials during pregnancy. Can Fam Physician. 2011 Nov;57(11):1279–81.

7. Magann EF, Chauhan SP, Dahlke JD, McKelvey SS, Watson EM, Morrison JC. Air travel and pregnancy outcomes: a review of pregnancy regulations and outcomes for passengers, flight attendants, and aviators. Obstet Gynecol Surv. 2010 Jun;65(6):396–402.

8. Mehta P, Smith-Bindman R. Airport full-body screening: what is the risk? Arch Intern Med. 2011 Jun 27;171(12):1112–5.

9. Rasmussen SA, Jamieson DJ, Honein MA, Petersen LR. Zika virus and birth defects—reviewing the evidence for causality. N Engl J Med. 2016 May 19;374(20):1981–7.

10. Rasmussen SA, Watson AK, Kennedy ED, Broder KR, Jamieson DJ. Vaccines and pregnancy: past, present, and future. Semin Fetal Neonatal Med. 2014 Jun;19(3):161–9.

11. Roggelin L, Cramer JP. Malaria prevention in the pregnant traveller: a review. Travel Med Infect Dis. 2014 May–Jun;12(3):229–36.

12. van der Linden V. Congenital Zika syndrome. Int J Infect Diseases. 2016 Dec;53(Suppl):6.

# TRAVEL & BREASTFEEDING

Erica H. Anstey, Katherine R. Shealy

The medical preparation of a traveler who is breastfeeding differs only slightly from that of other travelers and depends in part on whether the mother and child will be separated or together during travel. Most mothers should be advised to continue breastfeeding their infants throughout travel. Before departure, mothers may wish to compile a list of local breastfeeding resources at their destination to have on hand. Clinicians and travelers can use the Find a Lactation Consultant Tool (www.ilca.org/why-ibclc/falc) to find contact information for experts at their destination. Clinicians and travelers can use La Leche League International's interactive map (www.llli.org/get-help) to find specific location and contact information for breastfeeding support group leaders and groups worldwide.

## TRAVELING WITH A BREASTFEEDING CHILD

Breastfeeding provides unique benefits to mothers and children traveling together. Health care providers should explain clearly to breastfeeding mothers the value of continuing breastfeeding during travel. For the first 6 months of life, exclusive breastfeeding is recommended. This is especially important during travel because exclusive breastfeeding means feeding only breast milk, no other foods or drinks, which potentially protects infants from exposure to contamination and pathogens via foods or liquids. Additionally, feeding only at the breast protects infants from potential exposure to contamination from containers (bottles, cups, utensils).

Breastfeeding infants require no water supplementation, even in extreme heat environments. Breastfeeding protects children from eustachian tube pain and collapse during air travel, especially during ascent and descent, by allowing them to stabilize and gradually equalize internal and external air pressure.

Frequent, unrestricted breastfeeding opportunities ensure the mother's milk supply remains sufficient and the child's nutrition and hydration are ideal. Mothers who are concerned about breastfeeding away from home may feel more comfortable breastfeeding the child in a fabric carrier. In many countries around the world, breastfeeding in public places is more widely practiced than in the United States. US federal legislation protects mothers' and children's right to breastfeed anywhere they are otherwise authorized to be while on federal property, which includes US Customs areas, embassies, and consulates overseas.

## TRAVELING WITHOUT A BREASTFEEDING CHILD

Before departure, a breastfeeding mother traveling without her breastfeeding infant or child may wish to express and store a supply of milk to be fed to the infant or child during her absence. Building a supply to be fed in her absence takes time and patience and is most successful when begun gradually, many weeks in advance of the mother's departure. A mother's milk supply can diminish if she does not express milk while away from her nursing child, but this does not need to be a reason to stop breastfeeding. Clinicians should help mothers determine the best course for breastfeeding based on a variety of factors, including the amount of time she has to prepare for her trip, the flexibility of her time while traveling, her options for expressing and storing milk while traveling, the duration of her travel, and her destination. A mother who returns to her nursing infant or child can continue breastfeeding and, if necessary, supplement as needed until her milk supply returns to its prior level. Often, after a mother returns from travel, her nursing infant or child will help bring her milk supply to its prior level. However, nursing infants or children who are separated from their mother for an extended time may have difficulty transitioning back to breastfeeding. Support from a lactation provider may be helpful if a mother is experiencing breastfeeding challenges after reuniting with her infant or child.

7

## BREAST PUMP SAFETY

Mothers who plan to use an electric breast pump while traveling may need an electrical current adapter and converter and should have a back-up option available, including information on hand expression techniques (detailed hand expression instructions are available at https://healthychildren.org/English/ages-stages/baby/breastfeeding/Pages/Hand-Expressing-Milk.aspx) or a manual pump. Mothers using a breast pump should be sure to follow proper breast pump cleaning guidance (www.cdc.gov/healthywater/hygiene/healthychildcare/infantfeeding/breastpump.html) to minimize potential contamination. Related guidance for cleaning infant feeding items such as bottles and the nipples, rings, and caps that go with them is available at www.cdc.gov/healthywater/hygiene/healthychildcare/infantfeeding/cleansanitize.html. Handwashing (www.cdc.gov/handwashing/when-how-handwashing.html) with soap and water prior to pumping and handling expressed milk is best, but if safe water is not immediately available, an alcohol-based hand sanitizer that contains at least 60% alcohol may be used. If cleaning the pump parts between uses will not be possible, mothers should bring extra sets of pump parts (for example, flanges, membranes, valves, connectors) to use until thorough cleaning of used parts is possible. Mothers may also consider packing a cleaning kit for breast pump parts, including a cleaning brush, dish soap, and portable drying rack or mesh bag to hang items in to air dry.

## AIR TRAVEL

X-rays used in airport screenings have no effect on breastfeeding, breast milk, or the process of lactation. The Food and Drug Administration states that there are no known adverse effects from eating food, drinking beverages, or using medicine screened by x-ray. Airlines typically consider breast pumps as personal items to be carried onboard, similar to laptop computers, handbags, and diaper bags.

Before departure, people who will be traveling by air and expect to have expressed milk with them during travel need to carefully plan how they will transport the expressed milk.

Airport security regulations for passengers carrying expressed milk vary internationally and are subject to change. In the United States, expressed milk and related infant and child feeding items are exempt from Transportation Security Administration (TSA) regulations limiting quantities of other liquids and gels. The Infant and Child Nourishment Exemption permits passengers to carry with them all expressed milk, ice, gel packs (frozen or unfrozen), and other accessories required to transport expressed milk through airport security checkpoints and onboard flights, regardless of whether the breastfeeding child is also traveling. At the beginning of the screening process, travelers should inform the TSA officer and separate the expressed milk and related accessories from the liquids, gels, and aerosols that are limited to 3.4 oz (100 mL) each, as subject to TSA's Liquids Rule (available at www.tsa.gov/travel/security-screening/liquids-rule). Travelers may find that having on hand the related TSA regulations for expressed milk (available at www.tsa.gov/travel/special-procedures/traveling-children) facilitates the screening process.

Travelers carrying expressed milk in checked luggage should refer to cooler pack storage guidelines in "Proper Handling and Storage of Human Milk" on CDC's website (www.cdc.gov/breastfeeding/recommendations/handling_breastmilk.htm). Expressed milk is considered a food for individual use and is not considered a biohazard. International Air Transport Authority regulations for shipping category B biological substances (UN 3373) do not apply to expressed milk. Travelers shipping frozen milk should follow guidelines for shipping other frozen foods and liquids. Travelers planning to ship frozen milk may need to bring along supplies such as milk storage bags, coolers, shipping boxes, labels, packing tape, resealable bags, newspaper or brown lunch bags for wrapping frozen milk, and gloves or tongs for handling dry ice. Some shipping carriers provide temperature-controlled options that can be used for transporting expressed milk. Travelers should make sure in advance that transporting expressed milk will meet customs regulations, as these can vary by country. Expressed milk does not need to be declared at US Customs upon return to the United States.

## IMMUNIZATIONS AND MEDICATIONS

In almost all situations, clinicians can and should select immunizations and medications for the nursing mother that are compatible with breastfeeding. In most circumstances, it is inappropriate to counsel mothers to wean in order to be vaccinated or to withhold vaccination due to breastfeeding status.

Breastfeeding and lactation do not affect maternal or infant dosage guidelines for any immunization or medication; children always require their own immunization or medication, regardless of maternal dose. In the absence of documented risk to the breastfeeding child of a particular maternal medication, the known risks of stopping breastfeeding generally outweigh a theoretical risk of exposure via breastfeeding.

### Immunizations

Breastfeeding mothers and children should be vaccinated according to routine, recommended schedules. Administration of most live and inactivated vaccines does not affect breastfeeding, breast milk, or the process of lactation. Only 2 vaccines, vaccinia (smallpox) and yellow fever, require special consideration. Preventive vaccinia (smallpox) vaccine is contraindicated for use in breastfeeding mothers.

#### YELLOW FEVER VACCINE

Breastfeeding is a precaution for yellow fever vaccine administration. Three cases of yellow fever vaccine–associated neurologic disease (YEL-AND) have been reported in exclusively breastfed infants whose mothers were vaccinated with yellow fever vaccine. All 3 infants were diagnosed with encephalitis and aged <1 month at the time of exposure.

Until specific research data are available, yellow fever vaccine should be avoided in breastfeeding women. However, when nursing mothers must travel to a yellow fever–endemic area, these women should be vaccinated. Although there are no data,

some experts recommend that breastfeeding women who receive yellow fever vaccine should temporarily suspend breastfeeding, pump, and discard milk for at least 2 weeks after vaccination before resuming breastfeeding (see Chapter 4, Yellow Fever, for more information).

### Medications

According to the American Academy of Pediatrics (AAP) 2013 Clinical Report: The Transfer of Drugs and Therapeutics into Human Breast Milk, many mothers are inappropriately advised to discontinue breastfeeding or avoid taking essential medications because of fears of adverse effects on their infants. The AAP's Tips for Giving Accurate Information to Mothers (www.aap.org/en-us/advocacy-and-policy/aap-health-initiatives/Breastfeeding/Pages/Medications-and-Breastfeeding.aspx) advises that this is usually unnecessary because only a small proportion of medications are contraindicated in breastfeeding mothers or associated with adverse effects on their infants. The National Institutes for Health's database of information on drugs and lactation (LactMed) is an online database of clinical information about drugs and breastfeeding that is updated monthly (https://toxnet.nlm.nih.gov/newtoxnet/lactmed.htm). It provides information about the levels of substances in breast milk, levels in infant blood, potential effects in breastfeeding infants and on lactation itself, and alternate drugs to consider. The pharmaceutical reference guide, Medications and Mothers' Milk, is updated every 2 years and provides a comprehensive review of the compatibility or effects of approximately 1,100 drugs, vaccines, herbs, and chemicals on breastfeeding and includes risk categories, pharmacologic properties, interactions with other drugs, and suitable alternatives. The Medications and Mothers' Milk Online version is now available by subscription and is updated regularly and printable.

#### ANTIMALARIALS

Since chloroquine and mefloquine may be safely prescribed to infants, both are considered compatible with breastfeeding. Most experts consider short-term use of doxycycline compatible with breastfeeding. Primaquine may be used for breastfeeding mothers and children with normal G6PD levels. The mother and infant should both be tested for G6PD deficiency before primaquine is given to the breastfeeding mother. Because data are not yet available on the safety of atovaquone-proguanil prophylaxis in infants weighing <11 lb (5 kg), CDC does not recommend it to prevent malaria in women who are breastfeeding infants weighing <5 kg (see Chapter 4, Malaria, for more information).

The quantity of antimalarial drugs transferred to breast milk is not enough to provide protection against malaria for the infant. The breastfeeding infant needs his or her own antimalarial drug.

### TRAVELERS' DIARRHEA TREATMENT

Exclusive breastfeeding protects infants against travelers' diarrhea. Breastfeeding is ideal rehydration therapy. Children who are suspected of having travelers' diarrhea should breastfeed more frequently. Children in this situation should not be offered other fluids or foods that replace breastfeeding. Breastfeeding mothers with travelers' diarrhea should continue breastfeeding if possible and increase their own fluid intake. The organisms that cause travelers' diarrhea

do not pass through breast milk. Breastfeeding mothers should carefully check the labels of over-the-counter antidiarrheal medications to avoid using bismuth subsalicylate compounds, which can lead to the transfer of salicylate to the child via breast milk. Fluoroquinolones and macrolides, which are commonly used to treat travelers' diarrhea, are excreted in breast milk. The decision about the use of antibiotics such as fluoroquinolones and macrolides in nursing mothers should be made in consultation with the child's primary health care provider. Most experts consider the use of short-term azithromycin compatible with breastfeeding. Use of oral rehydration salts by breastfeeding mothers and their children is fully compatible with breastfeeding.

## SPECIAL CONSIDERATION: ZIKA VIRUS

CDC encourages mothers with Zika virus infection and living in or traveling to areas with ongoing Zika virus transmission to breastfeed their infants. Evidence suggests that the benefits of breastfeeding outweigh the risks of Zika virus transmission through breast milk. Updated information is available at www.cdc.gov/pregnancy/zika/testing-follow-up/zika-in-infants-children.html.

### BIBLIOGRAPHY

1. Academy of Breastfeeding Medicine (ABM) Protocol Committee. ABM clinical protocol #8: human milk storage information for home use for full-term infants, revised 2017. Breastfeed Med. 2017 Sept;12(7):390–5. Available from: http://online.liebertpub.com/doi/full/10.1089/bfm.2017.29047.aje

2. Fleming-Dutra KE, Nelson JM, Fischer M, Staples JE, Karwowski MP, Mead P, et al. Update: interim guidelines for health care providers caring for infants and children with possible Zika virus infection—United States, February 2016. MMWR Morb Mortal Wkly Rep 2016 Feb 26;65(7):182–7.

3. Hale TW, Rowe HE. Medications and Mothers' Milk 2017. New York: Springer Publishing Company, LLC; 2017.

4. Kuhn S, Twele-Montecinos L, MacDonald J, Webster P, Law B. Case report: probable transmission of vaccine

strain of yellow fever virus to an infant via breast milk. CMAJ. 2011 Mar 8;183(4):e243–5.

5. Sachdev HP, Krishna J, Puri RK, Satyanarayana L, Kumar S. Water supplementation in exclusively breastfed infants during summer in the tropics. Lancet. 1991 Apr 20;337(8747):929–33.

6. Section on Breastfeeding. Breastfeeding and the use of human milk. Pediatrics. 2012 Mar;129(3):e827–41.

7. Staples JE, Gershman M, Fischer M. Yellow fever vaccine: recommendations of the Advisory Committee on Immunization Practices (ACIP). MMWR Recomm Rep. 2010 Jul 30;59(RR-7):1–27.

8. CDC. Travel Recommendations for Nursing Families [cited 2019 Apr 1]. Available from: https://www.cdc.gov/nutrition/infantandtoddlernutrition/breastfeeding/travel-recommendations.html.

**7**

# TRAVELING SAFELY WITH INFANTS & CHILDREN

Michelle S. Weinberg, Nicholas Weinberg, Susan A. Maloney

## OVERVIEW

The number of children who travel or live outside their home countries has increased dramatically. In 2016, an estimated 2.81 million international travelers from the United States were children or adults traveling with children. Although data about the incidence of pediatric illnesses associated with international travel are limited, the risks that children face while traveling are likely similar to those their parents face. However, children are less likely to receive pretravel advice. In a review of children with posttravel illnesses seen at clinics in the GeoSentinel Global Surveillance Network, only 51% of all children and 32% of the children visiting friends and relatives (VFRs) had received pretravel medical advice, compared with 59% of adults. The most commonly reported health problems among child travelers are as follows:

- Diarrheal illnesses

- Dermatologic conditions, including animal and arthropod bites, cutaneous larva migrans, and sunburn

- Systemic febrile illnesses, especially malaria

- Respiratory disorders

Motor vehicle and water-related injuries, including drowning, are also major health and safety concerns for child travelers.

In assessing a child who is planning international travel, clinicians should:

- Review routine childhood and travel-related vaccinations. The pretravel visit is an opportunity to ensure that children are up-to-date on routine vaccinations.

- Assess all anticipated travel-related activities.

- Provide preventive counseling and interventions tailored to specific risks, including special travel preparations and treatment that may be required for infants and children with underlying conditions, chronic diseases, or immunocompromising conditions. Adolescents traveling in a student group or program may require counseling about disease prevention and the risks of sexually transmitted infections, empiric treatment and management of common travel-related illnesses, sexual assault, and drug and alcohol use during international travel (see Chapter 9, Study Abroad & Other International Student Travel).

- Give special consideration to the risks of children who are VFR travelers in developing countries. Conditions may include increased risk of malaria, intestinal parasites, and tuberculosis.

- Consider counseling adults traveling with children and older children to take a course in basic first aid before travel.

## DIARRHEA

Diarrhea and associated gastrointestinal illness are among the most common travel-related problems affecting children. Infants and children with diarrhea can become dehydrated more quickly than adults. The etiology of travelers' diarrhea (TD) in children is similar to that in adults (see Chapter 2, Travelers' Diarrhea).

### Prevention

For infants, breastfeeding is the best way to reduce the risk of foodborne and waterborne illness. Infant formulas available abroad may not have the same nutritional composition or be held to the same safety standards as in the United States; parents feeding their child formula should consider whether they need to bring formula from home.

Water served to young children, including water used to prepare infant formula, should be disinfected (see Chapter 2, Water Disinfection). In some parts of the world, bottled water may also be contaminated and should be disinfected before consumption.

Similarly, food precautions should be followed diligently. Foods served to children should be cooked thoroughly and eaten while still hot; fruits eaten raw should be peeled by the caregiver immediately before consumption. Additionally, caution should be used with fresh dairy products, which may not be pasteurized and/or diluted with untreated water. For short trips, parents may want to bring a supply of safe snacks from home for times when children are hungry and available food may not be appealing or safe. See Chapter 2, Food & Water Precautions, for more information.

Scrupulous attention should be paid to hand-washing and cleaning bottles, pacifiers, teething rings, and toys that fall to the floor or are handled by others; water used to clean these items should be potable. After diaper changes, parents should be particularly careful to wash hands well, especially for infants with diarrhea, to avoid spreading infection to themselves and other family members. When proper handwashing facilities are not available, an alcohol-based hand sanitizer (containing ≥60% alcohol) can be used as a disinfecting agent. However, because alcohol-based hand sanitizers are not effective against certain pathogens, hands should be washed with soap and water as soon as possible. Additionally, alcohol does not remove organic material; visibly soiled hands should be washed with soap and water.

Chemoprophylaxis with antibiotics is not generally used in children.

## Treatment

### ANTIEMETICS AND ANTIMOTILITY DRUGS

Because of potential side effects, antiemetics are generally not recommended for self- or family-administered treatment of children with vomiting and TD. Because of the association between salicylates and Reye syndrome, bismuth subsalicylate (BSS), the active ingredient in both Pepto-Bismol and Kaopectate, is not generally recommended to treat diarrhea in children aged <12 years. However, some clinicians use it off-label

with caution in certain circumstances. Caution should be taken in administering BSS to children with viral infections, such as varicella or influenza, because of the risk for Reye syndrome. BSS is not recommended for children aged <3 years.

A Cochrane Collaboration Review of the use of antiemetics for reducing vomiting related to acute gastroenteritis in children and adolescents showed some benefits with ondansetron, metoclopramide, or dimenhydrinate. Recent guidelines from the Infectious Disease Society of America suggest that an antinausea and antiemetic medication (such as ondansetron) may be given to facilitate tolerance of oral rehydration in children >4 years of age and in adolescents with acute gastroenteritis. However, the routine use of these medications as part of self-treatment for emesis associated with TD in children has not yet been determined and is not generally recommended.

Antimotility drugs, such as loperamide and diphenoxylate, should generally not be given to children <18 years of age with acute diarrhea. Loperamide is not recommended for children aged <6 years. Diphenoxylate and atropine combination tablets are not recommended for children aged <2 years. These drugs should be used with caution in children because of potential side effects (see Chapter 2, Travelers' Diarrhea).

### ANTIBIOTICS

Few data are available regarding empiric treatment of TD in children. The antimicrobial options for empiric treatment of TD in children are limited. In practice, when an antibiotic is indicated for moderate to severe diarrhea, some clinicians prescribe azithromycin as a single daily dose (10 mg/kg) for 3 days. Clinicians can prescribe unreconstituted azithromycin powder before travel, with instructions from the pharmacist for mixing it into an oral suspension if it becomes necessary to use it. Although resistance breakpoints have not yet been determined, elevated minimum inhibitory concentrations for azithromycin have been reported for some gastrointestinal pathogens. Therefore, parents should be counseled to seek medical attention for their children if they do not improve after empiric treatment. Clinicians should review possible contraindications, such as QT prolongation and cardiac arrhythmias with azithromycin, before prescribing medications for empiric treatment of TD.

Although fluoroquinolones are frequently used for the empiric treatment of TD in adults, they are not approved by the Food and Drug Administration for this purpose among children aged <18 years because of cartilage damage seen in animal studies. The American Academy of Pediatrics suggests that fluoroquinolones be considered for the treatment of children with severe infections caused by multidrug-resistant strains of *Shigella* species, *Salmonella* species, *Vibrio cholerae*, or *Campylobacter jejuni*. Clinicians should be aware that fluoroquinolone resistance in gastrointestinal organisms has been reported from some countries, particularly in Asia. The use of fluoroquinolones has been associated with tendinopathies, development of *Clostridium difficile* infection, and central nervous system side effects including confusion and hallucinations. Routine use of fluoroquinolones for prophylaxis or empiric treatment for TD among children is not recommended.

Rifaximin is approved for use in children aged ≥12 years but has limited use for empiric treatment since it is only approved to treat noninvasive strains of *Escherichia coli*. Children with bloody diarrhea should be advised to seek medical care since antibiotic treatment of enterohemorrhagic *E. coli*, a cause of bloody diarrhea, has been associated with increased risk of hemolytic uremic syndrome.

## Fluid and Nutrition Management

The biggest threat to the infant with diarrhea and vomiting is dehydration. Fever or increased ambient temperature increases fluid loss and speeds dehydration. Adults traveling with children should be counseled about the signs and symptoms of dehydration and the proper use of oral rehydration salts (ORS). Medical attention may be required for an infant or young child with diarrhea who has the following:

- Signs of moderate to severe dehydration

- Bloody diarrhea

- Temperature >101.5°F (38.6°C)

- Persistent vomiting (unable to maintain oral hydration)

The mainstay of management of TD is adequate hydration.

### ORS USE AND AVAILABILITY

Parents should be advised that dehydration is best prevented and treated by use of ORS in addition to the infant's usual food. ORS should be provided to the infant by bottle, cup, oral syringe (often available in pharmacies), or spoon while medical attention is being obtained. Low-osmolarity ORS is the most effective in preventing dehydration, although other formulations are available and may be used if they are more acceptable to young children. Homemade sugar-salt solutions are not recommended. Adults traveling with children should be counseled that sports drinks, which are designed to replace water and electrolytes lost through sweat, do not contain the same proportions of electrolytes as the solution recommended by the World Health Organization for rehydration during diarrheal illness. However, if ORS is not readily available, children should be offered whatever safe, palatable liquid they will take until ORS is obtained. Breastfed infants should continue to be breastfed.

ORS packets are available at stores or pharmacies in almost all developing countries. ORS is prepared by adding 1 packet to boiled or treated water (see Chapter 2, Water Disinfection for Travelers). Travelers should be advised to check packet instructions carefully to ensure that the salts are added to the correct volume of water. ORS solution should be consumed or discarded within 12 hours if held at room temperature or 24 hours if kept refrigerated. A dehydrated child will usually drink ORS avidly; travelers should be advised to give it to the child as long as the dehydration persists. As dehydration lessens, the child may refuse the salty-tasting ORS solution, and another safe liquid can be offered. An infant or child who has been vomiting will usually keep ORS down if it is offered by spoon or oral syringe in small sips; these small amounts must be offered frequently, however, so the child can receive an adequate volume of ORS. Older children will often drink well by sipping through a straw. Severely dehydrated children, however, often will be unable to drink adequately. Severe dehydration is a medical emergency that usually requires administration of fluids by intravenous or intraosseous routes.

In general, children weighing <22 lb (10 kg) who have mild to moderate dehydration should be administered 2–4 oz (60–120 mL) ORS for each diarrheal stool or vomiting episode. Children who weigh ≥22 lb (10 kg) should receive 4–8 oz (120–240 mL) of ORS for each diarrheal stool or vomiting episode. The American Academy of Pediatrics provides detailed guidance on rehydration for vomiting and diarrhea; see www.healthychildren.org/English/health-issues/conditions/abdominal/Pages/Treating-Dehydration-with-Electrolyte-Solution.aspx. ORS packets are available in the United States from Jianas Brothers Packaging Company (816-421-2880; http://rehydrate.org/resources/jianas.htm). ORS packets may also be available at stores that sell outdoor recreation and camping supplies. In addition, Cera Products (843-842-2600 or 706-221-1542; www.ceraproductsinc.com) markets a rice-based, rather than glucose-based, product.

### DIETARY MODIFICATION

Breastfed infants should continue nursing on demand. Formula-fed infants should continue their usual formula during rehydration. They should receive a volume sufficient to satisfy energy and nutrient requirements. Lactose-free or lactose-reduced formulas are usually unnecessary. Diluting formula may slow resolution of diarrhea and is not recommended. Older infants and children receiving semisolid or solid foods should continue to receive their usual diet during the illness. Recommended foods include starches, cereals, pasteurized yogurt, fruits, and vegetables. Foods high in simple sugars, such as soft drinks, undiluted apple juice, gelatins, and presweetened cereals, can exacerbate diarrhea by osmotic effects and should be avoided. In addition, foods high in fat may not be tolerated because of their tendency to delay gastric emptying.

The practice of withholding food for ≥24 hours is not recommended. Early feeding can decrease changes in intestinal permeability caused by infection, reduce illness duration, and improve nutritional outcome. Highly specific diets (such as the BRAT [bananas, rice, applesauce, and toast] diet) have been commonly recommended; however, similar to juice-based and clear fluid diets, such severely restrictive diets have no scientific basis and should be avoided.

## MALARIA

Malaria is among the most serious and life-threatening infections that can be acquired by pediatric international travelers. Pediatric VFR travelers are at particularly high risk for acquiring malaria if they do not receive prophylaxis.

Children with malaria can rapidly develop high levels of parasitemia. They are at increased risk for severe complications of malaria, including shock, seizures, coma, and death. Initial symptoms of malaria in children may mimic many other common causes of pediatric febrile illness and therefore may result in delayed diagnosis and treatment. Among 33 children with imported malaria diagnosed at 11 medical centers in New York City, 11 (32%) had severe malaria and 14 (43%) were initially misdiagnosed. Clinicians should counsel adults traveling with children in malaria-endemic areas to use preventive measures, be aware of the signs and symptoms of malaria, and seek prompt medical attention if they develop.

### Antimalarial Drugs

Pediatric doses for malaria prophylaxis are provided in Table 4-10. All dosing should be calculated on the basis of body weight. Medications used for infants and young children are the same as those recommended for adults, except under the following circumstances:

- Doxycycline should not be recommended for malaria prophylaxis for children aged <8 years. Although doxycycline has not been associated with dental staining when given as a routine treatment for some infections, other tetracyclines may cause teeth staining.

- Atovaquone-proguanil should not be used for prophylaxis in children weighing <11 lb (<5 kg) because of lack of data on safety and efficacy.

Chloroquine, mefloquine, and atovaquone-proguanil have a bitter taste. Pharmacists can

7

be asked to pulverize tablets and prepare gelatin capsules with calculated pediatric doses. Mixing the powder in a small amount of food or drink can facilitate the administration of antimalarial drugs to infants and children. Additionally, any compounding pharmacy can alter the flavoring of malaria medication tablets so that children are more willing to take them. Assistance with finding a compounding pharmacy is available on the Compounder Connect section of the International Academy of Compounding Pharmacists' website (www.iacprx.org; 800-927-4227). Because overdose of antimalarial drugs, particularly chloroquine, can be fatal, medication should be stored in childproof containers and kept out of the reach of infants and children.

## Personal Protective Measures and Repellent Use

Children should sleep in rooms with air conditioning or screened windows, or sleep under bed nets when air conditioning or screens are not available. Mosquito netting should be used over infant carriers. Children can reduce skin exposed to mosquitoes by wearing long pants and long sleeves while outdoors in areas where malaria is transmitted. Clothing and mosquito nets can be treated with insect repellents such as permethrin, a repellent and insecticide that repels and kills ticks, mosquitoes, and other arthropods. Permethrin remains effective through multiple washings. Clothing and bed nets should be retreated according to the product label. Permethrin should not be applied to the skin.

Although permethrin provides longer duration of protection, recommended repellents that can be applied to skin can also be used on clothing and mosquito nets. See Chapter 3, Mosquitoes, Ticks & Other Arthropods for more details about these protective measures. CDC recommends the use of Environmental Protection Agency (EPA)–registered repellents containing one of the following active ingredients: DEET (*N,N*-diethyl-*m*-toluamide), picaridin, oil of lemon eucalyptus (OLE) or PMD (para-menthane-3,8-diol), IR3535, and 2-undecanone (methyl nonyl ketone) (www.epa.gov/insect-repellents/find-repellent-right-you).

Most of the EPA-registered repellents can be used on children aged >2 months, with the following considerations:

- Products containing OLE or PMD specify that they should not be used on children aged <3 years.

- Repellent products must state any age restriction. If none is stated, the EPA has not required a restriction on the use of the product.

Many repellents contain DEET as the active ingredient. The concentration of DEET varies considerably among products. The duration of protection varies with the DEET concentration; higher concentrations protect longer. Products with DEET concentration >50% do not offer a marked increase in protection time. The American Academy of Pediatrics recommends that ≤30% DEET should be used on children aged >2 months.

Repellents can be applied to exposed skin and clothing; however, they should not be applied under clothing. Repellents should never be used over cuts, wounds, or irritated skin. Young children should not be allowed to handle the product. When using repellent on a child, an adult should apply it to his or her own hands and then rub them on the child, with the following considerations:

- Avoid the child's eyes and mouth, and apply sparingly around the ears.

- Do not apply repellent to children's hands, since children tend to put their hands in their mouths.

- Heavy application and saturation are generally unnecessary for effectiveness. If biting insects are not repelled by a thin film of repellent, then apply a bit more.

- After returning indoors, wash treated skin with soap and water or bathe. This is particularly important when repellents are used repeatedly in a day or on consecutive days.

Combination products containing repellents and sunscreen are generally not recommended, because instructions for use are different and sunscreen may need to be reapplied more often and

7

in larger amounts than repellent. In general, apply sunscreen first, and then apply repellent.

Mosquito coils should be used with caution in the presence of children to avoid burns and inadvertent ingestion. For more information about repellent use and other protective measures, see Chapter 3, Mosquitoes, Ticks & Other Arthropods.

## DENGUE AND OTHER ARBOVIRUSES

Pediatric VFR travelers with frequent or prolonged travel to areas where dengue or other arboviruses (such as chikungunya, Japanese encephalitis, yellow fever, or Zika viruses) are endemic or epidemic may be at increased risk for severe infection. Dengue can cause mild to severe illness. Most infections are asymptomatic, but some people with dengue virus infection can develop life-threatening illness. Among 8 children who were diagnosed with acute dengue virus infection after visiting friends and relatives in the Caribbean, 3 developed severe dengue.

Children traveling to areas with dengue or other arboviruses should use the same mosquito protection measures described for malaria. However, families should be counseled that, unlike the mosquitoes that transmit malaria, the *Aedes* mosquitoes that transmit dengue, chikungunya, yellow fever, and Zika are aggressive daytime biters and can also bite at night. Clinicians should consider dengue or other arboviral infections in children with fever if they have recently been in the tropics.

## INFECTION AND INFESTATION FROM SOIL CONTACT

Children are more likely than adults to have contact with soil or sand and therefore may be exposed to diseases caused by infectious stages of parasites present in soil, including ascariasis, hookworm, cutaneous or visceral larva migrans, trichuriasis, and strongyloidiasis. Children and infants should wear protective footwear and play on a sheet or towel rather than directly on the ground. Clothing should not be dried on the ground. In countries with a tropical climate, clothing or diapers dried in the open air should be ironed before use to prevent infestation with fly larvae.

## ANIMAL EXPOSURES AND RABIES

Worldwide, rabies is more common in children than adults. In addition to the potential for increased contact with animals, children are also more likely to be bitten on the head or neck, leading to more severe injuries. Children and their families should be counseled to avoid all stray or unfamiliar animals and to inform adults of any contact or bites. Bats throughout the world are considered to have the potential to transmit rabies virus. Animal bites and scratches should be washed thoroughly with water and soap (and povidone iodine if available); for mammal bites and scratches, the child should be evaluated promptly to assess the need for rabies postexposure prophylaxis. Because rabies vaccine and rabies immune globulin may not be available in certain destinations, families traveling to areas with high risk of rabies should seriously consider purchasing medical evacuation insurance.

## AIR TRAVEL

Although air travel is safe for most newborns, infants, and children, a few issues should be considered in preparation for travel. Children with chronic heart or lung problems may be at risk for hypoxia during flight, and a clinician should be consulted before travel. Making sure that children can be safely restrained during a flight is a safety consideration. Severe turbulence or a crash can create enough momentum that a parent cannot hold onto a child. The safest place for a child on an airplane is in a government-approved child safety restraint system/device (CRS). The Federal Aviation Administration (FAA) strongly urges that children be secured in a CRS for the duration of the flight. Car seats cannot be used in all seats or on all planes, and some airlines may have limited safety equipment available. Travelers should check with the airline about specific restrictions and approved child restraint options. FAA provides additional information at www.faa.gov/travelers/fly_children.

Ear pain can be troublesome for infants and children during descent. Pressure in the middle ear can be equalized by swallowing or chewing:

- Infants should nurse or suck on a bottle.
- Older children can try chewing gum.

7

- Antihistamines and decongestants have not been shown to be of benefit.

There is no evidence that air travel exacerbates the symptoms or complications associated with otitis media. Travel to different time zones, jet lag, and schedule disruptions can disturb sleep patterns in infants and children, as well as in adults (Chapter 2, Jet Lag).

## INJURIES

### Motor Vehicle-Related

Vehicle-related injuries are the leading cause of death in children who travel. While traveling in automobiles and other vehicles, children should be properly restrained in a car seat, booster seat, or with a seat belt, as appropriate for their weight, height, and age. Information about child passenger safety is available at www.healthychildren. org/English/safety-prevention/on-the-go/Pages/Car-Safety-Seats-Information-for-Families.aspx. Car/booster seats often must be carried from home, since availability of well-maintained and approved seats may be limited abroad.

In general, children ≤12 years of age are safest traveling properly buckled in the rear seat; no one should ever travel in the bed of a pickup truck. Families should be counseled that in many developing countries, cars may lack front or rear seatbelts. They should attempt to arrange transportation in vehicles or rent vehicles with seatbelts and other safety features. Helmets should be used when riding bicycles, scooters, or motorcycles. Pedestrians should take caution when crossing streets, particularly in those countries where cars drive on the left, as children may not be used to looking in that direction before crossing.

### Drowning and Water-Related Illness and Other Injuries

Drowning is the second leading cause of death in young travelers. Children may not be familiar with hazards in the ocean or in rivers. Swimming pools may not have protective fencing to keep toddlers from falling into the pool. Close supervision of children around water is essential. Because drowning occurs quickly and quietly, adults should not be involved in any other distracting activity while supervising children around water.

Water safety devices such as life vests may not be available abroad, and families should consider bringing these from home. Protective footwear is important to avoid injury in many marine environments. Schistosomiasis is a risk to children and adults in endemic areas. While in schistosomiasis endemic areas (Map 4-11), children should not swim in fresh, unchlorinated water such as lakes or ponds.

### Accommodations

Conditions at hotels and other lodging may not be as safe as those in the United States, and accommodations should be carefully inspected for exposed wiring, pest poisons, paint chips, or inadequate stairway or balcony railings.

Planning ahead can better equip caregivers to provide a safe sleeping environment for their infant during international travel. General recommendations from the American Academy of Pediatrics task force on preventing SIDS and other sleep-related causes of infant death are important to take into consideration during travel (http://pediatrics.aappublications.org/content/early/2016/10/20/peds.2016-2938). Cribs in some locations may not meet US safety standards. Additional information about crib safety is available from the US Consumer Product Safety Commission (www.cpsc.gov/en/Safety-Education/Safety-Education-Centers/cribs).

### ALTITUDE

Children are as susceptible to altitude illness as adults (see Chapter 3, High-Altitude Travel & Altitude Illness). Young children who cannot talk can show nonspecific symptoms, such as loss of appetite and irritability. They may have unexplained fussiness and changes in sleep and activity patterns. Older children may complain of headache or shortness of breath. If children demonstrate unexplained symptoms after an ascent, it may be necessary to descend to see if they improve. Acetazolamide is not approved for pediatric use for altitude illness, but it is generally safe in children when used for other indications.

### SUN EXPOSURE

Sun exposure, and particularly sunburn before age 15 years, is strongly associated with melanoma

7

and other forms of skin cancer (see Chapter 3, Sun Exposure). Exposure to UV light is highest near the equator, at high altitudes, during midday (10 AM–4 PM), and where light is reflected off water or snow. Sunscreens are generally recommended for use in children aged >6 months. Sunscreens (or sun blocks), either physical (such as titanium or zinc oxides) or chemical (sun protection factor [SPF] ≥15 and providing protection from both UVA and UVB), should be applied as directed, and reapplied as needed after sweating and water exposure. Babies aged <6 months require extra protection from the sun because of their thinner and more sensitive skin; severe sunburn for this age group is considered a medical emergency. Babies should be kept in the shade and wear clothing that covers the entire body. A minimal amount of sunscreen can be applied to small exposed areas, including the infant's face and hands. Sun-blocking shirts are available that are made for swimming and preclude having to rub sunscreen over the entire trunk. Hats and sunglasses also reduce sun injury to skin and eyes. If both sunscreen and a DEET-containing insect repellent are applied, the level of protection provided by the sunscreen may be diminished by as much as one-third, and covering clothing should be worn, sunscreen reapplied, or time in the sun decreased accordingly.

## OTHER CONSIDERATIONS

### Travel Stress

Changes in schedule, activities, and environment can be stressful for children. Including children in planning for the trip and bringing along familiar toys or other objects can decrease these stresses. For children with chronic illnesses, decisions regarding timing and itinerary should be made in consultation with the child's health care providers.

### Insurance

As for any traveler, insurance coverage for illnesses and injuries while abroad should be verified before departure. Consideration should be given to purchasing special medical evacuation insurance for airlifting or air ambulance to an area with adequate medical care (see Chapter 6, Travel Insurance, Travel Health Insurance & Medical Evacuation Insurance).

### Identification

In case family members become separated, each infant or child should carry identifying information and contact numbers in his or her own clothing or pockets. Because of concerns about illegal transport of children across international borders, if only 1 parent is traveling with the child, he or she may need to carry relevant custody papers or a notarized permission letter from the other parent.

BIBLIOGRAPHY

1. Ashkenazi S, Schwartz E, Ryan M. Travelers' diarrhea in children: what have we learnt? Pediatr Infect Dis J. 2016 Jun;35(6):698–700.

2. Bradley JS, Jackson MA, Committee on Infectious Diseases. The use of systemic and topical fluoroquinolones. Pediatrics. 2011 Oct;128(4):e1034–45.

3. Fedorowicz Z, Jagannath VA, Carter B. Antiemetics for reducing vomiting related to acute gastroenteritis in children and adolescents. Cochrane Database Syst Rev. 2011 Sep 7(9):1–71.

4. Goldman-Yassen AE, Mony VK, Arguin PM, Daily JP. Higher Rates of misdiagnosis in pediatric patients versus adults hospitalized with imported malaria. Pediatr Emerg Care. 2016 Apr;32(4):227–31.

5. Hagmann S, Neugebauer R, Schwartz E, Perret C, Castelli F, Barnett ED, et al. Illness in children after international travel: analysis from the GeoSentinel Surveillance Network. Pediatrics. 2010 May;125(5):e1072–80.

6. Herbinger KH, Drerup L, Alberer M, Nothdurft HD, Sonnenburg F, Loscher T. Spectrum of imported infectious diseases among children and adolescents returning from the tropics and subtropics. J Travel Med. 2012 May–Jun;19(3):150–7.

7. Hunziker T, Berger C, Staubli G, Tschopp A, Weber R, Nadal D, et al. Profile of travel-associated illness in children, Zurich, Switzerland. J Travel Med. 2012 May–Jun;19(3):158–62.

8. Kamimura-Nishimura K, Rudikoff D, Purswani M, Hagmann S. Dermatological conditions in international pediatric travelers: epidemiology, prevention and management. Travel Med Infect Dis. 2013 Nov–Dec;11(6):350–6.

9. Krishnan N, Purswani M, Hagmann S. Severe dengue virus infection in pediatric travelers visiting friends and relatives after travel to the Caribbean. Am J Trop Med Hyg. 2012 Mar;86(3):474–6.

10. Riddle MS, Connor BA, Beeching NJ, DuPont HL, Hamer DH, Kozarsky P, et al. Guidelines for the prevention and treatment of travelers' diarrhea: a graded expert panel report. J Travel Med. 2017 Apr;24(1):S63–80.

11. Shane AL, Mody RK, Crump JA, Tarr PI, Steiner TS, Kotloff K, et al. 2017 Infectious Diseases Society of America clinical practice guidelines for the diagnosis and management of infectious diarrhea. Clin Infect Dis. 2017 Nov;65(12):e45–80.

12. Sleet DA, Balaban V. Travel medicine: preventing injuries to children. Amer J Lifestyle Med. 2013 Mar;7(2):121–9.

13. van Rijn SF, Driessen G, Overbosch D, van Genderen PJ. Travel-related morbidity in children: a prospective observational study. J Travel Med. 2012 May–Jun;19(3):144–9.

# VACCINE RECOMMENDATIONS FOR INFANTS & CHILDREN

Michelle S. Weinberg

Vaccinating children for travel requires careful evaluation. Whenever possible, children should complete the routine immunizations of childhood on a normal schedule. However, travel at an earlier age may require accelerated schedules. **Not all travel-related vaccines are effective in infants, and some are specifically contraindicated.**

The recommended childhood and adolescent immunization schedule is available at www.cdc.gov/vaccines/schedules/hcp/imz/child-adolescent.html. The catch-up schedule for children and adolescents who start their vaccination schedule late or who are >1 month behind can be accessed at www.cdc.gov/vaccines/schedules/hcp/imz/catchup.html. These tables also describe the recommended minimum intervals between doses for children who need to be vaccinated on an accelerated schedule, which may be necessary before international travel.

Country-specific vaccination recommendations and requirements for departure and entry vary over time. For example, proof of yellow fever vaccination is required for entry into certain countries. Meningococcal vaccination is required for travelers entering Saudi Arabia for the annual Hajj and Umrah pilgrimages. The World Health Organization issued temporary vaccination recommendations for residents of and long-term visitors to countries with active circulation of wild or vaccine-derived poliovirus. Clinicians should check the CDC website for up-to-date requirements and recommendations (www.cdc.gov/travel).

Additional information about diseases and routine vaccination is available in the disease-specific sections in Chapter 4. Interactive tools for determining routine and catch-up childhood vaccination are available at www.cdc.gov/vaccines/schedules/hcp/child-adolescent.html.

## MODIFYING THE IMMUNIZATION SCHEDULE FOR INADEQUATELY IMMUNIZED INFANTS AND YOUNGER CHILDREN BEFORE INTERNATIONAL TRAVEL

Several factors influence recommendations for the age at which a vaccine is administered, including age-specific risks of the disease and its complications, the ability of people of a given age to develop an adequate immune response to the vaccine, and potential interference with the immune response by passively transferred maternal antibodies.

The immunization schedules for infants and children in the United States do not provide specific guidelines for those traveling internationally before the age when specific vaccines are routinely recommended. Recommended age limitations are based on potential adverse events (yellow fever vaccine), lack of efficacy data or inadequate immune response (polysaccharide vaccines and influenza vaccine), maternal antibody interference and immaturity of the immune system (measles-mumps-rubella [MMR] vaccine), or lack of safety data. In deciding when to travel

7

with a young infant or child, parents should be advised that the earliest opportunity to receive routinely recommended immunizations in the United States (except for the dose of hepatitis B vaccine at birth and age 1 month) is at age 6 weeks. In general, live-virus vaccines (MMR, varicella, yellow fever) should be administered on the same day or spaced ≥28 days apart.

## Routine Infant and Childhood Vaccinations

Children should receive routine vaccination for hepatitis A virus; hepatitis B virus; diphtheria, tetanus, pertussis; *Haemophilus influenzae* type b (Hib); human papillomavirus; influenza; MMR; *Neisseria meningitidis*; polio; rotavirus; *Streptococcus pneumoniae*; and varicella. In order to complete vaccine series before travel, vaccine doses can be administered at the minimum ages and dose intervals. Parents should be informed that infants and children who have not received all recommended doses might not be fully protected.

Rotavirus vaccine is unique among the routine vaccines given to US infants because it has maximum ages for the first and last doses; specific consideration should be given to the timing of an infant's travel so that the infant will still be able to receive the vaccine series, if at all possible.

Travel-specific vaccine considerations include the following:

- **Hepatitis A vaccine:** Although hepatitis A is usually mild or asymptomatic in infants and children aged <5 years, infected children may transmit the infection to older children and adults, who are at risk for severe disease. Vaccination should be ensured for all children traveling to areas where there is an intermediate or high risk of hepatitis A.

  Because of the potential interference by maternal antibodies, the hepatitis A vaccine is not approved for children aged <1 year. The vaccine series consists of 2 doses ≥6 months apart. One dose of monovalent hepatitis A vaccine administered at any time before departure can provide adequate protection for most healthy children. The second dose is necessary for long-term protection.

- **Immune globulin (IG) for hepatitis A protection:** Children aged <1 year or who are allergic to a vaccine component and who are traveling to high-risk areas can receive IG. One dose of 0.1 mL/kg intramuscularly provides protection for up to 1 month. Those who do not receive vaccination and plan to travel for up to 2 months should receive an IG dose of 0.2 mL/kg. IG (0.2 mL/kg) can be repeated every 2 months thereafter if the traveler remains in a high-risk setting, though hepatitis A vaccination should be encouraged if not contraindicated.

  For optimal protection, children aged ≥1 year who are immunocompromised or have chronic medical conditions and who are planning to depart to a high-risk area in <2 weeks should receive the initial dose of vaccine along with IG at a separate anatomic injection site.

  IG does not interfere with the response to yellow fever vaccine but can interfere with the response to other live injected vaccines (such as MMR and varicella vaccines). Administration of MMR and varicella vaccines should be delayed for >3 months after administration of IG for hepatitis A prophylaxis. IG should not be administered <2 weeks after MMR or varicella vaccines unless the benefits exceed those of vaccination. If IG is given during this time, the child should be revaccinated with the live MMR or varicella vaccines but not sooner than 3 months after IG administration. When travel plans do not allow adequate time to administer live vaccines and IG before travel, the severity of the diseases and their epidemiology at the destination will help determine the course of preparation.

- **Hepatitis B vaccine:** Vaccine can be administered with an accelerated schedule of 4 doses of vaccine given at 0, 1, 2, and 12 months; the last dose may be given on return from travel.

- **Influenza vaccine:** Influenza viruses circulate predominantly in the winter months in temperate regions (typically November– April in the Northern Hemisphere and April– September in the Southern Hemisphere) but can occur year-round in tropical climates. Since influenza viruses may be circulating at any time of the year, travelers aged ≥6 months who were not vaccinated during the influenza season of their country of residence should be vaccinated ≥2 weeks before departure if vaccine is available.

Children aged 6 months through 8 years who did not receive at least 2 doses of influenza vaccine before July 1 of the fall influenza season should receive 2 doses separated by at least 4 weeks. Check the CDC website annually for updated recommendations about seasonal influenza vaccination.

- **MMR or MMRV vaccine:** Children traveling abroad need to be vaccinated at an earlier age than is routinely recommended. Infants aged 6–11 months should receive 1 MMR dose. Infants vaccinated before age 12 months must be revaccinated on or after the first birthday with 2 doses of MMR or MMRV separated by ≥28 days. Children aged ≥12 months should be given 2 MMR or MMRV doses separated by ≥28 days.

- **Meningococcal vaccine:** Children aged 2 months to 18 years who travel to or reside in areas of sub-Saharan Africa known as the "meningitis belt" (see Map 4-10) during the dry season (December through June) should receive quadrivalent meningococcal conjugate (MenACWY) vaccine.

Meningococcal vaccination is a requirement to enter Saudi Arabia when traveling to Mecca during the annual Hajj or Umrah pilgrimages. Health requirements and recommendations for US travelers to the Hajj or Umrah are available each year on the CDC Travelers' Health website (www.cdc.gov/ travel).

The schedule for the primary series and booster doses varies depending on which meningococcal vaccine is administered (see CDC's Immunization Schedules website at www.cdc.gov/vaccines/schedules for additional information).

Vaccination with a serogroup B meningococcal (MenB) vaccine is not routinely recommended for travel to the meningitis belt or other regions of the world unless an outbreak of serogroup B disease has been reported. Although MenB vaccine is not licensed in the United States for children <10 years of age, some European countries have recently introduced MenB vaccine as a routine immunization for infants. Infants who will be residing in these countries may consider MenB vaccination according to the routine infant immunization recommendations of that country.

- **Polio vaccine:** Polio vaccine is recommended for travelers to countries with evidence of wild poliovirus (WPV) or vaccine-derived poliovirus circulation (during the last 12 months) and for travelers with a high risk of exposure to someone with imported WPV infection when traveling to some countries that border areas with WPV circulation. Refer to the CDC Travelers' Health website destination pages for the most up-to-date polio vaccine recommendations (wwwnc.cdc.gov/travel/destinations/list).

Clinicians should ensure that travelers have completed the recommended age-appropriate polio vaccine series and have received a single lifetime booster dose, if necessary. Infants and children should receive an accelerated schedule to complete the routine series. See Chapter 4, Poliomyelitis, and CDC's Immunization Schedules website (www.cdc.gov/vaccines/schedules) for information about accelerated schedules.

Young adults (≥18 years of age) who are traveling to areas where polio vaccine is recommended and who have received a routine series with either inactivated polio vaccine (IPV) or live oral polio vaccine in childhood should receive a single lifetime booster dose of IPV before departure. Available data do not indicate the need for more than a single lifetime booster dose with IPV. However, requirements for long-term travelers may apply when departing certain countries.

In May 2014, the World Health Organization (WHO) declared the international spread of polio to be a Public Health Emergency of International Concern (PHEIC) under the authority of the International

7

Health Regulations (2005). To prevent further spread of disease, WHO issued temporary polio vaccine recommendations for long-term travelers (staying >4 weeks) and residents departing from countries with WPV transmission ("exporting WPV" or "infected with WPV") or with circulating vaccine-derived polioviruses types 1 or 3. Clinicians should be aware that long-term travelers and residents may be required to show proof of polio vaccination when departing from these countries. All polio vaccination administration should be documented on an International Certificate of Vaccination or Prophylaxis (ICVP). The polio vaccine must be received between 4 weeks and 12 months before the date of departure from the polio-infected country.

Country requirements may change, so clinicians should check for updates on the CDC Travelers' Health website. Refer to the Clinical Update: Interim CDC Guidance for Travel to and from Countries Affected by the New Polio Vaccine Requirements (wwwnc.cdc.gov/travel/news-announcements/polio-guidance-new-requirements) for a list of affected countries, guidance on meeting the vaccination requirements, and instructions on how to order and fill out the ICVP.

## Other Vaccines

### JAPANESE ENCEPHALITIS

Japanese encephalitis (JE) virus is transmitted by mosquitoes and is endemic throughout most of Asia and parts of the western Pacific. The risk can be seasonal in temperate climates and year-round in more tropical climates. The risk to short-term travelers and those who confine their travel to urban centers is low. JE vaccine is recommended for travelers who plan to spend a month or longer in endemic areas during the JE virus transmission season. JE vaccine should be considered for short-term (<1 month) travelers whose itinerary or activities might increase their risk for exposure to JE virus. The decision to vaccinate a child should follow the more detailed recommendations in Chapter 4, Japanese Encephalitis.

An inactivated Vero cell culture–derived JE vaccine (Ixiaro [Valneva]) was licensed by the Food and Drug Administration in 2009 for use in the United States for travelers aged ≥17 years. In 2013, the recommendations were expanded and the vaccine was licensed for use in children starting at age 2 months.

For children aged 2 months through 17 years, the primary series consists of 2 intramuscular doses administered 28 days apart. For travelers who received their primary JE vaccine series ≥1 year prior to potential JE virus exposure, ACIP recommends providing them with a booster dose before departure. Information on age-appropriate dosing is available at www.cdc.gov/japaneseencephalitis/vaccine/vaccineChildren.html.

### RABIES

Rabies virus causes an acute viral encephalitis that is virtually 100% fatal. Traveling children may be at increased risk of rabies exposure, mainly from dogs that roam the streets in developing countries. Bat bites carry a potential risk of rabies throughout the world. There are 2 strategies to prevent rabies in humans:

- Avoiding animal bites or scratches.

- Use of preexposure and postexposure prophylaxis. A 3-dose preexposure immunization series may be given on days 0, 7, and 21 or 28. In the event of a subsequent possible rabies virus exposure, the child will require 2 more doses of rabies vaccine on days 0 and 3. The decision whether to obtain preexposure immunization for children should follow the recommendations in Chapter 4, Rabies. Children who have not received preexposure immunization and may have been exposed to rabies require a weight-based dose of human rabies immune globulin and a series of 4 rabies vaccine doses on days 0, 3, 7, and 14.

### TYPHOID

Typhoid fever is caused by the bacterium *Salmonella enterica* serotype Typhi. Vaccination is recommended for travelers to areas where there is a recognized risk of exposure to *Salmonella* Typhi. Two typhoid vaccines are available: Vi capsular polysaccharide vaccine (ViCPS) administered intramuscularly, and oral live attenuated vaccine (Ty21a). Both vaccines induce a protective response in 50%–80% of recipients. The ViCPS vaccine can be administered to children who are aged ≥2 years, with a booster dose 2 years later if continued protection is needed. The Ty21a vaccine, which consists of a series of 4 capsules (1 taken every other day) can be administered to children aged ≥6 years. A booster series for Ty21a should be taken every 5 years, if indicated. The capsule cannot be opened for administration and must be swallowed whole. All 4 doses should be taken ≥1 week before potential exposure.

## YELLOW FEVER

Yellow fever, a disease transmitted by mosquitoes, is endemic in certain areas of Africa and South America (see Maps 4-13 and 4-14). Proof of yellow fever vaccination is required for entry into some countries (see Chapter 2, Yellow Fever Vaccine & Malaria Prophylaxis Information, by Country). Infants and children aged ≥9 months can be vaccinated if they travel to countries within the yellow fever–endemic zone. In February 2015, the CDC Advisory Committee on Immunization Practices (ACIP) approved a new recommendation that a single dose of yellow fever vaccine provides long-lasting protection and is adequate for most travelers. The updated recommendations also identify specific groups of travelers who should receive additional doses and others for whom additional doses may be considered. More information, including how to access yellow fever vaccine in the United States, is available in Chapter 4, Yellow Fever.

Infants aged <9 months are at higher risk for developing encephalitis from yellow fever vaccine, which is a live-virus vaccine. Studies conducted during the early 1950s identified 4 cases of encephalitis out of 1,000 children aged <6 months vaccinated with yellow fever vaccine. An additional 10 cases of encephalitis associated with yellow fever vaccine administered to infants aged <4 months were reported worldwide during the 1950s. Travelers with infants aged <9 months should be advised against traveling to areas within the yellow fever–endemic zone. ACIP recommends that yellow fever vaccine *never* be given to infants aged <6 months. Infants aged 6–8 months should be vaccinated only if they must travel to areas of ongoing epidemic yellow fever and if a high level of protection against mosquito bites is not possible. Clinicians considering vaccinating infants aged 6–8 months may contact their respective state health departments or CDC toll-free at 800-CDC-INFO (800-232-4636) or wwwn.cdc.gov/dcs/ContactUs/Form.

**7**

## BIBLIOGRAPHY

1. CDC. General recommendations on immunization—recommendations of the Advisory Committee on Immunization Practices (ACIP). MMWR Recomm Rep. 2011 Jan 28;60(2):1–64.

2. CDC. Use of Japanese encephalitis vaccine in children: recommendations of the Advisory Committee on Immunization Practices, 2013. MMWR Morb Mortal Wkly Rep. 2013 Nov 15;62(45):898–900.

3. CDC. Prevention and control of meningococcal disease: recommendations of the Advisory Committee on Immunization Practices (ACIP). MMWR Recomm Rep. 2013 Mar 22;62(RR-2):1–28.

4. CDC. Interim CDC guidance for polio vaccination for travel to and from countries affected by wild poliovirus. MMWR Morb Mortal Wkly Rep. 2014 Jul 11;63(27):591–4.

5. CDC. Yellow fever vaccine: recommendations of the Advisory Committee on Immunization Practices (ACIP). MMWR Recomm Rep. 2015 Jun 19;64(23):647–50.

6. Global Polio Eradication Initiative. Public health emergency status: IHR public health emergency of international concern. Temporary recommendations to reduce international spread of poliovirus. Geneva: Global Polio Eradication Initiative; 2018 [cited 2018 Jul 16]. Available from: www.polioeradication.org/ Keycountries/ PolioEmergency.aspx.

7. Jackson BR, Iqbal S, Mahon B, Centers for Disease Control and Prevention (CDC). Updated recommendations for the use of typhoid vaccine—Advisory Committee on Immunization Practices, United States, 2015. MMWR Morb Mortal Wkly Rep. 2015 Mar 27;64(11):305–8.

8. MacNeil JR, Rubin L, Folaranmi T, Ortega-Sanchez IR, Patel M, Martin SW, et al. Use of serogroup B meningococcal vaccines in adolescents and young adults: recommendations of the Advisory Committee on Immunization Practices, 2015. MMWR Morb Mortal Wkly Rep. 2015 Oct 23;64(41):1171–6.

9. Red Book. 2018-2021 Report of the Committee on Infectious Diseases. 31st ed. Kimberlin DW, Brady MT, Jackson MA, editors. Elk Grove Village, IL: American Academy of Pediatrics; 2018.

# INTERNATIONAL ADOPTION

Mary Allen Staat, Simone Wien, Emily Jentes

## OVERVIEW

In the past 15 years, >260,000 children have come to the United States to join their families through international adoption. Families traveling to unite with their adopted child, siblings who wait at home for the child's arrival, extended family members, and childcare providers are all at risk for acquiring infectious diseases secondary to travel or resulting from contact with the newly arrived child. International adoptees may be underimmunized and are at increased risk for infections such as measles, hepatitis A, and hepatitis B because of crowded living conditions, malnutrition, lack of clean water, lack of immunizations, and exposure to endemic diseases not commonly seen in the United States. Challenges in providing care to internationally adopted children include the absence of a complete medical history, lack of availability of a biological family history, questionable reliability of immunization records, variation in preadoption living standards, varying disease epidemiology in the countries of origin, the presence of previously unidentified medical problems, and the increased risk for developmental delays and psychological issues in these children.

## TRAVEL PREPARATION FOR ADOPTIVE PARENTS AND THEIR FAMILIES

A pretravel clinic visit is strongly recommended for prospective adoptive parents. In preparation, the travel health provider must know the disease risks in the adopted child's country of origin and the medical and social histories of the adoptee (if available), as well as which family members will be traveling, their immunization and medical histories, the season of travel, the length of stay in the country, and the itinerary while in country.

Family members who remain at home, including extended family, should be current on their routine immunizations. Protection against measles, varicella, tetanus, diphtheria, pertussis, polio, and hepatitis A (HAV), as well as hepatitis

B (HBV) if the adoptee has known infection or if the family is traveling to a country with high or intermediate levels of endemic HBV infection, must be ensured for all age-eligible people who will be in the household or in close contact by providing care for the adopted child.

An accelerated schedule of doses may be used to complete a vaccine series as long as minimum ages and dose intervals are followed. Measles immunity or 2 doses of measles-mumps-rubella (MMR) vaccine separated by ≥28 days should be documented for all people born in or after 1957. Varicella vaccine should be given to those born in or after 1980 without a history of varicella disease, documented immunity (serology), or documentation of 2 doses of varicella vaccine. Adults who have not received the tetanus-diphtheria-acellular pertussis (Tdap) vaccine, including adults >65 years old, should receive a single dose of Tdap to protect against *Bordetella pertussis* in addition to tetanus and diphtheria. Unprotected family members and close contacts of the adopted child should be immunized against HAV before the child's arrival. Most adult family members and caretakers will need to be immunized with hepatitis B vaccine if the adoptee has a known HBV infection, since it has only been routinely given since 1991.

If the adopted child is from a polio-endemic area, family members and caretakers should ensure they have completed the recommended age-appropriate polio vaccine series. A one-time inactivated polio booster for adults who have completed the primary series in the past is recommended if they are traveling to these areas and can be considered for adults who remain at home but who will be in close contact caring for the child. Additional polio vaccination requirements for long-term travelers (staying >4 weeks) and residents departing from countries with polio transmission may affect travel (see Chapter 4, Poliomyelitis).

Prospective adoptive parents and any children traveling with them should receive advice on travel safety, food safety, immunization, malaria prophylaxis, diarrhea prevention and treatment, and other travel-related health issues, as outlined elsewhere in this book.

## OVERSEAS MEDICAL EXAMINATION OF THE ADOPTED CHILD

All immigrants, including children adopted internationally by US citizens, must undergo a medical examination in their country of origin, performed by a physician designated by the Department of State. Additional information about the medical examination for internationally adopted children is available on the Department of State website at https://travel.state.gov/content/travel/en/Intercountry-Adoption/Adoption-Process/how-to-adopt/medical-examination.html and https://eforms.state.gov/Forms/ds1981.pdf.

Prospective adoptive parents should not rely on this overseas medical examination to detect all possible disabilities and illnesses, as the purpose of the medical examination is to identify applicants with inadmissible health-related conditions. To understand more about possible health concerns for an individual child, prospective adoptive parents should consider a preadoption medical review with a pediatrician who is familiar with the health issues of internationally adopted children to review the available medical history and vaccination record for the child. This preadoption medical review can prepare parents and providers for potential health issues that may occur with internationally adopted children, whose living conditions in their country of origin may differ significantly from those in the United States. Prospective adoptive parents can then proactively arrange and schedule any recommended follow-up after arrival home, including the initial follow-up medical examination that is recommended within 2 weeks of arrival to the United States (for additional information, see www.cdc.gov/immigrantrefugeehealth/adoption/finding-doctor.html). Although the overseas medical examination is not a comprehensive medical review, adoptive parents may be able to provide the results of the overseas examination, recorded on the Department of State medical forms, to the clinicians at the initial follow-up medical examination.

## FOLLOW-UP MEDICAL EXAMINATION AFTER ARRIVAL IN THE UNITED STATES

Adopted children should have a complete medical examination within 2 weeks of arrival in the United States or earlier if the child has fever, anorexia, diarrhea, vomiting, or other medical concerns. In addition, all children should receive a developmental screening by an experienced clinician to determine if immediate referrals should be made for more detailed neurodevelopmental examination and therapies. Further evaluation will depend on the country of origin, the age of the child, previous living conditions, nutritional status, developmental status, and the adoptive family's specific questions. Concerns raised during the preadoption medical review may dictate further investigation.

## SCREENING FOR INFECTIOUS DISEASES

Screening recommendations for some infectious diseases vary by organization. The current panel of tests for infectious diseases recommended by the American Academy of Pediatrics (AAP) for screening internationally adopted children is as follows:

- Hepatitis A serologic testing (IgG and IgM)

- Hepatitis B serologic testing

- Hepatitis C serologic testing

- Syphilis serologic testing (treponemal and nontreponemal testing)

- HIV 1 and 2 serologic testing (antigen/antibody)

- Complete blood cell count with differential and red blood cell indices

- Stool examination for ova and parasites (3 specimens)

- Stool examination for *Giardia intestinalis* and *Cryptosporidium* antigen (1 specimen)

- TB testing:
  - > For children <2 years of age, tuberculin skin test (TST) is preferred
  - > For children ≥2 years of age, either interferon-γ release assay (IGRA) or TST can be used (for those previously vaccinated with BCG, IGRA is preferred)
  - > Repeat testing should be done 3–6 months later, if initial testing is negative

Additional screening tests may be useful, depending on the child's country of origin or specific risk factors. These screens may include Chagas disease serologic tests, malaria smears or PCR, and serologic testing for schistosomiasis, strongyloidiasis, and filariasis. Cases of reportable diseases should be reported to the state or local health department.

## Gastrointestinal Parasites

Gastrointestinal parasites are commonly seen in international adoptees, but the prevalence varies by birth country and age. The highest rates of infection have been reported from Ukraine and Ethiopia and increase with older age.

*Giardia intestinalis* is the most common parasite identified. Three stool samples collected in the early morning, 2–3 days apart, and placed in a container with preservative are recommended for ova and parasite analysis. Because routine examination of stool for ova and parasites is unlikely to include testing for *Cryptosporidium*, health care providers should specifically request *Cryptosporidium* testing.

Although theoretically possible, transmission of intestinal parasites from internationally adopted children to family and school contacts has not been reported; however, good hand hygiene is recommended to prevent infection. Stool samples should be tested for enteric pathogens for any child with fever and diarrhea. If a culturable enteric pathogen is detected, samples should be cultured to determine antimicrobial susceptibility. Unlike refugees, internationally adopted children are not treated for parasites before departure.

## Hepatitis A

Screening asymptomatic people for hepatitis A is generally not recommended; however, clinicians may decide to test internationally adopted children for anti-HAV IgG and IgM to identify those who may be acutely infected and shedding virus and to make decisions regarding hepatitis A vaccination.

In 2007 and early 2008, multiple cases of hepatitis A secondary to exposure to newly arrived internationally adopted children were reported in the United States. Some of these cases involved extended family members who were not living in the household. Identification of acutely infected toddlers new to the United States is necessary to prevent further transmission. If a child is found to have an acute infection, hepatitis A vaccine or immunoglobulin can be given to close contacts to prevent infection. In addition, it is cost effective to identify children with past infection with serologic testing, since they would not need to receive the hepatitis A vaccine.

## Hepatitis B

All internationally adopted children should be screened for HBV infection with serologic tests for hepatitis B surface antigen (HBsAg), hepatitis B surface antibody, and hepatitis B core antibody to determine past infection, current infection, or protection due to vaccination. Because of widespread use of the hepatitis B vaccine, the prevalence of HBV infection has decreased over the years. HBV infection has been reported in 1%– 5% of newly arrived adoptees. Children found to be positive for HBsAg should be retested 6 months later to determine if the child has a chronic infection. Results of a positive HBsAg test should be reported to the state health department.

HBV is highly transmissible within the household. All members of households adopting children with chronic HBV infection must be immunized. Children with chronic HBV infection should receive additional tests for HBV e antigen, HBV e antibody, hepatitis D virus antibody, viral load, and liver function. They should be vaccinated for hepatitis A if they are not immune. They should also have a consultation with a pediatric gastroenterologist.

Although not currently recommended by CDC or AAP, repeat screening at 6 months after arrival may be considered for all children who initially test negative for hepatitis B surface antibody.

## Hepatitis C

Routine screening for hepatitis C virus (HCV) may be considered, since most children with HCV infection are asymptomatic, screening for risk factors is not possible, and close follow-up of infected patients is needed to identify long-term complications. Antibody testing should be used for screening. Since maternal antibody may be present in children <18 months of age, PCR testing should be done if the antibody test is positive. Children with HCV infection should be referred to a gastroenterologist for further evaluation, management, and treatment.

## Syphilis

Screening for *Treponema pallidum* is recommended for all internationally adopted children. Initial screening is done with both nontreponemal and treponemal tests. Treponemal tests remain positive for life in most cases even after successful treatment, and are specific for treponemal diseases, which include syphilis and other diseases (such as yaws, pinta, and bejel) that can be seen in some countries. In children with a history of syphilis, the child's initial evaluation, treatment (antibiotic type and treatment duration), and follow-up testing are rarely available; therefore, a full evaluation for disease must be undertaken and antitreponemal treatment given depending upon the results.

## HIV

HIV screening is recommended for all internationally adopted children. Positive HIV antibodies in children aged <18 months may reflect maternal antibody and not infection. PCR assay for HIV DNA will confirm the diagnosis in the infant or child. Standard screening for HIV is with ELISA antibody testing, but some experts recommend PCR for any infant aged <6 months on arrival. If PCR testing is done, 2 negative results from assays administered 1 month apart, at least one of which is done after the age of 4 months, are necessary to exclude infection. Children with HIV infection should be referred to a specialist. Some experts recommend repeating the screen for HIV

antibodies 6 months after arrival if the initial testing is negative.

## Other Sexually Transmitted Infections

Although routine screening for sexually transmitted infections beyond syphilis and HIV is not recommended, some experts will screen all children older than 5 years of age for chlamydia and gonorrhea. In addition, if there is any question or concern of sexual abuse, chlamydia and gonorrhea screening should be done for a child of any age.

## Chagas Disease

Screening for Chagas should be considered for children arriving from countries endemic for the disease. Chagas disease is endemic throughout much of Mexico, Central America, and South America (see Chapter 4, Trypanosomiasis, American [Chagas Disease]).

The risk of Chagas disease varies by region within endemic countries. Although the risk of Chagas disease is likely low in adopted children from endemic countries, treatment of infected children is effective. Serologic testing when the child is aged 9–12 months will avoid possible false-positive results from maternal antibody. Testing by PCR can be done in children <9 months of age. Children testing positive for Chagas disease should be referred to a specialist for further evaluation and management.

## Malaria

Routine screening for malaria is not recommended for internationally adopted children. However, thick and thin malaria smears should be obtained immediately for any febrile child or child symptomatic with splenomegaly who has arrived from a malaria-endemic area (see Chapter 4, Malaria). Rapid diagnostic tests (RDTs) for malaria may be useful to decrease the amount of time that it takes to determine that a patient is infected with malaria, but microscopy should be used to confirm the results and determine the degree of parasitemia.

PCR testing may be useful to confirm the species of parasite after the diagnosis has been established by either smear microscopy or a RDT. Of note, asymptomatic children with splenomegaly need a workup for this condition. This workup should include antibody titers for malaria, since asymptomatic children with splenomegaly due to repeated malaria infections may have high titers but negative smears.

## Tuberculosis

Internationally adopted children are at 4–6 times the risk for TB than their US-born peers. Screening for TB is an integral part of the overseas medical examination, and positive results from this screening on the Department of State medical forms may be available from adoptive parents (if they retained a copy) or with the local health department. If overseas screening results are not available, all internationally adopted children should be screened for TB after arriving in the United States, and any cases should be reported to the state health department.

To screen for TB, AAP recommends a TST for children <2 years of age. For children ≥2 years of age, either IGRA or a TST can be used. For those previously vaccinated with BCG, IGRAs appear to be more specific than the TST for *Mycobacterium tuberculosis* infection. For children who initially test negative for TB, repeat testing is recommended 3–6 months after arrival.

If the TST or IGRA is positive for TB, the child has TB infection and an additional evaluation needs to be done to determine if the child has latent TB infection (LTBI) or TB disease. Additional information is available at www.cdc.gov/tb/topic/reatment/ltbi.htm.

If a child has evidence of TB disease, consultation with an infectious disease expert is recommended.

## Eosinophilia

A complete blood count with a differential should be drawn for all internationally adopted children. An eosinophil count >450 cells/mm³ in an internationally adopted child may warrant further evaluation. Intestinal parasite screening will identify some helminths that may cause eosinophilia. Further investigation of the eosinophilia might include serologic evaluation for *Strongyloides stercoralis*, *Toxocara canis*, *Ancylostoma* spp., and *Trichinella spiralis*. For children arriving from countries endemic for *Schistosoma* spp. and

filariasis, serologic testing should be done for these diseases as well.

## SCREENING FOR NONINFECTIOUS DISEASES

Several screening tests for noninfectious diseases should be performed in all or in select internationally adopted children. All children should have a complete blood count with a differential, hemoglobin electrophoresis, and G6PD deficiency screening. Serum levels of thyroid-stimulating hormone and lead should be measured in all internationally adopted children. Testing for serum levels of iron, iron-binding capacity, transferrin, ferritin, and total vitamin D 25-hydroxy should be considered. All children should have vision and hearing screening and a dental evaluation. In certain circumstances, neurologic and psychological testing may also be considered.

## IMMUNIZATIONS

The US Immigration and Nationality Act requires that any person seeking an immigrant visa for permanent residency must show proof of having received the Advisory Committee on Immunization Practices (ACIP)-recommended vaccines before immigration (www.cdc.gov/vaccines/schedules/hcp/imz/child-adolescent.html). This requirement applies to all immigrant infants and children entering the United States, but internationally adopted children aged <10 years are exempt from the overseas immunization requirements. Adoptive parents are required to sign an affidavit indicating their intention to comply with the immunization requirements within 30 days of the child's arrival in the United States. The vaccination affidavit can be found at https://eforms.state.gov/Forms/ds1981.pdf.

Most children throughout the developing world receive BCG, hepatitis B, polio, measles, diphtheria, tetanus, and pertussis vaccines. Upon arrival in the United States, >90% of newly arrived internationally adopted children need catch-up immunizations to meet ACIP guidelines since rotavirus, *Haemophilus influenzae* type b (Hib), pneumococcal conjugate, hepatitis A, mumps, rubella, varicella, meningococcal, and human papillomavirus vaccines are often not available or given in these countries. Reliability of vaccine records

7

appears to differ by, and even within, country of origin. Some children may have an immunization record with documentation of the vaccines and dates they were given, and others may have incomplete documentation or no records at all. MMR is not given in most countries of origin, as measles vaccine is often administered as a single antigen. In addition, some children may be immune to hepatitis A, measles, mumps, rubella, or varicella as a result of natural infection. A clinical diagnosis of any of these diseases, however, should not be accepted as evidence of immunity.

Providers can choose 1 of 2 approaches for vaccination of internationally adopted children. The first is to reimmunize regardless of immunization record. The second, applicable to children aged ≥6 months, is to test antibody titers to the vaccines reportedly administered and reimmunize only for those diseases to which the child has no protective titers. Immunity to *B. pertussis* is an exception; antibody titers do not correlate with immune status to *B. pertussis*. However, higher protective antibody levels to diphtheria and tetanus might imply protective antibody levels to *B. pertussis*. Immunity to hepatitis B is also an exception, as anti-HBs as a correlate of vaccine-induced protection has only been determined for people who have completed an approved vaccination series.

For children ≥6 months of age, testing can be done for diphtheria (IgG), tetanus (IgG), hepatitis B (as outlined above), and Hib. For children ≥12 months of age, testing can also be done for measles, mumps, rubella, hepatitis A, and varicella. Since April 2016, a bivalent polio vaccine has been used in many resource-poor countries. Thus, children born on or after this date who do not have documentation of US and WHO age-appropriate inactivated polio vaccine, vaccination should be given a series of IPV vaccine. Reimmunization with pneumococcal vaccine is recommended given that there are 13 serotypes in the vaccine. ACIP recommends that children with positive hepatitis B surface antibody should have documentation of 3 appropriately spaced doses of hepatitis B vaccine to be considered immune. For children with positive hepatitis B surface antibody and positive hepatitis B core antibody, vaccination is not required as they are considered to be immune after natural infection. Passively acquired maternal antibodies to HBV core antigen may be detected in an infant up to age 24 months.

Once the immunization record has been assessed and antibody level results are available, any indicated immunizations should be given according to the current ACIP schedule for catch-up vaccination. If the infant is <6 months old and there is uncertainty regarding immunization status or validity of the immunization record, the child should be immunized according to the ACIP schedule.

**7**

## BIBLIOGRAPHY

1. American Academy of Pediatrics. Medical evaluation for infectious diseases for internationally adopted, refugee, and immigrant children. In: Red Book: 2018–2021 Report of the Committee on Infectious Diseases. 31st ed. Elk Grove Village, IL: American Academy of Pediatrics; 2018. Available from: https://redbook.solutions.aap.org/chapter.aspx?sectionid=189640017&bookid=2205.

2. American Academy of Pediatrics Committee on Infectious Diseases. Recommendations for administering hepatitis A vaccine to contacts of international adoptees. Pediatrics. 2011 Oct;128(4):803–4.

3. CDC. Measles among adults associated with adoption of children in China—California, Missouri, and Washington, July–August 2006. MMWR Morb Mortal Wkly Rep. 2007 Feb 23;56(7):144–6.

4. CDC. CDC immigration requirements: technical instructions for tuberculosis screening and treatment: using cultures and directly observed therapy. 2009 [cited 2018 Jul 15]. Available from: www.cdc.gov/immigrantrefugeehealth/exams/ti/panel/tuberculosis-panel-technical-instructions.html.

5. CDC. Recommended immunization schedules for persons aged 0 through 18 years—United States, 2018. MMWR Morb Mortal Wkly Rep. 2018 Feb 6;67(5):156–7.

6. CDC, ACIP. Updated recommendations from the Advisory Committee on Immunization Practices (ACIP) for use of hepatitis A vaccine in close contacts of newly arriving international adoption. MMWR Morb Mortal Wkly Rep. 2009;58(36):1006–7.

7. Immigrant visas issued to orphans coming into the US. [database on the Internet]. US Department of State. 1999–2016 [cited 2018 Mar 29]. Available from: https://travel.state.gov/content/travel/en/Intercountry-Adoption/adopt_ref/adoption-statistics.html.

8. Lewinsohn, DM, Leonard MK, LoBue P, Cohn DL, Daley CL, Desmond E, et al. Official American Thoracic Society/Infectious Diseases Society of America/Centers for Disease Control and Prevention clinical practice guidelines: diagnosis of tuberculosis in adults and children. Clin Infect Dis. 2017;64(2):111–5.

9. Mandalakas AM, Kirchner HL, Iverson S, Chesney M, Spencer MJ, Sidler A, et al. Predictors of *Mycobacterium tuberculosis* infection in international adoptees. Pediatrics. 2007 Sep;120(3):e610–6.

10. Marin M, Patel M, Oberste S, Pallansch MA. Guidance for assessment of poliovirus vaccination status and vaccination of children who have received poliovirus vaccine outside the United States. MMWR Morb Mortal Wkly Rep. 2017 Jan 13;66(1):23–5.

11. Staat MA, Rice M, Donauer S, Mukkada S, Holloway M, Cassedy A, et al. Intestinal parasite screening in internationally adopted children: importance of multiple stool specimens. Pediatrics. 2011 Sep;128(3):e613–22.

12. Staat MA, Stadler LP, Donauer S, Trehan I, Rice M, Salisbury S. Serologic testing to verify the immune status of internationally adopted children against vaccine preventable diseases. Vaccine. 2010 Nov 23;28(50):7947–55.

13. Stadler LP, Donauer S, Rice M, Trehan I, Salisbury S, Staat MA. Factors associated with protective antibody levels to vaccine preventable diseases in internationally adopted children. Vaccine. 2010 Dec 10;29(1):95–103.

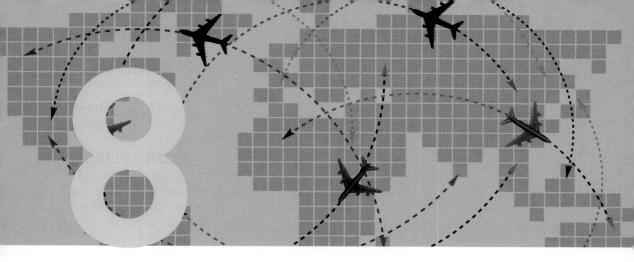

# Travel by Air, Land & Sea

## AIR TRAVEL

Paul J. Edelson, Phyllis E. Kozarsky, Clive Brown

Worldwide, an estimated 3.6 billion people travel by commercial aircraft every year, and this number continues to rise. Travelers often have concerns about the health risks of flying in airplanes. Those with underlying illness need to be aware that the entire point-to-point travel experience, including buses, trains, taxis, public waiting areas, and even movement within the airport, can pose challenges. Although illness may occur as a direct result of air travel, it is uncommon; the main concerns are:

- Exacerbations of chronic medical problems due to changes in air pressure and humidity

- Relative immobility during flights leading to thromboembolic disease (see Deep Vein Thrombosis & Pulmonary Embolism in this chapter)

- Close proximity to other passengers with communicable diseases

### PREFLIGHT MEDICAL CONSIDERATIONS

During flight, the aircraft cabin pressure is usually maintained at the equivalent of 6,000–8,000 ft (1,829–2,438 m) above sea level. Most healthy travelers will not notice any effects. However, for travelers with cardiopulmonary diseases (especially those who normally require supplemental oxygen), cerebrovascular disease, anemia, or sickle cell disease, conditions in an aircraft can exacerbate underlying medical conditions. Aircraft cabin air is typically dry, usually 10%–20% humidity, which can cause dryness of the mucous membranes of the eyes and airways.

The new Boeing 787 and Airbus A 350 have improved the cabin environment: a greater number of temperature zones, a higher humidity of 25%, a faster time to refresh cabin air, lower ambient noise, and multiple shades of LED lighting. These, along with a cabin air pressure equivalent to an altitude of only 2,000 ft, should provide more comfort and ease jet lag.

The Aerospace Medical Association (www.asma.org) recommends evaluating chronic medical conditions and addressing instabilities prior to travel, particularly in those who have underlying cardiovascular disease, a history of deep vein thrombosis or pulmonary embolism, chronic lung disease, surgical conditions, seizures, stroke, mental illness, or diabetes.

For information on contraindications and precautions related to flying during pregnancy, see Chapter 7, Pregnant Travelers. Specific information for travelers with disabilities and medical conditions that may affect security screening can be found at www.tsa.gov/travel/special-procedures. For those who require supplemental in-flight oxygen, the following must be taken into consideration:

- Travelers must arrange their own oxygen supplies while on the ground, at departure, during layovers, and upon arrival.

- Federal regulations prohibit airlines from allowing passengers to bring their own oxygen onboard; passengers requiring in-flight supplemental oxygen should notify the airline ≥72 hours before departure.

- Airlines might not offer in-flight supplemental oxygen on all aircraft or flights; some airlines permit only Federal Aviation Administration (FAA)-approved portable oxygen concentrators. Information to assist people who require supplemental oxygen during travel and FAA-approved portable oxygen concentrators can be found at the FAA website: www.faa.gov/about/initiatives/cabin_safety/portable_oxygen.

- Information regarding the screening of portable oxygen concentrators at airports in the United States can be

found at www.tsa.gov/blog/2014/04/08/tsa-travel-tips-traveling-portable-oxygen.

For more information, see Chapter 5, Travelers with Disabilities.

## BAROTRAUMA DURING FLIGHT

Barotrauma can occur when the pressure inside an air-filled, enclosed body space (such as the middle ear, sinuses, or abdomen) is not the same as the air pressure inside the aircraft cabin. It most commonly is the result of rapid changes in environmental pressure, such as during ascent, when cabin pressure rapidly falls, and during descent, when cabin pressure rapidly rises. Barotrauma most commonly affects the middle ear; it happens when the eustachian tube is blocked and thus unable to equalize the air pressure in the middle ear with the outside cabin pressure. Middle ear barotrauma is usually not severe or dangerous and can usually be prevented or self-treated. It may rarely cause complications such as a perforated tympanic membrane, dizziness, permanent tinnitus, or hearing loss. The following suggestions may help avoid potential barotrauma:

- People with ear, nose, and sinus infections or severe congestion may wish to postpone flying to prevent pain or injury.

- Oral or nasal decongestants may alleviate symptoms.

- Travelers with allergies should continue their regular allergy medications.

- Travelers should stay hydrated to help avoid irritation of nasal passages and pharynx and to promote better function of the eustachian tubes.

- Travelers sensitive to abdominal bloating should avoid carbonated beverages and foods that can increase gas production.

- People who have had recent surgery, particularly intra-abdominal, neurologic, intrapulmonary, or intraocular procedures, should consult with their physician before flying.

## VENTILATION AND AIR QUALITY

All commercial jet aircraft built after the late 1980s, and a few modified older aircraft, recirculate 10%–50% of the air in the cabin, mixed with outside air. The recirculated air passes through a series of filters 20–30 times per hour. In most newer-model airplanes, the recycled air passes through high-efficiency particulate air (HEPA) filters, which capture 99.9% of particles (bacteria, fungi, and larger viruses or virus clumps) 0.1–0.3 μm in diameter. Furthermore, air generally circulates in defined areas within the aircraft, thus limiting the radius of distribution of pathogens spread by small-particle aerosols. As a result, the cabin air environment is not conducive to the spread of most infectious diseases.

Some diseases may be spread by contact with infected secretions, such as when an ill person sneezes or coughs (and the secretions or droplets land on another person's face, mouth, nose, or eyes), or touches a communal surface (such as a door knob or rest room faucet) with contaminated hands. Other people handling those contaminated surfaces may then be inoculated with the contaminant. Practicing good handwashing and respiratory hygiene (covering mouth when coughing or sneezing) decreases the risk of disease spread by direct or indirect contact.

## IN-FLIGHT MEDICAL EMERGENCIES

The increasing number of travelers combined with an increase in the number of older passengers make the incidence of onboard medical emergencies likely to increase. Medical emergencies occur in approximately 1 in 600 flights or about 16 medical emergencies per 1 million passengers. The most commonly encountered in-flight medical events are:

- Syncope or presyncope (37%)
- Respiratory symptoms (12%)
- Nausea or vomiting (10%)
- Cardiac symptoms (8%)
- Seizures (6%)

Although in-flight medical emergencies occur, serious illness or death onboard a commercial aircraft is rare. Deaths onboard commercial aircraft have been estimated at 0.3 per 1 million passengers; approximately two-thirds of these are caused by cardiac conditions. Most commercial airplanes that fly within the United States are required to carry at least 1 approved automatic external defibrillator (AED) and an emergency medical kit.

Flight attendants are trained in basic first aid procedures such as CPR, and use of AED machines, but are generally not certified in emergency medical response. Many airlines use ground-based medical consultants to assist flight crew and volunteer passenger responders in managing medical cases. In nearly one-half of in-flight emergencies, physician volunteers have provided assistance. The Aviation Medical Assistance Act, passed in 1998, provides some protection from liability to providers who respond to in-flight medical emergencies.

The goal of managing in-flight medical emergencies is to stabilize the passenger until ground-based medical care can safely be reached. When considering diversion to a closer airport, the captain must consider the needs of the ill passenger, as well as other safety concerns such as weather, landing conditions, and terrain. Certain routes, such as transoceanic flights, and availability of definitive medical care may limit diversion options.

## IN-FLIGHT TRANSMISSION OF COMMUNICABLE DISEASES

Communicable diseases may be transmitted to other travelers during air travel; therefore, people who are acutely ill, or still within the infectious period for a specific disease, should delay their travel until they are no longer contagious. For example, otherwise healthy adults can transmit influenza to others for 5–7 days. Travelers should be up-to-date on routine vaccinations and receive destination-specific vaccinations before travel. Travelers should be reminded to wash their hands frequently and thoroughly (or use an alcohol-based hand sanitizer containing at least 60% alcohol), especially after using the toilet and before preparing or eating food, and to cover their noses and mouths when coughing or sneezing. For further information on control of communicable diseases, see Appendix D: Airplanes & Cruise

Ships: Illness & Death Reporting & Public Health Interventions.

## INFORMATION FOR AIRCREW

In preparation for a healthy journey, flight crew can refer to Chapter 9, Aircrews, and to the CDC Travelers' Health website (www.cdc.gov/travel). If flight crews encounter passengers with potentially infectious diseases, see the CDC Airline Guidance web page: www.cdc.gov/quarantine/air. Requirements and tools for reporting by aircrews are also provided there.

### BIBLIOGRAPHY

1. Aerospace Medical Association Air Transport Medicine Committee. Medical considerations for airline travel. Alexandria, VA: Aerospace Medical Association; 2018 [cited 2018 Oct 23]. Available from: www.asma.org/publications/medical-publications-for-airline-travel/medical-considerations-for-airline-travel.

2. Bagshaw M, Barbeau DN. The aircraft cabin environment. In: Keystone JS, Kozarsky PE, Freedman DO, Northdurft HO, Connor BA editors. Travel Medicine. 3rd ed. Philadelphia: Saunders Elsevier; 2013, pp. 405–12.

3. Huizer YL, Swaanm CM, Leitmeyer KC, Timen A. Usefulness and applicability of infectious disease control measures in air travel: a review. Travel Med Infect Dis. 2015 Jan–Feb;13(1):19–30.

4. Illig PA. Passenger health. In: Curdt-Christiansen C, Draeger J, Kriebel J, Antunano M, editors. Principles and Practice of Aviation Medicine. Hackensack, NJ: World Scientific; 2009. pp. 667–708.

5. Nable JV, Tupe CL, Gehle BD, Brady WJ. In-Flight medical emergencies during commercial travel. N Engl J Med 2015 Sep 3;375(10):939–45.

6. Peterson DC, Martin-Gill C, Guyette FX, Tobias AZ, McCarthy CE, Harrington ST, et al. Outcomes of medical emergencies on commercial airline flights. N Engl J Med. 2013 May 5;368(22):2075–83.

# DEEP VEIN THROMBOSIS & PULMONARY EMBOLISM

**8**

Nimia L. Reyes, Michele G. Beckman, Karon Abe

Deep vein thrombosis (DVT) is a condition in which a blood clot develops in the deep veins, most commonly in the lower extremities. A pulmonary embolism occurs when a part of the clot breaks off and travels to the lungs, a potential life threat. Venous thromboembolism (VTE) refers to DVT, PE, or both. VTE is often recurrent, and long-term complications, such as postthrombotic syndrome after a DVT or chronic thromboembolic pulmonary hypertension after a PE, are frequent.

Extended periods of limited mobility inherent to long-haul travel may increase a travelers' risk for DVT/PE; an association between VTE and air travel was first reported in the early 1950s. Since then, as prolonged air travel has become more common (>300 million people take long-distance flights each year) concerns about travel-related VTE have become more prevalent.

## PATHOGENESIS

Virchow's classic triad for thrombus formation is venous stasis, vessel wall damage, and a hypercoagulable state. Prolonged, cramped sitting during long-distance travel interferes with venous flow in the legs creating venous stasis. Seat-edge pressure to the popliteal area of the legs can aggravate venous stasis as well as contribute to vessel wall damage. Studies of the pathophysiologic mechanisms for the increased risk of VTE after long-distance travel have not produced consistent results, but venous stasis appears to play a major role.

Other factors specific to air travel may increase coagulation activation, particularly in travelers with preexisting risk factors for VTE. Coagulation activation may result from an interaction between cabin conditions (such as hypobaric hypoxia) and individual risk factors for VTE.

## INCIDENCE

There is no national surveillance for VTE; research estimates the annual incidence of VTE in the general population at 0.1% although it is higher in subpopulations with risk factors (Box 8-1). In the absence of national surveillance for VTE (as a whole), the incidence of travel-related VTE is even more difficult to determine and varies from study to study. Complicating the matter, no consensus exists on what constitutes a travel-related VTE, particularly duration of travel and period of observation after travel.

In general, the overall incidence of travel-related VTE is low. Two studies reported that the absolute risk of VTE for flights >4 hours is 1 in 4,656 flights and 1 in 6,000 flights. People who travel on long-distance flights are generally healthier and therefore at lower risk for VTE than the general population. Five prospective studies to assess the incidence of DVT among travelers at low to intermediate risk for VTE after travel >8 hours yielded an overall incidence of VTE of 0.5%, while the incidence of symptomatic VTE was 0.3%.

## ASSOCIATION WITH TRAVEL

Studies examining the association between long-range travel, particularly air travel, and VTE do not share common definitions. Flight duration, used both as the criteria for what constitutes long-range travel as well as a surrogate (albeit imprecise) measure of the length of time travelers are immobile, ranges from >3 hours to >10 hours. Duration of observation of travelers after flights also varies, ranging from a few hours after landing to ≥8 weeks posttravel. Furthermore, outcome measures differ—from asymptomatic DVT to symptomatic DVT/PE to severe or fatal PE.

In aggregate, the studies indicate that long-distance air travel may increase the risk for VTE by 2- to 4-fold; however, some studies found that long-distance travel increased the risk for VTE, while others found no definitive evidence of an increase in risk, perhaps because of the aforementioned differences in definitions used. Still others identified an increase in risk only if ≥1 additional risk factor was present. Asymptomatic DVT (which is of uncertain clinical significance and often resolves spontaneously) was estimated to be 5- to 20-fold more common than symptomatic events.

A similar increase in risk for VTE is seen with other modes of long-distance travel (car, bus, or train). This implies that the increase in risk is due mainly to prolonged limited mobility rather than by the air cabin environment, per se. Level of risk

**8**

---

**BOX 8-1.** Venous thromboembolism (VTE) risk factors

General risk factors for VTE include the following:

- Older age (increasing risk after age 40)
- Obesity (BMI ≥30 kg/m²)
- Estrogen use (hormonal contraceptives or hormone replacement therapy)

- Pregnancy and the postpartum period
- Thrombophilia (such as factor V Leiden mutation or antiphospholipid syndrome) or a family history of VTE
- Previous VTE

- Active cancer
- Serious medical illness (such as congestive heart failure or inflammatory bowel disease)
- Recent surgery, hospitalization, or trauma
- Limited mobility

correlates with duration of travel and with preexisting risk factors for VTE. Risk decreases with time after air travel and returns to baseline by 8 weeks; most air travel-related VTE occurs within the first 1–2 weeks after the flight.

## RISK FACTORS

Most travel-related VTE occurs in travelers with preexisting risk factors for VTE (Box 8-1). The combination of air travel with preexisting individual risk factors may synergistically increase risk. Some studies have shown that 75%–99.5% of those who developed travel-related VTE had ≥1 preexisting risk factor(s); one study showed that 20% had ≥5 risk factors. For travelers without preexisting risk factors, the risk of travel-related VTE is low. However, a person may not be aware that he or she has a risk factor such as inherited thrombophilia.

For airline passengers, risk of travel-related VTE varies depending on traveler height, with the lowest risk among adults of average height and the greatest risk among adults at both extremes. Because of the inability to adjust airline seats, adults <1.6 m (5 ft 3 in) may be more prone to pressure to the popliteal area, a phenomenon already identified as contributing to venous stasis in the legs and possibly vessel wall damage. Air travelers >1.9 m (6 ft 3 in) are also at increased risk for VTE, possibly because in the main cabin, in particular, there is typically less leg room for taller travelers.

## CLINICAL PRESENTATION

Signs and symptoms of DVT/PE are nonspecific:

- Typical signs or symptoms of DVT in the extremities include pain or tenderness, swelling, increased warmth in the affected area, and redness or discoloration of the overlying skin.

- The most common signs or symptoms of acute PE include unexplained shortness of breath, pleuritic chest pain, cough or hemoptysis, and syncope.

## DIAGNOSIS

Imaging studies needed for diagnosis:

- Duplex ultrasonography is the standard imaging procedure for DVT diagnosis.

- Computed tomographic pulmonary angiography is the standard imaging procedure for diagnosis of PE. Ventilation-perfusion scan is the second-line imaging procedure.

## TREATMENT

Anticoagulants are the medications most commonly used to treat DVT or PE. Bleeding can be a complication of anticoagulant therapy. The most frequently used injectable anticoagulants are unfractionated heparin, low molecular weight heparin (LMWH), and fondaparinux. Oral anticoagulants include warfarin, dabigatran, rivaroxaban, apixaban, and edoxaban.

## PREVENTIVE MEASURES FOR LONG-DISTANCE TRAVELERS

The American College of Chest Physicians published the 9th edition of their *Antithrombotic Therapy and Prevention of Thrombosis Evidence-Based Clinical Practice Guidelines* in February 2012. Recommendations for long-distance travelers (considered grade 2C: weak recommendation, low- or very low-quality evidence) are the following:

1. For long-distance travelers at increased risk of VTE (Box 8-1), frequent ambulation, calf muscle exercise, and sitting in an aisle seat if feasible are suggested.

2. For long-distance travelers at increased risk of VTE (Box 8-1), use of properly fitted, below-knee graduated compression stockings (GCS) providing 15–30 mm Hg of pressure at the ankle during travel is suggested. GCS appear to reduce asymptomatic DVT in travelers and are well tolerated, generally. For long-distance travelers not at increased risk of VTE, use of GCS is not recommended.

The guidelines do not recommend the use of aspirin or anticoagulants globally to prevent VTE in long-distance travelers. Decisions regarding use of pharmacologic prophylaxis for long-distance travelers at particularly high risk should be made on an individual basis. In cases where the potential benefits of pharmacologic

8

prophylaxis outweigh the possible adverse effects, anticoagulants rather than antiplatelet drugs (such as aspirin) are recommended. Patients at increased risk should be evaluated with enough time before departure so that they understand how to take the medication, and the health provider can evaluate whether there are any potential adverse effects of the combination of these medications with others that the travel health provider has prescribed.

There is no evidence of an association between dehydration and travel-related VTE. Furthermore, no direct evidence exists to support the concept that drinking plenty of nonalcoholic beverages to ensure adequate hydration or avoiding alcoholic beverages has a protective effect. Therefore, while maintaining hydration is reasonable and unlikely to cause harm, it cannot be recommended specifically to prevent travel-related VTE.

Immobility while flying is a risk for VTE. Indirect evidence suggests that maintaining mobility may prevent VTE. In view of the role that venous stasis plays in the pathogenesis of travel-related VTE, it would be reasonable to recommend frequent ambulation and calf muscle exercises for long-distance travelers.

Seat location within an aisle may also be a protective factor to reduce the risk of developing VTE. In one study, travelers seated in window seats, as compared to those in aisle seats, experienced an increase in the general risk of VTE by 2-fold; obese travelers had a 6-fold increase in risk. Conversely, aisle seats are reported to have a protective effect compared with window or middle seats, probably because travelers are freer to move around.

## RECOMMENDATIONS

1. General measures for long-distance travelers:
   a. Calf muscle exercises
   b. Frequent ambulation
   c. Aisle seating when feasible
2. Additional measures for long-distance travelers at increased risk of VTE:
   a. Properly fitted below-knee GCS
   b. Anticoagulant prophylaxis only in particularly high-risk cases where the potential benefits outweigh the risks

### BIBLIOGRAPHY

1. Aryal KR, Al-Khaffaf H. Venous thromboembolic complications following air travel: what's the quantitative risk? A literature review. Eur J Vasc Endovasc Surg. 2006 Feb;31(2):187–99.

2. Bartholomew JR, Schaffer JL, McCormick GF. Air travel and venous thromboembolism: minimizing the risk. Cleve Clin J Med. 2011 Feb;78(2):111–20.

3. Chandra D, Parisini E, Mozaffarian D. Meta-analysis: travel and risk for venous thromboembolism. Ann Intern Med. 2009 Aug 4;151(3):180–90.

4. Eklof B, Maksimovic D, Caprini JA, Glase C. Air travel-related venous thromboembolism. Disease-a-month: DM. 2005 Feb–Mar;51(2–3):200–7.

5. Gavish I, Brenner B. Air travel and the risk of thromboembolism. Intern Emerg Med. 2011 Apr;6(2):113–6.

6. Kahn SR, Lim W, Dunn AS, Cushman M, Dentali F, Akl EA, et al. Prevention of VTE in nonsurgical patients: antithrombotic therapy and prevention of thrombosis, 9th ed: American College of Chest Physicians evidence-based clinical practice guidelines. Chest. 2012 Feb;141(2 Suppl):e195S–226S.

7. Schobersberger W, Schobersberger B, Partsch H. Travel-related thromboembolism: mechanisms and avoidance. Expert Rev Cardiovasc Ther. 2009 Dec;7(12):1559–67.

8. Schreijer AJ, Cannegieter SC, Caramella M, Meijers JC, Krediet RT, Simons RM, et al. Fluid loss does not explain coagulation activation during air travel. Thromb Haemost. 2008 Jun;99(6):1053–9.

9. Schreijer AJ, Cannegieter SC, Doggen CJ, Rosendaal FR. The effect of flight-related behaviour on the risk of venous thrombosis after air travel. Br J Haematol. 2009 Feb;144(3):425–9.

10. Watson HG, Baglin TP. Guidelines on travel-related venous thrombosis. Br J Haematol. 2011 Jan;152(1):31–4.

8

# JET LAG

Greg Atkinson, Ronnie Henry, Alan M. Batterham, Andrew Thompson

## RISK FOR TRAVELERS

Jet lag results from a mismatch between a person's circadian (24-hour) rhythms and the time of day in the new time zone. When establishing risk, clinicians should first determine how many time zones the traveler will cross and what the discrepancy will be between time of day at home and at the destination. During the first few days after a flight to a new time zone, a person's circadian rhythms are still "anchored" to time of day at home. Rhythms then adjust gradually to the new time zone. A useful web-based tool for world time zone travel information can be found at www.timeanddate.com/worldclock/converter.html. If ≤3 time zones are being crossed, any symptoms such as tiredness are likely due to travel fatigue rather than significant jet lag, and will soon abate.

Many people traveling >3 time zones away for a vacation accept the risk of jet lag as a transient and mild inconvenience, while other people who are traveling on business or to compete in athletic events desire clear advice on prophylactic measures and treatments. If ≤2 days are spent in the new time zone, some people may prefer to anchor their sleep-wake schedule to time of day at home as much as is practical. Thereby, the total "burden" of jet lag resulting from the short round trip is minimized.

## CLINICAL PRESENTATION

The symptomatology of jet lag can often be difficult to define because of variation between people, but also because the same person can experience different symptoms after each flight. Jet-lagged travelers typically experience ≥1 of the following symptoms after a flight across >3 time zones:

- Poor sleep, including difficulty initiating sleep at the usual time of night (after eastward flights), early awakening (after westward flights), and fractionated sleep (after flights in either direction)

- Poor performance in physical and mental tasks during the new daytime

- Negative feelings such as fatigue, headache, irritability, anxiety, inability to concentrate, and depression

- Gastrointestinal disturbances and decreased interest in, and enjoyment of, meals

- Symptoms are difficult to distinguish from the general fatigue resulting from international travel itself, as well as from other travel factors such as the hypoxia in the aircraft cabin.

## TREATMENT

Since light and social contacts influence the timing of internal circadian rhythms, a traveler who is staying in the time zone for >2 days should try to follow the local people's sleep-wake habits as much as possible and as quickly as possible. This approach can be supplemented with the following information on specific treatments.

### Light

Exposure to bright light can advance or delay human circadian rhythms depending on when it is received relative to a person's body clock time. Consequently, schedules have been formulated for proposed "good" and "bad" times for exposure to light after arrival in a new time zone (www.caa.co.uk/Passengers/Before-you-fly/Am-I-fit-to-fly/Health-information-for-passengers/Jet-lag/).

After flights that cross a large number of time zones, the proposed best circadian time for exposure to light immediately after the flight may actually be when it is still dark in the new time zone, which raises the question of whether exposure to supplementary light from a "light box" is helpful. Unfortunately, to date, only 1 small randomized controlled trial on supplementary bright light for reducing jet lag has been conducted. No clinically relevant effects of supplementary light on jet lag symptoms were detected after a flight across 5 time zones going west.

## Diet and Physical Activity

Most dietary interventions have not been found to reduce jet lag symptoms. In a recent study, long-haul flight crews showed a small improvement in their general subjective rating of jet lag, but not the separate symptoms of jet lag or alertness, on their days off work when they adopted more regular meal times. Because gastrointestinal disturbance is a common symptom, smaller meals before and during the flight might be better tolerated than larger meals. Caffeine and physical activity may be used strategically at the destination to ameliorate any daytime sleepiness, but little evidence indicates that these interventions reduce overall feelings of jet lag. Any purported treatments that are underpinned by homeopathy, aromatherapy, and acupressure have no scientific basis.

## Hypnotic Medications

Prescription medications like temazepam, zolpidem, or zopiclone may reduce sleep loss during and after travel but do not necessarily help resynchronize circadian rhythms or improve overall jet lag symptoms. If indicated, the lowest effective dose of a short-to medium-acting compound should be prescribed for the initial few days, bearing in mind the adverse effects of these drugs.

Taking hypnotics during a flight should be considered with caution because the resulting immobility could increase the risk of deep vein thrombosis. Alcohol should not be used by travelers as a sleep aid, because it disrupts sleep and can provoke obstructive sleep apnea.

## Melatonin and Melatonin-Receptor Analogs

Melatonin is secreted at night by the pineal gland and is probably the most well-known treatment for jet lag. Melatonin delays circadian rhythms when taken during the rising phase of body temperature (usually the morning) and advances rhythms when ingested during the falling phase of body temperature (usually the evening). These effects are opposite to those of bright light.

The instructions on most melatonin products advise travelers to take it before nocturnal sleep in the new time zone, irrespective of number of time zones crossed or direction of travel. Studies published in the mid-1980s indicated a substantial benefit of melatonin (just before sleep) for reducing overall feelings of jet lag after flights. However, subsequent larger studies did not replicate the earlier findings.

Melatonin is considered a dietary supplement in the United States and is not regulated by the Food and Drug Administration. Therefore, the advertised concentration of melatonin has not been confirmed for most melatonin products on the market, and the presence of contaminants in the product cannot be ruled out.

Ramelteon, a melatonin-receptor agonist, is an FDA-approved treatment for insomnia. A dose of 1 mg taken just before bedtime can decrease sleep onset latency after eastward travel across 5 time zones. Higher doses do not seem to lead to further improvements, and the effects of the medication on other symptoms of jet lag and the timing of circadian rhythms are not as clear.

## Combination Treatments

Multiple therapies to decrease jet lag symptoms may be combined into treatment packages. Although marginal gains from multiple treatments may aggregate, evidence from robust randomized controlled trials is lacking for most of these treatment packages. One treatment package offering tailored advice via a mobile application was piloted to be used over several months of frequent flying. Participants reported reduced fatigue compared with the comparator group and improved aspects of health-related behavior such as physical activity, snacking, and sleep quality but not other measures of sleep (latency, duration, use of sleep-related medication).

In conclusion, there is still no "cure" for jet lag. Counseling should focus on the factors that are known, from laboratory simulations, to alter circadian timing. Nevertheless, more randomized controlled trials of treatments prescribed before, during, or after transmeridian flights are needed before the clinician can provide robust, evidence-based advice.

8

## BIBLIOGRAPHY

1. Atkinson G, Batterham AM, Dowdall N, Thompson A, Van Drongelen A. From animal cage to aircraft cabin: an overview of evidence translation in jet lag research. Eur J Appl Physiol. 2014 Dec;114(12):2459–68.

2. Herxheimer A. Jet lag. BMJ Clin Evid. 2014 Apr 29;2014. pii:2303.

3. Herxheimer A, Petrie KJ. Melatonin for the prevention and treatment of jet lag. Cochrane Database System Rev. 2002(2):CD001520.

4. Ruscitto C, Ogden J. The impact of an implementation intention to improve mealtimes and reduce jet lag in long-haul cabin crew. Psychol Health. 2016 Jan;32(1):61–77

5. Ruscitto C, Ogden J. Predicting jet lag in long-haul cabin crew: the role of illness cognitions and behaviour. Psychol Health. 2017 Sep;32(9):1055–81.

6. Samuels CH. Jet lag and travel fatigue: a comprehensive management plan for sport medicine physicians and high-performance support teams Clin J Sport Med. 2012 May;22(3):268–73.

7. Thompson A, Batterham AM, Jones H, Gregson W, Scott D, Atkinson G. The practicality and effectiveness of supplementary bright light for reducing jet-lag in elite female athletes. Int J Sports Med. 2013 Jul;34(7):582–9.

8. Van Drongelen A, Boot CR, Hlobil H, Twisk JW, Smid T, Van der Beek AJ. Evaluation of an mHealth intervention aiming to improve health-related behavior and sleep and reduce fatigue among airline pilots. Scand J Work Environ Health. 2014 Nov;40(6):557–68.

9. Waterhouse J, Reilly T, Atkinson G. Jet-lag. Lancet. 1997 Nov 29;350(9091):1611–6.

10. Waterhouse J, Reilly T, Atkinson G, Edwards B. Jet lag: trends and coping strategies. Lancet. 2007 Mar 31;369(9567):1117–29.

# ROAD & TRAFFIC SAFETY

Erin K. Sauber-Schatz, Erin M. Parker, David A. Sleet, Michael F. Ballesteros

**8**

Globally, an estimated 3,400 people, including more than 500 children, are killed each day in motor vehicle crashes involving cars, buses, motorcycles, bicycles, trucks, and pedestrians. Annually, about 1.3 million people are killed and an additional 20–50 million are injured in motor vehicle crashes. Although only 54% of the world's vehicles are in developing countries, 90% of the world's crash deaths occur in these countries. Nearly half of people who die on the world's roads each year are pedestrians, cyclists, and motorcyclists, also called "vulnerable road users."

According to US Department of State data, motor vehicle crashes are the leading cause of nonnatural death among US citizens who die in a foreign country (see Chapter 3, Injury & Trauma). From 2015 through 2016, 484 US citizens living or traveling internationally died as a result of a motor vehicle crash. Most crash deaths (63%) occurred in drivers and passengers of passenger vehicles (cars, trucks, or sport utility vehicles), followed by 18% in motorcycle drivers and passengers; 10% of traffic-related fatalities involved pedestrians.

Table 8-1 shows the top 29 countries visited by US citizens, based on the *Survey of International Air Travelers* from the Department of Commerce. For each country, the estimated "motor vehicle crash death rate per 100,000 population" is listed as an indicator for the risk of motor vehicle crash death, along with the number of US citizens who died in each country from a crash death from 2015 through 2016.

Motor vehicle crashes are common among foreign travelers for a number of reasons. In many developing countries, unsafe vehicles (vehicles sold in 80% of all countries worldwide fail to meet basic safety standards promoted by the United Nations World Forum for Harmonization of Vehicle Regulations) and an inadequate transportation environment contribute to the crash injury problem. Motor vehicles share the road with vulnerable road users. The mix of traffic including cars, buses, taxis, rickshaws, large trucks, and even animals increases the risk for crashes and injuries. Speed is another risk factor for vehicular crashes, injuries, and deaths. Just

**Table 8-1.** Twenty-nine most visited destinations for US citizens traveling abroad, 2015–2016: WHO estimated crash death rate (per 100,000 population) and number of US citizen crash deaths per country

| COUNTRY | COUNTRY VISITATION RANK[1] | WORLD HEALTH ORGANIZATION ESTIMATED CRASH DEATH RATE PER 100,000 POPULATION[2] | NUMBER OF US CITIZEN CRASH DEATHS[3,4] |
|---|---|---|---|
| Mexico | 1 | 12.3 | 159 |
| Canada | 2 | 6.0 | 10 |
| United Kingdom | 3 | 2.9 | 3 |
| Dominican Republic | 4 | 29.3 | 15 |
| Italy | 5 | 6.1 | 3 |
| France | 6 | 5.1 | 1 |
| Germany | 7 | 4.3 | 10 |
| Jamaica | 8 | 11.5 | 14 |
| Spain | 9 | 3.7 | 2 |
| China | 10 | 18.8 | 12 |
| India | 11 | 16.6 | 9 |
| Costa Rica | 12 | 13.9 | 12 |
| Bahamas | 13 | 13.8 | 0 |
| Japan | 14 | 4.7 | 2 |
| Ireland | 15 | 4.1 | 0 |
| Netherlands | 15 | 3.4 | 1 |
| Philippines | 17 | 10.5 | 10 |
| Colombia | 18 | 16.8 | 1 |
| Aruba | 18 | NA | 0 |
| Switzerland | 20 | 3.3 | 0 |
| Israel | 20 | 3.6 | 0 |
| Peru | 20 | 13.9 | 3 |

(continued)

## Table 8-1. Twenty-nine most visited destinations for US citizens traveling abroad, 2015–2016: WHO estimated crash death rate (per 100,000 population) and number of US citizen crash deaths per country (continued)

| COUNTRY | COUNTRY VISITATION RANK[1] | WORLD HEALTH ORGANIZATION ESTIMATED CRASH DEATH RATE PER 100,000 POPULATION[2] | NUMBER OF US CITIZEN CRASH DEATHS[3,4] |
|---|---|---|---|
| Hong Kong | 20 | NA | 1 |
| Thailand | 24 | 36.2 | 21 |
| Austria | 24 | 5.4 | 0 |
| Greece | 24 | 9.1 | 5 |
| South Korea | 27 | 12.0 | 6 |
| Taiwan | 27 | NA | 8 |
| Australia | 29 | 5.4 | 5 |

Abbreviation: NA, data not available.

[1] US Department of Commerce, National Travel & Tourism Office. Top destinations of US residents traveling abroad, 2015–2016. December 2017. [cited 2018 Apr 2]. Available from: http://travel.trade.gov/research/programs/ifs/index.html.
[2] World Health Organization. WHO global status report on road safety 2015. Geneva: World Health Organization; 2015 [cited 2018 Apr 2]. Available from: www.who.int/violence_injury_prevention/road_safety_status/2015/en.
[3] US Department of State. Deaths of US citizens abroad by nonnatural causes. Washington, DC: US Department of State; 2018 [cited 2018 Mar 1]. Available from: https://travel.state.gov/content/travel/en/international-travel/while-abroad/death-abroad1/death-statistics.htm.
[4] A total of 171 crash deaths occurred in countries not included in the list of top visited countries, including New Zealand (13 deaths); Honduras (11 deaths); Cuba and Cambodia (8 deaths each); Vietnam, Haiti, and Saudi Arabia (7 deaths each); and South Africa (6 deaths). All other countries not listed reported ≤5 deaths in 2015–2016.

47 countries, comprising 13% of the world's population, have laws that meet best practices on urban speed (≤50 km [31 mi] per hour). When driving, a lack of familiarity with the roads, driving on the opposite side of the road, the influence of alcohol, poorly made or inadequately maintained vehicles, travel fatigue, poor road surfaces without shoulders, unprotected curves and cliffs, and poor visibility due to lack of adequate lighting can also contribute to a crash.

When a crash occurs, the use of protective equipment significantly decreases the risk of injury and death. Seat belts, car seats, booster seats for children, and helmets (bike and motorcycle), are all proven ways to reduce crash-related injury and death, but this equipment may be scarce. In addition, timely and effective emergency and hospital care may be unavailable in some locations or not acceptable by US standards. Trauma centers capable of providing optimal care for serious injuries are uncommon outside urban areas in many international destinations.

Strategies to reduce the risk of motor vehicle crash injury are shown in Table 8-2. The Department of State has useful safety information for international travelers, including road safety and security alerts, international driving permits, travel insurance (www.travel.state.gov and https://travel.state.gov/content/

## Table 8-2. Recommended strategies to reduce road traffic crashes and injuries while abroad

| | |
|---|---|
| Seat belts and child safety seats | Always use seat belts and child safety seats. Whenever possible, rent vehicles with seat belts and ride in taxis with seat belts, opting for the rear seat. Bring car seats or booster seats from home for children. Remember you can refuse a taxi if seat belts are not available or the vehicle is in disrepair. |
| Driving hazards | When possible, avoid driving at night in developing countries (adequate lighting is limited in many countries). Always pay close attention to the correct side of the road when driving in countries that drive on the left. Speed is a major risk factor for crashes, injury, and death. Note speed limits, but you will also need to take into account the driving conditions (road quality, infrastructure, weather). |
| Country-specific driving hazards | Check the US Department of State Driving and Road Safety Abroad to learn more about driving in another country, and check the Association for Safe International Road Travel website for driving hazards or risks by country. |
| Helmet use | Always wear helmets when riding a motorcycle, motorbike, or bicycle. Consider bringing one from home to ensure it meets safety standards. A good-quality helmet can reduce the risk of death by 40% and severe injury by 70%. When possible, avoid driving or riding on motorcycles or motorbikes, including motorcycle and motorbike taxis. Traveling overseas is not the time to learn to drive a motorcycle/motorbike. |
| Alcohol-impaired driving | Alcohol increases the risk for all causes of injury. Do not drive after consuming alcohol or other drugs, and avoid riding with someone who has been drinking. Penalties for impaired driving (alcohol or drugs) can be severe overseas, and laws vary widely by country. |
| Cellular telephones | Do not use a cellular telephone or text while driving. Distracted driving increases your risk of a crash. Many countries have enacted laws banning cellular telephone use while driving, and some countries have made using any kind of telephone, including hands-free, illegal while driving. |
| Taxis or hired drivers | Ride only in marked taxis. Try to ride in taxis with seat belts. If no seat belt is available, wait for another taxi. Hire drivers familiar with the area and that have official status or credentials as taxis. Ask the US embassy or consulate for taxi company recommendations. |
| Bus travel | Avoid riding in overcrowded, overweight, or top-heavy buses or minivans, and avoid riding in mountainous terrain, at night, and with an impaired (alcohol or drugs) or distracted driver. |
| Pedestrian hazards | Be alert when crossing streets, especially in countries where motorists drive on the left side of the road. Walk with a companion or someone from the host country. When available use crosswalks and follow pedestrian signals. Pay full attention to your surroundings when crossing streets (don't walk distracted). |

8

travel/en/international-travel/before-you-go/driving-and-road-safety.html), and the Smart Traveler Enrollment Program (https://step.state.gov/step). The Association for International Road Travel (www.asirt.org) also has useful safety information for international travelers, including road safety checklists and country-specific driving risks.

## BIBLIOGRAPHY

1. 10 Facts on Global Road Safety. World Health Organization. [cited 2018 Apr 3]. Available from: www.who.int/features/factfiles/roadsafety/en/.

2. 2017 UN Global Road Safety Week. FIA Foundation. [cited 2018 Apr 2]. Available from: www.unroadsafetyweek.org/en/previous-weeks/2015-save-kids-lives.

3. National Center for Injury Prevention and Control: Motor Vehicle Safety. CDC. [cited 2018 Apr 3]. Available from: www.cdc.gov/motorvehiclesafety/index.html.

4. Violence and Injury Prevention: Road Traffic Injuries. World Health Organization. [cited 2018 Apr 2]. Available from: www.who.int/violence_injury_prevention/road_traffic/en/.

5. Violence and Injury Prevention: Developing Global Targets for Road Safety Risk Factors and Service Delivery Mechanisms. World Health Organization. [cited 2018 Apr 3]. Available from: www.who.int/violence_injury_prevention/road_traffic/road-safety-targets/en/.

6. WHO Global Status Report on Road Safety 2015. Geneva: World Health Organization; 2015.

# CRUISE SHIP TRAVEL

Kara Tardivel, Stefanie B. White, Krista Kornylo Duong

## INTRODUCTION

Cruise ship travel presents a unique combination of health concerns. Travelers from diverse regions brought together in the often crowded, semi-enclosed environments onboard ships can facilitate the spread of person-to-person, foodborne, or waterborne diseases. Outbreaks on ships can be sustained for multiple voyages by transmission among crew members who remain onboard or by persistent environmental contamination. Port visits can expose travelers to local vectorborne diseases. The remote location of the travelers at sea means that they may need to rely on the medical capabilities and supplies available onboard the ship for extended periods of time, and cruise travelers and their physicians should be aware of ships' medical limitations and prepare accordingly. Certain groups, such as pregnant women, the elderly, or those with chronic health conditions or who are immunocompromised, require special consideration when considering cruise travel.

## CRUISE SHIP MEDICAL CAPABILITIES

Medical facilities on cruise ships can vary widely depending on ship size, itinerary, length of cruise, and passenger demographics. Generally, shipboard medical centers can provide medical care comparable to that of ambulatory care centers; some can provide hospitalization services. Although no agency officially regulates medical practice aboard cruise ships, consensus-based guidelines for cruise ship medical facilities were published by the American College of Emergency Physicians (ACEP) in 1995 and most recently updated in 2013. ACEP guidelines (www.acep.org/Content.aspx?id=29980), which are followed by most major cruise lines, state that the cruise ship medical facilities should maintain the following minimum capabilities:

- Provide emergency medical care for passengers and crew

- Stabilize patients and initiate reasonable diagnostic and therapeutic interventions

- Facilitate the evacuation of seriously ill or injured patients

## ILLNESSES AND INJURY ABOARD CRUISE SHIPS

Cruise ship medical centers deal with a wide variety of illnesses and injuries. Approximately 3%–11% of conditions reported to cruise ship medical centers are urgent or an emergency. Approximately 95% of illnesses are treated or managed onboard, and 5% require evacuation and shoreside consultation for medical, surgical, or dental problems.

Roughly half of passengers who seek medical care are older than 65 years of age. Most medical center visits are due to acute illnesses, of which respiratory illnesses (19%–29%); seasickness (10%–25%); injuries from slips, trips, or falls (12%–18%); and gastrointestinal (GI) illness (9%–10%) are the most frequently reported diagnoses. Death rates for cruise ship passengers, most often from cardiovascular events, range from 0.6 to 9.8 deaths per million passenger-nights.

The most frequently reported cruise ship outbreaks involve respiratory infections, GI infections (such as norovirus), and vaccine-preventable diseases other than influenza, such as varicella (chickenpox). To reduce the risk of onboard introduction of communicable diseases by embarking passengers, ships may conduct medical screening during embarkation to identify ill passengers, preventing them from boarding or requiring isolation if they are allowed to board.

The following measures should be encouraged to limit the introduction and spread of communicable diseases on cruise ships:

- Passengers and their clinicians should consult CDC's Travelers' Health website (www.cdc.gov/travel) before travel for updates on outbreaks and travel health notices.

- Passengers ill with communicable diseases before a voyage should delay travel until they are no longer contagious. When booking a cruise, travelers should check to see what the trip cancellation policies are, as well as consider purchasing trip cancellation insurance.

- Passengers who become ill during the voyage should seek care in the ship's medical center to receive clinical management, facilitate infection-control measures, and maximize reporting of potential public health events.

## SPECIFIC HEALTH RISKS

### GI Illness

From 2008 through 2014, rates of GI illness among passengers on voyages lasting 3–21 days decreased from 27.2 to 22.3 cases per 100,000 travel days. Despite this decrease, GI illness outbreaks continue to occur. Updates on these outbreaks involving ships with US ports of call can be found at www.cdc.gov/nceh/vsp/surv/gilist.htm.

More than 90% of GI outbreaks with a confirmed cause are due to norovirus. Characteristics of norovirus that facilitate outbreaks are a low infective dose, easy person-to-person transmissibility, prolonged viral shedding, no long-term immunity, and the organism's ability to survive routine cleaning procedures. For international cruise ships porting in the United States from 2010 through 2015, 8–16 outbreaks of norovirus infections occurred each year.

GI outbreaks on cruise ships from food and water sources have also been associated with *Salmonella* spp., enterotoxigenic *Escherichia coli*, *Shigella* spp., *Clostridium perfringens*, and *Cyclospora cayetanensis*. To protect themselves from infections and reduce the spread of GI illnesses on cruise ships, passengers should be counseled on the following:

- Washing hands with soap and water often, especially before eating and after using the restroom.

- Promptly calling the ship's medical center and follow cruise ship guidance regarding isolation and other infection-control measures, even for mild symptoms of a GI illness (see Chapter 4, Norovirus).

- Additional information on cruise ship GI illnesses is available at www.cdc.gov/nceh/vsp/.

## Respiratory Illness

### INFLUENZA

Respiratory illnesses are the most common medical complaint, and influenza is the most commonly reported vaccine-preventable illness on cruise ships. Since passengers and crew originate from all regions of the world, shipboard outbreaks of influenza A and B can occur year-round, and travelers on cruise ships can be exposed to strains circulating in different parts of the world.

Given the cruise ship environment, population, and variable medical capabilities, the following measures are recommended year-round to protect travelers from influenza:

8

- All travelers planning a cruise should have the current seasonal influenza vaccine (as long as there is no contraindication and if available) at least 2 weeks before travel.

- Passengers at high risk for influenza complications should discuss antiviral treatment and chemoprophylaxis with their health care provider before travel.

- Passengers should practice good respiratory hygiene and cough etiquette.

- Passengers should report their respiratory illness to the medical center promptly and follow isolation recommendations, if indicated.

Additional guidance on the prevention and control of influenza on cruise ships is available at www.cdc.gov/quarantine/cruise/management/guidance-cruise-ships-influenza-updated.html. For more information, see Chapter 4, Influenza.

## LEGIONNAIRES' DISEASE

Although it is not a common cause of respiratory illness on cruise ships, Legionnaires' disease is a treatable infection that can result in severe pneumonia leading to death. Approximately 10%–15% of all Legionnaires' disease cases reported to CDC occur in people who have traveled during the 10 days before symptom onset. Clusters of Legionnaires' disease associated with hotel or cruise ship travel can be difficult to detect because travelers often disperse from the source of infection before symptoms begin. From 1977 through 2012, 8 ship-associated outbreaks of Legionnaires' disease were reported in the literature. These outbreaks included a total of 83 cases, with a median of 4 cases per outbreak (range, 2–50 cases); 6 cases resulted in death.

In general, Legionnaires' disease is contracted by inhaling warm, aerosolized water containing *Legionella*. Transmission can also sometimes occur through aspiration of water containing *Legionella*. A single episode of possible person-to-person transmission of Legionnaires' disease has been reported. Contaminated hot tubs are a commonly implicated source of shipboard *Legionella* outbreaks, although potable water supply systems have also been implicated. Improvements in ship design and standardization of water disinfection have reduced the risk of *Legionella* growth and colonization.

Most cruise ships have health care personnel who can perform *Legionella* urine antigen testing. People with suspected Legionnaires' disease require prompt antibiotic treatment. See Chapter 4, Legionellosis (Legionnaires' Disease & Pontiac Fever) for more information.

In evaluating cruise travelers for Legionnaires' disease, clinicians should do the following:

- Obtain a thorough travel history of all destinations during the 10 days before symptom onset (to assist in the identification of potential sources of exposure).

- Collect urine for antigen testing, which detects *L. pneumophila* serogroup 1 (the most common serogroup).

- Culture lower respiratory secretions on selective media, which is important for detection of non–*L. pneumophila* serogroup 1 species and serogroups and is useful for comparing clinical isolates to environmental isolates during an outbreak investigation.

- Inform CDC of any travel-associated Legionnaires' disease cases by sending an email to travellegionella@cdc.gov. Cases of Legionnaires' disease should be quickly reported to public health officials in order to determine if there are links to previously reported cases and to stop potential clusters and new outbreaks.

## Vaccine-Preventable Diseases (VPDs)

Although most cruise ship passengers are from countries with routine vaccination programs (such as the United States and Canada), many crew members originate from developing countries with low immunization rates. Outbreaks of measles, rubella, meningococcal disease and, most commonly, varicella, have been reported on cruise ships. Preventive measures to reduce the spread of VPDs onboard cruise ships should be followed:

- All passengers should be up-to-date with routine vaccinations before travel, as well as any

8

required or recommended vaccinations specific for their destinations.

- Women of childbearing age should be immune to measles, varicella and rubella before cruise ship travel.

- Crew members should have documented proof of immunity to VPDs (see Chapter 2, Vaccination & Immunoprophylaxis: General Recommendations).

## Vectorborne Diseases

Cruise ship port visits may include countries where vectorborne diseases such as malaria, dengue, yellow fever, Japanese encephalitis, and Zika are endemic. New diseases might surface in unexpected locations. For example, chikungunya was reported in late 2013 for the first time in the Caribbean (with subsequent spread throughout the Caribbean and numerous North, Central, and South American countries and territories). Zika virus was first reported in Brazil in 2015 and subsequently spread across the Caribbean and Latin America, sparking concern because of its association with microcephaly and other congenital abnormalities in the fetus. See Chapter 4 for additional information on specific vectorborne diseases.

Passengers should follow recommendations for avoiding mosquito bites and vectorborne infections:

- Use an Environmental Protection Agency (EPA)-registered insect repellent (see Chapter 3, Mosquitoes, Ticks & Other Arthropods).

- Treat clothing and gear with permethrin or purchase permethrin-treated items.

- While indoors, remain in well-screened or air-conditioned areas.

- When outdoors, wear long-sleeved shirts, long pants, boots, and hats.

- Obtain yellow fever vaccination if recommended or required.

- Take antimalarial chemoprophylaxis if needed (see Chapter 2, Yellow Fever Vaccine & Malaria Prophylaxis Information, by Country).

## OTHER HEALTH CONCERNS

Stresses of cruise ship travel include varying weather and environmental conditions, as well as unaccustomed changes in diet and physical activity. Foreign travel may increase the likelihood of risk-taking behaviors such as alcohol misuse, drug use, and unsafe sex. In spite of modern stabilizer systems, seasickness is a common complaint, affecting up to one-fourth of travelers (see Motion Sickness later in this chapter).

Because cruise may not allow women to board after the 24th week of pregnancy, pregnant women should contact the cruise line for specific policies recommendations before booking (for additional information, see Chapter 7, Pregnant Travelers).

For reporting travelers that have become ill with a suspect communicable disease after they have returned home from sailing on a cruise ship, please see Appendix D: Airplanes & Cruise Ships: Illness & Death Reporting & Public Health Interventions.

## PREVENTIVE MEASURES FOR CRUISE SHIP TRAVELERS

Cruise ship travelers often have complex itineraries due to multiple short port visits. Although most of these port visits do not include overnight stays off the cruise ship, some trips have options for travelers to venture off the ship for ≥1 night. Therefore, cruise ship travelers may be uncertain about potential exposures and which antimicrobial prophylaxis, immunizations, and preventive measures should be considered. Box 8-2 summarizes recommendations for cruise travelers and clinicians advising cruise travelers in pretravel preparation and healthy behaviors during travel.

Travelers with special medical needs, such as wheelchairs, oxygen tanks, or dialysis, should inform their cruise line before traveling. Travelers with health conditions should carry a written summary of essential health information (electrocardiogram; chest radiograph, if abnormal; blood type; chronic conditions; allergies; treating physician contact information; and medication list) that would facilitate their care during a medical emergency.

In addition, all prospective cruise travelers should verify coverage with their health

## BOX 8-2. Cruise travel health precautions

**ADVICE FOR CLINICIANS GIVING PRETRAVEL CRUISE CONSULTATIONS**

*Risk Assessment and Risk Communication*

- Discuss itinerary, including season, duration of travel, and activities at port stops.
- Review the traveler's medical and immunization history, allergies, and special health needs.
- Discuss relevant travel-specific health hazards and risk reduction.
- Provide the traveler with documentation of his or her medical history, immunizations, and medications.

*Immunization and Risk Management*

- Provide immunizations that are routinely recommended (age-specific), required (yellow fever), and recommended based on risk.
- Discuss food and water precautions and insect-bite prevention.
- Older travelers, especially those with a history of heart disease, should carry a baseline electrocardiogram to

facilitate onboard or overseas medical care.

*Medications Based on Risk and Need*

- Consider malaria chemoprophylaxis if itinerary includes port stops in malaria-endemic areas.
- Consider motion sickness medications for self-treatment (see Motion Sickness in this chapter).

**PRECAUTIONS FOR CRUISE SHIP TRAVELERS**

*Pretravel*

- Evaluate the type and length of the planned cruise in the context of personal health requirements.
- Consult medical and dental providers before cruise travel.
- Notify cruise line of special needs (such as wheelchair access, dialysis, oxygen tank).
- Consider additional insurance for overseas health care and medical evacuation.
- Carry prescription medications in original containers, with a copy of the prescription and accompanying physician's letter.
- Bring EPA-registered insect repellent and sunscreen, and

consider treating clothes and gear with permethrin.
- Defer travel while acutely ill.
- Consult wwwnc.cdc.gov/travel/notices for travel health notices.
- Check www.cdc.gov/nceh/vsp/surv/gilist.htm for gastrointestinal outbreaks.

*During Travel*

- Wash hands frequently with soap and water. If soap and water are not available, use an alcohol-based sanitizer that contains ≥60% alcohol.
- Follow safe food and water precautions when eating off the ship at ports of call.
- Use measures to prevent insect bites during port visits, especially in malaria- or dengue-endemic areas or areas where outbreaks of vectorborne diseases, such as chikungunya and Zika, are occurring.
- Use sun protection.
- Maintain good fluid intake, and avoid excessive alcohol consumption.
- Avoid contact with ill people.
- If sexually active, practice safe sex.
- Report illness to ship's medical center and follow medical recommendations.

---

insurance carriers and, if not included, consider purchasing additional insurance to cover medical evacuation and health services in foreign countries (see Chapter 6, Travel Insurance, Travel Health Insurance & Medical Evacuation Insurance).

### BIBLIOGRAPHY

1. Cramer EH, Slaten DD, Guerreiro A, Robbins D, Ganzon A. Management and control of varicella on cruise ships: a collaborative approach to promoting public health. J Travel Med. 2012 Jul;19(4):226–32.

2. Freeland AL, Vaughan GHJ, Banerjee SN. Acute gastroenteritis on cruise ships—United States, 2008–2014. MMWR Morb Mortal Wkly Rep. 2016 Jan 15;65(1):1–5.

3. Guyard C, Low DE. *Legionella* infections and travel associated legionellosis. Travel Med Infect Dis. 2011 Jul;9(4):176–86.

4. Hill CD. Cruise ship travel. In: Keystone JS, Freedman DO, Kozarsky PE, Connor BA, Nothdurft HD, editors. Travel Medicine. 3rd ed. Philadelphia: Saunders Elsevier; 2013. pp. 349–55.

5. Lanini S, Capobianchi MR, Puro V, Filia A, Del Manso M, Karki T, et al. Measles outbreak on a cruise ship in the western Mediterranean, February 2014, preliminary report. Euro Surveill. 2014 Mar 13;19(10):2–6.

6. Millman AJ, Kornylo Duong K, Lafond K, Green NM, Lippold SA, Jhung MA. Influenza outbreaks among passengers and crew on two cruise ships: a recent account of preparedness and response to an ever-present challenge. J Travel Med. 2015 Sep–Oct;22(5):306–11.

7. Mouchtouri VA, Rudge JW. Legionnaires' disease in hotels and passenger ships: a systematic review of evidence, sources, and contributing factors. J Travel Med. 2015 Sep–Oct;22(5):325–37.

8. Neri A, Fazio C, Ciammaruconi A, Anselmo A, Fortunato A, Palozzi A, et al. Draft genome sequence of C:P1.5-1,10-8:F3-6:ST-11 meningococcal clinical isolate associated with a cluster on a cruise ship. Genome Announc. 2014 Dec 4;2(6):e01263–14.

9. Peake DE, Gray CL, Ludwig MR, Hill CD. Descriptive epidemiology of injury and illness among cruise ship passengers. Ann Emerg Med. 1999 Jan;33(1):67–72.

10. Tomaszewski R, Nahorski WL. Interpopulation study of medical attendance aboard a cruise ship. Int Marit Health. 2008;59(1–4):61–8.

# MOTION SICKNESS

Stefanie K. Erskine

## RISK FOR TRAVELERS

Motion sickness is the term attributed to physiologic responses to travel by sea, car, train, air, and virtual reality immersion. Given sufficient stimulus, all people with functional vestibular systems can develop motion sickness. However, people vary in their susceptibility. Risk factors include the following:

- Age—children aged 2–12 years are especially susceptible, but infants and toddlers are generally immune. Adults >50 years are less susceptible to motion sickness.

- Sex—women are more likely to have motion sickness, especially when pregnant, menstruating, or on hormones.

- Migraines—people who get migraine headaches are more prone to motion sickness, especially during a migraine.

- Medication—some prescriptions can worsen the nausea of motion sickness.

## CLINICAL PRESENTATION

Travelers suffering from motion sickness commonly exhibit some or all of the following symptoms:

- Nausea

- Vomiting/retching
- Sweating
- Cold sweats
- Excessive salivation
- Apathy
- Hyperventilation
- Increased sensitivity to odors
- Loss of appetite
- Headache
- Drowsiness
- Warm sensation
- General discomfort

## PREVENTION

Nonpharmacologic interventions to prevent or treat motion sickness include the following:

- Being aware of and avoiding situations that tend to trigger symptoms.

- Optimizing position to reduce motion or motion perception—for example, driving a vehicle instead of riding in it, sitting in the front

8

seat of a car or bus, sitting over the wing of an aircraft, holding the head firmly against the back of the seat, and choosing a window seat on flights and trains.

- Reducing sensory input—lying prone, shutting eyes, sleeping, or looking at the horizon.

- Maintaining hydration by drinking water, eating small meals frequently, and limiting alcoholic and caffeinated beverages.

- Avoiding smoking—even short-term cessation reduces susceptibility to motion sickness.

- Adding distractions—controlling breathing, listening to music, or using aromatherapy scents such as mint or lavender. Flavored lozenges may also help.

- Using acupressure or magnets is advocated by some to prevent or treat nausea, although scientific data on efficacy of these interventions for preventing motion sickness are lacking.

- Gradually exposing oneself to continuous or repeated motion sickness triggers. Most people, in time, notice a reduction in motion sickness symptoms.

## TREATMENT

Antihistamines are the most frequently used and widely available medications for motion sickness; nonsedating ones appear to be less effective. Antihistamines commonly used for motion sickness include cyclizine, dimenhydrinate, meclizine, and promethazine (oral and suppository). Other common medications used to treat motion sickness are anticholinergics such as scopolamine (hyoscine—oral, intranasal, and transdermal), antidopaminergic drugs (such as prochlorperazine), metoclopramide, sympathomimetics, and benzodiazepines. Clinical trials have not shown that ondansetron, a drug commonly used as an antiemetic in cancer patients, is effective in the prevention of nausea associated with motion sickness.

## Medications in Children

Although using antihistamines to treat motion sickness in children is considered off-label, for children aged 2–12 years, dimenhydrinate (Dramamine), 1–1.5 mg/kg per dose, or diphenhydramine (Benadryl), 0.5–1 mg/kg per dose up to 25 mg, can be given 1 hour before travel and every 6 hours during the trip. Because some children have paradoxical agitation with these medicines, a test dose should be given at home before departure. Oversedation of young children with antihistamines can be life-threatening.

Scopolamine can cause dangerous adverse effects in children and should not be used; prochlorperazine and metoclopramide should be used with caution in children.

### BIBLIOGRAPHY

1. Golding JF, Gresty MA. Pathophysiology and treatment of motion sickness. Curr Opin Neurol. 2015 Feb;28(1):83–8.

2. Murdin L, Golding J, Bronstein A. Managing motion sickness. BMJ. 2011 Dec 2;343:d7430.

3. Priesol AJ. Motion sickness. Deschler DG, editor. Waltham MA: UpToDate; 2017.

4. Schmäl F. Neuronal mechanisms and the treatment of motion sickness. Pharmacology. 2013 May;91(3–4):229–41.

5. Shupak A, Gordon CR. Motion sickness: advances in pathogenesis, prediction, prevention, and treatment. Aviat Space Environ Med. 2006 Dec;77(12):1213–23.

6. Zhang L, Wang J, Qi R, Pan L, Li M, Cai Y. Motion sickness: current knowledge and recent advance. CNS Neurosci Ther. 2016 Jan;22(1):15–24.

8

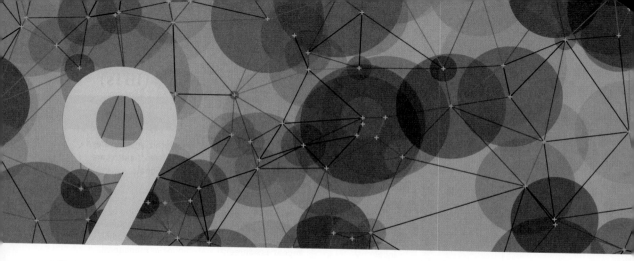

# 9

# Travel for Work & Other Reasons

## THE BUSINESS TRAVELER

William B. Bunn

In 2017, an estimated 4.8 million US residents traveled overseas for business, and with an increasingly global economy, this number is expected to increase. Business travelers (also known as occupational travelers) include people traveling for work-related training, conventions, research, and volunteer work. Business travelers may fall into any of several different categories according to duration and purpose of travel (Table 9-1).

For international business travelers (IBTs), the likelihood of an adverse health event increases with the number of trips made to at-risk areas and the time spent there. Since most IBTs take multiple trips each year, travel health consultants should consider the cumulative risk to the traveler and not just the risks of the current trip.

### HOW THE IBT DIFFERS FROM OTHER TRAVELERS

Unlike leisure travelers, IBTs are employees. Their employers have an interest and responsibility in protecting them from health threats. Employers should cover the cost for all vaccinations, required and recommended, either through a sponsored health plan or through direct reimbursement to the IBT.

In the United States, employers are liable for tort suits for negligence and workers' compensation claims. Adverse outcomes resulting from a failure to vaccinate or to provide "US-style" medical care to employees working overseas have led to legal settlements against companies. Employers must be prepared to evacuate IBTs traveling under their auspices;

## Table 9-1. Types of international business travelers (IBTs)

| IBT CATEGORY | TRAVEL DURATION | TRAVEL DESCRIPTION | ADDITIONAL TRAVEL DETAILS | REPRESENTATIVE PROFESSIONS |
|---|---|---|---|---|
| Short-term traveler | ≤2 weeks | Single destination for a specific meeting or event | Make presentations, attend conventions or association meetings | Academicians, business executives, health care professionals |
| Frequent traveler | 2 weeks on average | Multiple trips per year to different locations | Most often over a number of years to same site but may repeat assignment | Auditors, business executives, engineers, managers (including financial managers), researchers, technical trainers, volunteer workers |
| Commuter or recurrent traveler | Varies | Regular international travel, multiple times per year | Special projects | Managers (such as financial or engineering), researchers |
| Assignee | 3–12 months | Travels for specific, time-limited objectives | Does not relocate; may return home on a regular basis | Engineers, managers, specialists (such as legal or financial), volunteer workers |
| Expatriate | Long-term assignments (often 2–5 years or more) | Moves to host country | Usually relocates with family | Business executives, managers, researchers, technical experts |

this typically requires a preexisting contractual relationship with an air medical evacuation provider or some form of comprehensive travel health insurance that includes medical evacuation coverage.

To better prepare their employees for healthy travel, businesses have developed international travel health programs (ITHPs). Primarily an innovation of larger corporations, ITHPs focus on disease prevention and health promotion activities before, during, and after international travel. Healthier IBTs mean fewer instances of urgent repatriations (including emergency medical evacuations) and hospital admissions. Additional advantages include enhanced employee confidence, improved productivity overseas, and better public relations. Midsized and smaller businesses with significant numbers of IBTs may also benefit from the cost savings realized by an ITHP.

## SPECIAL CONSIDERATIONS FOR THE IBT

Traditionally, the risk of travel-related adverse health outcomes in IBTs was considered low, but as the number of people traveling for work (and the overall distance they travel) increases, and as the time allotted for adjustment after arrival at destination and following return decreases, this is no longer the case. Studies suggest that the profile of diseases an IBT encounters during travel and the likelihood of being injured or developing a travel-related illness is now similar to that of other international travelers. More than 60% of travelers going to areas within Asia considered "high risk" for infectious diseases listed a work-related reason for their travel. Whereas IBTs are just as likely as other travelers to develop some travel-related illnesses (among them, travelers' diarrhea, respiratory diseases, and malaria), they are more likely to become infected with

9

influenza, sexually transmitted pathogens, and hepatitis B.

Extensive business travel also correlates with a higher body mass index and increased cholesterol, hypertension, and mental stress. A World Bank study showed overall health plan expenditures were 70% higher for IBTs than for their nontraveling counterparts, and that the likelihood of developing a noncommunicable disease increased with frequency of travel. The study also showed increased incidence for 20 noncommunicable disease categories.

Although IBTs should receive all indicated vaccines and prophylaxis prior to travel, studies demonstrate gaps in practitioner adherence to the most current guidance, insufficient pretravel counseling, and the failure of travelers to follow recommendations when provided. Adequate prophylaxis against malaria, despite information and counseling, remains a challenge. A 2017 study showed that 89% of IBTs who contracted malaria while traveling, and 50% of those who died, did not take prophylaxis, although the authors did not specify the reasons for nonadherence.

## PRETRAVEL CONSIDERATIONS

The pretravel consultation should determine and document fitness for travel. Fitness for travel and, in particular, the risk of adverse health events overseas, depends on several factors: 1) how well underlying medical conditions are controlled, 2) how easily preexisting medical conditions can be managed during travel, 3) duration of time spent away from home, 4) destination-specific health risks, and 5) access to health care while away. As much as possible, IBTs (especially recurrent travelers, assignees, and expatriates) and their health care providers should attempt to improve those factors within their control and to minimize the risks presented by factors outside their control.

Making the decision that the risk to a person's health is too high for the assignment rests with the employer, not the IBT. Although almost all medical risks can be managed, it is up to the provider to ascertain whether a health condition (given the medical resources expected to be available) will prevent a traveler from fulfilling occupational obligations. Diabetic monitoring and care,

for example, may represent a challenge during international travel, particularly in more austere environments.

If, during the pretravel consultation, a provider identifies underlying medical conditions that cannot be accommodated reasonably at the destination, a full discussion with the IBT of the risks associated with travel, and careful documentation for the employer, must occur. Disability laws apply to all employees. Tort suits and workers' compensation liability are considerations for situations where a US standard of medical care is not readily available or when an increased risk of illness, accident, or injury is expected.

Structure the pretravel consultation to identify and address risks to both physical and mental health. Administering vaccines, prescribing prophylactic medication, and educating travelers about how to mitigate health threats while traveling are other key elements of the consultation. To best prepare an IBT for healthy travel, providers must have access to the traveler's full itinerary including all work sites, stopovers, likely side trips, and potential itinerary changes. Do not assume that IBTs will only visit major cities, stay in first-class hotels, and eat at 5-star restaurants.

Attempt to elicit information about conditions at worksites listed in the itinerary, going into as much detail as possible. IBTs include travelers to industrial sites where there may be exposures to chemical or physical toxins or poor air quality. Some work locations may pose slip, trip, and fall hazards or the possibility of other unintentional injuries. IBTs visiting hospitals or medical environments may require protection from biological hazards. Compared with those traveling internationally for other reasons, then, providing requisite personal protective equipment—including education regarding its proper use—is unique to the pretravel consultation for people preparing to work internationally.

A mental health assessment is another component of the pretravel consultation for IBTs. IBTs show more psychological stress than other travelers, which can manifest as sleep disorders, circadian rhythm disruption, and increased alcohol or substance abuse. Because IBTs must be able to perform effectively in a wide variety of business and social settings, the inability to adapt

9

to other cultures can reflect negatively not only on the traveler but also on the company he or she represents. The ramifications of sending an impaired or culturally inflexible person overseas for work can be serious and costly.

Testing can help predict whether an IBT has the skills to deal effectively with other cultures (cultural adaptability). Used more commonly as part of the pretravel assessment for those being sent to work overseas for extended periods (assignees and expatriates), cultural adaptability testing should be included as part of the pretravel consultation of frequent travelers, particularly when previous incidents have occurred. Attend to mental health and adaptability issues before the IBT embarks on international travel or assignment.

Once mental health issues and risks associated with a particular travel itinerary have been identified and addressed, the next step in the pretravel consultation involves evaluating the traveler for needed vaccines. This includes updating routine vaccines such as influenza, tetanus, and measles, where indicated. Unlike the leisure traveler, there is typically more of a need for the IBT to be fully productive when traveling overseas. The inability to perform one's job because of illness can have serious negative financial implications; for this reason, practitioners are encouraged to immunize IBTs against all potential vaccine-preventable health risks.

Administer vaccinations with a view toward the IBT's total travel over the course of a year or next several years, not just an individual trip. A single business trip of only 1 or 2 weeks' duration to a low-risk destination may not warrant immediate vaccination against a particular disease. However, future work trips may present a risk of exposure. Due deliberation should be given to initiating a vaccine course, even if the travel requiring it has not yet been planned. Because business travel is often last-minute, it is reasonable to begin vaccinating the IBT for later trips when immunity against specific diseases is required. This is true even if the traveler does not complete the full vaccine series in advance of the most current trip.

Simply providing prescriptions for necessary prophylaxis against travel-related diseases,

malaria in particular, is not enough. As noted above, in a recent study nearly 90% of IBTs who contracted malaria while traveling did not take their prescribed medication. Even though IBTs are aware of the need for prophylaxis, they demonstrate poor adherence that only worsens with the length of the trip. Reported reasons for nonadherence include the challenges posed by daily dosing, presumed immunity, busy schedules or forgetfulness, conflicting advice, and fear of side effects. The use of electronic reminders (such as apps on handheld devices) can help.

Travel plans often change. Before departing, IBTs should know where to access health and safety information for destinations not included on the original itinerary. Destination-specific health recommendations are available from www.cdc.gov/travel.

All family members accompanying the IBT should also visit a primary care provider for a pretravel physical and mental health screen; the inability of a spouse or a child to adjust to an international environment is often a cause for early repatriation. Each family member also requires his or her own consultation with a travel health specialist.

## TRAVEL HEALTH ISSUES DURING TRAVEL AND AT THE DESTINATION

Advance planning and adherence to guidance provided by medical and human resource personnel can mitigate health and wellness risks posed by lengthy flights. These risks include dehydration, deep vein thrombosis, motion sickness, and jet lag. Multiple-leg, complex itineraries can aggravate and increase the likelihood of these conditions. Counseling travelers to limit or refrain from in-flight alcohol consumption and to use hypnotics judiciously to facilitate sleep can decrease the chances of a hangover, which is particularly important when work duties are scheduled on or close to arrival.

Changing time zones can interfere with taking prescribed medicine on time, another potential threat to the health and wellness of international travelers. Adjusting the timing of regular medication during international travel

9

may be a challenge for the IBT; be prepared to help create schedules for travelers taking medication, both on the way overseas and when returning. Anticipating the possibility that checked luggage could be delayed or lost during international travel, IBTs should carry with them a travel health kit containing all necessary medications in sufficient quantities.

On arrival, IBTs should review with their hosts all safety, security, occupational, and environmental hazards specific to the destination. In developing countries in particular, IBTs may encounter occupational and environmental health risks significantly different from what they have at home; chemicals used in some locations may no longer be used (or were never approved for use) in the United States because of their hazardous properties. Foreign governments may lack or not enforce exposure limits, requirements for personal protective equipment use, or worker safety laws. Moreover, IBTs should know in advance what to do in case of a health emergency, as well as which hospitals and health clinics in the vicinity provide the highest levels of medical care. Details about how to access quality outpatient and inpatient care must be available to the IBT throughout the trip and updated as needed.

# POSTTRAVEL CARE

IHTPs provide IBTs with both pretravel and posttravel care. Studies show that, upon returning home, 22%–64% of people traveling internationally for work will have an unresolved health issue meriting careful case management with referral to specialists. Because an IBT could be a sentinel for a health risk at an overseas facility or workplace, a correct diagnosis is important not only to the health and well-being of the traveler but to that of the other workers at that jobsite.

The US Occupational Safety and Health Administration does not have jurisdiction or requirements to report illness or accidents for work done outside the United States. Nevertheless, an employer has a general duty to prevent occupational injuries. Returning workers can assist by notifying employers of any work-related incidents or on-the-job exposures. Such workplace hazards may require medical monitoring and referral to occupational health specialists for the person, and exposure mitigation by a hierarchy of controls at the location. IBTs should also provide intelligence about any changes in the quality of available medical care, accommodations, security, and any other medical or legal issues that may have a deleterious impact on the health of future travelers.

## BIBLIOGRAPHY

1. Burkholder J, Jaines R, Cunningham-Hill M, Xa B. Health and wellbeing factors associated with international business travel. J Travel Med. 2010;17:329–33.

2. Bunn W. Health and productivity in business/occupational travelers, assignees and expatriates. Int J Health Productivity. 2016;8(1):30–7.

3. Bunn WB. Assessing risk and improving travel vaccine programs for business travelers. J Occup Environ Med. 2014;56(11):1167–8.

4. Chen L, Leder K, Wilson M. Business travelers: vaccination considerations for this population. Expert Rev Vaccines. 2013;12(4):453–66.

5. Deshpande B, Rao S, Jentes E, Hills S, Fischer M. Use of Japanese vaccine in US travel medicine practices in Global TravEpiNet. Am J Trop Med Hyg. 2014;91(4):694–8.

6. Khan NM, Jentes ES, Brown C, Han P, Rao SR, Kozarsky P, et al. Pre-travel medical preparation of business and occupational travelers: an analysis of Global TravEpiNet Consortium, 2009 to 2012. J Occup Environ Med. 2016;58(1):76–82.

7. Liese B, Mundt K, Dell L, Nagy L, Demure B. Medical insurance claims associated with business travel. Occup Environ Med. 1997;54:499–503.

8. Richards C, Rundle A. Business travel and self-rated health, obesity, and cardiovascular disease risk factors. J Occup Environ Med. 2011;53(4):358–63.

9. Rogers B, Bunn W, Connor B. An update on travel vaccines and issues in travel and international medicine. Workplace Health Saf. 2016;64(7):462–8.

9

# ADVICE FOR AIRCREWS

Phyllis E. Kozarsky

## OVERVIEW

As airlines expand their reach and aircrews are asked to travel to more exotic destinations, often with short layovers, these frequent travelers need to prepare ahead of time for the exposures they may encounter. To some degree, aircrews are similar to all travelers to such destinations, but the differences require some modifications of travel health guidance for several reasons:

- Layovers are short, often 24–48 hours.

- Travel is frequent.

- Travel to new destinations may be on short notice.

- Despite short travel times, aircrews may be more adventuresome and thus have more risk than typical tourists.

- Aircrews may perceive themselves to be low-risk because of their generally healthy status and because their in-country exposure time is short.

Given these factors, it is worth noting some guidelines for this special group. In general, air carriers that fly to the developing world try to inform their crews about health issues they may face. However, airlines do not necessarily employ occupational health providers or experts in travel medicine; they may be unaware of special risks at the destinations they serve. Therefore, airlines may wish to avail themselves of professionals who are knowledgeable in the field and who can help make recommendations for their traveling employees.

Pilots are often aware of some of the medications and classes of medications that may interfere with their flight capacity. Providers should not prescribe for pilots medications that affect the central nervous system when flying. Pilots who take sedating antihistamines (including diphenhydramine [Benadryl] and chlorpheniramine) should not fly until more than 5 half-lives have elapsed since the last dose. For diphenhydramine, this equates to a 2-day "no fly" rule (9 days for chlorpheniramine). Trials of new medications or any drugs with potential side effects that could interfere with a pilot's abilities or judgment should take place between (not during) trips. Prescriptions or recommendations for nonsedating antihistamines (loratadine, desloratadine, and fexofenadine, for example) can be provided after an initial trial period demonstrates they can be taken without adverse effect.

Federal Aviation Authority (FAA)-certified aeromedical examiners (AMEs) examine pilots regularly and are responsible for certifying that they are fit to fly. For some common medications, AMEs might not certify pilots taking them without clearance from the FAA. For other medications, AMEs will advise pilots not to fly. The FAA provides a list of these medications at www.faa.gov/about/office_org/headquarters_offices/avs/offices/aam/ame/guide/pharm/dni_dnf. Sometimes medication decisions are made on a case-by-case basis. If questions arise, an AME should be consulted (www.faa.gov/pilots/amelocator).

Although any travel health provider can see and advise flight crews, it is important to ask each crewmember what the company requires, in addition to what is required or recommended to maintain health while traveling. If in doubt, the travel health provider should contact the airline medical director or occupational health department for guidance. For example, some aircrews primarily fly domestic routes or routes to Western Europe or Japan, so would not fly to a region of yellow fever risk in their normal daily work. However, an airline may require that crewmembers without contraindications be vaccinated against yellow fever, so that the airline has flexibility to shift crews and address any urgent needs.

# GENERAL HEALTH MEASURES

Although pilots are required to have periodic provider visits to ensure they are fit to fly, these do not address issues that may affect them when they travel internationally, particularly to destinations in the developing world. Flight attendants and others should also consider asking their health care providers about these recommendations:

- Administering a periodic tuberculin skin test if traveling frequently to destinations where the prevalence of tuberculosis is much higher than in the United States, where the incidence of antimicrobial resistance is higher, or where the crewmember will be in close contact with crowds (www.who.int/tb/areas-ofwork/drug-resistant-tb/en).

- Checking at each visit to make sure that routine immunizations are up-to-date (see below).

- Immunizing against seasonal influenza every year when the vaccine becomes available.

In addition, all medications for chronic conditions should be carried in extra quantities, as they may not be available at some locations, and, even if available and less costly, may be counterfeit or of poor quality (see Chapter 6, *Perspectives*: Avoiding Poorly Regulated Medicines and Medical Products during Travel). The manufacture of counterfeit medications in developing countries is a large and growing industry. It is impossible to tell from the packaging or pills if they are counterfeit. Some counterfeit drugs contain little or no active ingredient, and others contain toxic contaminants.

## Vaccinations

Because of their frequency of travel, aircrews may be exposed to various diseases that are not common in the United States. For example, measles can be a life-threatening illness for adults; it is more common in most of the world, including Europe, because of a lack of mandatory childhood immunization in some countries. In addition, flight crews may not have had varicella as children and, because of their age, may not have been immunized. This illness often occurs at a later age in the tropics; thus, if there is interaction with local populations in these destinations, risk for infection will be higher.

International flight crews should consider a travel health visit to ensure as complete protection as possible. Since some may have short notice before traveling to new destinations, ask aircrew members about this possibility during their visit so that vaccinations for upcoming trips may be given, or a series can be started early. Educate travelers about health risks in the various destinations; administration of certain vaccinations will depend on the traveler's tolerance for risk.

At a minimum, aircrew members should be up-to-date with routine vaccinations. These vaccines include measles-mumps-rubella (MMR), diphtheria-tetanus-pertussis, varicella, polio, and the seasonal influenza vaccine (see the separate sections on these diseases in Chapter 4).

Although there are no established guidelines or recommendations for the use of travel vaccinations in pilots and other aircrew members, for some it may be reasonable to offer meningococcal, Japanese encephalitis, yellow fever, and typhoid vaccines because of their frequent, short-stay, and at times unpredictable assignments. In addition, because some pilots do relief work or fly to areas of natural disasters, cholera vaccine may also be considered for them. Hepatitis A is advisable for all travelers and may be stressed for aircrews, since most adults in the United States have not been immunized. Hepatitis B is advisable for frequent travelers because of the unpredictability of exposure. Aircrews are generally a group who travel frequently beyond work, so they should always be asked during a consultation whether they are planning other travel that can be addressed at the same time.

## Malaria Prophylaxis

Airlines typically inform crewmembers as to which destinations harbor malaria. Some European and Asian air carriers have longer experience flying to destinations where malaria is endemic, and these airlines have various policies with respect to prevention of the disease. While there may be malaria transmission in some areas

**9**

of destination countries, sometimes there is none in the capitals or the larger urban areas to which the major American carriers fly (such as in China or the Philippines). This is generally not the case in sub-Saharan Africa, where there can be substantial exposure during a short 24-hour layover (although in Ethiopia, there is no malaria risk in Addis Ababa).

Although the risk of malaria transmission in hotels at the destination may be low, it may be increased at the international airports, during unpredictable delays in transit, and during outings on layovers. Even during short single stops ( for example, in West Africa on the way to South Africa), there is some risk when the aircraft doors are open. Little published data are available on the risk of malaria for flight crews with short layovers, but some information suggests that it is less than that for tourists.

Unfortunately, experience has shown that American and European aircrews going to malaria-endemic destinations continue to acquire malaria, as well as develop severe and complicated disease. Some illness may result from lack of awareness of airline recommendations, failure to take precautions against mosquito bites, lack of compliance with antimalarial prophylaxis, or inaccurate information regarding toxicity of medication. Transmission can be focal and intermittent, so prophylaxis for every trip to a highly endemic region should be stressed.

Flight crewmembers should have easy access to educational materials and prophylaxis and, if desired, should be able to have an individual risk assessment for preventive measures. For destinations where the prevalence of malaria is high (countries in West Africa, for example), crewmembers should take prophylaxis for layovers. For destinations where crews are thought to be at low risk based on local intensity of transmission, accommodations, and personal behaviors, providers may advise them to use insect repellents and to take other precautions to avoid mosquito bites (see Chapter 3, Mosquitoes, Ticks & Other Arthropods) but take no prophylaxis. Flight crews should always:

- Educate themselves as much as possible about malaria.

- Understand the importance of personal protective measures such as repellents, and use them properly.

- Take prophylaxis if recommended.

- Know that if fever or chills occur after exposure, it is a medical emergency.

- Know how they can get medical assistance at their destinations or at home in the event of symptoms or signs of malaria.

There are several options for malaria prophylaxis, depending on the destination city, although needed duration of prophylaxis and adverse effects profiles of some of the drugs make them less than desirable for aircrews. Country-specific recommendations can be accessed either in this text (see Chapter 2, Yellow Fever Vaccine & Malaria Prophylaxis Information, by Country) or on the CDC Travelers' Health website (www.cdc.gov/travel). International airlines generally prefer the combination drug atovaquone-proguanil; its adverse effect profile and its dosing make it the most suitable for aircrews.

Additional information on malaria prevention may be found in Chapter 4, Malaria.

## Other Vectorborne Diseases

In the last decade, several mosquitoborne viruses have emerged or reemerged, including dengue, chikungunya, and Zika (see the individual disease sections in Chapter 4). Preventing mosquito bites in tropical and subtropical destinations is critical to preventing disease. Because Zika virus infection during pregnancy can cause severe birth defects, airlines should develop flight destination policies for pilots and flight attendants who are pregnant, plan to become pregnant, or have a partner who is or may become pregnant.

## Food and Water Precautions and Travelers' Diarrhea

Advise pilots and aircrew members to follow the same safe food and water precautions and prevention and management of travelers' diarrhea as other travelers (see Chapter 2, Travelers' Diarrhea). They should also be well versed in the recognition and self-treatment of moderate to severe travelers' diarrhea to shorten the duration of illness that could affect their job performance. In addition, pilots should make sure that their preferred medication for self-treatment is compatible with flying.

## Bloodborne and Sexually Transmitted Infections

Although these risks and preventions are addressed in more detail in other sections, it is worth reiterating that frequent travelers have an increased likelihood of engaging in casual and unprotected sex, and travelers have higher rates of HIV and other sexually transmitted infections (see Chapter 9, Sex & Travel). The risk of acquisition may be higher not only for diseases such as gonorrhea and chlamydia but also for chronic illnesses such as hepatitis B and C. Dental procedures and activities such as acupuncture, tattooing, and piercing also are ill-advised during travel to developing countries.

### BIBLIOGRAPHY

1. Bagshaw M, Illig, P. The aircraft cabin environment. In: Keystone JS, Kozarsky PE, Connor BA, Nothdurft HD, Mendelson M, Leder K. editors. Travel Medicine. 4th ed: Elsevier. 2019:429–36.

2. Byrne N. Urban malaria risk in sub-Saharan Africa: where is the evidence? Travel Med Infect Dis. 2007 Mar;5(2):135–7.

3. Byrne NJ, Behrens RH. Airline crews' risk for malaria on layovers in urban sub-Saharan Africa: risk assessment and appropriate prevention policy. J Travel Med. 2004 Nov–Dec;11(6):359–63.

4. CDC. Notes from the field: malaria imported from West Africa by flight crews—Florida and Pennsylvania, 2010. MMWR Morb Mortal Wkly Rep. 2010 Nov 5;59(43):1412.

5. Schwartz MD, Macias-Moriarity LZ, Schelling J. Professional aircrews' attitudes toward infectious diseases and aviation medical issues. Aviat Space Environ Med. 2012 Dec;83(12):1167–70.

6. Selent M, de Rochars VMB, Stanek D, Bensyl D, Martin B, Cohen NJ, et al. Malaria prevention knowledge, attitudes, and practices (KAP) among international flying pilots and flight attendants of a US commercial airline. J Travel Med. 2012 Dec;19(6):366–72.

# HEALTH CARE WORKERS, INCLUDING PUBLIC HEALTH RESEARCHERS & MEDICAL LABORATORIANS

Henry M. Wu, Alan G. Czarkowski, Eric J. Nilles

## RISKS FOR HEALTH CARE WORKERS PRACTICING DURING TRAVEL OUTSIDE THE UNITED STATES

Health care workers practicing outside the United States face unique health hazards, including infectious disease risks associated with patient contact or handling clinical specimens. Any type of health care worker working in clinical areas or handling specimens may be at risk, including physicians, nurses, ancillary clinical staff, trainees (for example, students on international rotations), researchers, and public health workers.

Health care workers can be exposed to infections spread through blood and bodily fluids (such as HIV or hepatitis B) or through airborne or respiratory droplet routes (such as tuberculosis [TB] or influenza). Risks vary depending on the duties of the worker, the geographic location, and the practice setting. Of note, health care workers working overseas can have increased risk of exposure to patients with certain uncommon, highly pathogenic, or emerging infectious diseases such as extensively drug-resistant tuberculosis (XDR-TB), Middle East respiratory syndrome (MERS), and Ebola virus disease.

Risks encountered while performing medical work outside the United States can be due to multiple factors, including:

- Less stringent safety regulations or infection control standards.

- Limited availability of personal protective equipment (PPE), safety-engineered devices, or postexposure management resources.

- Unfamiliar practice conditions, equipment, or procedures.

- Challenging practice conditions that can prevent providers from adhering to standard precautions (such as extremely resource-limited settings, natural disasters, or conflict zones) (see Box 9-1).

- Higher prevalence of transmissible infections (such as HIV, hepatitis B virus [HBV],

---

**BOX 9-1.** Health care workers in extreme circumstances

Health care workers regularly provide care in a range of extreme circumstances, which may be characterized by: limited or absent medical and public health infrastructure; lack of fundamental hygiene supplies (such as soap and water for handwashing); increased infectious disease transmission; extreme environmental conditions; and high levels of violence. In 2016, there were 158 attacks against aid workers; 101 were killed.

Because of these increased risks and consequences of severe disease or injury, adequate prevention and preparation are essential. Health problems for the health care worker can have serious implications, both for the person and for those who depend on the health care worker for provision of health care. Detailed instructions on how to prepare for travel or work in developing countries or humanitarian environments is covered in detail in other sections, but additional key considerations for the health care worker include:

1. **Having reliable communication equipment:** usually satellite phone, ensuring service provider contract for duration of the mission. Consider portable solar recharging capabilities unless there is a guaranteed power supply, which is rare in most extreme circumstances.

2. **Acquiring evacuation insurance and having a plan if ill or injured:** deploying organizations may not provide evacuation insurance (see Chapter 6, Travel Insurance, Travel Health Insurance & Medical Evacuation Insurance) or a detailed evacuation contingency plan. However, both are critical, and the health care worker should be familiar with all details.

3. **Considering underlying health conditions:** the provider's health should be monitored closely and treatment initiated early, if necessary. Any indication that a potentially serious condition is not responding to treatment should

warrant rapid planning for potential medical evacuation.

4. **Being psychologically stable and knowing whom to contact if problems arise:** providers in conflict and disaster zones typically work long hours in dangerous conditions and are exposed to profound suffering. These experiences can be intensely stressful, leading to increased rates of depression, posttraumatic stress disorder, and anxiety. Before deployment, providers should think about coping strategies and, as much as possible, stay in contact with a support network of family and friends.

5. **Inquiring about availability of antidotes to chemical warfare:** although rare, health care workers may be exposed to chemical warfare agents while caring for patients, as recently documented in Syria. If exposure to these agents is a possibility, antidotes (such as atropine) should be immediately available.

hepatitis C virus [HCV], or TB), with potentially increased transmission risk from untreated source patients.

## PRETRAVEL VACCINATION AND SCREENING

In addition to vaccinations specifically indicated for the country visited and routine age-appropriate vaccines, all health care workers should be up-to-date on all recommended vaccinations for employment in health care settings. These include vaccinations (or documented immunity) for the following:

- Measles, mumps, and rubella
- Influenza
- Varicella
- Tetanus, diphtheria, and pertussis
- Hepatitis B

For hepatitis B, postvaccination serologic testing for antibody to hepatitis B surface antigen (anti-HBsAg) is recommended. Health care workers without documented response to vaccination should receive 1 more additional dose of hepatitis B vaccine followed by anti-HBsAg testing to assess protection.

Regular screening for latent TB infection with tuberculin skin test or interferon-γ release assay is recommended for health care workers at increased risk of TB exposure. Testing before and after travel should be considered when the provider is working in a country with a high prevalence of TB infection or in a setting of high TB exposure, such as in prisons, refugee camps, and health facilities (see Chapter 4, Tuberculosis). Routine vaccination of health care workers with bacillus Calmette-Guérin (BCG) is not recommended in the United States; however, BCG vaccination may be considered for some health care workers who will work in settings with high TB transmission risk and a high prevalence of strains resistant to isoniazid and rifampin.

Baseline testing for HIV and hepatitis C is not routinely recommended, although it should be considered if risk of exposure will be high and reliable testing will not be available locally in the event of an exposure. Inactivated polio vaccine (given as an adult booster dose) or meningococcal vaccine may be indicated for specific locations experiencing high incidence or outbreaks of these infections.

## PERSONAL PROTECTIVE EQUIPMENT AND INFECTION CONTROL

Health care workers should consistently follow standard precautions and, if possible, apply other precautions (contact, droplet, or airborne) as needed. For details, guidelines, and training materials on standard precautions and personal protective equipment (PPE), see https://www.cdc.gov/hai/prevent/ppe_train.html. PPE, including gloves, gowns, aprons, surgical masks, fit-tested N95 respirators, and protective eyewear, may be necessary to achieve personal protection. Workers untrained in infection-control practices should not participate in patient care or activities with risk of exposure to infectious materials. Specialized PPE and infection-control techniques might be indicated for certain infections that pose high risk to health care workers, such as MERS, avian influenza, and Ebola virus (see disease-specific websites at www.cdc.gov for the most up-to-date epidemiology and infection control recommendations).

Health care workers should be properly trained for all anticipated procedures, considering the locally available equipment. Health care workers should maintain strict safety standards, even if local practices are less stringent. Needlestick injuries are a common mode of percutaneous exposure to bloodborne pathogens, and practices known to increase risk of needlestick injuries, such as recapping syringes or using needles to transfer a bodily fluid between containers, should be avoided whenever possible. Safety-engineered medical devices and biosafety equipment such as sharps containers might not be available. Local infection-control practices and supplies should be determined in advance. If the local supply of PPE is questionable, bringing one's own supply can be important.

9

## INFECTIONS TRANSMITTED BY AIRBORNE OR DROPLET ROUTES

Although some airborne or respiratory droplet–transmitted infections are vaccine preventable (such as measles, seasonal influenza, and varicella), vaccines are not routine or available for many others, including TB, MERS, and pneumonic plague. TB is a particular concern for health care workers working overseas in high-incidence areas, and BCG vaccination might be considered for health care workers going to areas with high risk of exposure to multidrug resistant–TB.

Since equipment and facilities for airborne isolation are limited or unavailable in many countries, bringing a personal supply of PPE including N95 respirator masks might be prudent. However, identifying the situations where their use is indicated can be difficult, especially when TB is highly prevalent and isolation of patients is suboptimal. Enhanced PPE recommendations may apply for emerging respiratory pathogens, such as MERS or avian influenza.

## INFECTIONS TRANSMITTED THROUGH BLOOD OR BODILY FLUIDS

Health care workers are at risk for numerous infections transmitted through blood or body fluids via percutaneous, mucous membrane, or nonintact skin exposures. These include bloodborne pathogens such as HIV, HBV, and HCV. The risk of HIV transmission is approximately 0.3% after a percutaneous exposure to HIV-infected blood and approximately 0.09% after a mucous membrane exposure. Health care workers who have received hepatitis B vaccine and have developed immunity to the virus are at virtually no risk for infection. Based on limited studies, the estimated risk for HCV transmission after a needlestick or cut exposure to HCV-infected blood is approximately 1.8%. Other bodily fluids that may transmit HIV and hepatitis viruses include cerebrospinal fluid, synovial fluid, pericardial fluid, pleural fluid, peritoneal fluid, amniotic fluid, semen, and vaginal secretions. Saliva, urine, sputum, nasal secretions, tears, feces, vomitus, and sweat are not considered infectious for HIV and HCV unless they are visibly bloody. Numerous other infections have also been transmitted to health care workers via blood or bodily fluids, including many that are uncommon or not endemic to the United States, such as viral infections (including Ebola virus, dengue), parasitic infections (including malaria), and brucellosis.

Typically, exposures occur as a result of percutaneous exposure to contaminated sharps, including needles, lancets, scalpels, and broken glass (from capillary or test tubes). Infection risk is considered increased after percutaneous exposures to larger blood volumes (visible blood on the injuring device, hollow-bore needles, deeper injuries, or procedures that involved direct cannulation of an artery or vein). Skin exposures to potentially infectious bodily fluids are only considered to be at risk for bloodborne pathogen infection if there is evidence of compromised skin integrity (for example, dermatitis, abrasion, or open wound). Higher circulating viral load in the source patient is also thought to increase the risk of transmission, and this can be of particular concern in resource-poor settings where treatments for HIV and viral hepatitis are limited.

Health care workers with occupational exposures to blood or bodily fluids should perform the following steps immediately:

- Wash the exposed area with soap and water thoroughly. If mucous membrane exposure has occurred, flush the area with copious amounts of water or saline.

- If possible, assess the HIV and HCV status of the source patient. Rapid HIV testing of the source patient is preferred. Exposures originating from source patients who test HIV negative are considered not to pose HIV transmission risk, unless they have clinical evidence of primary HIV infection or HIV-related disease. HBV testing of the source patient may be indicated if the health care worker is not a documented responder to hepatitis B vaccination.

- Baseline HIV (and potentially HCV and HBV) testing of the exposed health care worker should be performed immediately after the exposure.

- Seek qualified medical evaluation as soon as possible to guide decisions on HIV PEP (see below).

## Postexposure Prophylaxis (PEP)

PEP after percutaneous and mucous membrane exposures to potentially infectious bodily fluids from patients with known or potential HIV infection is recommended to reduce the chance of transmission. A number of medication combinations are available for PEP (see the Updated US Public Health Service Guidelines for the Management of Occupational Exposures to HIV and Recommendations for Postexposure Prophylaxis at http://aidsinfo.nih.gov/guidelines).

The decision of whether or not to initiate PEP must weigh numerous factors. These include the timing, nature, and source of the exposure; regimen choice as affected by drug availability; the exposed person's medical history; potential drug interactions; and the possibility of exposure to a drug-resistant strain. Expert consultation is important when considering PEP. When expert advice is not immediately available, the National Clinicians' Postexposure Prophylaxis Hotline (PEPline) can be reached toll-free at 888-448-4911 (11 AM to 8 PM Eastern Time daily) for assistance in managing occupational exposures to HIV and HBV and HCV (http://nccc.ucsf.edu/clinician-consultation/pep-post-exposure-prophylaxis).

Other considerations when initiating HIV PEP include the following:

- Initiate HIV PEP as soon as possible after exposure.

- PEP can be stopped if new information changes the decision to treat.

- PEP recipients should be counseled regarding drug toxicities, drug interactions, and the importance of adherence.

Other potentially infectious exposures in the source material might require specific interventions. For example, if the health care worker is not a documented serologic responder to hepatitis B vaccination or is incompletely vaccinated, postexposure testing of the source patient and health care worker may be indicated, as well as PEP with hepatitis B immune globulin and vaccination.

## Postexposure Testing and Counseling

Postexposure testing and counseling are important follow-up measures for exposed health care workers, whether or not HIV or HBV PEP have been administered. This may include:

- Advice to take precautions to avoid secondary transmission (such as abstaining from sexual contact, using condoms or other barriers to prevent transmission, avoiding blood or tissue donations, and breastfeeding, if possible) during the first 12 weeks after exposure.

- Psychological counseling is considered essential since the emotional effect of occupational exposures can be substantial and exacerbated by stressors inherent to the overseas work environment.

- Baseline and follow-up testing for HIV at 6 weeks, 3 months, and 6 months ( follow-up at 6 weeks and 4 months is acceptable if a fourth-generation combination HIV p24 antigen-HIV antibody test is used). Extended HIV follow-up testing for up to 12 months is recommended for those who become infected with HCV after exposure to a source coinfected with HIV and HCV.

- Baseline and follow-up testing for HCV for those with known or potential exposure to HCV. Perform a baseline test for HCV antibody and if positive perform confirmatory RNA test. Follow-up testing should include either a test for HCV RNA at ≥3 weeks after exposure or a test for HCV antibody at ≥6 months after exposure with a confirmatory RNA test if positive.

- Baseline and follow-up testing for HBV for those with known or potential exposure to HBV if the health care worker is not a documented serologic responder to hepatitis B vaccination or is incompletely

9

vaccinated. Baseline testing of total antibodies to hepatitis B core antigen (anti-HBc) should be performed as soon as possible after exposure with follow-up testing HBsAg and anti-HBc 6 months after exposure.

## BIBLIOGRAPHY

1. Aid Worker Security Database (AWSD): figures at a glance [database on the Internet]. Humanitarian Outcomes; 2015 [cited 2018 Mar 29]. Available from: http://reliefweb.int/sites/reliefweb.int/files/resources/ho_aidworkersecuritypreview2015_0.pdf.

2. CDC. Healthcare-associated infections (HAIs). Atlanta: CDC; 2018 [cited 2018 May 13]. Available from: www.cdc.gov/HAI/prevent/ppe.html.

3. CDC. Hepatitis C and health care personnel. 2018 [cited 2018 May 13]. Available from: www.cdc.gov/hepatitis/hcv/hcvfaq.htm#section6.

4. CDC. Tuberculosis: testing health care workers. 2018 [cited 2018 May 13]. Available from: www.cdc.gov/tb/topic/testing/healthcareworkers.htm.

5. Clinicians Consultation Center. Post-exposure prophylaxis (PEP): timely answers for urgent exposure management. San Francisco: UCSF; 2014 [cited 2018 May 13]. Available from: http://nccc.ucsf.edu/clinician-consultation/pep-post-exposure-prophylaxis.

6. Connorton E, Perry MJ, Hemenway D, Miller M. Humanitarian relief workers and trauma-related mental illness. Epidemiol Rev. 2012 Jan;34(1):145–55.

7. Grinnell M, Dixon MG, Patton M, Fitter D, Bilivogui P, Johnson C, et al. Ebola virus disease in health care workers—Guinea, 2014. MMWR Morb Mortal Wkly Rep. 2015 Oct 2;64(38):1083–7.

8. Human Rights Watch, Safeguarding Health in Conflict Coalition. Under attack: violence against health workers, patients, and facilities. 2014 [cited 2016 Sep. 27]. Available from: www.msh.org/sites/msh.org/files/hhr0514_brochure_lowres.pdf.

9. Kuhar DT, Henderson DK, Struble KA, Heneine W, Thomas V, Cheever LW, et al. Updated US Public Health Service guidelines for the management of occupational exposures to human immunodeficiency virus and recommendations for postexposure prophylaxis. Infect Control Hosp Epidemiol. 2013 Sep;34(9):875–92.

10. Lee R. Occupational transmission of bloodborne diseases to healthcare workers in developing countries: meeting the challenges. J Hosp Infect. 2009 Aug;72(4):285–91.

11. Lyon RM, Wiggins CM. Expedition medicine—the risk of illness and injury. Wilderness Environ Med. 2010 Dec;21(4):318–24.

12. Mohan S, Sarfaty S, Hamer DH. Human immunodeficiency virus postexposure prophylaxis for medical trainees on international rotations. J Travel Med. 2010 Jul–Aug;17(4):264–8.

13. Schillie S, Vellozzi C, Reingold A, Harris A, Haber P, Ward JW, et al. Prevention of hepatitis B virus infection in the United States: recommendations of the Advisory Committee on Immunization Practices. MMWR Recomm Rep 2018;67(RR-1):1–31.

14. Vaid N, Langan KM, Maude RJ. Post-exposure prophylaxis in resource-poor settings: review and recommendations for pre-departure risk assessment and planning for expatriate healthcare workers. Trop Med Int Health. 2013 May;18(5):588–95.

**9**

# HUMANITARIAN AID WORKERS

Eric J. Nilles, Brian D. Gushulak, Stephanie Kayden

Humanitarian aid workers assist people forced from their homes because of conflict or natural disasters. This assistance begins within hours after a disaster and often continues for years. Humanitarian relief deployments themselves can last weeks to years. During these deployments, humanitarian aid workers must plan for self-sufficiency and for the unique challenges they will face, including insecure environments and emotional stress.

Each year tens of thousands of aid workers are deployed worldwide, and many more people (doctors, civic and religious groups) participate as amateur responders to international disasters. Professional aid workers often deploy with large specialist organizations like Doctors

## BOX 9-2. Voluntourism

Volunteer tourism, also called "voluntourism," describes tourists volunteering for a charity or development organization, usually for short periods, in developing countries. Although largely well intentioned, the impact of short-term visits—often by volunteers lacking specific understanding of the local context and lacking requisite skills—is variable and may be harmful in certain settings.

Voluntourism in humanitarian emergencies may be particularly problematic given dynamic and often dangerous humanitarian environments that require professional knowledge, organizational infrastructure, and understanding of the humanitarian response coordination system. Without the necessary individual competencies and organizational support, voluntourists in these settings expose themselves to unnecessary personal risks and can create a burden on the broader humanitarian response operations.

---

Without Borders that have infrastructure and resources to properly support their personnel. By contrast, amateur responders may deploy with smaller, less prepared groups with less experience in humanitarian work (Box 9-2).

## UNIQUE CHALLENGES FOR HUMANITARIAN AID WORKERS

Aid workers experience specific risks and situations related to the provision of humanitarian relief, such as:

- Safety and security
  > Exposure to the disaster or conflict environment that precipitated or sustained the crisis
  > Damaged or absent infrastructure, including sanitation facilities and living accommodations
  > High levels of insecurity
- Mental health
  > Stressful environments
  > Working long hours under adverse or extreme conditions

Humanitarian service can have an adverse effect on personal health. Studies of long-term humanitarian workers indicate that >35% report a deterioration in their personal health during the mission. Accidents and violence are risks for humanitarian aid workers and cause more deaths than disease or natural causes. Recent estimates place the risk of violence-related deaths, medical evacuations, and hospitalizations at approximately 6 per 10,000 person-years among aid workers. Conditions and outcomes vary by location, nature of the humanitarian event, and time spent in the field. A study of American Red Cross workers reported that 10% experienced injury or accident and 16% were exposed to violence. The same study demonstrated that >40% found the experience more stressful than expected.

## SAFETY AND SECURITY

Security risks and targeting of aid workers continues to be a concern for the humanitarian community. However, risks to staff are not uniformly distributed across the humanitarian landscape. Ongoing surveillance of violence directed against humanitarian and disaster relief aid workers continues to demonstrate that a small number of insecure locations (Afghanistan, Syria, South Sudan, Somalia, Yemen, and the Democratic Republic of Congo) account for most of these events.

Injuries and motor vehicle accidents are common risks for travelers throughout the world, and travelers should be sensitive to their surroundings and carefully select the type of transportation and hour of travel, if possible (see Chapter 8, Road & Traffic Safety).

In disaster and emergency situations, aid workers should be aware of physical hazards such as debris, unstable structures, downed power lines, and other environmental hazards. Workers in certain conflict and postconflict settings should be educated on improvised explosive devices, land mines, and other unexploded ordnance. Although less common, some environments may involve unusual exposures such as radiation exposure (for example, after the earthquake in Japan in 2011) or chemical agents (for example, sarin and mustard gas used on civilians in the Syrian conflict). Disaster relief and humanitarian aid workers who will be deployed to insecure areas including active conflict zones should undergo specialized security briefings by the deploying agency or private sources.

In situations associated with damage or destruction to local services and facilities, humanitarian aid workers should expect, anticipate, and plan for limited accommodations and logistical and personal support. Disaster relief and humanitarian aid workers destined for low-resource areas or situations may benefit from pretravel training and counseling regarding the moral complexities of providing service in these environments.

Travelers should enroll in the Department of State's Smart Traveler Enrollment Program (STEP, https://step.state.gov/step) to register with the US embassy in the destination country before departure. This will ensure that the local consulate is aware of their presence and can provide them with notifications, account for them, and include them in evacuation plans. Travelers providing humanitarian assistance should review and understand medical, evacuation, and life insurance provided by their employing agency. They should also consider supplemental travel, travel health, and medical evacuation insurance to cover medical care and evacuation should they become ill or injured (see Chapter 6, Travel Insurance, Travel Health Insurance & Medical Evacuation Insurance).

## MENTAL HEALTH

Studies suggest that aid workers returning from humanitarian missions, particularly missions that are characterized by high or chronic stress, have increased symptoms of anxiety, posttraumatic stress disorder, and depression. Preexisting psychological disorders including depression and anxiety predispose to worse outcomes. Generally, humanitarian aid and disaster relief workers demonstrate considerable resilience and adapt to the stressful environments, but elevated and chronic stress can lead to psychological deterioration and decompensation in certain people. Effective predeployment briefings can increase confidence a deployee's ability to cope with highly stressful environments; however, data are lacking on the effectiveness of postdeployment psychological debriefing to decrease adverse psychological impact of deployment.

A detailed evaluation of risk factors (psychiatric illness, family history, history of alcohol or substance abuse) may direct additional evaluation and identify previously unrecognized psychological problems or chronic conditions. Identifying alcohol or substance dependence, depression, or other psychiatric illness is particularly important, as stressful humanitarian environments frequently exacerbate these conditions; they are often the reason for emergency repatriation.

## PREPARATION

Careful attention to pretravel evaluation, both medical and psychological, can reduce the likelihood of illness and the need for emergency repatriation of humanitarian workers. Medical illness or injury among deployed staff, particularly serious conditions that require repatriation, are not only burdensome and potentially dangerous for the affected staff member, but these events redirect limited organizational resources from the beneficiaries.

Comprehensive medical examinations can prepare travelers by identifying previously unrecognized conditions, allowing for treatment before travel. Most of the core elements of the pretravel evaluation and counseling are discussed in detail elsewhere, including in The Pretravel Consultation (Chapter 2) and in the Health Care Workers section of this chapter. Providers should administer routine vaccinations and prescribe malaria prophylaxis (if appropriate). They should also give guidance on food and water precautions, self-treatment for travelers' diarrhea, protection from insect bites, behavioral risk avoidance, and injury prevention. Aid workers planning long-term assignments should have dental evaluations and address any problems identified before departure.

For health care workers providing medical care as part of their humanitarian activities, evaluation of occupational risk and the need for preventive preexposure or postexposure interventions is necessary. Medical humanitarian workers responding to outbreaks of communicable diseases are often at increased risk of exposure and infection by specific infectious pathogens, and meticulous attention to infection control and personal protective measures protocols may be required. Medical workers should ensure their organization provides personal protective equipment such as masks, gloves, gowns, and eye protection.

In humanitarian emergencies, direct infrastructure damage; lack of equipment, supplies, and human resources; or a surge in medical need can all contribute to a medical facility becoming compromised or overwhelmed. Volunteers with significant underlying medical conditions who are likely to require care themselves should be counseled against travel and encouraged to support the response in other ways. Similarly, pregnant women should discuss deployment with their obstetrician and should typically be encouraged to defer deployment.

Travelers planning to participate in animal rescue should review information available in Appendix E: Taking Animals & Animal Products across International Borders, and discuss rabies preexposure prophylaxis with a health care provider (see Chapter 4, Rabies).

## Health Kits

Aid workers should usually prepare a travel health kit that is more extensive than a typical kit (Chapter 6, Travel Health Kits). They should liaise with the deploying organization to tailor how extensive their packed supplies should be. For example, health care workers deployed by a medical organization will usually be able to access basic pharmacologic and other medical supplies for acute care treatment from the organization. They should also be familiar with basic first aid to self-treat any injury until they can obtain medical attention.

Conversely, people with chronic medical conditions requiring treatment should ensure they travel with prescriptions and medications sufficient for the duration of their service. They should also consider bringing along treatment for exacerbations of diseases or conditions that they may not usually experience, such as back pain or

asthma. Because not all pharmaceuticals are globally available, travelers on extended deployments should review alternative preparations or compounds should their normal formulations not be available. It is a good practice to separate and store medications in 2 separate allotments in case of loss or theft. See Chapter 6, Travel Health Kits, for additional information on preparing, storing, and traveling with medications.

People with dental crowns or bridgework should consider taking temporary dental adhesive for short-term management of a dislodged dental appliance. In addition to a basic travel health kit, humanitarian aid workers should consider bringing the following items:

- Menstrual supplies
- Long pants, shirts that cover the shoulders
- Boots (particularly in disaster or rudimentary settings)
- Gloves (leather gloves if physical labor will be performed)
- Safety goggles
- Sunglasses
- Sunscreen
- Insect repellent
- Headlamp with spare batteries
- Sewing kit
- Insecticide-impregnated bed net (if traveling to areas endemic for mosquitoborne diseases)
- Money belt
- Cash (new or crisp bills can often be exchanged at better rates)
- Cellular telephone, equipped to work internationally (or preferably unlocked)

## Personal Items

Loss of life, serious injuries, missing and separated families, and destruction of communities are often associated with humanitarian emergencies; aid workers should recognize that they are likely to encounter stressful situations as part of their work. Keeping a personal item nearby, such as a family photo, favorite music, or religious material, can offer comfort. Communicating with family members and close friends from time to time can be an important means of support. Access to mobile phones and Internet services are frequent challenges in humanitarian emergencies, and satellite telephones are small, function in most regions globally, and can be rented for <$10 per day. However, some government authorities may prohibit or limit the importation and use of satellite phones, particularly in conflict zones, and this should be clarified before rental.

## Documents

Aid workers should take extra passport-style photos, which may be required for certain types of visas, for work permits, and security passes. Travelers should bring photocopies of documents such as passports and credit cards, as well as copies of their medical, nursing, or other professional license if applicable. Medical information such as immunization records and blood type should be available. The traveler should carry physical copies of all of these documents, leave copies with their main contact at home, scan and email copies to their smart phones (if appropriate), and ensure the documents are securely stored and available in a cloud storage service. In addition, they should carry contact information for their designated emergency contacts.

## POSTTRAVEL

Returning disaster relief and humanitarian aid workers should be advised to seek medical care if they sustain injuries during their travel or become ill after returning home. To ensure a thorough assessment, they should advise their providers of the nature and location of their recent travel. Depending on the duration and nature of the deployment, including if they were providing direct medical care, returning aid workers may benefit from a comprehensive medical review. Those involved in responding to infectious disease outbreaks should be educated on posttravel illness monitoring recommendations or requirements, if applicable.

Homecoming can be psychologically challenging, and treatment or counseling should be sought if there are concerns about an individual's ability to transition to postdeployment life. Consider referring workers who witnessed or were involved in mass casualties, deaths, or serious injuries or who have been victims of violence (assault, kidnapping, or serious road traffic crash) for critical incident counseling. They should be educated that the onset of adverse psychological effects after exposure to traumatic experiences may be delayed, sometimes by several months or longer.

9

## BIBLIOGRAPHY

1. Aid Worker Security Report 2017: Behind the attacks—a look at the perpetrators of violence against aid workers. Humanitarian Outcomes; 2017 [cited 2018 Mar 19]. Available from: https://aidworkersecurity.org/sites/default/files/AWSR2017.pdf.

2. Brooks SK, Dunn R, Sage CA, Amlot R, Greenberg N, Rubin GJ. Risk and resilience factors affecting the psychological wellbeing of individuals deployed in humanitarian relief roles after a disaster. J Ment Health. 2015 Dec;24(6):385–413.

3. Callahan MV, Hamer DH. On the medical edge: preparation of expatriates, refugee and disaster relief workers, and Peace Corps volunteers. Infect Dis Clin North Am. 2005 Mar;19(1):85–101.

4. Costa M, Oberholzer-Riss M, Hatz C, Steffen R, Puhan M, Schlagenhauf P. Pre-travel health advice guidelines for humanitarian workers: A systematic review. Travel Med Infect Dis. 2015 Nov–Dec;13(6):449–65.

5. Kortepeter MG, Seaworth BJ, Tasker SA, Burgess TH, Coldren RL, Aronson NE. Health care workers and researchers traveling to developing-world clinical settings: disease transmission risk and mitigation. Clin Infect Dis. 2010 Dec 1;51(11):1298–305.

6. Lopes Cardozo B, Gotway Crawford C, Eriksson C, Zhu J, Sabin M, Ager A, et al. Psychological distress, depression, anxiety, and burnout among international humanitarian aid workers: a longitudinal study. PLoS ONE. 2012;7(9):e44948 [cited 2018 Mar 19]. Available from: https://doi.org/10.1371/journal.pone.0044948.

7. Peytremann I, Baduraux M, O'Donovan S, Loutan L. Medical evacuations and fatalities of United Nations High Commissioner for Refugees field employees. J Travel Med. 2001 May–Jun;8(3):117–21.

8. Substance abuse and Mental Health Services Administration. Disaster preparedness, response, and recovery [cited 2018 Mar 19]. Available from: www.samhsa.gov/disaster-preparedness.

# US MILITARY DEPLOYMENTS

Gregory A. Raczniak, Mark S. Riddle, Michael Forgione

In 2016, approximately 1.3 million US military members were on active-duty, and approximately 800,000 were in the reserve forces. The US military, as a matter of policy, follows most of the recommendations in the CDC Yellow Book. However, certain situations apply only to the US military, and some policies or recommendations differ from what is recommended in the Yellow Book for civilian travel. Active-duty military physicians generally manage predeployment medicine, but civilian physicians may interact with people who are on reserve status, home on leave, recently discharged from active duty, or veterans. Providers can find predeployment and postdeployment information, policies, and guidelines for clinicians, service members and their families, and veterans on the Deployment Health Clinical Center website (www.pdhealth.mil).

## FORCE HEALTH PROTECTION

Force health protection (FHP) is an important concept in military medicine. FHP is defined as all measures taken by commanders, supervisors, individual service members, and the military health system to promote, protect, improve, conserve, and restore the mental and physical well-being of service members across the range of military activities and operations. Delivery of vaccines and the use of malaria chemoprophylaxis agents are 2 aspects of FHP.

Medical interventions for FHP are the responsibility of the unit commander, with advice from the unit medical officer. When predeployment vaccines or malaria chemoprophylaxis are indicated, the commander includes such requirements in the mission plan. Service members are then required to receive these interventions under proper medical supervision. If a particular vaccine or drug is medically contraindicated, alternative agents may be employed if they are available. The unit medical officer documents which military personnel have not received standard preventive measures, so these people may receive additional monitoring or treatment if they become ill.

FHP policy positions in the Department of Defense (DoD) are issued as directives and instructions. All directives and instructions can be found online at www.dtic.mil/whs/directives. The Policy and Program for Immunizations to Protect the Health of Service Members and Military Beneficiaries is found in directive 6205.02E (September 19, 2006) at www.esd.whs.mil/Portals/54/Documents/DD/issuances/dodd/620502p.pdf.

Although policy may be made at higher levels in Washington, DC, the final decision to use vaccines or malaria chemoprophylaxis under FHP is made by commanders in the field, guided by their medical staff. In certain circumstances, individual service members may be exempt from vaccination. There are 2 types of exemptions from immunization: medical and administrative. Granting medical exemptions is a medical function that can be validated only by a health care professional. Granting administrative exemptions is a nonmedical function, usually controlled by the person's unit commander.

## ROUTINE AND TRAVEL-RELATED IMMUNIZATION

Department of Defense (DoD) policy states that the recommendations for immunization from CDC and the Advisory Committee for Immunization Practices shall generally be followed, consistent with requirements and guidance of the Food and Drug Administration (FDA) and with consideration for the unique needs of military settings and exposure risks. The specific vaccines given prior to deployment are dependent on the assignment and are summarized at the Military Health System website (https://health.mil/Military-Health-Topics/Health-Readiness/Immunization-Healthcare/Vaccine-Recommendations/Vaccine-Recommendations-by-AOR). The Defense Health Agency (DHA) Immunization Healthcare

**9**

Branch (IHB) [formerly the Military Vaccine Agency (MILVAX)] enhances military medical readiness by coordinating DoD immunization (vaccination) programs worldwide. A valuable source of service-specific information on immunizations for all branches of the US Armed Services is found at the DHA IHB website (www.health.mil/vaccines).

## MALARIA PROPHYLAXIS

Preventing malaria in military units deployed to endemic areas is essential. Medical commanders must designate trained staff to provide comprehensive malaria prevention counseling to military and civilian personnel considered at risk of contracting malaria.

Several features of malaria prophylaxis are unique to the US military because of the activities and stressors of military deployments. When antimalarial drugs are used, the military can only use FDA-approved agents in accordance with the specific FDA-approved indications. Off-label use of drugs is not allowed. If off-label use is felt to be in the best interest of the person or unit, trained and knowledgeable clinicians must provide one-on-one medical evaluations, document in the medical record the rationale for such use, and provide a prescription for the drug or vaccine to each person.

Atovaquone-proguanil (Malarone) is the recommended malaria prophylaxis option for all personnel for both short- and long-term deployments in high-transmission areas of Africa. For practical purposes, this includes most of sub-Saharan Africa. For people who are unable to receive atovaquone-proguanil because of intolerance or contraindication, doxycycline is the preferred second-line therapy. Use of mefloquine as prophylaxis is a third-line recommendation for those unable to receive either atovaquone-proguanil or doxycycline. Before prescribing mefloquine for prophylaxis, absolute and relative contraindications as described in the approved product label must be considered.

Atovaquone-proguanil and doxycycline are both first-line choices in areas other than sub-Saharan Africa. Mefloquine should be reserved for people with intolerance or contraindications to both first-line medications.

As a matter of policy, the US military routinely uses primaquine for presumptive antirelapse treatment (PART) in returning military populations to prevent the late relapse of *P. vivax* malaria or *P. ovale* malaria. PART is also referred to as "terminal prophylaxis." In PART, primaquine is given to otherwise healthy people on their departure from an endemic area. Primaquine is used for this indication much more frequently in the military than in most civilian travelers.

The FDA-approved regimen for PART is 15 mg (base) given daily for 14 days. In 2003, CDC recommended 30 mg (base) of primaquine daily for 14 days for PART based on available evidence, but the FDA-approved regimen remains the lower dose. Adherence to the daily 14-day regimen is poor unless primaquine is given under directly observed therapy, which is rarely done. As a result of noncompliance and subtherapeutic dosing with the 15-mg/day regimen, periodic outbreaks of relapsed *P. vivax* malaria continue to occur in returning military personnel. Use of the higher-dose primaquine regimen for PART is now recommended for military personnel.

Although primaquine is included as an acceptable alternative by CDC for primary prophylaxis in some countries where the risk of malaria is exclusively or mostly *P. vivax* malaria, primaquine is not FDA-approved for primary prophylaxis. Because use of primaquine for primary prophylaxis constitutes off-label use, it cannot be prescribed for a deploying group, but it can be prescribed by a licensed medical provider on an individual basis as part of medical practice.

The most important risk of using primaquine is hemolytic anemia in those who are deficient in G6PD. Current policy is for all US military personnel to be screened for G6PD deficiency on entry into military service. However, some people, such as reservists, may have deployed without testing, or clinicians may not be able to confirm results for all people in a unit requiring PART. Clinicians should be aware that hemolytic reactions to primaquine may occur in those with unrecognized G6PD deficiency.

A recurrent issue for military medicine is the correct timing of primaquine when given as PART in conjunction with the standard prescribed prophylaxis. Primaquine can be given at any time

9

after personnel leave an endemic area. For convenience and for enhancing adherence to the 14-day regimen, it is often best for military units to prescribe primaquine in the immediate 2 weeks after return. During this time, units are often still at their home base completing in-processing before block leave. Once personnel depart on leave, adherence and monitoring for side effects are more difficult.

In 2018, the US Food and Drug Administration approved tafenoquine for malaria prophylaxis and treatment, including PART for *P. vivax* and *P. ovale* malaria. As with primaquine, the most important risk of tafenoquine is hemolytic anemia in people who are G6PD deficient. As of press time, it is unclear whether and how the US military will adopt the use of tafenoquine. More information on tafenoquine is available in Chapter 4, Malaria.

## UNIQUE NEEDS FOR THE MILITARY

US military personnel may encounter threats, such as biological warfare agents, that are not usually considered for civilian travelers. Vaccines, immunoglobulins, drug prophylaxis, and drug treatment regimens can be given only in accordance with FDA-licensed products and regimens and for FDA-approved indications.

Products not approved by the FDA are given to soldiers only with voluntary informed consent under an institutional review board-approved protocol and in accordance with a current and FDA-approved investigational new drug application.

Only under exceptional circumstances would products not approved by the FDA be given to soldiers without informed consent. The FDA commissioner can authorize the use of an unapproved medical product or an unapproved use of an approved medical product during a declared emergency involving a heightened risk of attack on the public or US military forces or when national security may be affected.

## THE RETURNING SERVICE MEMBER WITH HEALTH CONCERNS

Symptoms and health concerns after a deployment may be similar to health issues reported from nonmilitary returning travelers. However, deployment presents a different set of circumstances from the civilian traveler such as differential vaccination recommendations, physical and psychological stress and trauma of combat, environmental exposures, and infections that may cause unique health concerns. The Post-Deployment Health Clinical Practice Guideline (PDH-CPG) is designed to help clinicians implement specific approaches to address these distinctive experiences and exposures and includes clinical tools and resources to evaluate and manage patients with the full spectrum of deployment-related concerns.

## DISCLOSURE

Drs. Forgione and Riddle are employees of the Department of Defense. The views expressed in this section are those of the authors and do not necessarily reflect the official policy or position of the Departments of the Air Force, Army, or Navy, nor the Department of Defense.

**9**

## BIBLIOGRAPHY

1. Armed Forces Health Surveillance Center. Update: Malaria, U.S. Armed Forces, 2015. MSMR. 2016 Jan;23(1):2–6.

2. Brisson M, Brisson P. Compliance with antimalaria chemoprophylaxis in a combat zone. Am J Trop Med Hyg. 2012 Apr;86(4):587–90.

3. Carr ME, Jr., Fandre MN, Oduwa FO. Glucose-6-phosphate dehydrogenase deficiency in two returning Operation Iraqi Freedom soldiers who developed hemolytic anemia while receiving primaquine prophylaxis for malaria. Mil Med. 2005 Apr;170(4):273–6.

4. Food and Drug Administration. Emergency use authorization of medical products. Rockville, MD: Food and Drug Administration; 2007 [cited 2016 Sep 27]. Available from: www.fda.gov/RegulatoryInformation/Guidances/ucm125127.htm.

5. Office of the Assistant Secretary of Defense (Health Affairs). HA-Policy 13-002. Guidance on medications for prophylaxis of malaria. Washington, DC 2013 Apr 15 [cited 2018 Oct 24] Available from: https://health.mil/Reference-Center/Policies/2013/04/15/Guidance-on-Medications-for-Prophylaxis-of-Malaria.

6. Townell N, Looke D, McDougall D, McCarthy JS. Relapse of imported *Plasmodium vivax* malaria is related to primaquine dose: a retrospective study. Malar J. 2012 Jun 22;11(1):214.

7. US Africa Command. Force Health Protection procedures for deployment and travel 2011 [cited 2016 Sep 27]. Available from: www.med.navy.mil/sites/nepmu2/Documents/threat_assessment/AFRICOM-FHP-Guidance-22SEP11.pdf.

8. US Department of Defense. Department of Defense directive: Force Health Protection (FHP), no. 6200.04. Washington, DC: US Department of Defense; 2004 [updated 2007 Apr 23; cited 2016 Sep 27]. Available from: www.dtic.mil/whs/directives/corres/pdf/620004p.pdf.

9. US Department of Defense. Department of Defense instruction: application of Food and Drug Administration (FDA) rules to Department of Defense Force Health Protection programs, no 6200.02. Washington, DC: US Department of Defense; 2008 [cited 2016 Sep 27]. Available from: www.dtic.mil/whs/directives/corres/pdf/620002p.pdf.

10. Whitman TJ, Coyne PE, Magill AJ, Blazes DL, Green MD, Milhous WK, et al. An outbreak of *Plasmodium falciparum* malaria in US Marines deployed to Liberia. Am J Trop Med Hyg. 2010 Aug;83(2):258–65.

# LONG-TERM TRAVELERS & EXPATRIATES

Lin H. Chen, Davidson H. Hamer

The risk of illness or injury increases with duration of travel, so special consideration should be given to travelers who are planning long-term visits (≥6 months is a common definition) to low- or middle-income countries, whether they are expatriates with definite plans or adventurers with open itineraries. Points to discuss in the pretravel consultation include accessing care at the destination, vaccines, infectious diseases not prevented by vaccines, injury prevention, and psychological and cultural issues that long-term travelers may encounter.

## ACCESSING CARE ABROAD

Before departure, all long-term travelers should undergo complete medical and dental examinations. For expatriates, it also may be beneficial to have a psychological evaluation, as early repatriation is often due to psychological issues that could be addressed prior to travel. Travelers should anticipate that they will need care at some point during their stay, and they should plan where they will obtain it and how they will pay for it. Those traveling for work or with an organization (such as a university, the Peace Corps, or a nongovernmental organization) may have a predetermined source of care and some may access advice from the international expatriate community. By contrast, other travelers should identify a source in advance (see Chapter 6,

Obtaining Health Care Abroad). Long-term travelers should also determine if they will need supplemental travel health insurance and evacuation insurance (see Chapter 6, Travel Insurance, Travel Health Insurance & Medical Evacuation Insurance).

In some countries, travelers are likely to encounter poor-quality (substandard, falsified, counterfeit, or expired) medications. Because the pills and packaging may be nearly indistinguishable from their legitimate counterparts, travelers should bring a sufficient supply of their routine medications (such as antihypertensive or antihyperlipidemic drugs) from the United States (see Chapter 6, *Perspectives*: Avoiding Poorly Regulated Medicines and Medical Products during Travel). Options for obtaining sufficient medications include 1) requesting an override from the insurance company to dispense the entire quantity of medication; 2) paying out of pocket for the full amount of medication needed and then submitting to the insurance company for reimbursement; 3) refilling prescriptions during trips home; or 4) relying on friends or family members who visit to bring refilled medication supplies.

## VACCINES

Routine vaccines, including influenza vaccine, should be updated. In addition, long-term travelers should be aware of any vaccine requirements at

9

their destination for employment, schooling, or entry. A number of travel-related vaccines warrant consideration:

- Hepatitis A and typhoid vaccines are appropriate given the cumulative risk, although the traveler should be aware that the latter does not provide full protection.

- Travel-associated hepatitis B infections are rare, but the risk for travelers may be higher than for nontravelers, and the vaccine should be considered for all long-term travelers and expatriates.

- Meningococcal disease is more likely in travelers with prolonged exposure to local populations in endemic or epidemic areas; quadrivalent vaccine should be considered for those at risk.

- Japanese encephalitis is associated with longer stays in endemic areas, and the vaccine is recommended for travelers who plan longer stays or residence in endemic areas, travelers anticipating outdoor activities in endemic areas after dusk, and travelers who are uncertain of specific destinations or activities. (see Chapter 4, Japanese Encephalitis).

- Rabies preexposure prophylaxis is an important consideration for people spending a prolonged time in endemic countries, especially in areas where rabies immune globulin is not available (which is true of many resource-limited countries). Vaccinating children who will be living in high-risk areas is a priority.

- Yellow fever vaccination may be required or recommended. Numerous unvaccinated Chinese expatriates have recently fallen ill from yellow fever while working in Angola, illustrating the importance of yellow fever vaccination for travelers who will be working in an endemic area.

In addition to the intended destination, consider disease risk in surrounding areas, since long-term travelers may be likely to travel locally. For example, a short-term traveler to Seoul would not be considered at risk for Japanese encephalitis, but an expatriate living in Seoul may have opportunities to visit the Korean countryside or other areas in Asia where he or she could be exposed. Similarly, yellow fever vaccination needs consideration as the location of posting may not be in an endemic area, but the traveler may journey to these areas when posted abroad.

## INFECTIOUS DISEASES NOT PREVENTED BY VACCINES

### Malaria

Data suggest that the incidence of malaria increases and the use of preventive measures decreases with increasing length of stay. For instance, malaria incidence in British travelers returning from West Africa after a stay of 6–12 months was 80 times that of the incidence in travelers who had stayed only 1 week. Among expatriate corporate employees in Ghana, adherence to malaria prophylaxis deteriorated with increasing duration of stay, and all those who had been on the site for >1 year had abandoned prophylaxis. About half of the cohort used insect repellent only intermittently, and more than one-third never used repellent. Even though most British expatriates from the UK Foreign and Commonwealth Office had good knowledge about malaria and its prevention strategies, they adhered to malaria prophylaxis <25% of the time; only 25% reported rigorous compliance, and 13% reported having contracted malaria. A recent GeoSentinel Global Surveillance Network analysis found that *Plasmodium falciparum* malaria was the most frequent diagnosis among ill returned expatriate workers, occurring in 6%, and was most commonly acquired in sub-Saharan Africa. Given the high relative risk of malaria for travelers in Africa, these data on long-term travelers and expatriates highlight worrisome risks and practices.

A traveler residing in an area of continuous malaria transmission should continue to use malaria prophylaxis for the entire stay. It is important to reassure the traveler that the drugs are safe and effective. Doxycycline has been well-tolerated for long-term malaria prophylaxis in the military, and CDC has no recommended limits on its duration of use for malaria prophylaxis. Peace Corps volunteers frequently use mefloquine during prolonged stays, with a discontinuation rate of 0.9%. Mefloquine may be appropriate for long-term prophylaxis in chloroquine-resistant areas because

9

of its convenient weekly dosing, but concern has increased regarding its neuropsychiatric side-effect profile, especially with the Food and Drug Administration label indicating that neurologic side effects may persist.

Atovaquone-proguanil has shown good long-term tolerability in postmarketing surveillance, with a discontinuation rate of only 1% because of diarrhea. Peace Corps Volunteers prescribed atovaquone-proguanil adhered to prophylaxis best, when compared to those given doxycycline and mefloquine. If long-term use (>5 years) of chloroquine is planned, a baseline ophthalmic examination with biannual follow-up is recommended to screen for potential retinal toxicity.

The possibility of pregnancy requires careful consideration for travelers to areas where malaria is endemic (see Chapter 7, Pregnant Travelers). Malaria infection during pregnancy can result in severe complications to both mother and fetus. When pregnancy is anticipated, prophylaxis options may need to be adjusted. Ideally, this possibility should be explored before travel with all female long-term travelers of childbearing age. For women who are pregnant or plan to become pregnant during long-term travel, mefloquine is considered safe in all trimesters. Data from published studies in pregnant women have shown no increase in the risk of teratogenic effects or adverse pregnancy outcomes after mefloquine prophylaxis during pregnancy. Chloroquine has also been used long-term without ill effect on pregnancy. If a woman traveling long-term is taking atovaquone-proguanil, doxycycline, or primaquine, she should discontinue her medication and begin weekly mefloquine (or chloroquine in those areas where it remains efficacious), and then wait at least 3–4 weeks to conceive so that a therapeutic blood level of mefloquine can build up.

Women who become pregnant while taking antimalarial drugs do not need a therapeutic abortion but should be advised during the pretravel consultation of potential risks. The effect of atovaquone-proguanil on the fetus is unknown, but doxycycline is associated with fetal toxicity in animals and is contraindicated in pregnant women. Primaquine and tafenoquine may harm a G6PD-deficient fetus, so should not be used in pregnancy.

French service members deployed to the Central African Republic for 4 months in 2013 experienced malaria at a rate of 150 cases/1,000 person-years. A survey found that prophylaxis compliance correlated positively with use of other prophylactic measures against malaria (bed net use, insecticide on clothing, taking prophylaxis at the same time every day), correct perception of malaria risk, favorable perception of prophylaxis effectiveness, and peer-to-peer reinforcement.

For long-term travelers, the need for adjuncts to prophylaxis should be stressed, such as personal protection measures to avoid mosquito bites (see Chapter 3, Mosquitoes, Ticks & Other Arthropods). Even with urging to adhere to personal protective measures and reassurance that long-term prophylaxis is safe and effective, adherence is likely to decline over time. Consequently, the pretravel consultation for a long-term traveler to areas where malaria is present should stress the severity of the disease, its signs and symptoms, and the need to seek care immediately if they develop. Travelers could consider bringing a reliable supply of drugs to treat malaria if they are diagnosed with the disease.

## Other Diseases

Because diarrhea and gastrointestinal diseases occur commonly, long-term travelers should be educated about their management (see Chapter 2, Travelers' Diarrhea). Measures include rehydration, use of antimotility agents, empiric antimicrobial therapy, and knowing when to seek care.

Tuberculosis risk in a traveler may rise to that of the local population if the traveler or expatriate has a longer stay and intimate contact with the local population. A baseline interferon-γ release assay or a tuberculin skin test, followed by the same test after travel, should be considered for long-term travelers. Tuberculosis screening is particularly important for health care workers or those who may be working in hospitals, refugee camps, or in prisons.

Likewise, dengue seroconversion occurred at a rate of 3.4/1,000 workers per month of stay in endemic areas. Other mosquitoborne viral illnesses (such as chikungunya and Zika) also pose potential risk, so advise long-term travelers and expatriates to protect themselves from mosquito vectors. Chapter 4 provides disease-specific information on dengue, chikungunya, and Zika virus infections.

Risk for HIV and sexually transmitted infections are increased in travelers and expatriates, and the consistent use of condoms in expatriates is low (approximately 20%). Long-term travelers should be educated about the risk of HIV and sexually transmitted infections at their destination, as well as preventive measures. The potential for occupational exposure to HIV is important to consider in health care workers; postexposure prophylaxis with antiretroviral therapy and risk avoidance should be included in the pretravel consultation (see the Health Care Workers section in this chapter).

Transfusion is a potential source of hepatitis C infection in expatriates. The risk of hepatitis E, spread by the fecal–oral route, is highest in Asia, although it has been transmitted in many different tropical locations. Pregnant women are at highest risk of fulminant disease.

Other infections vary with location and include giardiasis, amebiasis, strongyloidiasis, schistosomiasis, cutaneous leishmaniasis, and filariasis. Travelers can prevent *Strongyloides stercoralis* infections by not walking barefoot through soil and schistosomiasis by not swimming or wading in fresh water. This latter risk is difficult to communicate to long-term travelers who, for example, may be living in sub-Saharan Africa and who look forward to river rafting or vacationing at a lake. The risks of strongyloidiasis and schistosomiasis increase with long-term travel, so screening on return (and also during long-term expatriate assignments for those with access to health care) should also be discussed. Cutaneous leishmaniasis and filariasis should be reviewed if a traveler has the potential geographic exposure risk. Compared with short-term travelers, long-term travelers experience more chronic diarrhea and postinfectious irritable bowel syndrome (possibly because some become less adherent to food and water precautions over time) and should be advised to continue food and water precautions in order to reduce the risk for these conditions (see Chapter 2, Food & Water Precautions).

## INJURY

Since injuries are the leading cause of preventable death in travelers, educate long-term travelers about safety (see Chapter 8, Road & Traffic Safety). Stress the importance of road and vehicle safety and emphasize that travelers should choose the safest vehicle options available. Roads are often poorly constructed and maintained, traffic laws may not be enforced, vehicles may not have seatbelts or be properly maintained, and drivers may be reckless and poorly trained. See Chapter 3, Injury & Trauma, for strategies to reduce the risk of traffic and other injuries.

## PSYCHOLOGICAL ISSUES

Culture shock and the stress of long-term travel can trigger or exacerbate psychiatric reactions. A long-term traveler should be assessed for preexisting psychiatric diagnosis, depressed mood, recent major life stressors, and use of medications that may have psychiatric effects. Any of these conditions suggest a need for further screening. All long-term travelers should be warned about illicit drug use and urged to take care of their physical and mental health by exercising regularly and eating healthfully. They should be able to recognize signs of anxiety and depression and have a plan for coping with them. Having photographs or other mementos of friends and family at hand and staying in close contact with loved ones at home can alleviate the stress of long-term travel. For more information, see Chapter 3, Mental Health.

## LONG-TERM TRAVELERS WITH OPEN ITINERARIES

Offering pretravel care to long-term travelers, especially those with no itinerary or those who present with only vague travel plans, presents unique challenges. These travelers benefit from broad immunization coverage for all potential exposures to vaccine-preventable diseases. Because their plans are unclear, these travelers must understand that they may need to diagnose and treat themselves for common ailments, including travelers' diarrhea, upper respiratory tract infections, urinary tract infections, vaginitis, skin disorders, and musculoskeletal problems. For travelers such as backpackers who may go in and out of malarious areas, a sensible approach is to provide a supply of atovaquone-proguanil with instructions on how to take it when they do visit risk areas. In addition to strategies to prevent health problems and

9

injuries during their long sojourns, traveler education is imperative regarding health resources, signs and symptoms that require urgent medical evaluation, and medical evacuation.

## SCREENING LONG-TERM TRAVELERS AND EXPATRIATES AFTER RETURN

After returning to their country of origin, long-term travelers (expatriate workers, Peace Corps volunteers, or highly adventurous travelers) will ideally have a thorough medical interview to assess potential infectious exposures. A careful itinerary-specific history with detailed questioning about potential high-risk exposures including food, water,

animal, and human contact is the foundation of the posttravel evaluation. Returning travelers should have a physical examination focused on specific signs and symptoms and a selected array of tests. These tests include a complete blood count with differential, hepatic transaminases, and serologic markers depending on types of exposure (but most importantly for strongyloidiasis and schistosomiasis). Serologic testing can detect subclinical infections and determine whether seroconversion to the more common pathogens (where treatment would be advised) has occurred (see Chapter 11, Screening Asymptomatic Returned Travelers). A benefit of the posttravel evaluation is preventive counseling for potential future travel.

## BIBLIOGRAPHY

1. Chen LH, Leder K, Barbre KA, Schlagenhauf P, Libman M, Keystone J, et al. Business travel–associated illness: a GeoSentinel analysis. J Travel Med. 2018 Jan 1;25(1).

2. Chen LH, Wilson ME, Schlagenhauf P. Prevention of malaria in long-term travelers. JAMA. 2006 Nov 8;296(18):2234–44.

3. Clerinx J, Hamer DH, Libman M. Post-travel screening. In: Keystone JS, Kozarsky PE, Connor BA, Nothdurft HD, Mendelson M, Leder K, editors. Travel Medicine. 4th ed. Elsevier Limited: London; 487–94.

4. Créach M-A, Velut G, de Laval F, Briolant S, Aigle L, Marimoutou C, et al. Factors associated with malaria chemoprophylaxis compliance among French service members deployed in Central African Republic. Malaria J. 2016;15:174.

5. Cunningham J, Horsley J, Patel D, Tunbridge A, Lalloo DG. Compliance with long-term malaria prophylaxis in British expatriates. Travel Med Infect Dis. 2014 Jul–Aug;12(4):341–8.

6. Hamer DH, Ruffing R, Callahan MV, Lyons SH, Abdullah AS. Knowledge and use of measures to reduce health risks by corporate expatriate employees in western Ghana. J Travel Med. 2008 Jul–Aug;15(4):237–42.

7. Landman KZ, Tan KR, Arguin PM; Centers for Disease Control and Prevention (CDC). Knowledge, attitudes, and practices regarding antimalarial chemoprophylaxis in U.S. Peace Corps Volunteers—Africa, 2013. MMWR Morb Mortal Wkly Rep. 2014 Jun 13;63(23):516–7.

8. Lim PL, Han P, Chen LH, MacDonald S, Pandey P, Hale D, et al. Expatriates ill after travel: results from the Geosentinel Surveillance Network. BMC Infect Dis. 2012;12:386.

9. Pierre CM, Lim PL, Hamer DH. Expatriates: special considerations in pretravel preparation. Curr Infect Dis Rep. 2013 Aug;15(4):299–306.

10. Visser JT, Edwards CA. Dengue fever, tuberculosis, human immunodeficiency virus, and hepatitis C virus conversion in a group of long-term development aid workers. J Travel Med. 2013 Nov–Dec;20(6):361–7.

# STUDY ABROAD & OTHER INTERNATIONAL STUDENT TRAVEL

Kristina M. Angelo, Gary Rhodes, Inés DeRomaña

Students and their families are responsible for planning for and understanding health and safety risks. They are encouraged to contact study abroad program administrators before departure to discuss the local view and approach to health issues, legality of prescribed medications, and standards of health care in the country where they are going. Preparation can help reduce a student's chances of becoming ill overseas and engaging in behaviors that can put them at increased risk.

Study abroad programs vary in structure and staffing, resources and level of support provided, and obligations placed on students. Some institutions have several employees (study abroad professionals) dedicated to supporting study abroad programs—this includes people who have expertise on international health and safety issues and who have the background to make specific recommendations regarding insurance coverage; other programs have limited or no staff dedicated to such activities.

## PREDEPARTURE PREPARATION

The pretravel consultation with a health care provider should cover those items that any pretravel counseling session includes: risk assessment, risk mitigation, and preparation to respond effectively to health and safety issues while abroad (see Chapter 2, The Pretravel Consultation).

Travel health professionals can think about dividing risk mitigation practices for students traveling overseas into 2 categories: general and specific considerations. General risk mitigation activities—those that might apply to anyone traveling internationally—include:

- Ensuring appropriate immunizations for the destination: routine, recommended, and required vaccinations need to be reviewed and administered as necessary

- Providing recommended prophylactic and self-treatment medications and first aid kit (see Chapter 6, Travel Health Kits)

- Providing country- and region-specific environmental health and safety information

- Guidance for managing chronic health conditions, including compromised immunity

- Providing information about how to obtain routine and emergency medical and dental care while abroad

- Assisting travelers with finding out whether their medications can be brought into other countries legally

- Managing stress and other mental health issues associated with international travel, including culture shock, jet lag and altered sleep patterns

- Encouraging students to register with the Department of State's Smart Traveler Enrollment Program (STEP, https://step.state.gov/step/)

Travel health professionals are also encouraged to take the time to discuss with student travelers these additional, specific topics:

- The importance of purchasing a travel insurance policy that covers major medical, evacuation, and repatriation: student insurance options offered through the parent institution may be a reasonable, cost-effective option for the student traveler

- Gender-related health issues, including information for lesbian, gay, bisexual, and transgender (LGBT) students

- Good oral hygiene and dental care

- Proper nutrition and diet

- Alcohol and (illicit) drug use: this may include making arrangements for those with preexisting dependency issues

- Bloodborne pathogen precautions: avoiding needles, blood products, tattoos, piercing, surgeries, acupuncture

- Practicing safe sex, including what to do in the event of pregnancy

- Water and extreme sport risks

Providing support for students with special needs, disabilities, or preexisting health conditions may require travel health professionals to collaborate with study abroad professionals.

Study abroad professionals should share general instructions with students about how to locate physicians and mental health providers for emergency and non-emergency situations. They should also encourage students to familiarize themselves with the study-abroad codes of conduct for their home and host institutions, as well as local health and safety issues, cultural norms, laws, and political climate.

## SPECIFIC ISSUES

### Gender Identity
Students who self-identify as LGBT should familiarize themselves with local laws, cultural attitudes, and tolerance in their proposed host country. Identifying health care providers in the host country with experience working with LGBT people (if desired) may require additional research and planning; students should prepare accordingly. The Department of State website (http://travel.state.gov) and specific US Embassy or Consulate websites in the countries and cities around the world where they are located (www.usembassy.gov) are useful sources of information on host country laws.

### Mental Health
International travel can be stressful for anyone, particularly students away from their usual support systems. Culture shock, isolation, loneliness, fear, and insecurity can exacerbate existing mental health issues or unveil new ones (see Chapter 3, Mental Health). Students should consider their preexisting mental and physical well-being, and the availability of local resources, when deciding on a destination for study. Encourage students to take an active role in planning for transition support, as well as care abroad, by disclosing all chronic mental health conditions and support needs before departure.

### Alcohol and Illicit Drugs
Use and abuse of alcohol and illicit drugs pose serious health consequences, can increase the risk of accidents and injuries, and make students potential targets for crime and incarceration. Moreover, availability and/or use of drugs by citizens of host countries may not translate to legal use by international travelers.

Although marijuana may be legal under certain US state laws, its use continues to be illegal under US federal law. US airports and airlines operate under federal jurisdiction and, as such, do not recognize the medical marijuana laws or cards of any state. Even with a US prescription for marijuana use, students found in possession of marijuana in countries outside the US where it is illegal can be arrested, fined, prosecuted, or imprisoned and deported.

### Prescription Drugs
Some drugs legally prescribed for use in the US may be illegal abroad. Travel health providers and personal physicians should review whether prescribed drugs are legal at the destination. In some instances, where a drug prescribed for use in the US is not legal at the student's intended destination, a weaning period or changing prescriptions (with enough lead time before travel to identify any adverse effects) may be appropriate medical practice.

All prescriptions carried internationally must indicate the student's name, the name of the medication (brand name *and* generic), and the dosage and quantity prescribed. Treating physicians should provide a letter explaining the student's diagnosis and the recommended treatment. Translations of documents into local languages may be helpful and in some cases, required. Instruct students to pack a copy of the physician's letter along with all medications (in their original, labeled containers) in their carry-on baggage. Some destinations may require disclosure of prescription medications when clearing customs.

Most countries prohibit arriving travelers to import quantities of medication greater than what has been prescribed for personal use. For study abroad exceeding 90 days, students should—where possible—fill prescriptions in the US that will cover them for the full duration of their time away from home. Some medications may be unavailable for sale at the destination; if available, counterfeit or poor-quality medication purchased overseas poses another potential health risk (see Chapter 6, *Perspectives*: Avoiding Poorly Regulated Medicines and Medical Products during Travel).

9

Because pharmacies in other countries do not accept prescriptions written by US providers, students who anticipate needing to refill a prescription while abroad must be prepared to schedule an appointment to visit a local doctor to obtain a valid, accepted prescription. Students need to determine before travel whether their travel insurance policy covers such appointments; insurers may consider this to be preventive care and refuse coverage.

## Safe Sex

Travel health professionals should discuss safe sex practices (condom use, birth control, and emergency contraception) and provide information about the prevalence of sexually transmitted infections and diseases at the destination. Encourage students to learn about the social customs of their host city and country with regard to dating and public displays of affection.

## Water and Extreme Sports

Drowning is a leading cause of death, both at home and away. Students should know how to swim or avoid swimming while abroad. Warn students about the risks associated with swimming in unfamiliar bodies of water without a lifeguard present. Before venturing into the water, students should ask lifeguards about any known dangers. Advise students not to go into the water while intoxicated and to always have a swimming buddy. Discuss unforeseen risks in both fresh water (schistosomiasis) and salt water (marine envenomations). Students planning participation in extreme sports (e.g., skydiving, rafting, scuba diving) should be cautioned to reconsider; at the very least, they should be knowledgeable about the risks and encouraged to obtain extreme sport coverage as part of their international travel health insurance policy.

## Emergency Contact Information Card

Students should carry their personal information and important telephone numbers at all times, both in hard copy and entered into their mobile device. A sample emergency contact card can be found at http://studentsabroad.com/handbook/emergency-card.php?country=General. Travel health professionals can assist students with special physical or mental health needs by describing in writing all health issues and recommended care; in preparing to go abroad, students should ensure that this letter gets translated accurately into the local language(s).

## DURING AND AFTER TRAVEL CONSIDERATIONS

During their time abroad, students should seek health care immediately if they become ill, injured, or have a bloodborne pathogen exposure. Students should adhere to food and water precautions (see Chapter 2, Food & Water Precautions) and use insect repellent (see Chapter 3, Mosquitoes, Ticks & Other Arthropods) to prevent vectorborne diseases.

Students who become ill after study abroad should alert health care providers about their international travel. Fever within 1 year of return from a study abroad program in students who traveled to malaria-endemic countries mandates immediate testing for the disease (see Chapter 4, Malaria). Students with new sexual partners while abroad should be tested for sexually transmitted infections and diseases, including gonorrhea, chlamydia, and HIV, if they become symptomatic while abroad, but certainly following return home.

## RESOURCES

The US Department of State has online resources to assist both students and study abroad programs with considerations and advice for study abroad travel (https://travel.state.gov/content/travel/en/international-travel/before-you-go/travelers-with-special-considerations/students.html). Additional resources for study abroad are provided in Table 9-2.

9

## Table 9-2. Online health and safety information resources for study abroad students

| ORGANIZATION | HEALTH & SAFETY INFORMATION PROVIDED |
|---|---|
| US Department of State Bureau of Consular Affairs (https://travel.state.gov/) | • Country- and region-specific guidance<br>• Travel advisories with safety and security information<br>• Crime and transportation information<br>• Travel preparation health checklist<br>• Contact information for US embassies and consulates |
| Centers for Disease Control and Prevention (wwwnc.cdc.gov/travel) | • Country-specific health information<br>• Travel notices for specific diseases in a particular destination<br>• Infectious disease directory<br>• Links to mobile app downloads |
| Center for Global Education Safety Abroad First–Educational Travel Information (SAFETI) (http://globaled.us/safeti) | • Health and safety workshops<br>• Resources for program administrators, focusing on health and safety issues<br>• Student-focused videos on health and safety issues (e.g., alcohol awareness)<br>• A-to-Z Health and Safety Issue index |
| NAFSA: Association of International Educators (www.nafsa.org) | • LGBT student advising guide and student guide to studying abroad<br>• Student health and safety guidance |
| The Forum on Education Abroad (www.forumea.org) | • Training, workshops, and webinars on mental health, academic frameworks, health, and safety |
| International Narcotics Control Board (www.incb.org) US Department of State—Overseas Security Advisory Council (www.osac.gov/pages/contentreportdetails.aspx?cid=17386) | • Traveling with medications overseas |
| Pathways to Safety International, formerly Sexual Assault Support & Help for Americans Abroad (https://pathwaystosafety.org/) | • Sexual harassment and sexual violence |

## BIBLIOGRAPHY

1. Angelin M, Evengård B, Palmgren H. Illness and risk behavior in health care students studying abroad. Med Educ. 2015;49(7):684–91.

2. Aresi G, Moore S, Marta E. Drinking, drug use, and related consequences among university students completing study abroad experiences: a systematic review. Subst Use Misuse. 2016;51(14):1888–1904.

3. Institute of International Education. U.S. students study abroad 2015/2016 data; 2017. [cited 2018 Jan 10].

Available from: www.iie.org/Research-and-Insights/Open-Doors/Data/US-Study-Abroad.

4. NAFSA: Association of International Educators. Best practices in addressing mental health issues affecting education abroad participants. Washington, DC: NAFSA: Association of International Educators; 2006. [cited 2018 Jan 17]. Available from: www.nafsa.org/mentalhealth.

# VISITING FRIENDS & RELATIVES: VFR TRAVEL

Jay S. Keystone

## DEFINITION OF VFR

A traveler categorized as a VFR is an immigrant, ethnically and racially distinct from the majority population of the country of residence (a higher-income country), who returns to his or her home country (lower-income country) to visit friends or relatives. Included in the VFR category are family members, such as the spouse or children, who were born in the country of residence. Some experts have recommended that the term VFR refer to all those visiting friends and relatives regardless of the traveler's country of origin; however, this proposed definition may be too broad and not take into consideration cultural, economic, and attitudinal issues. Therefore, this review uses the more classic definition.

## DISPROPORTIONATE INFECTIOUS DISEASE RISKS IN THE VFR TRAVELER

Altered migration patterns to North America in the past 30 years have resulted in many immigrants originating from Asia, Southeast Asia, and Latin America instead of Europe. Although 14% of the US population is foreign born, in 2016, 44% of overseas international travelers from the United States listed VFR as a reason for travel. VFRs experience a higher incidence of travel-related infectious diseases, such as malaria, typhoid fever, tuberculosis, hepatitis A, and sexually transmitted diseases, than do other groups of international travelers, for a number of reasons:

- Lack of awareness of risk

- ≤30% have a pretravel health care encounter

- Financial barriers to pretravel health care

- Lack of access to providers with travel health expertise

- Cultural and language barriers with health care providers

- Lack of trust in the medical system

- Last-minute travel plans and longer trips

- Travel to higher-risk destinations

- High-risk trip characteristics, such as staying in homes and living the local lifestyle, which often includes lack of safe food and water and not using bed nets

### Malaria

In 2014, 67% of imported malaria cases in US civilians occurred among VFRs. Data collected from GeoSentinel Global Surveillance Network clinics from 2003–2016 showed that 53% of returned travelers diagnosed with malaria were VFRs, 83% of whom acquired their disease in sub-Saharan Africa. Although malaria disproportionately affects VFRs, severe disease and death from malaria in VFRs have historically been lower than in tourist and business travelers, possibly because of some preexisting immunity or increased awareness. However, in recent years, a number of VFRs have died of malaria after returning to North America. In the United States in 2014, 51% of those with severe malaria for whom the purpose of travel was known were VFRs, mostly returning from West Africa, and in the annual US malaria surveillance reports in 2014 and 2015, 5 of 5 and 5 of 11 reported deaths, respectively, were in VFRs.

### Other Infections

From 2008 through 2012 in the United States, 85% of typhoid and 88% of paratyphoid A cases occurred in VFRs, mostly from southern Asia. Most isolates were resistant or showed decreased susceptibility to fluoroquinolone antibiotics. Similar rates of resistant infections were noted in imported cases in Switzerland from the Indian subcontinent.

VFR children aged <15 years are at highest risk for hepatitis A, and many are asymptomatic. A Canadian study found that 65% of hepatitis A cases occurred in VFRs aged <20 years, and in a Swedish study of 636 cases of imported infection, 52% were in VFRs, of whom 90% were <14 years old. Other diseases, such as tuberculosis, hepatitis B, cholera, and measles, occur more commonly in VFRs after travel.

## PRETRAVEL HEALTH COUNSELING FOR THE VFR TRAVELER

Table 9-3 summarizes VFR health risks and prevention recommendations. It is important to increase awareness among VFR travelers regarding their unique risks for travel-related infections and the barriers to travel health services. If possible,

## Table 9-3. Diseases for which VFR travelers are at increased risk, proposed reasons for risk variance, and recommendations to reduce risks[1]

| DISEASES | REASON FOR RISK VARIANCE[2] | RECOMMENDATIONS TO STRESS WITH VFR TRAVELERS |
|---|---|---|
| Foodborne and waterborne illness | Social and cultural pressure (eat meals served by hosts). | Frequent handwashing. Avoid high-risk foods (dairy products, undercooked foods) and unpurified water. Simplify treatment regimens (single dose, such as azithromycin, 1,000 mg, or ciprofloxacin, 500 mg). Discuss food preparation. |
| Fish-related toxins and infections | Eating high-risk foods. Lack of pretravel counseling. | Avoidance counseling about specific foods (such as raw freshwater fish). |
| Malaria | Longer stays. Higher-risk destinations. Less pretravel advice leading to less use of prophylaxis and fewer personal protection measures. Belief that one is already immune. | Education on malaria, mosquito avoidance, and the need for prophylaxis. Consider cost of prophylaxis. Use of insecticide-treated bed nets. |
| Tuberculosis (particularly multidrug-resistant) | Increased close contact with local population. Increased contact with HIV-coinfected people. | Check TST 2–3 months after return if history of negative tuberculin skin test and long stay (>3 months); use IGRA if history of BCG vaccination. Educate about tuberculosis signs, symptoms, and avoidance. |
| Bloodborne and sexually transmitted infections | More likely to seek substandard local care. Cultural practices (tattoos, body modification practices). Longer stays and increased chance of blood transfusion. Higher likelihood of sexual encounters with local population. | Discuss high-risk behaviors, including tattoos, piercings, dental work, sexual encounters. Encourage purchase of condoms before travel. Consider providing syringes, needles for needed medications for long-term travel. Recommend hepatitis B immunization if nonimmune. |

9

## Table 9-3. Diseases for which VFR travelers are at increased risk, proposed reasons for risk variance, and recommendations to reduce risks[1] (continued)

| DISEASES | REASON FOR RISK VARIANCE[2] | RECOMMENDATIONS TO STRESS WITH VFR TRAVELERS |
|---|---|---|
| Schistosomiasis and soil-transmitted helminths | Limited access to piped-in water in rural areas for bathing and washing clothes. | Avoid freshwater exposure. Towel off quickly and use liposomal DEET preparation with freshwater exposures.[3] Discourage children from playing in dirt. Use ground cover. Use protective footwear. |
| Respiratory problems | Increased close exposure to fires, smoking, or pollution. | Prepare for asthma exacerbations by considering stand-by .bronchodilators and steroids. |
| Zoonotic diseases (such as rickettsial infections, leptospirosis, viral fevers, leishmaniasis, anthrax, Chagas disease) | Rural destinations. Staying with family where animals are kept. Increased exposure to insects. Increased exposure to rodents (mice and rats). Sleeping on floors. | Avoid animal contact. Wash hands. Wear protective clothing and use insect repellent. Check for ticks daily. Avoid thatched roofs and mud walled accommodations and fresh sugar cane juice in Latin America. Avoid sleeping at floor level. |
| Envenomation (snakes, spiders, scorpions) | Sleeping on floors. | Avoid sleeping at floor level. Wear protective footwear outdoors at night. |
| Toxin ingestion (medication adverse events, heavy metal ingestion) | Purchase of local medications. Use of traditional therapies. Use of contaminated products (such as pottery with lead glaze). Eating contaminated freshwater fish. | Anticipate need and purchase medications before travel. Counsel avoidance of known traditional medications (such as Hmong bark tea with aspirin) and high-risk items (such as large reef fish). |
| Yellow fever and Japanese encephalitis | Unclear, partial immunity from previous exposure or vaccination. | Avoid mosquitoes by taking protective measures and receiving vaccination when appropriate. |
| Dengue (especially risk of severe dengue) | Severe dengue occurs on repeat exposure to a different serotype of dengue; VFRs more likely to have had previous exposure. | Avoid mosquitoes by taking protective measures. |

Abbreviations: VFR, visiting friends and relatives; TST, tuberculin skin test; DEET, *N,N*-diethyl-*m*-toluamide.
[1] Adapted from: Bacaner N, Stauffer W, Boulware DR, Walker PF, Keystone JS. Travel medicine considerations for North American immigrants visiting friends and relatives. JAMA. 2004;291(23):2856–64.
[2] Hypothetical unless referenced to support assertions.
[3] In animal models, DEET (liposomal preparations) prevents *Schistosoma* cercariae from penetrating the skin.

9

clinics should provide culturally sensitive educational materials (in multiple languages) and have language translators available. However, studies in the United Kingdom aimed at preventing malaria among VFRs showed that increased awareness and availability of medications do not necessarily increase use of malaria chemoprophylaxis, highlighting the complex socioecological context in which VFRs make travel health decisions.

## Vaccinations

Travel immunization recommendations and requirements for VFRs are the same as those for US-born travelers. It is crucial, however, to first try to establish whether the immigrant traveler has had routine immunizations (such as measles and tetanus/diphtheria) or has a history of specific diseases. Adult travelers, in the absence of documentation of immunizations, may be considered susceptible. Age-appropriate vaccinations (or serologic studies to check for antibody status) should be provided, with 2 caveats:

- Immunity to hepatitis A should not be assumed; many young adults and adolescents from developing countries are still susceptible.

- Consider varicella immunization for people born outside the United States. Such travelers may be more susceptible because infection occurs at an older age in tropical than in temperate regions. Also, rates of death and complications from varicella disease are higher in adults than in children.

## Malaria Prevention

VFR travelers to endemic areas should not only be encouraged to take prophylactic medications but also should be reminded of the benefits of barrier methods of prevention, such as bed nets and insect repellents, particularly for children (see Chapter 3, Mosquitoes, Ticks & Other Arthropods). VFRs should be advised that drugs such as chloroquine and pyrimethamine, as well as proguanil monotherapy, are no longer effective in most areas, especially in sub-Saharan Africa. These medications are often readily available and inexpensive in their home countries but are not efficacious.

Encourage VFRs to purchase their medications before traveling to ensure good drug quality. Studies in Africa and Southeast Asia show that one-third to one-half of antimalarial drugs purchased locally are counterfeit or substandard.

## HEADING HOME HEALTHY

The CDC-supported Heading Home Healthy program (www.HeadingHomeHealthy.org) is focused on reducing travel-related illnesses in VFR travelers. The program contains videos, informational resources, and health tools in multiple languages and was developed to assist not only VFR travelers but also their primary care health providers.

BIBLIOGRAPHY

1. Angelo KM, Libman M, Caumes E, Hamer DH, Kain KC, Leder K, et al. Malaria after international travel: a GeoSentinel analysis, 2003–2016. Malar J. 2017 Jul 20;16(1):293.

2. Behrens RH, Neave PE, Jones CO. Imported malaria among people who travel to visit friends and relatives: is current UK policy effective or does it need a strategic change? Malar J. 2015;14:149.

3. Chaccour C, Kaur H, Del Pozo JL. Falsified antimalarials: a minireview. Expert review of anti-infective therapy. 2015 Apr;13(4):505–9.

4. Date KA, Newton AE, Medalla F, Blackstock A, Richardson L, McCullough A, et al. Changing patterns in enteric fever incidence and increasing antibiotic resistance of enteric fever isolates in the United States, 2008–2012. Clin Infect Dis. 2016 Aug 1;63(3):322–9.

5. Hendel-Paterson B, Swanson SJ. Pediatric travelers visiting friends and relatives (VFR) abroad: illnesses, barriers and pre-travel recommendations. Travel Med Infect Dis. 2011 Jul;9(4):192–203.

6. LaRocque RC, Deshpande BR, Rao SR, Brunette GW, Sotir MJ, Jentes ES, et al. Pre-travel health care of immigrants returning home to visit friends and relatives. Am J Trop Med Hyg. 2013 Feb;88(2): 376–80.

7. Leder K, Tong S, Weld L, Kain KC, Wilder-Smith A, von Sonnenburg F, et al. Illness in travelers visiting friends and relatives: a review of the GeoSentinel Surveillance Network. Clin Infect Dis. 2006 Nov 1;43(9):1185–93.

8. Monge-Maillo B, Norman FF, Perez-Molina JA, Navarro M, Diaz-Menendez M, Lopez-Velez R. Travelers visiting friends and relatives (VFR) and imported infectious disease: travelers, immigrants or both? A comparative analysis. Travel Med Infect Dis. 2014 Jan–Feb;12(1):88–94.

# TRAVEL TO MASS GATHERINGS

Joanna Gaines, Gary W. Brunette

## OVERVIEW

Mass gatherings are typically defined as large numbers of people (1,000 to >25,000) at a specific location, for a specific purpose. More practically speaking, a mass gathering can be thought of as any assembly of people large enough to strain local resources. Travelers to mass gatherings face unique risks because these events are associated with environmental hazards, increased infectious disease transmission due to the influx of attendees, crowding, poor hygiene from temporary food and sanitation facilities, and challenging security situations.

## CHARACTERISTICS OF MASS GATHERINGS

Medical providers preparing travelers for international travel and travelers themselves should understand the characteristics of mass gatherings. Some can be spontaneous, such as political protests; others are planned events. Some mass gatherings regularly occur at different locations, (the Olympic Games or the FIFA World Cup, for example) while others recur in the same location, such as the Hajj or Wimbledon. Table 9-4 provides a representative (albeit not comprehensive) list of scheduled, upcoming mass gatherings, including type (religious observance, sporting event, art and music festival), location, dates, and anticipated numbers of attendees.

Mass gatherings can be described effectively in terms of their location, venue, purpose, size, participants, duration, timing, activities, and capacity.

- **Location:** Factors to consider include the host country, available infrastructure, the local environment, and the adequacy of security arrangements.

- **Venue:** Facilities vary widely, and events may be held indoors or outdoors. Food, water, and sanitation, may be of varying quality.

- **Purpose:** Mass gatherings can be political, religious, social, or athletic; the purpose of an event can affect the activities and mood of participants.

- **Size:** The density of crowds at a mass gathering, rather than just the specific number of attendees, can further increase health risks. More densely packed crowds can facilitate disease spread or induce riots or crowd crush disasters.

- **Participants:** Attendees may represent a unique demographic, such as a religious or political group, or may vary by features such as sex or age ( for example, older adults attempting to complete a religious pilgrimage toward the end of their life).

- **Duration:** The longer an event lasts, the more likely it is that local resources will be depleted and become strained.

- **Timing:** Mass gatherings and local capacity are affected by the timing of an event. Weather, heavy tourism, and other factors can affect the ability of a host to organize a safe mass gathering.

- **Activities:** Understand the activities involved at the mass gathering. Some may be risky or strenuous (e.g., walking a long way in extreme temperatures) or may involve alcohol or drug use.

- **Capacity:** Hosts differ in terms of their ability to detect, respond to, and prevent public health emergencies. Understanding what health outcomes have been previously associated with recurring mass gatherings can help travelers prepare for future events.

9

## Table 9-4. International mass gathering events, 2019–2022

| EVENT TYPE | EVENT NAME | LOCATION | UPCOMING DATES | PROJECTED ATTENDANCE |
|---|---|---|---|---|
| Religious events | Kumbh Mela | Multiple locations in India: Allahbad, Haridwar, Madhya Pradesh, Maharashtra | 2019 in Allahbad 2022 in Haridwar | 40 million |
| | Arba'een Pilgrimage | Karbala, Iraq | October 2019 | 22 million |
| | Grand Magal of Touba | Touba, Senegal | October 2019 | 3 million |
| | Hajj | Mecca, Saudi Arabia | August 10, 2019 July 30, 2020 | 2.5 million |
| | Iztapalapa Passion Play | Mexico City, Mexico | Good Friday (annually) | 2 million |
| | Urs of Fariduddin Ganjshakar | Pakpattan, Pakistan | September 2019 | 500,000 |
| Sporting events | 2020 Summer Olympics | Tokyo, Japan | July 24–August 9, 2020 | 7.5 million |
| | FIFA World Cup | Qatar | November 21–December 18, 2022 | 3 million |
| | 2022 Winter Olympics | Beijing, China | February 4–20, 2022 | 1 million |
| Art and music festivals | Edinburgh Festival Fringe | Edinburgh, Scotland | August 2–26, 2019 | 2.5 million |
| | Street Parade | Zurich, Switzerland | 2nd Saturday in August | 1 million |

## HEALTH CONCERNS RELATED TO MASS GATHERINGS

Attendance at a mass gathering can exacerbate a traveler's existing medical conditions. Emergency medical services are often involved in preparations and are usually equipped to address acute medical conditions such as myocardial infarction and asthma. Planners usually handle conditions such as heat exhaustion, dehydration, hypothermia, or sunburn on site, as well.

Catastrophic incidents are of particular concern with mass gatherings, particularly with extremely dense crowds of people. Numerous casualties at mass gatherings have occurred as the result of poor crowd management, structural collapses, fires, and violence. Serious crush injuries and death can result from crowding and stampedes. In 2013, dozens of religious pilgrims were killed in India during a stampede at Kumbh Mela, the world's largest mass gathering. Thousands of pilgrims were killed in a stampede at the 2015 Hajj pilgrimage in Saudi Arabia.

Personal safety during mass gatherings is important. Although the risk for large-scale incidents

9

such as terror attacks are low, they are impossible to predict or eliminate. Travelers should be aware of their surroundings. More information is available in Chapter 3, Safety & Security Overseas.

Mass gathering attendees also are at risk for infections. Previous mass gatherings have been associated with outbreaks of influenza, meningococcal disease, and norovirus. Mass gatherings also have implications for global health security. Travelers to mass gatherings may import diseases to a host site as well as spread acquired diseases when they return home. An example was the emergence of Zika virus in 2015 in Brazil shortly before the Olympics and Paralympic Games. Visiting athletes and attendees to the Games were at risk for infection with Zika virus while attending the Games, as well as potentially exporting Zika virus to their home countries. This also posed a significant challenge to travel medicine providers, as little was known at that time about the timeline for risk to people of reproductive age.

## GUIDANCE FOR CLINICIANS

### Assessing Risk

- **Ask travelers about their itineraries and activities.** Verify a traveler's itinerary to identify risks beyond those associated with the event itself. Patients may add side trips or extend travel beyond the mass gathering.

- **Consider your patient's unique characteristics.** Chronic health conditions may be exacerbated by participation in a mass gathering. Counsel patients on the importance of having adequate supplies of medication for the duration of their trip as well as documentation for any prescriptions.

### Mitigating Risk

- **Identify requirements** for mass gathering attendees beyond those required for entry to a country. For example, all participants in the Hajj, the Islamic pilgrimage to Mecca, require vaccination against meningococcal disease, whereas other travelers to Saudi Arabia do not.

- **Identify recommendations** for attendees, as host sites may make additional

recommendations based on public health concerns. After the emergence of the Middle East Respiratory Syndrome (MERS) coronavirus, Saudi Arabia recommended that elderly or immunocompromised people delay their pilgrimage.

- **Educate travelers on preventive measures.** These may include things such as the regular use of insect repellent or advice on how to choose safe food and water from vendors. Educate all travelers on the importance of regular handwashing with soap and water and the use of alcohol-based sanitizer when sanitation facilities are not available.

- **Visit the CDC Travelers' Health website at** www.cdc.gov/travel. CDC regularly updates its website with travel health notices and notifications to the public of disease outbreaks in countries around the world; information may also be provided on mass gatherings such as the Hajj or Olympic Games.

## GUIDANCE FOR TRAVELERS

- **Consult a travel medicine provider at least 4–6 weeks before the departure date.** This should allow adequate time to receive most vaccinations. Discuss your itinerary and any planned activities with your provider so that he or she can make more accurate recommendations to ensure your health and safety. If a travel medicine provider is not locally available, a primary care provider should be able to assist you with ensuring you have the adequate vaccinations and health information necessary.

- **Register with the Department of State's Smart Traveler Enrollment Program (STEP, https://step.state.gov/step).** Subscribe for notifications on travel warnings, travel alerts, and other information for your specific destination(s), as well as ensure that the Department of State is aware of a your presence in the event of serious legal, medical, or financial difficulties while traveling. In the event of an emergency at home,

9

STEP can also help friends and family reach you abroad.

- **Ensure any existing medical conditions are well controlled before departure.** Discuss your medical history with your medical provider during your pretravel consultation, and ensure you have an adequate supply of any prescription medications you take regularly, prior to departure.

- **Visit the CDC Travelers' Health website at** www.cdc.gov/travel. Learn more about specific destinations and view any travel notices for your destination.

## BIBLIOGRAPHY

1. Abubakar I, Gautret P, Brunette GW, Blumberg L, Johnson D, Poumerol G, et al. Global perspectives for prevention of infectious diseases associated with mass gatherings. Lancet Infect Dis. 2012 Jan;12(1):66–74.

2. Arbon P. Mass-gathering medicine: a review of the evidence and future directions for research. Prehosp Disaster Med. 2007 Mar–Apr;22(2):131–5.

3. Emergency Management Australia. Safe and healthy mass gatherings: a health, medical and safety planning manual for public events. Fyshwick (Australia): Commonwealth of Australia; 1999 [cited 2016 Sep 28]. Available from: www.health.sa.gov.au/pehs/publications/ema-mass-gatheringsmanual.pdf.

4. Lombardo JS, Sniegoski CA, Loschen WA, Westercamp M, Wade M, Dearth S, et al. Public health surveillance for mass gatherings. Johns Hopkins APL Tech Dig. 2008;27(4):1–9.

5. McCloskey B, Endericks T. Learning from London 2012: a practical guide to public health and mass gatherings. London: Public Health England; 2013 [cited 2018 Oct 24]. Available from: http://webarchive.nationalarchives.gov.uk/20140714102440/http://www.hpa.org.uk/webc/HPAwebFile/HPAweb_C/1317138422305.

6. Milsten AM, Maguire BJ, Bissell RA, Seaman KG. Mass-gathering medical care: a review of the literature. Prehosp Disaster Med. 2002 Jul–Sep;17(3):151–62.

7. Steffen R, Bouchama A, Johansson A, Dvorak J, Isla N, Smallwood C, et al. Non-communicable health risks during mass gatherings. Lancet Infect Dis. 2012 Feb;12(2):142–9.

8. World Health Organization. Communicable disease alert and response for mass gatherings: key considerations. Geneva: World Health Organization; 2008 [cited 2016 Sep 28]. Available from: www.who.int/csr/Mass_gatherings2.pdf.

# ADVENTURE TRAVEL

9

Christopher Van Tilburg

Adventure travel is unique because of the challenging terrain, extreme weather, remote locales, and long durations involved. Popular destinations include trekking to Everest Base Camp, climbing Mount Kilimanjaro, hiking the Inca Trail, sailing the South Pacific, touring the Galapagos, and exploring the North and South poles. Adventure travel often includes mountaineering, backpacking, cycling, skiing, diving, surfing, and river rafting. Travelers may be working, providing humanitarian relief, or completing scientific research; they may be part of expeditions climbing mountains or driving overland.

Risk of injury and illness associated with adventure travel is increased significantly compared to other types of travel for several reasons:

- Destinations may be remote and lack access to care.

- Communication is often limited.

- Weather, climate, and terrain can be extreme.

- Travelers exert themselves physically, increasing caloric, fluid, and sleep requirements.

- Trips are often long, lasting: several weeks, months, or years.

- Trips are often goal oriented, which can cause travelers to exceed safety limits and take increased risk.

Risk usually involves 2 components: probability and consequence. The probability of a mishap occurring is based on frequency, duration, and severity of exposure to hazards. Hazards are categorized as objective—omnipresent natural hazards like weather and terrain—and subjective—human-controlled hazards like lack of sleep, poor nutrition, and dehydration. All 3 components of probability (frequency, duration, and severity) are increased in adventure travel.

The second component of risk, consequence, is the outcome of an accident. Consequence of an accident or illness is nearly always greater in adventure travel with increased distance to help and austere conditions. Therefore, travelers should know that even if the probability of a mishap is low, the consequence is almost always increased. Even a minor injury or illness in the wrong setting can be disastrous.

In addition, major accidents are rarely due to a single event; usually multiple events occur in sequence preceding an accident. Travelers should have heightened awareness of the probability and consequence of risk and try to make good decisions before they get into trouble.

## PRETRAVEL CONSIDERATIONS

In addition to routine travel medicine advice, providers should gather extra information and discuss precautions for wilderness and expedition travel.

## Trip Type

Obtain details about the type, length, and remoteness of the trip. Guided trips may eliminate some of the need for complex logistics planning on the part of the traveler. However, participants in guided trips should ask key questions of the trip organizers including:

- Guide experience and medical training.

- Type of medical kit and safety equipment carried by guides.

- Contingency plan for emergencies.

- Recommended medications and medical supplies to be carried by participants.

- Type of insurance recommended.

In a few cases, such as polar cruises and Mount Everest expeditions, a formal medical officer with a comprehensive medical kit may be available. For self-planned trips, the travel medicine practitioner may need to augment a comprehensive medical kit with prescription medication and offer more support with logistics, evacuation planning, and insurance.

Confirm if the skill level of the participant matches the trip type. Beginners in an activity such as diving, mountaineering, skiing, or sailing should participate in instructional trips. Those with less experience or visiting a location for the first time should be encouraged to go on a guided trip. Since most people will consult a travel medicine professional only after they have selected and paid for their adventure, they may need assistance in changing the trip to be more in line with their skill and experience.

## Personal Health Requirements

Adequate nutrition, hydration, and sleep may be in short supply, especially with increased demand because of weather, terrain, and exertion. Travelers should pay attention during the planning stages to how food and water will be obtained on the journey.

Screen travelers for conditions that can be exacerbated by high altitude, extreme heat, extreme cold, exertion, and other environmental hazards. These include diabetes, asthma, any cardiac disease, chronic pain treated with opiates, recent surgery, anaphylaxis-level allergy, oxygen-dependent emphysema, joint replacement, and sleep apnea. Caution travelers who have battery-operated devices, such as a continuous positive airway pressure machine or an insulin pump, about device failure, and discuss the need for a backup plan. A past history of environmental illness—altitude illness, hypothermia, frostbite, heat exhaustion, or anaphylaxis—likely puts one at increased risk for recurrence.

9

Travelers with chronic or major medical issues should carry a medication list, a copy of their most recent ECG and chest x-ray, and their medical history on their phone in PDF or JPG format.

Medical clearance for participation may be required for a guided trip. The traveler's primary care provider should complete medical clearance for those with chronic disease. Travel health practitioners can complete pretravel medical clearance if it is a usual function of their practice and the patient has no chronic disease or medications. If possible, travelers should get medications for chronic illness from their primary care provider.

## Money and Insurance

Rescue, evacuation, and repatriation may require upfront payment, especially with aeromedical transport from remote locations. Travelers should bring sufficient emergency cash and a credit card with high credit and cash advance limits.

Insurance is widely variable and comes in many forms, but insurance does not guarantee rescue (see Chapter 6, Travel Insurance, Travel Health Insurance & Medical Evacuation Insurance). Coverage may be contingent on preexisting conditions, deductibles, maximum expenditures, and medical control approval. Insurers may also not authorize aeromedical transport. Insurance companies may deny claims involving chronic illness, drugs, alcohol, pregnancy, mental health, and acts of war or civil unrest. Travelers should read policies carefully before purchasing and departing on their trip.

Types of insurance include:

- Domestic health insurance, which may or may not be effective outside a home country. Often, travelers need to pay up front for medical care and get reimbursed from health insurance once they return home.

- Travel insurance, which often includes medical, trip cancellation, evacuation, and repatriation benefits, but may exclude coverage for wilderness rescue and adventure sports like mountaineering, skiing, and diving. An adventure sports rider is available with some travel insurance policies.

- Wilderness rescue insurance (usually separate from travel insurance), such as policies through North American mountaineering clubs, outdoor and professional associations, and scuba dive organizations. Short-term rescue insurance is available in some destination countries, for example, through local helicopter rescue companies, ski resorts, and mountaineering clubs.

- Comprehensive expedition policies, which can include travel, medical, rescue, security, and repatriation services.

## Training

If travelers have time, they should consider completing a first aid and basic life support course (CPR) before departure. This may be particularly helpful for regular adventure travelers. Such courses can be found through local community colleges and fire departments.

## Emergency Resources

Before they go, travelers should know emergency escape routes, local rescue resources, embassy contacts, and local medical facilities.

If travel medicine practitioners are willing to accept phone calls, emails, and text messages from travelers abroad, make sure travelers understand this is not a substitute for local emergency care.

Travelers should keep their passport, money, credit card, and other documents on their person at all times, as they may need to seek medical care or evacuate urgently and without their luggage. Backup copies can be stored in PDF or JPG on a phone.

In a travel medicine encounter, physicians may only have a brief moment to educate travelers. Depending on the type, duration, and location of trip, a few key pearls may be worth discussing:

- Travelers should understand basic wound care, seek help with signs of infection—redness, swelling, pus, and warmth—and be educated on self-treatment with antibiotics.

- For hypothermia, cessation of shivering and mental status changes are dangerous signs.

9

- Frostbite is treated with rapid rewarming, but people with frozen extremities should be careful not to refreeze a thawed extremity (see Chapter 3, Extremes of Temperature).

- Heat stroke marked by a temperature of 40°C and mental status changes is a medical emergency.

- Snakes, spiders, scorpions, ticks, and jellyfish can deliver toxic venom, inoculate microbes, and cause anaphylaxis. Region-specific antivenoms may be found around the world for certain venomous snakes, spiders, scorpions, and jellyfish.

- Bites, stings, food, and other allergens can all cause anaphylaxis. Treatment with epinephrine and corticosteroids can be lifesaving if administered immediately.

- Travel to high altitude may require acetazolamide, dexamethasone, and other medications to prevent or treat altitude illness. Mental status changes and ataxia are ominous signs of high-altitude cerebral edema. Breathlessness at rest is the sign of life-threatening high-altitude pulmonary edema.

## WILDERNESS SUPPLIES

Travelers should pack and keep basic emergency supplies and equipment with them at all times.

### Communication and Route Finding

Travelers should carry a cell phone enabled with global positioning system (GPS), such as a smart phone. Phones can be used to store documents, including plane tickets, embassy and hospital contact information, insurance, passport copies, and medical data in email, JPG, or PDF format. Importantly, not all North American cell phones and service plans are compatible with international networks. Travelers should check with their cell carrier before departing.

Alternatively, an unlocked (not restricted to any carrier) global-compatible cell phone can be used with a local SIM card in the country of travel. Phones and SIM cards are usually available at stores in major cities and airports. In some countries, registration to obtain a local SIM card requires fingerprinting and a passport picture.

Where cell phone service is not available, travelers may consider an unlocked (no frequency restrictions) VHF/UHF radio or a satellite phone. Advise travelers that restrictions exist, and permits are required in many countries regarding use of handheld radios and satellite phones; they should check local restrictions prior to departing.

Remind travelers that electronics are not foolproof; often they are limited by battery power, dense cloud cover, deep canyons, government restrictions, and physical damage caused by impact, water, or extreme temperatures. A backup power pack and external power source, such as a solar or dynamo charger, is useful.

For extreme terrain and remote locations, adventurers should carry and know how to use a GPS unit (or have a GPS app installed on their phone), compass, altimeter, and local topographic map (the latter may need to be acquired in-country).

### Clothing

Remind travelers that clothing helps prevent heat and cold illness as well as bites and stings from insects and arthropods.

Cold weather clothing should be polyester, nylon, Merino wool, or, in some circumstances, down. Layering typically consists of a base layer, insulating layers of heavy-pile polyester or nylon-encased polyester (down suffices if traveling to a location that is dry and cold), and a windproof, waterproof outer layer of tightly woven nylon with a durable water-repellent coating. Gloves, hat, neck warmer, warm socks, and goggles are vital to cover all exposed skin.

For hot weather, sun- and insect-protective clothing is important including loose-fitting, lightweight clothing made from nylon, polyester, or a cotton blend. Long-sleeve shirts and long pants offer the most protection. A wide brim sun hat and a bandana protect the head and neck. Sunglasses protect eyes. Clothing should be sprayed with permethrin to ward off insects and arthropods.

Footwear should be activity-specific boots or shoes, equally important in a marine or mountain environment. Advise travelers to never go without footwear, as even a minor foot injury can be debilitating.

## Emergency Kits

Adventure travelers often require a comprehensive, yet compact, personal emergency kit for survival, medical care, and equipment repair. In addition to a basic travel health kit (see Chapter 6, Travel Health Kits), travelers should consider packing additional items due to the remote nature of their travel. Standard kits may need to be augmented for specific activities like undersea, open ocean, jungle, polar, and high-elevation travel.

If travelers are on guided trips, they may only need a small personal medical kit. Before they depart, travelers should determine whether guides provide group emergency equipment such as an automatic external defibrillator, a portable stretcher, portable hyperbaric chamber, oxygen, and comprehensive medical kit.

Be cautious if asked to prescribe medications for guides to stock in the expedition medical kit intended for clients. Third-party use of prescription medication is unlawful in most jurisdictions and best left for the guide company medical director. If prescribing to a guide as a patient, clarify that the medication is for the guide's personal use.

### MEDICATIONS

Consider prescribing anaphylaxis, antibiotic, and analgesic medications in addition to routine travel medications. Instruct travelers on self-treatment of anaphylaxis, as this can be lifesaving, and provide guidance on self-treatment for gastroenteritis, febrile illness, wound infections, and respiratory illness. Consider opioid and prescription NSAID pain medication, bearing in mind that in some countries, travelers may be restricted from bringing in opioid drugs, even for their own use. In addition, consider prescribing ophthalmologic antibiotics and anesthetic, antiemetic/motion sickness medication, nonsedating antihistamines, and altitude illness medicines.

### SAFETY SUPPLIES

Adventure travelers should consider packing additional safety equipment to supplement a travel health kit. These items can help in an emergency situation.

- Spare phone power pack or solar/dynamo charger
- Headlight with extra batteries
- Map, compass, GPS (or GPS app on phone)
- Perlon cord
- Emergency sleeping sack or tarp
- Earplugs and eyeshade
- Sun hat, bandana, and sunglasses
- Spare eyeglasses (if required)
- Duct tape
- Multi-tool
- Safety pins
- Polyurethane straps and plastic cable ties
- Chemical heat packs
- Whistle
- Water purification tablets
- Sunscreen and lip balm
- Oral rehydration powder
- Insect repellent
- Rain poncho and umbrella
- Hand sanitizer
- Toilet paper
- Antibacterial towelette
- Sewing kit
- Laundry detergent

### BIBLIOGRAPHY

1. Iserson KV. Medical planning for extended remote expeditions. Wilderness Environ Med. 2013 Dec;24(4):366–77.

2. Lipman GS, Eifling KP, Ellis MA, Gaudio FG, Otten EM, Grissom CK. Wilderness Medical Society practice guidelines for the prevention and treatment of

9

heat-related illness: 2014 update. Wilderness Environ Med. 2014 Dec;25(4 Suppl):S55–65.

3. Lipnick MS, Lewin M. Wilderness preparation, equipment, and medical supplies. In: Auerbach PS, editor. Auerbach's Wilderness Medicine. 7th ed. Philadelphia: Elsevier; 2017. pp. 2272–305.

4. McIntosh SE, Opacic M, Freer L, Grissom CK, Auerbach PS, Rodway GW, et al. Wilderness Medical Society practice guidelines for the prevention and treatment of frostbite: 2014 update. Wilderness Environ Med. 2014 Dec;25(4 Suppl):S43–54.

5. Mellor A, Dodds N, Joshi R, Hall J, Dhillon S, Hollis S, et al. Faculty of Prehospital Care, Royal College of Surgeons Edinburgh guidance for medical provision for wilderness medicine. Extrem Physiol Med. 2015;4:22.

6. Quinn RH, Wedmore I, Johnson EL, Islas AA, Anglim A, Zafren K, et al. Wilderness Medical Society practice guidelines for basic wound management in the austere environment: 2014 update. Wilderness Environ Med. 2014 Dec;25(4 Suppl):S118–33.

7. Zafren K, Giesbrecht GG, Danzl DF, Brugger H, Sagalyn EB, Walpoth B, et al. Wilderness Medical Society practice guidelines for the out-of-hospital evaluation and treatment of accidental hypothermia: 2014 update. Wilderness Environ Med. 2014 Dec;25(4 Suppl):S66–85.

# MEDICAL TOURISM

Isaac Benowitz, Joanna Gaines

Medical tourism is the term commonly used to describe international travel for the purpose of receiving medical care. Medical tourists may pursue medical care abroad for a variety of reasons, such as decreased cost, a recommendation from friends or family, the opportunity to combine medical care with a vacation destination, a preference for care from providers who share the traveler's culture, or to receive a procedure or therapy not available in their country of residence. Medical tourism is a worldwide, multibillion-dollar market that continues to grow. Surveillance data indicate that millions of US residents travel internationally for medical care each year. Ongoing reports of infections and other adverse events following medical or dental procedures abroad serve as reminders that medical tourism is not without risks.

Common categories of procedures that US medical tourists pursue include dental care, noncosmetic surgery (such as orthopedic surgery), cosmetic surgery, fertility treatments, organ and tissue transplantation, and cancer treatment. Medical tourism destinations for US residents include Argentina, Brazil, Costa Rica, Cuba, India, Malaysia, Mexico, Singapore, and Thailand. When reviewing the risks associated with medical tourism, travelers should consider both the procedure and destination.

Overseas facilities may not maintain accreditation or provider licensure, track patient outcome data, or maintain formal medical record privacy or security policies. Medical tourists should also be aware that the drugs and medical products and devices used in foreign countries might not be subject to the same regulatory scrutiny and oversight as in the United States. In addition, some drugs may be counterfeit or otherwise ineffective (for example, expired, contaminated, or improperly stored).

Most medical tourists pay for their care at time of service and often rely on private companies or medical concierge services to identify foreign health care facilities. Some US health insurance companies and large employers have formed alliances with health care facilities outside the United States to control costs.

## RISKS ASSOCIATED WITH MEDICAL TOURISM

All medical and surgical procedures carry some risk, and complications can occur regardless of where treatment is received. Possible infectious complications associated with medical procedures performed outside the United States include wound infections, bloodstream infections, donor-derived infections, and acquisition of bloodborne pathogens, including hepatitis B, hepatitis C, and HIV. The risk of acquiring antibiotic-resistant infections may be increased in certain countries or regions; some highly resistant pathogens (such as carbapenem-resistant Enterobacteriaceae) appear to be more common in some countries where US residents go for medical tourism (see Chapter 11, Antimicrobial Resistance).

Several outbreaks of infectious disease among medical tourists have been documented. Recent examples include surgical site infections caused by nontuberculous mycobacteria in patients who underwent cosmetic surgery in the Dominican Republic and Q fever in patients who received fetal sheep cell injections in Germany. Noninfectious complications among medical tourists are similar to those seen in patients who receive medical care in the United States and include surgical incision dehiscence, blood clots, or contour abnormalities after cosmetic surgery.

Medical or surgical complications may require follow-up care from a health care provider in the United States. Medical tourists should request a copy of their medical records and provide these to health care providers for any follow-up care.

Medical tourists should be aware of the additional risks associated with traveling while being treated for a medical condition or during recovery after surgery or other procedure. Air travel and surgery independently increase the risk of blood clots, including deep vein thrombosis and pulmonary emboli; travel and surgery together further increase the risks. Commercial aircraft cabin pressures are roughly equivalent to an outside air pressure at 6,000–8,000 ft. above sea level. Medical tourists should not fly for 10 days after chest or abdominal surgery to avoid risks associated with changes in atmospheric pressure.

Furthermore, the American Society of Plastic Surgeons advises people who have had cosmetic procedures of the face, eyelids, or nose, or who have had laser treatments, to wait 7–10 days before flying. The Aerospace Medical Association has published medical guidelines for airline travel that provide useful information on the risks of travel with certain medical conditions (www.asma.org/asma/media/asma/Travel-Publications/paxguidelines.pdf). Medical tourists are also advised to avoid typical vacation activities that can interfere with healing such as sunbathing, drinking alcohol, swimming, taking long tours, or engaging in strenuous activities or exercise after surgery.

## PRETRAVEL ADVICE FOR MEDICAL TOURISTS

Medical tourists should consult a travel medicine specialist for advice tailored to their specific health needs, preferably 4–6 weeks before travel. Medical tourists should also communicate with their primary care provider to discuss their plan to seek medical care outside the United States and to discuss any concerns they or their provider might have. Any current medical conditions should be well controlled, and medical tourists should make sure they have enough medication for the duration of their trip. All medical tourists should be up-to-date on all routine vaccinations and consider immunization against hepatitis B virus before travel.

Advise medical tourists to seek prompt medical care, while still traveling or after returning home, if they suspect any complication. Encourage them to disclose information about travel history, medical history, and recent surgeries or medical treatments received during their trip. Seeking prompt medical care may lead to early diagnosis and treatment and a better outcome.

## GUIDANCE FOR TRAVELERS PLANNING MEDICAL CARE ABROAD

Several professional organizations have developed guidance that includes template questions that medical tourists can use when discussing care abroad, with the facility providing the care, with the group facilitating the trip, and with their regular health care provider. Medical tourists should be aware of the guiding principles developed by the American Medical Association (Box 9-3). The American College of Surgeons (ACS) issued a similar statement on medical and surgical tourism, with the additional

The American Medical Association advocates that employers, insurance companies, and other entities that facilitate or incentivize medical care outside the United States adhere to the following principles:

a. Medical care outside the United States must be voluntary.

b. Financial incentives to travel outside the United States for medical care should not inappropriately limit the diagnostic and therapeutic alternatives that are offered to patients, or restrict treatment or referral options.

c. Patients should only be referred for medical care to institutions that have been accredited by recognized international accrediting bodies (such as the Joint Commission International or the International Society for Quality in Health Care).

d. Prior to travel, local follow-up care should be coordinated and financing should be arranged to ensure continuity of care when patients return from medical care outside the United States.

e. Coverage for travel outside the United States for medical care must include the costs of necessary follow-up care upon return to the United States.

f. Patients should be informed of their rights and legal recourse before agreeing to travel outside the United States for medical care.

g. Access to physician licensing and outcome data, as well as facility accreditation and outcomes data, should be arranged for patients seeking medical care outside the United States.

h. The transfer of patient medical records to and from facilities outside the United States should be consistent with Health Insurance Portability and Accountability Action (HIPAA) guidelines.

i. Patients choosing to travel outside the United States for medical care should be provided with information about the potential risks of combining surgical procedures with long flights and vacation activities.

From American Medical Association (AMA). New AMA Guidelines on Medical Tourism. Chicago: AMA; 2008. Available from: www.medretreat.com/templates/UserFiles/Documents/Whitepapers/AMAGuidelines.pdf

recommendation that travelers obtain a complete set of medical records before returning home to ensure that details of their care are available to providers in the United States. This helps facilitate continuity of care and proper follow-up, if needed.

Local standards for facility accreditation and provider certification vary and may not be the same as US standards. ACS recommends that medical tourists use internationally accredited facilities and seek care from providers certified in their specialties through a process equivalent to that established by the member boards of the American Board of Medical Specialties. ACS, the American Society for Aesthetic Plastic Surgery, the American Society of Plastic Surgeons, and the International Society of Aesthetic Plastic Surgery all accredit overseas physicians. However, accreditation does not necessarily ensure a good outcome, and medical tourists should be encouraged to do as much advance research as possible on a health care provider and facility they are considering using.

Many medical tourism websites market directly to travelers. These sites may not include comprehensive details on the qualifications or certifications of a facility or provider. For travelers seeking dental care while abroad, the Organization for Safety, Asepsis and Prevention provides the "Traveler's Guide to Safe Dental Care" (Box 9-4), which contains several questions to help travelers find a dental clinic and identify potential infection control concerns in a dental clinic. Additional resources exist to assist both providers and medical tourists (Box 9-5).

## TRANSPLANT TOURISM

"Transplant tourism" refers to travel for the purpose of receiving an organ or stem cells purchased from an unrelated human donor for

## BOX 9-4. Patient checklist for obtaining safe dental care during international travel[1]

**Before you leave:**

- Visit your dentist for a checkup to reduce the chances you will have a dental emergency.
- Consider appropriate vaccinations.

When seeking treatment for a dental emergency during your trip:

- Consult hotel staff or the American Embassy or consulate for assistance in finding a dentist.
- If possible, consider recommendations from Americans living in the area or from other trusted sources.

For the items below, if the answers to any of the asterisked (*) items are "No," you should have reservations about the office's infection-control standards. If the answer to a two-star item (**) is "No," consider making a gracious but swift exit.

When making the appointment, ask the following:

- Do you use new gloves for each patient?*
- Do you use an autoclave (steam sterilizer) or dry heat oven to sterilize your instruments between patients?**
- Do you sterilize your handpieces (drills)?* (If not, do you disinfect them?)**
- Do you use new needles for each patient?**[2]
- Is sterile (or boiled) water used for surgical procedures?** (In areas where drinking water is unsafe, the water also may cause illness if used for dental treatment.)

Upon arriving at the office, observe the following:

- Is the office clean and neat?
- Do staff wash their hands, with soap, between patients?**
- Do they wear gloves for all procedures?**
- Do they clean and disinfect or use disposable covers on surfaces touched during treatment?

Although it is important to be sensitive to cultural differences when making inquiries about the safety of dental care, remember that it is your health and well-being that are at stake.

[1] Excerpt from Organization for Safety, Asepsis, and Prevention. Traveler's guide to safe dental care. Annapolis, MD: Organization for Safety, Asepsis, and Prevention; 2001. Available from: www.osap.org/?page=TravelersGuide.

[2] CDC recommends a new needle and new syringe for each injection. For further information, see https://www.cdc.gov/injectionsafety/1anonly.html

**9**

transplantation. This practice may be motivated by cost or in effort to reduce the waiting period. Xenotransplantation refers to travel to receive other biomaterial (cell, tissue) from nonhuman species. It is regulated differently among countries; no scientific evidence supports its therapeutic benefit, and adverse events have been reported, including the outbreak of Q fever described above.

In 2004, to protect vulnerable populations from becoming victims of transplant tourism, the World Health Assembly Resolution 57.18 encouraged member countries to "take measures to protect the poorest and vulnerable groups [the donors] from 'transplant tourism' and the sale of tissues and organs." A meeting in 2008 in Istanbul addressed the issue of transplant tourism and organ trafficking, which resulted in a call for these activities to be prohibited. In view of those events, in 2009 the World Health Organization released the revised Guiding Principles on Human Cell, Tissue, and Organ Transplantation, emphasizing that cells, tissues, and organs should be donated freely without any form of financial incentive.

Several studies have identified potential medical issues associated with transplant tourism. Patients may receive fewer immunosuppressive drugs than is the current practice in the United States and might not receive antimicrobial prophylaxis. Immunocompromised travelers are more susceptible to infection, which can pose additional challenges while traveling.

## BOX 9-5. Helpful resources on medical tourism

- Aerospace Medical Association's Medical Guidelines for Airline Passengers (2002) provides useful information on the risks of travel with certain medical conditions: www.asma.org/asma/media/asma/Travel-Publications/paxguidelines.pdf
- American Academy of Orthopaedic Surgeons Bulletin, July 2007, discusses safety issues that patients should consider: www.aaos.org/news/bulletin/jul07/cover1.asp (requires paid access)
- American Academy of Orthopaedic Surgeons Bulletin, February 2008, discusses liability implications of medical tourism: www.aaos.org/news/aaosnow/feb08/managing7.asp (requires paid access)
- American College of Surgeons (ACS). Statement on medical and surgical tourism: www.facs.org/about-acs/statements/65-surgical-tourism
- American Society for Aesthetic Plastic Surgery (ASAPS). Guidelines for patients seeking cosmetic procedures abroad: www.surgery.org/consumers/consumer-resources/consumer-tips/guidelines-for-patients-seeking-cosmetic-procedures-abroad
- American Society of Plastic Surgeons (ASPS). Dangers of plastic surgery tourism: www.plasticsurgery.org/patient-safety/dangers-of-plastic-surgery-tourism
- ACS's Find a Surgeon tool helps identify ACS members including fellows and associate fellows: www.facs.org/search/find-a-surgeon
- ASAPS's Find a Plastic Surgeon tool helps identify ASAPS member surgeons in the United States and overseas: www.surgery.org/consumers/find-a-plastic-surgeon
- ASPS's plastic surgeon match tool helps identify ASPS member surgeons in the United States and overseas: https://find.plasticsurgery.org
- International Society for Aesthetic Plastic Surgery's Find-a-surgeon tool helps identify a surgeon: www.isaps.org/find-a-surgeon
- Joint Commission International list of its accredited facilities outside of the United States: www.jointcommissioninternational.org/JCI-Accredited-Organizations/
- Organization for Safety, Asepsis, and Prevention. Traveler's guide to safe dental care: www.osap.org/?page=TravelersGuide
- World Health Organization. Guiding principles on human cell, tissue and organ transplantation: https://www.who.int/transplantation/Guiding_PrinciplesTransplantation_WHA63.22en.pdf
- US Department of State: Your Health Abroad https://travel.state.gov/content/travel/en/international-travel/before-you-go/your-health-abroad.html

**9**

## BIBLIOGRAPHY

1. Adabi K, Stern C, Weichman K, Garfein ES, Pothula A, Draper L, et al. Population health implications of medical tourism. Plast Reconstr Surg. 2017 Jul;140(1):66–74.

2. Budiani-Saberi DA, Delmonico FL. Organ trafficking and transplant tourism: a commentary on the global realities. Am J Transplant. 2008 May;8(5): 925–9.

3. Chen LH, Wilson ME. The globalization of healthcare: implications of medical tourism for the infectious disease clinician. Clin Infect Dis. 2013 Dec;57(12): 1752–9.

4. Gaines J, Poy J, Musser KA, Benowitz I, Leung V, Carothers B, et al. Notes from the field: rapidly growing nontuberculous mycobacteria associated with plastic surgery in the Dominican Republic, 2017. MMWR Morb Mortal Wkly Rep. 2018 Mar 30;67(12).

5. Melendez MM, Alizadeh K. Complications from international surgery tourism. Aesthet Surg J. 2011 Aug;31(6):694–7.

6. Merion RM, Barnes AD, Lin M, Ashby VB, McBride V, Ortiz-Rios E, et al. Transplants in foreign countries among patients removed from the US transplant waiting list. Am J Transplant. 2008 Apr;8(4 Pt 2):988–96.

7. Organ Procurement and Transplantation Network, Scientific Registry of Transplant Recipients. United States organ transplantation annual data report, 2011. Rockville (MD): US Department of Health and Human Services; 2012 [cited 2016 Sep 22]. Available from: http://srtr.transplant.hrsa.gov/annual_reports/2011/default.aspx.

8. Reed CM. Medical tourism. Med Clin North Am. 2008 Nov;92(6):1433–46, xi.

9. Robyn MP, Newman AP, Amato M, Walawander M, Kothe C, Nerone JD, et al. Q fever outbreak among travelers to Germany who received live cell therapy—United States and Canada, 2014. MMWR Morb Mortal Wkly Rep. 2015 Oct;64(38):1071–3.

10. Schnabel D, Esposito DH, Gaines J, Ridpath A, Barry MA, Feldman KA, et al. Multistate US outbreak of rapidly growing mycobacterial infections associated with medical tourism to the Dominican Republic, 2013–2014. Emerg Infect Dis. 2016 Aug;22(8):1340–7.

# SEX & TRAVEL

Jay Keystone, Kimberly A. Workowski, Emily Meites

The World Health Organization estimates approximately 357 million infections with curable sexually transmitted pathogens (chlamydia, gonorrhea, trichomoniasis, and syphilis) per year, or nearly 1 million new infections per day. More than 30 different sexually transmitted infections (STIs) are caused by a range of pathogens, not all of which are curable or vaccine preventable. Travel health providers have a responsibility to educate their patients about what they can do to reduce the chances of acquiring an STI during travel. Targeted teaching and messaging to travelers at highest risk is a prudent approach.

Global distribution of sexually transmitted pathogens and their sensitivity to available treatment varies. International travelers having sex with new partners while abroad are exposed to different "sexual networks" than at home and can serve as a conduit for importation of novel or drug-resistant STIs into parts of the world where they are unknown or rare. Gonorrhea, for example, among the more common STIs globally (with an estimated 85 million new cases in 2012), has become extensively drug resistant in some parts of the world. Patients presenting with antimicrobial-resistant gonococcal infections should prompt providers to inquire about their travel history and the travel history of their sex partners.

## CASUAL SEX DURING TRAVEL

It is important to distinguish between casual sex and sex tourism. Sex tourism (see below) is travel for the specific purpose of having sex, typically with commercial sex workers. Casual sex during travel, by contrast, describes informal sexual encounters with fellow travelers or locals.

Although some travelers may expect to have casual sexual encounters, others who have sex do not.

Two meta-analyses (2010 and 2018) provide a range of how many international travelers engage in casual sex, approximately 20%–34%. Although crude—both the 2010 and 2018 pooled prevalence values are based on just a handful of studies, each with considerable variation in their own estimates—these numbers shed some light on how common casual sex during travel may be. These same studies also provide estimates on the number of travelers engaging in unprotected sex (i.e., sex without a condom). The 2010 report indicates that approximately half (49%) of all travelers participating in casual sex abroad have unprotected intercourse, although in the 2018 report, that number was slightly lower (43%).

Populations less well represented in the literature include female travelers and men who have sex with men (MSM). Limited data on the casual sexual activity of female travelers suggest that such activity occurs almost as frequently as it does in male travelers, and that the incidence of unprotected sex is nearly as high. Existing literature concerning MSM is conflicting. Some studies report MSM are more likely to have new sex partners and unprotected intercourse while abroad. A recent study from California, however, demonstrated that MSM who travel internationally are more likely to use condoms and engage in less risky behavior.

As travelers go places where they are not known, they may no longer feel obligated to observe the same moral standards as at home, or they may desire to create connection with others.

BOX 9-6 ## Factors associated with higher frequency of casual or unprotected sex abroad

- Male
- Single
- Younger age
- Traveling without a partner (either alone or with friends)
- ≥2 sex partners in the last 2 years

- History of previous sexually transmitted infection
- Illicit drug use, alcohol abuse, tobacco use
- Casual sex at home and during a previous travel experience

- Expectation of casual sex while abroad
- Long-term travel (expatriates, military, Peace Corps volunteers)

The act of travel itself may create the potential for casual sex. Disinhibition resulting from drug and alcohol use, a desire for adventure and excitement, peer pressure, and underlying psychological needs and personality traits may contribute, individually or in combination, to travelers having casual sex. Several studies (including the meta-analyses referenced above) have attempted to identify characteristics of travelers who are most likely to have casual sex during travel (Box 9-6). See Chapter 2, The Pretravel Consultation, for additional recommendations and guidance on preventing STIs.

## SEX TOURISM

"Sex tourism," as defined above, is travel specifically for the purposes of procuring sex. In one study, typical sex tourists were highly educated men, 30–40 years of age, going to economically disadvantaged countries to pay for sex with commercial sex workers. Fewer than half of these men reported regularly using condoms, even in destinations where the prevalence of STIs (including HIV disease) is high.

In some countries, commercial sex work is legal and culturally acceptable. In many other places, however, sex tourism supports sex trafficking, among the largest and most lucrative criminal industries in the world.

## SEXUAL ABUSE, CHILD PORNOGRAPHY, AND THE LAW

Although commercial sex work may be legal in some parts of the world, sex trafficking, sex with a minor, and child pornography are always

criminal activities according to US law; travelers can be prosecuted in the United States even if they participated in such activities overseas. The Trafficking Victims Protection Act makes it illegal to recruit, entice, or obtain a person of any age to engage in commercial sex acts or to benefit from such activities.

Federal law bars US residents traveling abroad from having sex with minors. This applies to all travelers, both adult and youth. Travel health providers should inform student travelers (and other young people going abroad) that according to US law, it is illegal for a US resident to have sex with a minor in another country. Bear in mind, however, that the legal age of consent varies around the world, from 11–21 years. In some countries, there is no legal age of consent: local law forbids all sexual relations outside of marriage.

Regardless of the local age of consent, participation in child pornography anywhere in the world is illegal in the United States. This includes sex with minors, as well as the purchase, procurement, holding, or storage of material depicting such acts. These crimes are subject to prosecution with penalties of up to 30 years in prison. Victims of child pornography suffer multiple forms of abuse (sexual, physical, emotional, and psychological), poverty and homelessness, and health problems, including physical injury, STIs, other infections and illnesses, addiction, and malnourishment.

A report published in 2016 by End Child Prostitution, Child Pornography, and Trafficking of Children for Sexual Purposes International (ECPAT) identified that most perpetrators of

9

child pornography are "situational" offenders, people who may have never considered sexually exploiting a child until given the opportunity to do so. Americans and US permanent residents account for an estimated 25% of child sex tourists worldwide and up to 80% in Latin America. They are typically white men aged ≥40 who have been traced visiting Mexico, Central and South America (Brazil, Colombia, Costa Rica, Dominican Republic), Southeast Asia (Cambodia, India, Laos, Philippines, Thailand), Eastern Europe (Estonia, Latvia, Lithuania, Russia), and other regions.

To combat child sexual abuse, some international hotels and other tourism services have voluntarily adopted a code of conduct that includes training and reporting suspicious activities. Tourist establishments supporting this initiative to protect children from sex tourism are listed online (www.thecode.org). Providers and travelers who suspect child sexual exploitation occurring overseas can report tips anonymously by:

- Using the Operation Predator smart-phone app (https://itunes.apple.com/us/app/operation-predator/id695130859).

- Calling the Homeland Security Investigations Tip Line (866-347-2423).

- Submitting information online (www.ice.gov/tips).

In the United States, the National Center for Missing & Exploited Children's CyberTipline collects reports of child prostitution and other crimes against children (toll-free at 800-843-5678, https://report.cybertip.org).

Since 2003, when Congress passed the federal PROTECT Act, at least 8,000 Americans have been arrested—and 99 convicted—for child sex tourism and exploitation. The PROTECT Act strengthens the US government's' ability to prosecute and punish crimes related to sex tourism, including incarceration of up to 30 years for acts committed at home or abroad. Cooperation of the host country is required to open an investigation of criminal activity, resulting in a much lower than hoped for conviction rate. Some countries are wary of working too closely with the United States. In others, the judicial system may be prone to bribery and corruption, or the government is otherwise willing to expand tourism (and the money it brings in) at the expense of children being trafficked for sex. For more ways you can help, see the Department of State list of 15 ways to fight human trafficking (www.state.gov/j/tip/id/help).

## BIBLIOGRAPHY

1. Abdullah AS, Ebrahim SH, Fielding R, Morisky DE. Sexually transmitted infections in travelers: implications for prevention and control. Clin Infect Dis. 2004 Aug 15;39(4):533–8.

2. CDC. Sexually transmitted diseases treatment guidelines, 2015. MMWR Recomm Rep. 2015 Jun 5;64(RR-03):1–137.

3. Marrazzo JM. Sexual tourism: implications for travelers and the destination culture. Infect Dis Clin North Am. 2005 Mar;19(1):103–20.

4. Newman WJ, Holt BW, Rabun JS, Phillips G, Scott CL. Child sex tourism: extending the borders of sexual offender legislation. Int J Law Psychiatry. 2011 Mar–Apr;34(2):116–21.

5. Offenders on the move: the global study report on sexual exploitation of children in travel and tourism, ECPAT International, Bangkok Thailand, May 2016. Available from: https://issuu.com/ecpat5/docs/global-report-offenders-on-the-move.

6. Svensson P, Sundbeck M, Persson KI, Stafstrn M, Östergren P-O, Mannheimer L, Agardh A. A meta-analysis and systematic literature review of factors associated with sexual risk-taking during international travel Travel Med Infect Dis. 2018 Mar 19;pii:S1477–8939(18)30045-0.

7. Vivancos R, Abubakar I, Hunter PR. Foreign travel, casual sex, and sexually transmitted infections: systematic review and meta-analysis. Int J Infect Dis. 2010 Oct;14(10):e842–51.

**9**

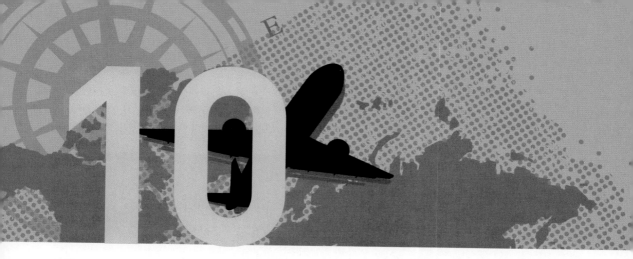

# 10

# Popular Itineraries

## THE RATIONALE FOR POPULAR ITINERARIES

Ronnie Henry

This chapter of the *Yellow Book* allows experts who have lived in or frequently visited particular destinations to share their insider's knowledge of these places. Consider each of these sections to be a personal perspective on the area discussed. Editorial in nature and containing the author's expressed opinions, they should not be taken as a prescription for pretravel care. Each section is intended to help a travel health provider feel more comfortable giving advice about a destination he or she may never have visited and to provide a level of detail about local attractions and risks not provided elsewhere in this book.

The following sections are among the most popular features of the *Yellow Book*. Space limitations prevent us from including all popular itineraries here, and the decision of which ones to add or remove is guided by volume of US travel, uniqueness of health risks, and other factors. In addition to the sections found in the print edition, readers can find more popular itineraries online: Cambodia, Egypt & Nile River Cruises, Guatemala and Belize, Iguaçu Falls, Jamaica, and Vietnam (www.cdc.gov/yellowbook).

# AFRICA & THE MIDDLE EAST

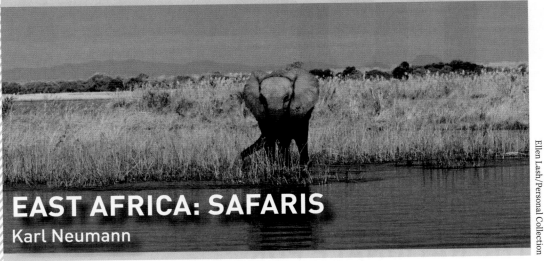

## EAST AFRICA: SAFARIS
### Karl Neumann

**10**

## DESTINATION OVERVIEW

Arguably the ultimate in adventure travel, an African safari is the experience of a lifetime. There are safaris for families, honeymooners, and people with similar interests (serious photographers, for example). Many safaris accept young children as participants and have special age-appropriate programs for children and adolescents aged 6–16 years. While the centerpiece of safari-going remains viewing majestic animals in their natural habitat, many tour operators now include programs on local culture, history, geology, and ecosystems, encouraging travelers to get to know the local people not merely as subjects of photos. Topography, vegetation, and bird life in the region also help differentiate safari types.

Animals can be viewed from open trucks, air-conditioned vans, private aircraft, or hot air balloons. Hiking with trained, licensed guides in well-scouted settings offers another opportunity to see wildlife up close. Safari accommodations can range from crawl-in tents to air-conditioned, walk-in canopy tents with full bathrooms. Luxurious 5-star lodges with floodlit water holes

enable patrons to view animals at night. Dining in the wilderness varies from eating prepackaged sandwiches while seated on a tree stump to formally served 3-course meals on tables with linen cloths and matching napkins. Some safaris include side trips to exotic places—to see or climb Mount Kilimanjaro, or to visit Zanzibar or Lake Victoria, for example.

Travelers often choose an East African game park in Kenya or Tanzania for their first safari. The most famous game park in Kenya is the Masai Mara National Reserve, the northern continuation of the Serengeti National Park game reserve in Tanzania. Together these parks are home to perhaps the grandest and most complete collection of the large wild animals for which Africa is famous. The Serengeti is the starting point of the annual migration of more than a million wildebeest and several hundred thousand zebras searching for pasture and water. Tanzania also has the Ngorongoro Crater, a 100-square-mile depression (caldera) formed when a giant volcano, perhaps the size of Mount Kilimanjaro, exploded and collapsed on itself millions of

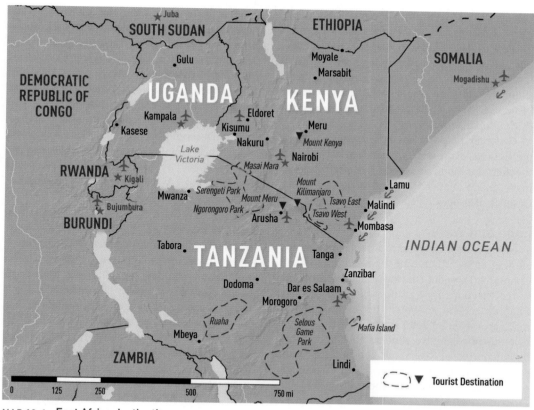

MAP 10-1. East Africa destination map

years ago. The major East African game parks are shown on Map 10-1.

Travelers should research the optimum time of the year for their safari. The wildebeest migration in the Serengeti is a seasonal event, for example, although the precise time of the migration may vary from year to year. Some parks have a dry season, offering better views of the animals as the vegetation is sparser, and animals gather where water is present, but roads are dustier. And many areas of Africa have times of the year that are more comfortable for visitors, with cooler weather, lower humidity, and less chance of rain.

## HEALTH ISSUES

Health and safety issues that safari-goers are likely to encounter are mostly predictable and largely avoidable. A pretravel consultation with a travel health care provider is essential. Multiple vaccinations as well as malaria prophylaxis may be required. Health advice must be specific to each itinerary and game park visited. Immunizations and preventive medications necessary for one park may not be so for others. Parks may be long distances apart and located in countries with different health standards and dissimilar climates. Some parks are located at higher elevations and close to the equator, making proper sun precautions imperative, including seeking shade when possible and avoiding the sun during midday hours. Significant sunburn can occur in less than an hour. Sunglasses are essential, in addition to protective clothing, hats, and use of a broad-spectrum sunscreen with SPF ≥15 that protects against both UVA and UVB (see Chapter 3, Sun Exposure).

Travelers should choose an experienced and sophisticated tour operator and take along a small, personal medical kit (see Chapter 6, Travel Health Kits). Experienced tour operators generally provide clients with ample literature describing local conditions and require that clients purchase medical evacuation insurance policies. In addition, they employ knowledgeable guides who carry first-aid kits and communication equipment to summon help, if necessary (see Chapter 6, Travel Insurance, Travel Health Insurance & Medical Evacuation Insurance).

Generally, proper preparations, commonsense precautions, experienced guides and drivers, and the short duration of most trips (usually <2 weeks), make safaris relatively low-risk undertakings for travelers of all ages.

## Food and Water

Travelers' diarrhea appears to be the most common ailment on safari, and most cases are mild (see Chapter 2, Travelers' Diarrhea). Sensible food and water selections may reduce the incidence (see Chapter 2, Food & Water Precautions). Illness may occur even on deluxe trips; self-treatment is recommended. Active cholera transmission has been reported in Kenya and Tanzania in recent years. Check the destination page at www.cdc.gov/travel for current recommendations.

## Animals

Wild animals are unpredictable. Travelers should follow verbal and written instructions provided by safari operators. Animal-related injuries are extremely uncommon and usually result when travelers disregard rules, for example, when they approach animals too closely to feed or photograph them (see Chapter 3, Animal Bites & Stings).

Rabies exists throughout Africa; dogs and bats are the primary animal reservoirs (see Chapter 4, Rabies). Bats transmit other infections to humans, such as viral hemorrhagic fevers. Warn travelers not to enter caves where bats roost and shelter; several cases of Marburg hemorrhagic fever have occurred in travelers visiting bat caves in Uganda.

## Malaria

Malaria transmission occurs in most game parks. Most infections are caused by *Plasmodium falciparum*, and all *P. falciparum* in sub-Saharan Africa should be considered chloroquine-resistant.

Safari activities often include sleeping in tents and observing animals at dusk or after dark, sometimes near water holes, all increasing the risk of being bitten by malaria-carrying mosquitoes. Preventive medication and personal protection—wearing long-sleeved shirts and pants, using insect repellents, and sleeping under permethrin-impregnated mosquito netting—are essential. Observing recommendations to prevent malaria helps minimize the risk of a host of other diseases spread by insects (see Chapter 2, Yellow Fever Vaccine & Malaria Prophylaxis Information, by Country, and Chapter 4, Malaria).

## Yellow Fever

Travelers going on an African safari should consult a travel medicine professional for the very latest information regarding yellow fever at their destination. The World Health Organization (WHO) and CDC update yellow fever activity and vaccination recommendations regularly. Currently, WHO and CDC recommend yellow fever vaccination for much of sub-Saharan Africa (see Chapter 2, Yellow Fever Vaccine & Malaria Prophylaxis Information, by Country).

In 2010, WHO and CDC reclassified a portion of East Africa as "low potential for exposure" to yellow fever virus and consequently downgraded the vaccination recommendation for these areas to "generally not recommended." This recommendation now limits vaccination to a small subset of travelers at increased risk for exposure to yellow fever virus (prolonged travel, heavy exposure to mosquitoes, and/or inability to avoid mosquito bites). Areas where vaccine is no longer generally recommended include (but are not limited to) eastern Kenya, the cities of Nairobi and Mombasa, and all of Tanzania.

Some countries require proof of yellow fever vaccination in the form of a valid International Certificate of Vaccination or Prophylaxis (ICVP) as a condition of entry. Moreover, some safaris cross international borders to include more than one country. Travelers must check the requirements of each country on their itinerary, including countries they only transit through on the way to their destination. Some countries may require a valid ICVP even if there is no yellow fever in the country they are leaving or entering.

10

## Other Health Risks

Day-biting tsetse flies (Glossina) transmit African trypanosomiasis (sleeping sickness), a disease only rarely seen in travelers (see Chapter 4, African Trypanosomiasis). Light-colored clothing (and not wearing blue) seems to deter the flies, whereas insect repellents are only partially effective. Symptoms include fever, eschar at the site of the bite, and headache. There may be signs of central nervous system involvement. Several reports document recent cases of trypanosomiasis (*rhodesiense*) in European tourists visiting the Masai Mara National Reserve in Kenya and wildlife reserves in Tanzania.

Zika virus, dengue, filariasis, leishmaniasis, and onchocerciasis (river blindness) are other diseases carried by insects found in East Africa. Entering freshwater ponds, lakes, and rivers can expose travelers to *Schistosoma* spp., a parasite found in freshwater snails (see Chapter 4, Schistosomiasis). Travelers should consider all freshwater sources to be contaminated. Swimming in the ocean or well-chlorinated pools is not a risk for schistosomiasis (bilharzia).

Myiasis and tungiasis are rare skin diseases among travelers. Caused by fly larvae penetrating the skin, myiasis is characterized by boil-like lesions with a central aperture. Adult flies lay eggs on clothing left to dry outdoors; when the traveler puts on the clothing, the larvae can enter the wearer's skin. Instruct travelers to dry their clothing indoors or press with a hot iron before wearing. Tungiasis, small, painful nodules, often on the foot adjacent to toenails, is caused by direct penetration of skin by sand fleas. Prevention includes wearing closed-toed footwear, not walking barefoot.

Symptoms of many diseases acquired in Africa may surface weeks and occasionally months after exposure, sometimes long after the traveler has returned home. Obtain a travel history from all patients presenting for care.

## SAFETY RISKS

Within the game parks themselves, crime is unusual. Robberies and carjackings are more common in urban areas (see Chapter 3, Safety & Security Overseas). Street muggings occur during the day and night. In sub-Saharan African countries, the rates of fatal motor vehicle crashes are among the highest in the world. Travelers should fasten seat belts when riding in cars, and wear a helmet when riding bicycles or motorbikes (see Chapter 8, Road & Traffic Safety). Within game parks, serious motor vehicle crashes are rare, as the poor roads discourage speeding. However, travel in rural areas between parks is high risk, especially after dark. If possible, travelers should avoid nighttime driving in sub-Saharan Africa, and pedestrians should take extra care for speeding vehicles. Travelers should also avoid boarding overcrowded buses.

### BIBLIOGRAPHY

1. Clerinx J, Van Gompel A. Schistosomiasis in travellers and migrants. Travel Med Infect Dis. 2011 Jan;9(1):6–24.

2. Gobbi F, Bisoffi Z. Human African trypanosomiasis in travellers to Kenya. Eurosurveillance. 2012 Mar 8;17(10):pii: 20109.

3. Schlagenhauf P, Weld L, Goorhuis A, Gautret P, Weber R, von Sonnenburg F, et al. Travel-associated infection presenting in Europe (2008–12): an analysis of EuroTravNet longitudinal, surveillance data, and evaluation of the effect of the pre-travel consultation. Lancet Infect Dis. 2015 Jan;15(1):55–64.

4. Warne B, Weld LH, Cramer JP, Field VK, Grobusch MP, Caumes E, et al. Travel-related infection in European travelers, EuroTravNet 2011. J Travel Med 2014 Jul–Aug;21(4):248–54.

5. World Health Organization. Vaccines and vaccination against yellow fever. WHO position paper—June 2013. Wkly Epidemiol Rec. 2013 Jul 5;88(27):269–83.

10

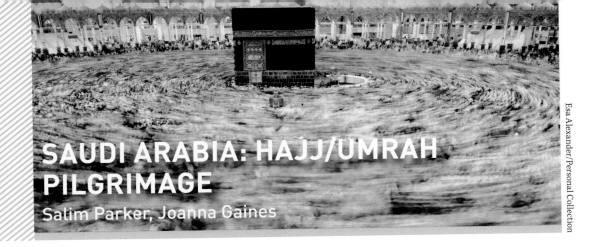

# SAUDI ARABIA: HAJJ/UMRAH PILGRIMAGE

Salim Parker, Joanna Gaines

## DESTINATION OVERVIEW

Hajj and Umrah are religious pilgrimages to Mecca, Saudi Arabia. Islamic religious doctrine dictates that every able-bodied adult Muslim who can afford to do so is obligated to make Hajj at least once in his or her lifetime. Hajj takes place from the 8th through the 12th day of the last month of the Islamic year (Dhul Hijah). The timing of Hajj (based on the lunar Islamic calendar) varies with respect to the Gregorian calendar, occurring about 11 days earlier each successive year ( for example, it was held August 19–24 in 2018 and in 2019, August 9–14). Muslims may perform Umrah, the "minor pilgrimage," any time of the year; unlike Hajj, Umrah is not compulsory.

Approximately 2 million Muslims from >183 countries make Hajj each year and the Kingdom of Saudi Arabia (KSA) continues its efforts to allow for an even greater number of pilgrims. Annually, over 11,000 pilgrims travel from the United States. Most international pilgrims fly into Jeddah or Medina and take a bus to Mecca. Pilgrims then travel by foot or by bus approximately 5 miles (8 km) to the tent city of Mina, the largest temporary city in the world, where most pilgrims stay in air-conditioned tents.

At dawn on the ninth day of Dhul Hijah, pilgrims begin a nearly 9 mile (14.4 km) trip (by foot, by bus or by train) to the Plain of Arafat (Map 10-2). During the summer months, in particular, daytime temperatures can reach 122°F (50°C). Though the route features mist sprinklers, the risk of heat-related illnesses is high, and ambulances and medical stations along the route provide needed medical assistance. Hajj climaxes on the Plain of Arafat, a few miles east of Mecca. Pilgrims spend the day in supplication, praying and reading the Quran. Being on Arafat on the ninth of Dhul Hijah, even if only for a few moments, is an absolute rite of Hajj. Any hajji who fails to reach the Plain of Arafat on that day must repeat his or her pilgrimage. After sunset, pilgrims begin a 5.5 mile (9 km) journey to Muzdalifah, where most sleep in the open air. Potential threats to health there include thick dust, inadequate and overcrowded washing and sanitation facilities, and the possibility of separation or becoming lost.

At sunrise on the 10th, pilgrims collect small pebbles to carry to Jamaraat, the site of multiple deadly crowd crush disasters. At Jamaraat, hajjis throw 7 tiny pebbles at the largest of 3 white pillars—the stoning of the effigy of the Devil. Afterwards, it is traditional for pilgrims to sacrifice an animal. Some purchase vouchers to have licensed abattoirs perform this ritual on their behalf, thereby limiting their potential exposure to zoonotic diseases. Others may visit farms where they sacrifice an animal themselves or have it done by an appointed representative.

The next morning, hajjis go to the Grand Mosque, which houses the Ka'aba ("The Cube"), which Muslims consider the house of God. Pilgrims perform *tawaf*, 7 complete counterclockwise circuits around the Ka'aba. Because each floor of the 3-level mosque can hold 750,000 people, performing *tawaf* can take hours. In addition to *tawaf*, pilgrims may perform *sa'i*, walking (sometimes running) 7 times between the hills of Safa and Marwah, then drinking water from the Well of Zamzam. Hajjis may travel between Safa and Marwah via air-conditioned tunnels, with separate sections for walkers, runners, and

10

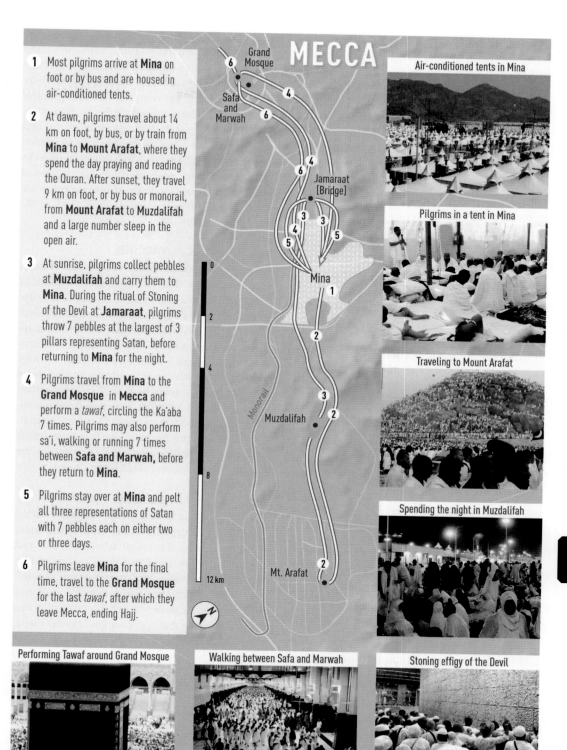

1. Most pilgrims arrive at **Mina** on foot or by bus and are housed in air-conditioned tents.

2. At dawn, pilgrims travel about 14 km on foot, by bus, or by train from **Mina** to **Mount Arafat**, where they spend the day praying and reading the Quran. After sunset, they travel 9 km on foot, or by bus or monorail, from **Mount Arafat** to Muzdalifah and a large number sleep in the open air.

3. At sunrise, pilgrims collect pebbles at **Muzdalifah** and carry them to **Mina**. During the ritual of Stoning of the Devil at **Jamaraat**, pilgrims throw 7 pebbles at the largest of 3 pillars representing Satan, before returning to **Mina** for the night.

4. Pilgrims travel from **Mina** to the **Grand Mosque** in **Mecca** and perform a *tawaf*, circling the Ka'aba 7 times. Pilgrims may also perform sa'i, walking or running 7 times between **Safa and Marwah,** before they return to **Mina**.

5. Pilgrims stay over at **Mina** and pelt all three representations of Satan with 7 pebbles each on either two or three days.

6. Pilgrims leave **Mina** for the final time, travel to the **Grand Mosque** for the last *tawaf*, after which they leave Mecca, ending Hajj.

MECCA

Grand Mosque

Safa and Marwah

Jamaraat [Bridge]

Mina

Monorail

Muzdalifah

Mt. Arafat

0 2 4 8 12 km

N

Air-conditioned tents in Mina

Pilgrims in a tent in Mina

Traveling to Mount Arafat

Spending the night in Muzdalifah

Performing Tawaf around Grand Mosque

Walking between Safa and Marwah

Stoning effigy of the Devil

**MAP 10-2.** Hajj destination map

10

disabled pilgrims. At the end of the day, pilgrims return to Mina (via Jamaraat) pelting all 3 pillars with pebbles along the way.

The following day, after performing a final *tawaf*, pilgrims leave Mecca, ending their Hajj. Although not required, hajjis may add a trip to Medina where they visit the Mosque of the Prophet, home to the tomb of Mohammed.

## HEALTH ISSUES

Travelers who become ill during Hajj have access to medical facilities strategically located in and around the holy sites. With an estimated 25,000 health care workers in attendance, medical services are offered free of charge to all pilgrims. For safety reasons, the KSA advises the elderly, the seriously ill, pregnant women, and children to postpone Hajj and Umrah. KSA may also choose to limit issuance of visas to travelers from countries experiencing infectious disease outbreaks. In 2012, for example, KSA did not permit anyone from Uganda to attend Hajj due to an Ebola outbreak in that country; the same restriction applied to Liberia, Guinea, and Sierra Leone in 2015.

### Vaccine-Preventable Diseases

The Saudi Arabian Ministry of Hajj (http://haj.gov.sa/english/pages/default.aspx) regularly updates vaccine requirements on its website; refer to this source for additional information. Current Hajj vaccination requirements are also available from these sources

- Saudi Arabian Embassy (http://embassies. mofa.gov.sa/sites/usa/AR/Pages/default.aspx)

- Saudi Arabian Ministry of Health (www. moh.gov.sa/en/Hajj/HealthGuidelines/ HealthGuidelinesBeforeHajj/Pages/default.asp)

KSA requires proof of vaccination as part of the Hajj and Umrah visa application process. Required vaccines include meningitis (see below) and—for anyone arriving from a yellow fever–endemic country—yellow fever. CDC recommends all travelers to Saudi Arabia be up-to-date with routine immunizations, including hepatitis A vaccine for most travelers. Hepatitis B vaccination is recommended for health care workers or other caretakers participating in Hajj.

Although KSA's requirement for polio vaccine does not include adult pilgrims from the United States, it is best to ensure full vaccination before travel. All pilgrims traveling from countries where polio is reported are required to show proof of vaccination at least 4 weeks prior to departure. KSA also administers a single dose of the oral polio vaccine to pilgrims coming from countries where polio has been reported; this in addition to any polio vaccine received in a hajji's country of origin. About 500,000 doses of polio vaccine are given at ports of entry, representing >90% of eligible pilgrims.

### MENINGOCOCCAL VACCINE

All pilgrims must have received a single dose of quadrivalent ACWY vaccine and show proof of vaccination on a valid International Certificate of Vaccination or Prophylaxis; KSA will not issue visas for Hajj or Umrah without it. Hajjis must receive their meningococcal conjugate vaccination no more than 5 years before arrival. The KSA Ministry of Health currently advises against travel to the Hajj for pregnant women or children; if they choose to travel, however, these groups should receive meningococcal vaccination according to licensed indications for their age. For more details on meningococcal disease and its prevention, see Chapter 4, Meningococcal Disease.

### Respiratory Infections

Respiratory tract infections are common during Hajj, with pneumonia being among the most common causes of hospital admission. This risk underscores the need to follow recommendations from the Advisory Committee on Immunization Practices for pneumococcal conjugate and polysaccharide vaccines for pilgrims aged ≥65 years and for younger travelers with comorbidities.

Although not a requirement, CDC strongly recommends that hajjis receive a seasonal influenza vaccine. Behavioral interventions (regular handwashing with soap and water, wearing a facemask, cough etiquette, and—if possible—social distancing and contact avoidance) can help mitigate the risk of respiratory illnesses among pilgrims. Assess travelers for respiratory fitness, administer necessary vaccines, and

**10**

prescribe adequate supplies of portable respiratory medications (inhalers are easier to transport than nebulizers), as needed.

Crowded conditions during Hajj (densities can reach 9 pilgrims per square meter) increase the probability of respiratory disease transmission, including tuberculosis and Middle East Respiratory Syndrome (MERS). Many pilgrims come from areas highly endemic for tuberculosis; some arrive for Hajj with active pulmonary disease. Educate pilgrims about this risk and instruct them to see their doctor if they develop symptoms of active tuberculosis.

MERS, caused by the MERS coronavirus, was identified first in Saudi Arabia in 2012. Domestic cases (in and around the Arabian Peninsula) and exported cases (including the United States) have ranged from mild to severe; approximately 40% of reported cases have been fatal. The role of animal-to-human transmission is unclear, but the virus has been isolated in camels in this region. More information is available in Chapter 4, Middle East Respiratory Syndrome (MERS). At the time of writing, there have been no reports of Hajj-associated cases of MERS.

## Other Infectious Diseases

Diarrheal disease is common during Hajj; a pretravel consultation with travelers should include discussions about prevention, oral rehydration strategies, proper use of antimotility agents, and self-treatment of travelers' diarrhea (TD) with antibiotics. Most TD in hajjis is bacterial (up to 83%), with smaller proportions due to viruses and parasites. More information can be found in Chapter 2, Travelers' Diarrhea.

The World Health Organization recommends travelers visiting farms (or other areas where animals are present) practice general hygiene measures: regular handwashing before and after touching animals and avoiding contact with sick animals. Travelers should avoid consuming raw or undercooked animal products (including milk and meat). Pilgrims bitten by an animal should seek immediate medical attention to address any potential rabies exposure (see Chapter 3, Animal Bites & Stings, and Chapter 4, Rabies).

Chafing caused by long periods of standing and walking in the heat can lead to fungal or bacterial skin infections. Clothing should be light, not restrictive, and changed often to maintain hygiene. Advise travelers to keep skin dry, use talcum powder, and to be aware of any pain or irritation caused by garments. Open sores and blisters should be disinfected and kept covered. As a sign of respect, pilgrims enter the Grand Mosque with bare feet; careful foot protection is therefore essential, especially in diabetics who are at increased risk of infection.

On completion of Hajj, Muslim men shave their heads. KSA tests licensed barbers for bloodborne pathogens (hepatitis B, hepatitis C, and human immunodeficiency viruses) and requires that they use only disposable, single-use blades. By contrast, unlicensed barbers reusing blades can transmit bloodborne pathogens between customers. Remind male travelers to patronize only officially licensed barbers whose establishments are clearly marked.

*Aedes* and *Anopheles* mosquitoes, vectors for dengue and malaria, respectively, are present in Saudi Arabia. Mosquito bite prevention measures are outlined in Chapter 3, Mosquitoes, Ticks & Other Arthropods. Dengue has been documented in Mecca but not during Hajj. Intensive insecticide spraying campaigns are undertaken before Hajj, and the housing units of pilgrims arriving from endemic areas are especially targeted before their arrival. Prophylaxis against malaria is not required.

## Noninfectious Health Threats and Other Hazards

Hajj is arduous even for young, healthy pilgrims. Because many Muslims wait until they are older before making Hajj, they are more likely to have chronic health conditions; travelers caught up in the experience of Hajj or Umrah may forget to take their usual medications. People with chronic medical conditions should undergo a functional assessment before leaving for Hajj. Medical providers should tailor a plan for each traveler's unique risks including adjusting the usual medical regimen (if necessary), ensuring an adequate supply of medications, and providing education

**10**

about symptoms that indicate a condition requiring urgent attention.

Diabetic pilgrims, in particular, should have a customized management plan that will enable them to meet the arduous physical challenges of the Hajj. Adequate amounts of all medications, plus syringes and needles, are a must. Diabetic travelers also need to carry with them on their pilgrimage an emergency kit that includes easily accessible carbohydrate sources, glucagon, a glucometer and test strips, urine ketone sticks to evaluate for ketoacidosis, and a list of medications and care plans. Durable and protective footwear is necessary to reduce the incidence of minor foot trauma that can lead to infections.

Heat is a threat to the health and well-being of all travelers, with both heat exhaustion and heatstroke causing incapacitation and death among pilgrims (see Chapter 3, Extremes of Temperature). Travelers are at risk particularly when Hajj occurs during summer months, when the average high temperatures between June and September are ≥110°F. High temperatures together with high humidity can lead to a heat index indicative of an extreme heat warning. High heat alone can exacerbate chronic conditions.

About 45% of pilgrims walk during the Hajj rituals, averaging 23.9 km over 5 days. Counsel pilgrims to stay well hydrated, wear sunscreen, and seek shade or use umbrellas when possible. Religious leaders have ruled that it is permissible for hajjis to perform some rituals after dark. In addition, except for a pilgrim's required presence on Arafat on the ninth, most other compulsory rituals can be postponed, done by proxy, or redeemed by paying a penalty.

Fire is a potential risk during Hajj. In 1997, open stoves set tents on fire, and the resulting blaze killed 343 pilgrims and injured more than 1,500. Since then, KSA no longer allows pilgrims to erect their own lodgings or prepare their own food; permanent fiberglass structures have replaced formerly makeshift accommodations. In 2015, a hotel caught fire; more than 1,000 pilgrims were evacuated.

### TRAUMA

Trauma is a major cause of injury and death during Hajj. Hajj is associated with dense crowding, leading to crush disasters or stampedes. Thousands of pilgrims were killed during a crush at Mina in 2015, making it the deadliest Hajj disaster on record. Death usually results from asphyxiation or head trauma, and large crowds limit the movement of emergency medical services, making prompt rescue and treatment difficult.

As in other countries, motor vehicle crashes are the primary risk for US travelers overseas; remind Hajj pilgrims of the importance of seatbelt use (see Chapter 8, Road & Traffic Safety). Encourage pilgrims to be mindful of their own safety as they walk long distances through or near dense traffic.

## SPECIAL HEALTH CONSIDERATIONS

### Menstruation

Muslim law prohibits menstruating women from performing *tawaf*. All other rituals are independent of menses. Because pilgrims generally know well in advance that they will be making Hajj/Umrah, a woman should consult with her physician 2–3 months before the journey if she intends to manipulate her periods before the pilgrimage.

### BIBLIOGRAPHY

1. Alsafadi H, Goodwin W, Syed A. Diabetes care during Hajj. Clin Med. 2011 Jun;11(3):218–21.

2. Alzahrani AG, Choudhry AJ, Al Mazroa MA, Turkistani AH, Nouman GS, Memish ZA. Pattern of diseases among visitors to Mina health centers during the Hajj season, 1429 H (2008 G). J Infect Public Health. 2012 Mar;5(1):22–34.

3. Assiri A, Al-Tawfiq JA, Al-Rabeeah AA, Al-Rabiah FA, Al-Hajjar S, Al-Barrak A, et al. Epidemiological,

demographic, and clinical characteristics of 47 cases of Middle East respiratory syndrome coronavirus disease from Saudi Arabia: a descriptive study. Lancet Infect Dis. 2013 Sep;13(9):752–61.

4. Balaban V, Stauffer WM, Hammad A, Afgarshe M, Abd-Alla M, Ahmed Q, et al. Protective practices and respiratory illness among US travelers to the 2009 Hajj. J Travel Med. 2012 May–Jun; 19(3):163–8.

5. Memish Z, Zumla A, Alhakeem R, Assiri A, Turkestani A, Al Harby KD, et al. Hajj: infectious disease surveillance and control. Lancet. 2014 Jun 14;383(9934):2073–82.

6. Memish ZA. The Hajj: communicable and noncommunicable health hazards and current guidance for pilgrims. Euro Surveill. 2010 Sep 30;15(39):19671.

7. Memish ZA. Saudi Arabia has several strategies to care for pilgrims on the Hajj. BMJ. 2011;343:d7731.

8. Memish ZA, Al-Rabeeah AA. Health conditions of travellers to Saudi Arabia for the pilgrimage to Mecca

(Hajj and Umra) for 1434 (2013). J Epidemiol Glob Health. 2013 Jun;3(2):59–61.

9. Shibl A, Tufenkeji H, Khalil M, Memish Z, Meningococcal Leadership Forum (MLF) Expert Group. Consensus recommendation for meningococcal disease prevention for Hajj and Umra pilgrimage/travel medicine. East Mediterr Health J 2013 Apr;19(4):389–92.

10. World Health Organization. Health conditions for travellers to Saudi Arabia pilgrimage to Mecca (Hajj). Wkly Epidemiol Rec. 2005 Dec 9;80(49-50): 431–2.

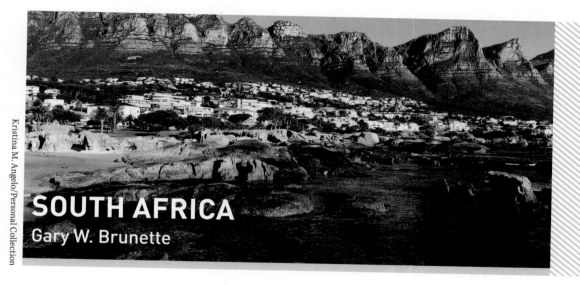

Kristina M. Angelo/Personal Collection

# SOUTH AFRICA
Gary W. Brunette

## DESTINATION OVERVIEW

South Africa is "a world in one country." Diverse geography (ranging from lush subtropical regions, old hardwood forests, and sweeping Highveld vistas to the deep desert of the Kalahari) and large animals (found throughout South Africa and in protected, expansive game reserves) are one part of this world. The people who live here (with their origins in Africa, Europe, India, and Southeast Asia) make up another; they bring a vibrant, global cultural, artistic, and culinary variety to the country. All this, combined with access to the conveniences of a developed infrastructure amid the challenges of Africa, make the country truly unique.

South Africa has experienced a surge in both business and pleasure travel in the past 2 decades, with visitors arriving from within the African continent and from Europe and North America. Business travelers typically head to the commercial centers of Johannesburg, Cape Town, and Durban.

Tourist itineraries are as diverse as the country itself. From Cape Town, for example, visitors can follow the wine route of the Western Cape exploring the many wineries along the way. Or they can take spectacular drives along the coast; going east, travelers can visit the southernmost point of Africa at Cape Agulhas—where the Indian and Atlantic Oceans meet in a roar of foam—continuing on to the small scenic towns of Knysna and Plettenberg Bay. Mpumalanga, home to half of Kruger National Park, has old

10

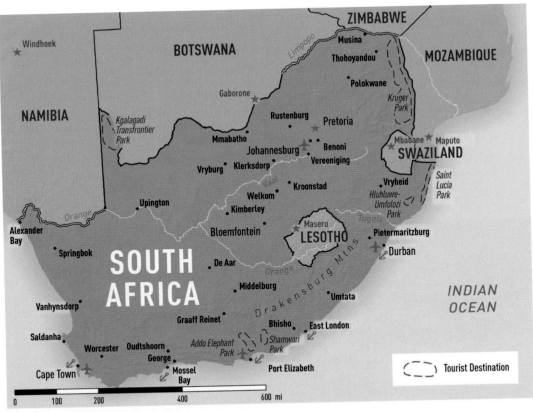

MAP 10-3. **South Africa destination map**

gold-mining towns, many of which are in near-original condition.

Game reserves located throughout the country attract many tourists. The largest, Kruger National Park, is located along the Mozambique border in the northeast (see Map 10-3). Kwa-Zulu Natal has a number of game parks (Hluhluwe-Umfolozi and Saint Lucia) set inland from Durban, and the Eastern Cape has parks (Addo Elephant Park and Shamwari) easily accessed from Port Elizabeth on the southern coast. Many smaller luxury reserves have emerged that cater to high-end travelers.

South Africa is also a common destination for humanitarian workers, missionaries, and students. A sizable number of South Africans live outside the country; those returning home for a visit are considered VFR travelers (see Chapter 9, Visiting Friends & Relatives: VFR Travel).

While there is a wide range of living standards in South Africa, most visitors experience standards comparable to those in developed countries. A smaller number of visitors may go to less developed areas, either to rural areas or to lower-income townships found outside most towns and cities. Hikers, adventure-seekers, and missionaries will experience a wider range of living standards. Similarly, the quality and availability of health care is variable. Middle- and upper-income South Africans live in low-risk environments, have a standard of health comparable to that of North Americans, and can access world-class medical facilities. Poorer South Africans live in areas with few amenities, are exposed to a wide range of diseases, and have limited access to adequate health care.

## HEALTH ISSUES

### Vaccine-Preventable Diseases

All travelers to South Africa should be up-to-date with their routine vaccinations. Infectious diseases such as measles and mumps are endemic to the region. In addition, hepatitis A vaccine is recommended for most travelers, and hepatitis B vaccine is recommended for travelers who may be exposed to blood or other body fluids, including through sexual contact. Travelers should also consider typhoid vaccine, especially more adventuresome eaters or those staying in less-than-sanitary surroundings.

### YELLOW FEVER VACCINE REQUIREMENTS

South Africa requires a valid International Certificate of Vaccination or Prophylaxis (ICVP) documenting yellow fever vaccination ≥10 days before arrival in South Africa for all travelers aged ≥1 year traveling from or transiting for >12 hours through the airport of a country with risk of yellow fever virus transmission. South Africa considers a one-time dose of yellow fever vaccine (properly documented with an ICVP) to be good for the life of the traveler. Any traveler not meeting this requirement can be refused entry to South Africa or quarantined for up to 6 days. Travelers may also be vaccinated on entry. Unvaccinated travelers presenting a medical waiver signed by a licensed health care provider are generally allowed entry.

Travelers going to or transiting through South Africa are advised to seek the most current information by consulting the CDC Travelers' Health website (www.cdc.gov/travel), the website of the US embassy and consulates in South Africa (https://za.usembassy.gov/), and the embassy of South Africa in Washington, DC (www.saembassy.org/).

## HIV and Sexually Transmitted Infections

South Africa has the largest estimated number of people living with HIV of any country in the world. The prevalence of HIV infection is approximately 19% among people aged 15–49 years, and the prevalence among sex workers is even higher. Other sexually transmitted infections (STIs) are also present at high rates in this population. Travelers should be aware of STI risks and use condoms when having sex with someone whose HIV or STI status is unknown.

## Vectorborne Diseases

Chloroquine-resistant *Plasmodium falciparum* malaria is found along the border with Zimbabwe and Mozambique in the following locations: 1) the Vembe and Mopane district municipalities of Limpopo Province; 2) Ehlanzeni district municipality in Mpumalanga Province; and 3) Umkhanyakude in KwaZulu-Natal Province. This region includes Kruger National Park (see Map 10-3). In addition, in March 2017, the CDC received reports of malaria in the western Waterberg District of Limpopo Province, an area not known previously to have malaria transmission. Visitors to all of these areas should take malaria chemoprophylaxis and use mosquito precautions; preventing mosquito bites is the first line of defense against malaria. The South African Department of Health recommends malaria chemoprophylaxis for travelers visiting malaria risk areas from September through May and reliance on mosquito-avoidance measures for the rest of the year. CDC, however, recommends chemoprophylaxis at all times of the year (see Chapter 2, Yellow Fever Vaccine & Malaria Prophylaxis Information, by Country).

Rickettsial tick-bite fever is common in South Africa (see Chapter 4, Rickettsial Diseases). The incidence rate for visitors from Europe is estimated to be 4%–5%. The disease is characterized by an eschar at the bite site, regional adenopathy, and a maculopapular or petechial rash. Hikers and campers in rural areas are especially at risk and should take measures to prevent tick bites (see Chapter 2, Mosquitoes, Ticks & Other Arthropods). Travelers taking doxycycline for malaria chemoprophylaxis may have some protection against tick-bite fever, but no studies exist to support or refute this viewpoint. Taking doxycycline solely as prophylaxis for tick-bite fever (as opposed to taking it for malaria chemoprophylaxis) is not recommended.

## Travelers' Diarrhea

As with most destinations, the risk of travelers' diarrhea depends on style of travel and food choices (see Chapter 2, Food & Water Precautions, and Travelers' Diarrhea). Consider dispensing a fluoroquinolone, such as ciprofloxacin, for travelers to use as self-treatment of moderate to severe diarrhea.

## Waterborne Diseases

*Schistosoma* spp., parasites found throughout Africa, may be present in any body of unchlorinated, fresh water (see Chapter 4, Schistosomiasis). Travelers should avoid swimming in lakes, streams, and ponds.

## Animal Avoidance

Although most travelers avoid wild animals in game reserves, rabies is common in dogs and other mammals throughout the country. The KwaZulu-Natal Province has the highest incidence of rabies. Travelers have no way of telling if a given animal is rabid and should avoid all contact with animals. Instruct travelers to wash any bite or scratch from an animal with soap and water immediately and to see a clinician as soon as possible (see Chapter 3, Animal Bites & Stings, and Chapter 4, Rabies).

Hospitals in South Africa are equipped to provide postexposure prophylaxis and medical care for rabies exposures. Rabies vaccine is available throughout South Africa, and rabies immune globulin (RIG) is available in major urban medical centers. Most of the new formulations of Equine RIG used in the public health system are potent, highly purified, and safe. Private medical centers stock human RIG.

## SAFETY AND SECURITY

Over the past several years, South Africa has experienced a rise in violent crime, including armed robberies, carjackings, home invasions, and rape (see Chapter 3, Safety & Security Overseas). Most incidents occur in lower-income residential areas and, as such, most visitors will not be targets or victims. However, awareness of personal safety and security should be stressed to all visitors. Travelers should rely on local guidance about what security precautions to take in specific areas.

Although South Africa has a modern road system, drivers should be alert for dangerous driving practices, stray animals, and poor roads in remote rural areas (see Chapter 8, Road & Traffic Safety).

### BIBLIOGRAPHY

1. Blumberg LH, de Frey A, Frean J, Mendelson M. The 2010 FIFA World Cup: communicable disease risks and advice for visitors to South Africa. J Travel Med. 2010 May–Jun;17(3):150–2.

2. Durrheim DN, Braack LE, Waner S, Gammon S. Risk of malaria in visitors to the Kruger National Park, South Africa. J Travel Med. 1998 Dec;5(4):173–7.

3. Frean J, Blumberg L, Ogunbanjo GA. Tick bite fever in South Africa. SA Fam Pract. 2008 Mar–Apr;50(2):33–5.

4. Maharaj R, Raman J, Morris N, Moonasar D, Durrheim DN, Seocharan I, et al. Epidemiology of malaria in South Africa: from control to elimination. S Afr Med J. 2013 Oct;103(10 Pt2):779–83.

5. Probst C, Parry CD, Rehm J. Socio-economic differences in HIV/AIDS mortality in South Africa. Trop Med Int Health. 2016 Jul;21(7):846–55.

6. South African National Travel Health Network. SaNTHNet [homepage on the Internet]. Dunvegan (South Africa): South African National Travel Health Network; 2013 [cited 2018 Sep 23]. Available from: www.santhnet.co.za/.

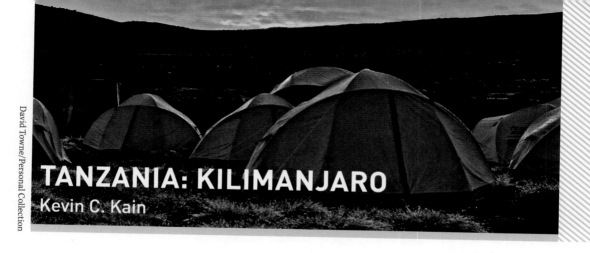

# TANZANIA: KILIMANJARO
Kevin C. Kain

## DESTINATION OVERVIEW

The tallest mountain on the African continent, and one of the largest freestanding volcanoes in the world, Kilimanjaro remains a revered and classic image. Its snow-capped peak rises 19,341 ft (5,895 m) above the tropical African savanna, an irresistible draw for trekkers and mountaineers from around the globe. Although no technical climbing is required to reach the summit, its challenges are often misjudged. Climbing Kilimanjaro is a serious undertaking, requiring advance planning. Unfortunately, large numbers of travelers are ill prepared, ascend too quickly, and consequently fail to reach the peak. With due preparation and more reasonable ascent rates, however, climbing "Kili" is an aspiration that many can accomplish successfully. Heart, lung, and other transplant recipients, for example, have summited Kilimanjaro safely.

Despite being higher than classic trekking destinations in Nepal, such as Kala Pattar (18,450 ft; 5,625 m) or Everest base camp (17,598 ft; 5,364 m), typical ascent rates on Kilimanjaro are considerably faster (4–6 days vs 8–12 days). The classic route up Kilimanjaro is the Marangu (40 miles; 64 km), often sold as a 5-day, 4-night trip. Nicknamed the "Coca-Cola" route, Marangu features bunkhouse accommodations and food; the trail is wide and relatively easy compared to other routes. There are at least 9 other routes up the mountain (Map 10-4), including the stunningly beautiful Machame (the so-called "whiskey" route) with its longer days and generally tougher climbs. Machame and other routes involve camping and are sold as 6- to 9-day packages, providing more opportunity to acclimatize and a greater chance to successfully summit.

Kilimanjaro can be climbed throughout the year. March–April are often the wettest months, but the weather is unpredictable, and climbers must be prepared for extreme weather and rain at any time. A 2011 review of UK companies arranging high-elevation trekking trips reported that only 16 of 93 (17%) companies offering Kilimanjaro treks complied with Wilderness Medical Society guidelines on ascending to elevation, compared with 92% of treks to Everest base camp. Moreover, fewer than half of these companies carry medications to prevent or treat altitude illness, so trekkers should be prepared to carry and understand how and when to use these medications.

## HEALTH ISSUES

The main medical issues for those attempting to climb Kilimanjaro include the prevention and treatment of altitude illness and the potential for drug interactions between medications used for altitude illness and antimalarial or antidiarrheal agents commonly used by travelers to Tanzania.

### Altitude Illness and Acute Mountain Sickness (AMS)

Altitude illness is a major reason why only about half of those attempting to summit Kilimanjaro via Marangu reach the crater rim, known as Gilman's Point (18,652 ft; 5,685 m), and as few as 10% reach the top, Uhuru (Freedom) Peak (19,341 ft; 5,895 m). Prevalence rates of AMS were 75%–77% in recent studies of 4- and 5-day ascents on Marangu. Those using the carbonic

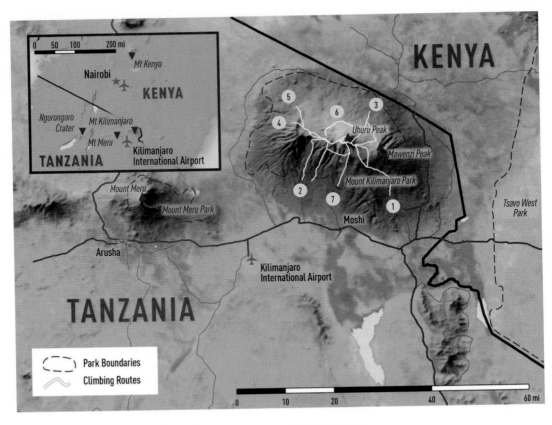

## SLEEPING ALTITUDE (FEET) PER NIGHT ALONG CLIMBING ROUTES

| | Route | Night 1 | Night 2 | Night 3 | Night 4 | Night 5 | Night 6 | Night 7 | Night 8 | Night 9 |
|---|---|---|---|---|---|---|---|---|---|---|
| 1 | MARANGU | 8,858 | 12,205 | 14,160 | 15,430 | 12,205 | 6,046 | n/a | n/a | n/a |
| 2 | MACHAME | 9,350 | 12,500 | 13,044 | 13,106 | 15,331 | 10,065 | 5,380 | n/a | n/a |
| 3 | RONGAI | 9,300 | 11,811 | 14,160 | 14,160 | 15,430 | 12,205 | 6,046 | n/a | n/a |
| 4 | LEMOSHO | 9,498 | 11,500 | 13,800 | 13,044 | 13,106 | 15,331 | 10,065 | 5,380 | n/a |
| 5 | SHIRA | 11,800 | 12,500 | 13,044 | 13,106 | 15,331 | 10,065 | 5,380 | n/a | n/a |
| 6 | NORTHERN | 9,498 | 11,500 | 12,500 | 13,580 | 13,200 | 12,700 | 15,600 | 10,065 | 5,380 |
| 7 | UMBWE | 9,514 | 13,044 | 13,106 | 15,331 | 10,065 | 5,380 | n/a | n/a | n/a |

MAP 10-4. Kilimanjaro destination map

anhydrase inhibitor acetazolamide were significantly less likely to develop acute mountain sickness (AMS) on the 5-day ascents, but 40% or more of those taking this medication still reported AMS symptoms.

Every hiker on Kilimanjaro should receive pretravel advice on AMS, be able to recognize symptoms, and know how to prevent and treat it (see Chapter 3, High-Altitude Travel & Altitude Illness). People with certain underlying medical conditions, including pregnancy, significant underlying lung or cardiac disease, and ocular or neurologic conditions, should consult a travel health provider with specialized knowledge of altitude illness. Such travelers may be more susceptible to problems associated with travel to high elevations, or they may be taking medications that can interact with medications taken to prevent AMS.

Climbers can enhance their enjoyment of the experience and increase their chances of successfully reaching the summit by allowing more time to acclimatize.

- If Ngorongoro crater (also in Tanzania) is part of a planned combined safari/Kilimanjaro hike itinerary, travelers should try to spend the last few nights of the safari there, because its elevation (7,500 ft; 2,286 m) will aid acclimatization for the Kilimanjaro trek.

- Before attempting Kilimanjaro, travelers may acclimatize by hiking nearby Mount Meru (14,978 ft; 4,565 m) or Mount Kenya (to Point Lenana, 16,355 ft; 4,895 m). Combined climbing trips for Mount Kenya and Kilimanjaro are now offered commercially.

- Adding at least an extra day or two to the ascent of Kilimanjaro facilitates acclimatization regardless of the route, but especially on routes normally promoted as 4- to 6-day trips.

Anyone with a history of AMS susceptibility and for those in whom adequate acclimatization is not possible (i.e., most "Kili" clients), use of medications such as acetazolamide to prevent altitude illness is recommended. Acetazolamide accelerates acclimatization. It is effective in preventing AMS (when started the day before ascent) and in treating AMS. Children may take it safely. Dexamethasone is an alternative for AMS prevention in people intolerant of or allergic to acetazolamide. Climbers may also use dexamethasone to prevent high-altitude pulmonary edema (HAPE) and to prevent and treat high-altitude cerebral edema (HACE).

Travelers with signs and symptoms of altitude illness must not continue to ascend and need to descend if symptoms are worsening at the same altitude. A flexible itinerary and having an extra guide who can accompany any members of the group down the mountain if they become ill are considerations.

## Malaria

Travel health providers must be aware of and consider possible interactions between antimalarials and drugs used to prevent or manage AMS. The tropical malaria-endemic location of Kilimanjaro means that many trekkers will be taking antimalarial drugs during their climb. And they will likely need to continue taking malaria prophylaxis after descent, particularly if they are visiting game parks or staying overnight at elevations below 6,562 ft (2,000 m).

Although the overall prevalence of malaria is falling in Tanzania, changes in climate have expanded the range of suitable habitats for *Anopheles* spp., making malaria transmission in the Kilimanjaro highlands a risk. Travelers flying directly into Kilimanjaro International Airport (2,932 ft; 894 m) and going the same day to an altitude above 6,562 ft (2,000 m), have little risk of malaria. Most people, however, will be on safari or traveling before or after their Kilimanjaro trip and will be on prophylaxis (see Chapter 2, Yellow Fever Vaccine & Malaria Prophylaxis Information, by Country).

## Remote Travel

Trekking Kilimanjaro is physically demanding, requiring a good level of fitness and preparation for the elements. Weather is characterized by extremes; travelers should be prepared for tropical heat, heavy rains, and bitter cold, and should store their gear (especially sleeping duffels) in waterproof bags. Travelers should have adequate health insurance, including medical evacuation insurance, and make sure their medical care and medical evacuation policies cover any potential costs for a rescue or evacuation from the top of the mountain.

Travelers should carry a first-aid kit that includes bandages, tape, a blister kit, antibacterial and antifungal cream, antibiotics for travelers' diarrhea, antimalarials, antiemetics, oral rehydration salts, antihistamines, analgesics, throat lozenges, and medications for altitude illness (see Chapter 6, Travel Health Kits).

10

## BIBLIOGRAPHY

1. Baumgartner RW, Siegel AM, Hackett PH. Going high with preexisting neurological conditions. High Alt Med Biol. 2007 Summer;8(2):108–16.

2. Davies AJ, Kalson NS, Stokes S, Earl MD, Whitehead AG, Frost H, et al. Determinants of summiting success and acute mountain sickness on Mt Kilimanjaro (5895 m). Wilderness Environ Med. 2009 Winter;20(4):311–7.

3. Jackson SJ, Varley J, Sellers C, Josephs K, Codrington L, Duke G, et al. Incidence and predictors of acute mountain sickness among trekkers on Mount Kilimanjaro. High Alt Med Biol. 2010 Fall;11(3):217–22.

4. Kulkarni MA, Desrochers RE, Kajeguka DC, Kaaya RD, Tomayer A, Kweka EJ, et al. 10 years of environmental change on the slopes of Mount Kilimanjaro and its associated shift in malaria vector distributions. Front Public Health. 2016 Dec 21;4:281.

5. Low EV, Avery AJ, Gupta V, Schedlbauer A, Grocott MP. Identifying the lowest effective dose of acetazolamide for the prophylaxis of acute mountain sickness: systematic review and meta-analysis. BMJ. 2012 Oct;345:e6779.

6. Luks AM, Swenson ER, Bartsch P. Acute high-altitude sickness. Eur Respir Rev 2017 Jan 31;26(143).

7. Luks AM, McIntosh SE, Grissom CK, Auerbach PS, Rodway GW, Schoene RB, et al. Wilderness Medical Society practice guidelines for the prevention and treatment of acute altitude illness: 2014 update. Wilderness Environ Med. 2014 Dec;25(4 Suppl):S4–14.

8. Luks AM, Swenson ER. Travel to high altitude with pre-existing lung disease. Eur Respir J. 2007 Apr;29(4):770–92.

9. Parati G, Agostoni P, Basnyat B, Bilo G, Brugger H, Coca A, et al. Clinical recommendations for high altitude exposure of individuals with pre-existing cardiovascular conditions. Eur Heart J. 2018 May 1;39(17):1546–54.

10. Ritchie ND, Baggott AV, Andrew Todd WT. Acetazolamide for the prevention of acute mountain sickness—a systematic review and meta-analysis. J Travel Med. 2012 Sep–Oct;19(5):298–307.

11. Shah NM, Windsor JS, Meijer H, Hillebrandt D. Are UK commercial expeditions complying with wilderness medical society guidelines on ascent rates to altitude? J Travel Med. 2011 May–Jun;18(3):214–6.

**10**

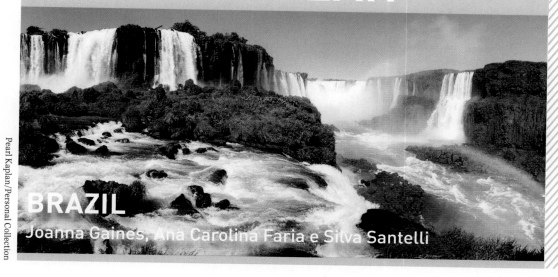

THE AMERICAS &
THE CARIBBEAN

BRAZIL
Joanna Gaines, Ana Carolina Faria e Silva Santelli

Pearl Kaplan/Personal Collection

## DESTINATION OVERVIEW

Brazil is the fifth largest country in the world and the largest country in South America, occupying nearly half the land area of the continent. With more than 200 million people, Brazil is home to the world's largest Portuguese-speaking population. It is the world's eighth largest economy and is classified as an upper-middle-income country. Nearly 85% of Brazilians live in urban areas.

In Brazil, tourism is a growing economic sector; it is the most popular tourist destination in South America, the second most popular in all Latin America. In 2016, more than 6 million international visitors traveled there. Brazil hosted the FIFA World Cup in 2014 and the Summer Olympic and Paralympic Games in 2016. Rio de Janeiro, Brazil's second-largest city (population >7 million) and most frequently visited tourist destination, is famous for its beaches, landmarks, and annual Carnival festivities. São Paulo, one of the world's largest cities (>21 million people in the greater metropolitan area), is the economic center of Brazil and the most visited destination for business travel. Brazilians prize many of their

major cities, including Salvador, Florianópolis, Fortaleza, Natal, and Recife for their coastlines and regional culture.

The country also boasts a number of UNESCO World Heritage sites. These include Iguaçu National Park in Paraná (home to the largest waterfalls in the Americas); the historic towns of Olinda (Pernambuco), Ouro Preto (Minas Gerais), Salvador (Bahia), and São Luis (Maranhão); the modern capital of Brasília; and natural areas of the Amazon forest, Pantanal Conservation Area (Mato Grosso and Mato Grosso do Sul). The Atlantic forests (Rio de Janeiro and São Paulo) and the archipelago of Fernando de Noronha in the Atlantic Ocean are also World Heritage sites (see Map 10-5).

## HEALTH ISSUES

### Vaccine-Preventable Diseases

Travelers to Brazil should be up-to-date on routine vaccines. Hepatitis A vaccination is recommended. Hepatitis B vaccination should be considered for most travelers and is recommended for anyone who could be exposed to blood or other body

10

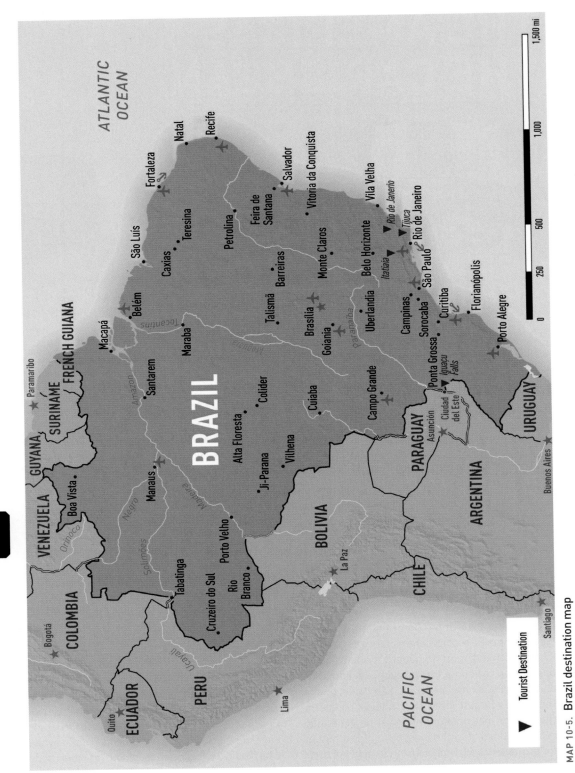

MAP 10-5. Brazil destination map

fluids, including through sexual contact. Consider vaccinating "adventurous eaters" and travelers who stay with friends or relatives, or who visit smaller cities, villages, or rural areas, against typhoid (see Chapter 4, Typhoid & Paratyphoid Fever). The World Health Organization and CDC recommend yellow fever vaccine for travelers going to certain areas of the country (see below for more details). Because of recent yellow fever outbreaks in previously unaffected areas, clinicians must ask patients about their itineraries and potential travel within Brazil and refer to the CDC Travelers' Health website (www.cdc.gov/travel) for the most recent recommendations.

## Vectorborne Diseases

Vectorborne (including mosquitoborne) diseases are present in many areas of Brazil; these infections are the leading causes of febrile illness among travelers returning from South America. *Aedes* mosquitoes transmit chikungunya, dengue, and Zika. More detailed information about each of these diseases can be found in Chapter 4. Risk of infection is high in many Brazilian states due to high indices of *Aedes* infestation. Some vectorborne diseases are new to Brazil: chikungunya was first detected there in 2014, Zika in 2015.

From 2000 through 2015, cases of dengue increased throughout Brazil, with epidemics reported in large cities including Rio de Janeiro and Salvador. In 2016, Brazil recorded 1.4 million probable cases of dengue, approximately 278,000 cases of chikungunya, and 216,000 cases of Zika virus infection. Travelers to Brazil should take measures to protect themselves from mosquito bites (see Chapter 3, Mosquitoes, Ticks & Other Arthropods). Because of the risk of birth defects in infants born to women infected with Zika during pregnancy, women who are pregnant or trying to become pregnant should research the most recent travel recommendations at www. cdc.gov/zika.

### MALARIA

Almost all malaria in Brazil occurs in the Amazon Basin, although the mosquito vector is present in much of the country. *Plasmodium vivax* is the main malaria species, although approximately 12% of cases are caused by *P. falciparum*.

Prophylactic treatment with antimalarial medication is recommended for travelers going to malaria-endemic areas (see Chapter 2, Yellow Fever Vaccine & Malaria Prophylaxis Information, by Country, and Map 4-21).

### YELLOW FEVER

Mosquitoes transmit the yellow fever virus throughout the Amazon Basin and in forested regions along all major river basins in Brazil, including Iguaçu Falls and as far south as Rio Grande do Sul. Vaccination against this potentially lethal disease is recommended for all travelers aged >9 months going to areas where there is risk of infection (see Chapter 2, Yellow Fever Vaccine & Malaria Prophylaxis Information, by Country).

### RICKETTSIAL DISEASES

Tickborne diseases have been identified in Brazil. Caused by the same etiologic agent (*Rickettsia rickettsii*) as Rocky Mountain spotted fever, these diseases include *febre maculosa* and Brazilian spotted fever. Travelers should take precautions to avoid flea and tick bites both indoors and outdoors. For more information, see Chapter 3, Mosquitoes, Ticks & Other Arthropods.

## Travelers' Diarrhea and Foodborne Infections

Travelers should take food and water precautions throughout Brazil (see Chapter 2, Food & Water Precautions). Travelers' diarrhea is the most common travel-related ailment; consuming raw fruits and/or vegetables or unpasteurized dairy products, or patronizing street vendors, increases the risk for foodborne infections. Oral rehydration salts are available from public health clinics and in almost all pharmacies in Brazil. Clinicians may prescribe an antibiotic for self-treatment of moderate to severe diarrhea (see Chapter 2, Travelers' Diarrhea).

## Other Infections

### SEXUALLY TRANSMITTED INFECTIONS

In Brazil, condoms are distributed free of charge by the government and are available in health clinics, tourist service centers, and other distribution points in many cities. Male condoms are available throughout Brazil in pharmacies, convenience

10

stores, and large supermarkets; female condoms are also available in some locations. Travelers, particularly those at high risk for acquiring HIV infection (men who have sex with men, for example) may wish to discuss preexposure prophylaxis with their health care provider (www.cdc.gov/hiv/prep).

## RESPIRATORY DISEASES

Peak influenza circulation occurs from April through September in most of Brazil but may occur throughout the year in tropical areas. CDC recommends seasonal influenza vaccination at least 2 weeks before travel and also pneumococcal vaccination for the elderly and younger adults with chronic medical conditions.

A number of fungal diseases are endemic to parts of Brazil. Inhaled fungal spores typically present in the soil (paracoccidioidomycosis, histoplasmosis, cryptococcosis, and coccidioidomycosis) cause respiratory illness and occasionally more severe disease such as meningitis or bone infections (see the sections on Histoplasmosis and Coccidioidomycosis in Chapter 4). Travelers should beware of bat guano in caves, and exercise caution before disturbing soil, particularly if contaminated by bird or bat feces.

## LEPTOSPIROSIS

Outbreaks of leptospirosis have occurred in urban areas in Brazil following heavy flooding (see Chapter 4, Leptospirosis). Travelers participating in recreational water activities are at increased risk, particularly after heavy rainfall.

## PARASITIC INFECTIONS

Most Brazilian states have eliminated Chagas disease (American trypanosomiasis) through insecticide spraying for the vector. Although the risk is extremely low, travelers and ecotourists staying in poor-quality housing may be at higher risk for this disease. Outbreaks have been associated with consuming foods or beverages containing açaí, an Amazonian fruit eaten throughout Brazil. Oral transmission occurs when people consume açaí contaminated with triatomines—the blood-sucking insects that transmit the etiologic agent of Chagas disease (*Trypanosoma cruzi*)—or their feces (see Chapter 4, American Trypanosomiasis).

*Schistosoma* spp. are parasites found in freshwater lakes and rivers in many states of Brazil, especially in the northeast. Swimming, bathing, and wading in fresh, unchlorinated water can result in schistosomiasis (see Chapter 4, Schistosomiasis). Swimming or bathing in saltwater (oceans or seas) is not a source of infection.

Both cutaneous and visceral leishmaniasis occur in Brazil and are most common in the Amazon and northeast regions (see Chapter 4, Cutaneous and Visceral Leishmaniasis). The risk is highest from dusk to dawn because the sand fly vector typically feeds (bites) at night and during twilight hours. Ecotourists and adventure travelers might have an increased risk, but even short-term travelers in endemic areas have developed leishmaniasis.

## RABIES

Preexposure rabies vaccination is recommended for travelers with extended itineraries, particularly children and those planning trips into rural areas. For shorter stays, rabies vaccination is recommended for adventure travelers, those who may be exposed to animals occupationally, and those staying in locations >24 hours away from access to rabies immune globulin (see Chapter 4, Rabies).

## TUBERCULOSIS (TB)

Tuberculosis is prevalent in Brazil, but short-term travelers are not considered high risk for infection unless visiting specific crowded environments. Travelers who anticipate prolonged exposure to people with TB (i.e., those whose travel plans include spending time in clinics, hospitals, prisons, or homeless shelters) should have a tuberculin skin test or TB blood test before leaving the United States. If the pretravel test is negative, travelers should undergo repeat testing 8–10 weeks after returning from Brazil. For more information, see Chapter 4, Tuberculosis.

## Other Health and Safety Risks

As in many foreign countries, motor vehicle accidents in Brazil are a leading cause of injury and death of US travelers (see Chapter 8, Road & Traffic Safety). Road conditions in Brazil differ significantly from those in the United States, and driving at night can be dangerous. The national toll-free number for emergency roadside assistance (193) is in Portuguese only. It is illegal to drive after drinking alcohol, even small quantities. Seatbelt use is mandatory, and motorcyclists are required to wear helmets.

Children aged ≤10 years must be seated in the back seat. Brazilian federal law requires infants up to 1 year of age to use rear-facing car seats, children 1–4 years of age to use forward-facing car seats, and children 4–7.5 years of age to use booster seats. Anyone traveling with small children should bring their own car or booster seats, in the event they are limited or unavailable.

Travelers to Brazil should familiarize themselves with climatic conditions at their destinations before travel. Temperatures >104°F (40°C) are common from October through January in some Brazilian cities (see Chapter 3, Extremes of Temperature).

Poisonous snakes are hazards in many locations in Brazil, although deaths from snakebites are rare (see Chapter 3, Animal Bites & Stings). Counsel travelers to seek immediate medical attention any time a bite wound breaks the skin or if a snake sprays venom into their eyes. In some areas of the country, specific antivenins are available; being able to identify the snake species may prove critical to delivery of optimal medical care. The national toll-free number for intoxication and poisoning assistance is 0800-722-6001 (in Portuguese only).

Travel in Brazil is generally safe, although crime remains a problem in urban areas and has spread to rural areas. The incidence of crime against tourists is higher in areas surrounding beaches, hotels, nightclubs, and other tourist destinations (see Chapter 3, Safety & Security Overseas). Drug-related violence has resulted in clashes with police in tourist areas. Political demonstrations may disrupt public and private transportation. Encourage travelers to register to receive Department of State advisories for alerts in areas they plan to visit (https://step.state.gov/step/). Several Brazilian cities have established specialized police units whose job is to patrol areas frequented by tourists.

## HEALTH CARE IN BRAZIL

Quality health care is available in most sizable Brazilian cities. Brazilian public health services are free. Foreign visitors can seek treatment in the emergency care network of Brazil's public health system, known as the Unified Health System or by its acronym, SUS, or through private facilities. The toll-free emergency number for ambulance services throughout Brazil is 192. The Brazilian Ministry of Health provides information in Portuguese for international visitors (http://portalms.saude.gov.br/saude-para-voce/saude-do-viajante/durante-sua-estadia), including a list of reference hospitals for mass events in Brazil.

Brazil has a growing number of private clinics that cater to international clientele and offer medical procedures using advanced technologies (see Chapter 9, Medical Tourism). Travel to Brazil for cosmetic surgery, assisted reproductive technology, or other elective medical procedures has increased in recent years, becoming a major part of the medical industry there. Although Brazil has many cosmetic surgery facilities on par with those found in the United States, quality of care can (and does) vary widely. Instruct patients seeking cosmetic surgery or other elective procedures to do their research and to make sure that emergency medical facilities are available at their clinic of choice.

**10**

## BIBLIOGRAPHY

1. Gaines J, Sotir MJ, Cunningham TJ, Harvey KA, Lee CV, Stoney RJ, et al. Health and safety issues for travelers attending the World Cup and Summer Olympic and Paralympic Games in Brazil, 2014 to 2016. JAMA Intern Med. 2014 Aug;174(8):1383–90.

2. Jentes ES, Poumerol G, Gershman MD, Hill DR, Lemarchand J, Lewis RF, et al. The revised global yellow fever risk map and recommendations for vaccination, 2010: consensus of the Informal WHO Working Group on Geographic Risk for Yellow Fever. Lancet Infect Dis. 2011 Aug;11(8):622–32.

3. Malaria Atlas Project. The spatial limits of *Plasmodium vivax* malaria transmission map in 2010 in Brazil. 2010 [cited 2016 Sep 23]. Available from: www.map.ox.ac.uk/explore/countries/BRA/.

4. Nobrega AA, Garcia MH, Tatto E, Obara MT, Costa E, Sobel J, et al. Oral transmission of Chagas disease by

consumption of acai palm fruit, Brazil. Emerg Infect Dis. 2009 Apr;15(4):653–5.

5. Oliveira-Ferreira J, Lacerda MV, Brasil P, Ladislau JL, Tauil PL, Daniel-Ribeiro CT. Malaria in Brazil: an overview. Malar J. 2010 Apr 30;9:115.

6. Teixeira MG, Siqueira JB Jr, Ferreira GL, Bricks L, Joint G. Epidemiological trends of dengue disease in Brazil

(2000–2010): a systematic literature search and analysis. PLoS Negl Trop Dis. 2013 Dec 19;7(12):e2520.

7. Wilson ME, Chen LH, Han PV, Keystone JS, Cramer JP, Segurado A, et al. Illness in travelers returned from Brazil: the GeoSentinel experience and implications for the 2014 FIFA World Cup and the 2016 Summer Olympics. Clin Infect Dis 2014 May;58(10):1347–56.

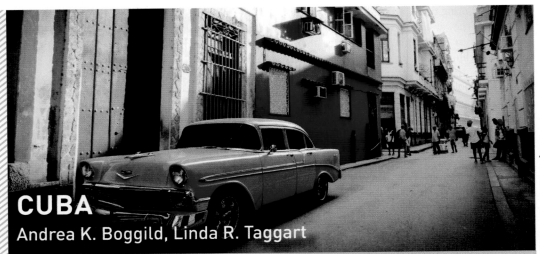

# CUBA
Andrea K. Boggild, Linda R. Taggart

Erica J. Sison/Personal Collection

## DESTINATION OVERVIEW

The Republic of Cuba is located between the Caribbean Sea and the North Atlantic Ocean, approximately 93 miles (150 km) south of Key West, Florida. The largest country in the Caribbean, it has a population of 11 million people. The official language is Spanish. The climate is tropical, with a dry season from November to April and a rainy season from May to October. Originally inhabited by a native Amerindian population, the Spanish colonized the island in the 15th century.

In 1898, Cuba gained independence from Spain, with the assistance of the United States. It then gained independence from the United States in 1902. In 1959, a revolutionary army under Fidel Castro overthrew the existing Cuban government and established a communist state. In response, the United States put in place an embargo against Castro and Cuba in 1961. More recently, the United

States initiated efforts to reestablish diplomatic relations, reopening the US embassy in Havana on July 20, 2015. Although tourist travel to Cuba is still prohibited under US law, 12 categories of travel are now authorized, including family visits, professional research and meetings, and humanitarian projects.

Out of reach of most US citizens for years, Cuba has long been a popular travel destination for Canadians and Europeans. The largest and most popular resort area is in Varadero, a peninsula with a vast, 13-mile stretch of sandy beach and more than 50 hotels. Those seeking to experience Cuban culture often travel to the capital city of Havana to explore the streets of La Habana Vieja (Old Havana) and to walk along the sea wall, the Malecon. Another popular destination is Trinidad, a colonial city known for its cobblestone streets (see Map 10-6). Throughout

10

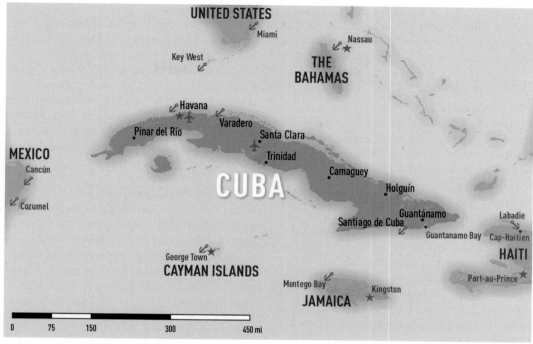

MAP 10-6. Cuba destination map

the country, tourists can enjoy the sight of vintage cars and sample Cuban cigars, rum, and mojitos.

## HEALTH ISSUES

### Vaccine-Preventable Diseases

Travelers should confirm that routine vaccinations are up-to-date, including seasonal influenza vaccine. Hepatitis A vaccine is recommended for non-immune travelers. Strongly encourage travelers anticipating blood or body fluid exposures—people intending to do medical work and those seeking medical treatment—to be vaccinated against hepatitis B. Travelers who obtain tattoos or piercings, users of injection drugs, and anyone who has sexual contact with the local population is also at risk for hepatitis B; because exposures such as these are often unanticipated, pretravel hepatitis B vaccination is a prudent choice for adult travelers.

Typhoid vaccination is recommended for most travelers, especially those visiting friends and relatives, people traveling to rural areas, and "adventurous eaters" (see Chapter 4, Typhoid

& Paratyphoid Fever). Rabies vaccine is recommended for travelers who may be in contact with dogs, bats, or other mammals at high risk for the disease; travelers who expect to have occupational exposure to animals; and long-term travelers.

### Vectorborne Diseases

Chikungunya, dengue, and Zika are mosquito-borne diseases that are present (or potentially present) in Cuba (see sections on chikungunya, dengue, and Zika in Chapter 4 for details on each). Travelers to this island nation should therefore take precautions against mosquitoes, using insect repellents and wearing pants and long-sleeved shirts (see Chapter 2, Mosquitoes, Ticks & Other Arthropods). Despite the large chikungunya outbreak that started in late 2013 and involved the entire Caribbean, Cuban authorities did not report any cases of local transmission. Dengue is a known risk, and the first cases of local vectorborne Zika virus transmission were reported in Cuba in 2016. Because of the risk of birth defects in infants born to women infected with Zika during pregnancy, women who are pregnant or trying to become pregnant should research the most recent travel recommendations at www.cdc.gov/zika.

## Other Health and Safety Risks

### FOOD AND WATER

Visitors to Cuba are at risk of developing travelers' diarrhea, even when staying at resorts. Remind travelers to refrain from eating raw or undercooked meat and seafood and any unpasteurized dairy products (see Chapter 2, Food & Water Precautions). Salads and uncooked vegetables should also be avoided, and fruit eaten only if washed in clean water or peeled by the traveler. Travelers should know to drink only bottled water or water that has been boiled and filtered or otherwise treated. Consider prescribing an antibiotic for self-treatment of moderate to severe diarrhea (see Chapter 2, Travelers' Diarrhea); these drugs are not readily available in Cuba.

Ciguatera fish poisoning is found in tropical and subtropical areas surrounded by coral reefs and is known to occur in Cuba. Counsel travelers to avoid or limit consumption of large reef fish, including their viscera, especially species such as grouper, snapper, barracuda, jack, sturgeon, sea bass, and moray eel (see Chapter 2, Food Poisoning from Marine Toxins).

### SUN, SAND, AND WATER HAZARDS

Care should be taken to avoid excess sun exposure: sunscreen of SPF ≥15 protects against both UVA and UVB; wearing protective clothing and seeking shade provide some respite from the tropical heat and sun (see Chapter 3, Sun Exposure).

In the Caribbean (and not unique to Cuba), travelers are at risk of a variety of other dermatological hazards. Cutaneous larva migrans is caused by dog and cat hookworms (see Chapter 4, Cutaneous Larva Migrans). Lying or walking on contaminated soil, including sandy beaches, exposes humans to hookworm larvae. Risk can be minimized by wearing shoes and by not lying directly on sand. Envenomation from jellyfish, microscopic cnidarians (sea bather's eruption), sea urchins, and stingrays can occur in the warm shallow waters surrounding many resort areas.

## SAFETY AND SECURITY

Road conditions are often dangerous (see Chapter 8, Road & Traffic Safety). The Carretera Central (main east–west highway) is in good condition, but hazards include unfenced livestock and farm vehicles. As many roads are unlit, travelers should avoid driving at night. Cars in Cuba are often old and may lack basic safety features such as turn signals. Tourist company buses and radio-dispatched taxis are generally safe and reliable; unlicensed taxis and yellow 3-wheeled "coco taxis" should be avoided. Advise travelers to fasten seat belts when riding in cars and to wear a helmet when riding bicycles or motorbikes. Petty theft may occur, especially in crowded tourist areas such as beaches and Old Town Havana. Typically nonviolent, there is some concern that violent crime is on the rise; travelers should not resist if confronted (see Chapter 3, Safety & Security Overseas).

## MEDICAL CARE

Health care does not meet American standards. Medical professionals are generally competent but medical supplies and certain medications may be in short supply or unavailable. Travelers should plan to bring adequate supplies of both prescription and nonprescription medications.

### BIBLIOGRAPHY

1. Boggild AK, Geduld J, Libman M, Ward BJ, McCarthy AE, Doyle PW, et al. Travel-acquired infections and illnesses in Canadians: surveillance report from CanTravNet surveillance data, 2009–2011. Open Med. 2014 Feb 11;8(1):e20–32.

2. Central Intelligence Agency. The World Factbook; 2017. [cited 2018 Mar 20]. Available from: www.cia.gov/library/publications/the-world-factbook/index.html.

3. Fillion K, Mileno MD. Cholera in travelers: shifting tides in epidemiology, management, and prevention. Curr Infect Dis Rep. 2015 Jan;17(1):455.

10

4. Morrison K, Aguiar Prieto P, Castro Domínguez A, Waltner-Toews D, FitzGibbon J. Ciguatera fish poisoning in La Habana, Cuba: a study of local social–ecological resilience. EcoHealth. 2008 Sep;5(3):346–59.

5. U.S. Department of State – Bureau of Consular Affairs. Country Information: Cuba. 2017. [cited 2018 Mar 20]. Available from: https://travel.state.gov/content/travel/en/international-travel/International-Travel-Country-Information-Pages/Cuba.html.

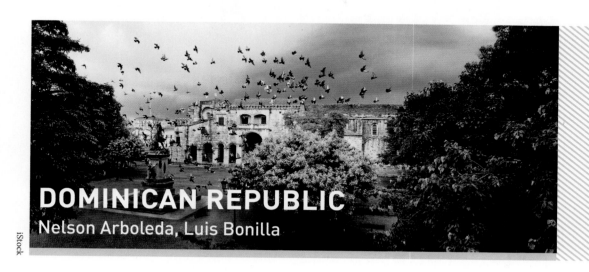

# DOMINICAN REPUBLIC
Nelson Arboleda, Luis Bonilla

iStock

## DESTINATION OVERVIEW

The Dominican Republic—the second-largest Caribbean nation, both by area and population—covers the eastern two-thirds of the Caribbean island of Hispaniola; Haiti comprises the western third. The capital city, Santo Domingo, is located on the southern coast of the island (see Map 10-7). Although English is spoken in most tourist areas (and approximately 250,000 US citizens call the Dominican Republic home), Spanish is the official language. Average temperatures range from 73.5°F (23°F) in January to 80°F (26.5°F) in August. The island receives more rain from May through November, and tropical storms or hurricanes are a possibility.

In 2017, more than 5 million foreign tourists (including approximately 3 million from the United States and Canada) visited the Dominican Republic, making it the most visited destination in the Caribbean. The Dominican Republic offers a diverse geography of beaches, mountain ranges (including the highest point in the Caribbean, Pico Duarte [10,164 ft; 3,098 m]), sugar cane and tobacco plantations, and farmland. Most tourism is concentrated in the east of the country around Bavaro and Punta Cana, which offer all-inclusive beach resorts. Whale watching is popular seasonally near the northeastern area in Samana, and kite- and windsurfing attract visitors to the northern areas of Puerto Plata, Sosua, and Cabarete. Santo Domingo has an attractive colonial district that contains many historical sites dating back to Christopher Columbus's arrival in the New World. A small number of travelers visit other parts of the country, where tourist infrastructure is limited or nonexistent.

## HEALTH ISSUES

### Vaccine-Preventable Diseases

All travelers should be up-to-date on routine vaccinations, including seasonal influenza. Cases of vaccine-preventable diseases have been reported among the local population and

10

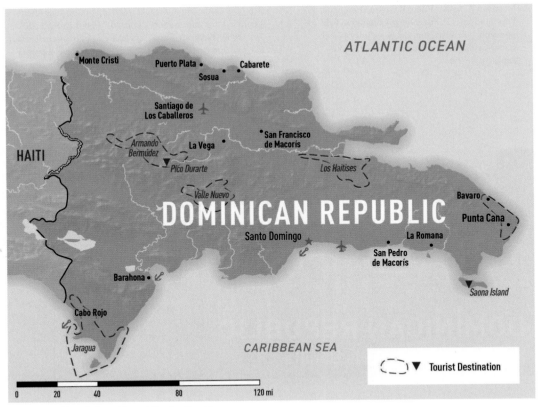

MAP 10-7. **Dominican Republic destination map**

unvaccinated tourists from Europe and other parts of the world.

Travelers should be vaccinated against hepatitis A and, depending upon itinerary and activities, typhoid—especially anyone staying with friends or family (see Chapter 4, Typhoid & Paratyphoid Fever). Hepatitis B vaccine is recommended for people who might be exposed to blood through needles or medical procedures, or body fluids during sexual intercourse with a new partner.

Reports of animal and human rabies in the Dominican Republic are not uncommon. In 2017, there were 41 cases of animal rabies and 1 human rabies case. Consider rabies preexposure vaccination for travelers potentially at risk for animal bites (those spending extended time outdoors or anyone who handles animals).

Cholera was reintroduced in 2010, although areas of active transmission are evolving. Visit the

Active cholera transmission has been reported in the Dominican Republic in recent years. Check the destination page at www.cdc.gov/travel for current recommendations.

## HIV and Other Sexually Transmitted Infections

Commercial sex workers (CSW) can be found throughout the Dominican Republic; Samana, Sosua, and Puerto Plata are known sex tourism destinations. HIV prevalence among female CSW is as high as 6% in some areas; syphilis (12%), hepatitis B virus (2.4%), and hepatitis C virus (0.9%) are also concerns. Among men who have sex with men, HIV prevalence is as high as 6.9% and active syphilis as high as 13.9%. Travelers should avoid sexual intercourse with CSW and always use condoms with any partner whose HIV or sexually transmitted disease status is unknown (see Chapter 9, Sex & Travel).

## Vectorborne Diseases

Malaria, dengue, Zika, and chikungunya are potential concerns for travelers to the Dominican Republic, and all travelers should take precautions to prevent mosquito bites by wearing long-sleeved shirts and long pants and using insect repellent (see Chapter 2, Mosquitoes, Ticks & Other Arthropods). Malaria is endemic to the Dominican Republic (see Chapter 4, Malaria). During 2017, a total of 395 cases of malaria were reported; 1 was fatal. Unless travelers are restricting their visit to the urban areas of Santiago or Santo Domingo only, CDC recommends taking malaria prophylaxis. This includes travel to the resort areas of Bavaro and Punta Cana; in 2015, several malaria cases were reported in US travelers returning from beach resort holidays. The malaria species found in the Dominican Republic (*Plasmodium falciparum*) remains sensitive to all known antimalarial drugs.

Dengue is also widespread; 1,359 cases were reported in 2017 with 1 death. Although cases of dengue are reported year-round, transmission frequently increases during the rainy season from May through November. The principal mosquito vector (*Aedes aegypti*) of the dengue virus is found in both urban and rural areas (see Chapter 4, Dengue).

Zika is a risk in the Dominican Republic (see Chapter 4, Zika). Because of the risk of birth defects in infants born to women infected with Zika during pregnancy, women who are pregnant or trying to become pregnant should research the most recent recommendations at www.cdc.gov/zika.

## Food and Water

Remind travelers to drink only purified, bottled water. Ice served in well-established tourist locations is usually made from purified water and safe to consume. However, ice may not be safe in remote or nontourist areas. Food hygiene at large, all-inclusive, and popular tourist locations has improved over the last few years. However, travelers' diarrhea continues to be the most common problem for visitors to the Dominican Republic (see Chapter 2, Travelers' Diarrhea). Food purchased on the street or sold on beaches by informal sellers presents a higher risk of illness (see Chapter 2, Food & Water Precautions). Advise travelers not to eat raw or undercooked seafood.

Leptospirosis is prevalent on the island, with 792 cases and 79 deaths reported in 2017. Leptospirosis contamination can be attributed to climatic conditions (heavy rainfall, flooding) and environmental factors (agricultural practices, animal husbandry, inadequate disposal of waste, poor sanitation). Travelers should avoid recreational activities in rivers and lakes or other unprotected exposures to fresh water bodies potentially contaminated with animal urine (see Chapter 4, Leptospirosis).

## Sun and Heat

Visitors to the Dominican Republic often underestimate the strength of the sun and the dehydrating effect of the humid environment. Encourage travelers to take precautions to avoid sunburn by wearing hats and suitable clothing, along with proper application of a broad-spectrum sunscreen with an SPF ≥15 that protects against both UVA and UVB (see Chapter 3, Sun Exposure). Travelers should be sure to drink plenty of hydrating fluids throughout the day.

## SAFETY AND SECURITY

Driving in the Dominican Republic is hazardous (see Chapter 8, Road & Traffic Safety). Traffic laws are rarely enforced, and drivers commonly drive while intoxicated, text while driving, exceed speed limits, do not respect red lights or stop signs, and drive without seatbelts or helmets. The Dominican Republic has among the highest number of traffic deaths per capita in the world (29.3 per 100,000 population in 2013). Many fatal or serious traffic crashes involve motorcycles and pedestrians. Motorcycle taxis, used throughout the country (including tourist areas), frequently carry 2 or more passengers riding without helmets. Remind visitors to avoid motorcycle taxis, to use only licensed taxis, and to always wear a seatbelt.

The risk of crime is similar to that of major US cities. Although most crime affecting tourists involves robbery or pickpocketing, more serious assaults occasionally occur, and perpetrators may react violently if resisted (see Chapter 3, Safety & Security Overseas). Visitors to the Dominican Republic should follow normal safety precautions such as going out in groups, especially at night; using only licensed taxi drivers; drinking alcohol in moderation; and being cautious of strangers. Criminal activity is often higher during the Christmas and New Year season. Additional caution during that time is warranted.

## MEDICAL TOURISM

The market for medical tourism, including plastic surgery and dental care, is growing in the Dominican Republic. It attracts thousands of patients each year who access medical services that cost a fraction of what they do in the United States. Several companies and clinics offer package deals that include postsurgical recovery at local tourist resorts. Most health care facilities catering to medical tourists have not met the standards required by international accrediting bodies, however.

Substandard quality of care, health care–associated infections, and deaths have been the experience of some medical tourists to the Dominican Republic. Anyone considering the Dominican Republic as a destination for medical procedures should consult with a health care provider before travel, and research whether foreign health care providers meet accepted standards of care (see Chapter 9, Medical Tourism).

### BIBLIOGRAPHY

1. Banco Central de la República Dominicana [Internet]. Estadísticas económicas: sector turismo. Santo Domingo (Dominican Republic): Banco Central de la República Dominicana; c2012 [cited 2016 Sep 23]. Available from: www.bancentral.gov.do/estadisticas_economicas/turismo/.

2. CDC. Dengue fever among US travelers returning from the Dominican Republic—Minnesota and Iowa, 2008. MMWR Morb Mortal Wkly Rep. 2010 Jun 4;59(21):654–6.

3. CONAVIHSIDA (Consejo Nacional para el VIH y sida). Segunda encuesta de vigilancia de comportamiento con vinculación serológica en poblaciones claves. Gais, trans y hombres que tienen sexo con hombres (GTH) trabajadoras sexuales (TRSX) usuarios de drogas (UD), 2012. Santo Domingo (Dominican Republic): CONAVIHSIDA; 2014 [cited 2016 Sep. 23]. Available from: http://countryoffice.unfpa.org/dominicanrepublic/drive/CONAVIHSIDASegundaEncuestaVigiliancia.pdf.

4. Dirección General de Epidemiología [Internet]. Sistema nacional de vigilancia epidemiológica, boletín semanal 2017. Santo Domingo (Dominican Republic) 2017 [updated Sep 2014; cited 2016 Sep 23]. Available from: http://digepisalud.gob.do/docs/Boletines%20epidemiologicos/Boletines%20semanales/2017/Boletin%20Semanal%2052-%202017.pdf.

5. Duijster JW, Goorhuis A, van Genderen PJ, Visser LG, Koopmans MP, Reimerink JH, et al. Zika virus infection in 18 travelers returning from Surinam and the Dominican Republic, The Netherlands, November 2015–March 2016. Infection. 2016 Dec;44(6):797–802.

6. Gaines J, Poy J, Musser KA, Benowitz I, Leung V, Carothers B, et al. Notes from the field: nontuberculous mycobacteria infections in U.S. medical tourists associated with plastic surgery—Dominican Republic, 2017. MMWR Morb Mortal Wkly Rep. 2018 Mar 30;67(12):369–70.

7. Millman AJ, Esposito DH, Biggs HM, Decenteceo M, Klevos A, Hunsperger E, et al. Chikungunya and dengue virus infections among United States community service volunteers returning from the Dominican Republic, 2014. Am J Trop Med Hyg. 2016 Jun 1;94(6):1336–41.

8. World Health Organization Global Health Observatory data repository. Road traffic deaths: Data by country. [cited 2018 Aug 22]. Available from: http://apps.who.int/gho/data/node.main.A997.

**10**

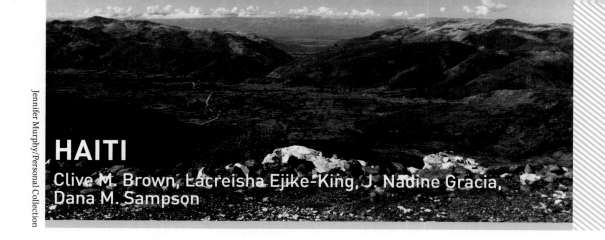

# HAITI

Clive M. Brown, Lacreisha Ejike-King, J. Nadine Gracia, Dana M. Sampson

## DESTINATION OVERVIEW

Nestled between the Caribbean Sea and the Atlantic Ocean, the Republic of Haiti occupies the western third of the island of Hispaniola, with the Dominican Republic on the eastern two-thirds (Map 10-8). Originally inhabited by the native Taíno, *Ayiti* ("land of high mountains") was introduced to European influence through periods of Spanish and French colonization from the 15th through 18th centuries. After a successful slave rebellion in 1804, Haiti became the first independent black republic in the Western Hemisphere, the first independent state in the Caribbean, and the second independent state in the Western Hemisphere after the United States.

The "Pearl of the Antilles," Haiti is home to a vibrant and diverse landscape that includes beaches, waterfalls, caves, and the most mountains of any nation in the Caribbean. Once rich in natural resources and products (sugar, rum, coffee, cotton, wood, and lumber), Haiti was the wealthiest French colony in the Caribbean. Deforestation, poor agricultural practices, and soil erosion have since contributed to considerable environmental degradation, however; it is now the poorest country in the Western Hemisphere.

Although Haiti has suffered from political and economic instability for most of its history, the people of Haiti are known for their resilience, strength, and warm and kind spirit, often leaving travelers to say that they have fallen in love with the country and its people. Because of the mix of indigenous, African, and European influences, Haiti possesses a "mosaic culture" reflected in its art, music, and cuisine. French and Creole are the official languages of the country. French is the principal written and administratively authorized language. It is the medium of instruction in most schools. Most (approximately 90%) of Haiti's 10.3 million people, however, use Creole as their primary language.

## HEALTH ISSUES

The environmental degradation described above has contributed to Haiti's poor sanitation and water quality. As a result, multiple public health risks exist for Haitians and for people traveling to Haiti.

### Vaccine-Preventable Diseases

Anyone traveling to Haiti should be up-to-date on routine vaccinations, including seasonal influenza and tetanus and diphtheria boosters. Diphtheria is endemic, and the number of reported cases has increased in recent years. Additionally, hepatitis A vaccine and typhoid vaccine are strongly recommended, especially for travelers staying with friends or relatives or visiting smaller cities or rural areas. Providers should also consider administering hepatitis B vaccine.

Rabies affects Haiti more than any other nation in the Americas. Prevention efforts have decreased the number of cases of human rabies transmitted by dogs, but deaths continue to be reported. Rabies vaccination is recommended for travelers anticipating contact with animals.

Active cholera transmission has been reported in Haiti in recent years. Check the

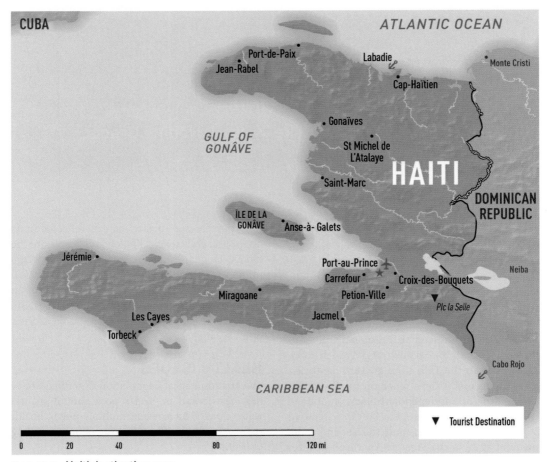

MAP 10-8. Haiti destination map

destination page at www.cdc.gov/travel for current recommendations.

Yellow fever vaccination is required for people traveling from countries where the disease is endemic.

## Vectorborne Diseases

Vectorborne diseases are common to Haiti and include *Plasmodium falciparum* malaria, dengue, chikungunya, and Zika. Travelers to Haiti should take measures to protect themselves from mosquito bites (see Chapter 3, Mosquitoes, Ticks & Other Arthropods).

### MALARIA

*P. falciparum* malaria is endemic to Haiti. The incidence of malaria in Haiti is approximately

1,278 per 100,000 people annually. The highest transmission rates are reported to occur after the rainy seasons from March through May and October through November. Instruct travelers to begin malaria prophylaxis before travel (see Chapter 4, Malaria).

### DENGUE, CHIKUNGUNYA, AND ZIKA

Dengue is endemic to Haiti, as it is throughout the Caribbean. Cases have been reported among military personnel and US missionaries; 240 cases were reported in 2014 alone. Chikungunya virus transmission was first reported in Haiti in May 2014, and the incidence rate is reported to be 627 per 100,000 population. For more information on these diseases, see Chapter 4.

Zika is a risk in Haiti. Because of the risk of birth defects in infants born to women infected with Zika during pregnancy, women who are pregnant or trying to become pregnant should research the most recent recommendations at www.cdc.gov/zika.

## Travelers' Diarrhea and Food- or Water-Related Diseases

Travelers wanting to experience the local, flavorful cuisine—rice with red beans, plantains, *griot* (seasoned fried pork), and a variety of fish and shellfish, including conch—should select food and beverages with care (see Chapter 2, Food & Water Precautions). Travelers' diarrhea is a significant risk; unvaccinated travelers are at additional risk of contracting hepatitis A and typhoid fever (see Chapter 4, Hepatitis A, and Typhoid & Paratyphoid Fever).

### CHOLERA

The cholera outbreak that followed the earthquake in 2010 caused 700,000 cases of illness and 8,500 deaths. The curve peaked in 2011, with incidence and mortality rates in decline every year since, a consequence of improved access to clean water and sanitation and the work of cholera treatment centers. In 2015, 5 years after the outbreak started, Haiti reported >30,000 cholera cases and about 325 deaths.

Cholera does remain a persistent public health threat (see Chapter 4, Cholera). Use of oral cholera vaccine has been implemented as part of a complementary set of ongoing treatment and control measures that include improved diarrheal disease surveillance and enhanced laboratory culture capacity. Urge all travelers to adhere to food and water precautions, and—depending on their planned itinerary—to consider cholera vaccine. See the Haiti destination page at www.cdc.gov/travel for current recommendations.

### LEPTOSPIROSIS

Leptospirosis is transmitted to humans who come into contact with the urine or tissues of an infected animal or with water or soil tainted by the urine of an infected animal (see Chapter 4, Leptospirosis). Travelers are advised to avoid freshwater (such as streams or lakes) that may be contaminated with animal urine. The incidence of leptospirosis is highest during the rainy season; because of recurring natural disasters like tropical storms and flooding, Haiti appears to be at greater risk for this disease than other places in the Caribbean (where it is endemic). Many cases have been reported since the 2010 earthquake.

## PHYSICAL CONCERNS FOR THE TRAVELER

### Motor Vehicle Safety

Motor vehicle injuries are the most common cause of death for healthy Americans traveling abroad (see Chapter 8, Road & Traffic Safety). The risk of death from road injuries in Haiti is high; the 2013 rate was 945 per 100,000 population, compared with an average rate of 721 for the region as a whole. Road conditions in Haiti differ significantly from those in the United States: roads and lanes are generally unmarked, speed limits are seldom posted or adhered to, right-of-way is not widely observed, and a variety of people and objects may appear on roads (such as carts, animals, and vendors). Roads may be unpaved or have large potholes. And, although the main roads have been cleared of rubble from the 2010 earthquake, debris still remains in some places.

Traffic is usually chaotic and congested in urban areas. Vibrantly painted *tap taps* are open-air vehicles (buses or pick-up trucks), mechanically unsound and often overloaded with passengers. A common form of public transportation for Haitians, tap taps are not recommended for visitors because of safety concerns (crashes, robberies, or kidnappings). Remind travelers to stay alert when walking, to choose safe vehicles, and to observe safety practices when operating vehicles. Travelers should fasten seat belts when riding in cars and wear a helmet when riding bicycles or motorbikes.

### Crime

The crime rate in Haiti is high, particularly in the capital of Port-au-Prince, presenting persistent safety concerns for travelers. Although much of the violent crime is perpetrated by Haitians on Haitians, American citizens have also been victims (see Chapter 3, Safety & Security Overseas). Travelers arriving on flights from the United States have been targeted for robbery and attack.

10

During Carnival, crime, disorderly conduct, and general congestion increase. Advise travelers to maintain awareness of their surroundings and recommend that they avoid nighttime travel, keep valuables well hidden (not left behind in parked vehicles), and lock closed all doors and windows.

## Civil Unrest

Civil unrest also poses a safety concern for visitors to Haiti. Frequent and sometimes spontaneous protests occur in Port-au-Prince. Demonstrations—which travelers should avoid, when possible—can turn violent. The US State Department's Smart Traveler Enrollment Program (https://step.state.gov/step/) sends enrolled travelers information about safety conditions at their destination and provides direct embassy contact in case of man-made emergencies (political unrest and demonstrations, rioting, terrorist activity) as well as natural disasters.

## Natural Disasters

Natural disasters common to Haiti include tropical storms, floods, hurricanes, and earthquakes. Haiti has two rainy seasons; the first runs from April to June and the second from October through November. Hurricane season lasts from June through November. In 2008, Haiti experienced a series of 4 hurricanes and tropical storms within 2 months.

In January 2010, Haiti experienced a 7.0 magnitude earthquake that killed more than 220,000 people and displaced 1.5 million from their homes. Multiple powerful aftershocks added to the widespread devastation and destruction, significantly weakening the health, emergency response, and safety infrastructure of the nation, which remains largely underdeveloped.

Hurricane Matthew, the first category 4 hurricane to hit the island since 1964, struck Haiti in October 2016. The storm took 546 lives and displaced more than 120,000. Strong winds and heavy rain caused flash floods, mudslides, river floods, crop and vegetation loss, and destruction of homes and businesses. One year later, rain and flooding from Hurricane Irma compounded the losses to Haiti's agricultural sector. These combined disasters have further weakened an already fragile infrastructure.

## DISCLOSURE

Lacreisha Ejike-King is an employee of the US Food and Drug Administration (FDA); views expressed in this chapter are those of the authors and do not necessarily reflect the official policy or position of the FDA.

### BIBLIOGRAPHY

1. Brown C, Ripp J, Kazura J. Perspectives on Haiti two years after the earthquake. Am J Trop Med Hyg. 2012 Jan;86(1):5–6.

2. CDC. Malaria in post-earthquake Haiti: CDC's recommendations for prevention and treatment. Atlanta: CDC; 2010 [cited 2016 Sep 23]. Available from: www.cdc.gov/malaria/resources/pdf/new_info/2010/malaria-1-pager_dec3v1_508.pdf.

3. Dowell SF, Tappero JW, Frieden TR. Public health in Haiti—challenges and progress. N Engl J Med. 2011 Jan 27;364(4):300–1.

4. Institute for Health Metrics and Evaluation. Country Profile: Haiti. IHME; [cited 2016 Mar 10]. Available from: www.healthdata.org/haiti.

5. National Oceanic and Atmospheric Administration. Hurricane Matthew. National Hurricane Center; 2017 [cited 2018 Mar 22]. Available from: www.nch.noaa.gov.

6. Pan American Health Organization/World Health Organization (PAHO/WHO), Health Information and Analysis Project (HSD/HA). Health situation in the Americas: basic indicators, 2014. Washington, DC: 2014. Available from: www.paho.org/hq/index.php?option=com_docman&task=doc_view&gid=27299&Itemid=721.

7. United Nations Development Programme (UNDP) Human Development Report Office. Human development report 2013. The rise of the South: human progress in a diverse world. New York: 2013 Sep 22. Available from: http://hdr.undp.org/en/2013-report.

8. United States Department of State. Haiti 2017 crime and safety report. Bureau of Diplomatic Security; 2007 [cited 2018 Mar 22]. Available from: www.osac.gov.

9. World Food Programme [Internet]. Haiti overview. Port au Prince (Haiti): World Food Programme; 2014 [cited 2016 Sep 23]. Available from: www.wfp.org/countries/haiti/overview.

10. World Health Organization. Countries: Haiti Country Profile. WHO; [cited 2016 Sep 23]. Available from: www.who.int/countries/hti/en/.

**10**

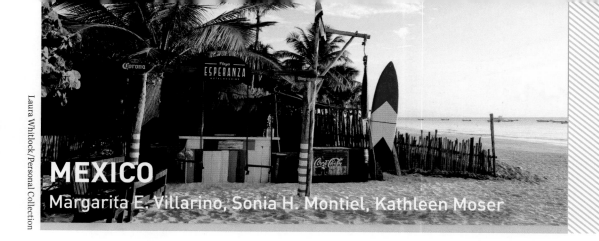

# MEXICO

Margarita E. Villarino, Sonia H. Montiel, Kathleen Moser

## DESTINATION OVERVIEW

Mexico, the second most populous country in Latin America, has a population of more than 120 million; 78% live in urban areas. The United States' second-largest agricultural trading partner and third-largest trading partner overall, Mexico ranks 15th in national wealth based on gross domestic product. The capital, Mexico City, is 1 of the world's largest cities (population >20 million) and is a frequent site for business and meetings, mass gathering events, and tourism travel.

One-fifth the size of the United States (about 3 times larger than Texas), Mexico has diverse geographic features throughout its 32 states. The Sonoran desert is in the northwest, beautiful beaches line both coasts, and forested mountain ranges traverse the western and eastern mainland. Impressive volcanic peaks rise up to 18,000 feet above the high central plateau. The Yucatán Peninsula and other southern and coastal regions are tropical. The Copper Canyon, in the state of Chihuahua, is larger than the Grand Canyon (see Map 10-9).

Mexico receives more foreign visitors than any other country in Latin America, and it is the country most frequently visited by US tourists. In 2017, there were 188 million border crossings at 25 land ports of entry between United States and Mexico. Beach resort travel (Acapulco, Ixtapa, Cancún, Puerto Peñasco, Playa del Carmen, Cozumel, Puerto Vallarta, Nuevo Vallarta, and Cabo San Lucas) and cruise ship tours make up a large portion of tourism to Mexico. On the Pacific Coast, travelers can go whale watching in Baja California or sport fishing in the Gulf of California.

The country's rich history and proud culture reflecting its pre-Columbian and Hispanic heritage attract many tourists, as well. Travelers to Mexico can visit World Heritage sites and pre-Columbian anthropologic destinations including Teotihuacan outside Mexico City, the Great Pyramid of Cholula in Puebla, Tulum and Cobá in Quintana Roo, El Tajín in Veracruz, Chichén Itzá in Yucatán, Monte Albán in Oaxaca, and Palenque in Chiapas.

A large number of US residents visit Mexico to receive health services. Only Thailand sees more medical tourists from the United States (see the Thailand section in this chapter). Services sought from providers in the northern border cities primarily include dental and eye care and cosmetic surgery. Increasingly, a complete range of services and specialized procedures for medical tourists are becoming available in Mexico City, Monterrey, Mérida, Cancún, and Guadalajara, cities that feature a more robust infrastructure (see Chapter 9, Medical Tourism).

## HEALTH ISSUES

### Vaccine-Preventable Diseases

All travelers should be up-to-date with their routine immunizations. Hepatitis A is endemic to Mexico; visitors should receive at least the first dose of the hepatitis A vaccine series before travel. Hepatitis B vaccine is also recommended, especially for those expecting to stay in Mexico ≥6 months, medical tourists, or anyone who might be exposed to blood or other body fluids (including through sexual contact). Discuss the need for typhoid and rabies vaccination with travelers going

**10**

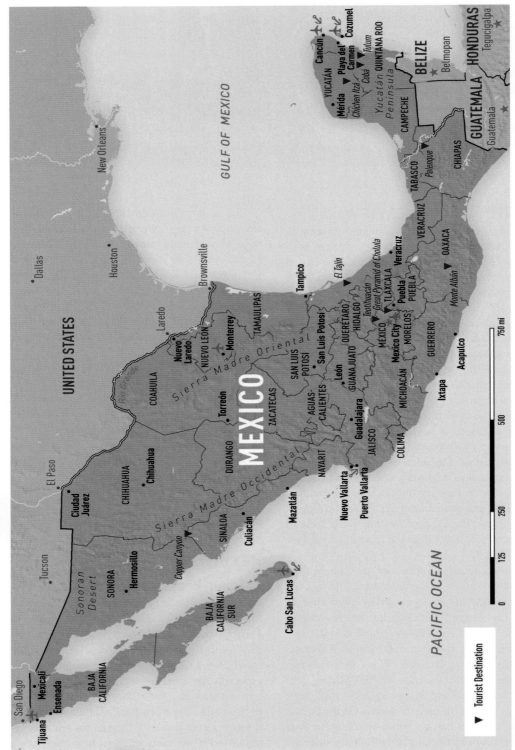

MAP 10-9. Mexico destination map

to less developed, remote areas of the country (field biologists and nature adventure tourists, for example) or anyone planning an extended visit to see friends or relatives (see Chapter 9, Visiting Friends & Relatives: VFR Travel).

## RABIES

Preexposure rabies prophylaxis is recommended for travelers likely to have contact with wild animals and for those traveling to areas with limited access to medical care (see Chapter 4, Rabies). In Mexico, the wild animal species that carry rabies include bats, coatis (also known as coatimundi, tejón, cholugo, or moncún), coyotes, foxes, and skunks; less commonly, unvaccinated dogs and cats are exposure sources.

## Travelers' Diarrhea and Other Foodborne and Waterborne Infections

Travelers' diarrhea is common among visitors to Mexico, and education is key. Provide traveler patients with instruction in proper food and water precautions (see Travelers' Diarrhea and Food & Water Precautions in Chapter 2). Remind travelers that tap water is not potable, to avoid consuming unpasteurized or unaged, artisanal dairy products, and not to eat raw or undercooked meat or fish, leafy greens, or raw vegetables. Foodborne infections in Mexico are due to a variety of pathogens (viral, bacterial, and parasitic) including, but in no particular order: *Salmonella enterica*, *Shigella* spp., *Escherichia coli*, *Campylobacter* spp., *Cyclospora cayetanensis*, *Entamoeba histolytica*, *Taenia solium* (cysticercosis), *Brucella* spp., *Listeria monocytogenes*, and *Mycobacterium bovis*. Prescribe antibiotics for self-treatment of diarrhea with careful and explicit directions for their use.

## Vectorborne Diseases

### DENGUE, CHIKUNGUNYA, AND ZIKA

Travelers should take steps to prevent mosquito bites by using insect repellent, wearing long-sleeved shirts and long pants, and staying in accommodations with screens or air conditioning (see Chapter 3, Mosquitoes, Ticks & Other Arthropods). Dengue is endemic throughout Mexico; virus transmission is a risk year-round, and large outbreaks occur periodically (see Chapter 4, Dengue). Chikungunya has been reported since 2014 (see Chapter 4, Chikungunya). Also, Zika is a risk in Mexico (see Chapter 4, Zika). Because of the risk of birth defects in infants born to women infected with Zika during pregnancy, women who are pregnant or trying to become pregnant should research the most recent recommendations at www.cdc.gov/zika.

### MALARIA

Dramatic decreases in malaria incidence in recent decades mean risk of infection to travelers to Mexico is low (see Chapter 4, Malaria). Major resorts are free of the disease, as is the US–Mexico border region. *Plasmodium vivax* malaria prophylaxis is currently recommended only for travelers going to Chiapas and the southern part of Chihuahua. Mosquito avoidance (but not prophylaxis) is recommended for travelers visiting Campeche, Durango, Jalisco, Nayarit, Quintana Roo, San Luis Potosí, Sinaloa, Sonora, and Tabasco.

### RICKETTSIAL DISEASE

In Mexico, rickettsial diseases (see Chapter 4, Rickettsial Diseases) include Rocky Mountain spotted fever (potentially fatal unless treated promptly with antibiotics) and fleaborne typhus (a severe disease with symptoms similar to dengue). The brown dog tick (*Rhipicephalus sanguineus*), associated with Mexico's large urban and rural stray dog population, is the vector for Rocky Mountain spotted fever. Provide travelers with information about how to avoid flea and tick bites, both indoors and outside.

### PARASITIC INFECTIONS

Transmitted by sand flies, cutaneous leishmaniasis is found in parts of coastal and southern Mexico (see Chapter 4, Cutaneous Leishmaniasis). The risk for this infection is greatest for ecotourists, field biologists, and long-term travelers. Travelers can reduce risk of sand fly bites by avoiding outdoor activities at night.

Beachgoers may be at risk for cutaneous larva migrans (CLM), a creeping skin eruption most commonly associated with dog hookworm infection. CLM is preventable by wearing shoes and avoiding direct skin contact with sand (see Chapter 4, Cutaneous Larva Migrans).

**10**

Chagas disease, transmitted by triatomine insects infected with *Trypanosoma cruzi*, is endemic throughout Mexico (see Chapter 4, American Trypanosomiasis).

## Other Infections

### RESPIRATORY DISEASES

Influenza virus strains similar to those in the United States circulate in Mexico, making pretravel flu vaccination a prudent health protection measure. Inhaled fungal spores have caused lung infections in returning travelers: *Coccidioides* is endemic to the soil of northwestern Mexico, and *Histoplasma* is found mainly in Mexico's central and southeast regions (see Chapter 4, Coccidioidomycosis and Histoplasmosis).

Legionellosis (Legionnaire's Disease) should be considered as part of the differential diagnosis in people developing pneumonia within 14 days of travel outside the United States, especially the elderly and immunocompromised (see Chapter 4, Legionellosis). Travel history surveillance periodically identifies associations between the disease and stays at particular hotels and resorts in Mexico.

### TUBERCULOSIS (TB)

Although 4 times what it is in the United States, Mexico's TB incidence is lower than that of Asia, Africa, and Eastern Europe. Providers should help travelers determine their potential for exposure to *M. tuberculosis*; risk of infection is greatest for those intending to remain in Mexico ≥6 months; travelers working in health care settings, homeless shelters, or prisons where they may be exposed to patients with untreated TB; or people planning an extended visit home to spend time with friends and relatives (see Chapter 4, Tuberculosis).

## OTHER HEALTH AND SAFETY RISKS

Good health care is available in most Mexican cities, and tourist hotels and resorts usually have well-trained physicians available. Payment (cash or credit card) may be required before any care is given, and most providers do not accept US health insurance or Medicare/Medicaid plans.

Injuries, not infectious diseases, pose the greatest life threat to healthy travelers in Mexico. In one review, about half (51%) of all US traveler deaths in Mexico were injury related; 18% due to motor vehicle crashes (see Chapter 8, Road & Traffic Safety). Mexico's highway system and roads are mostly modern, well maintained, and safe. Toll highways are often of high quality. Nevertheless, driving in city traffic and at night through the countryside can be dangerous. Remind travelers to use seat belts when riding in cars and to always wear a helmet when riding bicycles or motorbikes.

Although travel to Mexico is generally considered safe, thefts and robberies do occur, and drug-related violence does exist in some places (see Chapter 3, Safety & Security Overseas). Travelers should consult the US Department of State for relevant safety and security alerts pertaining to their intended destinations within Mexico.

Air pollution in Mexico City, while decreased in recent years, can be particularly severe during the dry winter months and can exacerbate asthma and aggravate chronic lung and heart conditions (see Chapter 3, Air Quality & Ionizing Radiation). Healthy travelers coming from lower elevations and people with lung and heart conditions should use caution while acclimating to Mexico City (elevation 7,382 ft; 2,250 m).

Injuries and deaths caused by poisonous *Centruroides* genus (bark) scorpions have been reported from states along the Pacific Coast (extending from Sonora down to Oaxaca) and in the center states of Durango, Guanajuato, State of Mexico, and Morelos. Travelers should be aware of scorpions, snakes, and other venomous creatures when visiting Mexico's rural areas and when participating in outdoor activities, especially during spring and summer (see Chapter 3, Animal Bites & Stings).

## BIBLIOGRAPHY

1. Brathwaite DO, San Martin JL, Montoya RH, del Diego J, Zambrano B, Dayan GH. The history of dengue outbreaks in the Americas. Am J Trop Med Hyg. 2012 Oct;87(4):584–93.

2. Bureau of Transportation Statistics. Border crossing/entry data. [cited 2018 Mar 26]. Available from: https://explore.dot.gov/t/BTS/views/BTSBorderCrossingAnnualData/BorderCrossingTableDashboard?:embed=y&:display_count=no&:showShareOptions=true&:showVizHome=no.

3. CDC. Human rabies from exposure to a vampire bat in Mexico—Louisiana, 2010. MMWR Morb Mortal Wkly Rep. 2011 Aug 12;60(31):1050–2.

4. CDC. Notes from the field: outbreak of *Vibrio cholerae* Serogroup O1, Serotype Ogawa, Biotype El Tor Strain—La Huasteca Region, Mexico, 2013. MMWR Morb Mortal Wkly Rep. 2013;63(25):552–3.

5. CDC. Update: novel influenza A (H1N1) virus infection—Mexico, March–May, 2009. MMWR Morb Mortal Wkly Rep. 2009 Jun 5;58(21):585–9.

6. Fitchett JR, Vallecillo AJ, Espitia C. Tuberculosis transmission across the United States–Mexico border. Rev Panam Salud Publica. 2011 Jan;29(1):57–60.

7. Flores-Figueroa J, Okhuysen PC, von Sonnenburg F, DuPont HL, Libman MD, Keystone JS, et al. Patterns of illness in travelers visiting Mexico and Central America: the GeoSentinel experience. Clin Infect Dis. 2011 Sep;53(6):523–31.

8. Laniado-Laborin R. Coccidioidomycosis and other endemic mycoses in Mexico. Rev Iberoam Micol. 2007 Dec 31;24(4):249–58.

9. Leparc-Goffart I, Nougairede A, Cassadou S, Prat C, de Lamballerie X. Chikungunya in the Americas. Lancet. 2014 Feb 8;383(9916):514.

10. Spradling PR, Xing J, Phippard A, Fonseca-Ford M, Montiel S, Guzman NL, et al. Acute viral hepatitis in the United States–Mexico border region: data from the Border Infectious Disease Surveillance (BIDS) Project, 2000–2009. J Immigr Minor Health. 2013 Apr;15(2):390–7.

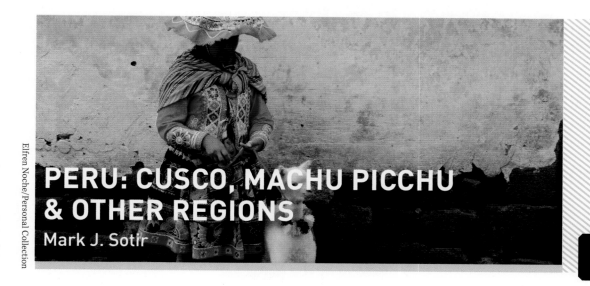

Elfren Noche/Personal Collection

# PERU: CUSCO, MACHU PICCHU & OTHER REGIONS

Mark J. Sotir

10

## DESTINATION OVERVIEW

Peru is a country almost twice the size of the state of Texas, with a population of 30 million people. Thousands of tourists are drawn to Peru every year to enjoy the country's magnificent geographic, biologic, and cultural diversity. A primary destination for most travelers are the remarkable Incan ruins of Machu Picchu, named a UNESCO World Heritage site in 1983 and voted one of the New Seven Wonders of the World in 2007. Located in southern Peru, in the middle of a tropical mountain forest on the eastern slopes of the Andes Mountains, Machu Picchu is extraordinarily picturesque. Considered perhaps the most amazing urban creation of the Inca Empire at its height, its giant walls, terraces, and ramps appear to be cut naturally from the continuous rock escarpment.

Lima, the capital city of Peru, is a sprawling megacity home to approximately one-third of Peru's population. Some mistakenly believe Lima is a high-altitude Incan city; it is actually located at sea level on the Pacific coast (Map 10-10). From Lima, it is an hour-long flight to get to Cusco, the gateway to Machu Picchu and a worthwhile

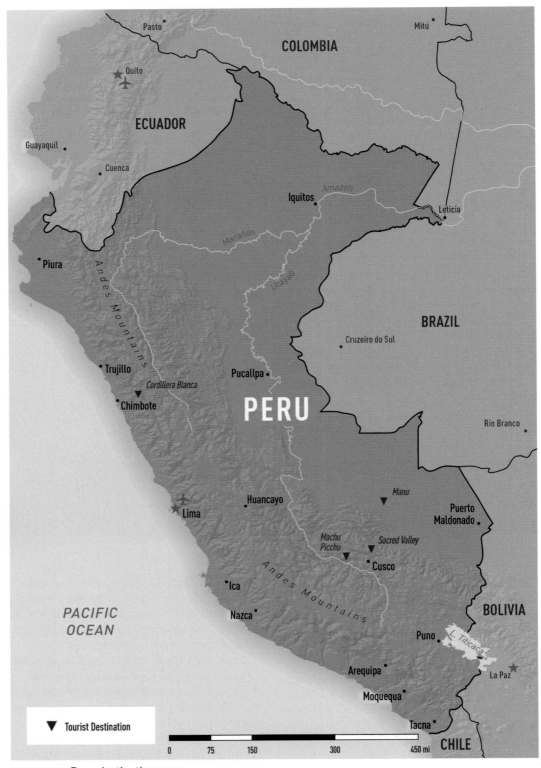

MAP 10-10.  Peru destination map

destination of its own. Visitors can see Inca-era ruins in Cusco and surrounding mountain villages, and shop in markets in the Valle Sagrado (Sacred Valley).

A train takes passengers from Cusco to several places where they can ascend to the actual site. From the town of Aguas Calientes, buses travel up the mountain to Machu Picchu. Multiple-day hikes across Andean mountain trails are also popular. One of the world's best-known treks, the Inca Trail, begins at an elevation of more than 8,000 ft (>2,500 m) on the Cusco-Machu Picchu railway. Most physically fit people should be able to complete this 26-mile (43-km) hike in 4 days and 3 nights. The route is quite challenging, however, traversing 3 high mountain passes—the highest is Warmiwañusca at 13,796 ft (4,205 m)—before it ends at the ruins of Machu Picchu (7,970 ft; 2,430 m).

Many people also choose to add a tropical rainforest experience to their Cusco trip and take the 30-minute flight from Cusco to Puerto Maldonado, 34 miles (55 km) west of the Bolivian border. Puerto Maldonado is at the confluence of the Rio Tambopata and the Madre de Dios River, a major tributary of the Amazon River. Most travelers take a boat up the Rio Tambopata to stay at one of several rustic lodges. Those wanting to see the Amazon rainforest can visit the more remote Manu National Park, also accessible from Cusco. Additional sites of interest in southern Peru include the Nazca Desert—home of the ancient geoglyphs known as the Nazca Lines—and Lake Titicaca, which overlaps Peru's border with Bolivia. It is called the highest navigable lake in the world.

Other natural wonders of this country include the Loreto Region and the Cordillera Blanca mountain range. Iquitos, the capital of the Loreto Region, can only be reached by boat or by plane; no roads lead to the city. From Iquitos, travelers can explore the northern Amazon rainforest by cruising upstream or downstream the Amazon River. The Cordillera Blanca, a hundred-mile range of spectacular snow-covered peaks, forms the backbone of the Andes Mountains in Peru. The Cordillera Blanca boasts 33 peaks >18,040 ft (5,500 m) and has earned a reputation for world-class trekking and mountaineering.

# HEALTH ISSUES

Important pretravel information for travelers going to Peru includes advice on preventing high-altitude illness, reducing risk for cutaneous leishmaniasis and vectorborne illnesses, including malaria, and—depending on the itinerary—the need for vaccination against yellow fever.

## Altitude Illness and Acute Mountain Sickness

Travelers to Machu Picchu will arrive and transit through Cusco, 11,200 ft (3,400 m) above sea level. A recent study of travelers to Cusco found that three-quarters flew directly from sea level. On arrival, most tourists will quickly notice they are short of breath when gathering luggage and making their way to local hotels on the hilly streets. Many, maybe as many as half, will find that Cusco's elevation leads to some degree of acute mountain sickness (AMS), with the initial symptoms of headache, nausea, and loss of appetite beginning 4–8 hours after arrival.

The hypoxemia that accompanies high-elevation travel can also affect the quality of sleep in the first few nights in Cusco, causing restless sleep, frequent awakening, and irregular respiratory patterns (alternating deep and shallow breathing), even in those who appear to be doing well during the day. Some travelers may progress to severe forms of altitude illness, including high-altitude pulmonary edema and high-altitude cerebral edema, life-threatening conditions that mandate immediate descent to a lower elevation. Even more mild symptoms of AMS can markedly impair the traveler and prevent enjoyment of the sights of Cusco. People with underlying lung disease may not be the best candidates for travel to this destination. Expert pretravel medical consultation is advised (see Chapter 3, High-Altitude Travel & Altitude Illness).

Surveys have shown that most travelers arrive in Cusco with limited or no knowledge of AMS or the fact that it can be prevented to a large degree by prophylactic use of acetazolamide. Pretravel counseling should include information about AMS and a prescription for medication to prevent or self-treat the condition. Travelers to other parts of Peru may also require counseling about AMS; common travel destinations at high elevation

**10**

include the city of Puno on the shore of Lake Titicaca (12,556 ft; 3,830 m), and the Cordillera Blanca (peaks >18,040 ft; 5,500 m).

Locals refer to AMS as *soroche* and may offer the new arrival a cup of hot coca tea (*mate de coca*) when checking in to the hotel. Although many believe *mate de coca* can prevent and treat *soroche*, no data support its use in the prevention or treatment of AMS. People who drink a single cup of coca tea will test positive for cocaine metabolites in standard drug toxicology screens for several days, a potential concern to anyone subject to random drug screens at work.

New arrivals may find it helpful to transit directly from Cusco to the Valle Sagrado of the Rio Urubamba to spend the first few days and nights at a somewhat lower elevation. This river valley begins 15 miles (24 km) northeast of Cusco in the town of Pisac (9,751 ft; 2,972 m), known for its colorful Sunday markets, continuing downstream toward the northwest for another 37 miles (60 km) to reach the town of Ollantaytambo (9,160 ft; 2,792 m). One can board the train to Machu Picchu in Ollantaytambo, at the northwest end of the Valle Sagrado, and visit Cusco on the return from Machu Picchu, when better acclimatized. The train follows the Rio Urubamba north and northwest (downstream) to Aguas Calientes (6,693 ft; 2,040 m). Machu Picchu (7,972 ft; 2,430 m) is located on a ridge above the town.

## Cutaneous Leishmaniasis

Many areas in the Pacific valleys of the Andes and the Amazon tropical rainforest are endemic for cutaneous leishmaniasis (CL), a parasitic infection transmitted by bites of sand flies (see Chapter 4, Cutaneous Leishmaniasis). While this disease is widespread in southeastern Peru, the highest risk for travelers seems to be in the Manu Park area in Madre de Dios. In Manu, CL is most often caused by *Leishmania braziliensis*, and there is a risk of both localized ulcerative CL and mucosal leishmaniasis. There is no visceral leishmaniasis in Peru. Counsel travelers to be meticulous about vector precautions, as there is no vaccine or prophylaxis to prevent this disease. Any person with a skin lesion persisting more than a few weeks after return from Peru should be evaluated for CL.

## Yellow Fever

Proof of yellow fever vaccination is not required for entry into Peru, and travelers limiting their itineraries to Lima, Cusco, Machu Picchu, and the Inca Trail do not need yellow fever vaccination. Many travelers, however, choose to acclimate and/or stay in Aguas Calientes before taking the bus to the Inca citadel. But because Aguas Calientes is in a region (Cusco Region) where yellow fever vaccine is recommended, and because it is at an elevation where yellow fever mosquitoes are potentially active (i.e., it is below 2,300 m), travel health providers should advise vaccination for any travel plans involving Aguas Calientes.

CDC recommends vaccination for all travelers ≥9 months of age who intend to visit areas of the country <7,546 ft (2,300 m) in the regions of Amazonas, Loreto, Madre de Dios, San Martin and Ucayali, Puno, Cusco, Junín, Pasco, and Huánuco, and designated areas of the following regions: far north of Apurimac, far northern Huancavelica, far northeastern Ancash, eastern La Libertad, northern and eastern Cajamarca, northern and northeastern Ayacucho, and eastern Piura (see Map 10-10). For complete CDC yellow fever vaccination recommendations for Peru, see Chapter 2, Yellow Fever Vaccine & Malaria Prophylaxis Information, by Country.

## Malaria

Both *Plasmodium vivax* and *P. falciparum* malaria are found in the Peruvian Amazon, as well as the central jungle and northern coastal regions. Except for the urban areas of Lima and its environs and the coastal areas south of Lima, malaria is presumed to be present in all departments of Peru <6,562 ft (2,000 m). This includes the cities of Iquitos (in the north) and Puerto Maldonado (in the south) and the remote eastern regions of La Libertad and Lambayeque. CDC recommends malaria prophylaxis when visiting any of these locations. There is no malaria risk for travelers visiting only the popular highland tourist areas of Cusco, Machu Picchu, and Lake Titicaca. For complete CDC malaria recommendations for Peru, see Chapter 2, Yellow Fever Vaccine & Malaria Prophylaxis Information, by Country.

The malaria-endemic areas of concern for most tourists are the neotropical rainforests of the Amazon, north and south (see Map 10-10). Although *P. falciparum* epidemics sometimes occur in the Loreto Region, routine malaria transmission in and around Iquitos happens throughout the year, with peak activity corresponding to the rainy season between January and May. In the south, Peruvian Ministry of Health data document that malaria transmission occurs in and around the city of Puerto Maldonado, the take-off point for travelers staying in rainforest lodges. Most cases reported in this region occur in local loggers and gold miners in the forests. Nevertheless, prophylaxis for travelers planning a visit to any rainforest areas should be strongly recommended.

## Other Infectious Diseases

Typical travelers' diarrhea is relatively common (see Chapter 2, Travelers' Diarrhea). Fluoroquinolone-resistant *Campylobacter* infections should be suspected in anyone with a gastrointestinal illness with fever, systemic symptoms, and failure to improve within 12–24 hours after beginning empiric fluoroquinolone treatment. Azithromycin can be used for people who do not respond to empiric treatment of acute gastroenteritis with a fluoroquinolone.

Cyclosporiasis, an intestinal illness caused by *Cyclospora cayetanensis*, is also common in Peru (see Chapter 4, Cyclosporiasis). The parasite, named for the Cayetano Heredia University in Lima, where early epidemiologic and taxonomic research was conducted, causes watery diarrhea, anorexia, weight loss, and cramping and bloating that persists for days to weeks. Treatment is trimethoprim-sulfamethoxazole.

In addition to yellow fever and malaria, several other mosquitoborne illnesses are found in Peru, and all travelers should be instructed on how to protect themselves from mosquito bites (see Chapter 3, Mosquitoes, Ticks & Other Arthropods). Dengue is common in the neotropical areas of Peru and the northern coast. Mayaro virus, an alphavirus transmitted by mosquitoes of the Amazon Basin, causes a dengue-like illness followed by, in some cases, long-lasting and debilitating arthralgias. Chikungunya, another alphavirus, has been reported. Most recently, Zika was identified in Peru. Because of the risk of birth defects in infants born to women infected with Zika during pregnancy, women who are pregnant or trying to become pregnant should research the most recent recommendations at www.cdc. gov/zika. Physicians treating patients with signs and symptoms of a dengue-like illness and a recent history of travel to the Amazon should include Mayaro, chikungunya, and Zika as part of their differential diagnosis. For more details, see sections on dengue, chikungunya, and Zika virus in Chapter 4.

### BIBLIOGRAPHY

1. Cabada MM, Maldonado F, Quispe W, Serrano E, Mozo K, Gonzales E, et al. Pretravel health advice among international travelers visiting Cuzco, Peru. J Travel Med. 2005 Mar–Apr;12(2):61–5.

2. Llanos-Chea F, Martínez D, Rosas A, Samalvides F, Vinetz JM, Llanos-Cuentas A. Characteristics of travel-related severe Plasmodium vivax and Plasmodium falciparum malaria in individuals hospitalized at a tertiary referral center in Lima, Peru. Am J Trop Med Hyg. 2015 Dec;93(6):1249–53.

3. Mazor SS, Mycyk MB, Wills BK, Brace LD, Gussow L, Erickson T. Coca tea consumption causes positive urine cocaine assay. Eur J Emerg Med. 2006 Dec;13(6):340–1.

4. Neumayr A, Gabriel M, Fritz J, Gunther S, Hatz C, Schmidt-Chanasit J, et al. Mayaro virus infection in traveler returning from Amazon Basin, northern Peru. Emerg Infect Dis. 2012 Apr;18(4):695–6.

5. Salazar H, Swanson J, Mozo K, White ACJ, Cabada MM. Acute mountain sickness impact among travelers to Cusco, Peru. J Travel Med 2012 Jul;19(4):220–5.

6. Shaw MT, Harding E, Leggat PA. Illness and injury to students on a school excursion to Peru. J Travel Med. 2014 May–Jun;21(3):183–8.

7. Steinhardt LC, Magill AJ, Arguin PM. Review: Malaria chemoprophylaxis for travelers to Latin America. Am J Trop Med Hyg. 2011 Dec;85(6):1015–24.

**10**

# ASIA

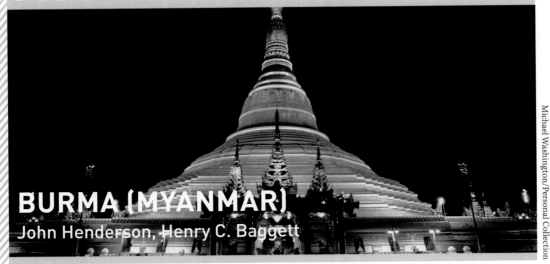

## BURMA (MYANMAR)
John Henderson, Henry C. Baggett

## DESTINATION OVERVIEW

Burma (also called Myanmar) offers travelers a mix of traditional and modern culture. Nearly all visitors to this country come to see the classic golden temples of Rangoon (Yangon), Burma's former capital and its largest city. Visitors here may also enjoy strolling colonial-era parks and shopping at Bogyoke Aung San Market. The city's influences include British, Chinese, and Indian. Those wanting a glimpse of rural life can get it with a short ferry ride across the Yangon River to Dala or by riding the circle train that makes a loop just north of the city.

Many tourists are now taking advantage of improving domestic bus and air service to explore other parts of the country. International flights to Mandalay are available from neighboring China, Singapore, and Thailand. Burma's varied geography includes highlands, plains, beaches, and more than 800 islands. Several climate zones are found along its river basins and mountain ranges. That diversity extends to languages, which number more than 100. Of the country's more than 56 million people, about two-thirds can speak or understand Burmese. English is widely spoken in popular visitor destinations, where visitors often remark on the hospitality and generosity of their hosts.

Religious sites and ancient cities, with their temples and festivals, attract many of Burma's tourists. Unique architecture and heritage combine at places like Bagan, Bago, Kyaiktiyo, and Mrauk U. Nature-based activities such as boating, trekking, and cycling are easily arranged around Inle or Hsipaw in hilly Shan State, home to a thrilling train ride across the Goteik Viaduct. River cruises along the Ayeyarwady begin or end in Mandalay (Map 10-11). Meditation retreats are also widespread.

Climate varies depending on season and elevation. During the dry months between November and February, Rangoon and southern Burma average 80°F (27°C) during the day. Further north in that season, nighttime temperatures can drop to 45°–50°F (8°–10°C). Hot season (March to May) and rainy season (June to October) are well named.

Local dishes such as *mohinga* (rice noodles in fish soup), curries, and salads appeal to many visitors, yet dietary caution is advised. Sanitation and clean water access may be inadequate, especially in secondary towns and rural areas.

After decades of authoritarian rule, economic isolation, and ethnic conflict, the country's governance and people remain mostly poor. While enjoying Burma's colorful and rustic aspects, visitors may do well to attempt an understanding of the country's society, human rights, and environment, and tourism's potential impact on them.

10

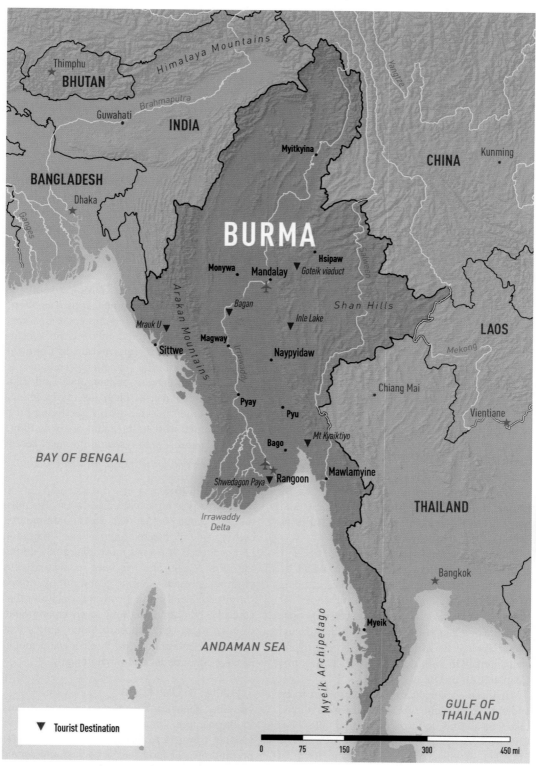

MAP 10-11. Burma (Myanmar) destination map

# HEALTH ISSUES

## Vaccine-Preventable Diseases

### ROUTINE IMMUNIZATIONS

Travelers to Burma should be up-to-date on routine vaccines, including measles-mumps-rubella (MMR), diphtheria-tetanus-pertussis, varicella (chickenpox), polio, and influenza. Influenza exhibits a seasonal pattern with peaks occurring from June through September, overlapping with the typical rainy season.

### OTHER VACCINATIONS

Hepatitis A is transmitted by contaminated food or water or person to person through the fecal–oral route and is endemic to Burma; susceptible travelers should be vaccinated (see Chapter 4, Hepatitis A). Travelers can also reduce the risk of hepatitis A infection by following recommendations for safe food and water (see Chapter 2, Food & Water Precautions).

The prevalence of hepatitis B infection in Burma has been estimated to be lower intermediate. Hepatitis B vaccination is recommended for travelers before departure, and it is especially important to vaccinate anyone engaging in activities that increase the risk of exposure to blood or body fluids: unprotected sexual contact, injection drug use, tattooing, or providing or receiving medical care. However, it can be difficult to predict which travelers will have such exposures.

Typhoid and other diseases transmitted by contaminated food and water are common, and typhoid vaccine is recommended (see Chapter 4, Typhoid & Paratyphoid Fever).

Rabies vaccination is recommended for travelers participating in outdoor activities that could increase their risk of animal bites, such as camping or caving. Vaccination is also recommended for travelers working with animals (e.g., veterinarians), people taking long trips or moving to Burma, and young children, for whom it can be difficult to prevent interaction with dogs or other animals (see Chapter 3, Animal Bites & Stings).

Japanese encephalitis (JE) is presumed to be endemic throughout Burma, so travelers should take precautions to avoid mosquito bites (see Chapter 3, Mosquitoes, Ticks & Other Arthropods). Travelers should consider vaccination for JE if they will be in country for >1 month or if their itineraries include higher-risk activities such as spending substantial time in rural areas; outdoor activities such as camping, hiking, or farming; or staying in accommodations without air conditioning, window or door screens, or bed nets (see Chapter 4, Japanese Encephalitis).

Active cholera transmission has been reported from Myanmar in recent years. Check the destination page at www.cdc.gov/travel for current recommendations.

## Malaria and Other Vectorborne Diseases

Malaria is present in all areas of Burma below 3,281 ft (1,000 m) elevation, including the ancient capital city of Bagan. Risk to travelers is considered moderate. Malaria incidence in Burma exceeds that of neighboring countries in the Greater Mekong Subregion and is concentrated in and around forested areas. Drug-resistant malaria has been and continues to be a concern, and chemoprophylaxis recommendations vary accordingly (see Chapter 2, Yellow Fever Vaccine & Malaria Prophylaxis Information, by Country).

Other vectorborne infections endemic to Burma include dengue, chikungunya, and Zika. Because of the risk of birth defects in infants born to women infected with Zika during pregnancy, women who are pregnant or trying to become pregnant should research the most recent recommendations at www.cdc.gov/zika.

## Leptospirosis

Leptospirosis is a bacterial disease usually transmitted through contact with water contaminated by the urine of infected animals (see Chapter 4, Leptospirosis). It occurs most commonly during the rainy season and has been associated with swimming, wading, kayaking, and rafting. Advise travelers to avoid contact with soil and water that could be contaminated and to cover any open wounds to prevent exposure. Skin wounds that have been contaminated with soil or water should be cleaned immediately and thoroughly.

## Travelers' Diarrhea

Travelers' diarrhea is common among visitors to Burma (see Chapter 2, Travelers' Diarrhea). Instruct travelers to follow safe food and water precautions: eat food that is cooked and served hot (avoiding raw or undercooked foods), and drink only bottled water (see Chapter 2, Food &

**10**

Water Precautions). Oral rehydration solution is helpful in case of severe diarrhea and is usually available in pharmacies.

## Avian Influenza

Live bird markets, common in Burma, can be a source of avian influenza virus. Travelers should avoid visiting poultry farms, bird markets, and other places where live poultry are raised, kept, or sold and avoid preparing or eating raw or undercooked poultry products.

## OTHER HEALTH AND SAFETY RISKS

### Road Traffic Injuries

Vehicular crashes are a leading cause of injury and death among travelers (see Chapter 8, Road & Traffic Safety). Remind people visiting Burma to use only reputable taxi or public transportation companies and to always wear seat belts. Motorcycles account for a high percentage of road traffic deaths and should be avoided. Pedestrians and bicyclists are also commonly victims of road traffic deaths and should exercise caution; right-of-way rules and infrastructure improvements (such as crosswalks or bike lanes) to protect these groups are often not followed or in place.

## Heat-Related Illnesses

Average high temperatures in the hot season (March to May) can exceed 95°F (35°C) in many parts of the country, including popular tourist destinations such as Yangon, Mandalay, and Bagan. Prolonged heat exposure, especially for travelers in poor physical condition, elderly or very young travelers, those undertaking strenuous activity, and those not accustomed to heat, poses a risk for heat-related illnesses such as heat exhaustion or heat stroke (see Chapter 3, Extremes of Temperature). During periods of high heat, travelers should seek shade, drink ample water, and wear lightweight, loose, and light-colored clothing.

## HEALTH CARE ACCESS

Travelers with chronic medical conditions should not rely on being able to purchase or refill medications in Burma; counterfeit and substandard medications are common. International-standard medical care is rarely available, so treatment of chronic disease exacerbations or severe injuries can be suboptimal. Travelers should strongly consider medical evacuation insurance (see Chapter 6, Travel Insurance, Travel Health Insurance & Medical Evacuation Insurance).

## BIBLIOGRAPHY

1. Cui L, Yan G, Sattabongkot J, Cao Y, Chen B, Chen X, et al. Malaria in the Greater Mekong Subregion: heterogeneity and complexity. Acta Trop. 2012 Mar;121(3):227–39.

2. Dapat C, Saito R, Kyaw Y, Naito M, Hasegawa G, Suzuki Y, et al. Epidemiology of human influenza A and B viruses in Myanmar from 2005 to 2007. Intervirology. 2009;52(6):310–20.

3. Hotez PJ, Bottazzi ME, Strych U, Chang LY, Lim YA, Goodenow MM, et al. Neglected tropical diseases among the Association of Southeast Asian Nations (ASEAN): overview and update. PLoS Negl Trop Dis. 2015;9(4):e0003575.

4. Lo E, Nguyen J, Oo W, Hemming-Schroeder E, Zhou G, Yang Z, et al. Examining *Plasmodium falciparum* and *P. vivax* clearance subsequent to antimalarial drug treatment in the Myanmar-China border area based on quantitative real-time polymerase chain reaction. BMC Infect Dis. 2016 Apr 16;16(1):154.

5. Ngwe Tun MM, Kyaw AK, Hmone SW, Inoue S, Buerano CC, Soe AM, et al. Detection of Zika virus infection in Myanmar. Am J Trop Med Hyg. 2018 Mar;98(3):868–71.

6. Republic of the Union of Myanmar. The 2014 Myanmar population and housing census: highlights of the main results. Census Report. Nay Pyi Taw: Department of Population MoIaP;2015 May. Available from: http://myanmar.unfpa.org/sites/asiapacific/files/pub-pdf/Census%20 Highlights%20Report%20-%20ENGLISH%20(1).pdf.

7. Schweitzer A, Horn J, Mikolajczyk RT, Krause G, Ott JJ. Estimations of worldwide prevalence of chronic hepatitis B virus infection: a systematic review of data published between 1965 and 2013. Lancet. 2015 Oct;386(10003):1546–55.

8. Tun Win Y, Gardner E, Hadrill D, Su Mon CC, Kyin MM, Maw MT, et al. Emerging Zoonotic Influenza A Virus Detection in Myanmar: Surveillance Practices and Findings. Health Secur. 2017 Sep/Oct;15(5):483–93.

9. World Health Organization. Global status report on road safety 2015. WHO; 2015 [cited 2018 April 27]. Available from: www.who.int/violence_injury_prevention/road_safety_status/2015/en/.

10

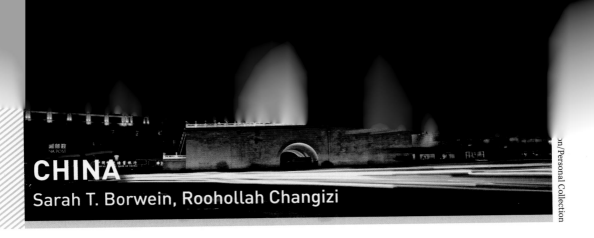

# CHINA
## Sarah T. Borwein, Roohollah Changizi

## DESTINATION OVERVIEW

China, the world's most populous country (>1.3 billion people), is the fourth largest geographically, behind Russia, Canada, and the United States. Divided into 23 provinces, 5 autonomous regions, and 4 municipalities (Map 10-12), it is home to diverse topographies, languages, and customs. The climate varies from tropical in the south to subarctic in the north, with wide variations between regions and seasons.

The long history and varied natural beauty of China can be traced through its 52 UNESCO World Heritage sites, including the Forbidden City and Temple of Heaven, the Great Wall, the terracotta warriors of Xi'an, and the spectacular mountainous sanctuaries of the west. Recent additions include the Tusi tribal domains in western China and the Grand Canal. The oldest (dating back to 468 BCE) and longest (1,115 miles; 1,794 km) man-made canal in the world, the Grand Canal, links the cities of Beijing and Hangzho and the island of Gulangyu, a historic pedestrian island settlement off the coast of Xiamen in southeastern China.

In 2017, more than 135 million tourists visited China. Tourism to China has grown at an extraordinary pace over the past decade, although numbers have leveled off slightly in the past few years. Travelers with special interests may go mountain climbing, tour small villages, or travel the Silk Road. More typical travel itineraries include sightseeing Beijing and the Great Wall, touring Shanghai, and cruising the Yangtze River (see Box 10-1 for information about Yangtze River cruises). Other tourist destinations include the following:

- Hong Kong, with its futuristic architecture and East-meets-West mystique

- Lijiang (Yunnan Province), with its many ethnic minorities

- Sichuan Province, home to China's iconic symbol, the panda

- Guilin, famous for its uniquely shaped limestone karst mountains, featured in paintings

- Tibet, accessible by the world's highest railroad (maximum elevation 16,640 ft [5,072 m])

- Xi'an, home to China's army of terracotta soldiers

- Hainan Island, home to tropical beaches and luxury resorts

Aside from tourism, increasing numbers of people travel to China to visit friends and relatives, to study, or to adopt children. These so-called "non-tourists" may be at an increased risk of becoming ill because they underestimate health hazards, are less likely to seek pretravel advice, and are more likely to stay in local or rural accommodations. People traveling to China to adopt often worry about the health of the child but neglect their own.

## HEALTH ISSUES

China is now the world's second-largest economy but, per capita income is still below the world average, with wide disparity in wealth and development between urban and rural, east and west. Health risks vary accordingly.

### Air Pollution

Although aggressive efforts are underway to control air pollution (a consequence of rapid economic

10

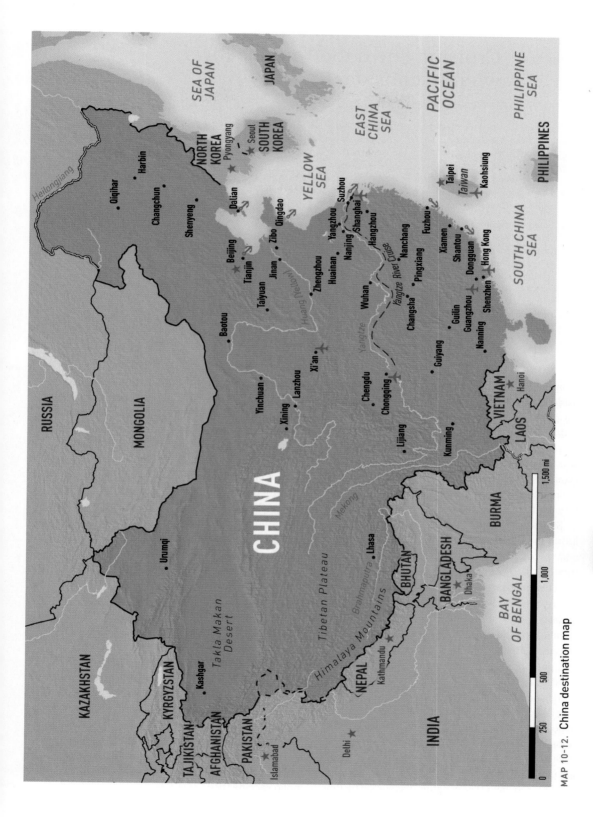

MAP 10-12. China destination map

## BOX 10-1. Cruising down the Yangtze River: what to consider

The Yangtze River is the third longest river in the world and one of the world's busiest and most polluted waterways. Yangtze River cruises are popular with tourists, and there are several health considerations for this trip:

- Japanese encephalitis (JE) is a risk; at least 1 case has been documented in a tourist whose 3-week trip to rural and urban China included a Yangtze River cruise.
- Malaria is not a substantial risk, although insect bite precautions are recommended.

- Schistosomiasis—*Schistosoma japonicum*—exists in the Yangtze River basin; swimming is ill-advised.
- Motion sickness is rare since much of the cruise takes place on a calm reservoir. However, susceptible travelers should carry antiemetic medication.
- Excursions off the boat often involve steep climbs, many stairs, and long walking distances that may not be accessible for infirm or less physically fit tourists.

- Air pollution on Yangtze River cruises can cause eye and throat irritation as well as respiratory problems in susceptible travelers. September and October are said to be the clearest months.
- Most non-Chinese-speaking tourists will prefer a 4- or 5-star "luxury" cruise. "First class" on Chinese tourist boats may not meet expectations for cleanliness, and English may not be spoken.
- Food and water precautions apply even on luxury cruises.

expansion), many of the most polluted cities in the world are in China; Beijing regularly tops the list. On peak pollution days, the levels of particulate matter (PM) in the air can exceed 40 times the limit considered safe by the World Health Organization (see Chapter 3, Air Quality & Ionizing Radiation). Haze has a negative impact on quality of life and indicates high concentrations of PM2.5, a respiratory, cardiovascular, and neuro toxin.

Short-term exposure to the levels of air pollution in China's megacities can irritate the eyes and throat. Travelers with underlying cardiorespiratory diseases, including asthma, chronic obstructive pulmonary disease, or congestive heart failure, may find their condition exacerbated. In addition, exposure to high levels of air pollution significantly increases the risk of respiratory tract infections, including sinusitis, otitis, bronchitis, and pneumonia. Children and the elderly are the most vulnerable to these effects.

Regional haze has triggered public anxiety and official concern. To tackle air pollution, a number of policies and measures targeted at reducing emissions and promoting alternative energy production have been implemented. Increased use of natural gas (and restrictions against burning coal) is key to these plans; China's use of natural gas surged by 19%

in 2017, as areas across northern China switched to this relatively clean fossil fuel and away from coal. This enabled those in Beijing and surrounding areas to enjoy many more days with clear, blue skies in the winter of 2017–2018. Other measures have included closing highly polluting factories and moving factories farther away from population centers.

Although surgical-style face masks have become fashionable in the big cities of China, especially Beijing and Shanghai, they afford wearers no protection from air pollution and are not recommended. Properly fitted N95 masks can filter out particulates but not gaseous pollutants and can sometimes actually compound breathing problems, so are not advisable for most people to wear.

## Vaccine-Preventable Diseases

Routine vaccinations should be up-to-date, including seasonal influenza. In addition, hepatitis A and B and typhoid vaccinations are recommended. The Xinjiang Uygur Autonomous Region borders Pakistan, a polio-endemic country. Adults traveling to this region who will be working in health care settings, refugee camps, or humanitarian aid settings should be vaccinated against polio, including a single lifetime booster dose of polio vaccine (IPV).

10

Measles and rubella immunity is particularly important. A massive vaccination campaign begun in September 2010 has decreased the number of reported measles cases; there were, however, still more than 100,000 cases of the disease reported in 2014. A few travelers have made news headlines by triggering outbreaks in their home countries after returning from China. Although limited data exist on rubella in China, it was not part of the national immunization program until 2008, and incidence is believed to be high.

China is making considerable advances in vaccination, with the objective of developing their own locally made vaccines or working with established pharmaceutical companies in a joint venture approach. One example is the recent introduction of quadrivalent human papilloma virus (HPV) vaccine. Strong demand has resulted in long waiting lists for this vaccine.

Unfortunately, there have been many issues with counterfeit and improperly stored vaccines. In addition, vaccine shortages are frequent; adult tetanus vaccines, for example, have been out of stock since 2014. Travelers cannot guarantee that they can complete an unfinished vaccination series once in China. Since tetanus vaccines are unavailable, ensure that all travelers going to China are up-to-date with their booster. Hong Kong, by contrast, functions under different rules; international vaccines are in use there and are generally available.

## HEPATITIS B

Hepatitis B infection is endemic to China. Nearly one-third of the 350 million people worldwide infected with the hepatitis B virus (HBV) reside in China. Hepatitis B vaccination is recommended for non-immune travelers.

## JAPANESE ENCEPHALITIS

Japanese encephalitis (JE) occurs in all regions except Qinghai, Xinjiang, and Xizang (Tibet) (see Map 4-7 and Table 4-7). China has successfully reduced the incidence of JE through vaccination and, as of 2008, included JE in its expanded national immunization program; however, the disease remains a potential threat to unvaccinated travelers.

Although the JE season varies by region, most cases in local residents occur from June through October. The risk of JE for most travelers to China varies based on season, destination, duration of stay, and activities. Risk is highest among travelers going to rural areas during the transmission season. JE vaccine is recommended for travelers who plan to spend ≥1 month in endemic areas during June through October.

Consider JE vaccine for shorter-term travelers (<1 month) planning visits to rural areas, or those at increased risk for JE virus exposure based on anticipated activities or itineraries (e.g., spending substantial time outdoors or staying in accommodations without air conditioning, screens, or bed nets). Sporadic cases have occurred on an unpredictable basis in short-term travelers, including in periurban Beijing and Shanghai. See Chapter 4, Japanese Encephalitis, for more detailed information.

## RABIES

Rabies is a serious problem in China, as in much of Asia. According to the World Health Organization, China has the second highest number of human rabies deaths in the world with more than 2,000 reported per year, every year for the past decade. Mammal bites in any area of China, including urban areas, must therefore be considered high risk for rabies (see Chapter 4, Rabies). As rabies immune globulin is generally unavailable, animal bites are often trip-enders, requiring evacuation to Hong Kong, Bangkok, or home for postexposure prophylaxis.

An analysis of data collected by the GeoSentinel Surveillance Network showed that bites from dogs are surprisingly common in tourists to China (see Chapter 3, Animal Bites & Stings). Include a discussion of rabies risk and prevention during pretravel consultations, and develop a strategy for dealing with possible exposure. Consider providing long-term travelers and expatriates going to live in China with the preexposure vaccination series.

# Vectorborne Diseases

## MALARIA

Malaria risk is very low for travelers to China, with the exception of those visiting rural parts of southern Yunnan Province. Consider prophylaxis for travelers to this region and reinforce the importance of mosquito prevention (see Chapter 3,

**10**

Mosquitoes, Ticks & Other Arthropods). Prescribe doxycycline or atovaquone-proguanil for travel to southern Yunnan, due to known mefloquine resistance (see Chapter 2, Yellow Fever Vaccine & Malaria Prophylaxis Information, by Country).

### DENGUE

In 2014, southern China experienced its worst dengue outbreak in decades; Guangdong province reported more than 40,000 cases in just 2 months. Travelers should practice daytime mosquito precautions in the summer months. See Chapter 4, Dengue, for more details on this disease.

## OTHER HEALTH RISKS

### Foodborne Illnesses

The risk for travelers' diarrhea appears to be low in deluxe accommodations in China but moderate elsewhere. Usual food and water precautions should apply, and travelers should consider bringing an antibiotic for self-treatment of moderate to severe diarrhea (see Chapter 2, Food & Water Precautions and Travelers' Diarrhea). Since highly quinolone-resistant *Campylobacter* is a problem in China, azithromycin may be a good choice.

Tap water is not safe to drink even in major cities. Most hotels provide bottled or boiled water, and bottled water is easily available. In addition, there have been several well-publicized episodes of contamination of food with pesticides and other substances. Travelers should strictly avoid undercooked fish and shellfish and unpasteurized milk.

### Sexually Transmitted Infections

Sexually transmitted infections (STIs), including syphilis, HIV, gonorrhea, and chlamydia, are a growing problem in China, particularly along the booming eastern seaboard. Travel is associated with loosened inhibitions and increased casual sexual liaisons (see Chapter 9, Sex & Travel). Travelers should be aware of STI risks and use condoms when having sex with anyone whose HIV or STI status is unknown. Hepatitis B vaccination before travel should be considered.

### Road Traffic Injuries

Traffic in China is often chaotic. The rate of traffic crashes, including fatal ones, is among the highest in the world (see Chapter 8, Road & Traffic Safety). Child safety seats, rear seat belts, and bicycle or motorcycle helmets are rarely seen and not widely available. Traffic crashes, even minor ones, can create major traffic jams and sometimes turn into violent altercations, particularly when foreigners are involved (see Chapter 3, Safety & Security Overseas).

China has not signed the convention that created the International Driving Permit, and travelers require a Chinese license to drive. Driving is on the right side of the road in mainland China but on the left in Hong Kong and Macau. In practice, many people drive down the middle of the road. It is advisable to avoid driving at night or when weather conditions are bad, and not to assume that traffic rules or right-of-way will be respected. For all of these reasons, it is often simpler and safer to hire a local driver than to drive oneself.

Electronic bicycles (E-bikes) are popular and do not have to be registered. They often travel in pedestrian and bicycle lanes as well as with traffic. Because there is no engine noise, it can be challenging for pedestrians to identify an oncoming E-bike. Motor vehicles and E-bikes often drive without lights, making night travel dangerous.

### Natural Disasters

Five of the 10 deadliest natural disasters in history have occurred in China. Natural hazards include dust storms in the north and typhoons along the southern and eastern seaboards. Torrential rain, floods, and landslides occur on a regular basis, most recently in the summer of 2017. Earthquakes cause significant death and destruction. The 1556 Shaanxi earthquake—thought to have killed more than 800,000 people—is the most lethal earthquake ever recorded and one of the 10 deadliest natural disasters. More recently, devastating earthquakes struck the western provinces of Sichuan in 2008 and Qinghai in 2010.

### High Elevation Travel

Western China is home to some of the highest mountains in the world. Some popular destinations are Lhasa (3,658 m), Shangri-La (3,280 m), Lijiang (2,418 m), and Xining (2,295 m). Preparation and gradual ascent to acclimatize are the mainstays travelers should follow to prevent the onset of altitude illness (see Chapter 3, High-Altitude Travel & Altitude Illness).

Travelers who cannot ascend gradually—or who develop acute mountain sickness (AMS)—should carry their own supply of acetazolamide; it is not available in China. Dexamethasone, a prevention for AMS and high-altitude pulmonary and cerebral edema (HAPE and HACE, respectively), is reportedly available in China. Similarly, nifedipine (as a prevention and treatment for HAPE) is reportedly available. The quality and ready availability of either of these drugs is unknown.

## Vitamin D Deficiency

Vitamin D deficiency is a major issue in the northern provinces of China, where smog blocks out sunlight, leading to inadequate vitamin D absorption, even in the summer months. To decrease the risk of osteomalacia and osteoporosis in travelers spending more than 6 months in China, prescribe vitamin D supplementation.

## MEDICAL CARE IN CHINA

Strongly encourage travelers to invest in travel health insurance, including medical evacuation insurance coverage (see Chapter 6, Travel Insurance, Travel Health Insurance & Medical Evacuation Insurance). Most hospitals do not accept foreign medical insurance, and patients are expected to pay a deposit to cover the expected cost of the treatment before care is delivered. Western-style medical facilities that meet international standards are available in Beijing, Shanghai, and Hong Kong.

Hospitals in other cities may have "VIP wards" (*gaogan bingfang*) with English-speaking staff. The standard of care in such facilities is somewhat unpredictable, however, and cultural and regulatory differences can cause difficulties for travelers. In rural areas, only rudimentary medical care may be available. Hepatitis B virus transmission from poorly sterilized medical equipment remains a risk outside major centers.

Ambulances are not staffed with trained paramedics and often have little or no medical equipment; rather than waiting for an ambulance to arrive, injured travelers may be better off taking a taxi or other immediately available vehicle to the nearest major hospital. Pharmacies often sell prescription medications over the counter; these may be counterfeit, substandard, or even contaminated. Travelers should bring all their regular medications in sufficient quantity. If more or other medications are required, visiting a reputable clinic or hospital is advised.

Most who wish to try traditional Chinese remedies do so uneventfully, although not without accepting some risk. Remind travelers that acupuncture needles may be a source of bloodborne and skin infections; acupressure may be preferable to acupuncture. Herbal medicine products may be contaminated with heavy metals or pharmaceutical agents.

Currently China is witnessing an influx of patients coming from Africa seeking treatment not available in their home countries. There is also a growing market of patients coming from more developed countries looking for as-yet unapproved experimental treatments (see Chapter 9, Medical Tourism).

### BIBLIOGRAPHY

1. Davis XM, MacDonald S, Borwein S, Freedman DO, Kozarsky PE, von Sonnenburg F, et al. Health risks in travelers to China: the GeoSentinel experience and implications for the 2008 Beijing Olympics. Am J Trop Med Hyg. 2008 Jul;79(1):4–8.

2. Hills SL, Griggs AC, Fischer M. Japanese encephalitis in travelers from non-endemic countries, 1973–2008. Am J Trop Med Hyg. 2010 May;82(5):930–6.

3. Shaw MT, Leggat PA, Borwein S. Travelling to China for the Beijing 2008 Olympic and Paralympic games. Travel Med Infect Dis. 2007 Nov;5(6):365–73.

4. United Nations World Tourism Organization. UNWTO tourism highlights. Madrid: United Nations World Tourism Organization; 2012 [cited 2016 Sep 24]. Available from: http://mkt.unwto.org/en/publication/unwto-tourism-highlights-2012-edition.

5. World Health Organization. Hepatitis B surveillance and control. WHO; [updated 2016 July; cited 2016 Sep 24]. Available from: www.who.int/mediacentre/factsheets/fs204/en/.

6. World Health Organization. Measles bulletin: Western Pacific region. Geneva: World Health Organization;

10

2010 [cited 2016 Sep 24]. Available from: www.wpro. who.int/entity/immunization/documents/docs/ MeasBulletinVol4Issue1_F840.pdf.

7. Xia J, Min L, Shu J. Dengue fever in China: an emerging problem demands attention. Emerg Microbes Infect. 2015 Jan;4(1):e3.

8. Zhang J, Jin Z, Sun GQ, Zhou T, Ruan S. Analysis of rabies in China: transmission dynamics and control. PLoS One. 2011;6(7):e20891.

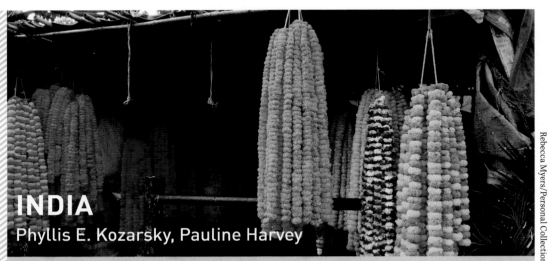

# INDIA

Phyllis E. Kozarsky, Pauline Harvey

## DESTINATION OVERVIEW

India is approximately one-third the size of the United States and has 4 times the population (almost 1.3 billion people). This makes it the second most populous country in the world, behind China. Rich in history, vibrant culture, and diversity, India is the birthplace of 4 world religions: Hinduism, Buddhism, Jainism, and Sikhism. Despite the growth of megacities such as Mumbai and Delhi (both more than 20 million people), India's rural population is still twice that of its urban population. Although India is one of the fastest-growing economies in the world, the literacy rate varies by state (64%–94%), the level of poverty is high, and the life expectancy is about 68 years.

The topography is varied, ranging from tropical beaches to foothills, deserts, and the Himalayan mountains. The north has a more temperate climate, while the south is more tropical year-round. Many travelers prefer India during the winter—November through March, when the temperatures are more agreeable—although some, particularly families with children, must travel during the summer vacation.

India is becoming more popular for US travelers, and rates of travel from the United States are increasing. Tourists are flocking to the temples, beaches, and the Taj Mahal, and international business is flourishing. For some new US residents, India remains their homeland, and they make frequent visits to see family and friends. In addition, India has a large and growing medical tourism sector.

Because tourists could not possibly visit all the sites in India during a 2-week holiday, they usually select a part of India for any given trip. A typical itinerary in the north of India includes Delhi, Agra, Varanasi, and cities in Rajasthan, such as Jaipur (the Pink City) and Udaipur. Agra is the home of the Taj Mahal, a breathtaking monument to lost love. Along the northern travel circle, one can stop to enjoy the magnificent bird sanctuary at Keoladeo Ghana and the tiger reserve at Ranthambore (see Map 10-13). Varanasi, sacred to Hindus, Buddhists,

10

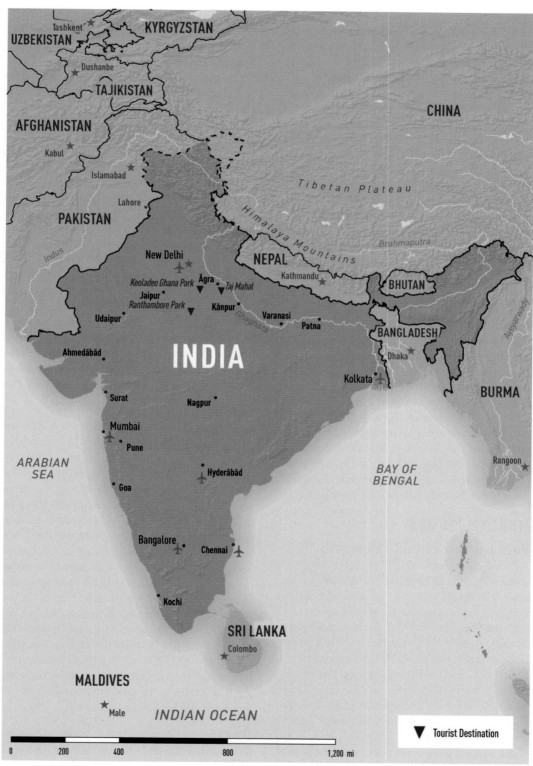

MAP 10-13. India destination map

and Jains, welcomes Hindu pilgrimages and boasts extraordinary experiences along the Ganges.

A more southern route might swing through Goa and its beautiful beaches along the western coast. What used to be the backdrop for great parties and old-time hippies, Goa has now become a haven for writers and artists, boasting a chic new culture. Mumbai, a common entry point to India, hosts Bollywood, the largest film industry in the world. Kolkata (Calcutta) is considered the cultural capital of the country. Bengaluru (Bangalore) in the south-central region is both the garden city and India's Silicon Valley. The old seaside town of Kochi (Cochin) shows evidence of its Portuguese heritage, and Hyderabad shows off its old granite fort, many mosques, and bazaars.

Despite the many and varied itineraries, most health recommendations for travelers to India are similar. The incidences of some illnesses, such as those transmitted by mosquitoes, increase during the monsoon season (May–October) with the high temperatures, heavy rains, and the risk of flooding. Some of the most important health considerations of travel to India are for travelers visiting friends and relatives (VFRs). They often do not seek pretravel health advice, since they are returning to their land of origin. But because they may stay in rural areas not often visited by tourists or business people, live in homes, and eat and drink with their families, they are at higher risk of many travel-related illnesses (see Chapter 9, Visiting Friends & Relatives: VFR Travel).

# HEALTH ISSUES

## Vaccine-Preventable Diseases

All travelers to India should be up-to-date with routine immunizations and are advised to consider hepatitis B vaccine. Particularly important is making sure that the traveler is immune to measles. India has not had a case of wild poliovirus since early 2011, obtained its polio-free certification from the World Health Organization in March 2014, and celebrated 7 years of being polio-free in January 2018. Polio vaccine is no longer recommended for US travelers to India. However, all travelers (residents and nationals) coming from countries reporting cases of polio should check to see if there is a requirement for a dose of polio vaccine prior to entry into India.

### HEPATITIS A

All travelers to India should be protected against hepatitis A (see Chapter 4, Hepatitis A). Although some assume that those born in India would have been exposed to hepatitis A in childhood and thus be immune, this may no longer be true, particularly for younger people. Consider serologic testing for hepatitis A IgG in VFR travelers, or immunize.

### TYPHOID

More than 80% of typhoid fever cases in the United States are in people who traveled to India or other countries in south Asia (see Chapter 4, Typhoid & Paratyphoid Fever). Thus, even for short-term travel, a typhoid vaccine is recommended. Patients hesitant to be vaccinated may be persuaded by learning that typhoid fever acquired in south Asia is becoming increasingly resistant to quinolone antibiotics, sometimes requiring parenteral therapy.

Paratyphoid fever, a similar disease caused by *Salmonella enterica* serovar Paratyphi A, B, and C, has become increasingly prevalent in south Asia, but typhoid vaccines are not protective against this infection.

### JAPANESE ENCEPHALITIS

Although there has never been a published case of a traveler acquiring Japanese encephalitis (JE) in India, the disease is present in many parts of the country (see Chapter 4, Japanese Encephalitis). Risk is highest during the monsoon season (from May through October) although the season may be extended or even year-round in some areas, especially in the south. Vaccination is not recommended for the typical 2-week trip most travelers take to see the major tourist sites in urban areas; publicized outbreaks in recent years have not been in typical tourist destinations. JE vaccine is recommended for those planning to spend ≥1 month in endemic areas during the JE virus transmission season. Consider giving JE vaccine to those planning repeated, short-term travel and to those planning short-term travel to periurban areas with an increased risk for JE virus exposure.

### RABIES

India has the highest burden of rabies in the world, with estimates of 18,000–20,000 human cases

10

per year (see Chapter 4, Rabies). Dogs roam in packs in many areas of the country. Unfortunately, human rabies immune globulin is not readily available except in some clinics in major cities. Information about such clinics can be obtained from the website of the International Society of Travel Medicine (www.istm.org).

A preexposure rabies vaccine series is not recommended for all travelers to India, and cost may be a consideration. Long-term travelers, expatriates, missionaries, and volunteers may, however, want to obtain preexposure immunization for themselves and their children. Without preexposure rabies vaccination, bitten travelers may have to leave the country to receive postexposure prophylaxis. Encouraging travelers to think about purchasing a medical evacuation insurance policy that will cover travel for recommended rabies postexposure prophylaxis and education about bite avoidance and management should be a part of every pretravel consultation.

## CHOLERA

Active cholera transmission has been reported from India in recent years. Check the destination page at www.cdc.gov/travel for current recommendations.

## Malaria

Unlike other countries in Asia, malaria is holoendemic in India (except at elevations >6,562 ft; 2,000 m) and occurs in both rural and urban areas. Rates of *Plasmodium falciparum* have increased in the last few decades, and chemoprophylaxis is recommended for all destinations. Remind travelers that malaria-transmitting mosquitoes primarily bite between dusk and dawn (see Chapter 2, Yellow Fever Vaccine & Malaria Prophylaxis Information, by Country; Chapter 3, Mosquitoes, Ticks & Other Arthropods; and Chapter 4, Malaria).

## Other Infections

### MULTIDRUG-RESISTANT BACTERIA

Strains of bacteria resistant to most antibiotics have been carried by travelers from India to many other countries, including the United States. High rates of resistance to multiple antibiotics have been shown among gram-negative (*Escherichia*

*coli*, *Klebsiella* spp., and *Salmonella* spp.) and gram-positive (*Staphylococcus aureus*) bacteria in India. In particular, bacterial resistance to carbapenems, third-generation cephalosporins, fluoroquinolones, and even colistin are becoming more common.

### DENGUE, CHIKUNGUNYA, AND ZIKA

Dengue is endemic to all of India except at high elevation in mountainous regions (see Chapter 4, Dengue). Poorly reported at the local and national levels, large outbreaks continue to occur, including in many urban areas. Incidence is highest during the wet summer season, which includes the monsoon season (May–October). Travelers to India should take measures to protect themselves from daytime mosquito bites to prevent dengue (see Chapter 3, Mosquitoes, Ticks & Other Arthropods).

During the last several years there have been outbreaks of chikungunya, transmitted by day- and night-biting mosquitoes. Symptoms are similar to those of dengue and malaria, although often with severe and persistent arthralgia (see Chapter 4, Chikungunya).

Zika is a risk in India. Because of the risk of birth defects in infants born to women infected with Zika during pregnancy, women who are pregnant or trying to become pregnant should research the most recent recommendations at www.cdc.gov/zika.

### HEPATITIS E

Hepatitis E is being recognized more frequently in travelers to India. A traveler who develops symptomatic hepatitis despite being immunized against hepatitis A will likely have hepatitis E.

### ANIMAL BITES AND WOUNDS

Diseases other than rabies can be transmitted by animal bites and wounds. Cellulitis, fasciitis, and wound infections can result from the scratch or bite of any animal. Potentially fatal to humans, B virus is carried by macaques (see Chapter 4, B Virus). These Old World monkeys inhabit many of the temples in India, scatter themselves in many tourist gathering places, and are kept as pets. Macaques can be aggressive and often seek food from travelers. When visiting temples, travelers should not carry any food in their hands, pockets, or bags. It is important to stress to travelers that monkeys and other animals should not be approached or handled. If bitten, travelers should seek immediate medical care.

## TRAVELERS' DIARRHEA

The risk for travelers' diarrhea is moderate to high in India, with an estimated 30%–50% likelihood of developing diarrhea during a 2-week journey. Discuss self-treatment for diarrheal illness (see Chapter 2, Travelers' Diarrhea), and remind travelers to practice safe food and water precautions (see Chapter 2, Food & Water Precautions).

## TUBERCULOSIS (TB)

India has among the highest prevalence of TB worldwide; approximately one-fourth of all TB cases worldwide occur there. An estimated 2%–3% of newly diagnosed cases are multidrug resistant; a smaller percentage are extensively drug resistant.

Travelers who plan to work in high-risk settings or in crowded institutions (e.g., medical clinics, hospital, prison, or homeless shelter populations) are at risk for TB exposure. Discuss with them the importance of testing before and after travel, and measures for disease prevention. Travelers should have a tuberculin skin test or TB blood test before leaving the United States. If the test is negative, repeat the test 8–10 weeks after the returning from India.

Use of bacillus Calmette-Guérin (BCG) vaccine in health care workers who will have increased risk of tuberculosis during travel has recently been proposed, although this recommendation remains controversial (see Chapter 4, Tuberculosis). Limited access to BCG and lack of expertise in administering the vaccine in the United States are also barriers.

## OTHER ISSUES

Travelers who have never before ventured into the developing world may be shocked when arriving in India for the first time. The crowds and the intense colors, heat, and smells are striking and invade all the senses at once. It is difficult to enjoy the beauty of the country without being touched by the enormity of its poverty. The close juxtaposition of the old and new is noteworthy. At times this culture shock can be overwhelming (see Chapter 3, Mental Health).

Transportation in India remains problematic. Recommend carrying food and beverages in the event of delays, which are almost inevitable no matter the mode of transport. Traveling by train can be particularly harrowing, having to force one's way through the crowd and onto the train. Travelers should make sure to keep passports and valuables safe while in crowds.

India's roadways are some of the most hazardous in the world, with large numbers of traffic-related—including pedestrian—deaths (see Chapter 8, Road & Traffic Safety). Animals, rickshaws, motor scooters, people, bicycles, trucks, and overcrowded buses compete for space in an unregulated free-for-all. Fasten seat belts when riding in cars and wear a helmet when riding bicycles or motorbikes. Advise travelers to avoid overcrowded buses and not to travel by bus into the interior of the country or on curving, mountainous roads. Discourage nighttime driving (in particular, long-distance travel), even when a paid driver has been hired. Air pollution is a problem in the major cities, so those with chronic lung disease or asthma may consider spending time outdoors when there is less traffic or staying in facilities outside major cities (see Chapter 3, Air Quality & Ionizing Radiation).

Medical tourism is a growing industry in India. Many newer medical facilities have opened recently for travelers desiring cardiac, orthopedic, dental, or plastic surgery or transplantations at a substantially lower cost than in the United States. The benefits and hazards require careful examination (see Chapter 9, Medical Tourism). The quality of health care is quite variable in India and depends on the location.

In general, travelers feel safe while in India, although peddlers and promoters are aggressive with tourists. Travelers may want to avoid making eye contact with a peddler or his goods, or they may risk having someone follow them down the street trying to sell them something. In such instances, a firm "no" should suffice. The stress of negotiating one's way through India makes it a place where having a close traveling companion is important. It is always wise to pay attention to US Department of State advisories in case of issues that arise at some borders, or occasional increases in religious tensions or terrorist activities.

## BIBLIOGRAPHY

1. Baggett HC, Graham S, Kozarsky PE, Gallagher N, Blumensaadt S, Bateman J, et al. Pretravel health preparation among US residents traveling to India to VFRs: importance of ethnicity in defining VFRs. J Travel Med. 2009 Mar–Apr;16(2):112–8.

2. Buhl MR, Lindquist L. Japanese encephalitis in travelers: review of cases and seasonal risk. J Travel Med. 2009 May;16:217–9.

3. Epelboin L, Robert J, Tsyrina-Kouyoumdjian E, Laouira S, Meyssonnier V, Caumes E, et al. High rate of multidrugresistant gram-negative bacilli carriage and infection in hospitalized returning travelers: a cross-sectional cohort study. J Travel Med. 2015 Sep–Oct;22(5):292–9.

4. Jensenius M, Han PV, Schlagenhauf P, Schwartz E, Parola P, Castelli F, et al. Acute and potentially life-threatening tropical diseases in western travelers—a GeoSentinel multicenter study, 1996–2011. Am J Trop Med Hyg. 2013 Feb;88(2):397–404.

5. Kumarasamy KK, Toleman MA, Walsh TR, Bagaria J, Butt F, Balakrishnan R, et al. Emergence of a new antibiotic resistance mechanism in India, Pakistan, and the UK: a molecular, biological, and epidemiological study. Lancet Infect Dis. 2010 Sep;10(9):597–602.

6. Laxminarayan R, Chaudhury RR. Antibiotic resistance in India: drivers and opportunities for action. PLoS Med. 2016 Mar 2;13(3):e1001974.

7. Leder K, Torresi J, Brownstein JS, Wilson ME, Keystone JS, Barnett E, et al. Travel-associated illness trends and clusters, 2000–2010. Emerg Infect Dis. 2013 Jul;19(7):1049–73.

8. Lynch MF, Blanton EM, Bulens S, Polyak C, Vojdani J, Stevenson J, et al. Typhoid fever in the United States, 1999–2006. JAMA. 2009 Aug 26;302(8): 859–65.

9. Shaw MT, Leggat PA, Chatterjee S. Travelling to India for the Delhi XIX Commonwealth Games 2010. Travel Med Infect Dis. 2010 May;8(3):129–38.

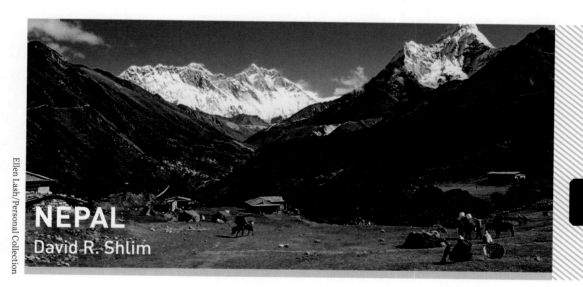

Ellen Lash/Personal Collection

# NEPAL
## David R. Shlim

**10**

## DESTINATION OVERVIEW

Home to more than 29 million people, Nepal stretches for 500 miles (805 km) along the Himalayan mountains that provide the natural border between it and China (see Map 10-14). The topography rises from low plains (elevation 200 ft; 70 m) to the highest point in the world at 29,029 ft (8,848 m), the summit of Mount Everest. Approximately 30% of tourists come to Nepal to trek into the mountains, while others come to experience the culture and stunning natural beauty. Kathmandu, the capital city with a population of more than 2 million people, sits in a lush valley at 4,344 ft (1,324 m) elevation.

Nepal's latitude of 28°N (the same as Florida) means that its nonmountainous areas are temperate year-round. Most annual rainfall comes during the monsoon season (June through

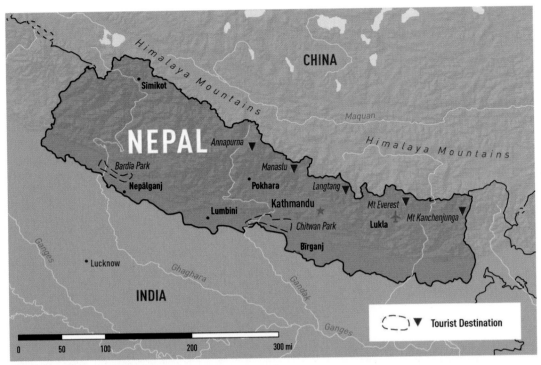

MAP 10-14. **Nepal destination map**

September). The main tourist seasons are the spring (March to May) and fall (October and November). The winter months, December through February, are pleasant in the lowlands but can be too cold to make trekking enjoyable in the high mountains.

In April 2015, a major earthquake caused extensive damage and killed more than 9,000 people. Most of the damage occurred in nontourist areas, and the infrastructure for tourists has largely been repaired. The Mount Everest region east of Kathmandu and the Annapurna region to the west are the destination for most trekkers. The Langtang trekking area, north of Kathmandu, was virtually destroyed by a major landslide caused by the 2015 earthquake; since then, many services have been rebuilt and tourism is returning to the area. The high point of the Langtang region is 14,000 ft (4,267 m).

Trekkers into the Mount Everest region routinely sleep at elevations of 14,000–16,000 ft (4,267–4,876 m) and hike to elevations >18,000 ft (5,486 m). This prolonged exposure to very high elevations means that tourists must be knowledgeable about the risks of altitude illness and

may need to carry specific medications to prevent and treat the problem (see Chapter 3, High-Altitude Travel & Altitude Illness). Most trekkers into the Mount Everest region arrive there by flying to a tiny airstrip at Lukla at 9,383 ft (2,860 m). The following day they reach Namche Bazaar at 11,290 ft (3,440 m). Acetazolamide prophylaxis can substantially decrease the chances of developing acute mountain sickness in Namche.

In the Annapurna region, short-term trekkers may choose to hike to viewpoints in the foothills without reaching any high elevations. Others may undertake a longer trek around the Annapurna massif, going over a 17,769 ft (5,416 m) pass (the Thorung La). Roads have been constructed up the 2 major valleys of this trek, shortening the overall trekking distance and changing the nature of the experience (buses, cars, and motorcycles may be encountered along the trek). However, new trails under development will allow trekkers to be off the roads for much of the way. The total exposure to high elevations is less in this region than in the Everest region. In recent years, trekkers have begun traveling to the Manaslu area, which offers a trekking experience with less-developed lodges and an extended time away from roads. Notable in this area is the Nubri Valley, with many sacred Buddhist sites.

In addition to trekking, Nepal has some of the best rafting and kayaking rivers in the world. Jungle lodges in Chitwan National Park allow tourists to view a wide range of wildlife, including tigers, rhinoceros, bears, and crocodiles, and a huge variety of exotic birds. For less adventurous travelers, it is possible to drive to comfortable hotels offering commanding views of the Himalayas, both near Kathmandu and near Pokhara.

Lumbini, in the Terai region of Nepal, is the birthplace of the Buddha. It has become an increasingly popular and beautifully developed pilgrimage destination for Buddhists from around the world. The airport near Lumbini is being upgraded to an international airport. Pokhara airport is also scheduled to become an international airport in the future, giving tourists more options for traveling in and out of Nepal.

## HEALTH ISSUES

### Vaccine-Preventable Diseases

Travelers to Nepal are at high risk for enteric diseases. Hepatitis A vaccine and typhoid vaccine are the 2 most important immunizations. The risk of typhoid fever and paratyphoid fever among travelers to Nepal is among the highest in the world, and the prevalence of fluoroquinolone resistance is high (see Chapter 4, Typhoid & Paratyphoid Fever).

#### JAPANESE ENCEPHALITIS

Japanese encephalitis (JE) is endemic to Nepal; the highest disease risk is in the Terai region during and immediately after monsoon season (June through October). JE has been identified in local residents of the Kathmandu Valley, but only 1 case of JE acquired in Nepal has been reported in a foreigner, a tourist who spent time in the Terai in August. JE vaccine is not routinely recommended for travelers trekking in high-elevation areas or spending time in Kathmandu or Pokhara en route to such treks (see Chapter 4, Japanese Encephalitis). JE vaccination is recommended for foreigners living in Nepal.

#### RABIES

Rabies is highly endemic to the dogs in Nepal, but in recent years there are fewer stray dogs in Kathmandu. Half of all tourist exposures to possibly rabid animals occur near Swayambunath, a beautiful hilltop shrine also known as the "monkey temple." Advise tourists to be extra cautious with the dogs and monkeys here. Monkeys can be aggressive if approached and will jump on a person's back if they smell food in a backpack. Clinics in Kathmandu specializing in the care of foreigners almost always have complete postexposure rabies prophylaxis, including human rabies immune globulin (see Chapter 4, Rabies). Trekkers bitten in the mountains should be able to return to Kathmandu within an average of 5 days.

### Malaria

Malaria is not a risk for most travelers to Nepal. There is no transmission of malaria in Kathmandu, and all the main trekking routes in Nepal are free of malaria transmission. Chitwan National Park is a popular tourist destination for wildlife viewing in the Terai. Although the Nepalese Ministry of Health and other regional organizations regard the Terai to be a malaria transmission area, this author, in 30 years of treating travelers in Nepal, has not seen a single case of malaria in a traveler to Chitwan, including foreign workers living in the park. Nepal has been targeted for the complete elimination of malaria within the next 10 years.

### Other Health and Safety Risks

#### GASTROINTESTINAL ISSUES

*Cyclospora cayetanensis*, an intestinal protozoal pathogen, is highly endemic to Nepal (see Chapter 4, Cyclosporiasis). Risk for infection is distinctly seasonal: transmission occurs almost exclusively from May through October, with a peak in June and July. Because this is outside the main tourist seasons, the primary effect is on expatriates who stay through the monsoon. In addition to watery diarrhea, profound anorexia and fatigue are the hallmark symptoms of *Cyclospora* infection. The treatment of choice is trimethoprim-sulfamethoxazole; no highly effective alternatives have been identified.

10

Travelers' diarrhea is a risk, and the risk in the spring trekking season (March through May) is double that in the fall trekking season (October and November). Since many tourists are heading to remote areas that do not have medical care available, they should be provided with medications for self-treatment (see Chapter 2, Travelers' Diarrhea). Extensive resistance to fluoroquinolones has been documented among bacterial diarrheal pathogens in Nepal, and moderate to severe diarrhea should be empirically treated with azithromycin. Hepatitis E virus is endemic to Nepal, and several cases each year are diagnosed in tourists or expatriates. There is no vaccine commercially available against hepatitis E.

## RESPIRATORY ISSUES

Air pollution problems in the Kathmandu Valley are frequent. People with underlying cardiorespiratory illness, including asthma, chronic obstructive pulmonary disease, or coronary heart failure may suffer exacerbations in Kathmandu, particularly after a viral upper respiratory infection. Short-term exposure to the levels of air pollution found there can irritate the eyes and throat. In addition, exposure to high levels of air pollution significantly increases the risk of respiratory tract infections, including sinusitis, otitis, bronchitis, and pneumonia (see Chapter 3, Air Quality & Ionizing Radiation).

Viral upper respiratory infections are extremely common, and the percentage of these that lead to bacterial sinusitis or bronchitis is high. Trekkers should consider carrying an antibiotic such as azithromycin to empirically treat a respiratory infection that lasts >7 days with no sign of improvement.

## EVACUATION AND MEDICAL CARE

Helicopter evacuation from most areas is readily available. Communication has improved from remote areas because of satellite and cellular telephones, and private helicopter companies accept credit cards and are eager to perform evacuations for profit. Evacuation can often take place on the same day as the request, weather permitting. Helicopter rescue is usually limited to morning hours because of afternoon winds in the mountains. Helicopter rescue is billed at $4,000 per hour, with an average total cost of $8,000 to $10,000.

New hospitals—being built at a rapid pace in Kathmandu—are competing for foreign patients. Overall, hospital facilities have improved steadily over the years; acute cardiac care, general surgery, and orthopedic surgery are all reliable and available in Kathmandu. The closest evacuation point for definitive care is Bangkok. Advise travelers of reliable sources of medical care in Nepal before their departure; clinics specializing in the care of foreigners can be found on the International Society of Travel Medicine website (www.istm.org).

## THE POLITICAL SITUATION

The political situation in Nepal has been in transition since 1990, when a mainly peaceful democratic revolution led to a multiparty parliamentary system under a constitutional monarch. Frustration with the rate of progress in rural areas led to a Maoist insurrection and 10 years of low-grade but violent civil war. A peace agreement was reached and the monarchy abolished in 2008. In 2017, the country was divided into 7 provinces, each with its own recognized local government. During election times, tourist schedules can be disrupted by demonstrations and strikes, but none of the political tension has been aimed at foreigners; Nepal remains a safe destination to visit. Visitors should, however, monitor the political situation while planning their journey.

## BIBLIOGRAPHY

1. Cave W, Pandey P, Osrin D, Shlim DR. Chemoprophylaxis use and the risk of malaria in travelers to Nepal. J Travel Med. 2003 Mar–Apr;10(2):100–5.

2. Hoge CW, Shlim DR, Echeverria P, Rajah R, Herrmann JE, Cross JH. Epidemiology of diarrhea among expatriate residents living in a highly endemic environment. JAMA. 1996 Feb 21;275(7):533–8.

10

3. Pandey P, Bodhidatta L, Lewis M, Murphy H, Shlim DR, Cave W, et al. Travelers' diarrhea in Nepal: an update on the pathogens and antibiotic resistance. J Travel Med. 2011;18(2):102–8.

4. Schwartz E, Shlim DR, Eaton M, Jenks N, Houston R. The effect of oral and parenteral typhoid vaccination on the rate of infection with *Salmonella typhi* and *Salmonella paratyphi* A among foreigners in Nepal. Arch Intern Med. 1990 Feb;150(2):349–51.

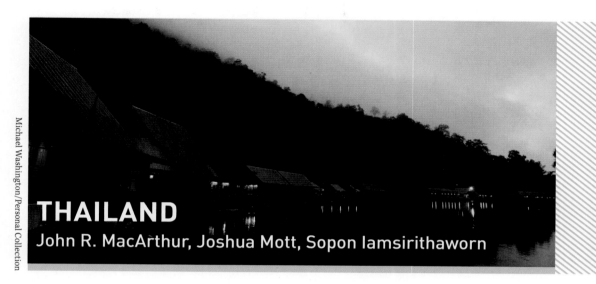

Michael Washington/Personal Collection

# THAILAND
## John R. MacArthur, Joshua Mott, Sopon Iamsirithaworn

## DESTINATION OVERVIEW

Known as "the Land of Smiles," Thailand is a popular destination for tourists, offering beautiful beaches, delicious cuisine, excellent shopping, fabulous golf courses, exciting nightlife, cultural diversity, and adventure opportunities. Thailand is also a regional business hub. In 2017, >35 million visitors spent more than 1 night in Thailand, and the number of visitors continues to grow. Thai is a melodic, tonal language that can be difficult to learn; however, English is commonly spoken at most popular destinations in Thailand. Road signs, maps, and tourist guides provide information in English and Thai.

Thailand is a geographically diverse country a little smaller than the state of Texas (Map 10-15). Because it is close to the equator, the climate is tropical and often hot and humid. Flooding is always a possibility, and various regions are prone to flash floods. Monsoon rains fall from July through October and can last until cooler, drier weather

comes in November, making November through February a popular time of year to visit. Thailand's central location and major international airports in Bangkok make it an easy access point for other destinations in Asia.

Out of a total population of nearly 70 million people, more than 10 million live in the capital city of Bangkok, a major metropolis and center of commerce. Tourists here visit historic sites of glittering grandeur such as the many Buddhist temples and the Grand Palace (to catch a glimpse of the Emerald Buddha). The main arteries of Bangkok are the Chao Phraya River and its canals, which provide access to tourist sites, the floating market, and restaurants. Bangkok is a paradise of culinary delights, from sidewalk noodle stands to exquisite 3-star restaurant meals.

Many visitors to Thailand also visit Chiang Mai in the north. The old city is surrounded by a moat and defensive wall; beyond the wall are

10

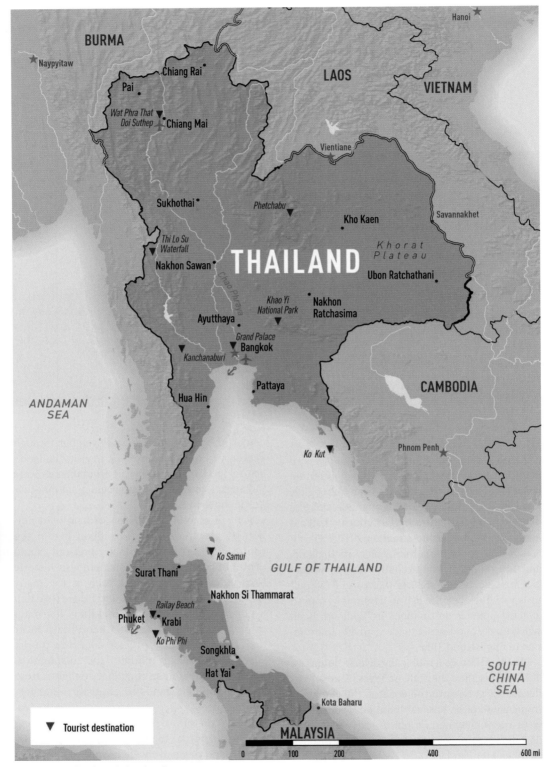

MAP 10-15. Thailand destination map

>300 temples, a popular night bazaar for shopping, and easy access to the handicraft villages, elephant nature parks, and popular outdoor adventures.

Over the years, medical tourism to Thailand has increased. Compared with the United States, the cost of medical or surgical treatment is much less, and the quality of care is generally good. In addition, the country has become a popular destination for retirees from around the world, including a large American expatriate community. The warm climate and low cost of living make Thailand an attractive place to live.

# HEALTH ISSUES

## Vaccine-Preventable Diseases

All travelers should be up-to-date on their routine vaccinations, including seasonal influenza. In addition, vaccination against hepatitis A and hepatitis B is strongly recommended. Typhoid and Japanese encephalitis vaccines should be considered based on potential risk.

### RABIES

Government-sponsored mass vaccination campaigns for dogs and cats have reduced the prevalence of rabies in Thailand, but a small risk persists. Preexposure vaccination is recommended only for travelers whose occupation puts them at risk for exposure (such as veterinarians) or for those who will be traveling in areas where it will be difficult to get immediate access to care, including biologics (see Chapter 4, Rabies). Rabies vaccine for preexposure and postexposure prophylaxis and human rabies immune globulin are readily available in all provincial and most district hospitals throughout Thailand.

### JAPANESE ENCEPHALITIS

Outside the capital, Japanese encephalitis (JE) is endemic to many parts of Thailand (see Chapter 4, Japanese Encephalitis). Transmission occurs year-round, with seasonal epidemics occurring in the northern provinces from May through October. Although the Chiang Mai Valley reports the highest rates of human disease, several cases have occurred in travelers who visited resort or coastal areas of southern Thailand. JE vaccine

is recommended for travelers who plan to visit Thailand for ≥1 month and should be considered for those visiting for a shorter period who have an increased risk of JE virus exposure due to their itineraries or activities.

## Vectorborne Diseases

### MALARIA

Malaria is endemic to specific areas in Thailand, particularly the rural, forested areas bordering Burma (Myanmar), Cambodia, and Laos and the provinces of the far south along the border with Malaysia. Transmission is year-round, peaking during the rainy season, with a second, smaller peak in December. More than 70% of cases are due to *Plasmodium vivax*, and the rest are due to *P. falciparum* or mixed infection. CDC recommends protection against mosquito bites and antimalarial prophylaxis for travelers visiting any of the endemic areas (see Chapter 2, Mosquitoes, Ticks & Other Arthropods and Chapter 4, Malaria). Atovaquone-proguanil, tafenoquine, or doxycycline are the recommended prophylactic antimalarial drugs for travelers going to Thailand.

### DENGUE

Dengue is endemic throughout Thailand, and large epidemics occur every several years (see Chapter 4, Dengue). Peak transmission is during the rainy season, although cases are reported year-round even in non-epidemic years. Travelers to Thailand should take measures to protect themselves from mosquito bites to prevent dengue (see Chapter 2, Mosquitoes, Ticks & Other Arthropods).

### ZIKA

Zika is a risk in Thailand. Because of the risk of birth defects in infants born to women infected with Zika during pregnancy, women who are pregnant or trying to become pregnant should research the most recent recommendations at www.cdc.gov/zika.

## Foodborne Disease

Thailand's street food is convenient, inexpensive, and delicious. Unfortunately, it can also be a source of "Bangkok belly," as the lack of running water at outdoor eateries precludes good hand and food preparation hygiene. Travelers can still enjoy the experience of street food, however, by following some basic food and water safety precautions: frequent only those restaurants or food stalls that cook food to order, avoid raw or undercooked food, and drink beverages only from sealed containers (see Chapter 2, Food & Water Precautions).

Although visitors can easily access hospitals, clinics, and laboratories in most cities, carrying antibiotics for self-treatment of moderate to severe diarrhea is prudent. Fluoroquinolone resistance is widespread in Thailand and other areas of Southeast Asia; therefore, azithromycin may be preferred (see Chapter 2, Travelers' Diarrhea).

Active cholera transmission has been reported from Thailand in recent years. Check the destination page at www.cdc.gov/travel for current recommendations.

## Water and Soil Diseases

Melioidosis is highly endemic in northeast Thailand, and most leptospirosis cases can be found in the southern and northeastern regions of the country. For both diseases, most cases occur during the rainy season from July through October. Because their activities expose them to soil and water, adventure travelers may be at increased risk for these diseases. Travelers visiting endemic areas should avoid contact with soil and water and ensure that any open wounds are covered to prevent exposure. When contact cannot be avoided, travelers should wear protective clothing and footwear to reduce the risk of exposure. Travelers should immediately and thoroughly clean skin lacerations, abrasions, or burns contaminated with soil or surface water.

## OTHER HEALTH AND SAFETY RISKS

### Medical Tourism

Thailand is among the top medical tourism destinations worldwide. Travelers intending to obtain medical care abroad should plan ahead by first researching the facilities at their destination, learning about health insurance coverage, and consulting with a travel medicine specialist in advance of their trip (see Chapter 9, Medical Tourism).

## Sexually Transmitted Infections and HIV/AIDS

Thailand is a destination for tourists seeking sex (see Chapter 9, Sex & Travel) and, although illegal, commercial sex work is practiced across the country. Visitors to Thailand's red-light district should be aware that these areas have been associated with human trafficking.

A 100% condom program with sex workers has helped slow the spread of HIV and other sexually transmitted diseases; however, approximately 450,000 people were living with HIV/AIDS in Thailand in 2014. Although the number of new HIV infections is decreasing, HIV remains concentrated in key populations. In Bangkok, for example, more than 28% of men who have sex with men are infected. Travelers should be aware of these risks, always use condoms during sex, and avoid injecting drugs or sharing needles. Travelers whose practices put them at high risk for HIV infection should discuss preexposure prophylaxis with their primary care and travel medicine providers.

## SAFETY AND SECURITY

Approximately 14,000 motor vehicle deaths occur in Thailand each year, with a substantial proportion (73% in 2012) due to motorcycle crashes. A cheap and popular mode of travel, motorcycles are among the most vulnerable vehicles on the road. Travelers should avoid riding motorcycles, including motorcycle taxis. If they must ride, they should wear a helmet. Travelers should also fasten seat belts when riding in cars (see Chapter 8, Road & Traffic Safety).

Thailand has experienced political unrest throughout the country and ethno-nationalist violence in the southern provinces. In 2014, a caretaker military government was established to maintain peace, develop a constitution, and facilitate democratic elections. However, the country remains politically divided. Travelers should be aware of the possibility of demonstrations, pay attention to the local news, and monitor the US embassy website (http://bangkok.usembassy.gov) and social media outlets to find out if, when, and where protests and demonstrations may occur. It may

10

be prudent to avoid these locations, since no one can predict whether protests will stay peaceful or turn violent (see Chapter 3, Safety & Security Overseas).

## BIBLIOGRAPHY

1. Central Intelligence Agency. The World Fact Book 2018; East and Southeast Asia: Thailand. Washington, DC: CIA; 2018 [updated 2018 Sep; cited 2018 Oct 3]. Available from: www.cia.gov/library/publications/the-world-factbook/geos/th.html.

2. Finch, S. Thailand top destination for medical tourists. CMAJ. 2014 Jan 7;186(1):E1–2.

3. National AIDS Committee, Royal Thai Government. Thailand ending AIDS: Thailand AIDS response progress report 2015. Geneva: UNAIDS, 2015 Apr 2. [cited 2018 Oct 3]. Available from: www.aidsdatahub.org/thailand-global-aids-response-progress-report-2015-national-aids-committee-2015.

4. Thailand Ministry of Public Health, Bureau of General Communicable Diseases. Rabies situation in Thailand. [cited 2018 Oct 2]. Available from: http://thaigcd.ddc.moph.go.th/en/health_issues/2.

5. World Health Organization. Global status report on road safety 2015. Geneva: 2015. 2016 Apr 9. Report No. 978 92 4 156506 6. [cited 2018 Oct 3]. Available from: www.who.int/violence_injury_prevention/road_safety_status/2015/en/.

**10**

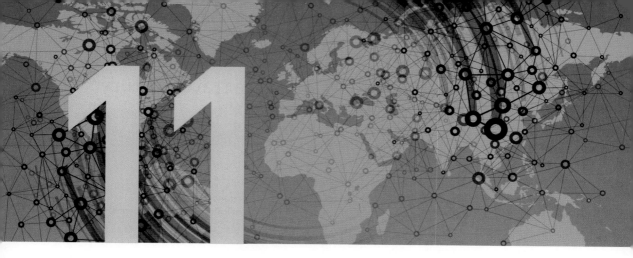

# 11

# Posttravel Evaluation

## GENERAL APPROACH TO THE RETURNED TRAVELER

Jessica K. Fairley

### THE POSTTRAVEL EVALUATION

As many as 43%–79% of travelers to low- and middle-income countries become ill with a travel-related health problem. Although most of these illnesses are mild, some travelers become sick enough to seek care from a health care provider. Most posttravel infections become apparent soon after returning from abroad, but incubation periods vary, and some syndromes can present months to years after initial infection. When evaluating a patient with a probable travel-related illness, the clinician should take a thorough medical and travel history, considering all the items summarized in Box 11-1. Salient points of the history, descriptions of common nonfebrile syndromes, and initial management steps are outlined below. The differential diagnosis and management for a traveler with fever

(or febrile syndrome) is discussed in detail in this chapter in Posttravel Evaluation: Fever.

### The Severity of Illness

As with any medical evaluation, the chief complaint and associated clinical factors are the first things to consider when approaching an ill returned traveler. Within this context, the severity of illness is not only important for patient triage but can help clinicians distinguish certain infections from one other. Is the traveler hemodynamically stable? Is the infection potentially life-threatening, such as malaria? Does the traveler have a severe respiratory syndrome or signs of hemorrhagic fever? Some suspected illnesses may also necessitate prompt involvement of public health authorities. See "Management" below for more details.

BOX 11-1. # Components of a complete travel history in an ill returned traveler

| | |
|---|---|
| Chief complaint | Main symptoms<br>Associated symptoms<br>Date of illness onset<br>Location where symptoms started (while away, in transit, or after return)<br>Health care received for this problem (such as medications or hospitalizations) while abroad and after return |
| Trip details | Countries visited<br>Itinerary in country<br>Duration of travel<br>Date of return from travel<br>Reason for travel<br>    Leisure<br>    Visiting friends and relatives<br>    Business<br>    Research/education<br>    Missionary/volunteer work<br>    Providing medical care<br>    Receiving medical care<br>Type of accommodations and sleeping arrangements<br>    Hotel (with or without air conditioning)<br>    Hostel<br>    Safari accommodations (for example, lodge, luxury tent)<br>    Camping<br>    Someone's home<br>Modes of transportation |
| Recreational activities | Safari<br>Hiking<br>Swimming<br>Ocean (scuba diving, marine life exposure)<br>Freshwater exposure (lake, river, stream)<br>Swimming pools and hot tubs<br>Rafting/boating<br>Sightseeing<br>Other adventuresome activities |
| Common exposures | Insect bites (for example, mosquito, tick, sand fly, tsetse fly)<br>Foods eaten<br>    Raw produce<br>    Undercooked meat<br>    Unpasteurized dairy products<br>    Seafood<br>Source of drinking water (for example, tap, bottled, purified, use of ice) |
| Other exposures | Sexual activity during travel (use of condoms, new partner)<br>Tattoos or piercings received while traveling<br>Animal or arthropod bites, stings, or scratches<br>Known outbreaks in the countries visited |

11

BOX 11-1.

# Components of a complete travel history in an ill returned traveler (continued)

| Use of travel precautions | Effective insect repellent (DEET 25%–40% or other EPA-registered product)<br>Bed nets<br>Adherence to malaria prophylaxis |
|---|---|
| Past medical history | Chronic medical conditions<br>    Diabetes<br>    Heart disease<br>    Autoimmune disease<br>    Immunosuppressive conditions<br>    Cancer<br>Recent illnesses or surgeries |
| Medications | Routine medications<br>Malaria prophylaxis<br>Antibiotics<br>Over-the-counter medications<br>Herbal, complementary, and alternative medicines |
| Pretravel and routine vaccinations received | Hepatitis A<br>Hepatitis B<br>Influenza<br>Japanese encephalitis<br>Meningococcal disease<br>Measles-mumps-rubella (MMR)<br>Polio<br>Rabies<br>Tetanus-diphtheria-acellular pertussis (Tdap)<br>Typhoid<br>Varicella<br>Yellow fever |
| Additional information | Smoking, alcohol, and illicit drug use<br>Recent domestic travel or prior international travel, especially within the prior 6 months<br>Family history |

11

## Travel Itinerary

The itinerary and activities in which the traveler participated are crucial to formulating a differential diagnosis, because potential exposures differ depending on the region of travel and behaviors. A febrile illness with nonspecific symptoms could be malaria, dengue, typhoid fever, or rickettsial disease, among others. Being able to exclude certain infections will avoid unnecessary testing. A 2013 study from the GeoSentinel Surveillance Network found that the frequency of certain diseases varied depending on the region of the world visited; among travelers with fevers, malaria was diagnosed most frequently among travelers returning from Africa, while dengue was diagnosed most frequently among travelers from Asia. The duration of travel is also important, since the risk of a travel-related illness increases with the length of the trip. A tropical medicine specialist can assist with the differential diagnosis and may be aware of outbreaks or the current prevalence of an infectious disease in an area. The 2014–2015 Ebola virus epidemic in West Africa highlighted the importance of epidemiologic factors and travel itineraries in managing patients and protecting staff and the community.

## Timing of Illness in Relation to Travel

Because most common travel-related infections have short incubation periods, a majority of ill travelers will seek medical attention within 1 month of return from their destination. Travelers' diarrhea, dengue, other arboviral infections, and influenza are examples of infections with shorter incubation periods (<2 weeks). Those with slightly longer incubation periods, up to 4–6 weeks, include malaria, typhoid fever, acute HIV, viral hepatitis, and leishmaniasis, among others. Occasionally, however, infections such as malaria, schistosomiasis, leishmaniasis, or tuberculosis can manifest months or even years later. In particular, malaria should be considered in the differential diagnosis of any traveler who traveled to a malaria-endemic area within a year of presentation. Therefore, a detailed history that extends beyond a few months before presentation can be helpful. The most common travel-related infections by incubation period are listed in Table 11-1.

## Underlying Medical Illness

Comorbidities can affect the susceptibility to infection, as well as the clinical manifestations and severity of illness. An increasing number of immunosuppressed people (due to organ transplants, immune-modulating medications, HIV infection, or other primary or acquired immunodeficiencies) are international travelers (see Chapter 8, Immunocompromised Travelers). In addition, a number of factors associated with travel can increase the likelihood of exacerbations of chronic conditions during or following travel such as ischemic heart disease, inflammatory bowel disease, or chronic lung disease.

## Vaccines Received and Prophylaxis Used

The history of vaccinations and malaria prophylaxis should be reviewed when evaluating an ill returned traveler. Fewer than half of US travelers to developing countries seek pretravel medical advice and may not have received vaccines or taken antimalarial drugs. Although adherence to malaria prophylaxis does not rule out the possibility of malaria, it reduces the risk and increases the likelihood of an alternative diagnosis. Fever and a rash in a traveler without measles vaccination would raise concern about measles. The most common vaccine-preventable diseases among returned travelers seeking care at a GeoSentinel clinic between 1997 and 2010 included typhoid fever, hepatitis A, hepatitis B, and influenza. More than half of these patients with vaccine-preventable diseases were hospitalized.

## Individual Exposure History

Knowledge of the patient's exposures during travel, including insect bites, contaminated food or water, or freshwater swimming, can also assist with the differential diagnosis. In addition to malarial parasites, mosquitoes transmit viruses (such as dengue, yellow fever, chikungunya, and Zika) and filarial parasites (such as *Wuchereria bancrofti*). Depending on the clinical syndrome, a history of a tick bite could suggest a diagnosis of tickborne encephalitis, African tick-bite fever, or other rickettsial infections. Tsetse flies are large, and their bites are painful and often recalled by the patient. They can carry *Trypanosoma brucei*, the protozoan that causes African sleeping sickness. Freshwater swimming or other water contact can put the patient at risk for schistosomiasis, leptospirosis, and other diseases.

Types of accommodations and activities can also influence the risk for acquiring certain diseases while abroad. Travelers who visit friends and relatives are at higher risk of malaria, typhoid fever, and certain other diseases, often because they stay longer, travel to more

11

# Table 11-1. Common travel-related infections by incubation period

| DISEASE | USUAL INCUBATION PERIOD (RANGE) | DISTRIBUTION |
|---|---|---|
| **Incubation <14 Days** | | |
| Chikungunya | 2–4 days (1–14 days) | Tropics, subtropics |
| Dengue | 4–8 days (3–14 days) | Tropics, subtropics |
| Encephalitis, arboviral (Japanese encephalitis, tickborne encephalitis, West Nile virus, other) | 3–14 days (1–20 days) | Specific agents vary by region |
| Enteric fever | 7–18 days (3–60 days) | Especially in Indian subcontinent |
| Acute HIV infection | 10–28 days (10 days to 6 weeks) | Worldwide |
| Influenza | 1–3 days | Worldwide, can also be acquired while traveling |
| Legionellosis | 5–6 days (2–10 days) | Widespread |
| Leptospirosis | 7–12 days (2–26 days) | Widespread, most common in tropical areas |
| Malaria, *Plasmodium falciparum* | 6–30 days (98% onset within 3 months of travel) | Tropics, subtropics |
| Malaria, *Plasmodium vivax* | 8 days to 12 months (almost half have onset >30 days after completion of travel) | Widespread in tropics and subtropics |
| Spotted fever rickettsiosis | Few days to 2–3 weeks | Causative species vary by region |
| Zika virus infection | 3–14 days | Widespread in Latin America, endemic through much of Africa, Southeast Asia, and Pacific Islands |
| **Incubation 14 Days to 6 Weeks** | | |
| Encephalitis, arboviral; enteric fever; acute HIV; leptospirosis; malaria | See above incubation periods for relevant diseases | See above distribution for relevant diseases |
| Amebic liver abscess | Weeks to months | Most common in resource-poor countries |
| Hepatitis A | 28–30 days (15–50 days) | Most common in resource-poor countries |
| Hepatitis E | 26–42 days (2–9 weeks) | Widespread |

(continued)

## Table 11-1. Common travel-related infections by incubation period (continued)

| DISEASE | USUAL INCUBATION PERIOD (RANGE) | DISTRIBUTION |
|---------|--------------------------------|--------------|
| Acute schistosomiasis (Katayama syndrome) | 4–8 weeks | Most common in sub-Saharan Africa |
| **Incubation >6 Weeks** | | |
| Amebic liver abscess, hepatitis E, malaria, acute schistosomiasis | See above incubation periods for relevant diseases | See above distribution for relevant diseases |
| Hepatitis B | 90 days (60–150 days) | Widespread |
| Leishmaniasis, visceral | 2–10 months (10 days to years) | Asia, Africa, Latin America, southern Europe, and the Middle East |
| Tuberculosis | Primary, weeks; reactivation, years | Global distribution, rates, and levels of resistance vary widely |

remote destinations, have more contact with local water sources, and do not seek pretravel advice (see Chapter 9, Visiting Friends & Relatives: VFR Travel). Travelers backpacking and camping in rural areas will also have a higher risk of certain diseases than those staying in luxury, air-conditioned hotels.

## COMMON SYNDROMES

The most common clinical syndromes after travel to developing countries include systemic febrile illness, diarrheal illness, and dermatologic conditions. These are described in more detail in the following sections of this chapter (Fever, Persistent Diarrhea in Returned Travelers, and Skin & Soft Tissue Infections). Fever in a traveler returning from a malaria-endemic country needs to be evaluated immediately.

Other common syndromes include respiratory illnesses, asymptomatic eosinophilia, animal bites and scratches, and anxiety- or stress-related conditions.

### Respiratory Complaints

Respiratory complaints are frequent among returned travelers and are typically associated with common respiratory viruses (see Chapter 2, Respiratory Infections). Influenza is the most common vaccine-preventable disease associated with international travel. Emerging respiratory infections such as Middle East respiratory syndrome (MERS) and H7N9 avian influenza from China should be in the differential diagnosis if the travel history is appropriate and respiratory symptoms do not have a clear alternative diagnosis. In these suspected cases, local public health authorities and CDC should be alerted immediately. See relevant sections in Chapter 4 for more information on these emerging infections, and Table 11-4 for a list of febrile respiratory illnesses among travelers.

Delayed-onset and chronic cough after travel could be tuberculosis, especially in a long-term traveler or health care worker. Helminth infections that may be associated with pulmonary symptoms include *Ascaris*, strongyloidiasis, paragonimiasis, schistosomiasis, and hookworms (*Necator* or *Ancylostoma*).

### Eosinophilia

Eosinophilia in a returning traveler suggests a possible helminth infection. Allergic diseases, hematologic disorders, and a few other viral, fungal, and protozoan infections can also cause eosinophilia. Eosinophilia can be present in some acute illnesses during pulmonary migration of parasites such as hookworm, *Ascaris*, schistosomiasis, and *Strongyloides*.

Other parasitic infections associated with eosinophilia include chronic strongyloidiasis, visceral larval migrans, lymphatic filariasis, and acute trichinellosis. These cases may be asymptomatic but could also have associated symptoms such as a rash, swelling, or other signs of the infection. For example, during an outbreak of sarcocystosis in travelers returning from Tioman Island, Malaysia, the affected travelers had eosinophilia and myalgias and were found to have eosinophilic myositis on muscle biopsy.

Last, since parasitic infections are rare in most travelers, it is still important to entertain other etiologies, since eosinophilia can be a sign of a hematologic malignancy. See Chapter 4 for more information on specific diseases.

## Animal Bites and Scratches

Travelers who report animal exposures during travel, including both bites and scratches, should be evaluated promptly for rabies exposure and provided rabies postexposure prophylaxis if indicated (see Chapter 4, Rabies). If the traveler was exposed to a macaque, herpes B virus postexposure prophylaxis may be considered (see Chapter 3, Animal Bites & Stings, and Chapter 4, B Virus).

## MANAGEMENT

**Triage:** Most posttravel illnesses can be managed on an outpatient basis, but some patients, especially those with systemic febrile illnesses, may need to be hospitalized. Furthermore, potentially severe, transmissible infections such as Ebola or MERS require enhanced infection control measures and may require higher levels of care. Severe presentations, such as acute respiratory distress, mental status change, and hemodynamic instability, require inpatient care.

Clinicians should have a low threshold for admitting febrile patients if malaria is suspected. Confirmation of diagnosis can be delayed, and complications can occur rapidly. Management in an inpatient setting is especially important for patients unlikely to follow up reliably or when no one is at home to assist if symptoms worsen quickly.

**Initial evaluation and common laboratory tests:** Although the chief complaint will direct diagnostic testing and management, common laboratory tests often help with the initial evaluation. These include a complete blood count with differential to look for leukocytosis, leukopenia, anemia, thrombocytopenia, and eosinophilia. A complete metabolic profile will identify electrolyte, renal, or liver dysfunction. Blood cultures and malaria rapid diagnostic tests may be needed depending on the presence of fever and travel itinerary. Last, depending on the differential diagnosis, serologic or PCR tests for arboviral infections, for example, as well as stool cultures and ova/parasite exams may be warranted.

**Consultation:** Consultation with an infectious diseases physician is recommended when managing severe and/or complicated travel-related infections, or when the diagnosis remains unclear. A tropical medicine or infectious disease specialist should be involved in cases that require specialized treatment, such as neurocysticercosis, severe malaria, and leishmaniasis, among others.

Public health authorities may need to be involved for transmissible, high-consequence infections. CDC provides on-call assistance with the diagnosis and management of parasitic infections at 404-718-4745 for parasitic infections other than malaria or 770-488-7788 (toll-free at 855-856-4713) for malaria, during business hours. After business hours, call the CDC Emergency Operations Center at 770-488-7100. See Chapter 1, Introduction to Travel Health & the CDC Yellow Book, for additional contact information.

BIBLIOGRAPHY

1. Angelo KM, Kozarsky PE, Ryan ET, Chen LH, Sotir MJ. What proportion of international travellers acquire a travel-related illness? A review of the literature. J Travel Med. 2017 Sep 1;24(5). doi: 10.1093/jtm/tax046.

2. Boggild AK, Castelli F, Gautret P, Torresi J, von Sonnenburg F, Barnett ED, et al. Vaccine preventable diseases in returned international travelers: results from the GeoSentinel Surveillance Network. Vaccine. 2010 Oct 28;28(46):7389–95.

3. CDC. Notes from the field: acute muscular sarcocystosis among returning travelers—Tioman Island, Malaysia, 2011. MMWR Morb Mortal Wkly Rep. 2012 Jan 20;61(2):37–8.

4. Chen LH, Wilson ME, Davis X, Loutan L, Schwartz E, Keystone J, et al. Illness in long-term travelers visiting GeoSentinel clinics. Emerg Infect Dis. 2009 Nov;15(11):1773–82.

5. Fairley JK, Kozarsky PE, Kraft CS, Guarner J, Steinberg JP, Anderson E, et al. Ebola or not? Evaluating the ill traveler from Ebola-affected countries in West Africa. Open Forum Infect Dis. 2016 Jan 18;3(1ofw005).

6. Hamer DH, Connor BA. Travel health knowledge, attitudes and practices among United States travelers. J Travel Med. 2004 Jan–Feb;11(1):23–6.

7. Hendel-Paterson B, Swanson SJ. Pediatric travelers visiting friends and relatives (VFR) abroad: illnesses, barriers and pre-travel recommendations. Travel Med Infect Dis. 2011 Jul;9(4):192–203.

8. Leder K, Torresi J, Libman MD, Cramer JP, Castelli F, Schlagenhauf P, et al. GeoSentinel surveillance of illness in returned travelers, 2007–2011. Ann Intern Med. 2013 Mar 19;158(6):456–68.

9. Ryan ET, Wilson ME, Kain KC. Illness after international travel. N Engl J Med. 2002 Aug 15;347(7):505–16.

10. Schulte C, Krebs B, Jelinek T, Nothdurft HD, von Sonnenburg F, Loscher T. Diagnostic significance of blood eosinophilia in returning travelers. Clin Infect Dis. 2002 Feb 1;34(3):407–11.

# SCREENING ASYMPTOMATIC RETURNED TRAVELERS

Michael Libman, Sapha Barkati

CDC has no official guidelines or recommendations for screening asymptomatic international travelers without other specific risk factors. (For recommendations regarding the screening of newly arrived immigrants and refugees, see Newly Arrived Immigrants & Refugees in this chapter.) Nevertheless, the screening of travelers returning from developing countries represents a substantial portion of the activity of many travel and tropical medicine clinics.

The scientific literature on the cost effectiveness of screening asymptomatic travelers is sparse. It is clear that asymptomatic travelers can harbor many infections acquired during travel, some of which have the potential to cause serious sequelae or have public health implications. In some cases, these will include pathogens rarely found in the traveler's country of origin. US medical practitioners may have little familiarity with the associated diseases, and specific diagnostic tests may not be readily available or may have poorly defined operating characteristics.

The decision to screen for particular pathogens partly will depend on the type of travel, itinerary, and exposure history. Screening short-term healthy travelers who do not report a particular exposure is often not necessary. On the other hand, special groups of travelers such as long-term travelers (expatriates, aid workers, and missionaries), travelers visiting friends and relatives, and adventure travelers may have prolonged or heavy exposure to particular pathogens, and specific tests may be considered. Clinicians should be aware that exposure history may be unreliable and may not be predictive of infection. Further, the value of a detailed itinerary can be limited by incomplete information on where pathogens are endemic. Finally, the type of travel may not provide a practical assessment of risk.

Screening traditionally has been viewed as a secondary prevention intervention, that is, an attempt to identify existing occult illnesses or health risks. The cost effectiveness of screening is dependent on the disease of interest and involves

11

several considerations. Before screening asymptomatic travelers, the physician should evaluate the potential outcomes associated with the disease and whether an early intervention may reduce morbidity or mortality.

Evaluate screening tests with respect to sensitivity and specificity, risk to the patient, and cost. The low prevalence of tropical infections in asymptomatic travelers will heavily influence the positive predictive value of the screening tests, leading to an increased likelihood of false-positive results. As a result, the asymptomatic traveler may be subjected to further investigations, generating higher costs, anxiety, and possible other harms related to diagnostic followup, and creating complex considerations when balancing risks and benefits.

Because of convenience and patient susceptibility to suggestion at the time of screening, the screening visit may offer an opportunity to promote primary prevention by discussing behavioral or other risk factors predisposing to ill health, such as exposure to contaminated food and water, arthropods, and fresh water, and behavioral risks such as drug use or high-risk sex. For many long-term travelers, visits for asymptomatic screening may also be their only hiatus from a continuing assignment abroad that allows for a general health evaluation. The usual recommendations for the periodic health exam, which may include screening for hypertension, diabetes, cardiovascular disorders, and malignancy, would apply. These visits also provide an opportunity to review vaccination status, malaria prophylaxis, and health behaviors.

## NONPARASITIC ILLNESS
### Sexually Transmitted Infections and Bloodborne Pathogens

High rates of sexual activity with new partners, including sex workers, have been documented in overseas volunteers, expatriate workers, backpackers, and military personnel. Of concern are the low rates of reported condom use. Moreover, travelers may engage in high-risk activities such as getting a tattoo or a piercing, using injection or intranasal drugs, or receiving medical or dental care. Returning travelers with acute HIV,

hepatitis B, hepatitis C, or syphilis infection pose public health risks and may be hesitant to volunteer a relevant history.

A detailed questionnaire on risk factors for sexually transmitted infections and bloodborne pathogens is recommended for all travelers, and screening according to published guidelines should always be considered. Screening for those with relevant exposures should include HIV and syphilis serologic tests as well as nucleic acid amplification testing for chlamydia and gonorrhea in urine and at sites of contact (rectum, pharynx). Hepatitis B and hepatitis C serology should be performed in travelers for whom a specific risk factor has been identified. All travelers born between 1945 and 1965 should be tested for hepatitis C if testing has not previously been done.

### Zika Virus

The prevalence of Zika virus infection in many countries has decreased dramatically since 2017, and, as a result, the likelihood of a false-positive test result has increased. Moreover, evidence of Zika virus IgM antibody persistence well beyond 12 weeks after infection makes it difficult to determine the date of infection. Screening guidelines for travelers, including pregnant women and their partners, can be found in Chapter 4 and at www.cdc.gov/zika/hc-providers/index.html.

### Tuberculosis

The incidence of tuberculosis (TB) infection related to travel is difficult to estimate. A history of work in high-prevalence settings such as in health care institutions or refugee camps merits screening. Traditionally performed using pretravel and posttravel TST, this process of screening is somewhat cumbersome, requiring as many as 4 visits (2 pretravel visits for a 2-step test and 2 posttravel visits after potential exposure) to a health care provider. This process can be simplified by using the interferon-γ release assay (IGRA), which is more expensive but also is less subject to false-positive results that can be related to previous bacillus Calmette-Guérin (BCG) vaccination. Studies assessing the use of IGRA for serial testing demonstrated a large variation in the rate of conversion and reversion. Fully investigate any positive TST or IGRA results,

11

assess for symptoms suggestive of active TB disease, and obtain a chest x-ray. For more information, see Chapter 4, *Perspectives*: Tuberculin Skin Testing of Travelers.

## PARASITIC INFECTION

Travelers are often most concerned with the possibility of an occult parasitic infection. Unfortunately, the literature shows that patient questionnaires and common laboratory testing used to screen for parasitic diseases possess poor sensitivity and specificity. Studies have shown that even an exhaustive risk factor history in asymptomatic patients is unable to reliably detect those who would or would not have evidence of parasitic infection. Physical examination is equally unrewarding.

Most commonly, a stool examination is performed, typically microscopy. Several molecular assays are commercially available; these detect a panel of viral, bacterial, and parasitic (limited to protozoal) pathogens. In some cases these panels are more sensitive than traditional testing methods, and even asymptomatic people are often found to harbor pathogens. The clinical implications of asymptomatic carriage, sometimes at a low level, are unknown for most of these agents, and the risks and benefits of treatment are not well studied.

A small number of helminthic infections, namely strongyloidiasis, schistosomiasis, and to a lesser extent filariasis, may be present in asymptomatic travelers and can be associated with significant morbidity if not screened and treated. Diagnostic methods to detect eggs and larvae directly may have poor sensitivity. Serologic tests are typically more sensitive, although some have performance limitations related to specificity and are usually preferred for screening asymptomatic travelers for these infections.

### Intestinal Protozoa

Symptomatic patients with intestinal protozoa should be treated, particularly in cases of *Entamoeba histolytica*, in which severe disease and ectopic infections such as liver abscess can develop. The finding of pathogenic protozoa in asymptomatic patients is of questionable significance (with the possible exception of *E. histolytica*, a rare finding in asymptomatic travelers).

The most common protozoa found in asymptomatic travelers is *Giardia duodenalis* and *Blastocystis* species. History of exposure to contaminated food or water has poor predictive value. There is no evidence to suggest that these asymptomatic carriers are likely to develop symptoms at a later time. Certainly, the medications used to treat pathogens may have their own adverse effects. In theory, these "carriers" (true carriers versus transient asymptomatic infection) pose a public health risk, although transmission by asymptomatic travelers appears to be rare. This is further complicated by the fact that stool microscopy for protozoa is expensive, not very sensitive, and not highly reproducible, and many laboratories have limited expertise.

*Entamoeba histolytica* cannot be distinguished from *E. dispar* by microscopy. Differentiation requires further specimen collection and testing. Studies reveal that most travelers with *Entamoeba* on microscopy are carrying *E. dispar*. Antigen testing for *E. histolytica* and *Giardia* (among others) is fairly reliable but lacks the potential to screen for all intestinal parasites with a single test, and only some antigen tests are able to differentiate *E. histolytica* from *E. dispar*.

Commercial molecular methods to screen stool specimens for multiple pathogens simultaneously typically include several protozoa, generally with better sensitivity than microscopy. These assays are also able to specifically detect the potentially pathogenic *E. histolytica* and not *E. dispar*. They also offer rapid turnaround times of several hours and, although costs remain high, these assays are increasingly being used in returned travelers with suspected protozoal disease. Some of these panels detect organisms for which pathogenicity remains controversial, such as *Blastocystis* and *Dientamoeba*. Identifying these may lead to patient anxiety and unnecessary treatment.

### Blood- and Tissue-Dwelling Protozoa

There is no justification for screening most asymptomatic travelers for malaria, whether by blood film, serologic tests, or molecular methods. No available tests can detect the latent hepatic forms (hypnozoites) of *Plasmodium vivax* or *P. ovale*. Travelers should be reminded to seek evaluation for unexplained fever and notify practitioners of any recent travel. Immigrants with frequent and regular exposure to malaria may gradually develop partial immunity. This may result in low-level parasitemia with few or no symptoms. They may later recrudesce with more severe illness. This phenomenon is rare in non-immigrant travelers. It should be noted that, in rare cases, travelers who have been compliant with prophylaxis may still acquire malaria and often these people will present with low parasitemia infections.

Occult trypanosomiasis in asymptomatic travelers (as opposed to immigrants) appears to be extremely rare. Screening tests, such as serology and molecular diagnostics, are of unknown value. For travelers to endemic areas of Latin America, testing for *Trypanosoma cruzi* might be considered in cases of prolonged residence in primitive housing, such as mud walls and thatched roofs, especially if reduviid bugs have been seen; in recipients of blood products; or in travelers with a convincing history of acute Chagas disease. East African trypanosomiasis has affected travelers but typically causes acute symptoms. West African trypanosomiasis is generally not reported in travelers. Refer patients suspected of having these infections (in the setting of clinical, biological, or radiologic abnormalities) to an infectious disease specialist.

## Helminths

Travelers are often concerned about "worms," by which they mean intestinal helminths. However, infections of travelers with large numbers of the common nematodes, such as *Ascaris, Trichuris,* or hookworm, are rare. Questioning returning expatriates infected with intestinal helminths has disclosed no attributable symptoms compared with uninfected controls. The life cycles of almost all helminths preclude any real risk of ongoing transmission from asymptomatic hosts in developed countries. Helminths generally have a natural lifespan of months to a few years, which ensures eventual spontaneous clearance. In addition, low-intensity infections are of limited clinical importance, though in rare cases aberrant migration of *Ascaris* spp. can result in clinical disease. The exception to this is *Strongyloides stercoralis.*

For *Strongyloides* infections, serious complications are well known, nonspecific symptoms may easily be overlooked, duration of carriage after infection is unlimited due to its autoinfection cycle, and the original burden of infection is irrelevant. Specific types of immune suppression, such as corticosteroid therapy, hematologic malignancy, hematopoietic stem cell transplant, solid organ transplant, and human T-lymphotropic virus type 1 infection, are the most important risk factors for a potentially lethal hyperinfection syndrome or disseminated strongyloidiasis. Unfortunately, diagnosis by stool examination is notoriously insensitive, and serologic methods are often required, as discussed below. Molecular detection of helminths is significantly more sensitive and specific compared with microscopy. However, molecular techniques are not widely available outside the reference laboratory and research setting.

Among the helminths capable of eventually causing illness in asymptomatic travelers, most emphasis in the literature has been given to *S. stercoralis* and the parasites that cause schistosomiasis and filariasis. There is no evidence that the low-burden schistosomal infections typically found in travelers are likely to lead to the types of complications commonly found in endemic areas, such as liver fibrosis or malignancy. Nevertheless, this possibility cannot be entirely ruled out, particularly in those who may have more intense exposures. Even brief exposures to freshwater lakes and rivers in known endemic areas in Africa are associated with substantial seroconversion rates. In addition, complications due to ectopic egg migration can occur in light infections and without warning.

On the other hand, reports of travelers with late complications from asymptomatic filarial infections are virtually nonexistent. Traditional tests for the parasites that cause these infections, including stool examination for *S. stercoralis* and *Schistosoma* spp., urine for *S. haematobium,* and blood or skin snips for microfilaria, all lack sensitivity, particularly in low-burden infection. For this reason, serologic testing has been advocated as the best screening tool. The problems with serologic screening include expense, lack of easy availability, and lack of standardization.

11

Serologic tests are often designed to maximize sensitivity, typically at the expense of specificity. Unfortunately, specificity is almost impossible to define. Seropositivity in the absence of direct pathogen detection is common, and its clinical significance can be difficult to determine.

Fortunately for patients with strongyloidiasis or schistosomiasis, treatment is cheap, easy, and effective. The common antihelminthic agents, such as ivermectin, albendazole, and praziquantel used for a short-course therapy, have excellent safety profiles. Clinicians should be aware of rare but severe adverse events that can occur when using common antihelminthics in patients who have occult, unsuspected coinfection with other parasites: ivermectin and *Loa loa* (can cause encephalopathy) or albendazole and *Taenia solium* (can cause seizures, increased intracranial pressure with focal signs, and retinal damage).

While it is not clear who should be screened for helminthic infections, it is logical to at least perform serologic tests on travelers with a high duration and risk of exposure and to treat all those found to be positive. Since asymptomatic filarial infections appear least likely to have sequelae, and treatment is often neither very effective nor easy, the threshold for filarial serology (and antigen testing in the case of *Wuchereria bancrofti*) should be higher. Serology usually only becomes positive after adult forms have matured, which means waiting for 3 months or so after exposure. Serology for these pathogens is available at the parasitic diseases laboratory at CDC (www.dpd. cdc.gov/dpdx; 404-718-4745; parasites@cdc.gov). Serology for filarial infection is available as well through the NIH laboratory (301-496-5398).

Other helminth parasitic infections rarely seen in returning travelers include neurocysticercosis, fascioliasis, paragonimiasis, and others. Screening asymptomatic travelers for these infections is generally not appropriate. Primary care providers should refer patients suspected of having these infections (in the setting of clinical, biological, or radiologic abnormalities) to an infectious diseases specialist.

## Eosinophilia

Screening for eosinophilia is a common test, since it is quick, universally available, and theoretically of value in detecting invasive helminths, if not protozoa. However, multiple studies have shown tests for eosinophilia to have poor sensitivity. Specificity can be high; however, the low prevalence of infection in asymptomatic travelers means positive predictive value is low. In addition, the finding of eosinophilia may lead to an extensive and often fruitless search for a cause, generating patient anxiety and high costs. Many cases of eosinophilia resolve spontaneously, possibly because of infection with nonpathogenic organisms or a noninfectious cause, such as allergy or drug reaction. Eosinophil counts may be repeated after several weeks or months before embarking on an extensive investigation. Counts may be highly variable, even within a single day, and are suppressed by endogenous or exogenous steroids. Evaluation of absolute counts, rather than by percentage of leukocytes, is more reproducible and predictive.

## GENERAL GUIDELINES

The following sections and Table 11-2 may serve as a general guideline for screening asymptomatic returned travelers.

### Short-Term Travelers (<3–6 months)

In this group of travelers, the yield of screening is low and should be directed by specific risk factors revealed in the history. A history of prolonged (>2 weeks) digestive symptoms during travel can suggest protozoal infection. Exposure to fresh water in a region endemic for schistosomiasis, especially in Africa, may merit serologic screening, with the addition of stool and urine examination in the case of high-intensity exposure. Serology for *Strongyloides* may be considered in those who have a high risk of skin exposure to soil likely to be contaminated with human feces, usually those with a history of frequently walking barefoot outdoors. A sexual history should be obtained, and screening for sexually transmitted and bloodborne infections may be warranted. Zika virus testing for asymptomatic travelers (including pregnant women) with potential exposure is generally not recommended unless there is ongoing Zika virus exposure (see Chapter 4, Zika).

# Table 11-2. Considerations for screening asymptomatic travelers

| RISK FACTOR OR EXPOSURE | SUGGESTED SCREENING TESTS |
|---|---|
| Short stay (<3–6 months), no identified risk factor/exposure | None |
| Long-stay (>3–6 months), poor sanitation or hygiene | CBC with eosinophil count, liver transaminases, creatinine, CRP; consider stool ova and parasite |
| Sexual contact | HIV, syphilis, chlamydia, gonorrhea; HBV for men who have sex with men or sex with unknown partners; HCV screening if risk factors present or born between 1945–1965 |
| Tattoo, piercing, injection or intranasal drug use, medical/dental care | HIV; HBV for injection drug use; HCV for injection or intranasal drug use or unregulated tattoos |
| Pregnant woman who traveled in Zika virus–endemic area or had sex with a partner who traveled in these areas | Screening asymptomatic female travelers with potential exposure (but without ongoing risk) is generally not recommended |
| Health care worker | TB screening (TST or IGRA) |
| Prolonged residence (>6 months) with population in a highly TB-endemic area | TB screening (TST or IGRA) |
| Walking barefoot on soil potentially contaminated with human feces or sewage | *Strongyloides* serology |
| Exposure to freshwater rivers, lakes, or irrigation canals | *Schistosoma* serology |

Abbreviations: CBC, complete blood count; CRP, C-reactive protein; HBV, hepatitis B virus; HCV, hepatitis C virus; TB, tuberculosis; TST, tuberculin skin test; IGRA, interferon-γ release assay.

Work in a health care setting or other area at high risk for TB may merit screening.

## Long-Term Travelers or Expatriates (>3–6 months)

For longer-stay travelers, as the overall yield of screening increases it becomes less useful to rely on history for selective testing. The emphasis should be on those with the longest stays and the most problematic sanitary conditions. In some cases employers may require certain tests, partly for reasons of liability. Stool examinations are usually done, although they serve mostly to provide psychological reassurance. Perform serologic testing for schistosomiasis and strongyloidiasis in those with recent or remote travel histories to endemic areas who report some level of risk.

A complete blood count with white blood cell differential, including eosinophil counts, liver transaminases, creatinine, and C-reactive protein are usually the basic set of tests performed. Interpret results cautiously as abnormalities may trigger further testing. Zika virus testing for asymptomatic travelers (including pregnant women) with potential exposure is generally not recommended unless there is ongoing exposure to Zika virus. TST or IGRA tests should be limited to those who have worked in a health care or similar setting or who have had intimate and prolonged contact with residents of a highly endemic area for ≥6 months. Any other screening should be guided by exceptional exposures or knowledge about local outbreaks.

## BIBLIOGRAPHY

1. Baaten GG, Sonder GJ, van Gool T, Kint JA, van den Hoek A. Travel-related schistosomiasis, strongyloidiasis, filariasis, and toxocariasis: the risk of infection and the diagnostic relevance of blood eosinophilia. BMC Infect Dis. 2011 Apr 5;11:84.

2. CDC. Zika Virus for health care providers. Available from: www.cdc.gov/zika/hc-providers.

3. MacLean JD, Libman M. Screening returning travelers. Infect Dis Clin North Am. 1998 Jun;12(2):431–43.

4. Smith BD, Morgan RL, Beckett GA, Falck-Ytter Y, et al. Recommendations for the identification of chronic hepatitis C virus infection among persons born during 1945–1965. MMWR Recomm Rep. 2012;61(RR04);1–18.

5. Soonawala D, van Lieshout L, den Boer MA, Claas EC, Verweij JJ, Godkewitsch A, et al. Post-travel screening of asymptomatic long-term travelers to the tropics for intestinal parasites using molecular diagnostics. Am J Trop Med Hyg. 2014 May;90(5):835–9.

6. US Preventive Services Task Force. Final Recommendation Statement. Hepatitis C: Screening. Available from: www.uspreventiveservicestaskforce.org/Page/Document/RecommendationStatementFinal/hepatitis-c-screening.

7. Weinbaum CM, Williams I, Mast EE, Wang SA, et al. Recommendations for identification and public health management of persons with chronic hepatitis B virus infection. MMWR Recomm Rep. 2008;57(RR08):1–20.

8. Yansouni CP, Merckx J, Libman MD, Ndao M. Recent advances in clinical parasitology diagnostics. Curr Infect Dis Rep 2014 Nov;16(11):434.

# FEVER

Mary Elizabeth Wilson

## INITIAL FOCUS

Fever commonly accompanies serious illness in returned travelers, and the most common life-threatening tropical disease associated with fever in returned travelers is malaria. Because an increased temperature can signal a rapidly progressive infection, clinicians must initiate early evaluation, especially in people who have visited areas with malaria in recent months (see Chapter 4, Malaria). The initial focus in evaluating a febrile returned traveler should be on identifying infections that are potentially life-threatening, treatable, or transmissible. In some instances, public health officials must be alerted if the traveler was possibly contagious while traveling or infected with a pathogen of public health importance (such as yellow fever or Ebola viruses) at the origin or destination. During an outbreak such as the Ebola epidemic in West Africa, special screening protocols may be needed. It is important to know that a specific cause for fever may not be identified in approximately 25% or more of returned travelers.

## USE OF HISTORY, LOCATION OF EXPOSURE, AND INCUBATION TO LIMIT DIFFERENTIAL DIAGNOSIS

A large proportion of illnesses in returned travelers are caused by common, cosmopolitan infections (such as diarrhea, pneumonia, or pyelonephritis), so these must be considered along with unusual infections. Because the geographic area of travel determines the relative likelihood of major causes of fever, it is essential to identify where the febrile patient has traveled and lived (Table 11-3). Details about activities (such as freshwater exposure in schistosomiasis-endemic areas, animal bites, sexual activities, tattoos, or local medical care with injections) and accommodations (bed nets, window screens, air conditioning, type of dwelling) during travel may provide useful clues. Preparation before travel (for example, vaccinations and malaria prophylaxis) will markedly reduce the likelihood of some infections, so this is also a relevant part of the history.

**11**

## Table 11-3. Common causes of fever in the tropics, by geographic area

| GEOGRAPHIC AREA | COMMON TROPICAL DISEASE CAUSING FEVER | OTHER INFECTIONS CAUSING OUTBREAKS OR CLUSTERS IN TRAVELERS |
|---|---|---|
| Caribbean | Chikungunya, dengue, malaria (Hispaniola), Zika | Acute histoplasmosis, leptospirosis |
| Central America | Chikungunya, dengue, malaria (primarily *Plasmodium vivax*), Zika, enteric fever | Leptospirosis, histoplasmosis, coccidioidomycosis, leishmaniasis |
| South America | Chikungunya, dengue, malaria (primarily *P. vivax*), Zika | Bartonellosis, leptospirosis, enteric fever, histoplasmosis |
| South-central Asia | Dengue, enteric fever, malaria (primarily non-falciparum) | Chikungunya, scrub typhus |
| Southeast Asia | Dengue, malaria (primarily non-falciparum) | Chikungunya, leptospirosis |
| Sub-Saharan Africa | Malaria (primarily *P. falciparum*), tickborne rickettsiae (main cause of fever in southern Africa), acute schistosomiasis (Katayama fever), dengue | African trypanosomiasis, chikungunya enteric fever, meningococcal meningitis |

Because each infection has a characteristic incubation period (although the range is extremely wide with some infections), the time of exposure needs to be defined in different geographic areas. This knowledge will allow the clinician to exclude some infections from the differential diagnosis. Most serious febrile infections manifest within the first month after return from tropical travel, yet infections related to travel exposures can occasionally occur months or even >1 year after return. In the United States, >90% of reported cases of *Plasmodium falciparum* malaria manifest within 30 days of return, but almost half of cases of *P. vivax* malaria manifest >30 days after return.

## FINDINGS REQUIRING URGENT ATTENTION

Presence of fever plus certain associated signs, symptoms, or laboratory findings can suggest specific infections (Table 11-4). Findings that should prompt urgent attention include hemorrhage, low blood pressure, altered consciousness, and high respiratory rate. Even if an initial physical examination is unremarkable, it should be repeated if diagnosis is not clear, as new findings may appear that will help in the diagnostic process (such as skin lesions or a tender liver). Although most febrile illnesses in returned travelers are related to infections, the clinician should bear in mind that other problems, including pulmonary emboli and drug hypersensitivity reactions, can also be associated with fever.

Fever accompanied by any of the following syndromes deserves further scrutiny, because it may indicate a disease of public health importance, where immediate infection control and containment measures are indicated:

- Skin rash with or without conjunctivitis (for example, measles, meningococcemia, hemorrhagic fevers such as Ebola)

## Table 11-4. Clinical findings and select associated infectious diseases

| CLINICAL FINDINGS | INFECTIONS TO CONSIDER AFTER TROPICAL TRAVEL |
| --- | --- |
| Fever and rash | Dengue, chikungunya, Zika, measles, spotted fever or typhus group rickettsioses, enteric fever (skin lesions may be sparse or absent), meningococcemia, acute HIV infection, varicella |
| Fever and abdominal pain | Enteric fever, amebic or pyogenic liver abscess |
| Fever and normal or low white blood cell count | Dengue, malaria, rickettsial infection, enteric fever, chikungunya, Zika, acute HIV |
| Fever and hemorrhage | Viral hemorrhagic fevers (for example, dengue, yellow fever, Ebola, Lassa fever), meningococcemia, leptospirosis, spotted fever group rickettsial infections |
| Fever and arthralgia or myalgia (sometimes persistent) | Chikungunya, dengue, Zika, Ross River virus, muscular sarcocystosis, trichinellosis |
| Fever and eosinophilia | Acute schistosomiasis, drug hypersensitivity reaction; fascioliasis, sarcocystosis, trichinellosis, angiostrongyliasis, and other parasitic infections (rare) |
| Fever and respiratory symptoms/pulmonary infiltrates | Influenza and other common bacterial and viral pathogens, legionellosis, tuberculosis, acute schistosomiasis, Q fever, leptospirosis, Middle East respiratory syndrome, acute histoplasmosis or coccidioidomycosis, psittacosis, melioidosis, pneumonic plague |
| Fever and altered mental status/central nervous system involvement | Cerebral malaria, arboviral encephalitides (for example, Japanese encephalitis, West Nile virus), meningococcal meningitis, rabies, African trypanosomiasis, scrub typhus, angiostrongyliasis, tickborne encephalitis, rabies |
| Fever and jaundice | Acute viral hepatitis (A, B, C, E), yellow fever and other viral hemorrhagic fevers, severe malaria, leptospirosis |
| Mononucleosis syndrome | Epstein-Barr virus infection, cytomegalovirus infection, toxoplasmosis, acute HIV infection |
| Fever persisting >2 weeks | Malaria, enteric fever, Epstein-Barr virus infection, cytomegalovirus infection, toxoplasmosis, acute HIV infection, acute schistosomiasis, brucellosis, tuberculosis, Q fever, visceral leishmaniasis (rare) |
| Fever with onset >6 weeks after travel | *Plasmodium vivax* or *ovale* malaria, acute hepatitis (B, C, or E), tuberculosis, amebic liver abscess, melioidosis, African trypanosomiasis |

- Rapid respiratory rate (for example, influenza, Middle East respiratory syndrome [MERS], pneumonic plague)

- Persistent cough (for example, tuberculosis, pertussis)

- Decreased consciousness (for example, meningococcal meningitis, rabies)

- Bruising or unusual bleeding without previous injury (for example, hemorrhagic fevers)

- Persistent voluminous diarrhea (for example, cholera)

- Persistent vomiting other than air or motion sickness (for example, norovirus infection)

11

- Jaundice (for example, hepatitis A)
- Flaccid paralysis of recent onset (for example, polio)

Travelers visiting friends and relatives (VFRs) often do not seek pretravel medical advice and are at higher risk for some diseases than other travelers. A review of GeoSentinel Surveillance Network data showed that a larger proportion of VFRs than tourist travelers presented with serious (requiring hospitalization), potentially preventable travel-related illnesses (see Chapter 9, Visiting Friends & Relatives: VFR Travel).

## CHANGE OVER TIME

Clinicians have access to resources on the Internet that provide information about geographic-specific risks, disease activity, and other useful information, such as drug-susceptibility patterns for pathogens. Infectious disease outbreaks are dynamic, as demonstrated by the Ebola epidemic in West Africa in 2014–2015, introduction and spread of chikungunya virus in the Americas beginning in late 2013, nosocomial spread from travel-associated MERS in Korea in 2015, and the rapid spread of Zika virus in the Americas in 2015 and 2016. In contrast, because of the wide use of vaccine, hepatitis A infection is now infrequently seen in US travelers.

Infections with typical seasonal transmission in the United States may occur at different times of the year (or throughout the year) in the tropics and subtropics. For example, influenza transmission can occur throughout the year in tropical areas, and the peak season in the Southern Hemisphere is April to September; clinicians in the Northern Hemisphere must be alert to the possibility of influenza outside the usual "winter" influenza season.

Travelers may acquire infections caused by bacteria resistant to commonly used antibiotics (see Antimicrobial Resistance in this chapter). Bacteria that produce extended-spectrum β-lactamases and carbapenem-resistant Enterobacteriaceae, including bacteria expressing the metalloprotease NDM-1, have been found in infections acquired during travel, most often related to medical care (both elective and emergency). Travelers to South and Southeast Asia are at high risk of acquiring multidrug-resistant Enterobacteriaceae. Enteric fever (typhoid or paratyphoid fever), has become increasingly resistant to fluoroquinolones and third-generation cephalosporins and azithromycin in some regions (see Chapter 4, Typhoid & Paratyphoid Fever).

## KEEP IN MIND
- Malaria is the most common cause of acute undifferentiated fever after travel to sub-Saharan Africa and some other tropical areas.

- Malaria, especially *P. falciparum*, can progress rapidly. Diagnostics should be done promptly and treatment instituted immediately if malaria is diagnosed (see Chapter 4, Malaria).

- A history of taking malaria prophylaxis does not exclude the possibility of malaria.

- Patients with malaria may be afebrile at the time of evaluation but typically give a history of fever or chills. They can have prominent respiratory (including acute respiratory distress syndrome), gastrointestinal, or central nervous system findings.

- Dengue is the most common cause of febrile illness among people who seek medical care after travel to Latin America or Asia.

- Other arboviral infections are emerging as causes of fever in travelers, including chikungunya and Zika viruses.

- Fever in returned travelers is often caused by common infections, such as diarrhea, pneumonia, and pyelonephritis, which should not be overlooked in the search for exotic diagnoses.

- The possibility that travelers may be infected or colonized with drug-resistant pathogens should be considered, especially among those who have been hospitalized abroad.

- Viral hemorrhagic fevers other than dengue ( for example, Ebola, Lassa fever, Marburg hemorrhagic fever) are important to identify but are rare in travelers; bacterial infections, such as leptospirosis, meningococcemia, and rickettsial infections, can also cause fever and hemorrhage and should always be considered because of the need to institute prompt, specific treatment.

- Sexually transmitted infections, including acute HIV, can cause acute febrile infections.

- Consider infection control, public health implications, and requirements for reportable diseases.

## BIBLIOGRAPHY

1. Bottieau E, Clerinx J, Schrooten W, Van den Enden E, Wouters R, Van Esbroeck M, et al. Etiology and outcome of fever after a stay in the tropics. Arch Intern Med. 2006 Aug 14-28;166(15):1642–8.

2. Date KA, Newton AE Medalla F, Blackstock A, Richardson L, McCullough A, et al. Changing patterns in enteric fever incidence and increasing antibiotic resistance of enteric fever isolates in the United States, 2008–2012. Clin Infect Dis. 2016;63(3):322–9.

3. Jensenius M, Han PV, Schlagenhauf P, et al. Acute and potentially life-threatening tropical diseases in western travelers—a GeoSentinel multicenter study, 1996–2011. Am J Trop Med Hyg. 2013;88:397–404.

4. Kantele A, Laaveri T, Mero S, et al. Antimicrobials increase travelers' risk of colonization by extended-spectrum beta-lactamase-producing Enterobacteriaceae. Clin Infect Dis. 2015;60:837–46.

5. Leder K, Torresi J, Libman MD, Cramer JP, Castelli F, Schlagenhauf P, et al. GeoSentinel surveillance of illness in returned travelers, 2007–2011. Ann Intern Med. 2013 Mar 19;158(6):456–68.

6. Mendelson M, Han PV, Vincent P, von Sonnenburg F, Cramer JP, Loutan L, et al. Regional variation in travel-related illness acquired in Africa, March 1997–May 2011. Emerg Infect Dis. 2014 Apr;20(4):532–41.

7. Ryan ET, Wilson ME, Kain KC. Illness after international travel. N Engl J Med. 2002 Aug 15;347(7):505–16.

8. Thwaites GE, Day PJ. Approach to fever in the returning traveler. N Engl J Med. 2017;376:548–60.

9. Wilson ME, Weld LH, Boggild A, Keystone JS, Kain KC, von Sonnenburg F, et al. Fever in returned travelers: results from the GeoSentinel Surveillance Network. Clin Infect Dis. 2007 Jun 15;44(12):1560–8.

# RAPID DIAGNOSTIC TESTS FOR INFECTIOUS DISEASES

Elizabeth Rabold, Jesse Waggoner

**11**

In the context of infectious diseases, the term rapid diagnostic test (RDT) most commonly refers to lateral-flow, immunochromatographic tests used to detect certain infections. More generally, such assays may be described as point-of-care (POC) tests. Although there are no accepted criteria for what constitutes an RDT or POC test, published definitions frequently focus on performance time and simplicity. Pathogen-specific or syndrome-based tests are considered RDTs if they meet either or both of the following criteria:

- The test can be incorporated into a POC testing protocol for a given infection or clinical syndrome. Such assays have relatively short performance times, yield results that will affect clinical decision making, and allow management decisions to be made during the same encounter.

- The test can be performed under a certificate of waiver under the Clinical Laboratory Improvement Amendments of 1988, so-called "waived" tests (Table 11-5).

Certain tests that meet this definition may not be used in a manner compatible with POC testing. For instance, an increasing number of waived, sample-to-answer molecular diagnostics (nucleic acid amplification tests, such as PCR or RT-PCR) are becoming available. At a given

## Table 11-5. Selected rapid diagnostic tests for pathogens in the returning traveler

| SYNDROME | PATHOGEN | SPECIMEN | ADDITIONAL INFORMATION |
|---|---|---|---|
| **Lateral-flow immunochromatographic tests and small panels** | | | |
| **Systemic febrile illness** | Ebola virus[1] | Whole blood | Received emergency use authorization by FDA and WHO. May not be appropriate for excluding illness in early infection. |
| | Dengue virus[1] | Serum | Not FDA-cleared. Highly variable diagnostic performance. Antibodies may cross-react with other flaviviruses. |
| | Malaria[1] | Whole blood | Best performance characteristics for *Plasmodium falciparum* infections. Many versions may be available in endemic areas. |
| **Gastrointestinal infections** | Norovirus, rotavirus, adenovirus[1] | Stool sample | Available in the United States individually or in combination. Adenovirus rapid tests are approved for ocular specimens. |
| **Respiratory infections** | Group A *Streptococcus* | Throat swab | Rapid antigen and molecular tests[2] available; both are specific but molecular tests have improved sensitivity. |
| | Influenza | NP or throat swab | Rapid test sensitivity 50%–70%; negative testing should not direct treatment. |
| | *Legionella pneumophila*[1] | Urine | Only detects serogroup 1. Recommended by IDSA for patients with more severe disease. |
| | Respiratory syncytial virus | NP or throat swab | Accurate antigen assays, recommended if results will affect management. |
| | *Streptococcus pneumoniae* | Urine | Recommended by IDSA for use in certain patient populations. |
| **Sexually transmitted infections** | *Chlamydia trachomatis* and *Neisseria gonorrhea*[1] | Urine, vaginal swab | Molecular tests remain gold standard; a sample-to-answer molecular assay is available.[1,2] |
| | HIV | Whole blood, oral fluids | Antibody and antibody/antigen kits available. Molecular testing preferred for acute infection. |
| | *Treponema pallidum* | Whole blood | Antibody detection, may not be appropriate for acute infections. |
| | *Trichomonas vaginalis* | Vaginal swab | Rapid antigen testing is specific with sensitivity approximately 90%. |
| | BV pathogens | Vaginal swab | Identifies increased sialidase activity, an enzyme associated with BV pathogens. |

(continued)

## Table 11-5. Selected rapid diagnostic tests for pathogens in the returning traveler (continued)

| SYNDROME | PATHOGEN | SPECIMEN | ADDITIONAL INFORMATION |
|---|---|---|---|
| **Multiplex molecular panels** | | | |
| **Gastrointestinal pathogens** | Includes common viruses, bacteria, and parasites[1,2] | Stool sample | Sensitive, certain positive results may be unrelated to active infection. |
| **Respiratory pathogens** | Includes common viruses and atypical bacteria[2] | NP swab | Pathogens may have prolonged shedding time; positive results may not rule out infection from other pathogens. |

Abbreviations: BV, bacterial vaginosis; FDA, US Food and Drug Administration; IDSA, Infectious Disease Society of America; NP, nasopharyngeal; WHO, World Health Organization.
[1] Not waived by Clinical Laboratory Improvement Amendments.
[2] Not immunochromatographic assay.

institution, though, such assays might only be performed in a central laboratory at specific times, thereby limiting their utility in a POC testing protocol. These assays typically require dedicated, bench-top equipment for performance. As such, adding capacity at individual clinical sites may not be feasible.

Assays that characterize a host response (such as C-reactive protein and procalcitonin) show promise in limiting unnecessary antibiotic use in certain clinical settings. However, their use and interpretation are complicated and can be confusing in the setting of returning travelers with potentially severe, nonbacterial tropical infectious diseases such as malaria and dengue.

## RAPID DIAGNOSTIC TESTING FOR CLINICAL SYNDROMES

Respiratory infections are among the most common travel-related diseases. Individual and multiplex tests using nasopharyngeal swab samples are widely available for influenza A, influenza B, and respiratory syncytial virus. The sensitivity of rapid antigen tests for influenza is notably poor; negative results should not dictate therapy decisions and should be confirmed with molecular testing. Influenza subtyping is primarily used for public health surveillance and is not commonly available with rapid testing. Subtyping does not affect clinical decision making; however, this may change if certain strains or subtypes become markers for resistance to antiviral medications.

Platforms for multiplex molecular testing are available that identify up to 11 respiratory viruses and 3 atypical bacteria (Table 11-5). These tests are often sensitive and can test for a large number of pathogens in a single sample. However, such multiplex panels are expensive, and results must be interpreted in light of prolonged shedding periods for certain pathogens, the possibility of multiple positive results or coinfections, and variable accuracy for different agents on the panel (such as adenovirus). In addition, currently available waived multiplex assays do not test for common bacterial causes of pneumonia or specific pathogens that may be included in the differential diagnosis for a returning traveler with a respiratory illness (such as Middle East respiratory syndrome coronavirus). Clinicians may prefer to order tests in a tiered approach to limit unnecessary results.

Although many travelers will develop gastrointestinal infections, patients may not present to travel clinics for short illnesses, or they may initiate treatment themselves with antibiotics provided to treat travelers' diarrhea. Rapid tests for rotavirus and norovirus have received US Food and Drug Administration (FDA) clearance, but not all assays received waived status. These are less sensitive than molecular tests, and for norovirus, rapid antigen testing has only been cleared for use in outbreaks. Multiplex molecular panels, which identify many common viral, bacterial, and parasitic diarrheal pathogens, are available (Table 11-5). These have the same limitations as the multiplex molecular panels described for respiratory pathogens, including the common detection of coinfections.

The undifferentiated acute febrile illness presents a diagnostic challenge in returning travelers, requiring prompt evaluation, diagnosis, and management. RDTs alone may not be sufficient in many settings. A commercial RDT for malaria is cleared for use in US hospitals and laboratories but not for individual clinics. Microscopy is still recommended in positive cases to identify the species and calculate parasitemia. Furthermore, patients with malaria can be coinfected with other pathogens contributing to and complicating their diagnosis and management. Rapid tests are not available in the United States for other common or widespread causes of an undifferentiated acute febrile illness in travelers, such as dengue or leptospirosis.

Sexually transmitted infections (STIs) may be acquired locally or abroad. Rapid HIV tests that use blood and cheek swab samples are widely available. These predominantly detect anti-HIV antibodies and perform well for patients with chronic infections, although not those with newly acquired HIV. Antigen/antibody combination tests are available that detect p24 antigen and anti-HIV antibodies. These remain less sensitive than molecular testing to detect acute HIV infection, and in high-risk patients, molecular testing or repeat testing is warranted. Rapid tests for syphilis, trichomonas, and vaginal bacterial infections are available and can help identify other common STIs (Table 11-5).

## DIAGNOSTIC TESTING PERFORMED DURING TRAVEL

People who become ill while traveling may seek medical care abroad; the development and availability of RDTs for tropical infectious diseases has expanded greatly in recent years. RDTs, in this context, are typically lateral-flow immunochromatographic tests that detect antigen from or antibodies to certain pathogens. Patients may, therefore, return home having received a diagnosis based on results from these tests. As only one such test has been cleared for use in the United States (for malaria), the diagnostic characteristics of these tests are unknown to most providers. Additionally, many different RDTs may be available for certain pathogens (such as dengue), with widely varying or poorly studied performance parameters. Institutions may not have continuous access to a single brand of test; as such, results even within a laboratory can be difficult to interpret.

Following are several common infections for which RDT or POC diagnostics may be available. This is intended to be an illustrative list but by no means exhaustive.

- **Malaria.** An FDA-cleared RDT for malaria is available, and malaria RDTs are in wide use throughout the endemic world. In general, these perform best in patients with malaria caused by *Plasmodium falciparum*, with variable or poor performance for other species.

- **Dengue.** Rapid, lateral-flow assays exist to detect the nonstructural protein 1 (NS1) antigen and anti-dengue IgM and IgG. Tests have widely variable performance, depending on the manufacturer, circulating dengue types in a region, a patient's past medical history, and duration of symptoms before presentation.

- **Emerging infections.** These pathogens represent a significant diagnostic challenge. Rapid assays became available after outbreaks of Ebola, chikungunya, and Zika viruses. However, such assays may not be available or well studied at the peak of an outbreak.

- **Visceral leishmaniasis.** Assays to detect antibodies against the rK39 antigen have demonstrated good performance characteristics in endemic regions.

- **Typhoid.** Rapid serologic tests have demonstrated only moderate accuracy to diagnose typhoid. Additionally, these are designed to detect *Salmonella enterica* serotype Typhi only.

- **Leptospirosis.** Serologic assays have been developed. Their use generally is limited by the large number of pathogenic and intermediate serotypes that result in human disease worldwide.

**11**

## SPECIAL CONSIDERATIONS

### Limitations

- Rapid diagnostic tests may require confirmatory or supplementary testing with more complex laboratory techniques.

- Tests are designed for specific targets and may not perform well in the setting of emerging pathogens or strains (such as rapid influenza diagnostics for avian influenza or malaria RDTs for *Plasmodium knowlesi*).

- Use of these tests does not provide biological material for additional studies, such as confirmatory testing, laboratory research and development, or strain characterization.

- Multiplex molecular panels may provide test results not requested by the clinician. How to interpret and make intelligent clinical use of such results needs to be clarified.

### Waived Tests

This designation is specific to the United States. Tests conducted under a certificate of waiver must be simple to perform with a low risk for yielding an incorrect result. Although mandated personnel requirements for waived tests are minimal, testers must be trained and have documented proficiency in assay performance. Additional considerations include the following:

- Waived tests can be performed only on unmodified specimens (saliva, urine, whole blood). Certain tests can be performed as both waived and moderate- or high-complexity tests, depending on the specimen type and protocol.

- Waived tests must be performed according to the most recent manufacturer recommendations. Deviation from the protocol defaults the test to a high-complexity test.

- Test volume and staffing should be considered. Reagents may have specific storage requirements and a relatively short shelf life, which can affect cost effectiveness.

- These tests require oversight and quality assessments to ensure performance.

## FUTURE DIRECTIONS

The number of assays compatible with POC testing will continue to increase, and implementation of these tests outside standard clinical diagnostic laboratories will no doubt expand. In the setting of returning travelers, where the breadth and diversity of infecting pathogens is greater, use of POC testing for nondomestic infectious diseases may not be practical for most centers when factors such as test volume, personnel training, and cost are taken into consideration. However, POC testing for common syndromes such as respiratory tract and gastrointestinal infections, which affect travelers and nontravelers alike, may provide a rapid diagnosis, inform triage decisions, and limit unnecessary laboratory testing.

### BIBLIOGRAPHY

1. Babady NE. The FilmArray respiratory panel: an automated, broadly multiplexed molecular test for the rapid and accurate detection of respiratory pathogens. Expert Rev Mol Diagn. 2013;13(8):779–88.

2. CDC. Ready? Set? Test! 2017 Oct 20. [cited 2018 Nov 6]. Available from: wwwn.cdc.gov/clia/resources/waivedtests/pdf/readysettestbooklet.pdf.

3. Gonzalez MD, McElvania E. New developments in rapid diagnostic testing for children. Infect Dis Clin North Am. 2018;32(1):19–34.

4. Hunsperger EA, Yoksan S, Buchy P, Nguyen VC, Sekaran SD, Enria DA, et al. Evaluation of commercially available diagnostic tests for the detection of dengue virus NS1 antigen and anti-dengue virus IgM antibody. PLoS Negl Trop Dis. 2014;8(10):e3171.

5. Infectious Disease Society of America. IDSA Practice Guidelines. Available at www.idsociety.org/PracticeGuidelines.

6. Pai NP, Vadnais C, Denkinger C, Engel N, Pai M. Point-of-care testing for infectious diseases: diversity, complexity, and barriers in low- and middle-income countries. PLoS Med. 2012;9(9):e1001306.

7. US Food and Drug Administration. CLIA—Clinical Laboratory Improvement Amendments—currently waived analytes. Available from: www.accessdata.fda.gov/scripts/cdrh/cfdocs/cfClia/analyteswaived.cfm.

**11**

# ANTIMICROBIAL RESISTANCE

D. Cal Ham, Joseph Lutgring, Aditya Sharma

Antimicrobial resistance enables microbes to avoid or diminish the effects of antimicrobial agents and is acquired either through mutation or the acquisition of resistance genes. Antimicrobial-resistant organisms can cause infections that are difficult to treat, often requiring the use of expensive, less effective, or more toxic alternative medications (www.cdc.gov/drugresistance/about.html). Resistance can occur in viral, bacterial, fungal, and parasitic pathogens. The epidemiology of resistant organisms often varies globally from that seen in the United States. Travelers and medical professionals should be aware of the risk of acquisition of resistant organisms during international travel and consider travel history when caring for patients, both to identify effective treatment for infections and to ensure infection control interventions are in place to prevent spread of antimicrobial resistance.

The focus of this section is on resistant bacteria and an emerging fungal pathogen; neither are covered in pathogen-specific chapters. These microbes can be acquired both from health care and community exposures during international travel, causing illness or asymptomatic colonization. Additional information about organism-specific resistance can be found in the disease specific sections of Chapter 4, Travel-Related Infectious Diseases, and in Chapter 9, Medical Tourism.

## INFECTIOUS AGENTS AND EPIDEMIOLOGY

### Antimicrobial-Resistant Organisms of Concern in the Community

Globally, use of health care services, use of antimicrobials in agriculture, and inadequate sanitation and water purification systems are associated with the emergence and spread of resistance at the community level. Resistance in the community can take many forms. Two categories of importance to travelers are the microorganisms that cause diarrhea and those that result in long-term intestinal colonization and sometimes extraintestinal infections.

Bacteria that cause diarrhea include a variety of enteric pathogens such as *Escherichia coli* O157, *Campylobacter jejuni*, *Salmonella* spp., and *Shigella* spp. Resistance to first-line antimicrobials among these enteric pathogens has risen worldwide in recent years, posing new challenges for treatment decisions. Please refer to Chapter 4, for further details of antimicrobial resistance in specific bacteria.

Intestinal colonization with bacteria is influenced by diet, exposure to agents (such as antibiotics) that disrupt the microbial flora, interaction with other humans or animals, and contact with the environment. Enterobacteriaceae, such as *Escherichia coli* and *Klebsiella pneumoniae*, commonly inhabit the human gut and can be transmitted silently between close contacts, including household members. Intestinal colonization with Enterobacteriaceae is usually asymptomatic; however, these bacteria may also cause a range of extraintestinal infections—most commonly urinary tract infections and less frequently bacteremia.

Enterobacteriaceae resistant to critically important antibiotics, such as extended-spectrum cephalosporins, carbapenems, and colistin, have been isolated from a wide range of community sources, including healthy people, animals, produce, meat, and drinking water. Consumption of foods prepared by street vendors, taking an antibiotic during travel, and travelers' diarrhea have been associated with intestinal colonization with antimicrobial-resistant Enterobacteriaceae. People with certain comorbidities, such as chronic bowel disease, are also more likely to become colonized with resistant Enterobacteriaceae during travel. Extraintestinal infections caused by Enterobacteriaceae resistant to extended-spectrum cephalosporins, carbapenems, or colistin may be more difficult to treat. Additionally, travelers colonized with antimicrobial-resistant

**11**

Enterobacteriaceae can transmit these bacteria or their mechanisms of antimicrobial resistance to close contacts upon return to their countries of origin. The duration of intestinal colonization with antimicrobial-resistant Enterobacteriaceae after travel ranges from 1 month to >1 year.

The risk of intestinal colonization with antimicrobial-resistant Enterobacteriaceae during travel is related to the prevalence of resistant organisms in the country visited. Studies of returning travelers have identified a high risk of colonization with Enterobacteriaceae resistant to extended-spectrum cephalosporins when returning from countries in South America, Southeast Asia, South Asia, East Africa, northern Africa, and the Middle East; the risk of acquisition was highest after travel to Vietnam, India, and Peru. Acquisition of carbapenem-resistant Enterobacteriaceae (CRE) has been reported in travelers returning from South Asia and Southeast Asia. Colonization with *E. coli* resistant to the last-resort antibiotic colistin has been reported from travelers returning from countries in Europe (Portugal), the Caribbean, the Middle East, South America, Southeast Asia, East Asia, and northwest Africa.

## Antimicrobial-Resistant Organisms of Concern in Health Care Settings

A patient history of recent hospitalization outside the United States has been associated with colonization or infection with antimicrobial-resistant organisms that are rare in the United States. This section describes organisms of concern for travelers with overseas health care exposures, such as hospitalization or surgery.

Gram-negative bacteria with resistance to broad-spectrum antibiotics, such as extended-spectrum cephalosporins, carbapenems, and colistin, cause infections that are difficult to treat and are of particular concern in health care settings because they have the potential for rapid spread to other patients. Resistance mechanisms of particular concern are extended-spectrum β-lactamases (ESBLs), carbapenemases, and mobile colistin resistance (MCR) genes, which confer resistance to extended-spectrum cephalosporins, carbapenems, and colistin, respectively. ESBL-producing gram-negative bacteria were originally described in health care settings but now have disseminated into communities globally, including in the United States. Carbapenemase-producing bacteria are often highly resistant to treatment. Although 1 carbapenemase, *K. pneumoniae* carbapenemase (KPC), emerged in the United States, other carbapenemases, which can be found in CRE, *Pseudomonas aeruginosa*, and *Acinetobacter baumannii*, have historically been associated with hospitalizations outside the United States.

Notably, there have been recent case reports of carbapenemase-producing CRE acquisition in travelers to South and Southeast Asia who did not have health care exposure; the rates of carbapenemase-producing CRE acquisition among healthy travelers are currently unknown. Bacteria harboring an MCR gene (such as *mcr*-1) appear to be primarily community associated and are often associated with ESBL-producing Enterobacteriaceae, although Enterobacteriaceae harboring MCR and carbapenemases have been reported from Asia and Europe.

Two hospital-based outbreaks of *K. pneumoniae* with MCR have been reported, from China and Portugal; the strain in the Portugal outbreak also produced a carbapenemase. Emergence of MCR in carbapenemase-producing CRE may result in rapid spread of strains with extremely limited treatment options in health care settings.

Antimicrobial-resistant gram-positive bacteria are a significant cause of health care–associated infections. Methicillin-resistant *Staphylococcus aureus* and vancomycin-resistant enterococci (VRE) are endemic in the United States, and travelers hospitalized outside the United States may also become colonized or infected by these organisms. Transmissible linezolid resistance has been identified in gram-positive bacilli, including *Staphylococcus aureus*, coagulase-negative *Staphylococcus*, and *Enterococcus* spp. from several countries worldwide, particularly in South America. This resistance is of particular concern in VRE, for which treatment options are limited.

The fungal pathogen *Candida auris* has rapidly emerged worldwide, and multiple US patients with *C. auris* have reported prior health care exposures in countries with documented *C. auris* transmission. Cases have been reported in >20 countries and broader spread is suspected (www.cdc.gov/

11

fungal/candida-auris/index.html). *C. auris* is distinct from other *Candida* species in its tendency to cause outbreaks in health care facilities, long duration of asymptomatic colonization of the skin, environmental persistence, and unusual levels of resistance to antifungals. Strains resistant to all 3 main classes of antifungal agents have been found in several countries but have not yet been identified in the United States. *C. auris* is frequently misidentified by routine laboratory diagnostics, which likely contributes to underdetection both domestically and outside the United States. Any *Candida* species isolated from patients who have received health care in the previous year in a country with documented *C. auris* transmission should be identified to the species level. Providers should notify public health agencies and implement infection control measures if suspected or confirmed *C. auris* is identified.

## PREVENTION DURING TRAVEL

### Community

In many countries, antibiotics may be readily available without prescription. Advise travelers seeking care for medical conditions while overseas, that although antibiotics may be procured easily, high-quality medical advice from a licensed practitioner is strongly suggested for assessing treatment options, including whether antibiotic treatment is indicated. Management of mild cough, upset stomach, diarrhea, and other simple ailments usually does not require an antibiotic. Over-the-counter medications for these minor health events should be included in the travel health kit for an international traveler. Use of antibiotics can predispose travelers to acquiring resistant bacteria.

Travelers and the clinicians treating them should be aware that common bacterial infections in destination countries may be resistant to first-line antimicrobials typically used in the United States. For example, enteric pathogens that cause travelers' diarrhea in the Caribbean and South Asia are commonly resistant to fluoroquinolones. Therefore, if antibiotics are needed for treatment, an alternative antibiotic may be required. Evidence regarding effective therapies to prevent colonization or infection with a resistant organism in travelers is lacking; probiotics and

bismuth-containing compounds are under investigation for this purpose.

Contaminated water may serve as a source of enteric bacteria, including *E. coli*, *Salmonella* spp., and *Shigella* spp. Drinking contaminated water confers a risk of transmission of enteric bacteria, including those that are resistant to antimicrobials. General safe water use recommendations apply to prevention of waterborne organisms. See Chapter 2, Water Disinfection, for CDC recommendations regarding water treatment.

Foods prepared under poor hygienic conditions may also be a source of enteric bacteria. Making safe food choices and paying careful attention to good hand hygiene can reduce the risk of exposure to these pathogens, including those that harbor antimicrobial resistance. See Chapter 2, Food & Water Precautions, for recommendations regarding food consumption and guidance on hand hygiene.

### Health Care Settings

Patients admitted to health care facilities outside the United States, especially in low- and middle-income countries, may be at higher risk for acquiring antimicrobial-resistant organisms. These exposures may be facilitated by inadequate hand hygiene practices, insufficient environmental cleaning of health facilities, and irregular supply or use of personal protective equipment by health care workers. These gaps are more common in low-resource settings.

Information about infection prevention and control services in international health care settings is often limited. However, patients and health care workers traveling overseas, particularly in low- and middle-income countries, may reduce risk by choosing health facilities with active infection prevention and control programs. Travelers may also consider visiting health care facilities that have been accredited for infection prevention and control by national and international bodies. A health care facility accredited by an external body may have better-developed infection control practices than a nonaccredited facility. However, accreditation does not guarantee absence of risk of pathogen transmission in health care.

11

## POSTTRAVEL CONSIDERATIONS

Some patients returning from international travel may be at higher risk for colonization and infection with resistant organisms depending on the location of their travel. Obtain an international travel history going back at least 12 months from all patients presenting for care. This information can play an important role in their clinical care and in the infection control practices employed during their clinical encounter.

### Health Care Provider Guidance for Returning Travelers

CDC has pathogen-specific guidance for CRE and *C. auris* in patients who had a recent overnight stay in a health care facility outside the United States. Recommendations for CRE include:

- When CRE is identified in a patient with a history of an overnight stay in a health care facility outside the United States in the past 6 months, the CRE isolate should be sent for confirmatory susceptibility testing and to determine the carbapenem resistance mechanism.

- For patients admitted to health care facilities in the United States after hospitalization in facilities outside the United States within the past 6 months, consider rectal screening to detect CRE colonization and place patients in contact precautions while awaiting these screening cultures.

Additional recommendations for patients infected or colonized with CRE can be found in the CRE Toolkit (www.cdc.gov/hai/pdfs/cre/CRE-guidance-508.pdf) and https://stacks.cdc.gov/view/cdc/25250/cdc_25250_DS1.pdf.

### Recommendations for *C. auris*

- All isolates of *Candida* collected from the bloodstream or other normally sterile sites should be identified to the species level. Species identification for *Candida* isolates from nonsterile sites should be considered when the patient has had an overnight stay in a health care facility outside the United States in the previous year in a country with documented *C. auris* transmission.

- Patients being treated for *C. auris* should be closely monitored for treatment failure.

Additional recommendations for providers caring for patients infected or colonized with *C. auris* can be found at www.cdc.gov/fungal/diseases/candidiasis/health-professionals.html.

## BIBLIOGRAPHY

1. Arcilla MS, van Hattem JM, Haverkate MR, Bootsma MCJ, van Genderen PJJ, Goorhuis A, et al. Import and spread of extended-spectrum β-lactamase-producing Enterobacteriaceae by international travellers (COMBAT study): a prospective, multicentre cohort study. Lancet Infect Dis 2017;17:78–85.

2. CDC. Antibiotic resistance threats in the United States, 2013. Atlanta, GA. Available from: www.cdc.gov/drugresistance/threat-report-2013.

3. Chen L, Todd R, Kiehlbauch J, Walters M, Kallen A. Notes from the field: pan-resistant New Delhi Metallo-beta-lactamase-producing *Klebsiella pneumoniae*—Washoe County, Nevada, 2016. MMWR Morb Mortal Wkly Rep. 2017;66:33.

4. Friedman DN, Carmeli Y, Walton AL, Schwaber MJ. Carbapenem-resistant Enterobacteriaceae: a strategic roadmap for infection control. Infect Control Hosp Epidemiol. 2017;38:580–94.

5. George DB, Manges AR. A systematic review of outbreak and non-outbreak studies of extraintestinal pathogenic *Escherichia coli* causing community-acquired infections. Epidemiol Infect. 2010;138:1679–90.

6. Liu YY, Wang Y, Walsh TR, Yi LX, Zhang R, Spencer J, et al. Emergence of plasmid-mediated colistin resistance mechanism MCR-1 in animals and human beings in China: a microbiological and molecular biological study. Lancet Infect Dis. 2016;16:161–8.

7. Peirano G, Bradford PA, Kazmierczak KM, Badal RE, Hackel M, Hoban DJ, et al. Global incidence of carbapenemase-producing Escherichia coli ST131. Emerg Infect Dis. 2014;20:1928–31.

8. Vincent C, Boerlin P, Daignault D, Dozois CM, Dutil L, Galanakis C, et al. Food reservoir for Escherichia coli causing urinary tract infections. Emerg Infect Dis. 2010;16:88–95.

11

9. Woerther PL, Andremont A, Kantele A. Travel-acquired ESBL-producing Enterobacteriaceae: impact of colonization at individual and community level. J Travel Med. 2017;24:S29–34.

10. World Health Organization. Antimicrobial resistance: global report on surveillance 2014. World Health Organization, Geneva, Switzerland. [cited 2018 Nov 6]. Available from: www.who.int/drugresistance/documents/surveillancereport/en.

# SEXUALLY TRANSMITTED INFECTIONS

Jodie Dionne-Odom, Kimberly Workowski

## INFECTIOUS AGENT

More than two dozen bacterial, viral, and parasitic pathogens can cause sexually transmitted infections (STIs).

## TRANSMISSION

This chapter focuses on infections transmitted from person to person during sexual activity with genital, anal, or oral mucosal contact.

## EPIDEMIOLOGY

STIs are among the most common infectious diseases reported worldwide. There were an estimated 20 million new cases of sexually transmitted infections in the United States in 2016 and 357 million cases globally in 2012.

Casual sex during travel is common (20% prevalence in a systematic review), and some people travel for sex tourism (see Chapter 9, Sex & Travel). Sex partners abroad may include male or female commercial sex workers with elevated STI prevalence. Documented risk factors for STI/HIV acquisition among travelers to low- and middle-income countries include male gender, men who have sex with men (MSM), single marital status, and longer duration of stay. Providers caring for returning travelers should know where to find up-to-date information about global epidemiology and antimicrobial resistance patterns of STI from national (CDC, www.cdc.gov/drugresistance/index.html) and international public health authorities (World Health Organization [WHO], www.who.int/gho/sti/en).

The epidemiology and clinical manifestations of common STIs are shown in Table 11-6. Returning travelers should be asked about sexual activity during their trip, with specific questions about region of travel, sexual partners, sites of sexual exposure, and condom use. Assessing risk in MSM is important because they have elevated rates of certain infections (syphilis, chlamydia, gonorrhea, and lymphogranuloma venereum). Screen travelers seeking an evaluation for STI or with evidence of STI for HIV infection. Provide anyone with HIV infection linkage to HIV care and treatment services if they are not already receiving care.

## CLINICAL PRESENTATION

Returning travelers should be assessed for chlamydia, gonorrhea, and syphilis, since many curable bacterial STIs are asymptomatic. Advise any traveler with sexual exposure who develops STI symptoms (vaginal, urethral, or rectal discharge, an unexplained rash or genital lesion, or genital or pelvic pain) to abstain from sex and seek prompt medical evaluation. Human papillomavirus (HPV) infection is commonly acquired within 2 years of sexual debut and usually clears spontaneously. Although most STIs involve the genital tract, some also cause disseminated disease (such as syphilis and herpes). Consider STI in returning travelers since infection can result in serious and long-term complications, including pelvic inflammatory disease, infertility, adverse birth outcomes, cervical cancer, anal cancer, and an increased risk of HIV acquisition and transmission.

11

# Table 11-6. Epidemiology and clinical manifestations of common STIs

| STI [CAUSE] | GEOGRAPHIC LOCATION | TYPICAL CLINICAL PRESENTATION (BUT OFTEN ASYMPTOMATIC) | INCUBATION PERIOD (DAYS) | DIAGNOSIS | FIRST-LINE THERAPY |
|---|---|---|---|---|---|
| **BACTERIAL** | | | | | |
| **Chancroid** (*Haemophilus ducreyi*) | Regional in Africa, Asia, Caribbean | Irregular, painful genital ulcer; tender, suppurative inguinal lymphadenopathy | 4–7 | Culture with specialized media | Azithromycin 1 g PO once OR Ceftriaxone 250 mg IM once |
| **Chlamydia** (*Chlamydia trachomatis*) | Widespread | Cervicitis, urethritis | 7–21 | NAAT | Azithromycin 1 g PO once OR Doxycycline 100 mg PO bid x 7 days |
| **Gonorrhea** (*Neisseria gonorrhoeae*) | Widespread | Cervicitis, urethritis | 1–14 | NAAT | Ceftriaxone 250 mg IM once AND Azithromycin 1 g PO once |
| **Granuloma inguinale or donovanosis** (*Klebsiella granulomatis*) | Southern Africa, India, Papua New Guinea, Australia | Extensive genital ulcerations with granulation and easy bleeding; tender lymphadenopathy | 4–28 days | Microscopy: donovan bodies in macrophages | Azithromycin 1 g PO weekly until resolution |
| **Lymphogranuloma venereum** (*Chlamydia trachomatis* serovar L1-3) | Widespread | Self-limited ulcer; tender inguinal lymphadenopathy, proctocolitis | 3–30 days | NAAT, serology | Doxycycline 100 mg PO bid x 21 days |
| **Syphilis** (*Treponema pallidum*) | Widespread | Primary: painless genital ulcer, regional lymphadenopathy; secondary: maculopapular skin rash | 10–90 days | Darkfield microscopy (primary infection), serology | Benzathine penicillin G 2.4 MU IM (once for primary, secondary, and early latent infection). 2.4 MU IM once weekly x 3 weeks for late latent infection or latent syphilis of unknown duration |

| | | | | | |
|---|---|---|---|---|---|
| **VIRAL** | | | | | |
| **Hepatitis A virus** | Widespread | Malaise, fatigue, anorexia, jaundice | 28 days | Serology | Supportive care |
| **Hepatitis B virus** | Widespread | Malaise, fatigue, anorexia, jaundice | 60–150 days | Serology | Several options, consult with expert |
| **Hepatitis C virus** | Widespread | Malaise, fatigue, anorexia, jaundice | 15–50 days | Serology | Several options, consult with expert |
| **Herpes simplex virus (HSV)** | Widespread | ≥1 painful genital ulcers | 2–7 days | Culture or PCR | Acyclovir 400 mg PO tid x 7–10 days OR valacyclovir 1 g PO bid x 7–10 days OR famciclovir 250 mg PO tid x 7–10 days |
| **Human papillomavirus** | Widespread | Warts | 14–240 days | Clinical or pathologic | Topical therapy or removal of lesion |
| **Zika virus** | Widespread | Fever, rash, joint pain, conjunctivitis | 3–14 days | Serology or PCR | Supportive care |
| **PARASITIC** | | | | | |
| **Trichomoniasis** (*Trichomonas vaginalis*) | Widespread | Vaginal discharge and itching | 5–28 days | NAAT | Metronidazole 2 g PO once OR tinidazole 2 g PO once; Metronidazole 500 mg bid x 7 days in women with HIV infection |

Abbreviations: STI, sexually transmitted infection; PO, orally; IM, intramuscularly; NAAT, nucleic acid amplification testing; bid, twice daily; tid, 3 times daily.

11

## TREATMENT

Base STI evaluation, management, and follow-up on the most recent national and international guidelines from CDC and WHO. In the United States, CDC guidelines are preferred since WHO follows a syndromic approach to STI management given limited availability of diagnostic testing in many countries. Treatment failure is a possibility if an infection does not respond, which is particularly relevant in a traveler with persistent gonococcal infection given the global spread of multidrug-resistant *Neisseria gonorrhoeae*.

## PREVENTION

Prevention and control of STIs is based on accurate risk assessment, education, counseling, early identification of asymptomatic infection, and effective treatment of travelers and their sex partners. Pretravel advice should include specific messages with strategies to avoid acquiring or transmitting STIs. Abstinence or mutual monogamy with an uninfected partner is the most reliable way to avoid acquiring and transmitting STIs.

For people whose sexual behaviors place them at risk for STIs, correct and consistent use of the male latex condom can reduce the risk of HIV infection and other STIs, including chlamydia, gonorrhea, and trichomoniasis. Preventing lower genital tract infections might reduce the risk of pelvic inflammatory disease in women. Correct and consistent use of male latex condoms also reduces the risk of HPV infection, genital herpes, syphilis, and chancroid, although data are limited. Only water-based lubricants, such as K-Y Jelly, should be used with latex condoms because oil-based lubricants (such as petroleum jelly, shortening, mineral oil, or massage oil) can weaken latex condoms. Spermicides containing nonoxynol-9 are not recommended for STI/HIV prevention. Contraceptive methods that are not mechanical barriers do not protect against HIV or other STIs.

Prompt evaluation of sex partners is necessary to prevent reinfection and disrupt STI transmission. Preexposure vaccination is among the most effective methods for preventing certain STIs. HPV vaccines are available and licensed for girls and boys to prevent transmission. Consider all travelers as candidates for hepatitis A and hepatitis B vaccines, as these infections can be sexually transmitted. Hepatitis B vaccine is recommended for all people being evaluated or treated for an STI. Hepatitis A and hepatitis B vaccines are also recommended for MSM. Travelers at risk of acquiring HIV infection may benefit from preexposure prophylaxis (see www.cdc.gov/hiv/prep and Chapter 4, HIV).

**CDC website:** www.cdc.gov/std

### BIBLIOGRAPHY

1. Crawford G, Lobo R, Brown G, Macri C, Smith H, Maycock B. HIV, other blood-borne viruses and sexually transmitted infections amongst expatriates and travellers to low- and middle-income countries: a systematic review. Int J Environ Res Public Health. 2016;13(12).

2. Meites E, Kempe A, Markowitz LE. Use of a 2-dose schedule for human papillomavirus vaccination—updated recommendations of the Advisory Committee on Immunization Practices. MMWR Morb Mortal Wkly Rep. 2016;65(49):1405–8.

3. Newman L, Rowley J, Vander Hoorn S, Wijesooriya NS, Unemo M, Low N, et al. Global estimates of the prevalence and incidence of four curable sexually transmitted infections in 2012 based on systematic review and global reporting. PLoS One. 2015;10(12):e0143304.

4. Vivancos R, Abubakar I, Hunter PR. Foreign travel, casual sex, and sexually transmitted infections: systematic review and meta-analysis. Int J Infect Dis. 2010;14(10):e842–51.

5. Weston EJ, Wi T, Papp J. Strengthening global surveillance for antimicrobial drug-resistant Neisseria gonorrhoeae through the Enhanced Gonococcal Antimicrobial Surveillance Program. Emerg Infect Dis. 2017;23(13).

6. Workowski KA, Bolan GA. Sexually transmitted diseases treatment guidelines, 2015. MMWR Recomm Rep. 2015;64(RR-03):1–137.

# SKIN & SOFT TISSUE INFECTIONS

Karolyn A. Wanat, Scott A. Norton

Skin problems are among the most frequent medical problems in returned travelers. A large case series of dermatologic problems in returned travelers showed that cutaneous larva migrans, insect bites, and bacterial infections were the most frequent skin problems in ill travelers seeking medical care, making up 30% of the 4,742 diagnoses (Table 11-7).

There are several ways to approach the diagnosis and management of skin conditions in returned travelers. A useful approach is to consider whether the skin condition is accompanied by fever. Skin eruptions and cutaneous lesions that are accompanied by fever constitute a minority of travelers' dermatoses, but fever may indicate a systemic infection, usually viral or bacterial, which may require prompt attention. A second consideration should focus on the geographic and exposure aspects of the travel history. A third consideration should focus on the morphology of the lesions as noted on physical examination. The most successful approach combines all of these considerations and may be supported by laboratory confirmation (skin biopsy, serology, cultures, microscopy) if required or indicated.

Diagnosis of skin problems in returned travelers should involve the following elements of the medical history and physical examination:

- Systemic diseases: cancer, allergy to penicillin

- Location and duration of travel

- Exposure history: freshwater, ocean, insects, animals, plant contact, human contact, occupational and recreational exposures, sexual contact

- Time of onset of lesions during or after travel

- Whether other travelers have similar findings

- Associated symptoms: fever, pain, pruritus

- Vaccination status and adherence to standard travel precautions (food, water, personal protection from insects)

## Table 11-7. Ten most common skin lesions in returned travelers, by cause

| SKIN LESION | PERCENTAGE OF ALL DERMATOLOGIC DIAGNOSES (N = 4,742) |
|---|---|
| Cutaneous larva migrans | 9.8 |
| Insect bite | 8.2 |
| Skin abscess | 7.7 |
| Superinfected insect bite | 6.8 |
| Allergic rash | 5.5 |
| Rash, unknown origin | 5.5 |
| Dog bite | 4.3 |
| Superficial fungal infection | 4.0 |
| Dengue | 3.4 |
| Leishmaniasis | 3.3 |
| Myiasis | 2.7 |
| Spotted fever group rickettsiosis | 1.5 |
| Scabies | 1.5 |
| Cellulitis | 1.5 |

Modified from Lederman ER, Weld LH, Elyazar IR, et al. Dermatologic conditions of the ill returned traveler: an analysis from the GeoSentinel Surveillance Network. Int J Infect Dis. 2008;12(6):593–602.

- Medications taken during travel (that may have side effects or may provide adequate prophylaxis for certain conditions)

11

- Existing skin conditions

- Shape of lesions, such as papules, plaques, nodules, macular lesions, or ulcerated lesions

- Number, pattern, and distribution of lesions

- Location of lesions: exposed versus unexposed skin surfaces

It is important to recognize that skin conditions in returned travelers may not have a travel-related cause or may represent worsening of a preexisting condition.

## PAPULAR LESIONS

**Arthropod bites** are probably the most common cause of papular lesions. Biting flies (such as mosquitoes, midges, and sandflies), bed bugs, headlice, and fleas are among the most common and universal biting arthropods. Itching associated with arthropod bites is due to hypersensitivity reactions to proteins and other components in the arthropod saliva. Individual bites usually appear as small (4–10 mm diameter) edematous, pink-to-red papules with a gentle "watch-glass" profile. The center of many bites will have a small, subtle break in the epidermis where the arthropod's mouth parts broke the surface. The pink-to-red color generally does not extend beyond the elevated part of the lesion. The lesions are almost invariably quite pruritic; scratching will often excoriate or erode the skin's surface. Such bites are vulnerable to secondary bacterial infections, usually with *Staphylococcus* spp. or *Streptococcus* spp. Many types of arthropods produce bite reactions with characteristic shapes, patterns, and distributions. For example, bites from bed bugs and fleas often appear as clustered papules (see Box 3-2, Bed bugs and international travel).

By contrast, scabies infestation usually manifests as a generalized or regional pruritic papular rash amidst erythema, abundant excoriations, and secondarily infected pustules. Scabies generally has regional symmetry, involving the volar wrists and finger web spaces. Most boys and men with scabies will have nodular lesions on the scrotum and penis. Scabies burrows are short linear lesions involving just the most superficial part of the epidermis and are pathognomonic but can be difficult to detect.

Other causes of widespread, extremely pruritic eruptions include allergic contact dermatitis (perhaps due to plants) and photosensitive dermatitis (often due to photosensitizing medications, such as doxycycline). Onchocerciasis (specifically onchocercal dermatitis due to microfilaria migrating through the skin) may occur in long-stay travelers living in endemic areas in sub-Saharan Africa and manifests as a generalized pruritic, papular dermatitis. Swimmer's itch and hookworm folliculitis are extremely itchy eruptions composed of papules on skin surfaces exposed to fresh water and contaminated soils, respectively.

## NODULAR OR SUBCUTANEOUS LESIONS, INCLUDING BACTERIAL SKIN INFECTIONS

**Bacterial skin infections** may occur more frequently after bites, minor scratches, or abrasions, particularly when maintaining good hygiene is difficult. Common organisms responsible are *Staphylococcus aureus* or *Streptococcus pyogenes*. Resulting infections are collectively called pyodermas ("pus skin") and can present as impetigo, folliculitis, ecthyma (ulcers or open sores), boils (also called furuncles and abscesses), cellulitis and erysipelas, lymphangitis, or ulceration. People whose skin or nasal mucosa is colonized with *S. aureus* are at risk for recurrent folliculitis or furunculosis. Boils may continue to occur weeks or months after a traveler returns, and, if associated with *S. aureus*, treatment usually involves a decolonization regimen with nasal mupirocin, a skin wash with an antimicrobial skin cleanser, and oral antibiotics. Many travelers who develop boils when abroad mistakenly attribute the tender lesions to spider bites; however, outside a few endemic areas, necrotizing spider bites are extremely rare. The lesions, in these cases, are far more likely to be abscesses caused by methicillin-resistant *S. aureus* and should be treated accordingly.

Cellulitis and erysipelas manifest as warm, red, edematous areas. They may start at the site of a minor injury or opening in the skin or without an obvious underlying suppurative focus. Unlike cellulitis, erysipelas tends to be raised, with a clear

11

line of demarcation at the edge of the lesion, and is more likely to be associated with fever. Cellulitis and erysipelas are usually caused by group A β-hemolytic streptococci. *S. aureus* (including methicillin-resistant strains) and gram-negative aerobic bacteria may also cause cellulitis.

Another common bacterial skin infection, especially in children in the tropics, is impetigo due to *S. aureus* or *S. pyogenes*. Impetigo is a highly contagious superficial skin infection that generally appears on the arms, legs, or face as "honey-colored" or golden crusting formed from dried serum. Streptococcal impetigo is usually the causative agent for the classic "honey-colored crust" seen in the mid-face of children. Staphylococcal impetigo often appears in body folds, especially the axillae, and may present with delicate pustules.

Soap and water should be used for local cleansing of skin infections. A topical antibiotic, such as bacitracin zinc and polymyxin sulfate, or mupirocin, may be used. In many developing countries gentian violet is the treatment of choice for impetigo. If the skin infection is extensive, expanding, or associated with systemic symptoms such as fever, parenteral antibiotics may be required. Antibiotic resistance among many bacterial species should be considered if the condition does not respond to therapy. Unusual gram-negative organisms and anaerobes may be involved in bites and scratches from animals, including domestic animals, and may require a specialist's care and debridement. See below and Chapter 3, Mosquitoes, Ticks & Other Arthropods, for more information.

**Myiasis** presents as a painful lesion, resembling a furuncle or boil, which is most often caused by infestation with larvae of the African tumbu fly (*Cordylobia anthropophaga*, found in much of sub-Saharan Africa) or the New World botfly (*Dermatobia hominis*, found from central Mexico to the northern half of South America). There can be single or multiple lesions; each lesion holds only 1 larva. The center of the lesion has a small punctum through which the larva can breathe. Extraction of the fly larva can be difficult and may be facilitated by first obstructing the breathing punctum with an occlusive dressing or covering (such as a bottle cap filled with petroleum jelly) for

several hours. Larvae may exit on their own or can be gently squeezed out. Treatment for secondary infection and updating tetanus vaccination may be required.

**Tungiasis** is caused by infestation by a sand flea (*Tunga penetrans*). A gestating female burrows into the usually thick skin on the sole or around the toes. Most people with tungiasis have multiple lesions. Individual lesions have a strikingly uniform appearance with a round, 5 mm diameter, white, slightly elevated surface. In the center of the lesion, there is a central minute opening, often black in color, through which the embedded flea breathes and eventually extrudes her eggs. Clustered lesions may appear as a dirty, crusty, draining plaque. Lesions are typically itchy, painful, and continue to expand as the female produces eggs in her uterus. Treatment involves flea extraction, treatment for secondary bacterial infection, and updating tetanus vaccination, if required. In many countries, extraction is performed at home by using a heat-sterilized needle to pluck out the mature flea and her eggs.

**Loiasis,** caused by *Loa loa*, a deerfly-transmitted nematode, occurs rarely in long-term travelers living in rural sub-Saharan Africa. The traveler may present with transient, migratory, subcutaneous, painful, or pruritic nodules (Calabar swelling) produced by adult nematode migration through the skin. Rarely, the worm can be visualized crossing the conjunctiva or eyelid. Peripheral eosinophilia is common. Loiasis can be diagnosed by finding microfilariae in blood collected during daytime; however, since microfilaremia may be absent, serologic tests may be helpful. Treatment of choice is diethylcarbamazine, but special consideration is warranted for areas endemic with both loiasis and onchocerciasis due to the relative contraindication for using diethylcarbamazine in onchocerciasis. Use of ivermectin to treat loiasis may cause neurological problems. Consultation with an expert is required for these cases (see Chapter 4, Filariasis, Lymphatic).

**Gnathostomiasis** is a nematode infection found primarily in Southeast Asia, the Pacific coast of Peru and Ecuador, parts of Mexico, and equatorial Africa. Infection results from eating undercooked or raw freshwater fish, amphibians, or reptiles. Infected travelers may experience transient, migratory, subcutaneous, pruritic and painful nodules that may occur weeks or even years after exposure. The symptoms are due to migration of the worm through the body, and the central nervous system may be involved. Eosinophilia is common, and serologic tests may be available for diagnosis. Treatment of cutaneous gnathostomiasis includes albendazole or ivermectin.

## MACULAR LESIONS

Macules and patches (flat lesions) are common and often nonspecific and are often due to drug reactions or viral exanthems. Purpura is typically macular—and any purpuric lesion associated with fever may indicate a life-threatening emergency such as meningococcemia.

**Tinea versicolor**, due to several species of fungi, *Malassezia* (for instance *M. furfur*, previously *Pityrosporum ovale*), is characterized by abundant, asymptomatic, hypopigmented or hyperpigmented oval skin patches. Individual lesions are often 1–3 cm in diameter, but dozens of lesions may coalesce to form a "maplike" appearance on the upper chest and back. The skin surface typically has a dry or dusty surface. The lesions may be skin colored, slightly hypopigmented, or slightly hyperpigmented (*versicolor* means "changed color"), but all lesions on a person have a uniform color.

Clinicians can make this diagnosis in various ways. Under the light of a Wood ultraviolet lamp, tinea versicolor produces a subtle yellowish-orange hue. Examination under a microscope can also identify tinea versicolor. Briefly apply a piece of clear cellophane tape to skin lesions to pick up superficial scales. Then place the tape (sticky side down) onto a glass slide. Next, put a drop of methylene blue at the edge of the tape allowing it to run between the tape and the slide. Detection of hyphae ("spaghetti") and spores ("meatballs") suggest the diagnosis. Often, however, a clinical diagnosis is made based on the appearance of the lesions.

Treatment with topical azoles (such as clotrimazole cream or ketoconazole shampoo used as a body wash), systemic azoles (such as fluconazole), or selenium sulfide shampoo is recommended. In many countries, the most common treatment is Whitfield ointment (salicylic acid 3% and benzoic acid 6%, mixed in a vehicle such as petrolatum). Antifungal agents such as griseofulvin and nystatin are ineffective.

**Tinea corporis** (ringworm) may be caused by a number of different superficial fungi. The lesion is often an expanding red, raised ring, with an area of central clearing. Treatment is usually several weeks' application of a topical antifungal agent or a short course of an oral antifungal agent (terbinafine, fluconazole, or griseofulvin).

**Lyme disease**, a tickborne infection with the spirochete *Borrelia burgdorferi* is common in North America, Europe, and Russia (see Chapter 3, Lyme Disease). An infected traveler may present with ≥1 large erythematous patches (erythema migrans). Lyme disease is transmitted by the bites of the hard tick, genus *Ixodes*, found mostly in temperate latitudes. If there are several lesions, the first to appear is where the tick bite occurred; subsequent lesions are due to a secondary, probably hematogenous, spread of *Borrelia*, not to multiple tick bites. Erythema migrans is often described as targetoid, but central clearing or red-and-white bands do not occur with every case. The lesions are generally asymptomatic; if a patient reports pruritus, it is usually intermittent and very mild.

**Leprosy** (Hansen disease) frequently presents with hypopigmented or erythematous patches frequently hypoesthetic to pin prick and associated with peripheral nerve enlargement. This condition is found almost exclusively in immigrants from developing countries. Diagnosis is made by biopsy of the lesions. The national Hansen disease clinical center in Baton Rouge, Louisiana, makes themselves available for consultations (e-mail nhdped@hrsa.gov; phone 800-642-2477).

## LINEAR LESIONS

**Cutaneous larva migrans**, a skin infestation with the larval stage of dog or cat hookworm (*Ancylostoma* spp.), manifests as an extremely pruritic, serpiginous, linear lesion that advances in the epidermis of the skin relatively slowly (see Chapter 4, Cutaneous Larva Migrans). A deeper lesion that resembles urticarial patches and that progresses rapidly may be due to **larva currens** ("running larva") caused by cutaneous migration of filariform larvae of *Strongyloides stercoralis*.

11

**Lymphocutaneous or sporotrichoid spread** of infection occurs when organisms ascend proximally along superficial cutaneous lymphatics, producing raised, linear, cordlike lesions. This is also called nodular lymphangitis. Another presentation is an ascending chain of discontinuous, sometimes ulcerated, nodules, after primary percutaneous inoculation of certain pathogens. Examples include sporotrichosis, atypical *Mycobacterium* (such as infection with *M. marinum* after exposure to brackish water or with rapidly growing *Mycobacteria* after pedicure footbaths), cutaneous leishmaniasis (particularly New World leishmaniasis), nocardiosis, tularemia, and coccidioidomycosis.

**Phytophotodermatitis** is a noninfectious condition resulting from interaction of natural psoralens, most commonly found in the juice of limes, and ultraviolet A radiation from the sun. The result is an exaggerated sunburn that creates a painful line of blisters, followed by asymptomatic hyperpigmented lines that may take weeks or months to resolve. Linear lesions caused by cnidarian envenomations, such as jellyfish stings, often resemble phytophotodermatitis.

## SKIN ULCERS

A skin ulcer forms when the epidermis, the skin's superficial layer, is damaged or absent, and the damaging process has entered the dermis, the skin's deeper, more leathery layer. The most common cutaneous ulcers are caused by the common pyogenic bacteria, staphylococci and streptococci, creating well-demarcated, shallow ulcers with sharp borders. These lesions are called bacterial or common ecthyma, and their treatment is described earlier in this chapter.

Cutaneous leishmaniasis (CL) can resemble bacterial ecthyma by forming shallow, although usually painless, ulcers. The surface of leishmanial ulcers can have a dried crust or a raw, fibrinous coat. The main areas of risk for CL are Latin America, the Mediterranean coastal areas, the Middle East, south and central Asia, and Africa's northeastern quadrant. Typically, CL forms a painless ulcer unless superinfected. It has heaped-up margins on exposed skin surfaces and is slow growing. Special diagnostic techniques are necessary to confirm the diagnosis. Both topical and systemic treatments may be effective; it is often necessary to speciate the pathogen to determine the proper treatment. When CL is suspected, clinicians may go to the CDC's web page, www.cdc.gov/parasites/leishmaniasis/index.html, or contact the CDC at 404-718-4745 or parasites@cdc.gov for recommendations on diagnosis and treatment (see Chapter 3, Cutaneous Leishmaniasis).

Cutaneous anthrax produces a large edematous swelling that, surprisingly, is painless. The surface develops a shallow ulcer that progresses into a necrotic black eschar. Nearly all cases of travel-associated anthrax will come from exposure to live cattle, sheep, or goats, or from handling unprocessed products made from their hides or wool (see Chapter 4, Anthrax).

Less common causes of ulcers include cutaneous diphtheria (*Corynebacterium diphtheriae*), Buruli ulcer (*Mycobacterium ulcerans*), and sexually transmitted infections of syphilis (*Treponema pallidum*) and chancroid (*Haemophilus ducreyi*). On several island groups in the southwestern Pacific, *H. ducreyi* causes nonvenereal cutaneous ulcers. Rarely, a painless destructive ulcer with undermined edges may arise from infection with *M. ulcerans* (Buruli ulcer), a freshwater bacterium found most commonly in equatorial Africa and in the Australian state of Victoria. The central African form of human African trypanosomiasis (due to *Trypanosoma brucei rhodesiense*) can produce a trypanosomal chancre at the bite site of the transmitting tsetse fly (*Glossina* spp.).

Necrotizing spider bites are usually caused by recluse spiders, of which the most common culprit is *Loxosceles reclusa*, the brown recluse found in the south-central part of the United States. Many studies have shown that outside a few endemic areas, most alleged spider bites are, in fact, infections with methicillin-resistant *S. aureus* and should be treated accordingly.

## MISCELLANEOUS SKIN INFECTIONS

### Skin Infections Associated with Water

Skin and soft tissue infections (SSTI) can occur after exposure to fresh, brackish, or saltwater, particularly if the skin's surface is compromised.

11

Abrasions or lacerations from submerged objects during wading and swimming, puncture wounds from fishhooks, and bites or stings from marine or aquatic creatures may be the source of the trauma leading to waterborne infections. The most virulent SSTIs associated with marine and estuarine exposures are due to *Vibrio vulnificus* (and related non-cholera *Vibrio*); for freshwater exposure, *Aeromonas hydrophila* is the most dangerous pathogen. A variety of skin and soft tissue manifestations may occur in association with these infections, including cellulitis, abscess formation, ecthyma gangrenosum, and necrotizing fasciitis.

Vibriosis infections may be acquired directly through the skin or by consumption of contaminated shellfish. The illness is especially severe in those with underlying liver disease and may manifest as a dramatic cellulitis with hemorrhagic bullae and sepsis. In general, infections caused by these organisms may be more severe in those who are immunosuppressed. Acute infections related to aquatic injury should be treated with an antibiotic that provides both gram-positive and gram-negative coverage (such as a fluoroquinolone or third-generation cephalosporin) until a specific organism has been identified.

*M. marinum* lesions are usually indolent and usually appear as solitary nodules or papules on an extremity, especially on the dorsum of feet and hands; subsequent progression to shallow ulceration and scar formation may occur. Occasionally, "sporotrichoid" spread may occur as the lesions spread proximally along superficial lymphatics.

"Hot tub folliculitis" due to *Pseudomonas aeruginosa* may result from the use of inadequately disinfected swimming pools and hot tubs. Folliculitis typically develops 8–48 hours after exposure to contaminated water and consists of tender or pruritic, folliculocentric red papules, papulopustules, or nodules. There are usually several dozen discrete lesions that occur only on skin surfaces submerged in the infectious waters. Most patients have malaise, and some have low-grade fever. The condition is self-limited in 2–12 days; typically no antibiotic therapy is required.

## Skin Infections Associated with Bites

Wound infections after dog and cat bites are caused by a variety of microorganisms. *S. aureus*; α-, β-, and γ-hemolytic streptococci; several genera of gram-negative organisms; and a number of anaerobic microorganisms have been isolated. *Pasteurella multocida* infection classically occurs after cat bites and may also occur after dog bites. Splenectomized patients are at particular risk of severe cellulitis and sepsis due to *Capnocytophaga canimorsus* after a dog bite. Management of dog and cat bites includes consideration of rabies postexposure prophylaxis, tetanus immunization, and antibiotic prophylaxis. Avoid primary closure of puncture wounds and dog bites to the hand.

Antibiotic prophylaxis after dog bites is controversial, although most experts would treat splenectomized patients with amoxicillin-clavulanate prophylactically. Since *P. multocida* is a common accompaniment of cat bites, consider prophylaxis with amoxicillin-clavulanate or a fluoroquinolone for 3–5 days. Management of monkey bites includes wound care, tetanus immunization, rabies postexposure prophylaxis, and consideration of antimicrobial prophylaxis. Bites and scratches from Old World macaque monkeys have also been associated with fatal encephalomyelitis due to B virus infection in humans (see Chapter 4, B Virus). Valacyclovir postexposure prophylaxis is recommended after a high-risk macaque exposure.

## FEVER AND RASH

Fever and rash in returned travelers are most often due to a viral infection.

**Dengue** is caused by 1 of 4 strains of dengue viruses (see Chapter 4, Dengue). The disease is transmitted by *Aedes* spp. mosquitoes often found in urban areas, and its incidence continues to increase. The disease is characterized by the abrupt onset of high fever, frontal headache (often accompanied by retro-orbital pain), myalgia, and a widespread but faint macular rash interrupted by islands of uninvolved pallid skin that becomes evident on the second to fourth day of illness. A petechial rash may be found in classic dengue as well as in severe dengue. Diagnostic modalities include antigen and antibody detection tests, as well as PCR assays; detecting IgM in the appropriate clinical scenario supports the diagnosis. Treatment is supportive; avoid using nonsteroidal anti-inflammatory drugs (NSAIDs) which may increase the risk of bleeding in patients with dengue.

**Chikungunya**, a virus also transmitted by *Aedes* spp. mosquitoes, has caused major outbreaks of illness in southeast Africa, South Asia, the Americas, and the Caribbean (see Chapter 3, Chikungunya). Chikungunya resembles dengue clinically, including the rash, although hemorrhage, shock, and death are not typical of chikungunya. A major distinguishing feature of chikungunya is its associated arthritis or arthralgia that may persist for months, whereas in dengue, myalgia is the major clinical feature. Similar to dengue, serologic tests are available. Chikungunya may resolve with persistent arthritis or tenosynovitis. After ruling out dengue, treatment of the arthritis is with NSAIDs.

**Zika**, a flavivirus also transmitted by *Aedes* spp. mosquitoes, caused major outbreaks in the Western Hemisphere beginning in 2015 (see Chapter 4, Zika). Sexual transmission has been documented up to several months after acquisition of the disease. Zika infection is generally subclinical or mild, characterized by fever, arthralgia, lymphadenopathy, morbilliform ("maculopapular") rash, and conjunctivitis. Infection of pregnant women can cause fetal loss or fetal microcephaly and neurological damage. Zika-associated Guillain-Barré syndrome has also been reported after infection. Zika virus infection is usually diagnosed by using molecular diagnostics and serologic testing. Treatment is supportive.

**Acute HIV** (acute retroviral syndrome) can present with a flulike syndrome including fever, malaise, generalized lymphadenopathy, and generalized skin eruption. Acute HIV infection associated skin findings are often nonspecific and present as pink to deeply red macules or papules, but urticarial and pustular eruptions have also been described. Oral ulcerations may be present.

**African tick-bite fever** or South African tick typhus, caused by *Rickettsia africae*, is a frequent cause of fever and rash in southern Africa. Travelers participating in safaris or who hike and camp outdoors are particularly at risk. Transmitted by ticks, the disease is characterized by fever and an eschar, called a *tache noire* (a mildly painful black necrotic lesion with a red rim), at the site of the tick bite. Within a few days, patients develop a fine petechial or papular rash, associated with localized lymphadenopathy. Several *taches noires* may be present, as people often suffer multiple tick bites. Diagnosis is usually through clinical recognition and is confirmed by serologic testing. Treatment is with doxycycline. Other rickettsial infections such as Mediterranean spotted fever, rickettsialpox, and scrub typhus may present with eschars or maculopapular, vesicular, and petechial rashes.

**Rocky Mountain spotted fever** (RMSF), although uncommon in travelers, is an important cause of fever and rash because of its potential severity and the need for early treatment. This tickborne infection is found in the United States, Mexico, and parts of Central and South America. Most patients with RMSF develop a rash between the third and fifth days of illness. The typical rash of RMSF begins on the ankles and wrists and spreads both centrally and to the palms and soles. The rash commonly starts as a blanching maculopapular eruption that becomes petechial, although in some patients it begins with petechiae. Doxycycline is the treatment of choice.

**Meningococcemia** represents invasive *Neisseria meningitidis* disease, occurs worldwide and is often associated with outbreaks, especially in the "meningitis belt" of sub-Saharan Africa. Meningococcemia is characterized by acute onset of fever and purpuric macules and patches, which can continue to spread, and is often associated with hypotension and multiorgan failure. Immediate treatment can be life-saving.

The category of fever with rash is large, and providers caring for ill travelers should also consider the following diagnoses: enteroviruses, such as echovirus and coxsackievirus; hepatitis B virus; measles; Epstein-Barr virus; cytomegalovirus; typhus; leptospirosis; histoplasmosis; and syphilis.

**11**

## BIBLIOGRAPHY

1. Aronson N, Herwaldt B, Libman M, Pearson R, Lopez-Velez R, Weina P, et al. Diagnosis and treatment of leishmaniasis: clinical practice guidelines by the Infectious Diseases Society of America (IDSA) and the American Society of Tropical Medicine and Hygiene (ASTMH). Clin Infect Dis. 2016 Dec 15;63(12):e202–64.

2. Bandino JP, Hang A, Norton SA. The infectious and non-infectious dermatological consequences of flooding: a field manual for the responding provider. Am J Clin Dermatol. 2015 Oct;16(5):399–424.

3. Hochedez P, Canestri A, Lecso M, Valin N, Bricaire F, Caumes E. Skin and soft tissue infections in returning travelers. Am J Trop Med Hyg. 2009 Mar;80(3):431–4.

4. Jensenius M, Davis X, von Sonnenburg F, Schwartz E, Keystone JS, Leder K, et al. Multicenter GeoSentinel analysis of rickettsial diseases in international travelers, 1996–2008. Emerg Infect Dis. 2009 Nov;15(11):1791–8.

5. Kamimura-Nishimura K, Rudikoff D, Purswania M, Hagmann S. Dermatological conditions in international pediatric travelers: epidemiology, prevention and management. Travel Med Infect Dis. 2013 Nov–Dec;11(6):350–6.

6. Klion AD. Filarial infections in travelers and immigrants. Curr Infect Dis Rep. 2008 Mar;10(1):50–7.

7. Lederman ER, Weld LH, Elyazar IR, von Sonnenburg F, Loutan L, Schwartz E, et al. Dermatologic conditions of the ill returned traveler: an analysis from the GeoSentinel Surveillance Network. Int J Infect Dis. 2008 Nov;12(6):593–602.

8. Nordlund JJ. Cutaneous ectoparasites. Dermatol Ther. 2009 Nov–Dec;22(6):503–17.

9. Nurjadi D, Friedrich-Jänicke B, Schäfer J, Van Genderen PJ, Goorhuis A, Perignon A, et al. Skin and soft tissue infections in intercontinental travellers and the import of multi-resistant *Staphylococcus aureus* to Europe. Clin Microbiol Infect. 2015 Jul;21(6):567.e1–10.

10. Stevens MS, Geduld J, Libman M, Ward BJ, McCarthy AE, Vincelette J, et al. Dermatoses among returned Canadian travellers and immigrants: surveillance report based on CanTravNet data, 2009–2012. CMAJ Open 2015 Jan 13;3(1):E119–26.

11. Zimmerman RF, Belanger ES, Pfeiffer CD. Skin infections in returned travelers: an update. Current infectious disease reports. 2015 Mar;17(3):467.

# RESPIRATORY INFECTIONS

Regina C. LaRocque, Edward T. Ryan

Among returning travelers, respiratory infections are a leading cause for seeking medical care. Upper respiratory infection is more common than lower respiratory infection. In general, the types of respiratory infections affecting travelers are similar to those in nontravelers, and exotic causes are rare. Clinicians should inquire about the details of travel (such as type of travel and travel destinations) when evaluating a returning traveler with a respiratory infection.

## INFECTIOUS AGENTS

Viral pathogens are the most common cause of respiratory infection in travelers; causative agents include rhinoviruses, respiratory syncytial virus, influenza virus, parainfluenza virus, human metapneumovirus, measles, mumps, adenovirus, and coronaviruses. Consider also viruses of special concern in travelers, including Middle East respiratory syndrome (MERS) coronavirus and highly pathogenic avian influenza viruses. Include MERS in the differential diagnosis of travelers who develop fever and pneumonia within 14 days after traveling from countries in or near the Arabian Peninsula. Contact with a confirmed or suspected MERS case, or with health care facilities with MERS transmission, is of special concern, even in the absence of confirmed pneumonia. Be aware that regions associated with MERS may expand or change (see Chapter 4, Middle East Respiratory Syndrome, and www.cdc.gov/coronavirus/mers).

Consider a diagnosis of highly pathogenic avian influenza viruses (such as H5N1 and H7N9) in patients with new-onset severe acute respiratory illness requiring hospitalization when no alternative cause has been identified. A history of recent travel (within 10 days) to a country with confirmed human or animal cases—especially if the traveler had contact with poultry or sick or dead birds—improves the likelihood of the diagnosis (see Chapter 4, Influenza, and www.cdc.gov/flu/avianflu/specific-flu-viruses.htm).

Bacterial pathogens are less common than viral but can include *Streptococcus pneumoniae*, *Mycoplasma pneumoniae*, *Haemophilus influenzae*, and *Chlamydophila pneumoniae*. *Coxiella burnetii* and *Legionella pneumophila* can cause outbreaks and sporadic cases of respiratory illness. Bacterial sinusitis, bronchitis, or pneumonia may also occur secondarily after a viral respiratory infection.

## EPIDEMIOLOGIC CONSIDERATIONS

Outbreaks may occur following common-source exposures in hotels, on cruise ships, or among tour groups. A few pathogens have been associated with outbreaks in travelers, including influenza virus, *L. pneumophila*, and *Histoplasma capsulatum*. The peak influenza season in the temperate Northern Hemisphere is December through February. In the temperate Southern Hemisphere, peak influenza season runs from June through August. There is no peak season for influenza in tropical climates; the risk of infection is present 12 months of the year. Exposure to an infected person traveling from another hemisphere, such as on a cruise ship or on a package tour, can lead to influenza outbreak at any time or place.

Air-pressure changes during ascent and descent of aircraft can facilitate the development of sinusitis and otitis media. Direct airborne transmission aboard commercial aircraft is unusual because recirculated air passes through a series of filters, and cabin air generally circulates within limited zones or areas of the aircraft. Despite this, influenza, tuberculosis, measles, and other diseases have resulted from transmission in aircraft. Transmission may occur via several pathways, including direct physical contact, fomites, direct droplet spread, and suspended small particles. Intermingling of large numbers of people in locations such as airports, cruise ships, and hotels can also facilitate transmission of respiratory pathogens.

The air quality at many travel destinations may be poor, and exposure to sulfur dioxide, nitrogen dioxide, carbon monoxide, ozone, and particulate matter is associated with a number of health risks, including respiratory tract inflammation, exacerbations of asthma and chronic obstructive pulmonary disease (COPD), impaired lung function, bronchitis, and pneumonia (see Chapter 3, Air Quality & Ionizing Radiation). Certain travelers have a higher risk for respiratory tract infection, including children, the elderly, and people with comorbid pulmonary conditions such as asthma or COPD.

Risk for tuberculosis among most travelers is low (see Chapter 4, Tuberculosis).

## CLINICAL PRESENTATION

Most respiratory infections, especially those of the upper respiratory tract, are mild and not incapacitating. Upper respiratory tract infections often cause rhinorrhea or pharyngitis. Lower respiratory tract infections, particularly pneumonia, can be more severe. Lower respiratory tract infections are more likely than upper respiratory tract infections to cause fever, dyspnea, or chest pain. Cough is often present in either upper or lower respiratory tract infections. People with influenza commonly have acute onset of fever, myalgia, headache, and cough. Consider pulmonary embolism in the differential diagnosis of travelers who present with dyspnea, cough, or pleurisy and fever, especially those who have recently been on long car or plane rides (see Chapter 8, Deep Vein Thrombosis & Pulmonary Embolism).

## DIAGNOSIS

Identifying a specific etiologic agent, especially in the absence of pneumonia or serious disease, is not always clinically necessary. If indicated, the following methods of diagnosis can be used:

- Molecular methods are available to detect a number of respiratory viruses, including influenza virus, parainfluenza virus, adenovirus, human metapneumovirus, and respiratory syncytial virus, and for certain nonviral pathogens.

- Rapid tests are also available to detect some pathogens such as respiratory syncytial virus, influenza virus, *L. pneumophila*, *Histoplasma capsulatum*, and group A *Streptococcus*.

11

- Microbiologic culturing of sputum and blood, although insensitive, can help identify a causative respiratory pathogen.

- Special consideration should be given to diagnosing patients with suspected MERS (www.cdc.gov/coronavirus/mers/interim-guidance.html) or avian influenza (www.cdc.gov/flu/avianflu/healthprofessionals.htm).

## TREATMENT

Travelers with respiratory infections are usually managed similarly to nontravelers, although travelers with progressive or severe illness should be evaluated for illnesses specific to their travel destinations and exposure history. Most respiratory infections are due to viruses, are mild, and do not require specific treatment or antibiotics. Travelers with pneumonia, as established by the presence of an infiltrate on chest radiography, can be treated with antibiotics in accordance with existing guidelines for community-acquired pneumonia. Antiviral treatment is recommended for travelers with influenza who have severe disease or who are at a higher risk for complications; it can be considered for others who present within 48 hours of symptom onset.

## PREVENTION

Vaccines are available to prevent a number of respiratory diseases, including influenza, *S. pneumoniae* infection, *H. influenzae* type B infection (in young children), pertussis, diphtheria, varicella, and measles. Unless contraindicated, travelers should be vaccinated against influenza and be up-to-date on other routine immunizations. Preventing respiratory illness while traveling may not be possible, but common-sense preventive measures include the following:

- Minimizing close contact with people who are coughing and sneezing

- Frequent handwashing, either with soap and water or alcohol-based hand sanitizers (containing ≥60% alcohol) when soap and water are not available

- Using a vasoconstricting nasal spray immediately before air travel if the traveler has a pre-existing eustachian tube dysfunction, which may help lessen the likelihood of otitis or barotrauma

Appropriate infection control measures should be used while managing any patient with a respiratory infection (www.cdc.gov/flu/professionals/infectioncontrol).

### BIBLIOGRAPHY

1. Camps M, Vilella A, Marcos MA, Letang E, Munoz J, Salvado E, et al. Incidence of respiratory viruses among travelers with a febrile syndrome returning from tropical and subtropical areas. J Med Virol. 2008 Apr;80(4):711–15.

2. Chen LH, Han PV, Wilson ME, Stoney RJ, Jentes ES, Benoit C, et al. Self-reported illness among Boston-area international travelers: a prospective study. Travel Med Infect Dis. 2016 Nov–Dec;14(6):604–13.

3. German M, Olsha R, Kristjanson E, Marchand-Austin A, Peci A, Winter AL, et al. Acute respiratory infections in travelers returning from MERS-CoV-affected areas. Emerg Infect Dis. 2015 Sep.;21(9):1654–6.

4. Hertzberg VS, Weiss H, Elon L, Si W, Norris SL, FlyHealthy Research Team. Behaviors, movements, and transmission of droplet-mediated respiratory diseases during transcontinental airline flights. Proc Natl Acad Sci. 2018 Apr 3;115(14):3623–7.

5. Jennings L, Priest PC, Psutka RA, Duncan AR, Anderson T, Mahagamasekera P, et al. Respiratory viruses in airline travellers with influenza symptoms: Results of an airport screening study. J Clin Virol. 2015 Jun;67:8–13.

6. Leder K, Sundararajan V, Weld L, Pandey P, Brown G, Torresi J. Respiratory tract infections in travelers: a review of the GeoSentinel surveillance network. Clin Infect Dis. 2003 Feb 15;36(4):399–406.

7. Leder K, Torresi J, Libman MD, Cramer JP, Castelli F, Schlagenhauf P, et al. GeoSentinel surveillance of illness in returned travelers, 2007–2011. Ann Intern Med. 2013 Mar 19;158(6):456–68.

8. Luna LK, Panning M, Grywna K, Pfefferle S, Drosten C. Spectrum of viruses and atypical bacteria in intercontinental air travelers with symptoms of acute respiratory infection. J Infect Dis. 2007 Mar 1;195(5):675–9.

9. Mandell LA, Wunderink RG, Anzueto A, Bartlett JG, Campbell GD, Dean NC, et al. Infectious Diseases Society of America/American Thoracic Society consensus guidelines on the management of community-acquired pneumonia in adults. *Clin Infect Dis*. 2007 Mar 1;44(Suppl 2):S2772,

11

# PERSISTENT DIARRHEA IN RETURNED TRAVELERS

Bradley A. Connor

Although most cases of travelers' diarrhea are acute and self-limited, a certain percentage of travelers will develop persistent (>14 days) gastrointestinal symptoms (see Chapter 2, Travelers' Diarrhea). The pathogenesis of persistent diarrhea in returned travelers generally falls into one of the following broad categories: 1) ongoing infection or coinfection with a second organism not targeted by initial therapy, 2) previously undiagnosed gastrointestinal disease unmasked by the enteric infection, or 3) a postinfectious phenomenon.

## ONGOING INFECTION

Most cases of travelers' diarrhea are the result of bacterial infection and are short-lived and self-limited. Prolonged diarrheal symptoms can be caused by immunosuppression, sequential infection with diarrheal pathogens, and infection with protozoan parasites. Parasites as a group are the pathogens most likely to be isolated from patients with persistent diarrhea; the probability of a traveler having a protozoal infection (relative to a bacterial infection) increases with increasing duration of symptoms. Parasites may also be the cause of persistent diarrhea in patients already treated for a bacterial pathogen.

*Giardia* is the most likely persistent parasitic pathogen to be encountered. Suspicion for giardiasis should be particularly high when upper gastrointestinal symptoms predominate. Untreated, symptoms may last for months, even in immunocompetent hosts. Stool microscopy, antigen detection, or immunofluorescence are used commonly to make the diagnosis. PCR-based diagnostics (particularly the multiplex DNA extraction PCR) are becoming the diagnostic method of choice to diagnose *Giardia* as well as other protozoan pathogens, including *Cryptosporidium*, *Cyclospora*, and *Entamoeba histolytica*. In the absence of diagnostics, however, and given the high prevalence of *Giardia* in persistent travelers' diarrhea, empiric therapy is a reasonable option in the clinical setting.

Other rare causes of persistent symptoms include the intestinal parasites *Microsporidia*, *Dientamoeba fragilis*, and *Cystoisospora*.

Individual bacterial infections rarely cause persistent symptoms, although ongoing diarrhea has been reported in travelers infected with enteroaggregative or enteropathogenic *Escherichia coli* and among people with diarrhea due to *Clostridioides difficile*. *C. difficile*–associated diarrhea may follow treatment of a bacterial pathogen with a fluoroquinolone or other antibiotic, or even malaria chemoprophylaxis. This is especially important to consider in the patient with persistent travelers' diarrhea that seems refractory to multiple courses of empiric antibiotic therapy. The initial workup of persistent travelers' diarrhea should always include a *C. difficile* stool toxin assay. Treatment of *C. difficile* infection is with oral vancomycin, fidaxomicin, or, less optimally, metronidazole.

Persistent travelers' diarrhea has also been associated with tropical sprue and Brainerd diarrhea. These syndromes are suspected to result from infectious diseases, but specific pathogens have not been identified. Tropical sprue is associated with deficiencies of vitamins absorbed in the proximal and distal small bowel and most commonly affects long-term travelers to, as the name implies, tropical areas. The incidence of tropical sprue appears to have declined dramatically over the past 2 decades and is diagnosed only rarely in travelers. Investigation of an outbreak of Brainerd diarrhea among passengers on a cruise ship to the Galápagos Islands of Ecuador revealed that diarrhea persisted from 7 to more than 42 months and did not respond to antimicrobial therapy. Brainerd diarrhea is one of the persistent mysteries of ongoing diarrhea.

## UNDERLYING GASTROINTESTINAL DISEASE

In some cases, persistence of gastrointestinal symptoms relates to chronic underlying gastrointestinal disease or to a susceptibility unmasked

11

by the enteric infection. Most prominent among these is celiac disease, a systemic disease manifesting primarily with small bowel changes. In genetically susceptible people, villous atrophy and crypt hyperplasia are seen in response to exposure to antigens found in wheat, leading to malabsorption. The diagnosis is made by obtaining serologic tests, including tissue transglutaminase antibodies. A biopsy of the small bowel showing villous atrophy confirms the diagnosis. Treatment is with a gluten-free diet.

Idiopathic inflammatory bowel disease, both Crohn's disease and ulcerative colitis, may be seen after acute bouts of travelers' diarrhea. One prevailing hypothesis is that an initiating exogenous pathogen changes microbiota of the gut, which triggers inflammatory bowel disease in genetically susceptible people. Microscopic colitis may be seen after travelers' diarrhea as well.

Depending on the clinical setting and age group, it may be necessary to do a more comprehensive search for other underlying causes of chronic diarrhea. Consider colorectal cancer in the differential diagnosis of patients passing occult or gross blood rectally or in those with new-onset iron-deficiency anemia.

## POSTINFECTIOUS PHENOMENA

In a certain percentage of patients who present with persistent gastrointestinal symptoms, no specific source will be found. Following an acute diarrheal infection, patients may experience temporary enteropathy characterized by villous atrophy, decreased absorptive surface area, and disaccharidase deficiencies. This can lead to osmotic diarrhea, particularly when large amounts of lactose, sucrose, sorbitol, or fructose are consumed. Use of antimicrobial medications during the initial days of diarrhea may also lead to alterations in intestinal flora and diarrhea symptoms.

Occasionally, the onset of irritable bowel syndrome (IBS) symptoms follows an acute bout of gastroenteritis, so-called postinfectious IBS (PI-IBS). To be labeled PI-IBS, symptoms should follow an episode of gastroenteritis or travelers' diarrhea if the workup for microbial pathogens and underlying gastrointestinal disease is negative. Whether the use of antibiotics to treat acute travelers' diarrhea decreases or increases the likelihood of PI-IBS is unknown.

## EVALUATION

Diagnostics to determine specific microbial etiologies in cases of persistent diarrhea have advanced in the past number of years. Among the most useful tools in microbial diagnosis is the high-throughput multiplex DNA extraction PCR. This technology uses a single stool specimen to detect multiple bacterial, parasitic, and viral enteropathogens simultaneously.

Except in the case of *Cryptosporidium*, these assays have high sensitivity and specificity; however, the clinical ramifications and the economic impact of using these diagnostic molecular panels has yet to be assessed fully. In some cases, molecular testing may detect colonization rather than infection, making it difficult for clinicians interpret and apply the results properly.

Traditional methods of microbial diagnosis have relied on the use of microscopy; 3 or more stool specimens should be examined for ova and parasites, including acid-fast stains for *Cryptosporidium, Cyclospora*, and *Cystoisospora*. Clinicians should also obtain *Giardia* antigen testing, a *C. difficile* toxin assay, and a D-xylose absorption test to determine if nutrients are being properly absorbed. If underlying gastrointestinal disease is suspected, an initial evaluation should include serologic tests for celiac and consideration of inflammatory bowel disease. Subsequently, other studies to visualize both the upper and lower gastrointestinal tracts, with biopsies, may be indicated.

## MANAGEMENT

Dietary modifications may help those with malabsorption. Avoid using antidiarrheal medications (e.g., loperamide or diphenoxylate) to treat children having bloody stools or disease caused by *C. difficile*; use these same drugs cautiously, if at all, in adults. Probiotic medications have been shown to reduce the duration of persistent diarrhea among children in some settings. Antimicrobial medications may be useful in treating persistent diarrhea caused by parasites. Nonabsorbable antibiotics may help if small intestinal bacterial overgrowth accompanies the symptom complex.

11

## BIBLIOGRAPHY

1. Connor BA. Sequelae of traveler's diarrhea: focus on postinfectious irritable bowel syndrome. Clin Infect Dis. 2005 Dec 1;41 (Suppl 8):S577–86.

2. Connor BA. Chronic diarrhea in travelers. Curr Infect Dis Rep. 2013 Jun;15(3):203–10.

3. Connor BA, Rogova M, Whyte O. Use of a multiplex DNA extraction PCR in the identification of pathogens in travelers' diarrhea. J Trav Med. 2018 Jun 1;25(1).

4. Duplessis CA, Gutierrez RL, Porter CK. Review: chronic and persistent diarrhea with a focus in the returning traveler. Trop Dis Travel Med Vaccines. 2017;3(9):1–17.

5. Hanevik K, Dizdar V, Langeland N, Hausken T. Development of functional gastrointestinal disorders after *Giardia lamblia* infection. BMC Gastroenterol 2009 Apr. 21;9:27.

6. Libman MD, Gyorkos TW, Kokoskin E, Maclean JD. Detection of pathogenic protozoa in the diagnostic laboratory: result reproducibility, specimen pooling, and competency assessment. J Clin Microbiol. 2008 Jul;76(7):2200–5.

7. Mintz ED, Weber JT, Guris D, Puhr N, Wells JG, Yashuk JC, et al. An outbreak of Brainerd diarrhea among travelers to the Galapagos Islands. J Infect Dis. 1998 Apr;177(4):1041–5.

8. Norman FF, Perez-Molina J, Perez de Ayala A, Jimenez BC, Navarro M, Lopez-Velez R. *Clostridium difficile*–associated diarrhea after antibiotic treatment for traveler's diarrhea. Clin Infect Dis. 2008 Apr 1;46(7):1060–3.

9. Porter CK, Tribble DR, Aliaga PA, Halvorson HA, Riddle MS. Infectious gastroenteritis and risk of developing inflammatory bowel disease. Gastroenterology. 2008 Sep;135(3):781–6.

10. Schwille-Kiuntke J, Mazurak N, Enck P. Systematic review with meta-analysis: post-infectious irritable bowel syndrome after travellers' diarrhoea. Aliment Pharmacol Ther 2015 Jul;41(11):1029–37.

# NEWLY ARRIVED IMMIGRANTS & REFUGEES

Michelle Russell Hollberg, Hope Pogemiller, Elizabeth D. Barnett

More than 1 million immigrants obtained legal permanent resident status in the United States during fiscal year (FY) 2016 (October 2015–September 2016). There were 5,378 children adopted internationally and 84,989 refugees admitted into the United States during FY 2016. In addition, more than 6 million people entered the United States as nonimmigrant, long-term visitors (including students, temporary workers, and exchange visitors staying longer than 6 months). Some will likely require some form of health care during their stay. US health care professionals are therefore very likely to interact with foreign-born people at some time in their career.

The Immigration and Nationality Act (INA) mandates that all immigrants and refugees undergo a medical screening examination to identify inadmissible health conditions. An authorized panel physician in the applicant's country of origin is responsible for performing the screening examination before departure. Applicants who adjust their immigration status after arriving in the United States undergo a medical screening by a civil surgeon.

A panel physician is a medical doctor practicing outside the United States who has an agreement with a US embassy or consulate general to conduct preimmigration medical screening examinations; >600 panel physicians perform these examinations internationally. A civil surgeon is a US physician authorized by US Citizenship and Immigration Services (USCIS) to perform official immigration medical examinations required for the adjustment of status after arrival in the United States (the process of becoming a permanent US resident). The CDC Division of Global Migration and Quarantine (DGMQ) issues *Technical Instructions* to panel physicians and civil surgeons and monitors the

**11**

quality of the premigration medical examination process.

CDC also issues recommendations for premigration health interventions for special populations, such as refugees (see www.cdc.gov/immigrantrefugeehealth/guidelines/overseas/overseas-guidelines.html). Recommended health interventions (such as treatment for parasitic diseases) are not required under the INA but may be implemented based on level of risk in the origin country.

Although refugees are not required by federal regulations to undergo a repeat medical examination upon arrival in the United States, systems are in place in all states for refugees to receive a health assessment shortly after arrival. CDC's screening guidelines for newly arrived refugees are available at www.cdc.gov/immigrantrefugeehealth/guidelines/domestic/domestic-guidelines.html. Specific protocols may vary by state and are usually available on the websites of the departments of health in the state or region. Any qualified health professional may conduct the health assessment, usually in coordination with resettlement volunteer agencies and local health departments.

In many other cases, health care providers in the United States have medical encounters with migrants who have not received any sort of formal predeparture medical screening examination. These individuals do not hold an immigrant or refugee visa and fall into other categories of temporary visitors and undocumented migrants.

## BEFORE ARRIVAL IN THE UNITED STATES

### Overseas Medical Screening Examination and Treatment

The purpose of the mandated medical screening examination is to detect inadmissible conditions, including communicable diseases of public health significance, mental disorders associated with harmful behavior, and substance-use or substance-induced disorders (www.cdc.gov/immigrantrefugeehealth/exams/ti/panel/technical-instructions-panel-physicians.html). For certain refugee populations, a visit to the panel physician also provides an opportunity for health interventions such as presumptive therapy for parasitic diseases, including intestinal parasite infections and malaria (www.cdc.gov/immigrantrefugeehealth/guidelines/refugee-guidelines.html).

The medical screening examination includes a brief physical exam, a mental health evaluation, serologic testing for syphilis, nucleic acid amplification testing for gonorrhea, a review of vaccination records, and chest radiography followed by acid-fast bacillus smears and sputum cultures if the chest radiograph is consistent with tuberculosis (TB). Chest radiographs are required for all applicants ≥15 years of age. Applicants 2–14 years old from high-TB-burden countries (incidence rate ≥20 cases per 100,000 population as estimated by the World Health Organization) must be tested for TB infection using an interferon-γ release assay (IGRA); chest radiographs are required for those who have a positive IGRA. For people diagnosed with active TB, CDC's *Technical Instructions* require *Mycobacterium tuberculosis* culture, drug-susceptibility testing, and directly observed therapy through the end of treatment before immigration. Treatment is also required before immigration for certain other inadmissible conditions, including syphilis, gonorrhea, and Hansen's disease.

### Proof of Vaccination

#### IMMIGRANTS

Applicants from outside the United States who apply for a US immigrant visa are required to receive all age-appropriate immunizations before immigration. Panel physicians administer vaccines according to CDC's *Vaccine Technical Instructions*. These instructions are based on the Advisory Committee on Immunization Practices (ACIP) recommendations, with some modifications for immigrant populations. For example, immigrants are not required to complete all doses of a multidose vaccine series as long as they have received the next dose in the series before arrival in the United States. Encourage new immigrant arrivals to complete their vaccination schedules according

11

to ACIP recommendations after arrival in the United States. CDC's *Vaccine Technical Instructions* are available at www.cdc.gov/immigrantrefugeehealth/exams/ti/panel/vaccination-panel-technical-instructions.html.

### CHILDREN ADOPTED INTERNATIONALLY

Parents adopting children internationally may request a delay in immunizing children <10 years of age by agreeing to begin immunizations within 30 days of arrival in the United States. Adopting families should be aware that vaccinating children before arrival in the United States reduces the risk of importing diseases of public health concern, such as measles, which was reported in unvaccinated children adopted from China in 2004, 2006, and 2013. For more on the topic of adopting children overseas, see Chapter 7, International Adoption.

### REFUGEES

Refugees are not required to meet the INA immunization requirements before entry into the United States; however, CDC is working with domestic and international migration partners to implement a vaccination program for US refugees. Program updates and population-specific schedules can be found at www.cdc.gov/immigrantrefugeehealth/guidelines/overseas/interventions/immunizations-schedules.html. When applying for permanent US residence, refugees are required to show proof of vaccination to a US civil surgeon during their adjustment of status exam. This occurs typically 1 year after arrival.

### OTHER IMMIGRANTS

Many people will arrive in the United States without having undergone any predeparture medical screening or vaccinations. Ask each patient for his or her health records. Unless documentation is available, do not assume that migrants presenting for care underwent a physical or mental health assessment, laboratory screening for diseases, or are up to date with immunizations.

## Classification of Medical Conditions

Medical conditions of public health significance are categorized into those that preclude an immigrant or refugee from entering the United States (class A) or those that indicate a departure from normal well-being and for which follow-up after arrival is recommended (class B). An immigrant or refugee who has an inadmissible class A condition may still be issued a visa after the illness has been treated or after a waiver of the visa ineligibility has been approved by the Department of Homeland Security United States Citizenship and Immigration Services.

## Notifications and Follow-Up on Arrival

CDC uses the medical screening examination reports and results (collected at US ports of entry when immigrants and refugees arrive) to notify state or local health departments of all arriving refugees and immigrants who have notifiable class A (with waiver) and class B conditions that require follow-up. State and local health departments are asked to report their findings back to CDC, and to provide information about any serious conditions of public health concern identified among recently arrived immigrants and refugees. Such reporting enables CDC to track epidemiologic patterns of disease in recently arrived immigrants and refugees and allows for monitoring of the quality of the overseas medical examinations.

## AFTER ARRIVAL IN THE UNITED STATES: THE NEW ARRIVAL HEALTH ASSESSMENT

A comprehensive new arrival health assessment is an additional opportunity to screen for communicable and noncommunicable diseases, to provide preventive services and individual counseling, to establish ongoing primary care and a medical home, and to orient new arrivals to the US health care system.

Challenges for health professionals in providing comprehensive health assessments for new arrivals include lack of familiarity with predeparture processes and the diseases endemic to a migrant's country of origin, lack of access to trained interpreters, and lack of knowledge of social and cultural beliefs of new migrant groups. Immigrants and refugees often have other priorities related to their new environment,

**11**

such as English classes, school, housing, and work, which may take precedence over accessing health care services. Several organizations can facilitate health assessments for refugees (such as the Association of Refugee Health Coordinators [ARHC]), and networks of clinicians who serve refugees and immigrants are growing.

## Medical Screening

Ideally, each new migrant should receive a complete health assessment that includes screening for migration-associated illnesses plus the age-appropriate screening and health care recommended for anyone residing in the United States. Ensure that migrants who are not recently arrived have completed the screenings associated with the new arrival health assessment, especially for diseases of long latency such as TB, hepatitis B, and HIV; if not, complete any missing tests. It would also be ideal to be able to screen each person for diseases specific to his or her country of origin, migration route, and individual epidemiologic risk. Described below are guidelines available for the 2 populations for which there are the most data to guide screening efforts (refugees and children adopted internationally), followed by an approach to performing health assessments for other categories of immigrants (see Newly Arrived Immigrants & Refugees in this chapter).

### HEALTH ASSESSMENT OF REFUGEES

CDC has developed evidence-based guidelines for health assessments in collaboration with the Department of Health and Human Services Administration for Children and Families' Office of Refugee Resettlement (ORR), clinical and subject matter experts outside of CDC, and representatives of ARHC. The full guidelines and a summary checklist of the new arrival exam components and recommended testing are available at www.cdc.gov/immigrantrefugeehealth/guidelines/domestic/domestic-guidelines.html. CDC has also developed population-specific health profiles for certain populations (e.g., Bhutanese and Congolese refugees); these are available at www.cdc.gov/immigrantrefugeehealth/profiles/index.html.

A function of the new arrival health assessment is to arrange and coordinate ongoing primary care. Many refugees have not had age-appropriate screening for chronic diseases such as heart disease, diabetes, cancer, or hearing, vision, or dental problems; address these needs at early follow-up visits. Several cancers are more prevalent in migrant populations, such as cervical, liver, stomach, and nasopharyngeal cancers. Introduce refugees to age-appropriate cancer screening tests, such as mammography, colonoscopy, and Papanicolaou tests during the new arrival exam. Integrate mental health screening into the new arrival health assessment, as it is an opportunity to screen for acute risk factors and triage refugees in need of urgent mental health treatment.

Refugees may qualify for state Medicaid programs that cover medical screening and any needed ongoing medical care. Refugees determined ineligible for Medicaid are eligible for Refugee Medical Assistance in many states, which provides for their medical care needs for up to 8 months from their date of arrival. For more information, clinicians and refugees can contact their state health departments and can access more information through the ORR, which administers this program (www.acf.hhs.gov/programs/orr/programs/cma).

Other published resources available to clinicians include consensus documents on evidence-based screening for newly arriving refugees to Canada, provided by the Canadian Collaboration for Immigrant and Refugee Health. A list of other resources is available in the online edition of the Yellow Book (see Box 11-2).

### HEALTH ASSESSMENT OF CHILDREN ADOPTED INTERNATIONALLY

There are many similarities in the health conditions found in international adoptees and in refugees. One difference is that refugees generally remain in their own cultural group for some time after arrival and may have limited interactions with the wider community, whereas international adoptees frequently enter households and communities that are clinically naïve to infections common in resource-poor settings. This distinction is particularly pertinent for conditions that may continue to be infectious for

11

BOX 11-2.

# Additional migrant health resources for clinicians

Visit this section in the online edition of the Yellow Book at www.cdc.gov/travel for a comprehensive list of resources for

clinicians and organizations that serve immigrants, refugees, asylum seekers, and international adoptees, including up-to-date

patient care guidelines, online education materials, and print resources.

weeks to months after arrival (such as hepatitis A or B and giardiasis).

Ensure that prospective parents, close family members, and caregivers have all been immunized properly prior to the adoption; this applies equally to those who will travel internationally to meet and bring home the adopted child/children and to those who will be waiting at home. In the *Red Book: Report of the Committee on Infectious Diseases*, the American Academy of Pediatrics (AAP) offers guidance for clinicians who will serve this population after their arrival in the United States. The Red Book may be accessed by AAP members free-of-charge at http://aapredbook.aappublications.org. Most families who adopt children internationally are required to have health insurance for the child effective upon arrival, so funding for the new arrival health assessment poses fewer problems than for other immigrant groups.

## HEALTH ASSESSMENT FOR OTHER IMMIGRANTS

Newly arrived immigrants derive important benefits from their participation in a comprehensive new arrival health assessment and introduction to the US health system. Because immigrants enter the country in so many different ways, they access health care at multiple different points and with providers who have differing levels of expertise in immigrant medicine. There is no formal mechanism or funding source available to cover the costs of a standard comprehensive health assessment. Immigrants may never receive any health assessment that targets conditions they may have acquired in their country of birth or during their migration process unless every health

professional assumes the responsibility and has the knowledge to assess these issues when caring for patients born outside the United States. A list of screening tests that should be considered for immigrant health assessments is included in Table 11-8.

Record all known medical and family history, and discuss medications and treatments received prior to migration. Most experts agree that testing for TB, hepatitis B, and HIV should be performed for all new arrivals to the United States who do not have documentation of prior screening. Make a habit of ensuring that this screening is completed for every new foreign-born patient seen, regardless of time since that person's arrival in this country.

Obtain any records, laboratory evidence of immunity, and history of vaccine-preventable diseases; give, and age-appropriate vaccines be given as indicated. Vaccine series do not need to be restarted if documentation of prior doses is available.

Adding a basic mental health screening to the assessment (including gathering information about coping strategies and support systems) permits appropriate and timely referral to resources, if necessary. A complete blood count with differential for most new arrivals facilitates making a diagnosis of anemia or eosinophilia, or finding evidence of hemoglobinopathy. A urinalysis and basic metabolic panel may be indicated, especially for those of appropriate age or with evidence of conditions such as renal disease or diabetes. Immigrant health care providers should continue to follow the age- and risk-based guidelines provided by the United States Preventive Services Task Force (USPSTF) for the

## Table 11-8. Recommended new arrival laboratory screening tests for immigrants receiving medical care in the United States

| TEST | AGE | POPULATION | COMMENTS |
|------|-----|------------|----------|
| Tuberculosis:IGRA TST | >5 years <br> <5 years | All | Test based on standard guidelines. |
| HIV | >13 years[1] | All | Test based on standard guidelines. |
| Hepatitis B: surface antigen | All | Where prevalence of hepatitis B infection in home country is >2% | Consider surface antibody if unimmunized. May consider core antibody. Follow current recommendations for refugees. |
| STDs (syphilis, gonorrhea, chlamydia, others as indicated) | 15–65 years or <15 if sexually active | All | Test choice based on standard guidelines. Consider for all immigrants, taking into account the migration history and if it adds increased risk. |
| CBC with differential and MCV | All | All | Screen for chronic anemias; look for absolute eosinophilia (possibly evidence of parasitic infection). |
| Serology for parasites: schistosomiasis strongyloidiasis other soil transmitted helminths | All | Where endemic if high risk of exposure | Consider screening with exposure history, unexplained eosinophilia. Some experts choose to treat empirically. Empiric treatment is recommended when at-risk immigrant is about to receive steroids or become immunocompromised, if testing is unavailable or when there is insufficient time to obtain results. |
| Malaria | All | Where malaria is endemic | Consider malaria if from highly endemic area within 3–6 months of arrival. |
| Blood lead level | <16 years or if clinical indication | All | Consider if never had a lead test and have additional risks: lived in a highly industrialized city with potential exposure to industrial waste, has a developmental delay, or has medical conditions consistent with lead exposure. |
| Varicella antibody | >5 years | All (especially if history of varicella and older children and adults) | |
| Urinalysis, basic metabolic panel | All adults or if clinical | All | Screening for renal failure and schistosomiasis (if from an endemic area). |

Abbreviations: IGRA, interferon-γ release assay; TST, tuberculin skin test; STD, sexually transmitted disease; CBC, complete blood count; MCV, mean corpuscular volume
[1] Consider in younger children who have signs or symptoms of disease, risk factors for transmission, or mother is missing or deceased or has illness compatible with HIV.

11

general US population when continuing to care for immigrant patients over time. Consider diagnostic testing if an immigrant presents with symptoms consistent with a particular parasite endemic to their country of origin (e.g., malaria, intestinal parasites). STD screening (syphilis, gonorrhea, chlamydia, HIV) beyond what may be recommended for the US general population should be considered for immigrants if their migration history places them at significant risk.

Immigrants who travel back to their country of origin may be at higher risk of travel-related infectious diseases (see Chapter 9, Visiting Friends & Relatives: VFR Travel). Thus, travel vaccines can be considered in addition to age-appropriate vaccinations for these immigrants.

## BIBLIOGRAPHY

1. Barnett ED. Immunizations and infectious disease screening for internationally adopted children. Pediatr Clin North Am. 2005 Oct;52(5):1287–309, vi.

2. CDC. Vitamin B12 deficiency in resettled Bhutanese refugees—United States, 2008–2011. MMWR Morb Mortal Wkly Rep. 2011 Mar 25;60(11):343–6.

3. CDC. Technical instructions for panel physicians. Atlanta: CDC; 2018 [cited 2018 Mar 17]. Available from: www.cdc.gov/immigrantrefugeehealth/exams/ti/panel/technical-instructions-panelphysicians.html.

4. Lowenthal P, Westenhouse J, Moore M, Posey DL, Watt JP, Flood J. Reduced importation of tuberculosis after the implementation of an enhanced pre-immigration screening protocol. Int J Tuberc Lung Dis. 2011 Jun;15(6):761–6.

5. Maloney SA, Fielding KL, Laserson KF, Jones W, Nguyen TN, Dang QA, et al. Assessing the performance of overseas tuberculosis screening programs: a study among US-bound immigrants in Vietnam. Arch Intern Med. 2006 Jan 23;166(2):234–40.

6. Miller LC. International adoption: infectious diseases issues. Clin Infect Dis. 2005 Jan 15;40(2):286–93.

7. Minnesota Department of Health. Lead poisoning in Minnesota refugee children, 2000–2002. Disease Control Newsletter [Internet]; 2004 [cited 2016 Sep 28]; 32(2):13–15. Available from: www.health.state.mn.us/divs/idepc/newsletters/dcn/2004/0402dcn.pdf.

8. Nyangoma EN, Olson CK, Benoit SR, Bos J, Debolt C, Kay M, et al. Measles outbreak associated with adopted children from China—Missouri, Minnesota, and Washington, July 2013. MMWR Morb Mortal Wkly Rep. 2014 Apr 11;63(14):301–4.

9. Office of Immigration Statistics. Yearbook of immigration statistics: 2016. Washington, DC: US Department of Homeland Security; 2016. [cited 2018 Mar 17]. Available from: www.dhs.gov/yearbook-immigration-statistics.

10. Posey DL, Blackburn BG, Weinberg M, Flagg EW, Ortega L, Wilson M, et al. High prevalence and presumptive treatment of schistosomiasis and strongyloidiasis among African refugees. Clin Infect Dis. 2007 Nov 15;45(10):1310–15.

11. Posey DL, Naughton MP, Willacy EA, Russell M, Olson CK, Godwin CM, et al. Implementation of new TB screening requirements for U.S.-bound immigrants and refugees—2007–2014. MMWR Morb Mortal Wkly Rep. 2014 Mar 21;63(11):234–6.

12. Pottie K, Greenaway C, Feightner J, Welch V, Swinkels H, Rashid M, et al. Evidence-based clinical guidelines for immigrants and refugees. CMAJ. 2011 Sep 6;183(12):E824–925.

13. Walker PF, Barnett ED, editors. Immigrant Medicine. Philadelphia: Saunders Elsevier; 2007.

**11**

# Appendices

## APPENDIX A: PROMOTING QUALITY IN THE PRACTICE OF TRAVEL MEDICINE

Keun Lee, Stephen M. Ostroff

Travel medicine remains a young area of medical practice, even as the field continues to mature based on a growing body of scientific and medical information. There is only a limited number of recognized travel medicine specialty or subspecialty programs around the world and none in the United States. Thus, clinicians offering travel medicine services are not "board certified" in travel medicine and are instead certified in other disciplines such as infectious diseases, internal medicine, pediatrics, nursing, pharmacy, and family practice. Clinics in the United States that offer travel medicine services are also not specifically credentialed for this activity. However, training opportunities and certification programs are available for interested clinicians through travel medicine professional organizations.

Although research on quality of travel health care is limited, several studies suggest that travelers who visit a clinician with training in travel medicine are more likely to receive pretravel and posttravel advice and care than those who see clinicians without such training. The 2006 guidelines on travel medicine published by the Infectious Diseases Society of America also recommend travelers seek pretravel and posttravel care from a clinician with expertise in travel medicine. This is especially important for travelers who are going to exotic destinations, engaging in adventure travel, or have special needs or preexisting medical conditions.

Providers can pursue training in travel medicine through a number of professional organizations. Providers may also look to the courses hosted by members of the International Society of Travel Medicine (ISTM), notably those in the United States, Canada, Ireland, Scotland, and Switzerland. They vary in length from days to a year, depending upon the depth of the course and credential offered. Many people looking for training beyond the textbook may do so informally by spending time in a travel clinic learning how to provide a pretravel consultation. Posttravel care typically involves infectious disease and tropical medicine training.

Below is a partial list of resources for clinicians who wish to enhance their knowledge of travel medicine. People seeking travel-related medical services may want to inquire whether their provider or clinic participates in these organizations or activities.

# TRAVEL MEDICINE–RELATED PROFESSIONAL ORGANIZATIONS

## International Society of Travel Medicine (ISTM)

Founded in 1991, ISTM (www.istm.org) is a multinational organization dealing exclusively with travel medicine. ISTM has >3,500 members worldwide.

ISTM activities include the following:

- *Journal of Travel Medicine*

- An active listserv (TravelMed) where members share information and can ask questions

- Special-interest groups that include travel medicine nurses and travel medicine pharmacists

- A biennial travel medicine meeting and annual regional submeetings

- A directory of domestic and international travel clinics affiliated with ISTM members in 65 countries

- An online learning curriculum of >60 programs that cover a wide range of topics and webinars on selected topics

- ISTM Travel Medicine Continuing Professional Development Program

- An examination leading to a Certificate of Knowledge in Travel Medicine, available to physicians, nurses, pharmacists, and other professionals offering travel advice

The ISTM Body of Knowledge, which covers the scope of the specialty of travel medicine, forms the basis for Certificate of Knowledge in Travel Medicine examination questions. It is regularly updated by the ISTM Exam Committee. Content areas in the Body of Knowledge include the following:

- Epidemiology related to travel medicine

- Immunology and vaccinology (including travel-related vaccines)
  - Pretravel consultation and management
  - Patient evaluation
  - Travelers with special needs
  - Special itineraries
  - Prevention and self-treatment
  - Risk communication

- Diseases contracted during travel
  - Vectorborne diseases
  - Diseases transmitted from person to person
  - Foodborne and waterborne diseases
  - Diseases related to bites and stings
  - Diseases due to environmental hazards

- Other conditions associated with travel
  - Conditions occurring during or after travel
  - Conditions due to environmental factors
  - Threats to personal safety and security
  - Psychocultural issues

- Posttravel assessment

- General travel medicine issues
  - Medical care abroad
  - Travel clinic management
  - Travel medicine information resources

The Certificate of Knowledge in Travel Medicine examination has been administered since 2003. The society hosts periodic 2-day intensive exam preparation courses open to all qualified professionals (such as physicians, nurses, pharmacists, and physician assistants) who provide travel health–related services. Those who successfully pass the examination are awarded a Certificate in Travel Health (CTH). Beginning with CTHs awarded in 2011, the certificate is good for 10 years, and the awardee must be recertified either through professional development activities or by retaking the examination. Currently there are >2,500 CTH holders from 67 countries. Practitioners offering travel medicine services or interested in the subject should consider membership in ISTM. ISTM member practitioners are listed on the organization's website, and those who have the CTH are designated as such. More than 1,000 members who have passed the exam are listed on the ISTM website

ISTM also offers research programs. These include research grants, travel awards, and support for such efforts as the GeoSentinel Global Surveillance Network (see Chapter 1, Travel Epidemiology).

A

## American Society of Tropical Medicine and Hygiene (ASTMH)

Formed in 1951 through the merger of predecessor organizations dating back to 1903, ASTMH (www.astmh.org) has a subsection that deals exclusively with tropical and travel medicine, known as the American Committee on Clinical Tropical Medicine and Travelers' Health.

ASTMH activities include the following:

- *The American Journal of Tropical Medicine and Hygiene*

- An annual meeting

- An electronic distribution list

- A tropical and travel medicine consultant directory

- A biennial examination leading to a Certificate of Knowledge in Clinical Tropical Medicine and Travelers' Health, available to those with a current professional health care license and who have passed an ASTMH-approved tropical medicine diploma course or have sufficient tropical medicine experience

The content areas of the ASTMH Certificate of Knowledge in Clinical Tropic Medicine and Travelers' Health are as follows:

- Basic science and fundamentals

- Infectious and tropical diseases (including parasites, bacteria, fungi, and viruses)

- Other diseases and conditions

- Diagnostic and therapeutic approach to clinical syndromes

- Travelers' health

- Public health in the tropics

- Epidemiology and control of disease

- Laboratory diagnosis

More than 900 people have passed the ASTMH examination and have received their CTropMed certificate. The society offers an annual intensive update course in clinical tropical medicine and travelers' health designed to prepare those planning to take the Certificate of Knowledge examination.

## Wilderness Medical Society

Organized in 1983, this society (www.wms.org) focuses on adventure travel, including wilderness travel and diving medicine. Its activities include the following:

- The journal *Wilderness and Environmental Medicine*

- Practice guidelines for emergency care in wilderness settings

- Annual meetings, a world congress, and subspecialty meetings

- Courses leading to certification in advanced wilderness life support

- Participation in courses that lead to a diploma in mountain medicine

- A wilderness medical curriculum that, when successfully completed, qualifies members for fellowship in the Academy of Wilderness Medicine

## Infectious Diseases Society of America (IDSA)

IDSA (www.idsociety.org) is the largest organization representing infectious disease clinicians in the United States. Although IDSA deals with all infectious diseases, it has many active members with expertise in tropical and travel medicine or strong interests in these disciplines. In 2006, IDSA published extensive evidence-based guidelines on the practice of travel medicine in the United States. IDSA also publishes travel-related research in its journals: *The Journal of Infectious Diseases, Clinical Infectious Diseases*, and *Open Forum Infectious Diseases.*

## International Society for Infectious Diseases (ISID)

ISID (www.isid.org) was formed in 1986 and has approximately 90,000 members in 155 countries around the world. Like IDSA, ISID does not specifically focus on travel medicine. However, its international reach, particularly in low-resource countries, makes travel medicine an important topic in ISID and a valuable source of information for infectious diseases clinicians in many overseas travel destinations. Activities relevant to travel medicine that are supported by ISID include the following:

- *International Journal of Infectious Diseases*

- The biennial meeting International Congress on Infectious Diseases

- International Meeting on Emerging Diseases and Surveillance

- The Program for Monitoring Emerging Diseases (ProMED), an open-source electronic reporting system for reports of emerging infectious diseases and toxins, including outbreaks (www.promedmail.org)

- EpiCore global outbreak surveillance system

## Aerospace Medical Association (ASMA)

This organization (www.asma.org) represents professionals in the fields of aviation, space, and environmental medicine who deal with air and space travelers. Its activities include the following:

- The journal *Aviation, Space, and Environmental Medicine*

- Annual scientific meeting

- Continuing medical education and certification in topics related to aerospace medicine

In addition to these professional societies, the World Health Organization maintains a list of regional and national societies of travel medicine on its website (www.who.int/ith/links/national_societies/en/).

### BIBLIOGRAPHY

1. Boddington NL, Simons H, Launders N, Hill DR. Quality improvement in travel medicine: a programme for yellow fever vaccination centres in England, Wales and Northern Ireland. Qual Prim Care 2011 Jan;19(6):391–8.

2. Chiodini JH, Anderson E, Driver C, Field VK, Flaherty GT, Grieve AM, et al. Recommendations for the practice of travel medicine. Travel Med Infect Dis. 2012 May;10(3):109–28.

3. Hill DR, Ericsson CD, Pearson RD, Keystone JS, Freedman DO, Kozarsky PE, et al. The practice of travel medicine: guidelines by the Infectious Diseases Society of America. Clin Infect Dis. 2006 Dec 15;42(12):1499–539.

4. Kozarsky P. The Body of Knowledge for the practice of travel medicine—2006. J Travel Med 2006 Sep–Oct;13(5):251–4.

5. Kozarsky PE, Steffen R. Travel medicine education-what are the needs? J Travel Med. 2016 Jul;23(5); doi: 10.1093/jtm/taw039.

6. LaRocque RC, Jentes ES. Health recommendations for international travel: a review of the evidence base of travel medicine. Curr Opin Infect Dis. 2011 Oct;24(5):403–9.

7. Leder K, Bouchard O, Chen LH. Training in travel medicine and general practitioners: a long-haul journey! J Travel Med. 2015 Nov–Dec;22(6):357–60.

8. Ruis JR, van Rijckevorsel GG, van den Hoek A, Koeman SC, Sonder GJ. Does registration of professionals improve the quality of travelers' health advice? J Travel Med. 2009 Jun–Aug;16(4):263–6.

9. Schlagenhauf P, Santos-O'Connor F, Parola P. The practice of travel medicine in Europe. Clin Microbiol Infect. 2010 Mar;16(3):203–8.

10. Sistenich V. International emergency medicine: how to train for it. Emerg Med Australas. 2012 Aug;24(4):435–41.

A

# APPENDIX B: TRAVEL VACCINE SUMMARY TABLE

Johanzynn Gatewood

Table B-1 is a quick reference for administering or prescribing travel-related vaccines. Before administering any vaccine, please pay particular attention to the dose and whether it is to be administered intramuscularly or subcutaneously. Also review detailed instructions, contraindications, precautions, and side effects under the specific vaccines discussed in this book or in the manufacturer's prescribing information. For other immunizations, refer to the corresponding disease section in Chapter 4.

## Table B-1. Travel vaccine summary

| VACCINE | TRADE NAME (MANUFACTURER) | AGE | DOSE | ROUTE | SCHEDULE | BOOSTER |
|---|---|---|---|---|---|---|
| Cholera CVD 103-HgR vaccine | Vaxchora (PaxVax) | 18–64 y | 100 mL (reconstituted) | Oral | 1 dose[1] | Undetermined[2] |
| Hepatitis A vaccine, inactivated | Havrix (GlaxoSmithKline) | 1–18 y<br>≥19 y | 0.5 mL (720 ELISA units)<br>1 mL (1,440 ELISA units) | IM<br>IM | 0 and 6–12 mo<br>0 and 6–12 mo | None<br>None |
| Hepatitis A vaccine, inactivated | Vaqta (Merck & Co., Inc.) | 1–18 y<br>≥19 y | 0.5 mL (25 U)<br>1 mL (50 U) | IM<br>IM | 0 and 6–18 mo<br>0 and 6–18 mo | None<br>None |
| Hepatitis B vaccine, recombinant with novel adjuvant (1018) | Heplisav-B (Dynavax Technologies Corp.) | >18 | 0.5 mL (20 μg HBsAg and 3,000 μg of 1018) | IM | 0, 1 mo | None |
| Hepatitis B vaccine, recombinant[3] | Engerix-B (GlaxoSmithKline) | 0–19 y<br>0–10 y (accelerated)<br>11–19 y (accelerated)<br>≥20 y (primary)<br>≥20 y (accelerated) | 0.5 mL (10 μg HBsAg)<br>0.5 mL (10 μg HBsAg)<br>1 mL (20 μg HBsAg)<br>1 mL (20 μg HBsAg)<br>1 mL (20 μg HBsAg) | IM<br>IM<br>IM<br>IM<br>IM | 0, 1, 6 mo<br>0, 1, 2 mo<br>0, 1, 2 mo<br>0, 1, 6 mo<br>0, 1, 2 mo | None<br>12 mo<br>12 mo<br>None<br>12 mo |
| Hepatitis B vaccine, recombinant[3] | Recombivax HB (Merck & Co., Inc.) | 0–19 y (primary)<br>11–15 y (adolescent accelerated)<br>≥20 y (primary) | 0.5 mL (5 μg HBsAg)<br>1 mL (10 μg HBsAg)<br>1 mL (10 μg HBsAg) | IM<br>IM<br>IM | 0, 1, 6 mo<br>0, 4–6 mo<br>0, 1, 6 mo | None<br>None<br>None |
| Combined hepatitis A and hepatitis B vaccine | Twinrix (GlaxoSmithKline) | ≥18 y (primary)<br>≥18 y (accelerated) | 1 mL (720 ELU HAV + 20 μg HBsAg)<br>1 mL (720 ELU HAV + 20 μg HBsAg) | IM<br>IM | 0, 1, 6 mo<br>0, 7, and 21–30 d | None<br>12 mo |

A

| Vaccine | Product | Age | Dose | Route | Schedule | Booster |
|---|---|---|---|---|---|---|
| Japanese encephalitis vaccine, inactivated | Ixiaro (Valneva) | 2 mo–2 y<br>3–17 y<br>18–65 y<br>>65 y | 0.25 mL<br>0.5 mL<br>0.5 mL<br>0.5 mL | IM<br>IM<br>IM<br>IM | 0, 28 d<br>0, 28 d<br>0, 7–28 d<br>0, 28 d | ≥1 year after primary series[4]<br>≥1 year after primary series[4]<br>≥1 year after primary series[4]<br>≥1 year after primary series[4] |
| Meningococcal (serogroups A, C, W, and Y) polysaccharide diphtheria toxoid conjugate vaccine (MenACWY-D)[5] | Menactra (Sanofi Pasteur) | 9–23 mo<br>≥2 y | 0.5 mL<br>0.5 mL | IM<br>IM | 0, 3 mo<br>1 dose[6] | If at continued risk[7] |
| Meningococcal (serogroups A, C, W, and Y) oligosaccharide diphtheria CRM197 conjugate vaccine (MenACWY-CRM)[5] | Menveo (GSK) | 2 mo<br>7–23 mo<br>≥2 y | 0.5 mL<br>0.5 mL<br>0.5 mL | IM<br>IM<br>IM | 0, 2, 4, 10 mo<br>0, 3 mo (2nd dose administered in 2nd year of life)<br>1 dose[6] | If at continued risk[7] |
| Polio vaccine, inactivated | Ipol (Sanofi Pasteur) | ≥18 y | 0.5 mL | SC or IM | 1 dose if patient has completed a pediatric series | Repeat boosters may be needed for long-term travelers to polio-affected countries; see Chapter 4, Polio |
| Rabies vaccine (human diploid cell) | Imovax (Sanofi Pasteur) | Any | 1 mL | IM | Preexposure series: days 0, 7, and 21 or 28 d | None; see Chapter 4, Rabies for postexposure immunization |
| Rabies vaccine (purified chick embryo cell) | RabAvert (Novartis) | Any | 1 mL | IM | Preexposure series: days 0, 7, and 21 or 28 d | None; see Chapter 4, Rabies for postexposure immunization |

(continued)

# Table B-1. Travel vaccine summary (continued)

| VACCINE | TRADE NAME (MANUFACTURER) | AGE | DOSE | ROUTE | SCHED-ULE | BOOSTER |
|---|---|---|---|---|---|---|
| Typhoid vaccine (oral, live, attenuated) | Vivotif (PaxVax) | ≥6 y | 1 capsule[8] | Oral | 0, 2, 4, 6 d | Repeat primary series after 5 y |
| Typhoid vaccine (Vi capsular polysaccharide) | Typhim Vi (Sanofi Pasteur) | ≥2 y | 0.5 mL | IM | 1 dose | 2 y |
| 17D yellow fever vaccine | YF-Vax (Sanofi Pasteur) | ≥9 mo[9] | 0.5 mL[10] | SC | 1 dose | Not recommended for most[11] |

Abbreviations: ACIP, Advisory Committee on Immunization Practices; ELU, ELISA units of inactivated HAV; HAV, hepatitis A virus; HBsAg, hepatitis B surface antigen; IM, intramuscular; U, units HAV antigen; SC, subcutaneous.

[1] Must be administered in a health care setting.

[2] In a clinical trial, vaccine efficacy was 90% at 10 days postvaccination and declined to 80% at 3 months postvaccination in prevention of severe diarrhea after oral cholera challenge. Long-term immunogenicity is unknown. Clinicians advising travelers who are at continued or repeated risk over an extended period may consider revaccination, although the appropriate interval and efficacy are unknown.

[3] Consult the prescribing information for differences in dosing for hemodialysis and other immunocompromised patients.

[4] If potential for Japanese encephalitis virus exposure continues.

[5] If an infant is receiving the vaccine before travel, 2 doses may be administered as early as 8 weeks apart.

[6] For people with HIV, anatomic or functional asplenia, and people with persistent complement component deficiencies (C3, C5-9, properdin, factor D, and factor H or people taking eculizumab [Soliris]) should receive a 2-dose primary series 8–12 weeks apart.

[7] Revaccination with meningococcal conjugate vaccine (MenACWY-D or MenACWY-CRM) is recommended after 3 years for children who received their last dose at <7 years of age. Revaccination with meningococcal conjugate vaccine is recommended after 5 years for people who received their last dose at ≥7 years of age, and every 5 years thereafter for people who are at continued risk.

[8] Must be kept refrigerated at 35.6°F–46.4°F (2°C–8°C); administer with cool liquid no warmer than 98.6°F (37°C).

[9] Ages 6–8 months and ≥60 years are precautions and age <6 months is a contraindication to the use of yellow fever vaccine.

[10] YF-Vax is available in single-dose and multiple-dose (5-dose) vials.

[11] For full details regarding revaccination, see "Vaccine Administration" in Chapter 4, Yellow Fever.

A

# APPENDIX C: DEATH DURING TRAVEL

Francisco Alvarado-Ramy, Kendra E. Stauffer

Death of a friend, relative, or coworker can be immensely distressing. The situation is aggravated when death occurs abroad, where grieving people may be unfamiliar with local processes, language, and culture. Whether dealing with the death locally or from their home country, next of kin could face large, unanticipated costs, and labor-intensive administrative steps. Depending on the circumstances surrounding the dead, some countries may require an autopsy. Besides relatives, sources of support include the local consulate or embassy, travel insurance provider, tour operator, faith-based and aid organizations, and the deceased's employer. There likely will need to be an official identification of the body. A body can be identified by witness statements of those who knew the person well, analyzing DNA samples, checking fingerprints, reviewing dental radiographs, or inspecting surgical implants.

## DEATH ONBOARD A CONVEYANCE

The Federal Aviation Administration requires that flight attendants receive training in cardiopulmonary resuscitation (CPR) and in proper use of an automated external defibrillator (AED) at least once every 2 years. Under federal law, there are Good Samaritan protections for actions brought in a federal or state court resulting out of acts or omissions when people assist in a medical emergency during flight unless there is gross negligence or willful misconduct. If CPR is performed in the aircraft cabin, once it has been continued for 30 minutes or longer with no signs of life within this period, and no shocks advised by an AED, the person may be presumed dead and resuscitation efforts halted. Airlines may choose to specify additional criteria, depending upon the availability of ground-to-air medical consultation service or a physician aboard.

Cruise ships are usually better equipped than aircraft and carry medical professionals to provide clinical care. If the death occurs on a cruise ship despite medical interventions, the crew are usually able to provide logistic support to repatriate the body. Cruise ships are equipped with morgues and carry body bags.

US regulations require that all deaths aboard commercial flights and ships destined for the United States be reported to CDC.

## OBTAINING DEPARTMENT OF STATE ASSISTANCE

When a US citizen dies outside the United States, the deceased person's next of kin or legal representative should notify US consular officials at the Department of State. Consular personnel are available 24 hours a day, 7 days a week, to provide assistance to US citizens for overseas emergencies.

- If the next of kin or legal representative is in the foreign country with the deceased US citizen, he or she should contact the nearest US embassy or consulate for assistance. Contact information for US embassies, consulates, and consular agencies overseas may be found at the Department of State website (www.usembassy.gov).

- If a family member, domestic partner, or legal representative is in a different country from the deceased person, he or she should call the Department of State's Office of Overseas Citizens Services in Washington, DC, from 8 AM to 5 PM Eastern time, Monday through Friday, at 888-407-4747 (toll-free) or 202-501-4444. For emergency assistance after working hours or on weekends and holidays, call the Department of State switchboard at 202-647-4000 and ask to speak with the Overseas Citizens Services duty officer. In addition, the US embassy closest to or in the country where the US citizen died can provide assistance (www.usembassy.gov).

The Department of State has no funds to assist in the return of remains of US citizens who die abroad. US consular officers assist the next of kin by conveying instructions to the appropriate offices within the foreign country and providing information to the family on how to transmit the necessary private funds to cover the costs of preparing and repatriating human remains. The process can be expensive and lengthy. Upon issuance of a local (foreign) death certificate, the nearest US embassy or consulate may prepare a consular report of the death of an American abroad. Copies of that report are provided to the next of kin or legal representative and may be used in US courts to settle estate matters. If there is no next of kin or legal representative in-country, a consular officer will act as a provisional conservator of the deceased's personal effects.

## IMPORTATION OF HUMAN REMAINS FOR INTERMENT OR CREMATION

### General Guidance

Except for cremated remains, human remains intended for interment (placement in a grave or tomb) or cremation after entry into the United States must be accompanied by a death certificate stating the cause of death. A death certificate is an official document signed by a coroner, health care provider, or other official authorized to make a declaration of cause of death. Death certificates written in a language other than English must be accompanied by an English translation. If a death certificate is not available in time for returning the remains, the US embassy or consulate should provide a consular mortuary certificate stating whether the person died from a disease classified as quarantinable in the United States (www.cdc.gov/quarantine/aboutlawsregulationsquarantineisolation.html). Any requirements of the country of origin, air carrier, US Customs and Border Protection, and the Transportation Security Administration must also be met (https://help.cbp.gov/app/answers/detail/a_id/237/~/requirements-for-importing-bodies-in-coffins-%2F-ashes-in-urns). CDC regulates the importation of human remains and provides guidance for their importation (www.cdc.gov/quarantine/human-remains.html). The requirements are more stringent if the person died from a disease classified as quarantinable in the United States.

## EXPORTATION OF HUMAN REMAINS

CDC does not regulate the exportation of human remains outside the United States, although other state and local regulations may apply. The United States Postal Service is the only courier authorized to ship cremated remains. Exporters of human remains and travelers taking human remains out of the United States should be aware that the importation requirements of the destination country and the air carrier must be met. Information regarding these requirements may be obtained from the foreign embassy or consulate (www.state.gov/s/cpr/rls) and the air carrier.

### BIBLIOGRAPHY

1. Advisory circular: emergency medical equipment training. AC No. 121-34B. Washington, DC: Federal Aviation Administration, 2006. Available from: www.faa.gov/documentLibrary/media/Advisory_Circular/AC121-34B.pdf.

2. Bureau of Consular Affairs, US State Department. Death abroad. Washington, DC: US Department of State; 2014 [cited 2018 Feb 23]. Available from: https://travel.state.gov/content/passports/en/abroad/events-and-records/death.html.

3. Bureau of Consular Affairs, US State Department. Return of remains of deceased US citizens.

Washington, DC: US Department of State; 2014 [cited 2018 Feb 23]. Available from: https://travel.state.gov/content/travel/en/international-travel/while-abroad/death-abroad1/return-of-remains-of-deceased-us-citizen.html.

4. CDC. Quarantine station contact list, map, and fact sheets. Atlanta: CDC; 2013 [cited 2018 Feb 23]. Available from: www.cdc.gov/quarantine/quarantinestationcontactlistfull.html.

5. CDC. Guidance for importation of human remains into the United States for interment or subsequent cremation. Atlanta: CDC; 2014 [cited 2018 Feb 23].

A

Available from: www.cdc.gov/quarantine/human-remains.html.

6. CDC. Specific laws and regulations governing the control of communicable diseases. Atlanta: CDC; 2014 [cited 2018 Feb 23]. Available from: www.cdc.gov/quarantine/specificlawsregulations.html.

7. Connolly R, Prendiville R, Cusack D, Flaherty G. Repatriation of human remains following death in international travelers. J Travel Med. 2017 Mar 1;24(2):1–6.

8. International Air Transport Association. Death on Board; 2016 [cited 2018 Feb 28]. Available from: www.iata.org/whatwedo/safety/health/Documents/death-on-board-guidelines.pdf.

9. National Funeral Directors Association. Shipping remains from the United States to a foreign country. Brookfield, WI: National Funeral Directors Association; c2014 [cited 2018 Feb 23]. Available from: www.nfda.org/resources/operations-management/shipping-remains.

10. U.S. Customs and Border Protection. Requirements for importing bodies in coffins/ashes in urns. Washington, DC: US Department of Homeland Security; 2015 [cited 2018 Feb 23]. Available from: https://help.cbp.gov/app/answers/detail/a_id/237/~/requirements-for-importing-bodies-in-coffins-%2F-ashes-in-urns.

**A**

# APPENDIX D: AIRPLANES & CRUISE SHIPS: ILLNESS & DEATH REPORTING & PUBLIC HEALTH INTERVENTIONS

Rebecca Hall, Kara Tardivel, Robynne Jungerman, Clive Brown

## FEDERAL REGULATIONS GOVERNING THE CONTROL OF COMMUNICABLE DISEASES

CDC has a regulatory mission to protect US public health by preventing the introduction, transmission, and spread of communicable diseases from foreign countries into and within the states or territories of the United States. As part of a range of authorized public health activities, presidential executive orders specify the diseases for which CDC may issue a federal public health order; that is, a federal quarantine, isolation, or conditional release order (cholera, diphtheria, infectious tuberculosis, plague, smallpox, yellow fever, viral hemorrhagic fevers, new or emerging types of influenza, and severe acute respiratory syndromes). The list of federally quarantinable diseases can be revised by executive order if an emerging infectious disease that is not on the list becomes a public health threat.

For more information on specific laws and regulations governing the control of communicable diseases, see www.cdc.gov/quarantine/specificlawsregulations.html.

## CDC ACTIONS BEFORE, DURING, AND AFTER TRAVEL TO PROTECT THE PUBLIC'S HEALTH

CDC conducts public health actions before, during, and after commercial aviation and maritime travel to prevent and mitigate the introduction and spread of diseases of public health concern into communities in the United States. Many of these actions are carried out by CDC staff working at quarantine stations located at or near the US ports of entry through which the majority of travelers transit.

### Before Travel

A health authority may notify CDC that a person with a communicable disease of public health concern is planning to travel on commercial flight. In 2007, CDC and the US Department of Homeland Security developed a public health do not board (DNB) list that prevents issuance of a boarding pass to any flight originating or landing at a US airport. US and international public health officials can recommend adding a person to the list if he or she has (or has been exposed to) a communicable disease that poses a public health threat during travel and meets specific criteria.

### During Travel

Regulations mandate that the person in charge of a conveyance destined for a US port report before arrival any death or "ill person" (as defined in the regulation) among passengers or crew members to the CDC quarantine station at or nearest the port of entry. The definition of an ill person on an airplane or maritime vessel—which applies to all travelers, including crew and passengers, US citizens or non-US citizens—is detailed in Table 12-2.

CDC quarantine station staff receives most illness and death reports during travel on airplanes from the airlines or from emergency medical personnel at the arrival airport. Most non-gastrointestinal illness and death reports on cruise ships are received directly from the vessel's medical staff. Reports for both airplane and cruise ship illnesses and deaths may also originate from federal partners or state and local health departments.

CDC provides guidance and tools to facilitate reporting of ill travelers on aviation and maritime conveyances at www.cdc.gov/quarantine.

**Regulatory definition of an "ill traveler" for the purposes of reporting illness on commercial airplanes and ships**

Fever[1] plus ≥1 of the following:

- Skin rash, difficulty breathing (or, for maritime conveyances, suspected or confirmed pneumonia), persistent cough (or, for maritime conveyances, cough with bloody sputum), decreased consciousness or confusion of recent onset, new unexplained bruising or bleeding (without previous injury), persistent diarrhea (air conveyances only), persistent vomiting (other than air or sea sickness), headache with stiff neck, or appears obviously unwell (air conveyances only); OR

Fever for >48 hours; OR

Acute gastroenteritis[2] (maritime conveyances only); OR

Symptoms or other indications of communicable disease, as the CDC may announce through posting of a notice in the federal register.

[1] Measured temperature ≥100.4°F (≥38°C); feels warm to the touch; or a history of feeling feverish

[2] Diarrhea (≥3 episodes of loose stools in a 24-hour period or what is above normal for the person) OR vomiting accompanied by ≥1 of the following: ≥1 episode of loose stools in a 24-hour period, abdominal cramps, headache, muscle aches, or fever (temperature ≥100.4°F [≥38°C])

## AIRPLANE RESPONSE

CDC's goals in responding to illness reports during air travel are to determine if the illness is a public health threat and to take public health actions. The 3 possible outcomes of a response during travel are to:

1. Recommend that the ill traveler seek medical care or delay further commercial travel until noninfectious if the traveler has a suspected communicable disease;

2. Require the ill traveler to be medically evaluated if he or she is suspected of having a quarantinable communicable disease; or

3. Allow the ill traveler to resume travel if the illness does not pose a risk of spreading to others onboard.

CDC may board an arriving airplane with airport/public health response partners (e.g., emergency medical services, local public health authorities) to undertake a public health assessment of the ill traveler and to make recommendations regarding the potentially exposed passengers. Potentially exposed travelers may be asked to provide their contact information before disembarking, so that health authorities can follow up and provide additional health information if the ill traveler is diagnosed with a disease of public health concern.

CDC provides guidance to airlines on managing ill travelers onboard on its website at www.cdc.gov/quarantine/air/managing-sick-travelers/index.html.

## CRUISE SHIP RESPONSE

For public health responses to ill cruise ship travelers, most control measures are initiated while the ship is at sea. CDC quarantine station staff obtains clinical, medical, and epidemiologic information about the ill or deceased traveler, determine public health risk, and provide guidance to the ship's clinicians about case findings, infection control measures, and contact investigations.

The CDC quarantine station staff may respond by meeting a ship at the port of entry to further investigate or assist a local health department with surveillance and control measures. On-site response is usually done for outbreaks or clusters of disease, quarantinable communicable diseases, and some vaccine-preventable diseases (such as measles or rubella). CDC's Vessel Sanitation Program (www.cdc.gov/nceh/vsp/default.htm) is responsible for responding to reports of acute gastroenteritis on cruise ships.

**A**

CDC provides guidance to cruise ships on managing ill passengers and crew at www.cdc.gov/quarantine/cruise/management/index.html.

## After Travel

If CDC is notified by a US or foreign health authority of an illness of public health concern in an airplane or cruise ship traveler after the traveler has reached his or her final destination, CDC may conduct a public health contact investigation. The primary purpose of the contact investigation is to identify and notify the potentially exposed passengers and crew, so that clinical evaluation, postexposure prophylaxis (when indicated), and health education can be offered. CDC provides information about potentially exposed to travelers to public health authorities in the states or countries where the travelers live, in order to facilitate these interventions.

# REPORTING ILLNESS AFTER TRAVEL

Travelers who become ill after returning home should inform their health care providers of where they have traveled. Clinicians should report cases of communicable diseases of public health concern in returning travelers to their local public health authority according to state-specific reportable disease requirements. Health departments may notify CDC of situations with risk of communicable disease transmission during travel by contacting the quarantine station with jurisdiction for their region (www.cdc.gov/quarantine/quarantinestations.html) or the Emergency Operations Center at 770-488-7100 or eocreport@cdc.gov. CDC may be notified of legionellosis cases associated with travel by sending an email to travellegionella@cdc.gov.

## BIBLIOGRAPHY

1. CDC. Criteria for requesting federal travel restrictions for public health purposes, including for viral hemorrhagic fevers. Fed Regist. 2015:16400e2. 80 FR 1640. [cited 2018 Aug 15]. Available from: www.federalregister.gov/documents/2015/03/27/2015-07118/criteria-for-requesting-federal-travel-restrictions-for-public-health-purposes-including-for-viral.

2. CDC. Vessel Sanitation Program Operations Manual. 2018. [cited 2018 Jun 15]. Available from: www.cdc.gov/nceh/vsp/pub/pub.htm.

3. Department of Health and Human Services. 42 Code of Federal Regulations Parts 70 (Interstate Quarantine) and 71 (Foreign Quarantine). [cited 2018 Aug 15]. Available from: www.ecfr.gov/cgi-bin/text-idx?tpl=/ecfrbrowse/Title42/42tab_02.tpl.

4. Jungerman MR, Vonnahme LA, Washburn F, Alvarado-Ramy F. Federal travel restrictions to prevent disease transmission in the United States: An analysis of requested travel restrictions. Travel Med Infect Dis. 2017 Jun;18:30–5.

5. World Health Organization. Report of the WHO Ad-hoc Advisory Group on aircraft disinsection for controlling the international spread of vector-borne diseases. Geneva, Switzerland, April 2016. [cited 2018 Mar 21]. Available from: www.who.int/ihr/publications/WHO_HSE_GCR_2016_12/en/.

6. World Health Organization. Guide to Hygiene and Sanitation in Aviation, 3rd Ed. WHO, Geneva; 2009. [cited 2018 Mar 21]. Available from: www.who.int/ihr/ports_airports/guide_hygiene_sanitation_aviation_3_edition_wcov.pdf.

A

# APPENDIX E: TAKING ANIMALS & ANIMAL PRODUCTS ACROSS INTERNATIONAL BORDERS

G. Gale Galland, Robert J. Mullan, Kendra E. Stauffer

## TRAVELING ABROAD WITH A PET

Travelers planning to take a companion animal to a foreign country must meet the entry requirements of that country and transportation guidelines of the airline. To get destination country information, travelers should contact the country's embassy in Washington, DC, or the nearest consulate (see www.usembassy.gov/). The US Department of Agriculture (USDA) pet travel website is another resource for destination country requirements (see www.aphis.usda.gov/aphis/pet-travel). Additionally, travelers can check with airline companies for their guidelines. Travelers should be aware that long flights can be hard on pets, particularly older animals with chronic health conditions, very young animals, and short-nosed breeds, such as bulldogs and Persian cats, which may be predisposed to respiratory stress. Additionally, upon reentering the United States, pets that traveled abroad are subject to the same import requirements as animals that never lived in the United States.

## REQUIREMENTS FOR ENTERING THE UNITED STATES

CDC restricts the importation of animals and animal products that might pose a public health threat. Any animal or animal product can be restricted from entry if there is reasonable knowledge or suspicion that it poses a human health risk. CDC has explicit restrictions for specific animals: dogs, cats, turtles, nonhuman primates, African rodents, civets, and bats, as well as products made from them. Importers must comply with certain requirements in order to import these animals or items into the United States. Many of these animals are also regulated by other federal agencies or by state governments. Travelers should check with the USDA, the US Fish and Wildlife Service (FWS), and their destination state for their rules about importation.

## ANIMAL HEALTH CERTIFICATES

CDC regulations do not require general health certificates for animals entering the United States. However, some states may require health certificates for entry, and some airlines may require these certificates for transport. Before departure, travelers should check with the departments of health and of agriculture in their destination states and with the airline for any health certificate requirements. The department of environmental protection or department of natural resources of some states and local governments may have additional requirements.

## INTERNATIONAL PET RESCUE AND ADOPTION

Although done with the best of intentions, rescuing and importing stray animals from foreign countries can create human health risks in the United States. Travelers are at an increased risk for bites and scratches from fearful and stressed animals, which may result in injury or exposure to infectious disease, such as rabies. Animals that are infected with zoonotic diseases might not show any outward signs of being ill but can still spread these harmful germs to people. Therefore, all rescued animals should be examined by a licensed veterinarian both before departure and after arrival in the United States. If the intent of travel is to rescue animals, participants should discuss rabies preexposure prophylaxis with their health care providers.

# IMPORTATION OF LIVE ANIMALS

## Dogs

Dogs are subject to inspection upon entry into the United States if they have evidence of being infected with a communicable disease or if they have not been vaccinated against rabies. If a dog appears to be ill, further examination by a licensed veterinarian may be required before entry is permitted. If it is necessary, this examination will be at the owner's expense.

Rabies vaccination is required for all dogs entering the United States from a country that is considered at high risk for canine variant rabies virus as determined by CDC's rabies experts. For more information, see www.cdc.gov/importation/bringing-an-animal-into-the-united-states/dogs.html. Dogs from high-risk countries must be accompanied by a current, valid rabies vaccination certificate that includes the following information:

- Name and address of owner
- Breed, sex, age, color, markings, and other identifying information for the dog
- Date of rabies vaccination and vaccine product information
- Date of expiration of vaccination
- Name, license number, address, and signature of veterinarian

Rabies certificates have expiration dates that range from 1 to 3 years from the date of vaccination, depending on the type of vaccine. All dogs must be ≥12 weeks of age before receiving their first rabies vaccination. Rabies vaccinations must occur at least 28 days before arrival, as it takes 28 days for these vaccines to be fully effective.

CDC recommends, and most state and local authorities in the United States require, routine rabies vaccination of dogs. Check with state and local authorities at the final destination to determine any state requirements for rabies vaccination. State-specific information is found at www.avma.org/Advocacy/StateAndLocal/Documents/Rabies%20state%20law%20chart.pdf.

## Cats

Cats are subject to inspection at US ports of entry and may be denied entry into the United States if they have evidence of being infected with a disease of public health concern. If a cat appears ill, examination by a licensed veterinarian may be required before entry is permitted. This examination, if necessary, is conducted at the owner's expense. Although CDC does not require cats to have proof of rabies vaccination for importation into the United States, CDC does recommend vaccination. In addition, many states have rabies vaccination requirements for cats. Check with state and local health authorities at the final destination to determine any state requirements for rabies vaccination of cats. For more information about importing cats, see www.cdc.gov/importation/bringing-an-animal-into-the-united-states/cats.html.

All dogs and cats arriving in the state of Hawaii or the territory of Guam, even from the US mainland, are subject to locally imposed quarantine requirements. For more information about animal importation in Hawaii, consult http://hdoa.hawaii.gov, or call 808-483-7151. For more information about animal importation in Guam, see www.guamcourts.org/CompilerofLaws/GAR/09GAR/09GAR001-1.pdf.

## Nonhuman Primates

Nonhuman primates can transmit a variety of serious diseases to humans, including Ebola virus disease and tuberculosis. Nonhuman primates may be imported into the United States only by a CDC-registered importer and only for scientific, educational, or exhibition purposes. All nonhuman primates also are considered endangered or threatened and require FWS permits for importation. Nonhuman primates may not be imported as pets. Nonhuman primates that are kept as pets in the United States and travel outside the United States will not be allowed to reenter the United States as pets. For more information on CDC's importation requirements, see www.cdc.gov/importation/bringing-an-animal-into-the-united-states/monkeys.html.

## Turtles

Although often kept as pets, turtles can transmit *Salmonella* to humans. CDC restricts the importation of some turtles. A person may import up to 6 viable turtle eggs or live turtles with a shell length of <4 in (10 cm) for noncommercial purposes. More live turtles or viable turtle eggs may be imported with CDC permission but only for science, education, or exhibition. CDC does not restrict the importation of live turtles with a shell length ≥4 inches. Check with USDA and FWS regarding additional requirements to import turtles. More information is available at www.cdc.gov/importation/bringing-an-animal-into-the-united-states/turtles.html.

## African Rodents

African rodents are a known source of communicable diseases, such as monkeypox. CDC does not allow the importation of these animals. Exceptions may be made for animals imported for science, education, or exhibition, with permission from CDC. Check with USDA and FWS regarding additional requirements to import African rodents. For more information, see www.cdc.gov/importation/bringing-an-animal-into-the-united-states/african-rodents.html.

## Civets and Related Animals

To reduce the risk of introducing severe acute respiratory syndrome (SARS) coronavirus, civets and related animals in the family Viverridae may not be imported into the United States. Exceptions may be made for animals imported for science, education, or exhibition purposes, with permission from CDC. Check with USDA and FWS regarding additional requirements to import civets and related animals. For more information, see www.cdc.gov/importation/bringing-an-animal-into-the-united-states/civets.html.

## Bats and Other Vectors

Bats are reservoirs of many viruses that can infect humans, including rabies virus, Nipah virus, and SARS coronavirus. To reduce the risk of introducing these viruses, the importation of all live bats requires a CDC permit. The application for a CDC bat import permit can be found at www.cdc.gov/importation/bringing-an-animal-into-the-united-states/bats.html. Bats may not be imported as pets. Many bats require additional permits issued by FWS.

In some circumstances, known vectors of human disease such as ticks or mosquitoes may be imported into the United States with a permit from CDC. For additional information, see www.cdc.gov/phpr/ipp/index.htm.

## Other Animals

Travelers planning to import horses, ruminants, swine, poultry or other birds, or dogs used for handling livestock should contact National Import Export Services, a part of USDA's Animal and Plant Health Inspection Service, at 301-851-3300, or visit www.aphis.usda.gov/aphis/ourfocus/animalhealth/animal-and-animal-product-import-information to learn about additional requirements.

Travelers planning to import fish, reptiles, spiders, wild birds, rabbits, bears, wild members of the cat family, or other wild or endangered animals should contact FWS at 800-344-9453 (toll-free general number) or 703-358-1949 (FWS Office of Law Enforcement), or visit www.fws.gov/le/travelers.html.

# IMPORTATION OF ANIMAL PRODUCTS

## Trophies and Animal Products

Travelers often want to import animal skins, hunting trophies, or other items made from animals when returning from a trip. These items must either be rendered noninfectious (see www.cdc.gov/importation/animal-products.html) or be accompanied by an import permit. CDC restricts products made from nonhuman primates, African rodents, civets and related animals (in the family Viverridae), and bats. These products may also be regulated by other US federal agencies. CDC has the right to restrict other items known to carry infectious diseases. For example, CDC restricts goatskin souvenirs, such as Haitian goatskin drums, from entry into the United States because they have been associated with cases of anthrax in humans. Travelers who want to import hunting trophies or other products made from animals should check with CDC, USDA, and FWS to make sure they are complying with federal regulations.

## Bushmeat

Animal products may also include items intended for human consumption. Bushmeat, generally raw, smoked, or partially processed meat from wild animals, might harbor infectious or zoonotic agents that can cause human or animal disease. As people have migrated around the world, bushmeat has become a growing commodity in the global wildlife trade. CDC prohibits the importation into the United States of bushmeat from CDC-restricted species. Bushmeat from other species is also restricted under USDA or FWS regulations. In addition to the human and animal health risks, many of the wild animals commonly hunted for bushmeat are threatened or endangered species protected by international wildlife laws and treaties such as the Convention on International Trade of Endangered Species (CITES). For additional information about importing animals and animal products into the United States and for permit applications, travelers should visit www.cdc.gov/importation/index.html or contact 1-800-CDC INFO (1-800-232-4636). To request CDC permission to import a CDC-regulated animal or product, send a message to CDCanimalimports@cdc.gov.

## BIBLIOGRAPHY

1. Bair-Brake H, Bell T, Higgins A, Bailey N, Duda M, Shapiro S, et al. Is that a rodent in your luggage? A mixed method approach to describe bushmeat importation into the United States. Zoonoses Public Health. 2014 Mar;61(2):97–104.

2. CDC. Multistate outbreak of monkeypox—Illinois, Indiana, and Wisconsin, 2003. MMWR Morb Mortal Wkly Rep. 2003 Jun 13;52(23):537–40.

3. CDC. Multistate outbreak of Salmonella infections associated with exposure to turtles—United States, 2007–2008. MMWR Morb Mortal Wkly Rep. 2008 Jan;57(3):69–72.

4. DeMarcus TA, Tipple MA, Ostrowski SR. US policy for disease control among imported nonhuman primates. J Infect Dis. 1999 Feb;179 Suppl 1:S281–2.

5. Hayman DTS, Bowen RA, Cryan PM, McCracken GF, O'Shea TJ, Peel AJ, et al. Ecology of zoonotic infectious diseases in bats: current knowledge and future directions. Zoonoses Public Health. 2013 Feb:60(1):2–21.

6. Lankau EW, Cohen NJ, Jentes ES, Adam LE, Bell TR, Blanton JD, et al. Prevention and control of rabies in an age of global travel: a review of travel- and trade-associated rabies events—United States, 1986–2012. Zoonoses Public Health. 2014 Aug;61(5):305–16.

7. McQuiston JH, Wilson T, Harris S, Bacon RM, Shapiro S, Trevino I, et al. Importation of dogs into the United States: risks from rabies and other zoonotic diseases. Zoonoses Public Health. 2008 Oct;55(8–10):421–6.

8. National Association of State Public Health Veterinarians, Inc. Compendium of animal rabies prevention and control, JAVMA. 2016 Mar 1;245(5):505–17.

9. Wu D, Tu C, Xin C, Xuan H, Meng Q, Liu Y, et al. Civets are equally susceptible to experimental infection by two different severe acute respiratory syndrome coronavirus isolates. J Virol. 2005 Feb;79(4):2620–5.

**A**

# Index

# Photography Credits

BANNER IMAGES FOR SELECT DESTINATIONS

East Africa (Safaris): Ellen Lash/Personal Collection

Saudi Arabia (Hajj/Umrah Pilgrimage): Esa Alexander/Personal Collection

South Africa: Kristina M. Angelo/Personal Collection

Tanzania (Kilimanjaro): David Towne/Personal Collection

Brazil: Pearl Kaplan/Personal Collection

Cuba: Erica J. Sison/Personal Collection

Dominican Republic: iStock

Haiti: Jennifer Murphy/Personal Collection

Mexico: Laura Whitlock/Personal Collection

Peru (Cusco, Machu Picchu & Other Regions): Elfren Noche/Personal Collection

Burma (Myanmar): Michael Washington/Personal Collection

China: Michael Washington/Personal Collection

India: Rebecca Myers/Personal Collection

Nepal: Ellen Lash/Personal Collection

Thailand: Michael Washington/Personal Collection